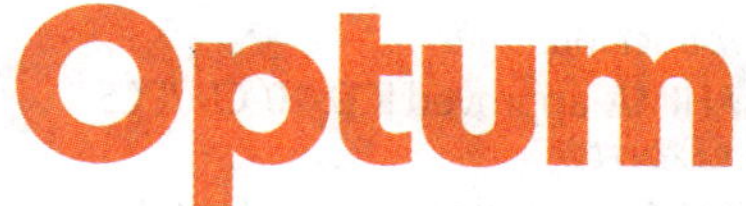

ICD-10-PCS

The complete official code set

Codes valid from October 1, 2023 through September 30, 2024

2024

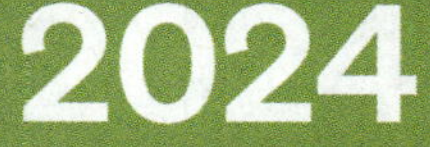

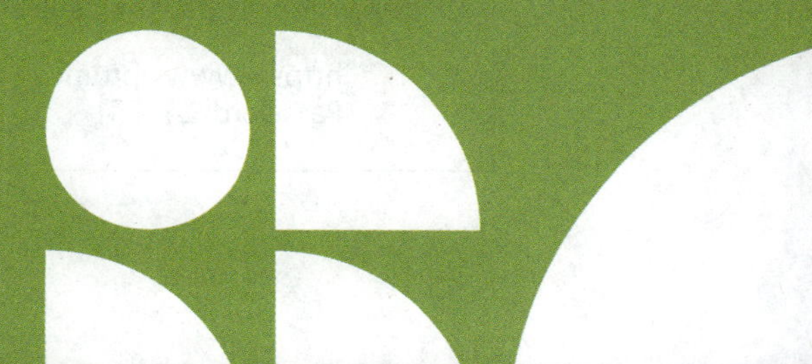

Notice

ICD-10-PCS: The Complete Official Code Set is designed to be an accurate and authoritative source regarding coding and every reasonable effort has been made to ensure accuracy and completeness of the content. However, Optum makes no guarantee, warranty, or representation that this publication is accurate, complete, or without errors. It is understood that Optum is not rendering any legal or other professional services or advice in this publication and that Optum bears no liability for any results or consequences that may arise from the use of this book. Please address all correspondence to:

Optum
2525 Lake Park Blvd
Salt Lake City, UT 84120

Our Commitment to Accuracy

Optum is committed to producing accurate and reliable materials.

To report corrections, please email customerassistance@optum.com. You can also reach customer service by calling 1.800.464.3649, option 1.

Copyright

Made in the USA
ISBN 978-1-62254-888-0 (Spiral)
ISBN 978-1-62254-889-7 (Softbound)

Acknowledgments

Marianne Randall, CPC, *Product Manager*
Anita Schmidt, BS, RHIA, AHIMA-approved ICD-10-CM/PCS Trainer, *Subject Matter Expert*
Laura M. Anderson, RN, BSN, CCDS, *Subject Matter Expert*
Stacy Perry, *Manager, Desktop Publishing*
Tracy Betzler, *Senior Desktop Publishing Specialist*
Hope M. Dunn, *Senior Desktop Publishing Specialist*
Katie Russell, *Desktop Publishing Specialist*
Kate Holden, *Editor*

Anita Schmidt, BS, RHIA, AHIMA-approved ICD-10-CM/PCS Trainer

Ms. Schmidt has expertise in ICD-10-CM/PCS, DRG, and CPT with more than 15 years' experience in coding in multiple settings, including inpatient, observation, and same-day surgery. Her experience includes analysis of medical record documentation, assignment of ICD-10-CM and PCS codes, and DRG validation. She has conducted training for ICD-10-CM/PCS and electronic health record. She has also collaborated with clinical documentation specialists to identify documentation needs and potential areas for physician education. Most recently she has been developing content for resource and educational products related to ICD-10-CM, ICD-10-PCS, DRG, and CPT. Ms. Schmidt is an AHIMA-approved ICD-10-CM/PCS trainer and is an active member of the American Health Information Management Association (AHIMA) and the Minnesota Health Information Management Association (MHIMA).

Laura M. Anderson, RN, BSN, CCDS

Ms. Anderson is a Registered Nurse and CDI Specialist/Educator with more than 20 years of experience in the healthcare profession. She obtained her BSN at the University of Minnesota and spent most of her bedside nursing career on Medical-Surgical care units. Her clinical documentation experience began in 2007, covering CDI specialist training, education development, and physician engagement. She has served as a CDI Team Lead and consultant, working with senior leadership to incorporate CDI work into documentation compliance and quality metrics. Ms. Anderson also has a BS degree in Biology (Winthrop University), with research experience in liver cancer and radiation-induced leukemia. She has presented at the state and national levels for the Association of Clinical Documentation Integrity Specialists (ACDIS) and serves as a co-lead for the Minnesota state chapter.

Product Updates

Significant updates to this manual, including April 1, 2024, updates, will be provided on our product updates page at Optumcoding.com, which can be accessed at the following:

https://www.optumcoding.com/ProductUpdates/
Password: 24PCS

Contents

What's New for 2024 iii

Introduction 1
- ICD-10-PCS Manual 1
- Medical and Surgical Section (Ø) 4
- Obstetrics Section (1) 7
- Placement Section (2) 7
- Administration Section (3) 8
- Measurement and Monitoring Section (4) 8
- Extracorporeal or Systemic Assistance and Performance Section (5) 9
- Extracorporeal or Systemic Therapies Section (6) 10
- Osteopathic Section (7) 10
- Other Procedures Section (8) 11
- Chiropractic Section (9) 11
- Imaging Section (B) 11
- Nuclear Medicine Section (C) 12
- Radiation Therapy Section (D) 13
- Physical Rehabilitation and Diagnostic Audiology Section (F) 13
- Mental Health Section (G) 14
- Substance Abuse Treatment Section (H) 15
- New Technology Section (X) 15

ICD-10-PCS Index and Tabular Format 17
- Index 17
- Code Tables 17

ICD-10-PCS Additional Features 19
- Use of Official Sources 19
- Table Notations 19
- Appendixes 20

ICD-10-PCS Official Guidelines for Coding and Reporting 2024 23
- Conventions 23
- Medical and Surgical Section Guidelines (section Ø) 24
- Obstetric Section Guidelines (section 1) 29
- Radiation Therapy Section Guidelines (section D) 29
- New Technology Section Guidelines (section X) 30

ICD-10-PCS Index 31

ICD-10-PCS Tables 131
- Central Nervous System and Cranial Nerves 131
- Peripheral Nervous System 153
- Heart and Great Vessels 171
- Upper Arteries 193
- Lower Arteries 219
- Upper Veins 243
- Lower Veins 263
- Lymphatic and Hemic Systems 283
- Eye 301
- Ear, Nose, Sinus 319
- Respiratory System 339
- Mouth and Throat 355
- Gastrointestinal System 373
- Hepatobiliary System and Pancreas 401
- Endocrine System 415
- Skin and Breast 427
- Subcutaneous Tissue and Fascia 445
- Muscles 465
- Tendons 487
- Bursae and Ligaments 501
- Head and Facial Bones 523
- Upper Bones 543
- Lower Bones 563
- Upper Joints 583
- Lower Joints 603
- Urinary System 627
- Female Reproductive System 643
- Male Reproductive System 663
- Anatomical Regions, General 679
- Anatomical Regions, Upper Extremities 691
- Anatomical Regions, Lower Extremities 701
- Obstetrics 711
- Placement 715
- Administration 721
- Measurement and Monitoring 735
- Extracorporeal or Systemic Assistance and Performance 739
- Extracorporeal or Systemic Therapies 741
- Osteopathic 743
- Other Procedures 745
- Chiropractic 747
- Imaging 749
- Nuclear Medicine 779
- Radiation Therapy 789
- Physical Rehabilitation and Diagnostic Audiology 807
- Mental Health 819
- Substance Abuse Treatment 821
- New Technology 823

Appendixes 835
- Appendix A: Components of the Medical and Surgical Approach Definitions 835
- Appendix B: Root Operation Definitions 838
- Appendix C: Comparison of Medical and Surgical Root Operations 843
- Appendix D: Body Part Key 845
- Appendix E: Body Part Definitions 860
- Appendix F: Device Classification 870
- Appendix G: Device Key and Aggregation Table 872
- Appendix H: Device Definitions 881
- Appendix I: Substance Key/Substance Definitions 887
- Appendix J: Sections B–H Character Definitions 892
- Appendix K: Hospital Acquired Conditions 900
- Appendix L: Procedure Combination Tables 919
- Appendix M: Coding Exercises and Answers 935
- Answers to Coding Exercises 941

What's New for 2024

The Centers for Medicare and Medicaid Services is the agency charged with maintaining and updating ICD-10-PCS. CMS released the most current revisions, a summary of which may be found on the CMS website at https://www.cms.gov/medicare/icd-10/2024-icd-10-pcs.

Due to the unique structure of ICD-10-PCS, a change in a character value may affect individual codes and several code tables.

Change Summary Table

2023 Total	New Codes	Revised Titles	Deleted Codes	2024 Total
78,530	78	14	5	78,603

ICD-10-PCS Code Totals, By Section

Medical and Surgical	68,058
Obstetrics	304
Placement	861
Administration	1,271
Measurement and Monitoring	422
Extracorporeal or Systemic Assistance and Performance	54
Extracorporeal or Systemic Therapies	46
Osteopathic	100
Other Procedures	88
Chiropractic	90
Imaging	2,978
Nuclear Medicine	463
Radiation Therapy	2,056
Physical Rehabilitation and Diagnostic Audiology	1,380
Mental Health	30
Substance Abuse Treatment	59
New Technology	343
Total	78,603

Table Addenda Highlights

- Device value Short-term External Heart Assist System was added to the root operation tables Insertion, Removal, and Revision in the Heart and Great Vessels body system for the body part Thoracic Aorta, Descending.
- Approach value Open was added to the root operation table Occlusion in the Heart and Great Vessels body system for the body part Thoracic Aorta, Descending.
- Approach value Open was added to the root operation table Occlusion in the Lower Arteries body system for the body part Abdominal Aorta, device value Intraluminal Device, and qualifier values Temporary and No Qualifier.
- Body part value Larynx was added to root operation table Reposition in the Mouth and Throat body system.
- Device value Magnetic Lengthening Device was added to the root operation table Insertion in the Gastrointestinal System body system for body part values Esophagus, Upper; Esophagus, Middle; and Esophagus, Lower.
- Qualifier value Laser Interstitial Thermal Therapy was added to root operation table Destruction in the Upper Bones body system for body parts Cervical Vertebra and Thoracic Vertebra.
- Qualifier value Laser Interstitial Thermal Therapy was added to root operation table Destruction in the Lower Bones body system for body parts Lumbar Vertebra and Sacrum.
- Device value Defibrillator Lead was added to the root operation tables Insertion, Removal, and Revision in the Anatomical Regions, General body system for the body part value Mediastinum.
- New row was added to the root operation table Transfusion to capture transfusion of whole blood, serum albumin, frozen plasma, fresh plasma, red blood cells, frozen red cells, and platelets into bone marrow.
- New row was added to the root operation table Assistance to capture ventilation of patients who are intubated in a prone position.
- New qualifier value Pafolacianine was added to the root operation table Other Procedures for the body region values Female Reproductive System and Trunk Region.
- Five new tables were added to the New Technology section:
  - — XØ5 Nervous System, Destruction
  - — X2H Cardiovascular System, Insertion
  - — X2U Cardiovascular System, Supplement
  - — XNR Bones, Replacement
  - — XX2 Physiological Systems, Monitoring
- Root operation table XV5 Male Reproductive System, Destruction was deleted from the New Technology section

Definitions Addenda

Section Ø – Medical and Surgical
Body Part Definitions

ICD-10-PCS Value	Definition	
Appendix	Add	Appendiceal Orifice
Intracranial Artery	Add	Middle meningeal artery, intracranial portion
	Add	Vertebral artery, intracranial portion
Pelvic Cavity	Add	Space of Retzius
Subcutaneous Tissue and Fascia, Face	Add	Chin

Section Ø – Medical and Surgical Device Definitions

ICD-10-PCS Value	Definition
Add Defibrillator Lead in Anatomical Regions, General	Add EV ICD System (Extravascular implantable defibrillator lead)
Internal Fixation Device, Sustained Compression for Fusion in Lower Joints	Delete DynaNail® (Hybrid)(Mini) Add DynaNail® (Helix)(Hybrid)(Mini)
Internal Fixation Device, Sustained Compression for Fusion in Upper Joints	Delete DynaNail® (Hybrid)(Mini) Add DynaNail® (Helix)(Hybrid)(Mini)
Add Intracardiac Pacemaker in Heart and Great Vessels	Add Aveir™ VR, as single chamber
Add Magnetic Lengthening Device in Gastrointestinal System	Add Flourish® Pediatric Esophageal Atresia Device
Short-term External Heart Assist System in Heart and Great Vessels	Add Aortix™ System
Stimulator Generator, Multiple Array for Insertion in Subcutaneous Tissue and Fascia	Add Vanta™ PC neurostimulator
Stimulator Generator, Multiple Array Rechargeable for Insertion in Subcutaneous Tissue and Fascia	Add Intellis™ neurostimulator

Section 3 – Administration Substance Definitions

ICD-10-PCS Value	Definition
Other Anti-infective	Add Plazomicin
Add Vasopressor	Add Angiotensin II Add GIAPREZA™ Add Human angiotensin II, synthetic

Section X – New Technology Device/Substance/Technology Definitions

ICD-10-PCS Value	Definition
Add Anacaulase-bcdb	Add Bromelain-enriched Proteolytic Enzyme Add NexoBrid™
Betibeglogene Autotemcel	Add ZYNTEGLO®
Delete Bromelain-enriched Proteolytic Enzyme	Delete NexoBrid™
Add Conduit through Femoral Vein to Popliteal Artery in New Technology	Add DETOUR® System
Add Conduit through Femoral Vein to Superficial Femoral Artery in New Technology	Add DETOUR® System
Add Conduit to Short-term External Heart Assist System in New Technology	Add Impella® 5.5 with SmartAssist® System
Add COVID-19 Vaccine	Add COMIRNATY® Add SPIKEVAX™
Add COVID-19 Vaccine Booster	Add COMIRNATY® Add SPIKEVAX™
Add COVID-19 Vaccine Dose 1	Add COMIRNATY® Add SPIKEVAX™
Add COVID-19 Vaccine Dose 2	Add COMIRNATY® Add SPIKEVAX™
Add COVID-19 Vaccine Dose 3	Add COMIRNATY® Add SPIKEVAX™
Add Exagamglogene Autotemcel	Add CTX001™
Delete Interbody Fusion Device, Customizable in New Technology	Delete aprevo™
Add Interbody Fusion Device, Custom-made Anatomically Designed in New Technology	Add aprevo™
Add Internal Fixation Device, Open-truss Design in New Technology	Add Ankle Truss System™ (ATS)
Add Intracardiac Pacemaker, Dual-Chamber in New Technology	Add Aveir™ AR, as dual chamber Add Aveir™ DR, dual chamber
Add Intraluminal Device, Bioprosthetic Valve in New Technology	Add TricValve® Transcatheter Bicaval Valve System Add VenoValve®
Add Melphalan Hydrochloride Antineoplastic	Add HEPZATO™ KIT (melphalan hydrochloride Hepatic Delivery System)
Add Mosunetuzumab Antineoplastic	Add LUNSUMIO™
Add Sulbactam-Durlobactam	Add SUL-DUR
Delete Synthetic Human Angiotensin II	Delete Angiotensin II Delete GIAPREZA™ Delete Human angiotensin II, synthetic
Add Synthetic Substitute, Extraluminal Support Device in New Technology	Add VasQ™ External Support device
Add Synthetic Substitute, Talar Prosthesis in New Technology	Add Total Ankle Talar Replacement™ (TATR)
Add Synthetic Substitute, Ultrasound Penetrable in New Technology	Add Longeviti ClearFit® Cranial Implant Add Longeviti ClearFit® OTS Cranial Implant
Add Tibial Extension with Motion Sensors in New Technology	Add Canturio™ te (Tibial Extension)
Add Vein Graft Extraluminal Support Device(s) in New Technology	Add VEST™ Venous External Support device

List of Updated Files

2024 Official ICD-10-PCS Coding Guidelines

- Guidelines B5.2b and B6.1a revised in response to public comment and internal review.
- Downloadable PDF

2024 ICD-10-PCS Code Tables and Index (Zip file)

- Code tables for use beginning October 1, 2024.
- Downloadable PDF, file name is pcs_2024.pdf
- Downloadable xml files for developers, file names are icd10pcs_tables_2024.xml, icd10pcs_index_2024.xml, icd10pcs_definitions_2024.xml
- Accompanying schema for developers, file names are icd10pcs_tables.xsd, icd10pcs_index.xsd, icd10pcs_definitions.xsd

2024 ICD-10-PCS Codes File (Zip file)

- ICD-10-PCS Codes file is a simple format for non-technical uses, containing the valid FY 2024 ICD-10-PCS codes and their long titles.
- File is in text file format, file name is icd10pcs_codes_2024.txt
- Accompanying documentation for codes file, file name is icd10pcsCodesFile.pdf
- Codes file addenda in text format, file name is codes_addenda_2024.txt

2024 ICD-10-PCS Order File (Long and Abbreviated Titles) (Zip file)

- ICD-10-PCS order file is for developers, provides a unique five-digit "order number" for each ICD-10-PCS table and code, as well as a long and abbreviated code title.
- ICD-10-PCS order file name is icd10pcs_order_2024.txt
- Accompanying documentation for tabular order file, file name is icd10pcsOrderFile.pdf
- Tabular order file addenda in text format, file name is order_addenda_2024.txt

2024 ICD-10-PCS Final Addenda (Zip file)

- Addenda files in downloadable PDF, file names are tables_addenda_2024.pdf, index_addenda_2024.pdf, definitions_addenda_2024.pdf
- Addenda files also in machine readable text format for developers, file names are tables_addenda_2024.txt, index_addenda_2024.txt, definitions_addenda_2024.txt

2024 ICD-10-PCS Conversion Table (Zip file)

- ICD-10-PCS code conversion table is provided to assist users in data retrieval, in downloadable Excel spreadsheet, file name is icd10pcs_conversion_table_2024.xlsx
- Conversion table also in machine readable text format for developers, file name is icd10pcs_conversion_table_2024.txt
- Accompanying documentation for code conversion table, file name is icd10pcsConversionTable.pdf

Introduction

ICD-10-PCS: The Complete Official Code Set is your definitive coding resource for procedure coding in acute inpatient hospitals. In addition to the official ICD-10-PCS Coding System Files, revised and distributed by the Centers for Medicare and Medicaid Services (CMS), Optum's coding experts have incorporated Medicare-related coding edits and proprietary features, such as coding tools and appendixes, into a comprehensive and easy-to-use reference.

This manual provides the most current information that was available at the time of publication. For updates to official source documents that may have occurred after this manual was published, please refer to the following:

- **CMS International Classification of Disease, 10th Revision, Procedural Coding System (ICD-10-PCS):**

  https://www.cms.gov/medicare/icd-10/2024-icd-10-pcs
- **CMS Inpatient Prospective Payment System (IPPS) and v41 MS-DRG Data Files, FY 2024**

  https://www.cms.gov/medicare/acute-inpatient-pps/fy-2024-ipps-proposed-rule-home-page

  https://www.cms.gov/Medicare/Medicare-Fee-for-Service-Payment/AcuteInpatientPPS/MS-DRG-Classifications-and-Software
- **American Hospital Association (AHA) Coding Clinics**

  https://www.codingclinicadvisor.com/

ICD-10-PCS Code Structure

All codes in ICD-10-PCS are seven characters long. Each character in the seven-character code represents an aspect of the procedure, as shown in the following diagram of characters from the main section of ICD-10-PCS, called the Medical and Surgical section.

	Section	Body System	Root Operation	Body Part	Approach	Device	Qualifier
Characters:	1	2	3	4	5	6	7

One of 34 possible alphanumeric values—using the digits Ø–9 and letters A–H, J–N, and P–Z—can be assigned to each character in a code. The letters O and I are not used so as to avoid confusion with the digits Ø and 1. A code is derived by choosing a specific value for each of the seven characters, based on details about the procedure performed. Because the definition of each character is a function of its physical position in the code, the same value placed in a different position means something different; the value Ø as the first character means something different from Ø as the second character or as the third character, and so on.

The first character always determines the broad procedure category, or section. The second through seventh characters have the same meaning within a specific section, but these meanings can change in a different section. For example, the sixth character means "device" in the Medical and Surgical section but "qualifier" in the Imaging section.

ICD-10-PCS Manual

Index

Codes may be found in the index based on the general type of procedure (e.g., resection, transfusion, fluoroscopy), or a more commonly used term (e.g., appendectomy). For example, the code for percutaneous intraluminal dilation of the coronary arteries with an intraluminal device can be found in the Index under *Dilation*, or a synonym of *Dilation* (e.g., angioplasty). The Index then specifies the first three or four values of the code or directs the user to see another term.

Example:

Dilation
  Artery
    Coronary
      One Artery Ø27Ø

Based on the first three values of the code provided in the Index, the corresponding table can be located. In the example above, the first three values indicate table Ø27 is to be referenced for code completion.

The tables and characters are arranged first by number and then by letter for each character (tables for ØØ-, Ø1-, Ø2-, etc., are followed by those for ØB-, ØC-, ØD-, etc., followed by ØB1, ØB2, etc., followed by ØBB, ØBC, ØBD, etc.).

Note: The Tables section must be used to construct a complete and valid code by specifying the last three or four values.

Tables

The tables in ICD-10-PCS provide the valid combination of character values needed to build a unique procedure code. Each table is preceded by the first three characters of the code, along with their descriptions. In the Medical and Surgical section, for example, the first three characters contain the name of the section (character 1), the body system (character 2), and the root operation performed (character 3).

Listed underneath the first three characters is a table comprising four columns and one or more rows. The four columns in the table specify the last four characters needed to complete the ICD-10-PCS code. Depending on the section, the labels for each column may be different. In the Medical and Surgical section, they are labeled body part (character 4), approach (character 5), device (character 6), and qualifier (character 7). Each row in the table specifies the valid combination of values for characters 4 through 7.

Table 1: Row from table Ø27

Ø Medical and Surgical
2 Heart and Great Vessels
7 Dilation Definition: Expanding an orifice or the lumen of a tubular body part
Explanation: The orifice can be a natural orifice or an artificially created orifice. Accomplished by stretching a tubular body part using intraluminal pressure or by cutting part of the orifice or wall of the tubular body part.

Body Part Character 4	Approach Character 5	Device Character 6	Qualifier Character 7
Ø Coronary Artery, One Artery 1 Coronary Artery, Two Arteries 2 Coronary Artery, Three Arteries 3 Coronary Artery, Four or More Arteries	Ø Open 3 Percutaneous 4 Percutaneous Endoscopic	4 Intraluminal Device, Drug-eluting 5 Intraluminal Device, Drug-eluting, Two 6 Intraluminal Device, Drug-eluting, Three 7 Intraluminal Device, Drug-eluting, Four or More D Intraluminal Device E Intraluminal Device, Two F Intraluminal Device, Three G Intraluminal Device, Four or More T Intraluminal Device, Radioactive Z No Device	6 Bifurcation Z No Qualifier

For instance, table 1 above shows the first row from table Ø27 in ICD-10-PCS. The values Ø27 specify the section *Medical and Surgical (Ø)*, the body system *Heart and Great Vessels (2)*, and the root operation *Dilation (7)*. As shown, the root operation (Dilation) is also accompanied by its corresponding definition and explanation. Note, a definition of the root operation is provided for every table in ICD-10-PCS; however, an explanation may not always be applicable.

In total, this single row can be used to construct 240 unique procedure codes. The valid codes shown in table 2 (below) are constructed using the body part (character 4) value of Ø, Coronary artery, one artery, combined with all valid approach (character 5) values, device (character 6) values, and a qualifier (character 7) value of Z, No Qualifier.

Table 2: Code titles for dilation of one coronary artery (Ø27Ø)

Ø27ØØ4Z	Dilation of Coronary Artery, One Artery with Drug-eluting Intraluminal Device, Open Approach
Ø27ØØ5Z	Dilation of Coronary Artery, One Artery with Two Drug-eluting Intraluminal Devices, Open Approach
Ø27ØØ6Z	Dilation of Coronary Artery, One Artery with Three Drug-eluting Intraluminal Devices, Open Approach
Ø27ØØ7Z	Dilation of Coronary Artery, One Artery with Four or More Drug-eluting Intraluminal Devices, Open Approach
Ø27ØØDZ	Dilation of Coronary Artery, One Artery with Intraluminal Device, Open Approach
Ø27ØØEZ	Dilation of Coronary Artery, One Artery with Two Intraluminal Devices, Open Approach
Ø27ØØFZ	Dilation of Coronary Artery, One Artery with Three Intraluminal Devices, Open Approach
Ø27ØØGZ	Dilation of Coronary Artery, One Artery with Four or More Intraluminal Devices, Open Approach
Ø27ØØTZ	Dilation of Coronary Artery, One Artery with Radioactive Intraluminal Device, Open Approach
Ø27ØØZZ	Dilation of Coronary Artery, One Artery, Open Approach
Ø27Ø34Z	Dilation of Coronary Artery, One Artery with Drug-eluting Intraluminal Device, Percutaneous Approach
Ø27Ø35Z	Dilation of Coronary Artery, One Artery with Two Drug-eluting Intraluminal Devices, Percutaneous Approach
Ø27Ø36Z	Dilation of Coronary Artery, One Artery with Three Drug-eluting Intraluminal Devices, Percutaneous Approach
Ø27Ø37Z	Dilation of Coronary Artery, One Artery with Four or More Drug-eluting Intraluminal Devices, Percutaneous Approach
Ø27Ø3DZ	Dilation of Coronary Artery, One Artery with Intraluminal Device, Percutaneous Approach
Ø27Ø3EZ	Dilation of Coronary Artery, One Artery with Two Intraluminal Devices, Percutaneous Approach
Ø27Ø3FZ	Dilation of Coronary Artery, One Artery with Three Intraluminal Devices, Percutaneous Approach
Ø27Ø3GZ	Dilation of Coronary Artery, One Artery with Four or More Intraluminal Devices, Percutaneous Approach
Ø27Ø3TZ	Dilation of Coronary Artery, One Artery with Radioactive Intraluminal Device, Percutaneous Approach
Ø27Ø3ZZ	Dilation of Coronary Artery, One Artery, Percutaneous Approach
Ø27Ø44Z	Dilation of Coronary Artery, One Artery with Drug-eluting Intraluminal Device, Percutaneous Endoscopic Approach
Ø27Ø45Z	Dilation of Coronary Artery, One Artery with Two Drug-eluting Intraluminal Devices, Percutaneous Endoscopic Approach
Ø27Ø46Z	Dilation of Coronary Artery, One Artery with Three Drug-eluting Intraluminal Devices, Percutaneous Endoscopic Approach
Ø27Ø47Z	Dilation of Coronary Artery, One Artery with Four or More Drug-eluting Intraluminal Devices, Percutaneous Endoscopic Approach
Ø27Ø4DZ	Dilation of Coronary Artery, One Artery with Intraluminal Device, Percutaneous Endoscopic Approach
Ø27Ø4EZ	Dilation of Coronary Artery, One Artery with Two Intraluminal Devices, Percutaneous Endoscopic Approach
Ø27Ø4FZ	Dilation of Coronary Artery, One Artery with Three Intraluminal Devices, Percutaneous Endoscopic Approach
Ø27Ø4GZ	Dilation of Coronary Artery, One Artery with Four or More Intraluminal Devices, Percutaneous Endoscopic Approach
Ø27Ø4TZ	Dilation of Coronary Artery, One Artery with Radioactive Intraluminal Device, Percutaneous Endoscopic Approach
Ø27Ø4ZZ	Dilation of Coronary Artery, One Artery, Percutaneous Endoscopic Approach

Table 3: Rows from table ØØH

Ø Medical and Surgical
Ø Central Nervous System and Cranial Nerves
H Insertion Definition: Putting in a nonbiological appliance that monitors, assists, performs, or prevents a physiological function but does not physically take the place of a body part

Explanation: None

Body Part Character 4	Approach Character 5	Device Character 6	Qualifier Character 7
Ø Brain Cerebrum Corpus callosum Encephalon	**Ø Open**	**1 Radioactive Element** **2 Monitoring Device** **3 Infusion Device** **4 Radioactive Element, Cesium-131 Collagen Implant** **M Neurostimulator Lead** **Y Other Device**	**Z No Qualifier**
Ø Brain Cerebrum Corpus callosum Encephalon	**3 Percutaneous** **4 Percutaneous Endoscopic**	**1 Radioactive Element** **2 Monitoring Device** **3 Infusion Device** **M Neurostimulator Lead** **Y Other Device**	**Z No Qualifier**
6 Cerebral Ventricle Aqueduct of Sylvius Cerebral aqueduct (Sylvius) Choroid plexus Ependyma Foramen of Monro (intraventricular) Fourth ventricle Interventricular foramen (Monro) Left lateral ventricle Right lateral ventricle Third ventricle **E Cranial Nerve** **U Spinal Canal** Epidural space, spinal Extradural space, spinal Subarachnoid space, spinal Subdural space, spinal Vertebral canal **V Spinal Cord** Dorsal root ganglion	**Ø Open** **3 Percutaneous** **4 Percutaneous Endoscopic**	**1 Radioactive Element** **2 Monitoring Device** **3 Infusion Device** **M Neurostimulator Lead** **Y Other Device**	**Z No Qualifier**

Table 3 is split into three rows; values of characters must all be selected from within the same row of the table. Rows 1 and 2 have the same body part (character 4) value of Ø Brain and the same qualifier value (character 7) of Z No Qualifier. However, the approach (character 5) values are not the same for these two rows, and there is one additional device (character 6) value in row 1 that is not included in row 2. As shown in row 1, body part value Brain (Ø) with device value Radioactive Element, Cesium-131 Collagen Implant (4) can only be used with approach value Open (Ø). In other words, code ØØHØ34Z would be invalid as the approach value 3 is only applicable to row 2 and the device value 4 is only applicable to row 1. It would be inappropriate to build a code for body part Ø if all of the values are not contained in its own row.

Note: In this manual, there are instances in which some tables due to length must be continued on the next page. Each section must be used separately and value selection must be made within the same row of the table.

Character Meanings

In each section, each character has a specific meaning, and this character meaning remains constant within that section. Character meaning tables have been provided at the beginning of each body system in the Medical and Surgical section (Ø) and the Obstetric section (1) to help the user identify the character members available within that section. These tables have purple headers, unlike the official code tables that have green headers and **SHOULD NOT** be used to build a PCS code. Following is an excerpt of a character meaning table.

Table 4: Rows from Central Nervous System and Cranial Nerves - Character Meanings Table

Operation–Character 3	Body Part–Character 4	Approach–Character 5	Device–Character 6	Qualifier–Character 7
1 Bypass	Ø Brain	Ø Open	Ø Drainage Device	Ø Nasopharynx
2 Change	1 Cerebral Meninges	3 Percutaneous	1 Radioactive Element	1 Mastoid Sinus
5 Destruction	2 Dura Mater	4 Percutaneous Endoscopic	2 Monitoring Device	2 Atrium
7 Dilation	3 Epidural Space, Intracranial	X External	3 Infusion Device	3 Blood Vessel
8 Division	4 Subdural Space, Intracranial		4 Radioactive Element, Cesium-131 Collagen Implant	4 Pleural Cavity
9 Drainage	5 Subarachnoid Space, Intracranial		7 Autologous Tissue Substitute	5 Intestine
B Excision	6 Cerebral Ventricle		J Synthetic Substitute	6 Peritoneal Cavity
C Extirpation	7 Cerebral Hemisphere		K Nonautologous Tissue Substitute	7 Urinary Tract
D Extraction	8 Basal Ganglia		M Neurostimulator Lead	8 Bone Marrow
F Fragmentation	9 Thalamus		Y Other Device	9 Fallopian Tube
H Insertion	A Hypothalamus		Z No Device	A Subgaleal space
J Inspection	B Pons			B Cerebral Cisterns

Introduction

Sections

The first character of the procedure code always specifies the section. There are 17 sections within the PCS manual, listed below.

Medical and Surgical Section

Ø Medical and Surgical

Medical and Surgical-related Sections

1 Obstetrics
2 Placement
3 Administration
4 Measurement and Monitoring
5 Extracorporeal or Systemic Assistance and Performance
6 Extracorporeal or Systemic Therapies
7 Osteopathic
8 Other Procedures
9 Chiropractic

Ancillary Sections

B Imaging
C Nuclear Medicine
D Radiation Therapy
F Physical Rehabilitation and Diagnostic Audiology
G Mental Health
H Substance Abuse Treatment

New Technology Section

X New Technology

Medical and Surgical Section (0)

The Medical and Surgical section contains codes for the vast majority of procedures typically reported in an inpatient setting.

Character Meaning

The seven characters for Medical and Surgical procedures have the following meaning:

Character	Meaning
1	Section
2	Body System
3	Root Operation
4	Body Part
5	Approach
6	Device
7	Qualifier

Section (Character 1)

Medical and Surgical procedure codes all have a first character value of Ø.

Body Systems (Character 2)

The second character represents the body system—the general physiological system or anatomical region where the procedure is being performed.

Body Systems

Ø Central Nervous System and Cranial Nerves
1 Peripheral Nervous System
2 Heart and Great Vessels
3 Upper Arteries
4 Lower Arteries
5 Upper Veins
6 Lower Veins
7 Lymphatic and Hemic Systems
8 Eye
9 Ear, Nose, Sinus
B Respiratory System
C Mouth and Throat
D Gastrointestinal System
F Hepatobiliary System and Pancreas
G Endocrine System
H Skin and Breast
J Subcutaneous Tissue and Fascia
K Muscles
L Tendons
M Bursae and Ligaments
N Head and Facial Bones
P Upper Bones
Q Lower Bones
R Upper Joints
S Lower Joints
T Urinary System
U Female Reproductive System
V Male Reproductive System
W Anatomical Regions, General
X Anatomical Regions, Upper Extremities
Y Anatomical Regions, Lower Extremities

Root Operations (Character 3)

The third character represents the root operation, or the primary objective, of the procedure. There are 31 different root operations in this section, each with its own precise definition.

- *Alteration:* Modifying the natural anatomic structure of a body part without affecting the function of the body part
- *Bypass:* Altering the route of passage of the contents of a tubular body part
- *Change:* Taking out or off a device from a body part and putting back an identical or similar device in or on the same body part without cutting or puncturing the skin or a mucous membrane
- *Control:* Stopping, or attempting to stop, postprocedural or other acute bleeding
- *Creation:* Putting in or on biological or synthetic material to form a new body part that to the extent possible replicates the anatomic structure or function of an absent body part
- *Destruction:* Physical eradication of all or a portion of a body part by the direct use of energy, force, or a destructive agent

- *Detachment:* Cutting off all or a portion of the upper or lower extremities
- *Dilation:* Expanding an orifice or the lumen of a tubular body part
- *Division:* Cutting into a body part without draining fluids and/or gases from the body part in order to separate or transect a body part
- *Drainage:* Taking or letting out fluids and/or gases from a body part
- *Excision:* Cutting out or off, without replacement, a portion of a body part
- *Extirpation:* Taking or cutting out solid matter from a body part
- *Extraction:* Pulling or stripping out or off all or a portion of a body part by the use of force
- *Fragmentation:* Breaking solid matter in a body part into pieces
- *Fusion:* Joining together portions of an articular body part rendering the articular body part immobile
- *Insertion:* Putting in a nonbiological appliance that monitors, assists, performs, or prevents a physiological function but does not physically take the place of a body part
- *Inspection:* Visually and/or manually exploring a body part
- *Map:* Locating the route of passage of electrical impulses and/or locating functional areas in a body part
- *Occlusion:* Completely closing an orifice or lumen of a tubular body part
- *Reattachment:* Putting back in or on all or a portion of a separated body part to its normal location or other suitable location
- *Release:* Freeing a body part from an abnormal physical constraint by cutting or by use of force
- *Removal:* Taking out or off a device from a body part
- *Repair:* Restoring, to the extent possible, a body part to its normal anatomic structure and function
- *Replacement:* Putting in or on biological or synthetic material that physically takes the place and/or function of all or a portion of a body part
- *Reposition:* Moving to its normal location or other suitable location all or a portion of a body part
- *Resection:* Cutting out or off, without replacement, all of a body part
- *Restriction:* Partially closing an orifice or lumen of a tubular body part
- *Revision:* Correcting, to the extent possible, a portion of a malfunctioning device or the position of a displaced device
- *Supplement:* Putting in or on biological or synthetic material that physically reinforces and/or augments the function of a portion of a body part
- *Transfer:* Moving, without taking out, all or a portion of a body part to another location to take over the function of all or a portion of a body part
- *Transplantation:* Putting in or on all or a portion of a living body part taken from another individual or animal to physically take the place and/or function of all or a portion of a similar body part

The standardized level of specificity designed into ICD-10-PCS restricts the use of broadly applicable "not otherwise specified (NOS)" or "unspecified code" options in the system. A minimal level of specificity is required to construct a valid code. "Not elsewhere classified (NEC)" options are provided in ICD-10-PCS but only for specific, limited use. The root operation Repair in the Medical and Surgical section functions as a "not elsewhere classified" option. Repair is used only when the procedure performed is not one of the other specific root operations in the Medical and Surgical section.

Appendixes B and C provide additional subcategorization, explanations, and representative examples of the Medical and Surgical section root operations.

Body Part (Character 4)

The fourth character represents the body part, or specific anatomical site where the procedure was performed. The body system (second character) provides only a general indication of the procedure site. The body part and body system values, together, provide a precise description of the procedure site.

Approach (Character 5)

The fifth character represents the approach, or the technique used to reach the procedure site. There are seven different approach values in this section.

- *Open*: Cutting through the skin or mucous membrane and any other body layers necessary to expose the site of the procedure
- *Percutaneous*: Entry, by puncture or minor incision, of instrumentation through the skin or mucous membrane and any other body layers necessary to reach the site of the procedure
- *Percutaneous Endoscopic*: Entry, by puncture or minor incision, of instrumentation through the skin or mucous membrane and any other body layers necessary to reach and visualize the site of the procedure
- *Via Natural or Artificial Opening*: Entry of instrumentation through a natural or artificial external opening to reach the site of the procedure
- *Via Natural or Artificial Opening Endoscopic*: Entry of instrumentation through a natural or artificial external opening to reach and visualize the site of the procedure
- *Via Natural or Artificial Opening with Percutaneous Endoscopic Assistance:* Entry of instrumentation through a natural or artificial external opening and entry, by puncture or minor incision, of instrumentation through the skin or mucous membrane and any other body layers necessary to aid in the performance of the procedure
- *External*: Procedures performed directly on the skin or mucous membrane and procedures performed indirectly by the application of external force through the skin or mucous membrane

Appendix A provides definitions and comparisons of the components (access location, method, and type of instrumentation) for each approach and provides an example and illustration.

Device (Character 6)

The sixth character represents a device. Broad categories of devices found in this section include:

- Grafts (e.g., skin)
- Prostheses (e.g., hip joint)
- Implants (e.g., internal fixation device, mesh)
- Simple or Mechanical Appliances (e.g., drainage device, IUD)
- Electronic Appliances (e.g., pacemaker, monitoring device)

Depending on the procedure performed, there may or may not be a device left in place at the end of the procedure. For procedures that do not utilize a device, the value of *No Device* is available. For devices that cannot be categorized into one of the current values, many tables also have a device value of *Other Device.* This value is intended to be used temporarily until a more specific value can be added to the classification. No categories of medical or surgical devices are permanently classified to *Other Device.*

Instruments used to visualize the procedure site are specified in the fifth-character approach, not the sixth-character device value. Materials that are incidental to a procedure such as clips, ligatures, and sutures are not specified in the device character.

Appendix F compares the general device types and provides examples of each.

Appendix G provides an aggregation table that crosswalks specific device character values used for specific root operations to more general device character values used when the root operation represents an entire family of devices.

Qualifier (Character 7)

The seventh character is a qualifier that captures additional attributes of the procedure, where applicable.

Medical and Surgical Section Principles

In developing the Medical and Surgical procedure codes, several specific principles were followed.

Composite Terms Are Not Root Operations

Composite terms such as colonoscopy, sigmoidectomy, or appendectomy do not describe root operations, but they do specify multiple components of a specific root operation. In ICD-10-PCS, the components of a procedure are defined separately by the characters making up the complete code. The only component of a procedure specified in the root operation is the objective of the procedure. With each complete code the underlying objective of the procedure is specified by the root operation (third character), the precise part is specified by the body part (fourth character), and the method used to reach and visualize the procedure site is specified by the approach (fifth character). While colonoscopy, sigmoidectomy, and appendectomy are included in the Index, they do not constitute root operations in the Tables section. The objective of colonoscopy is the visualization of the colon and the root operation (character 3) is *Inspection*. Character 4 specifies the body part, which in this case is part of the colon. These composite terms, like colonoscopy or appendectomy, are included as cross-reference only. The index provides the correct root operation reference. Examples of other types of composite terms not representative of root operations are *partial* sigmoidectomy, *total* hysterectomy, and *partial* hip replacement. Always refer to the correct root operation in the Index and Tables section.

Root Operation Based on Objective of Procedure

The root operation is based on the objective of the procedure, such as *Resection* of transverse colon or *Dilation* of an artery. The assignment of the root operation is based on the procedure actually performed, which may or may not have been the intended procedure. If the intended procedure is modified or discontinued (e.g., excision instead of resection is performed), the root operation is determined by the procedure actually performed. If the desired result is not attained after completing the procedure (i.e., the artery does not remain expanded after the dilation procedure), the root operation is still determined by the procedure actually performed.

Examples:

- Dilating the urethra is coded as *Dilation* since the objective of the procedure is to dilate the urethra. If dilation of the urethra includes putting in an intraluminal stent, the root operation remains *Dilation* and not *Insertion* of the intraluminal device because the underlying objective of the procedure is dilation of the urethra. The stent is identified by the intraluminal device value in the sixth character of the dilation procedure code.
- If the objective is solely to put a radioactive element in the urethra, then the procedure is coded to the root operation *Insertion*, with the radioactive element identified in the sixth character of the code.
- If the objective of the procedure is to correct a malfunctioning or displaced device, then the procedure is coded to the root operation *Revision*. In the root operation *Revision*, the original device being revised is identified in the device character. *Revision* is typically performed on mechanical appliances (e.g., pacemaker) or materials used in replacement procedures (e.g., synthetic substitute). Typical revision procedures include adjustment of pacemaker position and correction of malfunctioning knee prosthesis.

Combination Procedures Are Coded Separately

If multiple procedures as defined by distinct objectives are performed during an operative episode, then multiple codes are used. For example, obtaining the vein graft used for coronary bypass surgery is coded as a separate procedure from the bypass itself.

Redo of Procedures

The complete or partial redo of the original procedure is coded to the root operation that identifies the procedure performed rather than *Revision*.

Example:

A complete redo of a hip replacement procedure that requires putting in a new prosthesis is coded to the root operation *Replacement* rather than *Revision*.

The correction of complications arising from the original procedure, other than device complications, is coded to the procedure performed. Correction of a malfunctioning or displaced device would be coded to the root operation *Revision*.

Example:

A procedure to control hemorrhage arising from the original procedure is coded to *Control* rather than *Revision*.

Examples of Procedures Coded in the Medical Surgical Section

The following are examples of procedures from the Medical and Surgical section, coded in ICD-10-PCS.

- Suture of skin laceration, left lower arm: ØHQEXZZ
- Laparoscopic appendectomy: ØDTJ4ZZ
- Sigmoidoscopy with biopsy: ØDBN8ZX
- Tracheostomy with tracheostomy tube: ØB11ØF4

Obstetrics Section (1)

The Obstetrics section includes codes for procedures performed on the products of conception only. Procedures on pregnant females are coded in the Medical and Surgical section (e.g., episiotomy). The term "products of conception" refers to all physical components of a pregnancy, including the fetus, amnion, umbilical cord, and placenta. There is no differentiation of the products of conception based on gestational age. Thus, the diagnosis code, not the procedure code, specifies the products of conception as a zygote, embryo, or fetus, or of the trimester of the pregnancy.

Character Meanings

The seven characters in the Obstetrics section have the same meaning as in the Medical and Surgical section.

Character	Meaning
1	Section
2	Body System
3	Root Operation
4	Body Part
5	Approach
6	Device
7	Qualifier

Section (Character 1)

Obstetrics procedure codes have a first character value of *1*.

Body System (Character 2)

The second character represents the body system. There is only one value used in this section: *Pregnancy.*

Root Operation (Character 3)

The third character represents the root operation, or the primary objective, of the procedure. There are 12 values available in this section. Ten of these values specify root operations as defined in the Medical and Surgical section and include *Change, Drainage, Extraction, Insertion, Inspection, Removal, Repair, Reposition, Resection,* and *Transplantation.* The other two values are specific to this section only and are defined as follows:

- *Abortion*: Artificially terminating a pregnancy
- *Delivery*: Assisting the passage of the products of conception from the genital canal

A cesarean section is not a separate root operation because the underlying objective is *Extraction* (i.e., pulling out all or a portion of a body part).

Body Part (Character 4)

The fourth character represents the body part, which in this section is specific to the products of conception. The three values available are as follows:

- *Products of conception*
- *Products of conception, retained*
- *Products of conception, ectopic*

Approach (Character 5)

The fifth character represents the approach, as defined in the Medical and Surgical section.

Device (Character 6)

The sixth character represents a device used during the procedure, where applicable.

Qualifier (Character 7)

The seventh character is a qualifier that captures additional attributes of the procedure, where applicable.

Placement Section (2)

The Placement section includes codes for procedures that put a device in an orifice or on a body region, without making an incision or a puncture.

Character Meanings

The seven characters in the Placement section have the following meaning:

Character	Meaning
1	Section
2	Body System
3	Root Operation
4	Body Region
5	Approach
6	Device
7	Qualifier

Section (Character 1)

Placement procedure codes have a first character value of *2*.

Body System (Character 2)

The second character contains two values specifying either *Anatomical Regions* or *Anatomical Orifices*.

Root Operation (Character 3)

The third character represents the root operation, or the primary objective, of the procedure. There are seven values available in this section. Two of the values specify root operations as defined in the Medical and Surgical section and include *Change* and *Removal*. The other five values are specific to this section only and are defined as follows:

- *Compression*: Putting pressure on a body region
- *Dressing*: Putting material on a body region for protection
- *Immobilization*: Limiting or preventing motion of an external body region
- *Packing*: Putting material in a body region or orifice
- *Traction*: Exerting a pulling force on a body region in a distal direction

Body Region (Character 4)

The fourth character represents the specific body region or orifice. The body system (second character) provides only a general indication of the procedure site. The body region values and body system values, together, precisely describe the procedure site.

Approach (Character 5)

The fifth character represents the approach. Since all placement procedures are performed directly or indirectly on the skin or mucous membrane, the approach value is always *External*.

Device (Character 6)

The sixth character represents a device placed during the procedure, where applicable.

Except for devices used for fractures and dislocations, devices in this section are off the shelf and do not require any extensive design, fabrication, or fitting.

Qualifier (Character 7)

The seventh character is a qualifier. Because there are currently no specific qualifier values in this section, the value is always *No Qualifier.*

Administration Section (3)

The Administration section includes infusions, injections, and transfusions, as well as other related procedures, such as irrigation and tattooing. All codes in this section define procedures in which a diagnostic or therapeutic substance is given to the patient.

Character Meanings

The seven characters in the Administration section have the following meaning:

Character	Meaning
1	Section
2	Body System
3	Root Operation
4	Body System/Region
5	Approach
6	Substance
7	Qualifier

Section (Character 1)

Administration procedure codes have a first character value of *3*.

Body System (Character 2)

The second character can represent the general physiological system, anatomical region, or device to which a substance is being administered. The three values available in this section are *Indwelling Device, Physiological Systems and Anatomical Regions,* and *Circulatory System.*

Root Operation (Character 3)

The third character represents the root operation, or the primary objective, of the procedure. There are three values available in this section.

- *Introduction*: Putting in or on a therapeutic, diagnostic, nutritional, physiological, or prophylactic substance except blood or blood products
- *Irrigation*: Putting in or on a cleansing substance
- *Transfusion*: Putting in blood or blood products

Body/System Region (Character 4)

The fourth character represents the body system/region. The fourth character identifies the site where the substance is administered, not the site where the substance administered takes effect. Sites include *Skin and Mucous Membranes, Subcutaneous Tissue,* and *Muscle.* These differentiate intradermal, subcutaneous, and intramuscular injections, respectively. Other sites include *Eye, Respiratory Tract, Peritoneal Cavity,* and *Epidural Space.*

The body systems/regions for arteries and veins are *Peripheral Artery, Central Artery, Peripheral Vein,* and *Central Vein.* The *Peripheral Artery* or *Vein* is typically used when a substance is introduced locally into an artery or vein. For example, chemotherapy is the introduction of an antineoplastic substance into a peripheral artery or vein by a percutaneous approach. In general, the substance introduced into a peripheral artery or vein has a systemic effect.

The *Central Artery* or *Vein* is typically used when the site where the substance is introduced is distant from the point of entry into the artery or vein. For example, the introduction of a substance directly at the site of a clot within an artery or vein using a catheter is coded as an introduction of a thrombolytic substance into a central artery or vein by a percutaneous approach. In general, the substance introduced into a central artery or vein has a local effect.

Approach (Character 5)

The fifth character represents the approach, as defined in the Medical and Surgical section. The approach for intradermal, subcutaneous, and intramuscular introductions (i.e., injections) is *Percutaneous.* If a catheter is placed to introduce a substance into an internal site within the circulatory system, then the approach is also *Percutaneous.* For example, if a catheter is used to introduce contrast directly into the heart for angiography, then the procedure would be coded as a percutaneous introduction of contrast into the heart.

Substance (Character 6)

The sixth character represents the substance being introduced. Most of the values capture broad categories of substances to which several specific substances may be categorized.

Qualifier (Character 7)

The seventh character is a qualifier. The substance value (second character) provides the broad category to which a substance is classified. The qualifier and substance values, together, precisely describe the substance administered. Not every substance administered has its own unique qualifier.

Measurement and Monitoring Section (4)

The Measurement and Monitoring section represents procedures for determining the level of a physiological or physical function.

Character Meanings

The seven characters in the Measurement and Monitoring section have the following meaning:

Character	Meaning
1	Section
2	Body System
3	Root Operation
4	Body System
5	Approach
6	Function/Device
7	Qualifier

Section (Character 1)

Measurement and Monitoring procedure codes have a first character value of *4*.

Body System (Character 2)
The second character represents the body system or device being measured or monitored. There are two values available in this section, *Physiological Systems* and *Physiological Devices.*

Root Operation (Character 3)
The third character represents the root operation, or the primary objective, of the procedure. There are two values available in this section.

- *Measurement*: Determining the level of a physiological or physical function at a point in time
- *Monitoring*: Determining the level of a physiological or physical function repetitively over a period of time

Body System (Character 4)
The fourth character represents the specific body system measured or monitored.

Approach (Character 5)
The fifth character represents the approach, as defined in the Medical and Surgical section.

Function/Device (Character 6)
The sixth character represents the physiological or physical function, or the device function being measured or monitored.

Qualifier (Character 7)
The seventh character is a qualifier, which captures additional attributes of the procedure, where applicable.

Extracorporeal or Systemic Assistance and Performance Section (5)
The Extracorporeal or Systemic Assistance and Performance section describes procedures performed in a critical care setting, such as mechanical ventilation and cardioversion. It also includes other procedures, such as hemodialysis and hyperbaric oxygen treatment.

The procedures described in this section are meant to be temporary; that is, the equipment is used only for the duration of the procedure. The equipment resides primarily outside the body, though it may interface with the body via a tube or other means. Although parts of the equipment may be attached or inserted into the patient, such as lines or catheters, these are not coded as separate device insertion procedures.

Character Meanings
The seven characters in the Extracorporeal or Systemic Assistance and Performance section have the following meaning:

Character	Meaning
1	Section
2	Body System
3	Root Operation
4	Body System
5	Duration
6	Function
7	Qualifier

Section (Character 1)
Extracorporeal or Systemic Assistance and Performance procedure codes have a first character value of *5.*

Body System (Character 2)
The second character represents the body system. There is one value available in this section, *Physiological Systems.*

Root Operation (Character 3)
The third character represents the root operation, or the primary objective, of the procedure. There are three values available in this section.

- *Assistance*: Taking over a portion of a physiological function by extracorporeal means
- *Performance*: Completely taking over a physiological function by extracorporeal means
- *Restoration*: Returning, or attempting to return, a physiological function to its natural state by extracorporeal means

The root operation *Restoration* contains a single procedure code that identifies extracorporeal cardioversion.

Body System (Character 4)
The fourth character represents the body system for which support of a physiological function is required.

Duration (Character 5)
The fifth character specifies the duration of the procedure.

Function (Character 6)
The sixth character represents the physiological function assisted or performed (e.g., oxygenation, ventilation) during the procedure.

Qualifier (Character 7)
The seventh character is a qualifier, which captures additional attributes of the procedure, where applicable, such as the type of equipment used to support or assist a physiological function.

Introduction

Extracorporeal or Systemic Therapies Section (6)

The Extracorporeal or Systemic Therapies section describes procedures in which equipment outside the body is used for a therapeutic purpose that does not involve the assistance or performance of a physiological function. For procedures such as hypothermia, for which the therapy is not applied to a specific body system but the entire body, a fourth character for *None* is used.

Character Meanings

The seven characters in the Extracorporeal or Systemic Therapies section have the following meaning:

Character	Meaning
1	Section
2	Body System
3	Root Operation
4	Body System
5	Duration
6	Qualifier
7	Qualifier

Section (Character 1)

Extracorporeal or Systemic Therapy procedure codes have a first character value of *6*.

Body System (Character 2)

The second character represents the body system. There is one value available in this section, *Physiological Systems*.

Root Operation (Character 3)

The third character represents the root operation, or the primary objective, of the procedure. There are 11 values available in this section.

- *Atmospheric Control*: Extracorporeal control of atmospheric pressure and composition
- *Decompression*: Extracorporeal elimination of undissolved gas from body fluids

  Decompression involves only one type of procedure: treatment for decompression sickness (the bends) in a hyperbaric chamber.
- *Electromagnetic Therapy*: Extracorporeal treatment by electromagnetic rays
- *Hyperthermia*: Extracorporeal raising of body temperature

  The term hyperthermia is used to describe both a temperature imbalance treatment and also as an adjunct radiation treatment for cancer. When treating the temperature imbalance, it is coded to this section; for the cancer treatment, it is coded in the Radiation Therapy section.
- *Hypothermia*: Extracorporeal lowering of body temperature
- *Perfusion*: Extracorporeal treatment by diffusion of therapeutic fluid
- *Pheresis*: Extracorporeal separation of blood products

  Pheresis may be used for two main purposes: to treat diseases when too much of a blood component is produced (e.g., leukemia) and to remove a blood product such as platelets from a donor, for transfusion into another patient.
- *Phototherapy*: Extracorporeal treatment by light rays

  Phototherapy involves using a machine that exposes the blood to light rays outside the body, recirculates it, and then returns it to the body.
- *Shock Wave Therapy*: Extracorporeal treatment by shock waves
- *Ultrasound Therapy*: Extracorporeal treatment by ultrasound
- *Ultraviolet Light Therapy*: Extracorporeal treatment by ultraviolet light

Body System (Character 4)

The fourth character represents the body system on which the extracorporeal or systemic therapy is performed (e.g., skin, circulatory).

Duration (Character 5)

The fifth character specifies the duration of the procedure. There are two values available in this section, *Single* or *Multiple*.

Qualifier (Characters 6 and 7)

The sixth and seventh characters are qualifiers. The qualifier captures additional attributes of the procedure, where applicable.

Osteopathic Section (7)

Character Meanings

The seven characters in the Osteopathic section have the following meaning:

Character	Meaning
1	Section
2	Body System
3	Root Operation
4	Body Region
5	Approach
6	Method
7	Qualifier

Section (Character 1)

Osteopathic procedure codes have a first character value of *7*.

Body System (Character 2)

The second character represents the body system. There is one value available in this section, *Anatomical Regions*.

Root Operation (Character 3)

The third character represents the root operation, or the primary objective, of the procedure. There is one value available in this section.

- *Treatment*: Manual treatment to eliminate or alleviate somatic dysfunction and related disorders

Body Region (Character 4)

The fourth character represents the body region. The body system (second character) indicates only the anatomical region involved in the procedure. The body region values and body system value, together, precisely describe the procedure site.

Approach (Character 5)

The fifth character represents the approach. There is only one value available in this section, *External*.

Method (Character 6)

The sixth character represents the method used to carry out the osteopathic treatment.

Qualifier (Character 7)

The seventh character is a qualifier. Because there are currently no specific qualifier values in this section, the value is always *None*.

Other Procedures Section (8)

The Other Procedures section contains codes for procedures not included in the other medical and surgical-related sections, including computer- and robotic-assisted procedures.

Character Meanings

The seven characters in the Other Procedures section have the following meaning:

Character	Meaning
1	Section
2	Body System
3	Root Operation
4	Body Region
5	Approach
6	Method
7	Qualifier

Section (Character 1)

Other Procedures section codes have a first character value of *8*.

Body System (Character 2)

The second character represents the body system/region or a device. There are two values available in this section, *Physiological Systems and Anatomical Regions* and *Indwelling Device.*

Root Operation (Character 3)

The third character represents the root operation, or the primary objective, of the procedure. There is one value available in this section.

- *Other Procedures*: Methodologies that attempt to remediate or cure a disorder or disease.

Body Region (Character 4)

The fourth character contains specified body-region values, and also the body-region value *None*.

Approach (Character 5)

The fifth character represents the approach, as defined in the Medical and Surgical section.

Method (Character 6)

The sixth character specifies the method (e.g., *Acupuncture, Therapeutic Massage*).

Qualifier (Character 7)

The seventh character is a qualifier. The qualifier is used to capture additional attributes of the procedure, where applicable.

Chiropractic Section (9)

Character Meanings

The seven characters in the Chiropractic section have the following meaning:

Character	Meaning
1	Section
2	Body System
3	Root Operation
4	Body Region
5	Approach
6	Method
7	Qualifier

Section (Character 1)

Chiropractic section procedure codes have a first character value of *9*.

Body System (Character 2)

The second character represents the body region. There is one value available in this section, *Anatomical Regions*.

Root Operation (Character 3)

The third character represents the root operation, or the primary objective, of the procedure. There is one value available in this section.

- *Manipulation:* Manual procedure that involves a directed thrust to move a joint past the physiological range of motion, without exceeding the anatomical limit.

Body Region (Character 4)

The fourth character represents the body region on which the chiropractic manipulation is performed.

Approach (Character 5)

The fifth character represents the approach. There is only one value available in this section, *External*.

Method (Character 6)

The sixth character represents the method by which the manipulation is accomplished.

Qualifier (Character 7)

The seventh character is a qualifier. Because there are currently no specific qualifier values in this section, the value is always *None*.

Imaging Section (B)

The Imaging section contains codes for procedures such as plain radiography, fluoroscopy, CT, MRI, and ultrasound.

Procedures such as PET, uptakes, and scans are in the Nuclear Medicine section. Therapeutic radiation, for the treatment of cancer, is in the Radiation Therapy section.

Character Meanings

The seven characters in Imaging procedures have the following meaning:

Character	Meaning
1	Section
2	Body System
3	Root Type
4	Body Part
5	Contrast
6	Qualifier
7	Qualifier

Section (Character 1)

Imaging procedure codes have a first character value of *B*.

Body System (Character 2)

The second character represents the general body system where the imaging is being performed. The available values mimic those that are found in the Medical and Surgical section but may not be exact matches.

Root Type (Character 3)

The third character represents the root type. The section title, *Imaging,* essentially identifies the root operation, while the values for the third character describe the type of imaging being performed. There are six root types in this section.

- *Computerized Tomography (CT Scan)*: Computer reformatted digital display of multiplanar images developed from the capture of multiple exposures of external ionizing radiation
- *Fluoroscopy*: Single plane or bi-plane real time display of an image developed from the capture of external ionizing radiation on a fluorescent screen. The image may also be stored by either digital or analog means
- *Magnetic Resonance Imaging (MRI)*: Computer reformatted digital display of multiplanar images developed from the capture of radiofrequency signals emitted by nuclei in a body site excited within a magnetic field
- *Other Imaging:* Other specified modality for visualizing a body part
- *Plain Radiography*: Planar display of an image developed from the capture of external ionizing radiation on photographic or photoconductive plate
- *Ultrasonography*: Real time display of images of anatomy or flow information developed from the capture of reflected and attenuated high frequency sound waves

Body Part (Character 4)

The fourth character represents the body part, or specific anatomical site where the procedure was performed. The body system (second character) provides only a general indication of the procedure site. The body part and body system values, together, precisely describe the procedure site.

Contrast (Character 5)

The fifth character represents the type of contrast or enhancing material utilized to facilitate the procedure, when applicable.

Qualifier (Character 6)

The sixth character is a qualifier. The most common qualifier, *Unenhanced and Enhanced,* describes an image taken without contrast (unenhanced) followed by an image with contrast (enhanced). Other qualifier values describe other noncontrast material or technology used to facilitate the imaging.

Qualifier (Character 7)

The seventh character is a qualifier. The qualifier is used to capture additional attributes of the procedure, where applicable.

Nuclear Medicine Section (C)

The Nuclear Medicine section is organized like the Imaging section. Procedures captured in this section describe the introduction of radioactive material into the body to create an image, to diagnose or treat pathological conditions, or to assess metabolic functions.

The introduction of encapsulated radioactive material for the treatment of cancer is included in the Radiation Therapy section.

Character Meanings

The seven characters in the Nuclear Medicine section have the following meaning:

Character	Meaning
1	Section
2	Body System
3	Root Type
4	Body Part
5	Radionuclide
6	Qualifier
7	Qualifier

Section (Character 1)

Nuclear Medicine procedure codes have a first character value of *C*.

Body System (Character 2)

The second character represents the general body system or anatomical region to which the nuclear medicine procedure is performed.

Root Type (Character 3)

The third character represents the root type. The section title, *Nuclear Medicine*, essentially identifies the root operation, while the third character value describes the type of nuclear medicine being performed. There are seven root types available in this section.

- *Nonimaging Nuclear Medicine Assay:* Introduction of radioactive materials into the body for the study of body fluids and blood elements, by the detection of radioactive emissions
- *Nonimaging Nuclear Medicine Probe:* Introduction of radioactive materials into the body for the study of distribution and fate of certain substances by the detection of radioactive emissions; or alternatively, measurement of absorption of radioactive emissions from an external source
- *Nonimaging Nuclear Medicine Uptake:* Introduction of radioactive materials into the body for measurements of organ function, from the detection of radioactive emissions

- *Planar Nuclear Medicine Imaging*: Introduction of radioactive materials into the body for single-plane display of images developed from the capture of radioactive emissions
- *Positron Emission Tomography (PET) Imaging:* Introduction of radioactive materials into the body for three dimensional display of images developed from the simultaneous capture, 180 degrees apart, of radioactive emissions
- *Systemic Nuclear Medicine Therapy:* Introduction of unsealed radioactive materials into the body for treatment
- *Tomographic (Tomo) Nuclear Medicine Imaging*: Introduction of radioactive materials into the body for three dimensional display of images developed from the capture of radioactive emissions

Body Part (Character 4)

The fourth character represents the specific body part or region being studied, imaged, or treated. The body system (second character) provides only a general indication of the procedure site. The body part and body system values, together, provide a precise description of the procedure site.

Radionuclide (Character 5)

The fifth character represents the type of radioactive material utilized to facilitate the procedure, when applicable. The *Other Radionuclide* value is used for radioactive material that has been newly approved but does not yet have its own unique value in the coding system.

If more than one radioactive material is given to perform the procedure, more than one code is used.

Qualifier (Characters 6 and 7)

The sixth and seventh characters are qualifiers. Because there are currently no specific qualifier values in this section, the value is always *None*.

Radiation Therapy Section (D)

The Radiation Therapy section contains procedures performed for cancer treatment.

Character Meanings

The seven characters in the Radiation Therapy section have the following meaning:

Character	Meaning
1	Section
2	Body System
3	Modality
4	Treatment Site
5	Modality Qualifier
6	Isotope
7	Qualifier

Section (Character 1)

Radiation therapy procedure codes have a first character value of *D*.

Body System (Character 2)

The second character represents the general body system or anatomical region to which radiation therapy is being applied.

Modality (Character 3)

The third character represents the type of radiation, or modality, being used. There are four values available in this section.

- *Beam Radiation*
- *Brachytherapy*
- *Stereotactic Radiosurgery*
- *Other Radiation*

Treatment Site (Character 4)

The fourth character represents the specific body part or region being irradiated. The body system (second character) provides only a general indication of the procedure site. The treatment site and body system values, together, precisely describe the procedure site.

Modality Qualifier (Character 5)

The fifth character represents specific methods or materials unique to a particular type of radiation therapy. The modality (third character) and modality qualifier values, together, precisely describe the therapy performed.

Isotope (Character 6)

The sixth character represents the specific radioactive isotope introduced into the body, if applicable.

Qualifier (Character 7)

The seventh character is a qualifier. Besides the value of *None*, this section contains two other values, *Intraoperative* and *Unidirectional Source*.

Physical Rehabilitation and Diagnostic Audiology Section (F)

Character Meanings

The seven characters in the Physical Rehabilitation and Diagnostic Audiology section have the following meaning:

Character	Meaning
1	Section
2	Section Qualifier
3	Root Type
4	Body System/Region
5	Type Qualifier
6	Equipment
7	Qualifier

Section (Character 1)

Physical Rehabilitation and Diagnostic Audiology procedure codes have a first character value of *F*.

Section Qualifier (Character 2)

The second character qualifies which of the two services described in the section (character 1) is being represented. Therefore, only two values are available, *Rehabilitation* or *Diagnostic Audiology*.

Root Type (Character 3)

The third character represents the root type. The section qualifier (second character) identifies the root operation, while the third-character value describes the type of rehabilitation or diagnostic audiology being performed. There are 14 root types available in this section, each classified into four general categories.

Assessment: Used to evaluate a patient's level of function to determine the type and timing of treatment required. Assessment procedures focus on the faculties of hearing and speech, on various aspects of body function, and on the patient's quality of life, such as muscle performance, neuromotor development, and reintegration skills.

There are six root type values available for assessment.

- *Speech Assessment:* Measurement of speech and related functions
- *Motor and/or Nerve Function Assessment:* Measurement of motor, nerve, and related functions
- *Activities of Daily Living Assessment:* Measurement of functional level for activities of daily living
- *Hearing Assessment:* Measurement of hearing and related functions
- *Hearing Aid Assessment:* Measurement of the appropriateness and/or effectiveness of a hearing device
- *Vestibular Assessment:* Measurement of the vestibular system and related functions

Treatment: Use of specific activities or methods to develop, improve, and/or restore the performance of necessary functions, compensate for dysfunction and/or minimize debilitation. Procedures include swallowing dysfunction exercises, bathing and showering techniques, wound management, gait training, and a host of activities typically associated with rehabilitation.

There are six root type values available for treatment.

- *Speech Treatment:* Application of techniques to improve, augment, or compensate for speech and related functional impairment
- *Motor Treatment:* Exercise or activities to increase or facilitate motor function
- *Activities of Daily Living Treatment:* Exercise or activities to facilitate functional competence for activities of daily living
- *Hearing Treatment:* Application of techniques to improve, augment, or compensate for hearing and related functional impairment
- *Cochlear Implant Treatment:* Application of techniques to improve the communication abilities of individuals with cochlear implant
- *Vestibular Treatment:* Application of techniques to improve, augment, or compensate for vestibular and related functional impairment

Caregiver Training: Educating a caregiver with the skills and knowledge needed to interact with and assist the patient.

There is only one root type value available for caregiver training.

- *Caregiver Training:* Training in activities to support patient's optimal level of function

Fitting(s): Design, fabrication, modification, selection, and/or application of splint, orthosis, prosthesis, hearing aids, and/or other rehabilitation device. The fifth character used in Device Fitting procedures describes the device being fitted rather than the method used to fit the device. Definitions of devices, when provided, are in the definitions portion of the ICD-10-PCS tables and index, under section F, character 5.

There is only one root type value available for fittings.

- *Device Fitting:* Fitting of a device designed to facilitate or support achievement of a higher level of function

Body System/Region (Character 4)

The fourth character represents the body system and body region, where applicable, that requires rehabilitation. For diagnostic audiology procedures, this value is always *None*.

Type Qualifier (Character 5)

The fifth character represents a type qualifier. The root type (third character) and type qualifier values, together, precisely describe the procedure performed.

Equipment (Character 6)

The sixth character represents any equipment used to facilitate the procedure. The values provided are broad categories that may capture several specific types of equipment.

Qualifier (Character 7)

The seventh character is a qualifier. As there are currently no specific qualifier values in this section, the value is always *None*.

Mental Health Section (G)

Character Meanings

The seven characters in the Mental Health section have the following meaning:

Character	Meaning
1	Section
2	Body System
3	Type
4	Qualifier
5	Qualifier
6	Qualifier
7	Qualifier

Section (Character 1)

Mental health procedure codes have a first character value of *G*.

Body System (Character 2)

The second character is always represented by the value of *None*. As mental health care manages the psychological aspects of a patient's health, there is no specific body system or region that can be represented in this section.

Type (Character 3)

The third character represents the type of procedure. There are 12 values available in this section.

- *Psychological Tests:* The administration and interpretation of standardized psychological tests and measurement instruments for the assessment of psychological function
- *Crisis Intervention:* Treatment of a traumatized, acutely disturbed, or distressed individual for the purpose of short-term stabilization
- *Medication Management:* Monitoring and adjusting the use of medications for the treatment of a mental health disorder

- *Individual Psychotherapy:* Treatment of an individual with a mental health disorder by behavioral, cognitive, psychoanalytic, psychodynamic, or psychophysiological means to improve functioning or well-being
- *Counseling:* The application of psychological methods to treat an individual with normal developmental issues and psychological problems in order to increase function, improve well-being, alleviate distress, maladjustment, or resolve crises
- *Family Psychotherapy:* Treatment that includes one or more family members of an individual with a mental health disorder by behavioral, cognitive, psychoanalytic, psychodynamic, or psychophysiological means to improve functioning or well-being
- *Electroconvulsive Therapy:* The application of controlled electrical voltages to treat a mental health disorder
- *Biofeedback:* Provision of information from the monitoring and regulating of physiological processes in conjunction with cognitive-behavioral techniques to improve patient functioning or well-being
- *Hypnosis:* Induction of a state of heightened suggestibility by auditory, visual, and tactile techniques to elicit an emotional or behavioral response
- *Narcosynthesis:* Administration of intravenous barbiturates in order to release suppressed or repressed thoughts
- *Group Psychotherapy:* Treatment of two or more individuals with a mental health disorder by behavioral, cognitive, psychoanalytic, psychodynamic, or psychophysiological means to improve functioning or well-being
- *Light Therapy:* Application of specialized light treatments to improve functioning or well-being

Qualifier (Character 4)
The fourth character is a qualifier. This value represents the specific technique used to evaluate or treat a patient's mental health. In conjunction with the type (third character), the qualifier value precisely describes the procedure.

Qualifier (Characters 5, 6, and 7)
The fifth, sixth, and seventh characters are qualifiers. As there are currently no specific qualifier values in this section, the value is always *None*.

Substance Abuse Treatment Section (H)

Character Meanings
The seven characters in the Substance Abuse Treatment section have the following meaning:

Character	Meaning
1	Section
2	Body System
3	Type
4	Qualifier
5	Qualifier
6	Qualifier
7	Qualifier

Section (Character 1)
Substance Abuse Treatment codes have a first character value of *H*.

Body System (Character 2)
The second character is always represented by the value of *None*. As the substance abuse treatment section describes management of the psychological aspects of a patient's health, there is no specific body system or region that can be represented in this section.

Type (Character 3)
The third character represents the specific type of treatment. There are seven values available in this section.

- *Detoxification Services:* Detoxification from alcohol and/or drugs
- *Individual Counseling:* The application of psychological methods to treat an individual with addictive behavior
- *Group Counseling:* The application of psychological methods to treat two or more individuals with addictive behavior
- *Individual Psychotherapy:* Treatment of an individual with addictive behavior by behavioral, cognitive, psychoanalytic, psychodynamic, or psychophysiological means
- *Family Counseling:* The application of psychological methods that includes one or more family members to treat an individual with addictive behavior
- *Medication Management:* Monitoring and adjusting the use of replacement medications for the treatment of addiction
- *Pharmacotherapy:* The use of replacement medications for the treatment of addiction

Qualifier (Character 4)
The fourth character is a qualifier. The qualifier value further characterizes the type (character 3) of treatment being rendered, where applicable.

Qualifier (Characters 5, 6, and 7)
The fifth, sixth, and seventh characters are qualifiers. As there are currently no specific qualifier values in this section, the value is always *None*.

New Technology Section (X)

General Information
Section X New Technology is a section added to ICD-10-PCS beginning October 1, 2015. The new section provides a place for codes that uniquely identify procedures requested via the New Technology Application Process or that capture other new technologies not currently classified in ICD-10-PCS.

Section X does not introduce any new coding concepts or unusual guidelines for correct coding. In fact, Section X codes maintain continuity with the other sections in ICD-10-PCS by using the same root operation and body part values as their closest counterparts in other sections of ICD-10-PCS. For example, the codes for the infusion of Sarilumab, use the same root operation (Introduction) and body part values (Central Vein and Peripheral Vein) in section X as the infusion codes in section 3 Administration, which are their closest counterparts in the other sections of ICD-10-PCS.

Introduction

Character Meanings

The seven characters in the new technology section have the following meaning:

Character	Meaning
1	Section
2	Body System
3	Root Operation
4	Body Part
5	Approach
6	Device/Substance/Technology
7	Qualifier

Section (Character 1)

New technology procedure codes have a first character value of *X*.

Body System (Character 2)

The second character values for body system combine the uses of body system, body region, and physiological system as specified in other sections in ICD-10-PCS.

Root Operation (Character 3)

The third character utilizes the same root operation values as their counterparts in other sections of ICD-10-PCS.

Body Part (Character 4)

The fourth character represents the same body part values as their closest counterparts in other sections of ICD-10-PCS.

Approach (Character 5)

The fifth character represents the approach, as defined in the Medical and Surgical section.

Device/Substance/Technology (Character 6)

The sixth character represents the key feature of the new technology procedure. It may be specified as a new device, a new substance, or other new technology. Examples of sixth character values are *Robotic Waterjet Ablation, Interbody Fusion Device, Customizable, and Nafamostat Anticoagulant.*

Qualifier (Character 7)

The seventh character qualifier is used exclusively to specify the new technology group, a number or letter that changes each year that new technology codes are added to the system. For example, Section X codes added for the first year have the seventh character value 1, *New Technology Group 1*, and the next year that Section X codes are added have the seventh character value 2, *New Technology Group 2*, and so on. Changing the seventh character value to a unique letter or number every year that there are new codes in the new technology section allows the ICD-10-PCS to "recycle" the values in the third, fourth, and sixth characters as needed.

New Technology Coding Instruction

Section X codes are standalone codes. They are not supplemental codes. Section X codes fully represent the specific procedure described in the code title, and do not require any additional codes from other sections of ICD-10-PCS. When section X contains a code title which describes a specific new technology procedure, only that X code is reported for the procedure. There is no need to report a broader, non-specific code in another section of ICD-10-PCS.

For example, code XW033G5 Introduction of Sarilumab into Peripheral Vein, Percutaneous Approach, New Technology Group 5, would be reported to indicate that Sarilumab was administered via peripheral vein. A separate code from table 3EØ in the Administration section of ICD-10-PCS would not be reported in addition to this code. The X section code fully identifies the administration of the sarilumab, and no additional code is needed.

The New Technology section codes are easily found by looking in the ICD-10-PCS Index or the Tables. In the Index, the name of the new technology device, substance or technology for a section X code is included as a main term. In addition, all codes in section X are listed under the main term New Technology. The new technology code index entry for sarilumab is shown below.

Sarilumab XWØ

New Technology
Sarilumab XWØ

ICD-10-PCS Index and Tabular Format

The *ICD-10-PCS: The Complete Official Code Set* is based on the official version of the International Classification of Diseases, 10th Revision, Procedure Classification System, issued by the U.S. Department of Health and Human Services, Centers for Medicare and Medicaid Services. This book is consistent with the content of the government's version of ICD-10-PCS and follows their official format.

Index

The Alphabetic Index can be used to locate the appropriate table containing all the information necessary to construct a procedure code, however, the PCS tables should always be consulted to find the most appropriate valid code. Users may choose a valid code directly from the tables—he or she need not consult the index before proceeding to the tables to complete the code.

Main Terms

The Alphabetic Index reflects the structure of the tables. Therefore, the index is organized as an alphabetic listing. The index:

- Is based on the value of the third character
- Contains common procedure terms
- Lists anatomic sites
- Uses device terms

The main terms in the Alphabetic Index are root operations, root procedure types, or common procedure names. In addition, anatomic sites from the Body Part Key and device terms from the Device Key have been added for ease of use.

Examples:

Resection (root operation)

Fluoroscopy (root type)

Prostatectomy (common procedure name)

Brachiocephalic artery (body part)

Bard® Dulex™ mesh (device)

The index provides at least the first three or four values of the code, and some entries may provide complete valid codes. However, the user should always consult the appropriate table to verify that the most appropriate valid code has been selected.

Root Operation and Procedure Type Main Terms

For the *Medical and Surgical* and related sections, the root operation values are used as main terms in the index. The subterms under the root operation main terms are body parts. For the Ancillary section of the tables, the main terms in the index are the general type of procedure performed.

Examples:

Biofeedback GZC9ZZZ
Destruction
  Acetabulum
    Left ØQ55
    Right ØQ54
  Adenoids ØC5Q
  Ampulla of Vater ØF5C

Planar Nuclear Medicine Imaging
  Abdomen CW1Ø

See Reference

The second type of term in the index uses common procedure names, such as "appendectomy" or "fundoplication." These common terms are listed as main terms with a "see" reference noting the PCS root operations that are possible valid code tables based on the objective of the procedure.

Examples:

Tendonectomy
  see Excision, Tendons ØLB
  see Resection, Tendons ØLT

Use Reference

The index also lists anatomic sites from the Body Part Key and device terms from the Device Key. These terms are listed with a "use" reference. The purpose of these references is to act as an additional reference to the terms located in the Appendix Keys. The term provided is the Body Part value or Device value to be selected when constructing a procedure code using the code tables. This type of index reference is not intended to direct the user to another term in the index, but to provide guidance regarding character value selection. Therefore, "use" references generally do not refer to specific valid code tables.

Examples:

CoAxia NeuroFlo catheter
  use Intraluminal Device
Epitrochlear lymph node
  use Lymphatic, Left Upper Extremity
  use Lymphatic, Right Upper Extremity
SynCardia Total Artificial Heart
  use Synthetic Substitute

Code Tables

ICD-10-PCS contains 17 sections of Code Tables organized by general type of procedure. The first three characters of a procedure code define each table. The tables consist of columns providing the possible last four characters of codes and rows providing valid values for each character. Within a PCS table, valid codes include all combinations of choices in characters 4 through 7 contained in the same row of the table. All seven characters must be specified to form a valid code.

There are three main sections of tables:

- Medical and Surgical section:
  - *Medical and Surgical* (Ø)
- Medical and Surgical-related sections:
  - *Obstetrics* (1)
  - *Placement* (2)
  - *Administration* (3)
  - *Measurement and Monitoring* (4)
  - *Extracorporeal or Systemic Assistance and Performance* (5)
  - *Extracorporeal or Systemic Therapies* (6)
  - *Osteopathic* (7)

- *Other Procedures* (8)
- *Chiropractic* (9)

- Ancillary sections:
  - *Imaging* (B)
  - *Nuclear Medicine* (C)
  - *Radiation Therapy* (D)
  - *Physical Rehabilitation and Diagnostic Audiology* (F)
  - *Mental Health* (G)
  - *Substance Abuse Treatment* (H)
- New Technology section:
  - *New Technology* (X)

The first three character values define each table. The root operation or root type designated for each table is accompanied by its official definition.

Example:

Table ØØF provides codes for procedures on the central nervous system that involve breaking up of solid matter into pieces:

Character 1, Section	Ø: Medical and Surgical
Character 2, Body System	Ø: Central Nervous System and Cranial Nerves
Character 3, Root Operation	F: Fragmentation: Breaking solid matter in a body part into pieces

Tables are arranged numerically, then alphabetically.

When reviewing tables, the user should keep in mind that:

- Some tables may cover multiple pages in the code book—to ensure maximum clarity about character choices, valid entries do not split rows between pages. For instance, the entire table of valid characters completing a code beginning with 4A1 is split between two pages, but the split is between, not within, rows. This means that all the valid sixth and seventh characters for, say, body system *Arterial* (3) and approach *External* (X) are contained on one page.
- Individual entries may be listed in several horizontal "selection" lines.
- When a table is continued onto another page, a note to this effect has been added in red.

Body Part Definitions:

An exclusive Optum feature in the tables is the incorporation of the body part definitions provided in appendix E into the Medical and Surgical section (Ø) tables under their appropriate body part characters in the first column (character 4). This provides the user a direct reference to all anatomical descriptions, terms, and sites that could be coded to that particular body part value.

Paired body parts typically have values for the right and left side and in some cases a value for bilateral. These paired body parts often have the same list of inclusive body part definitions. When there are paired body parts with the same body part definitions, the first listed body part (usually the right side) contains the list of body part definitions while the second listed body part (usually the left side) contains a ***See*** instruction. This ***See*** instruction references the body part value that contains the body part definitions. In the table below, body part value P – Upper Eyelid, Left is followed by a ***See*** instruction that states ***See*** *N Upper Eyelid, Right*. All body part descriptions under value N also apply to body part value P.

Example:

Ø Medical and Surgical
8 Eye
M Reattachment Definition: Putting back in or on all or a portion of a separated body part to its normal location or other suitable location
Explanation: Vascular circulation and nervous pathways may or may not be reestablished

Body Part Character 4	Approach Character 5	Device Character 6	Qualifier Character 7
N Upper Eyelid, Right Lateral canthus Levator palpebrae superioris muscle Orbicularis oculi muscle Superior tarsal plate **P Upper Eyelid, Left** *See N Upper Eyelid, Right* **Q Lower Eyelid, Right** Inferior tarsal plate Medial canthus **R Lower Eyelid, Left** *See Q Lower Eyelid, Right*	**X External**	**Z No Device**	**Z No Qualifier**

ICD-10-PCS Additional Features

Use of Official Sources

Color-coding, icons, and other annotations in this manual identify coding and reimbursement edits derived from the inpatient prospective payment system (IPPS) official tables and data files and from the MS-DRG Grouper software.

In most instances, FY 2024 data from the above sources were not available at the time this book was printed. In an effort to make available the most current source information, Optum has provided a document identifying FY 2024 changes to edit designations for ICD-10-PCS codes. Edit changes identified in this document may include:

- Sex
- Hospital-acquired condition
- Noncovered procedures
- Limited coverage procedures
- Valid operating room procedures
- DRG nonoperating room procedures
- Nonoperating room procedures
- New-technology add-on payment

This document can be accessed at the following:

https://www.optumcoding.com/ProductUpdates/
Title: "2024 ICD-10-PCS Edit Changes"
Password: 24PCS

Table Notations

Many tables in ICD-10-PCS contain color or symbol annotations that may aid in code selection, provide clinical or coding information, or alert the coder to reimbursement issues affected by the PCS code assignment. These annotations may be displayed on or next to a character 4, character 6, or character 7 value. Please note that some values may have more than one annotation; this is true most often with the character 4 value.

Refer to the color/symbol legend at the bottom of each page in the tables section for an abridged description of each color and symbol.

Annotation Box

An annotation box has been appended to all tables that contain color-coding or symbol annotations. The color bar or symbol attached to a character value is provided in the box, as well as a list of the valid PCS code(s) to which that edit applies. The box may also list conditional criteria that must be met to satisfy the edit.

For example, see Table ØØF. Four character 4 body part values have a gray color bar. In the annotation box below the table, the gray color bar is defined as "Non-OR," or a nonoperating room procedure edit. Following the Non-OR annotation are the PCS codes that are considered nonoperating room procedures from that row of Table ØØF.

Bracketed Code Notation

The use of bracketed codes is an efficient convention to provide all valid character value alternatives for a specific set of circumstances. The character values in the brackets correspond to the valid values for the character in the position the bracket appears.

Examples:
In the annotation box for Table ØØF the Noncovered Procedure edit (NC) applies to codes represented in the bracketed code ØØF[3,4,5,6]XZZ.

ØØF[3,4,5,6]XZZ Fragmentation in (Central Nervous System and Cranial Nerves), External Approach

The valid fourth character values (body part) that may be selected for this specific circumstance are as follows:

3 Epidural Space, Intracranial
4 Subdural Space, Intracranial
5 Subarachnoid Space, Intracranial
6 Cerebral Ventricle

The fragmentation of matter in the spinal canal, Body Part value U, is not included in the noncovered procedure code edit.

Color-Coding/Symbols

New and Revised Text

Changes within the ICD-10-PCS tables, since the last published edition of this manual, are highlighted in two ways:

- **Red font** identifies new or revised text effective April 1, 2023.
- **Green font** identifies new or revised text effective October 1, 2023.

Medicare Code Edits

Medicare administrative contractors (MACs) and many payers use Medicare code edits to check the coding accuracy on claims. The coding edits provided in this manual include only those directly related to ICD-10-PCS codes used for acute care hospital inpatient admissions.

Sex Edit Symbols

The sex edit symbols below are used to detect inconsistencies between the patient's sex and the procedure. The symbols below most often appear to the right of the body part (character 4) value but may also be found to the right of the qualifier (character 7) value:

♂ Male procedure only
♀ Female procedure only

QA Questionable Obstetric Admission

An inpatient admission is considered questionable when a vaginal or cesarean delivery code is assigned without a corresponding secondary diagnosis code describing the outcome of delivery. Both a delivery (ICD-10-PCS) code and an outcome-of-delivery (ICD-10-CM) code must be present to avoid errors in MS-DRG assignment. This symbol is found only in the Obstetrics Section, appearing to the right of the body part (character 4) value.

NC Noncovered Procedure

Medicare does not cover all procedures. However, some noncovered procedures, due to the presence of certain diagnoses, are reimbursed.

LC **Limited Coverage**

For certain procedures whose medical complexity and serious nature incur extraordinary associated costs, Medicare limits coverage to a portion of the cost. The limited coverage edit indicates the type of limited coverage.

ICD-10 MS-DRG Definitions Manual Edits

An MS-DRG is assigned based on specific patient attributes, such as principal diagnosis, secondary diagnoses, procedures, and discharge status. The attributes (edits) provided in this manual include only those directly related to ICD-10-PCS codes used for acute care hospital inpatient admissions.

Non-Operating Room Procedures Not Affecting MS-DRG Assignment

In the Medical and Surgical section (ØØ1-ØYW) and the Obstetric section (1Ø2-1ØY) tables **only,** ICD-10-PCS procedures codes that DO NOT affect MS-DRG assignment are identified by a **gray color bar** over the body part (character 4) value and are considered non-operating room (non-OR) procedures.

Note: The majority of the ICD-10-PCS codes in the Medical and Surgical-Related, Ancillary and New Technology section tables are non-operating room procedures that do not typically affect MS-DRG assignment. Only the Valid Operating Room and DRG Non-Operating Room procedures are highlighted in these sections, *see* Non-Operating Room Procedures Affecting MS-DRG Assignment and Valid OR Procedure description below.

Non-Operating Room Procedures Affecting MS-DRG Assignment

Some ICD-10-PCS procedure codes, although considered non-operating room procedures, may still affect MS-DRG assignment. In all sections of the ICD-10-PCS book, these procedures are identified by a **purple color bar** over the body part (character 4) value.

Valid OR Procedure

In the Medical and Surgical-Related (2WØ-9WB), Ancillary (BØØ-HZ9) and New Technology (X2A-XYØ) section tables **only**, any codes that are considered a valid operating room procedure are identified with a **blue color bar** over the body part (character 4) value and will affect MS-DRG assignment. All codes without a color bar (blue or purple) are considered non-operating room procedures.

Hospital-Acquired Condition Related Procedures

Procedures associated with hospital-acquired conditions (HAC) are identified with the **yellow color bar** over the body part (character 4) value. Appendix K provides each specific HAC category and its associated ICD-10-CM and ICD-10-PCS codes.

Combination Only

Some ICD-10-PCS procedure codes that describe non-operating room procedures can group to a specific MS-DRG but only when used in combination with certain other ICD-10-PCS procedure codes. Such codes are designated by a **red color bar** over the body part (character 4) value.

⊞ Combination Member

A combination member, which can be either a valid operating room procedure or a non-operating room procedure, is an ICD-10-PCS procedure code that can influence MS-DRG assignment either on its own or in combination with other specific ICD-10-PCS procedure codes. Combination member codes are designated by a plus sign (⊞) to the right of the body part (character 4) value.

Note: In the few instances when a code is both a combination member and a non-operating room procedure affecting the MS-DRG assignment, the body part (character 4) value will have a purple color bar and the combination member icon.

See Appendix L for Procedure Combinations

Under certain circumstances, more than one procedure code is needed in order to group to a specific MS-DRG. When codes within a table have been identified as a Combination Only (**red color bar**) or Combination Member (⊞) code, there is also a footnote instructing the coder to *see Appendix L*. Appendix L contains tables that identify the other procedure codes needed in the combination and the title and number of the MS-DRG to which the combination will group.

Other Table Notations

AHA Coding Clinic:

Official citations from AHA's *Coding Clinic for ICD-10-CM/PCS* have been provided at the beginning of each section, when applicable. Each specific citation is listed below a header identifying the table to which that particular *Coding Clinic* citation applies. The citations appear in purple type with the year, quarter, and page of the reference as well as the title of the question as it appears in that *Coding Clinic's* table of contents. *Coding Clinic* citations included in this edition have been updated through second quarter 2023.

NT New Technology Add-on Payment

This symbol identifies procedure codes that involve new technologies or medical services that have qualified for a new technology add-on payment (NTAP). CMS provides incremental payment, in addition to the DRG payment, for technologies that have received the NTAP designation. This symbol appears to the right of the sixth character value.

Note: Only specific brand or trade named devices, substances, or technologies receive NTAP approval. The sixth character value in the PCS table provides a generalized description that may be applicable to several brand or trade names. Unless otherwise specified in the annotation box, refer to appendix H or I to determine the specific brand or trade name of the device, substance, or technology that is applicable to the new technology add-on payment. New technology add-on payments are not exclusive to the New Technology (X) section.

Appendixes

The resources described below have been included as appendixes for *ICD-10-PCS The Complete Official Code Set*. These resources further instruct the coder on the appropriate application of the ICD-10-PCS code set.

Appendix A: Components of the Medical and Surgical Approach Definitions

This resource further defines the approach characters used in the Medical and Surgical (Ø) section. Complementing the detailed definition of the approach, additional information includes whether or not instrumentation is a part of the approach, the typical access location, the method used to initiate the approach, related procedural examples, and illustrations all of which will help the user determine the appropriate approach value.

Appendix B: Root Operation Definitions

This resource is a compilation of all root operations found in the Medical and Surgical-related sections (Ø-9) of this PCS manual. It provides a definition and in some cases a more detailed explanation of the root operation, to better reflect the purpose or objective. Examples of related procedure(s) may also be provided.

Appendix C: Comparison of Medical and Surgical Root Operations

The Medical and Surgical (Ø) section root operations are divided into groups that share similar attributes. These groups, and the root operations in each group, are listed in this resource along with information identifying the target of the root operation, the action used to perform the root operation, any clarification or further explanation on the objective of the root operation, and procedure examples.

Appendix D: Body Part Key

When an anatomical term or description is provided in the documentation but does not have a specific body part character within a table, the user can reference this resource to search for the anatomical description or site noted in the documentation to determine if there is a specific PCS body part character (character 4) to which the anatomical description or site could be coded.

Appendix E: Body Part Definitions

This resource is the reverse look-up of the Body Part Key. Each table in the Medical and Surgical section (Ø) of the PCS manual contains anatomical terms linked to a body part character or value, for example, in Table ØBB the Body Part (character 4) of 1 is Trachea. The body part Trachea may have anatomical structures or descriptions that may be used in procedure documentation instead of the term trachea. The Body Part Definitions list other anatomical structures or synonyms that are included in specific ICD-10-PCS body part values. According to the body part definitions, in the example above, cricoid cartilage is included in the Trachea (character 1) body part.

Appendix F: Device Classification

This resource provides an explanation of how a device is defined in the ICD-10-PCS classification along with two tables. The first table groups devices used in the ICD-10-PCS tables into general categories, including a definition of each device type and related examples. The second table provides definitions of transplant and grafting tissue types and associated terminology that may be found in the documentation.

Appendix G: Device Key and Aggregation Table

The Device Key helps users code the appropriate PCS sixth character for device. Devices are listed alphabetically by brand name or commonly used medical terminology and are translated to the appropriate PCS language or value. The key also reflects the body system where the device is located. For example, a SAPIEN valve used for transaortic valve replacement translates to Zooplastic Tissue in Heart and Great Vessels.

The following symbol NT has been placed next to those devices that have received an NTAP (new technology add-on payment) designation. When the code for this device is applied to an inpatient encounter, CMS provides incremental payment in addition to the DRG payment.

The Aggregation Table crosswalks specific device character value definitions for specific root operations in a specific body system to the more general device character value to be used when the root operation covers a wide range of body parts and the device character represents an entire family of devices.

Appendix H: Device Definitions

This resource is a reverse look-up to the Device Key. The user may reference this resource to see all the specific devices that may be grouped to a particular device character (character 6).

Example:
The operative report states, "An internal fixation device was used to repair a fractured femur. Kirschner wire, bone screws and neutralization plate all used and left in the bone at the end of the procedure. "

Although PCS requires all devices left in the body to be coded and the operative report lists three different devices, a check in the device definitions shows that all of these devices are included in the PCS value "Internal Fixation Device" and require only one code.

The following symbol NT has been placed next to those devices that have received an NTAP (new technology add-on payment) designation. When the code for this device is applied to an inpatient encounter, CMS provides incremental payment in addition to the DRG payment.

Appendix I: Substance Key/Substance Definitions

The Substance Key lists substances by trade name or synonym and relates them to a PCS character in the Administration (3) or New Technology (X) section in the Substance (sixth character) or Qualifier (seventh character) column.

The Substance Definitions table is the reverse look-up of the substance key, relating all substance categories, the sixth- or seventh character values, to all trade name or synonyms that may be classified to that particular character.

The following symbol NT has been placed next to those substances/technologies that have received an NTAP (new technology add-on payment) designation. When the code for this substance/technology is applied to an inpatient encounter, CMS provides incremental payment in addition to the DRG payment.

Appendix J: Sections B-H Character Definitions

In each ancillary section (B-H) the characters in a particular column may have different meanings depending on which section the user is working from. This resource provides the values for the characters in these sections as well as a definition of the character value.

Appendix K: Hospital Acquired Conditions

Hospital acquired conditions (HACs) are conditions that are considered reasonably preventable when occurring during the hospital admission and may prevent a case from grouping to a higher-paying MS-DRG. In certain instances the HACs are conditional, requiring a specific ICD-10-CM diagnosis code in combination with a specific ICD-10-PCS procedure code. This resource identifies these conditional HACs, listing the diagnosis and procedure codes that, in combination, may trigger a HAC edit. All codes, ICD-10-CM and ICD-10-PCS, are listed with their full descriptions.

Appendix L: Procedure Combination Tables

The procedure combination tables provided in this resource illustrate certain procedure combinations that must occur in order to assign a specific MS-DRG.

Appendix M: Coding Exercises and Answers

This resource provides the coding exercises with answers, and in some cases a brief explanation as to the reason that particular code was used.

ICD-10-PCS Official Guidelines for Coding and Reporting 2024

Narrative changes appear in **bold** text.

The Centers for Medicare and Medicaid Services (CMS) and the National Center for Health Statistics (NCHS), two departments within the U.S. Federal Government's Department of Health and Human Services (DHHS) provide the following guidelines for coding and reporting using the International Classification of Diseases, 10th Revision, Procedure Coding System (ICD-10-PCS). These guidelines should be used as a companion document to the official version of the ICD-10-PCS as published on the CMS website. The ICD-10-PCS is a procedure classification published by the United States for classifying procedures performed in hospital inpatient health care settings.

These guidelines have been approved by the four organizations that make up the Cooperating Parties for the ICD-10-PCS: the American Hospital Association (AHA), the American Health Information Management Association (AHIMA), CMS, and NCHS.

These guidelines are a set of rules that have been developed to accompany and complement the official conventions and instructions provided within the ICD-10-PCS itself. They are intended to provide direction that is applicable in most circumstances. However, there may be unique circumstances where exceptions are applied. The instructions and conventions of the classification take precedence over guidelines. These guidelines are based on the coding and sequencing instructions in the Tables, Index and Definitions of ICD-10-PCS, but provide additional instruction. Adherence to these guidelines when assigning ICD-10-PCS procedure codes is required under the Health Insurance Portability and Accountability Act (HIPAA). The procedure codes have been adopted under HIPAA for hospital inpatient healthcare settings. A joint effort between the healthcare provider and the coder is essential to achieve complete and accurate documentation, code assignment, and reporting of diagnoses and procedures. These guidelines have been developed to assist both the healthcare provider and the coder in identifying those procedures that are to be reported. The importance of consistent, complete documentation in the medical record cannot be overemphasized. Without such documentation accurate coding cannot be achieved.

Conventions

A1. ICD-10-PCS codes are composed of seven characters. Each character is an axis of classification that specifies information about the procedure performed. Within a defined code range, a character specifies the same type of information in that axis of classification.

> *Example:*
> The fifth axis of classification specifies the approach in sections Ø through 4 and 7 through 9 of the system.

A2. One of 34 possible values can be assigned to each axis of classification in the seven-character code: they are the numbers Ø through 9 and the alphabet (except I and O because they are easily confused with the numbers 1 and Ø). The number of unique values used in an axis of classification differs as needed.

> *Example:*
> Where the fifth axis of classification specifies the approach, seven different approach values are currently used to specify the approach.

A3. The valid values for an axis of classification can be added to as needed.

> *Example:*
> If a significantly distinct type of device is used in a new procedure, a new device value can be added to the system.

A4. As with words in their context, the meaning of any single value is a combination of its axis of classification and any preceding values on which it may be dependent.

> *Example:*
> The meaning of a body part value in the Medical and Surgical section is always dependent on the body system value. The body part value Ø in the Central Nervous body system specifies Brain and the body part value Ø in the Peripheral Nervous body system specifies Cervical Plexus.

A5. As the system is expanded to become increasingly detailed, over time more values will depend on preceding values for their meaning.

> *Example:*
> In the Lower Joints body system, the device value 3 in the root operation Insertion specifies Infusion Device and the device value 3 in the root operation Replacement specifies Ceramic Synthetic Substitute.

A6. The purpose of the alphabetic index is to locate the appropriate table that contains all information necessary to construct a procedure code. The PCS Tables should always be consulted to find the most appropriate valid code.

A7. It is not required to consult the index first before proceeding to the tables to complete the code. A valid code may be chosen directly from the tables.

A8. All seven characters must be specified to be a valid code. If the documentation is incomplete for coding purposes, the physician should be queried for the necessary information.

A9. Within a PCS table, valid codes include all combinations of choices in characters 4 through 7 contained in the same row of the table. In the example below, ØJHT3VZ is a valid code, and ØJHW3VZ is *not* a valid code.

Section: Ø **Medical and Surgical**
Body System: J **Subcutaneous Tissue and Fascia**
Operation: H **Insertion** Putting in a nonbiological appliance that monitors, assists, performs, or prevents a physiological function but does not physically take the place of a body part

Body Part	Approach	Device	Qualifier
S Subcutaneous Tissue and Fascia, Head and Neck V Subcutaneous Tissue and Fascia, Upper Extremity W Subcutaneous Tissue and Fascia, Lower Extremity	Ø Open 3 Percutaneous	1 Radioactive Element 3 Infusion Device Y Other Device	Z No Qualifier
T Subcutaneous Tissue and Fascia, Trunk	Ø Open 3 Percutaneous	1 Radioactive Element 3 Infusion Device V Infusion Pump Y Other Device	Z No Qualifier

A10. "And," when used in a code description, means "and/or," except when used to describe a combination of multiple body parts for which separate values exist for each body part (e.g., Skin and Subcutaneous Tissue used as a qualifier, where there are separate body part values for "Skin" and "Subcutaneous Tissue").

Example:
Lower Arm and Wrist Muscle means lower arm and/or wrist muscle.

A11. Many of the terms used to construct PCS codes are defined within the system. It is the coder's responsibility to determine what the documentation in the medical record equates to in the PCS definitions. The physician is not expected to use the terms used in PCS code descriptions, nor is the coder required to query the physician when the correlation between the documentation and the defined PCS terms is clear.

Example:
When the physician documents "partial resection" the coder can independently correlate "partial resection" to the root operation Excision without querying the physician for clarification.

Medical and Surgical Section Guidelines (section Ø)

B2. Body System

General guidelines

B2.1a. The procedure codes in Anatomical Regions, General, Anatomical Regions, Upper Extremities and Anatomical Regions, Lower Extremities can be used when the procedure is performed on an anatomical region rather than a specific body part, or on the rare occasion when no information is available to support assignment of a code to a specific body part.

Examples:
Chest tube drainage of the pleural cavity is coded to the root operation Drainage found in the body system Anatomical Regions, General.

Suture repair of the abdominal wall is coded to the root operation Repair in the body system Anatomical Regions, General.

Amputation of the foot is coded to the root operation Detachment in the body system Anatomical Regions, Lower Extremities.

B2.1b. Where the general body part values "upper" and "lower" are provided as an option in the Upper Arteries, Lower Arteries, Upper Veins, Lower Veins, Muscles and Tendons body systems, "upper" or "lower" specifies body parts located above or below the diaphragm respectively.

Example:
Vein body parts above the diaphragm are found in the Upper Veins body system; vein body parts below the diaphragm are found in the Lower Veins body system.

B3. Root Operation

General guidelines

B3.1a. In order to determine the appropriate root operation, the full definition of the root operation as contained in the PCS Tables must be applied.

B3.1b. Components of a procedure specified in the root operation definition or explanation as integral to that root operation are not coded separately. Procedural steps necessary to reach the operative site and close the operative site, including anastomosis of a tubular body part, are also not coded separately.

Examples:
Resection of a joint as part of a joint replacement procedure is included in the root operation definition of Replacement and is not coded separately.

Laparotomy performed to reach the site of an open liver biopsy is not coded separately.

In a resection of sigmoid colon with anastomosis of descending colon to rectum, the anastomosis is not coded separately.

Multiple procedures

B3.2. During the same operative episode, multiple procedures are coded if:

a. The same root operation is performed on different body parts as defined by distinct values of the body part character.

Examples:
Diagnostic excision of liver and pancreas are coded separately.

Excision of lesion in the ascending colon and excision of lesion in the transverse colon are coded separately.

b. The same root operation is repeated in multiple body parts, and those body parts are separate and distinct body parts classified to a single ICD-10-PCS body part value.

Examples:
Excision of the sartorius muscle and excision of the gracilis muscle are both included in the upper leg muscle body part value, and multiple procedures are coded.

Extraction of multiple toenails are coded separately.

c. Multiple root operations with distinct objectives are performed on the same body part.

Example:
Destruction of sigmoid lesion and bypass of sigmoid colon are coded separately.

d. The intended root operation is attempted using one approach but is converted to a different approach.

Example:
Laparoscopic cholecystectomy converted to an open cholecystectomy is coded as percutaneous endoscopic Inspection and open Resection.

Discontinued or incomplete procedures

B3.3. If the intended procedure is discontinued or otherwise not completed, code the procedure to the root operation performed. If a procedure is discontinued before any other root operation is performed, code the root operation Inspection of the body part or anatomical region inspected.

Example:
A planned aortic valve replacement procedure is discontinued after the initial thoracotomy and before any incision is made in the heart muscle, when the patient becomes hemodynamically unstable. This procedure is coded as an open Inspection of the mediastinum.

Biopsy procedures

B3.4a. Biopsy procedures are coded using the root operations Excision, Extraction, or Drainage and the qualifier Diagnostic.

Examples:
Fine needle aspiration biopsy of fluid in the lung is coded to the root operation Drainage with the qualifier Diagnostic.

Biopsy of bone marrow is coded to the root operation Extraction with the qualifier Diagnostic.

Lymph node sampling for biopsy is coded to the root operation Excision with the qualifier Diagnostic.

Biopsy followed by more definitive treatment

B3.4b. If a diagnostic Excision, Extraction, or Drainage procedure (biopsy) is followed by a more definitive procedure, such as Destruction, Excision or Resection at the same procedure site, both the biopsy and the more definitive treatment are coded.

Example:
Biopsy of breast followed by partial mastectomy at the same procedure site, both the biopsy and the partial mastectomy procedure are coded.

Overlapping body layers

B3.5. If root operations such as Excision, Extraction, Repair or Inspection are performed on overlapping layers of the musculoskeletal system, the body part specifying the deepest layer is coded.

Example:
Excisional debridement that includes skin and subcutaneous tissue and muscle is coded to the muscle body part.

Bypass procedures

B3.6a. Bypass procedures are coded by identifying the body part bypassed "from" and the body part bypassed "to." The fourth character body part specifies the body part bypassed from, and the qualifier specifies the body part bypassed to.

Example:
Bypass from stomach to jejunum, stomach is the body part and jejunum is the qualifier.

B3.6b. Coronary artery bypass procedures are coded differently than other bypass procedures as described in the previous guideline. Rather than identifying the body part bypassed from, the body part identifies the number of coronary arteries bypassed to, and the qualifier specifies the vessel bypassed from.

Example:
Aortocoronary artery bypass of the left anterior descending coronary artery and the obtuse marginal coronary artery is classified in the body part axis of classification as two coronary arteries, and the qualifier specifies the aorta as the body part bypassed from.

B3.6c. If multiple coronary arteries are bypassed, a separate procedure is coded for each coronary artery that uses a different device and/or qualifier.

Example:
Aortocoronary artery bypass and internal mammary coronary artery bypass are coded separately.

Control vs. more specific root operations

B3.7. The root operation Control is defined as, "Stopping, or attempting to stop, postprocedural or other acute bleeding." Control is the root operation coded when the procedure performed to achieve hemostasis, beyond what would be considered integral to a procedure, utilizes techniques (e.g. cautery, application of substances or pressure, suturing or ligation or clipping of bleeding points at the site) that are not described by a more specific root operation definition, such as Bypass, Detachment, Excision, Extraction, Reposition, Replacement, or Resection. If a more specific root operation definition applies to the procedure performed, then the more specific root operation is coded instead of Control.

Example:
Silver nitrate cautery to treat acute nasal bleeding is coded to the root operation Control.

Example:
Liquid embolization of the right internal iliac artery to treat acute hematoma by stopping blood flow is coded to the root operation Occlusion.

Example:
Suctioning of residual blood to achieve hemostasis during a transbronchial cryobiopsy is considered integral to the cryobiopsy procedure and is not coded separately.

Excision vs. Resection

B3.8. PCS contains specific body parts for anatomical subdivisions of a body part, such as lobes of the lungs or liver and regions of the intestine. Resection of the specific body part is coded whenever all of the body part is cut out or off, rather than coding Excision of a less specific body part.

Example:
Left upper lung lobectomy is coded to Resection of Upper Lung Lobe, Left rather than Excision of Lung, Left.

Excision for graft

B3.9. If an autograft is obtained from a different procedure site in order to complete the objective of the procedure, a separate procedure is coded, except when the seventh character qualifier value in the ICD-10-PCS table fully specifies the site from which the autograft was obtained.

Examples:
Coronary bypass with excision of saphenous vein graft, excision of saphenous vein is coded separately.

Replacement of breast with autologous deep inferior epigastric artery perforator (DIEP) flap, excision of the DIEP flap is not coded separately. The seventh character qualifier value Deep Inferior Epigastric Artery Perforator Flap in the Replacement table fully specifies the site of the autograft harvest.

Fusion procedures of the spine

B3.10a. The body part coded for a spinal vertebral joint(s) rendered immobile by a spinal fusion procedure is classified by the level of the spine (e.g. thoracic). There are distinct body part values for a single vertebral joint and for multiple vertebral joints at each spinal level.

Example:
Body part values specify Lumbar Vertebral Joint, Lumbar Vertebral Joints, 2 or More and Lumbosacral Vertebral Joint.

B3.10b. If multiple vertebral joints are fused, a separate procedure is coded for each vertebral joint that uses a different device and/or qualifier.

Example:
Fusion of lumbar vertebral joint, posterior approach, anterior column and fusion of lumbar vertebral joint, posterior approach, posterior column are coded separately.

B3.10c. Combinations of devices and materials are often used on a vertebral joint to render the joint immobile. When combinations of devices are used on the same vertebral joint, the device value coded for the procedure is as follows:

- If an interbody fusion device is used to render the joint immobile (containing bone graft or bone graft substitute), the procedure is coded with the device value Interbody Fusion Device
- If bone graft is the *only* device used to render the joint immobile, the procedure is coded with the device value Nonautologous Tissue Substitute or Autologous Tissue Substitute
- If a mixture of autologous and nonautologous bone graft (with or without biological or synthetic extenders or binders) is used to render the joint immobile, code the procedure with the device value Autologous Tissue Substitute

Examples:
Fusion of a vertebral joint using a cage style interbody fusion device containing morsellized bone graft is coded to the device Interbody Fusion Device.

Fusion of a vertebral joint using a bone dowel interbody fusion device made of cadaver bone and packed with a mixture of local morsellized bone and demineralized bone matrix is coded to the device Interbody Fusion Device.

Fusion of a vertebral joint using both autologous bone graft and bone bank bone graft is coded to the device Autologous Tissue Substitute.

Inspection procedures

B3.11a. Inspection of a body part(s) performed in order to achieve the objective of a procedure is not coded separately.

Example:
Fiberoptic bronchoscopy performed for irrigation of bronchus, only the irrigation procedure is coded.

B3.11b. If multiple tubular body parts are inspected, the most distal body part (the body part furthest from the starting point of the inspection) is coded. If multiple non-tubular body parts in a region are inspected, the body part that specifies the entire area inspected is coded.

Examples:
Cystoureteroscopy with inspection of bladder and ureters is coded to the ureter body part value.

Exploratory laparotomy with general inspection of abdominal contents is coded to the peritoneal cavity body part value.

B3.11c. When both an Inspection procedure and another procedure are performed on the same body part during the same episode, if the Inspection procedure is performed using a different approach than the other procedure, the Inspection procedure is coded separately.

Example:
Endoscopic Inspection of the duodenum is coded separately when open Excision of the duodenum is performed during the same procedural episode.

Occlusion vs. Restriction for vessel embolization procedures

B3.12. If the objective of an embolization procedure is to completely close a vessel, the root operation Occlusion is coded. If the objective of an embolization procedure is to narrow the lumen of a vessel, the root operation Restriction is coded.

Examples:
Tumor embolization is coded to the root operation Occlusion, because the objective of the procedure is to cut off the blood supply to the vessel.

Embolization of a cerebral aneurysm is coded to the root operation Restriction, because the objective of the procedure is not to close off the vessel entirely, but to narrow the lumen of the vessel at the site of the aneurysm where it is abnormally wide.

Release procedures

B3.13. In the root operation Release, the body part value coded is the body part being freed and not the tissue being manipulated or cut to free the body part.

Example:
Lysis of intestinal adhesions is coded to the specific intestine body part value.

Release vs. Division

B3.14. If the sole objective of the procedure is freeing a body part without cutting the body part, the root operation is Release. If the sole objective of the procedure is separating or transecting a body part, the root operation is Division.

Examples:
Freeing a nerve root from surrounding scar tissue to relieve pain is coded to the root operation Release.

Severing a nerve root to relieve pain is coded to the root operation Division.

Reposition for fracture treatment

B3.15. Reduction of a displaced fracture is coded to the root operation Reposition and the application of a cast or splint in conjunction with the Reposition procedure is not coded separately. Treatment of a nondisplaced fracture is coded to the procedure performed.

Examples:
Casting of a nondisplaced fracture is coded to the root operation Immobilization in the Placement section.

Putting a pin in a nondisplaced fracture is coded to the root operation Insertion.

Transplantation vs. Administration

B3.16. Putting in a mature and functioning living body part taken from another individual or animal is coded to the root operation Transplantation. Putting in autologous or nonautologous cells is coded to the Administration section.

Example:
Putting in autologous or nonautologous bone marrow, pancreatic islet cells or stem cells is coded to the Administration section.

Transfer procedures using multiple tissue layers

B3.17. The root operation Transfer contains qualifiers that can be used to specify when a transfer flap is composed of more than one tissue layer, such as a musculocutaneous flap. For procedures involving transfer of multiple tissue layers including skin, subcutaneous tissue, fascia or muscle, the procedure is coded to the body part value that describes the deepest tissue layer in the flap, and the qualifier can be used to describe the other tissue layer(s) in the transfer flap.

Example:
A musculocutaneous flap transfer is coded to the appropriate body part value in the body system Muscles, and the qualifier is used to describe the additional tissue layer(s) in the transfer flap.

Excision/Resection followed by replacement

B3.18. If an excision or resection of a body part is followed by a replacement procedure, code both procedures to identify each distinct objective, except when the excision or resection is considered integral and preparatory for the replacement procedure.

Examples:
Mastectomy followed by reconstruction, both resection and replacement of the breast are coded to fully capture the distinct objectives of the procedures performed.

Maxillectomy with obturator reconstruction, both excision and replacement of the maxilla are coded to fully capture the distinct objectives of the procedures performed.

Excisional debridement of tendon with skin graft, both the excision of the tendon and the replacement of the skin with a graft are coded to fully capture the distinct objectives of the procedures performed.

Esophagectomy followed by reconstruction with colonic interposition, both the resection and the transfer of the large intestine to function as the esophagus are coded to fully capture the distinct objectives of the procedures performed.

Examples:
Resection of a joint as part of a joint replacement procedure is considered integral and preparatory for the replacement of the joint and the resection is not coded separately.

Resection of a valve as part of a valve replacement procedure is considered integral and preparatory for the valve replacement and the resection is not coded separately.

Detachment procedures of extremities

B3.19. The root operation Detachment contains qualifiers that can be used to specify the level where the extremity was amputated. These qualifiers are dependent on the body part value in the "upper extremities" and "lower extremities" body systems. For procedures involving the detachment of all or part of the upper or lower extremities, the procedure is coded to the body part value that describes the site of the detachment.

Example:
An amputation at the proximal portion of the shaft of the tibia and fibula is coded to the Lower leg body part value in the body system Anatomical Regions, Lower Extremities, and the qualifier High is used to specify the level where the extremity was detached.

The following definitions were developed for the Detachment qualifiers

Body Part	Qualifier	Definition
Upper arm and upper leg	1	High: Amputation at the proximal portion of the shaft of the humerus or femur
	2	Mid: Amputation at the middle portion of the shaft of the humerus or femur
	3	Low: Amputation at the distal portion of the shaft of the humerus or femur
Lower arm and lower leg	1	High: Amputation at the proximal portion of the shaft of the radius/ulna or tibia/fibula
	2	Mid: Amputation at the middle portion of the shaft of the radius/ulna or tibia/fibula
	3	Low: Amputation at the distal portion of the shaft of the radius/ulna or tibia/fibula
Hand and Foot	Ø	Complete*
	4	Complete 1st Ray
	5	Complete 2nd Ray
	6	Complete 3rd Ray
	7	Complete 4th Ray
	8	Complete 5th Ray
	9	Partial 1st Ray
	B	Partial 2nd Ray
	C	Partial 3rd Ray
	D	Partial 4th Ray
	F	Partial 5th Ray
Thumb, finger, or toe	Ø	Complete: Amputation at the metacarpophalangeal/metatarsal-phalangeal joint
	1	High: Amputation anywhere along the proximal phalanx
	2	Mid: Amputation through the proximal interphalangeal joint or anywhere along the middle phalanx
	3	Low: Amputation through the distal interphalangeal joint or anywhere along the distal phalanx

*When coding amputation of Hand and Foot, the following definitions are followed:

- Complete: Amputation through the carpometacarpal joint of the hand, or through the tarsal-metatarsal joint of the foot.
- Partial: Amputation anywhere along the shaft or head of the metacarpal bone of the hand, or of the metatarsal bone of the foot.

B4. Body Part

General guidelines

B4.1a. If a procedure is performed on a portion of a body part that does not have a separate body part value, code the body part value corresponding to the whole body part.

Example:
A procedure performed on the alveolar process of the mandible is coded to the mandible body part.

B4.1b. If the prefix "peri" is combined with a body part to identify the site of the procedure, and the site of the procedure is not further specified, then the procedure is coded to the body part named. This guideline applies only when a more specific body part value is not available.

Examples:
A procedure site identified as perirenal is coded to the kidney body part when the site of the procedure is not further specified.

A procedure site described in the documentation as peri-urethral, and the documentation also indicates that it is the vulvar tissue and not the urethral tissue that is the site of the procedure, then the procedure is coded to the vulva body part.

A procedure site documented as involving the periosteum is coded to the corresponding bone body part.

B4.1c. If a single vascular procedure is performed on a continuous section of an arterial or venous body part, code the body part value corresponding to the anatomically most proximal (closest to the heart) portion of the arterial or venous body part.

Example:
A procedure performed on a continuous section of artery from the femoral artery to the external iliac artery with the point of entry at the femoral artery is coded to the external iliac body part.

A procedure performed on a continuous section of artery from the femoral artery to the external iliac artery with the point of entry at the external iliac artery is also coded to the external iliac artery body part.

Branches of body parts

B4.2. Where a specific branch of a body part does not have its own body part value in PCS, the body part is typically coded to the closest proximal branch that has a specific body part value. In the cardiovascular body systems, if a general body part is available in the correct root operation table, and coding to a proximal branch would require assigning a code in a different body system, the procedure is coded using the general body part value.

Examples:
A procedure performed on the mandibular branch of the trigeminal nerve is coded to the trigeminal nerve body part value.

Occlusion of the bronchial artery is coded to the body part value Upper Artery in the body system Upper Arteries, and not to the body part value Thoracic Aorta, Descending in the body system Heart and Great Vessels.

Bilateral body part values

B4.3. Bilateral body part values are available for a limited number of body parts. If the identical procedure is performed on contralateral body parts, and a bilateral body part value exists for that body part, a single procedure is coded using the bilateral body part value. If no bilateral body part value exists, each procedure is coded separately using the appropriate body part value.

Examples:
The identical procedure performed on both fallopian tubes is coded once using the body part value Fallopian Tube, Bilateral.

The identical procedure performed on both knee joints is coded twice using the body part values Knee Joint, Right and Knee Joint, Left.

Coronary arteries

B4.4. The coronary arteries are classified as a single body part that is further specified by number of arteries treated. One procedure code specifying multiple arteries is used when the same procedure is performed, including the same device and qualifier values.

Examples:
Angioplasty of two distinct coronary arteries with placement of two stents is coded as Dilation of Coronary Artery, Two Arteries with Two Intraluminal Devices.

Angioplasty of two distinct coronary arteries, one with stent placed and one without, is coded separately as Dilation of Coronary Artery, One Artery with Intraluminal Device, and Dilation of Coronary Artery, One Artery with no device.

Tendons, ligaments, bursae and fascia near a joint

B4.5. Procedures performed on tendons, ligaments, bursae and fascia supporting a joint are coded to the body part in the respective body system that is the focus of the procedure. Procedures performed on joint structures themselves are coded to the body part in the joint body systems.

Examples:
Repair of the anterior cruciate ligament of the knee is coded to the knee bursa and ligament body part in the bursae and ligaments body system.

Knee arthroscopy with shaving of articular cartilage is coded to the knee joint body part in the Lower Joints body system.

Skin, subcutaneous tissue and fascia overlying a joint

B4.6. If a procedure is performed on the skin, subcutaneous tissue or fascia overlying a joint, the procedure is coded to the following body part:

- Shoulder is coded to Upper Arm
- Elbow is coded to Lower Arm
- Wrist is coded to Lower Arm
- Hip is coded to Upper Leg
- Knee is coded to Lower Leg
- Ankle is coded to Foot

Fingers and toes

B4.7. If a body system does not contain a separate body part value for fingers, procedures performed on the fingers are coded to the body part value for the hand. If a body system does not contain a separate body part value for toes, procedures performed on the toes are coded to the body part value for the foot.

Example:
Excision of finger muscle is coded to one of the hand muscle body part values in the Muscles body system.

Upper and lower intestinal tract

B4.8. In the Gastrointestinal body system, the general body part values Upper Intestinal Tract and Lower Intestinal Tract are provided as an option for the root operations such as Change, Insertion, Inspection, Removal and Revision. Upper Intestinal Tract includes the portion of the gastrointestinal tract from the esophagus down to and including the duodenum, and Lower Intestinal Tract includes the portion of the gastrointestinal tract from the jejunum down to and including the rectum and anus.

Example:
In the root operation Change table, change of a device in the jejunum is coded using the body part Lower Intestinal Tract.

B5. Approach

Open approach with percutaneous endoscopic assistance

B5.2a. Procedures performed using the open approach with percutaneous endoscopic assistance are coded to the approach Open.

Example:
Laparoscopic-assisted sigmoidectomy is coded to the approach Open.

Percutaneous endoscopic approach with ***hand-assistance or*** *extension of incision*

B5.2b. Procedures performed using the percutaneous endoscopic approach, **with hand-assistance, or with an** incision or extension of an incision to assist in the removal of all or a portion of a body part, or to anastomose a tubular body part **with or without the temporary exteriorization of a body structure,** are coded to the approach value Percutaneous Endoscopic.

Examples:
Hand-assisted laparoscopic sigmoid colon resection with exteriorization of a segment of the colon for removal of specimen with return of colon back into abdominal cavity is coded to the approach value percutaneous endoscopic.

Laparoscopic sigmoid colectomy with extension of stapling port for removal of specimen and direct anastomosis is coded to the approach value percutaneous endoscopic.

Laparoscopic nephrectomy with midline incision for removing the resected kidney is coded to the approach value percutaneous endoscopic.

Robotic-assisted laparoscopic prostatectomy with extension of incision for removal of the resected prostate is coded to the approach value percutaneous endoscopic.

External approach

B5.3a. Procedures performed within an orifice on structures that are visible without the aid of any instrumentation are coded to the approach External.

> *Example:*
> Resection of tonsils is coded to the approach External.

B5.3b. Procedures performed indirectly by the application of external force through the intervening body layers are coded to the approach External.

> *Example:*
> Closed reduction of fracture is coded to the approach External.

Percutaneous procedure via device

B5.4. Procedures performed percutaneously via a device placed for the procedure are coded to the approach Percutaneous.

> *Example:*
> Fragmentation of kidney stone performed via percutaneous nephrostomy is coded to the approach Percutaneous.

B6. Device

General guidelines

B6.1a. A device is coded only if a device remains after the procedure is completed. If no device remains, the device value No Device is coded. In limited root operations, the classification provides the qualifier values Temporary and Intraoperative, for specific procedures involving clinically significant devices, where the purpose of the device is to be utilized for a brief duration during the procedure or current inpatient stay. If a device that is intended to remain after the procedure is completed requires removal before the end of the operative episode in which it was inserted, both the insertion and removal of the device should be coded.

B6.1b. Materials such as sutures, ligatures, radiological markers and temporary post-operative wound drains are considered integral to the performance of a procedure and are not coded as devices.

B6.1c. Procedures performed on a device only and not on a body part are specified in the root operations Change, Irrigation, Removal and Revision, and are coded to the procedure performed.

> *Example:*
> Irrigation of percutaneous nephrostomy tube is coded to the root operation Irrigation of indwelling device in the Administration section.

Drainage device

B6.2. A separate procedure to put in a drainage device is coded to the root operation Drainage with the device value Drainage Device.

Obstetric Section Guidelines (section 1)

C. Obstetrics Section

Products of conception

C1. Procedures performed on the products of conception are coded to the Obstetrics section. Procedures performed on the pregnant female other than the products of conception are coded to the appropriate root operation in the Medical and Surgical section.

> *Examples:*
> Amniocentesis is coded to the products of conception body part in the Obstetrics section.
>
> Repair of obstetric urethral laceration is coded to the urethra body part in the Medical and Surgical section.

Procedures following delivery or abortion

C2. Procedures performed following a delivery or abortion for curettage of the endometrium or evacuation of retained products of conception are all coded in the Obstetrics section, to the root operation Extraction and the body part Products of Conception, Retained.

Diagnostic or therapeutic dilation and curettage performed during times other than the postpartum or post-abortion period are all coded in the Medical and Surgical section, to the root operation Extraction and the body part Endometrium.

Radiation Therapy Section Guidelines (section D)

D. Radiation Therapy Section

Brachytherapy

D1.a. Brachytherapy is coded to the modality Brachytherapy in the Radiation Therapy section. When a radioactive brachytherapy source is left in the body at the end of the procedure, it is coded separately to the root operation Insertion with the device value Radioactive Element.

> *Example:*
> Brachytherapy with implantation of a low dose rate brachytherapy source left in the body at the end of the procedure is coded to the applicable treatment site in section D, Radiation Therapy, with the modality Brachytherapy, the modality qualifier value Low Dose Rate, and the applicable isotope value and qualifier value. The implantation of the brachytherapy source is coded separately to the device value Radioactive Element in the appropriate Insertion table of the Medical and Surgical section. The Radiation Therapy section code identifies the specific modality and isotope of the brachytherapy, and the root operation Insertion code identifies the implantation of the brachytherapy source that remains in the body at the end of the procedure.
>
> *Exception:*
> Implantation of Cesium-131 brachytherapy seeds embedded in a collagen matrix to the treatment site after resection of brain tumor is coded to the root operation Insertion with the device value Radioactive Element, Cesium-131 Collagen Implant. The procedure is coded to the root operation Insertion only, because the device value identifies both the implantation of the radioactive element and a specific brachytherapy isotope that is not included in the Radiation Therapy section tables.

D1.b. A separate procedure to place a temporary applicator for delivering the brachytherapy is coded to the root operation Insertion and the device value Other Device.

> *Examples:*
> Intrauterine brachytherapy applicator placed as a separate procedure from the brachytherapy procedure is coded to Insertion of Other Device, and the brachytherapy is coded separately using the modality Brachytherapy in the Radiation Therapy section.
>
> Intrauterine brachytherapy applicator placed concomitantly with delivery of the brachytherapy dose is coded with a single code using the modality Brachytherapy in the Radiation Therapy section.

New Technology Section Guidelines (section X)

E. New Technology Section

General guidelines

E1.a. Section X codes fully represent the specific procedure described in the code title, and do not require additional codes from other sections of ICD-10-PCS. When section X contains a code title which fully describes a specific new technology procedure, and it is the only procedure performed, only the section X code is reported for the procedure. There is no need to report an additional code in another section of ICD-10-PCS.

> *Example:*
> XWØ43A6 Introduction of Cefiderocol Anti-infective into Central Vein, Percutaneous Approach, New Technology Group 6, can be coded to indicate that Cefiderocol Anti-infective was administered via a central vein. A separate code from table 3EØ in the Administration section of ICD-10-PCS is not coded in addition to this code.

E1.b. When multiple procedures are performed, New Technology section X codes are coded following the multiple procedures guideline.

> *Examples:*
> Dual filter cerebral embolic filtration used during transcatheter aortic valve replacement (TAVR), X2A5312 Cerebral Embolic Filtration, Dual Filter in Innominate Artery and Left Common Carotid Artery, Percutaneous Approach, New Technology Group 2, is coded for the cerebral embolic filtration, along with an ICD-10-PCS code for the TAVR procedure.
>
> An extracorporeal flow reversal circuit for embolic neuroprotection placed during a transcarotid arterial revascularization procedure, a code from table X2A, Assistance of the Cardiovascular System is coded for the use of the extracorporeal flow reversal circuit, along with an ICD-10-PCS code for the transcarotid arterial revascularization procedure.

F. Selection of Principal Procedure

The following instructions should be applied in the selection of principal procedure and clarification on the importance of the relation to the principal diagnosis when more than one procedure is performed:

1. Procedure performed for definitive treatment of both principal diagnosis and secondary diagnosis
   a. Sequence procedure performed for definitive treatment most related to principal diagnosis as principal procedure.
2. Procedure performed for definitive treatment and diagnostic procedures performed for both principal diagnosis and secondary diagnosis.
   a. Sequence procedure performed for definitive treatment most related to principal diagnosis as principal procedure
3. A diagnostic procedure was performed for the principal diagnosis and a procedure is performed for definitive treatment of a secondary diagnosis.
   a. Sequence diagnostic procedure as principal procedure, since the procedure most related to the principal diagnosis takes precedence.
4. No procedures performed that are related to principal diagnosis; procedures performed for definitive treatment and diagnostic procedures were performed for secondary diagnosis
   a. Sequence procedure performed for definitive treatment of secondary diagnosis as principal procedure, since there are no procedures (definitive or nondefinitive treatment) related to principal diagnosis.

3f (Aortic) Bioprosthesis valve *use* Zooplastic Tissue in Heart and Great Vessels

Abdominal aortic plexus *use* Abdominal Sympathetic Nerve
Abdominal cavity *use* Peritoneal Cavity
Abdominal esophagus *use* Esophagus, Lower
Abdominohysterectomy *see* Resection, Uterus ØUT9
Abdominoplasty
  see Alteration, Abdominal Wall ØWØF
  see Repair, Abdominal Wall ØWQF
  see Supplement, Abdominal Wall ØWUF
Abductor hallucis muscle
  use Foot Muscle, Left
  use Foot Muscle, Right
ABECMA® *use* Idecabtagene Vicleucel Immunotherapy
AbioCor® Total Replacement Heart *use* Synthetic Substitute
Ablation
  see Control bleeding in
  see Destruction
Abortion
  Abortifacient 1ØAØ7ZX
  Laminaria 1ØAØ7ZW
  Products of Conception 1ØAØ
  Vacuum 1ØAØ7Z6
Abrasion *see* Extraction
Absolute Pro Vascular (OTW) Self-Expanding Stent System *use* Intraluminal Device
Accelerate PhenoTest™ BC XXE5XN6
Accessory cephalic vein
  use Cephalic Vein, Left
  use Cephalic Vein, Right
Accessory obturator nerve *use* Lumbar Plexus
Accessory phrenic nerve *use* Phrenic Nerve
Accessory spleen *use* Spleen
Acculink (RX) Carotid Stent System *use* Intraluminal Device
Acellular Hydrated Dermis *use* Nonautologous Tissue Substitute
Acetabular cup *use* Liner in Lower Joints
Acetabulectomy
  see Excision, Lower Bones ØQB
  see Resection, Lower Bones ØQT
Acetabulofemoral joint
  use Hip Joint, Left
  use Hip Joint, Right
Acetabuloplasty
  see Repair, Lower Bones ØQQ
  see Replacement, Lower Bones ØQR
  see Supplement, Lower Bones ØQU
Achilles tendon
  use Lower Leg Tendon, Left
  use Lower Leg Tendon, Right
Achillorrhaphy *see* Repair, Tendons ØLQ
Achillotenotomy, achillotomy
  see Division, Tendons ØL8
  see Drainage, Tendons ØL9
Acoustic Pulse Thrombolysis *see* Fragmentation, Artery
Acromioclavicular ligament
  use Shoulder Bursa and Ligament, Left
  use Shoulder Bursa and Ligament, Right
Acromion (process)
  use Scapula, Left
  use Scapula, Right
Acromionectomy
  see Excision, Upper Joints ØRB
  see Resection, Upper Joints ØRT
Acromioplasty
  see Repair, Upper Joints ØRQ
  see Replacement, Upper Joints ØRR
  see Supplement, Upper Joints ØRU
ACTEMRA® *use* Tocilizumab
Activa PC neurostimulator *use* Stimulator Generator, Multiple Array in ØJH
Activa RC neurostimulator *use* Stimulator Generator, Multiple Array Rechargeable in ØJH
Activa SC neurostimulator *use* Stimulator Generator, Single Array in ØJH
Activities of Daily Living Assessment FØ2
Activities of Daily Living Treatment FØ8
ACUITY™ Steerable Lead
  use Cardiac Lead, Defibrillator in Ø2H
  use Cardiac Lead, Pacemaker in Ø2H
Acupuncture
  Breast
    Anesthesia 8EØH3ØØ
    No Qualifier 8EØH3ØZ
  Integumentary System
    Anesthesia 8EØH3ØØ
    No Qualifier 8EØH3ØZ
Adductor brevis muscle
  use Upper Leg Muscle, Left
  use Upper Leg Muscle, Right
Adductor hallucis muscle
  use Foot Muscle, Left
  use Foot Muscle, Right
Adductor longus muscle
  use Upper Leg Muscle, Left
  use Upper Leg Muscle, Right
Adductor magnus muscle
  use Upper Leg Muscle, Left
  use Upper Leg Muscle, Right
Adenohypophysis *use* Pituitary Gland
Adenoidectomy
  see Excision, Adenoids ØCBQ
  see Resection, Adenoids ØCTQ
Adenoidotomy *see* Drainage, Adenoids ØC9Q
Adhesiolysis *see* Release
Administration
  Blood products *see* Transfusion
  Other substance *see* Introduction of substance in or on
Adrenalectomy
  see Excision, Endocrine System ØGB
  see Resection, Endocrine System ØGT
Adrenalorrhaphy *see* Repair, Endocrine System ØGQ
Adrenalotomy *see* Drainage, Endocrine System ØG9
Advancement
  see Reposition
  see Transfer
Advisa (MRI) *use* Pacemaker, Dual Chamber in ØJH
afami-cel *use* Afamitresgene Autoleucel Immunotherapy
Afamitresgene Autoleucel Immunotherapy XWØ
AFX® Endovascular AAA System *use* Intraluminal Device
Aidoc Briefcase for PE (pulmonary embolism) XXE3X27
AIGISRx Antibacterial Envelope *use* Anti-Infective Envelope
Alar ligament of axis *use* Head and Neck Bursa and Ligament
Alfapump® system *use* Other Device
Alfieri Stitch Valvuloplasty *see* Restriction, Valve, Mitral Ø2VG
Alimentation *see* Introduction of substance in or on
ALPPS (Associating liver partition and portal vein ligation)
  see Division, Hepatobiliary System and Pancreas ØF8
  see Resection, Hepatobiliary System and Pancreas ØFT
Alteration
  Abdominal Wall ØWØF
  Ankle Region
    Left ØYØL
    Right ØYØK
  Arm
    Lower
      Left ØXØF
      Right ØXØD
    Upper
      Left ØXØ9
      Right ØXØ8
  Axilla
    Left ØXØ5
    Right ØXØ4
  Back
    Lower ØWØL
    Upper ØWØK
  Breast
    Bilateral ØHØV
    Left ØHØU
    Right ØHØT
  Buttock
    Left ØYØ1
Alteration — *continued*
  Buttock — *continued*
    Right ØYØØ
  Chest Wall ØWØ8
  Ear
    Bilateral Ø9Ø2
    Left Ø9Ø1
    Right Ø9ØØ
  Elbow Region
    Left ØXØC
    Right ØXØB
  Extremity
    Lower
      Left ØYØB
      Right ØYØ9
    Upper
      Left ØXØ7
      Right ØXØ6
  Eyelid
    Lower
      Left Ø8ØR
      Right Ø8ØQ
    Upper
      Left Ø8ØP
      Right Ø8ØN
  Face ØWØ2
  Head ØWØØ
  Jaw
    Lower ØWØ5
    Upper ØWØ4
  Knee Region
    Left ØYØG
    Right ØYØF
  Leg
    Lower
      Left ØYØJ
      Right ØYØH
    Upper
      Left ØYØD
      Right ØYØC
  Lip
    Lower ØCØ1X
    Upper ØCØØX
  Nasal Mucosa and Soft Tissue Ø9ØK
  Neck ØWØ6
  Perineum
    Female ØWØN
    Male ØWØM
  Shoulder Region
    Left ØXØ3
    Right ØXØ2
  Subcutaneous Tissue and Fascia
    Abdomen ØJØ8
    Back ØJØ7
    Buttock ØJØ9
    Chest ØJØ6
    Face ØJØ1
    Lower Arm
      Left ØJØH
      Right ØJØG
    Lower Leg
      Left ØJØP
      Right ØJØN
    Neck
      Left ØJØ5
      Right ØJØ4
    Upper Arm
      Left ØJØF
      Right ØJØD
    Upper Leg
      Left ØJØM
      Right ØJØL
  Wrist Region
    Left ØXØH
    Right ØXØG
Alveolar process of mandible
  use Mandible, Left
  use Mandible, Right
Alveolar process of maxilla *use* Maxilla
Alveolectomy
  see Excision, Head and Facial Bones ØNB
  see Resection, Head and Facial Bones ØNT
Alveoloplasty
  see Repair, Head and Facial Bones ØNQ
  see Replacement, Head and Facial Bones ØNR
  see Supplement, Head and Facial Bones ØNU
Alveolotomy
  see Division, Head and Facial Bones ØN8

Alveolotomy — *continued*
see Drainage, Head and Facial Bones ØN9
Ambulatory cardiac monitoring 4A12X45
Amivantamab Monoclonal Antibody XWØ
Amniocentesis *see* Drainage, Products of Conception 1Ø9Ø
Amnioinfusion *see* Introduction of substance in or on, Products of Conception 3EØE
Amnioscopy 1ØJØ8ZZ
Amniotomy *see* Drainage, Products of Conception 1Ø9Ø
AMPLATZER® Muscular VSD Occluder *use* Synthetic Substitute
Amputation *see* Detachment
AMS 8ØØ® Urinary Control System *use* Artificial Sphincter in Urinary System
Anacaulase-bcdb XWØ
Anal orifice *use* Anus
Analog radiography *see* Plain Radiography
Analog radiology *see* Plain Radiography
Anastomosis *see* Bypass
Anatomical snuffbox
use Lower Arm and Wrist Muscle, Left
use Lower Arm and Wrist Muscle, Right
Andexanet Alfa, Factor Xa Inhibitor Reversal Agent *use* Coagulation Factor Xa, Inactivated
Andexxa *use* Coagulation Factor Xa, Inactivated
AneuRx® AAA Advantage® *use* Intraluminal Device
Angiectomy
see Excision, Heart and Great Vessels Ø2B
see Excision, Lower Arteries Ø4B
see Excision, Lower Veins Ø6B
see Excision, Upper Arteries Ø3B
see Excision, Upper Veins Ø5B
Angiocardiography
Combined right and left heart *see* Fluoroscopy, Heart, Right and Left B216
Left Heart *see* Fluoroscopy, Heart, Left B215
Right Heart *see* Fluoroscopy, Heart, Right B214
SPY system intravascular fluorescence *see* Monitoring, Physiological Systems 4A1
Angiography
see Computerized Tomography (CT Scan), Artery
see Fluoroscopy, Artery
see Magnetic Resonance Imaging (MRI), Artery
see Plain Radiography, Artery
Angioplasty
see Dilation, Heart and Great Vessels Ø27
see Dilation, Lower Arteries Ø47
see Dilation, Upper Arteries Ø37
see Repair, Heart and Great Vessels Ø2Q
see Repair, Lower Arteries Ø4Q
see Repair, Upper Arteries Ø3Q
see Replacement, Heart and Great Vessels Ø2R
see Replacement, Lower Arteries Ø4R
see Replacement, Upper Arteries Ø3R
see Supplement, Heart and Great Vessels Ø2U
see Supplement, Lower Arteries Ø4U
see Supplement, Upper Arteries Ø3U
Angiorrhaphy
see Repair, Heart and Great Vessels Ø2Q
see Repair, Lower Arteries Ø4Q
see Repair, Upper Arteries Ø3Q
Angioscopy Ø2JY4ZZ, Ø3JY4ZZ, Ø4JY4ZZ
Angiotensin II *use* Vasopressor
Angiotripsy
see Occlusion, Lower Arteries Ø4L
see Occlusion, Upper Arteries Ø3L
Angular artery *use* Face Artery
Angular vein
use Face Vein, Left
use Face Vein, Right
Ankle Truss System™ (ATS) *use* Internal Fixation Device, Open-truss Design in New Technology
Annular ligament
use Elbow Bursa and Ligament, Left
use Elbow Bursa and Ligament, Right
Annuloplasty
see Repair, Heart and Great Vessels Ø2Q
see Supplement, Heart and Great Vessels Ø2U
Annuloplasty ring *use* Synthetic Substitute
Anoplasty
see Repair, Anus ØDQQ
see Supplement, Anus ØDUQ
Anorectal junction *use* Rectum
Anoscopy ØDJD8ZZ
Ansa cervicalis *use* Cervical Plexus
Antabuse therapy HZ93ZZZ
Antebrachial fascia
use Subcutaneous Tissue and Fascia, Left Lower Arm
use Subcutaneous Tissue and Fascia, Right Lower Arm
Anterior cerebral artery *use* Intracranial Artery
Anterior cerebral vein *use* Intracranial Vein
Anterior choroidal artery *use* Intracranial Artery
Anterior circumflex humeral artery
use Axillary Artery, Left
use Axillary Artery, Right
Anterior communicating artery *use* Intracranial Artery
Anterior cruciate ligament (ACL)
use Knee Bursa and Ligament, Left
use Knee Bursa and Ligament, Right
Anterior crural nerve *use* Femoral Nerve
Anterior facial vein
use Face Vein, Left
use Face Vein, Right
Anterior intercostal artery
use Internal Mammary Artery, Left
use Internal Mammary Artery, Right
Anterior interosseous nerve *use* Median Nerve
Anterior lateral malleolar artery
use Anterior Tibial Artery, Left
use Anterior Tibial Artery, Right
Anterior lingual gland *use* Minor Salivary Gland
Anterior (pectoral) lymph node
use Lymphatic, Left Axillary
use Lymphatic, Right Axillary
Anterior medial malleolar artery
use Anterior Tibial Artery, Left
use Anterior Tibial Artery, Right
Anterior spinal artery
use Vertebral Artery, Left
use Vertebral Artery, Right
Anterior tibial recurrent artery
use Anterior Tibial Artery, Left
use Anterior Tibial Artery, Right
Anterior ulnar recurrent artery
use Ulnar Artery, Left
use Ulnar Artery, Right
Anterior vagal trunk *use* Vagus Nerve
Anterior vertebral muscle
use Neck Muscle, Left
use Neck Muscle, Right
Antibacterial Envelope (TYRX) (AIGISRx) *use* Anti-Infective Envelope
Antibiotic-eluting Bone Void Filler XWØVØP7
Antigen-free air conditioning *see* Atmospheric Control, Physiological Systems 6AØ
Antihelix
use External Ear, Bilateral
use External Ear, Left
use External Ear, Right
Antimicrobial envelope *use* Anti-Infective Envelope
Anti-SARS-CoV-2 hyperimmune globulin *use* Hyperimmune Globulin
Antitragus
use External Ear, Bilateral
use External Ear, Left
use External Ear, Right
Antrostomy *see* Drainage, Ear, Nose, Sinus Ø99
Antrotomy *see* Drainage, Ear, Nose, Sinus Ø99
Antrum of Highmore
use Maxillary Sinus, Left
use Maxillary Sinus, Right
Aortic annulus *use* Aortic Valve
Aortic arch *use* Thoracic Aorta, Ascending/Arch
Aortic intercostal artery *use* Upper Artery
Aortix™ System *use* Short-term External Heart Assist System in Heart and Great Vessels
Aortography
see Fluoroscopy, Lower Arteries B41
see Fluoroscopy, Upper Arteries B31
see Plain Radiography, Lower Arteries B4Ø
see Plain Radiography, Upper Arteries B3Ø
Aortoplasty
see Repair, Aorta, Abdominal Ø4QØ
see Repair, Aorta, Thoracic, Ascending/Arch Ø2QX
see Repair, Aorta, Thoracic, Descending Ø2QW
see Replacement, Aorta, Abdominal Ø4RØ
see Replacement, Aorta, Thoracic, Ascending/Arch Ø2RX
Aortoplasty — *continued*
see Replacement, Aorta, Thoracic, Descending Ø2RW
see Supplement, Aorta, Abdominal Ø4UØ
see Supplement, Aorta, Thoracic, Ascending/Arch Ø2UX
see Supplement, Aorta, Thoracic, Descending Ø2UW
Apalutamide Antineoplastic XWØDXJ5
Apical (subclavicular) lymph node
use Lymphatic, Left Axillary
use Lymphatic, Right Axillary
ApiFix® Minimally Invasive Deformity Correction (MID-C) System *use* Posterior (Dynamic) Distraction Device in New Technology
Apneustic center *use* Pons
Appendectomy
see Excision, Appendix ØDBJ
see Resection, Appendix ØDTJ
Appendiceal orifice *use* Appendix
Appendicolysis *see* Release, Appendix ØDNJ
Appendicotomy *see* Drainage, Appendix ØD9J
Application *see* Introduction of substance in or on
aprevo™ *use* Interbody Fusion Device, Custom-Made Anatomically Designed in New Technology
Aquablation therapy, prostate ØV5Ø8ZZ
Aquapheresis 6A55ØZ3
Aqueduct of Sylvius *use* Cerebral Ventricle
Aqueous humour
use Anterior Chamber, Left
use Anterior Chamber, Right
Arachnoid mater, intracranial *use* Cerebral Meninges
Arachnoid mater, spinal *use* Spinal Meninges
Arcuate artery
use Foot Artery, Left
use Foot Artery, Right
Areola
use Nipple, Left
use Nipple, Right
AROM (artificial rupture of membranes) 1Ø9Ø7ZC
Arterial canal (duct) *use* Pulmonary Artery, Left
Arterial pulse tracing *see* Measurement, Arterial 4AØ3
Arteriectomy
see Excision, Heart and Great Vessels Ø2B
see Excision, Lower Arteries Ø4B
see Excision, Upper Arteries Ø3B
Arteriography
see Fluoroscopy, Heart B21
see Fluoroscopy, Lower Arteries B41
see Fluoroscopy, Upper Arteries B31
see Plain Radiography, Heart B2Ø
see Plain Radiography, Lower Arteries B4Ø
see Plain Radiography, Upper Arteries B3Ø
Arterioplasty
see Repair, Heart and Great Vessels Ø2Q
see Repair, Lower Arteries Ø4Q
see Repair, Upper Arteries Ø3Q
see Replacement, Heart and Great Vessels Ø2R
see Replacement, Lower Arteries Ø4R
see Replacement, Upper Arteries Ø3R
see Supplement, Heart and Great Vessels Ø2U
see Supplement, Lower Arteries Ø4U
see Supplement, Upper Arteries Ø3U
Arteriorrhaphy
see Repair, Heart and Great Vessels Ø2Q
see Repair, Lower Arteries Ø4Q
see Repair, Upper Arteries Ø3Q
Arterioscopy
see Inspection, Artery, Lower Ø4JY
see Inspection, Artery, Upper Ø3JY
see Inspection, Great Vessel Ø2JY
Arteriovenous Fistula, Extraluminal Support Device, Supplement X2U
Arthrectomy
see Excision, Lower Joints ØSB
see Excision, Upper Joints ØRB
see Resection, Lower Joints ØST
see Resection, Upper Joints ØRT
Arthrocentesis
see Drainage, Lower Joints ØS9
see Drainage, Upper Joints ØR9
Arthrodesis
see Fusion, Lower Joints ØSG
see Fusion, Upper Joints ØRG
Arthrography
see Plain Radiography, Non-Axial Lower Bones BQØ

Arthrography — *continued*
see Plain Radiography, Non-Axial Upper Bones BPØ
see Plain Radiography, Skull and Facial Bones BNØ
Arthrolysis
see Release, Lower Joints ØSN
see Release, Upper Joints ØRN
Arthropexy
see Repair, Lower Joints ØSQ
see Repair, Upper Joints ØRQ
see Reposition, Lower Joints ØSS
see Reposition, Upper Joints ØRS
Arthroplasty
see Repair, Lower Joints ØSQ
see Repair, Upper Joints ØRQ
see Replacement, Lower Joints ØSR
see Replacement, Upper Joints ØRR
see Supplement, Lower Joints ØSU
see Supplement, Upper Joints ØRU
Arthroplasty, radial head
see Replacement, Radius, Left ØPRJ
see Replacement, Radius, Right ØPRH
Arthroscopy
see Inspection, Lower Joints ØSJ
see Inspection, Upper Joints ØRJ
Arthrotomy
see Drainage, Lower Joints ØS9
see Drainage, Upper Joints ØR9
Articulating Spacer (Antibiotic) *use* Articulating Spacer in Lower Joints
Artificial anal sphincter (AAS) *use* Artificial Sphincter in Gastrointestinal System
Artificial bowel sphincter (neosphincter) *use* Artificial Sphincter in Gastrointestinal System
Artificial Sphincter
Insertion of device in
Anus ØDHQ
Bladder ØTHB
Bladder Neck ØTHC
Urethra ØTHD
Removal of device from
Anus ØDPQ
Bladder ØTPB
Urethra ØTPD
Revision of device in
Anus ØDWQ
Bladder ØTWB
Urethra ØTWD
Artificial urinary sphincter (AUS) *use* Artificial Sphincter in Urinary System
Aryepiglottic fold *use* Larynx
Arytenoid cartilage *use* Larynx
Arytenoid muscle
use Neck Muscle, Left
use Neck Muscle, Right
Arytenoidectomy *see* Excision, Larynx ØCBS
Arytenoidopexy *see* Repair, Larynx ØCQS
Ascenda Intrathecal Catheter *use* Infusion Device
Ascending aorta *use* Thoracic Aorta, Ascending/Arch
Ascending palatine artery *use* Face Artery
Ascending pharyngeal artery
use External Carotid Artery, Left
use External Carotid Artery, Right
aScope™ Duodeno *see* New Technology, Hepatobiliary System and Pancreas XFJ
Aspiration, fine needle
Fluid or gas *see* Drainage
Tissue biopsy
see Excision
see Extraction
Assessment
Activities of daily living *see* Activities of Daily Living Assessment, Rehabilitation FØ2
Hearing *see* Hearing Assessment, Diagnostic Audiology F13
Hearing aid *see* Hearing Aid Assessment, Diagnostic Audiology F14
Intravascular perfusion, using indocyanine green (ICG) dye *see* Monitoring, Physiological Systems 4A1
Motor function *see* Motor Function Assessment, Rehabilitation FØ1
Nerve function *see* Motor Function Assessment, Rehabilitation FØ1
Speech *see* Speech Assessment, Rehabilitation FØØ
Vestibular *see* Vestibular Assessment, Diagnostic Audiology F15
Assessment — *continued*
Vocational *see* Activities of Daily Living Treatment, Rehabilitation FØ8
Assistance
Cardiac
Continuous
Output
Balloon Pump 5AØ221Ø
Impeller Pump 5AØ221D
Other Pump 5AØ2216
Pulsatile Compression 5AØ2215
Oxygenation, Supersaturated 5AØ222C
Intermittent
Balloon Pump 5AØ211Ø
Impeller Pump 5AØ211D
Other Pump 5AØ2116
Pulsatile Compression 5AØ2115
Circulatory
Continuous, Oxygenation, Hyperbaric 5AØ5221
Intermittent, Oxygenation, Hyperbaric 5AØ5121
Respiratory
24-96 Consecutive Hours
Continuous Negative Airway Pressure 5AØ9459
Continuous Positive Airway Pressure 5AØ9457
High Nasal Flow/Velocity 5AØ945A
Intermittent Negative Airway Pressure 5AØ945B
Intermittent Positive Airway Pressure 5AØ9458
No Qualifier 5AØ945Z
8-24 Consecutive Hours, Ventilation, Intubated Prone Positioning 5AØ9C5K
Continuous, Filtration 5AØ92ØZ
Greater than 24 Consecutive Hours, Ventilation, Intubated Prone Positioning 5AØ9D5K
Greater than 96 Consecutive Hours
Continuous Negative Airway Pressure 5AØ9559
Continuous Positive Airway Pressure 5AØ9557
High Nasal Flow/Velocity 5AØ955A
Intermittent Negative Airway Pressure 5AØ955B
Intermittent Positive Airway Pressure 5AØ9558
No Qualifier 5AØ955Z
Less than 24 Consecutive Hours
Continuous Negative Airway Pressure 5AØ9359
Continuous Positive Airway Pressure 5AØ9357
High Nasal Flow/Velocity 5AØ935A
Intermittent Negative Airway Pressure 5AØ935B
Intermittent Positive Airway Pressure 5AØ9358
No Qualifier 5AØ935Z
Less than 8 Consecutive Hours, Ventilation, Intubated Prone Positioning 5AØ9B5K
Associating liver partition and portal vein ligation (ALPPS)
see Division, Hepatobiliary System and Pancreas ØF8
see Resection, Hepatobiliary System and Pancreas ØFT
Assurant (Cobalt) stent *use* Intraluminal Device
Atezolizumab Antineoplastic XWØ
Atherectomy
see Extirpation, Heart and Great Vessels Ø2C
see Extirpation, Lower Arteries Ø4C
see Extirpation, Upper Arteries Ø3C
Atlantoaxial joint *use* Cervical Vertebral Joint
Atmospheric Control 6AØZ
AtriClip LAA Exclusion System *use* Extraluminal Device
Atrioseptoplasty
see Repair, Heart and Great Vessels Ø2Q
see Replacement, Heart and Great Vessels Ø2R
see Supplement, Heart and Great Vessels Ø2U
Atrioventricular node *use* Conduction Mechanism
Atrium dextrum cordis *use* Atrium, Right
Atrium pulmonale *use* Atrium, Left
Attain Ability® lead Ø2H
Attain Ability® lead — *continued*
use Cardiac Lead, Defibrillator in Ø2H
use Cardiac Lead, Pacemaker in Ø2H
Attain Starfix® (OTW) lead
use Cardiac Lead, Defibrillator in Ø2H
use Cardiac Lead, Pacemaker in Ø2H
Audiology, diagnostic
see Hearing Aid Assessment, Diagnostic Audiology F14
see Hearing Assessment, Diagnostic Audiology F13
see Vestibular Assessment, Diagnostic Audiology F15
Audiometry *see* Hearing Assessment, Diagnostic Audiology F13
Auditory tube
use Eustachian Tube, Left
use Eustachian Tube, Right
Auerbach's (myenteric) plexus *use* Abdominal Sympathetic Nerve
Auricle
use External Ear, Bilateral
use External Ear, Left
use External Ear, Right
Auricularis muscle *use* Head Muscle
Autograft *use* Autologous Tissue Substitute
AutoLITT® System *see* Destruction
Autologous artery graft
use Autologous Arterial Tissue in Heart and Great Vessels
use Autologous Arterial Tissue in Lower Arteries
use Autologous Arterial Tissue in Lower Veins
use Autologous Arterial Tissue in Upper Arteries
use Autologous Arterial Tissue in Upper Veins
Autologous vein graft
use Autologous Venous Tissue in Heart and Great Vessels
use Autologous Venous Tissue in Lower Arteries
use Autologous Venous Tissue in Lower Veins
use Autologous Venous Tissue in Upper Arteries
use Autologous Venous Tissue in Upper Veins
Automated Chest Compression (ACC) 5A1221J
AutoPulse® Resuscitation System 5A1221J
Autotransfusion *see* Transfusion
Autotransplant
Adrenal tissue *see* Reposition, Endocrine System ØGS
Kidney *see* Reposition, Urinary System ØTS
Pancreatic tissue *see* Reposition, Pancreas ØFSG
Parathyroid tissue *see* Reposition, Endocrine System ØGS
Thyroid tissue *see* Reposition, Endocrine System ØGS
Tooth *see* Reattachment, Mouth and Throat ØCM
Aveir™ AR, as dual chamber *use* Intracardiac Pacemaker, Dual-Chamber in New Technology
Aveir™ DR, dual chamber *use* Intracardiac Pacemaker, Dual-Chamber in New Technology
Aveir™ VR, as single chamber *use* Intracardiac Pacemaker in Heart and Great Vessels
Avulsion *see* Extraction
AVYCAZ® (ceftazidime-avibactam) *use* Other Anti-infective
Axial Lumbar Interbody Fusion System *use* Interbody Fusion Device in Lower Joints
AxiaLIF® System *use* Interbody Fusion Device in Lower Joints
Axicabtagene Ciloleucel *use* Axicabtagene Ciloleucel Immunotherapy
Axicabtagene Ciloleucel Immunotherapy XWØ
Axillary fascia
use Subcutaneous Tissue and Fascia, Left Upper Arm
use Subcutaneous Tissue and Fascia, Right Upper Arm
Axillary nerve *use* Brachial Plexus
AZEDRA® *use* Iobenguane I-131 Antineoplastic

B

BAK/C® Interbody Cervical Fusion System *use* Interbody Fusion Device in Upper Joints
BAL (bronchial alveolar lavage), diagnostic *see* Drainage, Respiratory System ØB9
Balanoplasty
see Repair, Penis ØVQS

Balanoplasty — *continued*
see Supplement, Penis ØVUS
Balloon atrial septostomy (BAS) Ø2163Z7
Balloon Pump
Continuous, Output 5AØ221Ø
Intermittent, Output 5AØ211Ø
Bamlanivimab Monoclonal Antibody XWØ
Bandage, Elastic *see* Compression
Banding
see Occlusion
see Restriction
Banding, esophageal varices *see* Occlusion, Vein, Esophageal Ø6L3
Banding, laparoscopic (adjustable) gastric
Initial procedure ØDV64CZ
Surgical correction *see* Revision of device in, Stomach ØDW6
Bard® Composix® Kugel® patch *use* Synthetic Substitute
Bard® Composix® (E/X) (LP) mesh *use* Synthetic Substitute
Bard® Dulex™ mesh *use* Synthetic Substitute
Bard® Ventralex™ hernia patch *use* Synthetic Substitute
Baricitinib XWØ
Barium swallow *see* Fluoroscopy, Gastrointestinal System BD1
Baroreflex Activation Therapy® (BAT®)
use Stimulator Generator in Subcutaneous Tissue and Fascia
use Stimulator Lead in Upper Arteries
Barricaid® Annular Closure Device (ACD) *use* Synthetic Substitute
Bartholin's (greater vestibular) gland *use* Vestibular Gland
Basal (internal) cerebral vein *use* Intracranial Vein
Basal metabolic rate (BMR) *see* Measurement, Physiological Systems 4AØZ
Basal nuclei *use* Basal Ganglia
Base of Tongue *use* Pharynx
Basilar artery *use* Intracranial Artery
Basis pontis *use* Pons
Beam Radiation
Abdomen DWØ3
Intraoperative DWØ33ZØ
Adrenal Gland DGØ2
Intraoperative DGØ23ZØ
Bile Ducts DFØ2
Intraoperative DFØ23ZØ
Bladder DTØ2
Intraoperative DTØ23ZØ
Bone
Intraoperative DPØC3ZØ
Other DPØC
Bone Marrow D7ØØ
Intraoperative D7ØØ3ZØ
Brain DØØØ
Intraoperative DØØØ3ZØ
Brain Stem DØØ1
Intraoperative DØØ13ZØ
Breast
Left DMØØ
Intraoperative DMØØ3ZØ
Right DMØ1
Intraoperative DMØ13ZØ
Bronchus DBØ1
Intraoperative DBØ13ZØ
Cervix DUØ1
Intraoperative DUØ13ZØ
Chest DWØ2
Intraoperative DWØ23ZØ
Chest Wall DBØ7
Intraoperative DBØ73ZØ
Colon DDØ5
Intraoperative DDØ53ZØ
Diaphragm DBØ8
Intraoperative DBØ83ZØ
Duodenum DDØ2
Intraoperative DDØ23ZØ
Ear D9ØØ
Intraoperative D9ØØ3ZØ
Esophagus DDØØ
Intraoperative DDØØ3ZØ
Eye D8ØØ
Intraoperative D8ØØ3ZØ
Femur DPØ9
Intraoperative DPØ93ZØ
Fibula DPØB

Beam Radiation — *continued*
Fibula — *continued*
Intraoperative DPØB3ZØ
Gallbladder DFØ1
Intraoperative DFØ13ZØ
Gland
Adrenal DGØ2
Intraoperative DGØ23ZØ
Parathyroid DGØ4
Intraoperative DGØ43ZØ
Pituitary DGØØ
Intraoperative DGØØ3ZØ
Thyroid DGØ5
Intraoperative DGØ53ZØ
Glands
Intraoperative D9Ø63ZØ
Salivary D9Ø6
Head and Neck DWØ1
Intraoperative DWØ13ZØ
Hemibody DWØ4
Intraoperative DWØ43ZØ
Humerus DPØ6
Intraoperative DPØ63ZØ
Hypopharynx D9Ø3
Intraoperative D9Ø33ZØ
Ileum DDØ4
Intraoperative DDØ43ZØ
Jejunum DDØ3
Intraoperative DDØ33ZØ
Kidney DTØØ
Intraoperative DTØØ3ZØ
Larynx D9ØB
Intraoperative D9ØB3ZØ
Liver DFØØ
Intraoperative DFØØ3ZØ
Lung DBØ2
Intraoperative DBØ23ZØ
Lymphatics
Abdomen D7Ø6
Intraoperative D7Ø63ZØ
Axillary D7Ø4
Intraoperative D7Ø43ZØ
Inguinal D7Ø8
Intraoperative D7Ø83ZØ
Neck D7Ø3
Intraoperative D7Ø33ZØ
Pelvis D7Ø7
Intraoperative D7Ø73ZØ
Thorax D7Ø5
Intraoperative D7Ø53ZØ
Mandible DPØ3
Intraoperative DPØ33ZØ
Maxilla DPØ2
Intraoperative DPØ23ZØ
Mediastinum DBØ6
Intraoperative DBØ63ZØ
Mouth D9Ø4
Intraoperative D9Ø43ZØ
Nasopharynx D9ØD
Intraoperative D9ØD3ZØ
Neck and Head DWØ1
Intraoperative DWØ13ZØ
Nerve
Intraoperative DØØ73ZØ
Peripheral DØØ7
Nose D9Ø1
Intraoperative D9Ø13ZØ
Oropharynx D9ØF
Intraoperative D9ØF3ZØ
Ovary DUØØ
Intraoperative DUØØ3ZØ
Palate
Hard D9Ø8
Intraoperative D9Ø83ZØ
Soft D9Ø9
Intraoperative D9Ø93ZØ
Pancreas DFØ3
Intraoperative DFØ33ZØ
Parathyroid Gland DGØ4
Intraoperative DGØ43ZØ
Pelvic Bones DPØ8
Intraoperative DPØ83ZØ
Pelvic Region DWØ6
Intraoperative DWØ63ZØ
Pineal Body DGØ1
Intraoperative DGØ13ZØ
Pituitary Gland DGØØ
Intraoperative DGØØ3ZØ
Pleura DBØ5

Beam Radiation — *continued*
Pleura — *continued*
Intraoperative DBØ53ZØ
Prostate DVØØ
Intraoperative DVØØ3ZØ
Radius DPØ7
Intraoperative DPØ73ZØ
Rectum DDØ7
Intraoperative DDØ73ZØ
Rib DPØ5
Intraoperative DPØ53ZØ
Sinuses D9Ø7
Intraoperative D9Ø73ZØ
Skin
Abdomen DHØ8
Intraoperative DHØ83ZØ
Arm DHØ4
Intraoperative DHØ43ZØ
Back DHØ7
Intraoperative DHØ73ZØ
Buttock DHØ9
Intraoperative DHØ93ZØ
Chest DHØ6
Intraoperative DHØ63ZØ
Face DHØ2
Intraoperative DHØ23ZØ
Leg DHØB
Intraoperative DHØB3ZØ
Neck DHØ3
Intraoperative DHØ33ZØ
Skull DPØØ
Intraoperative DPØØ3ZØ
Spinal Cord DØØ6
Intraoperative DØØ63ZØ
Spleen D7Ø2
Intraoperative D7Ø23ZØ
Sternum DPØ4
Intraoperative DPØ43ZØ
Stomach DDØ1
Intraoperative DDØ13ZØ
Testis DVØ1
Intraoperative DVØ13ZØ
Thymus D7Ø1
Intraoperative D7Ø13ZØ
Thyroid Gland DGØ5
Intraoperative DGØ53ZØ
Tibia DPØB
Intraoperative DPØB3ZØ
Tongue D9Ø5
Intraoperative D9Ø53ZØ
Trachea DBØØ
Intraoperative DBØØ3ZØ
Ulna DPØ7
Intraoperative DPØ73ZØ
Ureter DTØ1
Intraoperative DTØ13ZØ
Urethra DTØ3
Intraoperative DTØ33ZØ
Uterus DUØ2
Intraoperative DUØ23ZØ
Whole Body DWØ5
Intraoperative DWØ53ZØ
Bedside swallow FØØZJWZ
Berlin Heart Ventricular Assist Device *use* Implantable Heart Assist System in Heart and Great Vessels
Betibeglogene Autotemcel XW1
beti-cel *use* Betibeglogene Autotemcel
Bezlotoxumab infusion *see* Introduction with qualifier Other Therapeutic Monoclonal Antibody
Biceps brachii muscle
use Upper Arm Muscle, Left
use Upper Arm Muscle, Right
Biceps femoris muscle
use Upper Leg Muscle, Left
use Upper Leg Muscle, Right
Bicipital aponeurosis
use Subcutaneous Tissue and Fascia, Left Lower Arm
use Subcutaneous Tissue and Fascia, Right Lower Arm
Bicuspid valve *use* Mitral Valve
Bili light therapy *see* Phototherapy, Skin 6A6Ø
Bioactive embolization coil(s) *use* Intraluminal Device, Bioactive in Upper Arteries
Bioengineered Allogeneic Construct, Skin XHRPXF7
Biofeedback GZC9ZZZ
BioFire® FilmArray® Pneumonia Panel XXEBXQ6

Biopsy
see Drainage with qualifier Diagnostic
see Excision with qualifier Diagnostic
see Extraction with qualifier Diagnostic
BiPAP *see* Assistance, Respiratory 5A09
Bisection *see* Division
Biventricular external heart assist system *use* Short-term External Heart Assist System in Heart and Great Vessels
Blepharectomy
see Excision, Eye Ø8B
see Resection, Eye Ø8T
Blepharoplasty
see Repair, Eye Ø8Q
see Replacement, Eye Ø8R
see Reposition, Eye Ø8S
see Supplement, Eye Ø8U
Blepharorrhaphy *see* Repair, Eye Ø8Q
Blepharotomy *see* Drainage, Eye Ø89
Blinatumomab *use* Other Antineoplastic
BLINCYTO® (blinatumomab) *use* Other Antineoplastic
Block, Nerve, anesthetic injection 3EØT3BZ
Blood glucose monitoring system *use* Monitoring Device
Blood pressure *see* Measurement, Arterial 4AØ3
BMR (basal metabolic rate) *see* Measurement, Physiological Systems 4AØZ
Body of femur
use Femoral Shaft, Left
use Femoral Shaft, Right
Body of fibula
use Fibula, Left
use Fibula, Right
Bone anchored hearing device
use Hearing Device, Bone Conduction in Ø9H
use Hearing Device in Head and Facial Bones
Bone bank bone graft *use* Nonautologous Tissue Substitute
Bone Growth Stimulator
Insertion of device in
Bone
Facial ØNHW
Lower ØQHY
Nasal ØNHB
Upper ØPHY
Skull ØNHØ
Removal of device from
Bone
Facial ØNPW
Lower ØQPY
Nasal ØNPB
Upper ØPPY
Skull ØNPØ
Revision of device in
Bone
Facial ØNWW
Lower ØQWY
Nasal ØNWB
Upper ØPWY
Skull ØNWØ
Bone marrow transplant *see* Transfusion, Circulatory 3Ø2
Bone morphogenetic protein 2 (BMP 2) *use* Recombinant Bone Morphogenetic Protein
Bone screw (interlocking) (lag) (pedicle) (recessed)
use Internal Fixation Device in Head and Facial Bones
use Internal Fixation Device in Lower Bones
use Internal Fixation Device in Upper Bones
Bony labyrinth
use Inner Ear, Left
use Inner Ear, Right
Bony orbit
use Orbit, Left
use Orbit, Right
Bony vestibule
use Inner Ear, Left
use Inner Ear, Right
Botallo's duct *use* Pulmonary Artery, Left
Bovine pericardial valve *use* Zooplastic Tissue in Heart and Great Vessels
Bovine pericardium graft *use* Zooplastic Tissue in Heart and Great Vessels
BP (blood pressure) *see* Measurement, Arterial 4AØ3
Brachial (lateral) lymph node
use Lymphatic, Left Axillary
use Lymphatic, Right Axillary
Brachialis muscle
use Upper Arm Muscle, Left
use Upper Arm Muscle, Right
Brachiocephalic artery *use* Innominate Artery
Brachiocephalic trunk *use* Innominate Artery
Brachiocephalic vein
use Innominate Vein, Left
use Innominate Vein, Right
Brachioradialis muscle
use Lower Arm and Wrist Muscle, Left
use Lower Arm and Wrist Muscle, Right
Brachytherapy
Abdomen DW13
Adrenal Gland DG12
Back
Lower DW1LBB
Upper DW1KBB
Bile Ducts DF12
Bladder DT12
Bone Marrow D71Ø
Brain DØ1Ø
Brain Stem DØ11
Breast
Left DM1Ø
Right DM11
Bronchus DB11
Cervix DU11
Chest DW12
Chest Wall DB17
Colon DD15
Cranial Cavity DW1ØBB
Diaphragm DB18
Duodenum DD12
Ear D91Ø
Esophagus DD1Ø
Extremity
Lower DW1YBB
Upper DW1XBB
Eye D81Ø
Gallbladder DF11
Gastrointestinal Tract DW1PBB
Genitourinary Tract DW1RBB
Gland
Adrenal DG12
Parathyroid DG14
Pituitary DG1Ø
Thyroid DG15
Glands, Salivary D916
Head and Neck DW11
Hypopharynx D913
Ileum DD14
Jejunum DD13
Kidney DT1Ø
Larynx D91B
Liver DF1Ø
Lung DB12
Lymphatics
Abdomen D716
Axillary D714
Inguinal D718
Neck D713
Pelvis D717
Thorax D715
Mediastinum DB16
Mouth D914
Nasopharynx D91D
Neck and Head DW11
Nerve, Peripheral DØ17
Nose D911
Oropharynx D91F
Ovary DU1Ø
Palate
Hard D918
Soft D919
Pancreas DF13
Parathyroid Gland DG14
Pelvic Region DW16
Pineal Body DG11
Pituitary Gland DG1Ø
Pleura DB15
Prostate DV1Ø
Rectum DD17
Respiratory Tract DW1QBB
Sinuses D917
Spinal Cord DØ16
Spleen D712
Stomach DD11
Testis DV11
Brachytherapy — *continued*
Thymus D711
Thyroid Gland DG15
Tongue D915
Trachea DB1Ø
Ureter DT11
Urethra DT13
Uterus DU12
Brachytherapy, CivaSheet®
see Brachytherapy with qualifier Unidirectional Source
see Insertion with device Radioactive Element
Brachytherapy seeds *use* Radioactive Element
Brain Electrical Activity
Computer-aided Detection and Notification XX2ØX89
Computer-aided Semiologic Analysis XXEØX48
Breast procedures, skin only *use* Skin, Chest
Brexanolone XWØ
Brexucabtagene Autoleucel *use* Brexucabtagene Autoleucel Immunotherapy
Brexucabtagene Autoleucel Immunotherapy XWØ
Breyanzi® *use* Lisocabtagene Maraleucel Immunotherapy
Broad Consortium Microbiota-based Live Biotherapeutic Suspension XWØH7X8
Broad ligament *use* Uterine Supporting Structure
Bromelain-enriched Proteolytic Enzyme *use* Anacaulase-bcdb
Bronchial artery *use* Upper Artery
Bronchography
see Fluoroscopy, Respiratory System BB1
see Plain Radiography, Respiratory System BBØ
Bronchoplasty
see Repair, Respiratory System ØBQ
see Supplement, Respiratory System ØBU
Bronchorrhaphy *see* Repair, Respiratory System ØBQ
Bronchoscopy ØBJØ8ZZ
Bronchotomy *see* Drainage, Respiratory System ØB9
Bronchus Intermedius *use* Main Bronchus, Right
BRYAN® Cervical Disc System *use* Synthetic Substitute
Buccal gland *use* Buccal Mucosa
Buccinator lymph node *use* Lymphatic, Head
Buccinator muscle *use* Facial Muscle
Buckling, scleral with implant *see* Supplement, Eye Ø8U
Bulbospongiosus muscle *use* Perineum Muscle
Bulbourethral (Cowper's) gland *use* Urethra
Bundle of His *use* Conduction Mechanism
Bundle of Kent *use* Conduction Mechanism
Bunionectomy *see* Excision, Lower Bones ØQB
Bursectomy
see Excision, Bursae and Ligaments ØMB
see Resection, Bursae and Ligaments ØMT
Bursocentesis *see* Drainage, Bursae and Ligaments ØM9
Bursography
see Plain Radiography, Non-Axial Lower Bones BQØ
see Plain Radiography, Non-Axial Upper Bones BPØ
Bursotomy
see Division, Bursae and Ligaments ØM8
see Drainage, Bursae and Ligaments ØM9
BVS 5ØØØ Ventricular Assist Device *use* Short-term External Heart Assist System in Heart and Great Vessels
Bypass
Anterior Chamber
Left Ø8133
Right Ø8123
Aorta
Abdominal Ø41Ø
Thoracic
Ascending/Arch Ø21X
Descending Ø21W
Artery
Anterior Tibial
Left Ø41Q
Right Ø41P
Axillary
Left Ø316Ø
Right Ø315Ø
Brachial
Left Ø318
Right Ø317
Common Carotid
Left Ø31JØ
Right Ø31HØ

- **Bypass** — *continued*
  - Artery — *continued*
    - Common Iliac
      - Left Ø41D
      - Right Ø41C
    - Coronary
      - Four or More Arteries Ø213
      - One Artery Ø21Ø
      - Three Arteries Ø212
      - Two Arteries Ø211
    - External Carotid
      - Left Ø31NØ
      - Right Ø31MØ
    - External Iliac
      - Left Ø41J
      - Right Ø41H
    - Femoral
      - Left Ø41L
      - Right Ø41K
    - Foot
      - Left Ø41W
      - Right Ø41V
    - Hepatic Ø413
    - Innominate Ø312Ø
    - Internal Carotid
      - Left Ø31LØ
      - Right Ø31KØ
    - Internal Iliac
      - Left Ø41F
      - Right Ø41E
    - Intracranial Ø31GØ
    - Peroneal
      - Left Ø41U
      - Right Ø41T
    - Popliteal
      - Left Ø41N
      - Right Ø41M
    - Posterior Tibial
      - Left Ø41S
      - Right Ø41R
    - Pulmonary
      - Left Ø21R
      - Right Ø21Q
    - Pulmonary Trunk Ø21P
    - Radial
      - Left Ø31C
      - Right Ø31B
    - Splenic Ø414
    - Subclavian
      - Left Ø314Ø
      - Right Ø313Ø
    - Temporal
      - Left Ø31TØ
      - Right Ø31SØ
    - Ulnar
      - Left Ø31A
      - Right Ø319
  - Atrium
    - Left Ø217
    - Right Ø216
  - Bladder ØT1B
  - Cavity, Cranial ØW11ØJ
  - Cecum ØD1H
  - Cerebral Ventricle ØØ16
  - Colon
    - Ascending ØD1K
    - Descending ØD1M
    - Sigmoid ØD1N
    - Transverse ØD1L
  - Conduit through Femoral Vein to Popliteal Artery X2K
  - Conduit through Femoral Vein to Superficial Femoral Artery X2K
  - Duct
    - Common Bile ØF19
    - Cystic ØF18
    - Hepatic
      - Common ØF17
      - Left ØF16
      - Right ØF15
    - Lacrimal
      - Left Ø81Y
      - Right Ø81X
    - Pancreatic ØF1D
      - Accessory ØF1F
  - Duodenum ØD19
  - Ear
    - Left Ø91EØ
    - Right Ø91DØ
- **Bypass** — *continued*
  - Esophagus ØD15
    - Lower ØD13
    - Middle ØD12
    - Upper ØD11
  - Fallopian Tube
    - Left ØU16
    - Right ØU15
  - Gallbladder ØF14
  - Ileum ØD1B
  - Intestine
    - Large ØD1E
    - Small ØD18
  - Jejunum ØD1A
  - Kidney Pelvis
    - Left ØT14
    - Right ØT13
  - Pancreas ØF1G
  - Pelvic Cavity ØW1J
  - Peritoneal Cavity ØW1G
  - Pleural Cavity
    - Left ØW1B
    - Right ØW19
  - Spinal Canal ØØ1U
  - Stomach ØD16
  - Trachea ØB11
  - Ureter
    - Left ØT17
    - Right ØT16
  - Ureters, Bilateral ØT18
  - Vas Deferens
    - Bilateral ØV1Q
    - Left ØV1P
    - Right ØV1N
  - Vein
    - Axillary
      - Left Ø518
      - Right Ø517
    - Azygos Ø51Ø
    - Basilic
      - Left Ø51C
      - Right Ø51B
    - Brachial
      - Left Ø51A
      - Right Ø519
    - Cephalic
      - Left Ø51F
      - Right Ø51D
    - Colic Ø617
    - Common Iliac
      - Left Ø61D
      - Right Ø61C
    - Esophageal Ø613
    - External Iliac
      - Left Ø61G
      - Right Ø61F
    - External Jugular
      - Left Ø51Q
      - Right Ø51P
    - Face
      - Left Ø51V
      - Right Ø51T
    - Femoral
      - Left Ø61N
      - Right Ø61M
    - Foot
      - Left Ø61V
      - Right Ø61T
    - Gastric Ø612
    - Hand
      - Left Ø51H
      - Right Ø51G
    - Hemiazygos Ø511
    - Hepatic Ø614
    - Hypogastric
      - Left Ø61J
      - Right Ø61H
    - Inferior Mesenteric Ø616
    - Innominate
      - Left Ø514
      - Right Ø513
    - Internal Jugular
      - Left Ø51N
      - Right Ø51M
    - Intracranial Ø51L
    - Portal Ø618
    - Renal
      - Left Ø61B
      - Right Ø619
- **Bypass** — *continued*
  - Vein — *continued*
    - Saphenous
      - Left Ø61Q
      - Right Ø61P
    - Splenic Ø611
    - Subclavian
      - Left Ø516
      - Right Ø515
    - Superior Mesenteric Ø615
    - Vertebral
      - Left Ø51S
      - Right Ø51R
  - Vena Cava
    - Inferior Ø61Ø
    - Superior Ø21V
  - Ventricle
    - Left Ø21L
    - Right Ø21K
- **Bypass, cardiopulmonary** 5A1221Z

C

- **Caesarean section** *see* Extraction, Products of Conception 1ØDØ
- **Calcaneocuboid joint**
  - *use* Tarsal Joint, Left
  - *use* Tarsal Joint, Right
- **Calcaneocuboid ligament**
  - *use* Foot Bursa and Ligament, Left
  - *use* Foot Bursa and Ligament, Right
- **Calcaneofibular ligament**
  - *use* Ankle Bursa and Ligament, Left
  - *use* Ankle Bursa and Ligament, Right
- **Calcaneus**
  - *use* Tarsal, Left
  - *use* Tarsal, Right
- **Cannulation**
  - *see* Bypass
  - *see* Dilation
  - *see* Drainage
  - *see* Irrigation
- **Canthorrhaphy** *see* Repair, Eye Ø8Q
- **Canthotomy** *see* Release, Eye Ø8N
- **Canturio™ te (Tibial Extension)** *use* Tibial Extension with Motion Sensors in New Technology
- **Capitate bone**
  - *use* Carpal, Left
  - *use* Carpal, Right
- **Caplacizumab** XWØ
- **Capsulectomy, lens** *see* Excision, Eye Ø8B
- **Capsulorrhaphy, joint**
  - *see* Repair, Lower Joints ØSQ
  - *see* Repair, Upper Joints ØRQ
- **Caption Guidance system** X2JAX47
- **Cardia** *use* Esophagogastric Junction
- **Cardiac contractility modulation lead** *use* Cardiac Lead in Heart and Great Vessels
- **Cardiac event recorder** *use* Monitoring Device
- **Cardiac Lead**
  - Defibrillator
    - Atrium
      - Left Ø2H7
      - Right Ø2H6
    - Pericardium Ø2HN
    - Vein, Coronary Ø2H4
    - Ventricle
      - Left Ø2HL
      - Right Ø2HK
  - Insertion of device in
    - Atrium
      - Left Ø2H7
      - Right Ø2H6
    - Pericardium Ø2HN
    - Vein, Coronary Ø2H4
    - Ventricle
      - Left Ø2HL
      - Right Ø2HK
  - Pacemaker
    - Atrium
      - Left Ø2H7
      - Right Ø2H6
    - Pericardium Ø2HN
    - Vein, Coronary Ø2H4
    - Ventricle
      - Left Ø2HL
      - Right Ø2HK

Cardiac Lead — *continued*
Removal of device from, Heart Ø2PA
Revision of device in, Heart Ø2WA
Cardiac plexus *use* Thoracic Sympathetic Nerve
Cardiac Resynchronization Defibrillator Pulse Generator
Abdomen ØJH8
Chest ØJH6
Cardiac Resynchronization Pacemaker Pulse Generator
Abdomen ØJH8
Chest ØJH6
Cardiac resynchronization therapy (CRT) lead
use Cardiac Lead, Defibrillator in Ø2H
use Cardiac Lead, Pacemaker in Ø2H
Cardiac Rhythm Related Device
Insertion of device in
Abdomen ØJH8
Chest ØJH6
Removal of device from, Subcutaneous Tissue and Fascia, Trunk ØJPT
Revision of device in, Subcutaneous Tissue and Fascia, Trunk ØJWT
Cardiocentesis *see* Drainage, Pericardial Cavity ØW9D
Cardioesophageal junction *use* Esophagogastric Junction
Cardiolysis *see* Release, Heart and Great Vessels Ø2N
CardioMEMS® pressure sensor *use* Monitoring Device, Pressure Sensor in Ø2H
Cardiomyotomy *see* Division, Esophagogastric Junction ØD84
Cardioplegia *see* Introduction of substance in or on, Heart 3EØ8
Cardiorrhaphy *see* Repair, Heart and Great Vessels Ø2Q
Cardioversion 5A22Ø4Z
Caregiver Training FØFZ
Carmat total artificial heart (TAH) *use* Biologic with Synthetic Substitute, Autoregulated Electrohydraulic in Ø2R
Caroticotympanic artery
use Internal Carotid Artery, Left
use Internal Carotid Artery, Right
Carotid glomus
use Carotid Bodies, Bilateral
use Carotid Body, Left
use Carotid Body, Right
Carotid sinus
use Internal Carotid Artery, Left
use Internal Carotid Artery, Right
Carotid (artery) sinus (baroreceptor) lead *use* Stimulator Lead in Upper Arteries
Carotid sinus nerve *use* Glossopharyngeal Nerve
Carotid WALLSTENT® Monorail® Endoprosthesis *use* Intraluminal Device
Carpectomy
see Excision, Upper Bones ØPB
see Resection, Upper Bones ØPT
Carpometacarpal ligament
use Hand Bursa and Ligament, Left
use Hand Bursa and Ligament, Right
CARVYKTI™ *use* Ciltacabtagene Autoleucel
Casirivimab (REGN1Ø933) and Imdevimab (REGN1Ø987) *use* REGN-COV2 Monoclonal Antibody
Casting *see* Immobilization
CAT scan *see* Computerized Tomography (CT Scan)
Catheterization
see Dilation
see Drainage
see Insertion of device in
see Irrigation
Heart *see* Measurement, Cardiac 4AØ2
Umbilical vein, for infusion Ø6HØ33T
Cauda equina *use* Lumbar Spinal Cord
Cauterization
see Destruction
see Repair
Cavernous plexus *use* Head and Neck Sympathetic Nerve
Cavoatrial junction *use* Superior Vena Cava
CBMA (Concentrated Bone Marrow Aspirate) *use* Other Substance
CBMA (Concentrated Bone Marrow Aspirate) injection *see* Introduction of substance in or on, Muscle 3EØ2
CD24Fc Immunomodulator XWØ
Cecectomy
see Excision, Cecum ØDBH
see Resection, Cecum ØDTH
Cecocolostomy
see Bypass, Gastrointestinal System ØD1
see Drainage, Gastrointestinal System ØD9
Cecopexy
see Repair, Cecum ØDQH
see Reposition, Cecum ØDSH
Cecoplication *see* Restriction, Cecum ØDVH
Cecorrhaphy *see* Repair, Cecum ØDQH
Cecostomy
see Bypass, Cecum ØD1H
see Drainage, Cecum ØD9H
Cecotomy *see* Drainage, Cecum ØD9H
Cefiderocol Anti-infective XWØ
Ceftazidime-avibactam *use* Other Anti-infective
Ceftolozane/Tazobactam Anti-infective XWØ
Celiac ganglion *use* Abdominal Sympathetic Nerve
Celiac lymph node *use* Lymphatic, Aortic
Celiac (solar) plexus *use* Abdominal Sympathetic Nerve
Celiac trunk *use* Celiac Artery
Central axillary lymph node
use Lymphatic, Left Axillary
use Lymphatic, Right Axillary
Central venous pressure *see* Measurement, Venous 4AØ4
Centrimag® Blood Pump *use* Short-term External Heart Assist System in Heart and Great Vessels
Cephalogram BNØØZZZ
CERAMENT® G *use* Antibiotic-eluting Bone Void Filler
Ceramic on ceramic bearing surface *use* Synthetic Substitute, Ceramic in ØSR
Cerclage *see* Restriction
Cerebral aqueduct (Sylvius) *use* Cerebral Ventricle
Cerebral Embolic Filtration
Dual Filter X2A5312
Extracorporeal Flow Reversal Circuit X2A
Single Deflection Filter X2A6325
Cerebrum *use* Brain
Ceribell® Monitor XX2ØX89
Cervical esophagus *use* Esophagus, Upper
Cervical facet joint
use Cervical Vertebral Joint
use Cervical Vertebral Joint, 2 or more
Cervical ganglion *use* Head and Neck Sympathetic Nerve
Cervical interspinous ligament *use* Head and Neck Bursa and Ligament
Cervical intertransverse ligament *use* Head and Neck Bursa and Ligament
Cervical Ligamentum Flavum *use* Head and Neck Bursa and Ligament
Cervical Lymph Node
use Lymphatic, Left Neck
use Lymphatic, Right Neck
Cervicectomy
see Excision, Cervix ØUBC
see Resection, Cervix ØUTC
Cervicothoracic facet joint *use* Cervicothoracic Vertebral Joint
Cesarean section *see* Extraction, Products of Conception 1ØDØ
Cesium-131 Collagen Implant *use* Radioactive Element, Cesium-131 Collagen Implant in ØØH
Change Device in
Abdominal Wall ØW2FX
Back
Lower ØW2LX
Upper ØW2KX
Bladder ØT2BX
Bone
Facial ØN2WX
Lower ØQ2YX
Nasal ØN2BX
Upper ØP2YX
Bone Marrow Ø72TX
Brain ØØ2ØX
Breast
Left ØH2UX
Right ØH2TX
Bursa and Ligament
Lower ØM2YX
Upper ØM2XX
Cavity, Cranial ØW21X
Chest Wall ØW28X
Change Device in — *continued*
Cisterna Chyli Ø72LX
Diaphragm ØB2TX
Duct
Hepatobiliary ØF2BX
Pancreatic ØF2DX
Ear
Left Ø92JX
Right Ø92HX
Epididymis and Spermatic Cord ØV2MX
Extremity
Lower
Left ØY2BX
Right ØY29X
Upper
Left ØX27X
Right ØX26X
Eye
Left Ø821X
Right Ø82ØX
Face ØW22X
Fallopian Tube ØU28X
Gallbladder ØF24X
Gland
Adrenal ØG25X
Endocrine ØG2SX
Pituitary ØG2ØX
Salivary ØC2AX
Head ØW2ØX
Intestinal Tract
Lower Intestinal Tract ØD2DXUZ
Upper Intestinal Tract ØD2ØXUZ
Jaw
Lower ØW25X
Upper ØW24X
Joint
Lower ØS2YX
Upper ØR2YX
Kidney ØT25X
Larynx ØC2SX
Liver ØF2ØX
Lung
Left ØB2LX
Right ØB2KX
Lymphatic Ø72NX
Thoracic Duct Ø72KX
Mediastinum ØW2CX
Mesentery ØD2VX
Mouth and Throat ØC2YX
Muscle
Lower ØK2YX
Upper ØK2XX
Nasal Mucosa and Soft Tissue Ø92KX
Neck ØW26X
Nerve
Cranial ØØ2EX
Peripheral Ø12YX
Omentum ØD2UX
Ovary ØU23X
Pancreas ØF2GX
Parathyroid Gland ØG2RX
Pelvic Cavity ØW2JX
Penis ØV2SX
Pericardial Cavity ØW2DX
Perineum
Female ØW2NX
Male ØW2MX
Peritoneal Cavity ØW2GX
Peritoneum ØD2WX
Pineal Body ØG21X
Pleura ØB2QX
Pleural Cavity
Left ØW2BX
Right ØW29X
Products of Conception 1Ø2Ø7
Prostate and Seminal Vesicles ØV24X
Retroperitoneum ØW2HX
Scrotum and Tunica Vaginalis ØV28X
Sinus Ø92YX
Skin ØH2PX
Skull ØN2ØX
Spinal Canal ØØ2UX
Spleen Ø72PX
Subcutaneous Tissue and Fascia
Head and Neck ØJ2SX
Lower Extremity ØJ2WX
Trunk ØJ2TX
Upper Extremity ØJ2VX

Change Device in — *continued*
Tendon
Lower ØL2YX
Upper ØL2XX
Testis ØV2DX
Thymus Ø72MX
Thyroid Gland ØG2KX
Trachea ØB21
Tracheobronchial Tree ØB2ØX
Ureter ØT29X
Urethra ØT2DX
Uterus and Cervix ØU2DXHZ
Vagina and Cul-de-sac ØU2HXGZ
Vas Deferens ØV2RX
Vulva ØU2MX
Change Device in or on
Abdominal Wall 2WØ3X
Anorectal 2YØ3X5Z
Arm
Lower
Left 2WØDX
Right 2WØCX
Upper
Left 2WØBX
Right 2WØAX
Back 2WØ5X
Chest Wall 2WØ4X
Ear 2YØ2X5Z
Extremity
Lower
Left 2WØMX
Right 2WØLX
Upper
Left 2WØ9X
Right 2WØ8X
Face 2WØ1X
Finger
Left 2WØKX
Right 2WØJX
Foot
Left 2WØTX
Right 2WØSX
Genital Tract, Female 2YØ4X5Z
Hand
Left 2WØFX
Right 2WØEX
Head 2WØØX
Inguinal Region
Left 2WØ7X
Right 2WØ6X
Leg
Lower
Left 2WØRX
Right 2WØQX
Upper
Left 2WØPX
Right 2WØNX
Mouth and Pharynx 2YØØX5Z
Nasal 2YØ1X5Z
Neck 2WØ2X
Thumb
Left 2WØHX
Right 2WØGX
Toe
Left 2WØVX
Right 2WØUX
Urethra 2YØ5X5Z
Chemoembolization *see* Introduction of substance in or on
Chemosurgery, Skin 3EØØXTZ
Chemothalamectomy *see* Destruction, Thalamus ØØ59
Chemotherapy, Infusion for Cancer *see* Introduction of substance in or on
Chest compression (CPR), external
Manual 5A12Ø12
Mechanical 5A1221J
Chest x-ray *see* Plain Radiography, Chest BWØ3
Chin *use* Subcutaneous Tissue and Fascia, Face
Chiropractic Manipulation
Abdomen 9WB9X
Cervical 9WB1X
Extremities
Lower 9WB6X
Upper 9WB7X
Head 9WBØX
Lumbar 9WB3X
Pelvis 9WB5X
Rib Cage 9WB8X
Chiropractic Manipulation — *continued*
Sacrum 9WB4X
Thoracic 9WB2X
Choana *use* Nasopharynx
Cholangiogram
see Fluoroscopy, Hepatobiliary System and Pancreas BF1
see Plain Radiography, Hepatobiliary System and Pancreas BFØ
Cholecystectomy
see Excision, Gallbladder ØFB4
see Resection, Gallbladder ØFT4
Cholecystojejunostomy
see Bypass, Hepatobiliary System and Pancreas ØF1
see Drainage, Hepatobiliary System and Pancreas ØF9
Cholecystopexy
see Repair, Gallbladder ØFQ4
see Reposition, Gallbladder ØFS4
Cholecystoscopy ØFJ44ZZ
Cholecystostomy
see Bypass, Gallbladder ØF14
see Drainage, Gallbladder ØF94
Cholecystotomy *see* Drainage, Gallbladder ØF94
Choledochectomy
see Excision, Hepatobiliary System and Pancreas ØFB
see Resection, Hepatobiliary System and Pancreas ØFT
Choledocholithotomy *see* Extirpation, Duct, Common Bile ØFC9
Choledochoplasty
see Repair, Hepatobiliary System and Pancreas ØFQ
see Replacement, Hepatobiliary System and Pancreas ØFR
see Supplement, Hepatobiliary System and Pancreas ØFU
Choledochoscopy ØFJB8ZZ
Choledochotomy *see* Drainage, Hepatobiliary System and Pancreas ØF9
Cholelithotomy *see* Extirpation, Hepatobiliary System and Pancreas ØFC
Chondrectomy
see Excision, Lower Joints ØSB
see Excision, Upper Joints ØRB
Knee *see* Excision, Lower Joints ØSB
Semilunar cartilage *see* Excision, Lower Joints ØSB
Chondroglossus muscle *use* Tongue, Palate, Pharynx Muscle
Chorda tympani *use* Facial Nerve
Chordotomy *see* Division, Central Nervous System and Cranial Nerves ØØ8
Choroid plexus *use* Cerebral Ventricle
Choroidectomy
see Excision, Eye Ø8B
see Resection, Eye Ø8T
Ciliary body
use Eye, Left
use Eye, Right
Ciliary ganglion *use* Head and Neck Sympathetic Nerve
Ciltacabtagene Autoleucel XWØ
cilta-cel *use* Ciltacabtagene Autoleucel
Circle of Willis *use* Intracranial Artery
Circumcision ØVTTXZZ
Circumflex iliac artery
use Femoral Artery, Left
use Femoral Artery, Right
CivaSheet® *use* Radioactive Element
CivaSheet® Brachytherapy
see Brachytherapy with qualifier Unidirectional Source
see Insertion with device Radioactive Element
Clamp and rod internal fixation system (CRIF)
use Internal Fixation Device in Lower Bones
use Internal Fixation Device in Upper Bones
Clamping *see* Occlusion
Claustrum *use* Basal Ganglia
Claviculectomy
see Excision, Upper Bones ØPB
see Resection, Upper Bones ØPT
Claviculotomy
see Division, Upper Bones ØP8
see Drainage, Upper Bones ØP9
Clipping, aneurysm
see Occlusion using Extraluminal Device
see Restriction using Extraluminal Device
Clitorectomy, clitoridectomy
see Excision, Clitoris ØUBJ
see Resection, Clitoris ØUTJ
Clolar *use* Clofarabine
Closure
see Occlusion
see Repair
Clysis *see* Introduction of substance in or on
Coagulation *see* Destruction
Coagulation Factor Xa, Inactivated XWØ
Coagulation Factor Xa, (Recombinant) Inactivated *use* Coagulation Factor Xa, Inactivated
COALESCE® radiolucent interbody fusion device
use Interbody Fusion Device in Lower Joints
use Interbody Fusion Device in Upper Joints
CoAxia NeuroFlo catheter *use* Intraluminal Device
Cobalt/chromium head and polyethylene socket *use* Synthetic Substitute, Metal on Polyethylene in ØSR
Cobalt/chromium head and socket *use* Synthetic Substitute, Metal in ØSR
Coccygeal body *use* Coccygeal Glomus
Coccygeus muscle
use Trunk Muscle, Left
use Trunk Muscle, Right
Cochlea
use Inner Ear, Left
use Inner Ear, Right
Cochlear implant (CI), multiple channel (electrode) *use* Hearing Device, Multiple Channel Cochlear Prosthesis in Ø9H
Cochlear implant (CI), single channel (electrode) *use* Hearing Device, Single Channel Cochlear Prosthesis in Ø9H
Cochlear Implant Treatment FØBZØ
Cochlear nerve *use* Acoustic Nerve
COGNIS® CRT-D *use* Cardiac Resynchronization Defibrillator Pulse Generator in ØJH
COHERE® radiolucent interbody fusion device
use Interbody Fusion Device in Lower Joints
use Interbody Fusion Device in Upper Joints
Colectomy
see Excision, Gastrointestinal System ØDB
see Resection, Gastrointestinal System ØDT
Collapse *see* Occlusion
Collection from
Breast, Breast Milk 8EØHX62
Indwelling Device
Circulatory System
Blood 8CØ2X6K
Other Fluid 8CØ2X6L
Nervous System
Cerebrospinal Fluid 8CØ1X6J
Other Fluid 8CØ1X6L
Integumentary System, Breast Milk 8EØHX62
Reproductive System, Male, Sperm 8EØVX63
Colocentesis *see* Drainage, Gastrointestinal System ØD9
Colofixation
see Repair, Gastrointestinal System ØDQ
see Reposition, Gastrointestinal System ØDS
Cololysis *see* Release, Gastrointestinal System ØDN
Colonic Z-Stent® *use* Intraluminal Device
Colonoscopy ØDJD8ZZ
Colopexy
see Repair, Gastrointestinal System ØDQ
see Reposition, Gastrointestinal System ØDS
Coloplication *see* Restriction, Gastrointestinal System ØDV
Coloproctectomy
see Excision, Gastrointestinal System ØDB
see Resection, Gastrointestinal System ØDT
Coloproctostomy
see Bypass, Gastrointestinal System ØD1
see Drainage, Gastrointestinal System ØD9
Colopuncture *see* Drainage, Gastrointestinal System ØD9
Colorrhaphy *see* Repair, Gastrointestinal System ØDQ
Colostomy
see Bypass, Gastrointestinal System ØD1
see Drainage, Gastrointestinal System ØD9
Colpectomy
see Excision, Vagina ØUBG
see Resection, Vagina ØUTG
Colpocentesis *see* Drainage, Vagina ØU9G
Colpopexy
see Repair, Vagina ØUQG

Colpopexy — *continued*
see Reposition, Vagina ØUSG
Colpoplasty
see Repair, Vagina ØUQG
see Supplement, Vagina ØUUG
Colporrhaphy *see* Repair, Vagina ØUQG
Colposcopy ØUJH8ZZ
Columella *use* Nasal Mucosa and Soft Tissue
COMIRNATY®
use COVID-19 Vaccine
use COVID-19 Vaccine Booster
use COVID-19 Vaccine Dose 1
use COVID-19 Vaccine Dose 2
use COVID-19 Vaccine Dose 3
Common digital vein
use Foot Vein, Left
use Foot Vein, Right
Common facial vein
use Face Vein, Left
use Face Vein, Right
Common fibular nerve *use* Peroneal Nerve
Common hepatic artery *use* Hepatic Artery
Common iliac (subaortic) lymph node *use* Lymphatic, Pelvis
Common interosseous artery
use Ulnar Artery, Left
use Ulnar Artery, Right
Common peroneal nerve *use* Peroneal Nerve
Complete (SE) stent *use* Intraluminal Device
Compression
see Restriction
Abdominal Wall 2W13X
Arm
Lower
Left 2W1DX
Right 2W1CX
Upper
Left 2W1BX
Right 2W1AX
Back 2W15X
Chest Wall 2W14X
Extremity
Lower
Left 2W1MX
Right 2W1LX
Upper
Left 2W19X
Right 2W18X
Face 2W11X
Finger
Left 2W1KX
Right 2W1JX
Foot
Left 2W1TX
Right 2W1SX
Hand
Left 2W1FX
Right 2W1EX
Head 2W1ØX
Inguinal Region
Left 2W17X
Right 2W16X
Leg
Lower
Left 2W1RX
Right 2W1QX
Upper
Left 2W1PX
Right 2W1NX
Neck 2W12X
Thumb
Left 2W1HX
Right 2W1GX
Toe
Left 2W1VX
Right 2W1UX
Computer Assisted Procedure
Extremity
Lower
No Qualifier 8EØYXBZ
With Computerized Tomography 8EØYXBG
With Fluoroscopy 8EØYXBF
With Magnetic Resonance Imaging 8EØYXBH
Upper
No Qualifier 8EØXXBZ

Computer Assisted Procedure — *continued*
Extremity — *continued*
Upper — *continued*
With Computerized Tomography 8EØXXBG
With Fluoroscopy 8EØXXBF
With Magnetic Resonance Imaging 8EØXXBH
Head and Neck Region
No Qualifier 8EØ9XBZ
With Computerized Tomography 8EØ9XBG
With Fluoroscopy 8EØ9XBF
With Magnetic Resonance Imaging 8EØ9XBH
Trunk Region
No Qualifier 8EØWXBZ
With Computerized Tomography 8EØWXBG
With Fluoroscopy 8EØWXBF
With Magnetic Resonance Imaging 8EØWXBH
Computer-aided Assessment
Cardiac Output XXE2X19
Intracranial Vascular Activity XXEØXØ7
Computer-aided Guidance, Transthoracic Echocardiography X2JAX47
Computer-aided Mechanical Aspiration X2C
Computer-aided Triage and Notification, Pulmonary Artery Flow XXE3X27
Computer-aided Valve Modeling and Notification, Coronary Artery Flow XXE3X68
Computer-assisted Intermittent Aspiration *see* New Technology, Cardiovascular System X2C
Computer-assisted Transcranial Magnetic Stimulation XØZØX18
Computerized Tomography (CT Scan)
Abdomen BW2Ø
Chest and Pelvis BW25
Abdomen and Chest BW24
Abdomen and Pelvis BW21
Airway, Trachea BB2F
Ankle
Left BQ2H
Right BQ2G
Aorta
Abdominal B42Ø
Intravascular Optical Coherence B42ØZ2Z
Thoracic B32Ø
Intravascular Optical Coherence B32ØZ2Z
Arm
Left BP2F
Right BP2E
Artery
Celiac B421
Intravascular Optical Coherence B421Z2Z
Common Carotid
Bilateral B325
Intravascular Optical Coherence B325Z2Z
Coronary
Bypass Graft
Intravascular Optical Coherence B223Z2Z
Multiple B223
Multiple B221
Intravascular Optical Coherence B221Z2Z
Internal Carotid
Bilateral B328
Intravascular Optical Coherence B328Z2Z
Intracranial B32R
Intravascular Optical Coherence B32RZ2Z
Lower Extremity
Bilateral B42H
Intravascular Optical Coherence B42HZ2Z
Left B42G
Intravascular Optical Coherence B42GZ2Z
Right B42F
Intravascular Optical Coherence B42FZ2Z
Pelvic B42C
Intravascular Optical Coherence B42CZ2Z

Computerized Tomography (CT Scan) — *continued*
Artery — *continued*
Pulmonary
Left B32T
Intravascular Optical Coherence B32TZ2Z
Right B32S
Intravascular Optical Coherence B32SZ2Z
Renal
Bilateral B428
Intravascular Optical Coherence B428Z2Z
Transplant B42M
Intravascular Optical Coherence B42MZ2Z
Superior Mesenteric B424
Intravascular Optical Coherence B424Z2Z
Vertebral
Bilateral B32G
Intravascular Optical Coherence B32GZ2Z
Bladder BT2Ø
Bone
Facial BN25
Temporal BN2F
Brain BØ2Ø
Calcaneus
Left BQ2K
Right BQ2J
Cerebral Ventricle BØ28
Chest, Abdomen and Pelvis BW25
Chest and Abdomen BW24
Cisterna BØ27
Clavicle
Left BP25
Right BP24
Coccyx BR2F
Colon BD24
Ear B92Ø
Elbow
Left BP2H
Right BP2G
Extremity
Lower
Left BQ2S
Right BQ2R
Upper
Bilateral BP2V
Left BP2U
Right BP2T
Eye
Bilateral B827
Left B826
Right B825
Femur
Left BQ24
Right BQ23
Fibula
Left BQ2C
Right BQ2B
Finger
Left BP2S
Right BP2R
Foot
Left BQ2M
Right BQ2L
Forearm
Left BP2K
Right BP2J
Gland
Adrenal, Bilateral BG22
Parathyroid BG23
Parotid, Bilateral B926
Salivary, Bilateral B92D
Submandibular, Bilateral B929
Thyroid BG24
Hand
Left BP2P
Right BP2N
Hands and Wrists, Bilateral BP2Q
Head BW28
Head and Neck BW29
Heart
Intravascular Optical Coherence B226Z2Z
Right and Left B226
Hepatobiliary System, All BF2C

Computerized Tomography (CT Scan) — *continued*
Hip
Left BQ21
Right BQ2Ø
Humerus
Left BP2B
Right BP2A
Intracranial Sinus B522
Intravascular Optical Coherence B522Z2Z
Joint
Acromioclavicular, Bilateral BP23
Finger
Left BP2DZZZ
Right BP2CZZZ
Foot
Left BQ2Y
Right BQ2X
Hand
Left BP2DZZZ
Right BP2CZZZ
Sacroiliac BR2D
Sternoclavicular
Bilateral BP22
Left BP21
Right BP2Ø
Temporomandibular, Bilateral BN29
Toe
Left BQ2Y
Right BQ2X
Kidney
Bilateral BT23
Left BT22
Right BT21
Transplant BT29
Knee
Left BQ28
Right BQ27
Larynx B92J
Leg
Left BQ2F
Right BQ2D
Liver BF25
Liver and Spleen BF26
Lung, Bilateral BB24
Mandible BN26
Nasopharynx B92F
Neck BW2F
Neck and Head BW29
Orbit, Bilateral BN23
Oropharynx B92F
Pancreas BF27
Patella
Left BQ2W
Right BQ2V
Pelvic Region BW2G
Pelvis BR2C
Chest and Abdomen BW25
Pelvis and Abdomen BW21
Pituitary Gland BØ29
Prostate BV23
Ribs
Left BP2Y
Right BP2X
Sacrum BR2F
Scapula
Left BP27
Right BP26
Sella Turcica BØ29
Shoulder
Left BP29
Right BP28
Sinus
Intracranial B522
Intravascular Optical Coherence B522Z2Z
Paranasal B922
Skull BN2Ø
Spinal Cord BØ2B
Spine
Cervical BR2Ø
Lumbar BR29
Thoracic BR27
Spleen and Liver BF26
Thorax BP2W
Tibia
Left BQ2C
Right BQ2B
Toe
Left BQ2Q

Computerized Tomography (CT Scan) — *continued*
Toe — *continued*
Right BQ2P
Trachea BB2F
Tracheobronchial Tree
Bilateral BB29
Left BB28
Right BB27
Vein
Pelvic (Iliac)
Left B52G
Intravascular Optical Coherence B52GZ2Z
Right B52F
Intravascular Optical Coherence B52FZ2Z
Pelvic (Iliac) Bilateral B52H
Intravascular Optical Coherence B52HZ2Z
Portal B52T
Intravascular Optical Coherence B52TZ2Z
Pulmonary
Bilateral B52S
Intravascular Optical Coherence B52SZ2Z
Left B52R
Intravascular Optical Coherence B52RZ2Z
Right B52Q
Intravascular Optical Coherence B52QZ2Z
Renal
Bilateral B52L
Intravascular Optical Coherence B52LZ2Z
Left B52K
Intravascular Optical Coherence B52KZ2Z
Right B52J
Intravascular Optical Coherence B52JZ2Z
Spanchnic B52T
Intravascular Optical Coherence B52TZ2Z
Vena Cava
Inferior B529
Intravascular Optical Coherence B529Z2Z
Superior B528
Intravascular Optical Coherence B528Z2Z
Ventricle, Cerebral BØ28
Wrist
Left BP2M
Right BP2L

Concerto II CRT-D *use* Cardiac Resynchronization Defibrillator Pulse Generator in ØJH
Conduit through Femoral Vein to Popliteal Artery, Bypass X2K
Conduit through Femoral Vein to Superficial Femoral Artery, Bypass X2K
Conduit to Short-term External Heart Assist System, Insertion X2H
Condylectomy
see Excision, Head and Facial Bones ØNB
see Excision, Lower Bones ØQB
see Excision, Upper Bones ØPB
Condyloid process
use Mandible, Left
use Mandible, Right
Condylotomy
see Division, Head and Facial Bones ØN8
see Division, Lower Bones ØQ8
see Division, Upper Bones ØP8
see Drainage, Head and Facial Bones ØN9
see Drainage, Lower Bones ØQ9
see Drainage, Upper Bones ØP9
Condylysis
see Release, Head and Facial Bones ØNN
see Release, Lower Bones ØQN
see Release, Upper Bones ØPN
Conization, cervix *see* Excision, Cervix ØUBC
Conjunctivoplasty
see Repair, Eye Ø8Q
see Replacement, Eye Ø8R
CONSERVE® PLUS Total Resurfacing Hip System *use* Resurfacing Device in Lower Joints

Construction
Auricle, ear *see* Replacement, Ear, Nose, Sinus Ø9R
Ileal conduit *see* Bypass, Urinary System ØT1
Consulta CRT-D *use* Cardiac Resynchronization Defibrillator Pulse Generator in ØJH
Consulta CRT-P *use* Cardiac Resynchronization Pacemaker Pulse Generator in ØJH
Contact Radiation
Abdomen DWY37ZZ
Adrenal Gland DGY27ZZ
Bile Ducts DFY27ZZ
Bladder DTY27ZZ
Bone, Other DPYC7ZZ
Brain DØYØ7ZZ
Brain Stem DØY17ZZ
Breast
Left DMYØ7ZZ
Right DMY17ZZ
Bronchus DBY17ZZ
Cervix DUY17ZZ
Chest DWY27ZZ
Chest Wall DBY77ZZ
Colon DDY57ZZ
Diaphragm DBY87ZZ
Duodenum DDY27ZZ
Ear D9YØ7ZZ
Esophagus DDYØ7ZZ
Eye D8YØ7ZZ
Femur DPY97ZZ
Fibula DPYB7ZZ
Gallbladder DFY17ZZ
Gland
Adrenal DGY27ZZ
Parathyroid DGY47ZZ
Pituitary DGYØ7ZZ
Thyroid DGY57ZZ
Glands, Salivary D9Y67ZZ
Head and Neck DWY17ZZ
Hemibody DWY47ZZ
Humerus DPY67ZZ
Hypopharynx D9Y37ZZ
Ileum DDY47ZZ
Jejunum DDY37ZZ
Kidney DTYØ7ZZ
Larynx D9YB7ZZ
Liver DFYØ7ZZ
Lung DBY27ZZ
Mandible DPY37ZZ
Maxilla DPY27ZZ
Mediastinum DBY67ZZ
Mouth D9Y47ZZ
Nasopharynx D9YD7ZZ
Neck and Head DWY17ZZ
Nerve, Peripheral DØY77ZZ
Nose D9Y17ZZ
Oropharynx D9YF7ZZ
Ovary DUYØ7ZZ
Palate
Hard D9Y87ZZ
Soft D9Y97ZZ
Pancreas DFY37ZZ
Parathyroid Gland DGY47ZZ
Pelvic Bones DPY87ZZ
Pelvic Region DWY67ZZ
Pineal Body DGY17ZZ
Pituitary Gland DGYØ7ZZ
Pleura DBY57ZZ
Prostate DVYØ7ZZ
Radius DPY77ZZ
Rectum DDY77ZZ
Rib DPY57ZZ
Sinuses D9Y77ZZ
Skin
Abdomen DHY87ZZ
Arm DHY47ZZ
Back DHY77ZZ
Buttock DHY97ZZ
Chest DHY67ZZ
Face DHY27ZZ
Leg DHYB7ZZ
Neck DHY37ZZ
Skull DPYØ7ZZ
Spinal Cord DØY67ZZ
Sternum DPY47ZZ
Stomach DDY17ZZ
Testis DVY17ZZ
Thyroid Gland DGY57ZZ
Tibia DPYB7ZZ
Tongue D9Y57ZZ

Contact Radiation — *continued*
- Trachea DBYØ7ZZ
- Ulna DPY77ZZ
- Ureter DTY17ZZ
- Urethra DTY37ZZ
- Uterus DUY27ZZ
- Whole Body DWY57ZZ

ContaCT software (Measurement of intracranial arterial flow) 4AØ3X5D

CONTAK RENEWAL® 3 RF (HE) CRT-D *use* Cardiac Resynchronization Defibrillator Pulse Generator in ØJH

Contegra Pulmonary Valved Conduit *use* Zooplastic Tissue in Heart and Great Vessels

CONTEPO™ *use* Fosfomycin Anti-Infective

Continent ileostomy *see* Bypass, Ileum ØD1B

Continuous Glucose Monitoring (CGM) device *use* Monitoring Device

Continuous Negative Airway Pressure
- 24-96 Consecutive Hours, Ventilation 5AØ9459
- Greater than 96 Consecutive Hours, Ventilation 5AØ9559
- Less than 24 Consecutive Hours, Ventilation 5AØ9359

Continuous Positive Airway Pressure
- 24-96 Consecutive Hours, Ventilation 5AØ9457
- Greater than 96 Consecutive Hours, Ventilation 5AØ9557
- Less than 24 Consecutive Hours, Ventilation 5AØ9357

Continuous renal replacement therapy (CRRT) 5A1D9ØZ

Contraceptive Device
- Change device in, Uterus and Cervix ØU2DXHZ
- Insertion of device in
  - Cervix ØUHC
  - Subcutaneous Tissue and Fascia
    - Abdomen ØJH8
    - Chest ØJH6
    - Lower Arm
      - Left ØJHH
      - Right ØJHG
    - Lower Leg
      - Left ØJHP
      - Right ØJHN
    - Upper Arm
      - Left ØJHF
      - Right ØJHD
    - Upper Leg
      - Left ØJHM
      - Right ØJHL
  - Uterus ØUH9
- Removal of device from
  - Subcutaneous Tissue and Fascia
    - Lower Extremity ØJPW
    - Trunk ØJPT
    - Upper Extremity ØJPV
  - Uterus and Cervix ØUPD
- Revision of device in
  - Subcutaneous Tissue and Fascia
    - Lower Extremity ØJWW
    - Trunk ØJWT
    - Upper Extremity ØJWV
  - Uterus and Cervix ØUWD

Contractility Modulation Device
- Abdomen ØJH8
- Chest ØJH6

Control bleeding in
- Abdominal Wall ØW3F
- Ankle Region
  - Left ØY3L
  - Right ØY3K
- Arm
  - Lower
    - Left ØX3F
    - Right ØX3D
  - Upper
    - Left ØX39
    - Right ØX38
- Axilla
  - Left ØX35
  - Right ØX34
- Back
  - Lower ØW3L
  - Upper ØW3K
- Buttock
  - Left ØY31
  - Right ØY3Ø

Control bleeding in — *continued*
- Cavity, Cranial ØW31
- Chest Wall ØW38
- Elbow Region
  - Left ØX3C
  - Right ØX3B
- Extremity
  - Lower
    - Left ØY3B
    - Right ØY39
  - Upper
    - Left ØX37
    - Right ØX36
- Face ØW32
- Femoral Region
  - Left ØY38
  - Right ØY37
- Foot
  - Left ØY3N
  - Right ØY3M
- Gastrointestinal Tract ØW3P
- Genitourinary Tract ØW3R
- Hand
  - Left ØX3K
  - Right ØX3J
- Head ØW3Ø
- Inguinal Region
  - Left ØY36
  - Right ØY35
- Jaw
  - Lower ØW35
  - Upper ØW34
- Knee Region
  - Left ØY3G
  - Right ØY3F
- Leg
  - Lower
    - Left ØY3J
    - Right ØY3H
  - Upper
    - Left ØY3D
    - Right ØY3C
- Mediastinum ØW3C
- Nasal Mucosa and Soft Tissue Ø93K
- Neck ØW36
- Oral Cavity and Throat ØW33
- Pelvic Cavity ØW3J
- Pericardial Cavity ØW3D
- Perineum
  - Female ØW3N
  - Male ØW3M
- Peritoneal Cavity ØW3G
- Pleural Cavity
  - Left ØW3B
  - Right ØW39
- Respiratory Tract ØW3Q
- Retroperitoneum ØW3H
- Shoulder Region
  - Left ØX33
  - Right ØX32
- Wrist Region
  - Left ØX3H
  - Right ØX3G

Control bleeding using Tourniquet, External *see* Compression, Anatomical Regions 2W1

Control, Epistaxis *see* Control bleeding in, Nasal Mucosa and Soft Tissue Ø93K

Conus arteriosus *use* Ventricle, Right

Conus medullaris *use* Lumbar Spinal Cord

Convalescent Plasma (Nonautologous) *see* New Technology, Anatomical Regions XW1

Conversion
- Cardiac rhythm 5A22Ø4Z
- Gastrostomy to jejunostomy feeding device *see* Insertion of device in, Jejunum ØDHA

Cook Biodesign® Fistula Plug(s) *use* Nonautologous Tissue Substitute

Cook Biodesign® Hernia Graft(s) *use* Nonautologous Tissue Substitute

Cook Biodesign® Layered Graft(s) *use* Nonautologous Tissue Substitute

Cook Zenapro™ Layered Graft(s) *use* Nonautologous Tissue Substitute

Cook Zenith AAA Endovascular Graft *use* Intraluminal Device

Cook Zenith® Fenestrated AAA Endovascular Graft
- *use* Intraluminal Device, Branched or Fenestrated, One or Two Arteries in Ø4V

Cook Zenith® Fenestrated AAA Endovascular Graft — *continued*
- *use* Intraluminal Device, Branched or Fenestrated, Three or More Arteries in Ø4V

Coracoacromial ligament
- *use* Shoulder Bursa and Ligament, Left
- *use* Shoulder Bursa and Ligament, Right

Coracobrachialis muscle
- *use* Upper Arm Muscle, Left
- *use* Upper Arm Muscle, Right

Coracoclavicular ligament
- *use* Shoulder Bursa and Ligament, Left
- *use* Shoulder Bursa and Ligament, Right

Coracohumeral ligament
- *use* Shoulder Bursa and Ligament, Left
- *use* Shoulder Bursa and Ligament, Right

Coracoid process
- *use* Scapula, Left
- *use* Scapula, Right

Cordotomy *see* Division, Central Nervous System and Cranial Nerves ØØ8

Core needle biopsy *see* Biopsy

CoreValve transcatheter aortic valve *use* Zooplastic Tissue in Heart and Great Vessels

Cormet Hip Resurfacing System *use* Resurfacing Device in Lower Joints

Corniculate cartilage *use* Larynx

CoRoent® XL *use* Interbody Fusion Device in Lower Joints

Coronary arteriography
- *see* Fluoroscopy, Heart B21
- *see* Plain Radiography, Heart B2Ø

Corox (OTW) Bipolar Lead
- *use* Cardiac Lead, Defibrillator in Ø2H
- *use* Cardiac Lead, Pacemaker in Ø2H

Corpus callosum *use* Brain

Corpus cavernosum *use* Penis

Corpus spongiosum *use* Penis

Corpus striatum *use* Basal Ganglia

Corrugator supercilii muscle *use* Facial Muscle

Cortical strip neurostimulator lead *use* Neurostimulator Lead in Central Nervous System and Cranial Nerves

Corvia IASD® *use* Synthetic Substitute

COSELA™ *use* Trilaciclib

Costatectomy
- *see* Excision, Upper Bones ØPB
- *see* Resection, Upper Bones ØPT

Costectomy
- *see* Excision, Upper Bones ØPB
- *see* Resection, Upper Bones ØPT

Costocervical trunk
- *use* Subclavian Artery, Left
- *use* Subclavian Artery, Right

Costochondrectomy
- *see* Excision, Upper Bones ØPB
- *see* Resection, Upper Bones ØPT

Costoclavicular ligament
- *use* Shoulder Bursa and Ligament, Left
- *use* Shoulder Bursa and Ligament, Right

Costosternoplasty
- *see* Repair, Upper Bones ØPQ
- *see* Replacement, Upper Bones ØPR
- *see* Supplement, Upper Bones ØPU

Costotomy
- *see* Division, Upper Bones ØP8
- *see* Drainage, Upper Bones ØP9

Costotransverse joint *use* Thoracic Vertebral Joint

Costotransverse ligament *use* Rib(s) Bursa and Ligament

Costovertebral joint *use* Thoracic Vertebral Joint

Costoxiphoid ligament *use* Sternum Bursa and Ligament

Counseling
- Family, for substance abuse, Other Family Counseling HZ63ZZZ
- Group
  - 12-Step HZ43ZZZ
  - Behavioral HZ41ZZZ
  - Cognitive HZ4ØZZZ
  - Cognitive-Behavioral HZ42ZZZ
  - Confrontational HZ48ZZZ
  - Continuing Care HZ49ZZZ
  - Infectious Disease
    - Post-Test HZ4CZZZ
    - Pre-Test HZ4CZZZ
  - Interpersonal HZ44ZZZ

Counseling — *continued*
Group — *continued*
Motivational Enhancement HZ47ZZZ
Psychoeducation HZ46ZZZ
Spiritual HZ4BZZZ
Vocational HZ45ZZZ
Individual
12-Step HZ33ZZZ
Behavioral HZ31ZZZ
Cognitive HZ30ZZZ
Cognitive-Behavioral HZ32ZZZ
Confrontational HZ38ZZZ
Continuing Care HZ39ZZZ
Infectious Disease
Post-Test HZ3CZZZ
Pre-Test HZ3CZZZ
Interpersonal HZ34ZZZ
Motivational Enhancement HZ37ZZZ
Psychoeducation HZ36ZZZ
Spiritual HZ3BZZZ
Vocational HZ35ZZZ
Mental Health Services
Educational GZ60ZZZ
Other Counseling GZ63ZZZ
Vocational GZ61ZZZ
Countershock, cardiac 5A2204Z
COVID-19 Vaccine XW0
COVID-19 Vaccine Booster XW0
COVID-19 Vaccine Dose 1 XW0
COVID-19 Vaccine Dose 2 XW0
COVID-19 Vaccine Dose 3 XW0
Cowper's (bulbourethral) gland *use* Urethra
CPAP (continuous positive airway pressure) *see* Assistance, Respiratory 5A09
Craniectomy
see Excision, Head and Facial Bones 0NB
see Resection, Head and Facial Bones 0NT
Cranioplasty
see Repair, Head and Facial Bones 0NQ
see Replacement, Head and Facial Bones 0NR
see Supplement, Head and Facial Bones 0NU
Craniotomy
see Division, Head and Facial Bones 0N8
see Drainage, Central Nervous System and Cranial Nerves 009
see Drainage, Head and Facial Bones 0N9
Creation
Perineum
Female 0W4N0
Male 0W4M0
Valve
Aortic 024F0
Mitral 024G0
Tricuspid 024J0
Cremaster muscle *use* Perineum Muscle
CRESEMBA® (isavuconazonium sulfate) *use* Other Anti-infective
Cribriform plate
use Ethmoid Bone, Left
use Ethmoid Bone, Right
Cricoid cartilage *use* Trachea
Cricoidectomy *see* Excision, Larynx 0CBS
Cricothyroid artery
use Thyroid Artery, Left
use Thyroid Artery, Right
Cricothyroid muscle
use Neck Muscle, Left
use Neck Muscle, Right
Crisis Intervention GZ2ZZZZ
CRRT (Continuous renal replacement therapy) 5A1D90Z
Crural fascia
use Subcutaneous Tissue and Fascia, Left Upper Leg
use Subcutaneous Tissue and Fascia, Right Upper Leg
Crushing, nerve
Cranial *see* Destruction, Central Nervous System and Cranial Nerves 005
Peripheral *see* Destruction, Peripheral Nervous System 015
Cryoablation *see* Destruction
Cryotherapy *see* Destruction
Cryptorchidectomy
see Excision, Male Reproductive System 0VB
see Resection, Male Reproductive System 0VT
Cryptorchiectomy
see Excision, Male Reproductive System 0VB
see Resection, Male Reproductive System 0VT
Cryptotomy
see Division, Gastrointestinal System 0D8
see Drainage, Gastrointestinal System 0D9
CT scan *see* Computerized Tomography (CT Scan)
CT sialogram *see* Computerized Tomography (CT Scan), Ear, Nose, Mouth and Throat B92
CTX001™ *use* Exagamglogene Autotemcel
Cubital lymph node
use Lymphatic, Left Upper Extremity
use Lymphatic, Right Upper Extremity
Cubital nerve *use* Ulnar Nerve
Cuboid bone
use Tarsal, Left
use Tarsal, Right
Cuboideonavicular joint
use Tarsal Joint, Left
use Tarsal Joint, Right
Culdocentesis *see* Drainage, Cul-de-sac 0U9F
Culdoplasty
see Repair, Cul-de-sac 0UQF
see Supplement, Cul-de-sac 0UUF
Culdoscopy 0UJH8ZZ
Culdotomy *see* Drainage, Cul-de-sac 0U9F
Culmen *use* Cerebellum
Cultured epidermal cell autograft *use* Autologous Tissue Substitute
Cuneiform cartilage *use* Larynx
Cuneonavicular joint
use Joint, Tarsal, Left
use Joint, Tarsal, Right
Cuneonavicular ligament
use Foot Bursa and Ligament, Left
use Foot Bursa and Ligament, Right
Curettage
see Excision
see Extraction
Cutaneous (transverse) cervical nerve *use* Cervical Plexus
CVP (central venous pressure) *see* Measurement, Venous 4A04
Cyclodiathermy *see* Destruction, Eye 085
Cyclophotocoagulation *see* Destruction, Eye 085
CYPHER® Stent *use* Intraluminal Device, Drug-eluting in Heart and Great Vessels
Cystectomy
see Excision, Bladder 0TBB
see Resection, Bladder 0TTB
Cystocele repair *see* Repair, Subcutaneous Tissue and Fascia, Pelvic Region 0JQC
Cystography
see Fluoroscopy, Urinary System BT1
see Plain Radiography, Urinary System BT0
Cystolithotomy *see* Extirpation, Bladder 0TCB
Cystopexy
see Repair, Bladder 0TQB
see Reposition, Bladder 0TSB
Cystoplasty
see Repair, Bladder 0TQB
see Replacement, Bladder 0TRB
see Supplement, Bladder 0TUB
Cystorrhaphy *see* Repair, Bladder 0TQB
Cystoscopy 0TJB8ZZ
Cystostomy *see* Bypass, Bladder 0T1B
Cystostomy Tube *use* Drainage Device
Cystotomy *see* Drainage, Bladder 0T9B
Cystourethrography
see Fluoroscopy, Urinary System BT1
see Plain Radiography, Urinary System BT0
Cystourethroplasty
see Repair, Urinary System 0TQ
see Replacement, Urinary System 0TR
see Supplement, Urinary System 0TU
CYTALUX® (Pafolacianine), in Fluorescence Guided Procedure *see* Fluorescence Guided Procedure
Cytarabine and Daunorubicin Liposome Antineoplastic XW0

D

Daratumumab and Hyaluronidase-fihj XW01318
Darzalex Faspro® *use* Daratumumab and Hyaluronidase-fihj
DBS lead *use* Neurostimulator Lead in Central Nervous System and Cranial Nerves
DeBakey Left Ventricular Assist Device *use* Implantable Heart Assist System in Heart and Great Vessels
Debridement
Excisional *see* Excision
Non-excisional *see* Extraction
Decompression, Circulatory 6A15
Decortication, lung
see Extirpation, Respiratory System 0BC
see Release, Respiratory System 0BN
Deep brain neurostimulator lead *use* Neurostimulator Lead in Central Nervous System and Cranial Nerves
Deep cervical fascia
use Subcutaneous Tissue and Fascia, Left Neck
use Subcutaneous Tissue and Fascia, Right Neck
Deep cervical vein
use Vertebral Vein, Left
use Vertebral Vein, Right
Deep circumflex iliac artery
use External Iliac Artery, Left
use External Iliac Artery, Right
Deep facial vein
use Face Vein, Left
use Face Vein, Right
Deep femoral artery
use Femoral Artery, Left
use Femoral Artery, Right
Deep femoral (profunda femoris) vein
use Femoral Vein, Left
use Femoral Vein, Right
Deep Inferior Epigastric Artery Perforator Flap
Replacement
Bilateral 0HRV077
Left 0HRU077
Right 0HRT077
Transfer
Left 0KXG
Right 0KXF
Deep palmar arch
use Hand Artery, Left
use Hand Artery, Right
Deep transverse perineal muscle *use* Perineum Muscle
DefenCath™ *use* Taurolidine Anti-infective and Heparin Anticoagulant
Deferential artery
use Internal Iliac Artery, Left
use Internal Iliac Artery, Right
Defibrillator Generator
Abdomen 0JH8
Chest 0JH6
Defibrillator Lead
Insertion of device in, Mediastinum 0WHC
Removal of device from, Mediastinum 0WPC
Revision of device in, Mediastinum 0WWC
Defibtech Automated Chest Compression (ACC) device 5A1221J
Defitelio *use* Other Substance
Defitelio® infusion *see* Introduction of substance in or on, Physiological Systems and Anatomical Regions 3E0
Delivery
Cesarean *see* Extraction, Products of Conception 10D0
Forceps *see* Extraction, Products of Conception 10D0
Manually assisted 10E0XZZ
Products of Conception 10E0XZZ
Vacuum assisted *see* Extraction, Products of Conception 10D0
Delta frame external fixator
use External Fixation Device, Hybrid in 0PH
use External Fixation Device, Hybrid in 0PS
use External Fixation Device, Hybrid in 0QH
use External Fixation Device, Hybrid in 0QS
Delta III Reverse shoulder prosthesis *use* Synthetic Substitute, Reverse Ball and Socket in 0RR
Deltoid fascia
use Subcutaneous Tissue and Fascia, Left Upper Arm
use Subcutaneous Tissue and Fascia, Right Upper Arm
Deltoid ligament
use Ankle Bursa and Ligament, Left

Deltoid ligament — *continued*
  use Ankle Bursa and Ligament, Right
Deltoid muscle
  use Shoulder Muscle, Left
  use Shoulder Muscle, Right
Deltopectoral (infraclavicular) lymph node
  use Lymphatic, Left Upper Extremity
  use Lymphatic, Right Upper Extremity
Denervation
  Cranial nerve *see* Destruction, Central Nervous System and Cranial Nerves ØØ5
  Peripheral nerve *see* Destruction, Peripheral Nervous System Ø15
Dens *use* Cervical Vertebra
Densitometry
  Plain Radiography
    Femur
      Left BQØ4ZZ1
      Right BQØ3ZZ1
    Hip
      Left BQØ1ZZ1
      Right BQØØZZ1
    Spine
      Cervical BRØØZZ1
      Lumbar BRØ9ZZ1
      Thoracic BRØ7ZZ1
      Whole BRØGZZ1
  Ultrasonography
    Elbow
      Left BP4HZZ1
      Right BP4GZZ1
    Hand
      Left BP4PZZ1
      Right BP4NZZ1
    Shoulder
      Left BP49ZZ1
      Right BP48ZZ1
    Wrist
      Left BP4MZZ1
      Right BP4LZZ1
Denticulate (dentate) ligament *use* Spinal Meninges
Depressor anguli oris muscle *use* Facial Muscle
Depressor labii inferioris muscle *use* Facial Muscle
Depressor septi nasi muscle *use* Facial Muscle
Depressor supercilii muscle *use* Facial Muscle
Dermabrasion *see* Extraction, Skin and Breast ØHD
Dermis *use* Skin
Descending genicular artery
  use Femoral Artery, Left
  use Femoral Artery, Right
Destruction
  Acetabulum
    Left ØQ55
    Right ØQ54
  Adenoids ØC5Q
  Ampulla of Vater ØF5C
  Anal Sphincter ØD5R
  Anterior Chamber
    Left Ø8533ZZ
    Right Ø8523ZZ
  Anus ØD5Q
  Aorta
    Abdominal
    Thoracic
      Ascending/Arch Ø25X
      Descending Ø25W
  Aortic Body ØG5D
  Appendix ØD5J
  Artery
    Anterior Tibial
      Left Ø45Q
      Right Ø45P
    Axillary
      Left Ø356
      Right Ø355
    Brachial
      Left Ø358
      Right Ø357
    Celiac Ø451
    Colic
      Left Ø457
      Middle Ø458
      Right Ø456
    Common Carotid
      Left Ø35J
      Right Ø35H
    Common Iliac
      Left Ø45D

Destruction — *continued*
  Artery — *continued*
    Common Iliac — *continued*
      Right Ø45C
    External Carotid
      Left Ø35N
      Right Ø35M
    External Iliac
      Left Ø45J
      Right Ø45H
    Face Ø35R
    Femoral
      Left Ø45L
      Right Ø45K
    Foot
      Left Ø45W
      Right Ø45V
    Gastric Ø452
    Hand
      Left Ø35F
      Right Ø35D
    Hepatic Ø453
    Inferior Mesenteric Ø45B
    Innominate Ø352
    Internal Carotid
      Left Ø35L
      Right Ø35K
    Internal Iliac
      Left Ø45F
      Right Ø45E
    Internal Mammary
      Left Ø351
      Right Ø35Ø
    Intracranial Ø35G
    Lower Ø45Y
    Peroneal
      Left Ø45U
      Right Ø45T
    Popliteal
      Left Ø45N
      Right Ø45M
    Posterior Tibial
      Left Ø45S
      Right Ø45R
    Pulmonary
      Left Ø25R
      Right Ø25Q
    Pulmonary Trunk Ø25P
    Radial
      Left Ø35C
      Right Ø35B
    Renal
      Left Ø45A
      Right Ø459
    Splenic Ø454
    Subclavian
      Left Ø354
      Right Ø353
    Superior Mesenteric Ø455
    Temporal
      Left Ø35T
      Right Ø35S
    Thyroid
      Left Ø35V
      Right Ø35U
    Ulnar
      Left Ø35A
      Right Ø359
    Upper Ø35Y
    Vertebral
      Left Ø35Q
      Right Ø35P
  Atrium
    Left Ø257
    Right Ø256
  Auditory Ossicle
    Left Ø95A
    Right Ø959
  Basal Ganglia ØØ58
  Bladder ØT5B
  Bladder Neck ØT5C
  Bone
    Ethmoid
      Left ØN5G
      Right ØN5F
    Frontal ØN51
    Hyoid ØN5X
    Lacrimal
      Left ØN5J

Destruction — *continued*
  Bone — *continued*
    Lacrimal — *continued*
      Right ØN5H
    Nasal ØN5B
    Occipital ØN57
    Palatine
      Left ØN5L
      Right ØN5K
    Parietal
      Left ØN54
      Right ØN53
    Pelvic
      Left ØQ53
      Right ØQ52
    Sphenoid ØN5C
    Temporal
      Left ØN56
      Right ØN55
    Zygomatic
      Left ØN5N
      Right ØN5M
  Brain ØØ5Ø
  Breast
    Bilateral ØH5V
    Left ØH5U
    Right ØH5T
  Bronchus
    Lingula ØB59
    Lower Lobe
      Left ØB5B
      Right ØB56
    Main
      Left ØB57
      Right ØB53
    Middle Lobe, Right ØB55
    Upper Lobe
      Left ØB58
      Right ØB54
  Buccal Mucosa ØC54
  Bursa and Ligament
    Abdomen
      Left ØM5J
      Right ØM5H
    Ankle
      Left ØM5R
      Right ØM5Q
    Elbow
      Left ØM54
      Right ØM53
    Foot
      Left ØM5T
      Right ØM5S
    Hand
      Left ØM58
      Right ØM57
    Head and Neck ØM5Ø
    Hip
      Left ØM5M
      Right ØM5L
    Knee
      Left ØM5P
      Right ØM5N
    Lower Extremity
      Left ØM5W
      Right ØM5V
    Perineum ØM5K
    Rib(s) ØM5G
    Shoulder
      Left ØM52
      Right ØM51
    Spine
      Lower ØM5D
      Upper ØM5C
    Sternum ØM5F
    Upper Extremity
      Left ØM5B
      Right ØM59
    Wrist
      Left ØM56
      Right ØM55
  Carina ØB52
  Carotid Bodies, Bilateral ØG58
  Carotid Body
    Left ØG56
    Right ØG57
  Carpal
    Left ØP5N
    Right ØP5M

Subterms under main terms may continue to next column or page

- **Destruction** — *continued*
  - Cecum ØD5H
  - Cerebellum ØØ5C
  - Cerebral Hemisphere ØØ57
  - Cerebral Meninges ØØ51
  - Cerebral Ventricle ØØ56
  - Cervix ØU5C
  - Chordae Tendineae Ø259
  - Choroid
    - Left Ø85B
    - Right Ø85A
  - Cisterna Chyli Ø75L
  - Clavicle
    - Left ØP5B
    - Right ØP59
  - Clitoris ØU5J
  - Coccygeal Glomus ØG5B
  - Coccyx ØQ5S
  - Colon
    - Ascending ØD5K
    - Descending ØD5M
    - Sigmoid ØD5N
    - Transverse ØD5L
  - Conduction Mechanism Ø258
  - Conjunctiva
    - Left Ø85TXZZ
    - Right Ø85SXZZ
  - Cord
    - Bilateral ØV5H
    - Left ØV5G
    - Right ØV5F
  - Cornea
    - Left Ø859XZZ
    - Right Ø858XZZ
  - Cul-de-sac ØU5F
  - Diaphragm ØB5T
  - Disc
    - Cervical Vertebral ØR53
    - Cervicothoracic Vertebral ØR55
    - Lumbar Vertebral ØS52
    - Lumbosacral ØS54
    - Thoracic Vertebral ØR59
    - Thoracolumbar Vertebral ØR5B
  - Duct
    - Common Bile ØF59
    - Cystic ØF58
    - Hepatic
      - Common ØF57
      - Left ØF56
      - Right ØF55
    - Lacrimal
      - Left Ø85Y
      - Right Ø85X
    - Pancreatic ØF5D
      - Accessory ØF5F
    - Parotid
      - Left ØC5C
      - Right ØC5B
  - Duodenum ØD59
  - Dura Mater ØØ52
  - Ear
    - External
      - Left Ø951
      - Right Ø95Ø
    - External Auditory Canal
      - Left Ø954
      - Right Ø953
    - Inner
      - Left Ø95E
      - Right Ø95D
    - Middle
      - Left Ø956
      - Right Ø955
  - Endometrium ØU5B
  - Epididymis
    - Bilateral ØV5L
    - Left ØV5K
    - Right ØV5J
  - Epiglottis ØC5R
  - Esophagogastric Junction ØD54
  - Esophagus ØD55
    - Lower ØD53
    - Middle ØD52
    - Upper ØD51
  - Eustachian Tube
    - Left Ø95G
    - Right Ø95F
  - Eye
    - Left Ø851XZZ
- **Destruction** — *continued*
  - Eye — *continued*
    - Right Ø85ØXZZ
  - Eyelid
    - Lower
      - Left Ø85R
      - Right Ø85Q
    - Upper
      - Left Ø85P
      - Right Ø85N
  - Fallopian Tube
    - Left ØU56
    - Right ØU55
  - Fallopian Tubes, Bilateral ØU57
  - Femoral Shaft
    - Left ØQ59
    - Right ØQ58
  - Femur
    - Lower
      - Left ØQ5C
      - Right ØQ5B
    - Upper
      - Left ØQ57
      - Right ØQ56
  - Fibula
    - Left ØQ5K
    - Right ØQ5J
  - Finger Nail ØH5QXZZ
  - Gallbladder ØF54
  - Gingiva
    - Lower ØC56
    - Upper ØC55
  - Gland
    - Adrenal
      - Bilateral ØG54
      - Left ØG52
      - Right ØG53
    - Lacrimal
      - Left Ø85W
      - Right Ø85V
    - Minor Salivary ØC5J
    - Parotid
      - Left ØC59
      - Right ØC58
    - Pituitary ØG5Ø
    - Sublingual
      - Left ØC5F
      - Right ØC5D
    - Submaxillary
      - Left ØC5H
      - Right ØC5G
    - Vestibular ØU5L
  - Glenoid Cavity
    - Left ØP58
    - Right ØP57
  - Glomus Jugulare ØG5C
  - Humeral Head
    - Left ØP5D
    - Right ØP5C
  - Humeral Shaft
    - Left ØP5G
    - Right ØP5F
  - Hymen ØU5K
  - Hypothalamus ØØ5A
  - Ileocecal Valve ØD5C
  - Ileum ØD5B
  - Intestine
    - Large ØD5E
      - Left ØD5G
      - Right ØD5F
    - Small ØD58
  - Iris
    - Left Ø85D3ZZ
    - Right Ø85C3ZZ
  - Jejunum ØD5A
  - Joint
    - Acromioclavicular
      - Left ØR5H
      - Right ØR5G
    - Ankle
      - Left ØS5G
      - Right ØS5F
    - Carpal
      - Left ØR5R
      - Right ØR5Q
    - Carpometacarpal
      - Left ØR5T
      - Right ØR5S
    - Cervical Vertebral ØR51
- **Destruction** — *continued*
  - Joint — *continued*
    - Cervicothoracic Vertebral ØR54
    - Coccygeal ØS56
    - Elbow
      - Left ØR5M
      - Right ØR5L
    - Finger Phalangeal
      - Left ØR5X
      - Right ØR5W
    - Hip
      - Left ØS5B
      - Right ØS59
    - Knee
      - Left ØS5D
      - Right ØS5C
    - Lumbar Vertebral ØS5Ø
    - Lumbosacral ØS53
    - Metacarpophalangeal
      - Left ØR5V
      - Right ØR5U
    - Metatarsal-Phalangeal
      - Left ØS5N
      - Right ØS5M
    - Occipital-cervical ØR5Ø
    - Sacrococcygeal ØS55
    - Sacroiliac
      - Left ØS58
      - Right ØS57
    - Shoulder
      - Left ØR5K
      - Right ØR5J
    - Sternoclavicular
      - Left ØR5F
      - Right ØR5E
    - Tarsal
      - Left ØS5J
      - Right ØS5H
    - Tarsometatarsal
      - Left ØS5L
      - Right ØS5K
    - Temporomandibular
      - Left ØR5D
      - Right ØR5C
    - Thoracic Vertebral ØR56
    - Thoracolumbar Vertebral ØR5A
    - Toe Phalangeal
      - Left ØS5Q
      - Right ØS5P
    - Wrist
      - Left ØR5P
      - Right ØR5N
  - Kidney
    - Left ØT51
    - Right ØT5Ø
  - Kidney Pelvis
    - Left ØT54
    - Right ØT53
  - Larynx ØC5S
  - Lens
    - Left Ø85K3ZZ
    - Right Ø85J3ZZ
  - Lip
    - Lower ØC51
    - Upper ØC5Ø
  - Liver ØF5Ø
    - Left Lobe ØF52
    - Right Lobe ØF51
    - Ultrasound-guided Cavitation XF5
  - Lung
    - Bilateral ØB5M
    - Left ØB5L
    - Lower Lobe
      - Left ØB5J
      - Right ØB5F
    - Middle Lobe, Right ØB5D
    - Right ØB5K
    - Upper Lobe
      - Left ØB5G
      - Right ØB5C
  - Lung Lingula ØB5H
  - Lymphatic
    - Aortic Ø75D
    - Axillary
      - Left Ø756
      - Right Ø755
    - Head Ø75Ø
    - Inguinal
      - Left Ø75J

Destruction — *continued*
Lymphatic — *continued*
Inguinal — *continued*
Right Ø75H
Internal Mammary
Left Ø759
Right Ø758
Lower Extremity
Left Ø75G
Right Ø75F
Mesenteric Ø75B
Neck
Left Ø752
Right Ø751
Pelvis Ø75C
Thoracic Duct Ø75K
Thorax Ø757
Upper Extremity
Left Ø754
Right Ø753
Mandible
Left ØN5V
Right ØN5T
Maxilla ØN5R
Medulla Oblongata ØØ5D
Mesentery ØD5V
Metacarpal
Left ØP5Q
Right ØP5P
Metatarsal
Left ØQ5P
Right ØQ5N
Muscle
Abdomen
Left ØK5L
Right ØK5K
Extraocular
Left Ø85M
Right Ø85L
Facial ØK51
Foot
Left ØK5W
Right ØK5V
Hand
Left ØK5D
Right ØK5C
Head ØK5Ø
Hip
Left ØK5P
Right ØK5N
Lower Arm and Wrist
Left ØK5B
Right ØK59
Lower Leg
Left ØK5T
Right ØK5S
Neck
Left ØK53
Right ØK52
Papillary Ø25D
Perineum ØK5M
Shoulder
Left ØK56
Right ØK55
Thorax
Left ØK5J
Right ØK5H
Tongue, Palate, Pharynx ØK54
Trunk
Left ØK5G
Right ØK5F
Upper Arm
Left ØK58
Right ØK57
Upper Leg
Left ØK5R
Right ØK5Q
Nasal Mucosa and Soft Tissue Ø95K
Nasopharynx Ø95N
Nerve
Abdominal Sympathetic Ø15M
Abducens ØØ5L
Accessory ØØ5R
Acoustic ØØ5N
Brachial Plexus Ø153
Cervical Ø151
Cervical Plexus Ø15Ø
Facial ØØ5M
Femoral Ø15D

Destruction — *continued*
Nerve — *continued*
Glossopharyngeal ØØ5P
Head and Neck Sympathetic Ø15K
Hypoglossal ØØ5S
Lumbar Ø15B
Lumbar Plexus Ø159
Lumbar Sympathetic Ø15N
Lumbosacral Plexus Ø15A
Median Ø155
Oculomotor ØØ5H
Olfactory ØØ5F
Optic ØØ5G
Peroneal Ø15H
Phrenic Ø152
Pudendal Ø15C
Radial Ø156
Sacral Ø15R
Sacral Plexus Ø15Q
Sacral Sympathetic Ø15P
Sciatic Ø15F
Thoracic Ø158
Thoracic Sympathetic Ø15L
Tibial Ø15G
Trigeminal ØØ5K
Trochlear ØØ5J
Ulnar Ø154
Vagus ØØ5Q
Nipple
Left ØH5X
Right ØH5W
Omentum ØD5U
Orbit
Left ØN5Q
Right ØN5P
Ovary
Bilateral ØU52
Left ØU51
Right ØU5Ø
Palate
Hard ØC52
Soft ØC53
Pancreas ØF5G
Para-aortic Body ØG59
Paraganglion Extremity ØG5F
Parathyroid Gland ØG5R
Inferior
Left ØG5P
Right ØG5N
Multiple ØG5Q
Superior
Left ØG5M
Right ØG5L
Patella
Left ØQ5F
Right ØQ5D
Penis ØV5S
Pericardium Ø25N
Peritoneum ØD5W
Phalanx
Finger
Left ØP5V
Right ØP5T
Thumb
Left ØP5S
Right ØP5R
Toe
Left ØQ5R
Right ØQ5Q
Pharynx ØC5M
Pineal Body ØG51
Pleura
Left ØB5P
Right ØB5N
Pons ØØ5B
Prepuce ØV5T
Prostate ØV5Ø
Radius
Left ØP5J
Right ØP5H
Rectum ØD5P
Renal Sympathetic Nerve(s), Ultrasound Ablation XØ51329
Retina
Left Ø85F3ZZ
Right Ø85E3ZZ
Retinal Vessel
Left Ø85H3ZZ
Right Ø85G3ZZ

Destruction — *continued*
Ribs
1 to 2 ØP51
3 or More ØP52
Sacrum ØQ51
Scapula
Left ØP56
Right ØP55
Sclera
Left Ø857XZZ
Right Ø856XZZ
Scrotum ØV55
Septum
Atrial Ø255
Nasal Ø95M
Ventricular Ø25M
Sinus
Accessory Ø95P
Ethmoid
Left Ø95V
Right Ø95U
Frontal
Left Ø95T
Right Ø95S
Mastoid
Left Ø95C
Right Ø95B
Maxillary
Left Ø95R
Right Ø95Q
Sphenoid
Left Ø95X
Right Ø95W
Skin
Abdomen ØH57XZ
Back ØH56XZ
Buttock ØH58XZ
Chest ØH55XZ
Ear
Left ØH53XZ
Right ØH52XZ
Face ØH51XZ
Foot
Left ØH5NXZ
Right ØH5MXZ
Hand
Left ØH5GXZ
Right ØH5FXZ
Inguinal ØH5AXZ
Lower Arm
Left ØH5EXZ
Right ØH5DXZ
Lower Leg
Left ØH5LXZ
Right ØH5KXZ
Neck ØH54XZ
Perineum ØH59XZ
Scalp ØH5ØXZ
Upper Arm
Left ØH5CXZ
Right ØH5BXZ
Upper Leg
Left ØH5JXZ
Right ØH5HXZ
Skull ØN5Ø
Spinal Cord
Cervical ØØ5W
Lumbar ØØ5Y
Thoracic ØØ5X
Spinal Meninges ØØ5T
Spleen Ø75P
Sternum ØP5Ø
Stomach ØD56
Pylorus ØD57
Subcutaneous Tissue and Fascia
Abdomen ØJ58
Back ØJ57
Buttock ØJ59
Chest ØJ56
Face ØJ51
Foot
Left ØJ5R
Right ØJ5Q
Hand
Left ØJ5K
Right ØJ5J
Lower Arm
Left ØJ5H
Right ØJ5G

Destruction — *continued*
Subcutaneous Tissue and Fascia — *continued*
Lower Leg
Left ØJ5P
Right ØJ5N
Neck
Left ØJ55
Right ØJ54
Pelvic Region ØJ5C
Perineum ØJ5B
Scalp ØJ5Ø
Upper Arm
Left ØJ5F
Right ØJ5D
Upper Leg
Left ØJ5M
Right ØJ5L
Tarsal
Left ØQ5M
Right ØQ5L
Tendon
Abdomen
Left ØL5G
Right ØL5F
Ankle
Left ØL5T
Right ØL5S
Foot
Left ØL5W
Right ØL5V
Hand
Left ØL58
Right ØL57
Head and Neck ØL5Ø
Hip
Left ØL5K
Right ØL5J
Knee
Left ØL5R
Right ØL5Q
Lower Arm and Wrist
Left ØL56
Right ØL55
Lower Leg
Left ØL5P
Right ØL5N
Perineum ØL5H
Shoulder
Left ØL52
Right ØL51
Thorax
Left ØL5D
Right ØL5C
Trunk
Left ØL5B
Right ØL59
Upper Arm
Left ØL54
Right ØL53
Upper Leg
Left ØL5M
Right ØL5L
Testis
Bilateral ØV5C
Left ØV5B
Right ØV59
Thalamus ØØ59
Thymus Ø75M
Thyroid Gland ØG5K
Left Lobe ØG5G
Right Lobe ØG5H
Tibia
Left ØQ5H
Right ØQ5G
Toe Nail ØH5RXZZ
Tongue ØC57
Tonsils ØC5P
Tooth
Lower ØC5X
Upper ØC5W
Trachea ØB51
Tunica Vaginalis
Left ØV57
Right ØV56
Turbinate, Nasal Ø95L
Tympanic Membrane
Left Ø958
Right Ø957

Destruction — *continued*
Ulna
Left ØP5L
Right ØP5K
Ureter
Left ØT57
Right ØT56
Urethra ØT5D
Uterine Supporting Structure ØU54
Uterus ØU59
Uvula ØC5N
Vagina ØU5G
Valve
Aortic Ø25F
Mitral Ø25G
Pulmonary Ø25H
Tricuspid Ø25J
Vas Deferens
Bilateral ØV5Q
Left ØV5P
Right ØV5N
Vein
Axillary
Left Ø558
Right Ø557
Azygos Ø55Ø
Basilic
Left Ø55C
Right Ø55B
Brachial
Left Ø55A
Right Ø559
Cephalic
Left Ø55F
Right Ø55D
Colic Ø657
Common Iliac
Left Ø65D
Right Ø65C
Coronary Ø254
Esophageal Ø653
External Iliac
Left Ø65G
Right Ø65F
External Jugular
Left Ø55Q
Right Ø55P
Face
Left Ø55V
Right Ø55T
Femoral
Left Ø65N
Right Ø65M
Foot
Left Ø65V
Right Ø65T
Gastric Ø652
Hand
Left Ø55H
Right Ø55G
Hemiazygos Ø551
Hepatic Ø654
Hypogastric
Left Ø65J
Right Ø65H
Inferior Mesenteric Ø656
Innominate
Left Ø554
Right Ø553
Internal Jugular
Left Ø55N
Right Ø55M
Intracranial Ø55L
Lower Ø65Y
Portal Ø658
Pulmonary
Left Ø25T
Right Ø25S
Renal
Left Ø65B
Right Ø659
Saphenous
Left Ø65Q
Right Ø65P
Splenic Ø651
Subclavian
Left Ø556
Right Ø555
Superior Mesenteric Ø655

Destruction — *continued*
Vein — *continued*
Upper Ø55Y
Vertebral
Left Ø55S
Right Ø55R
Vena Cava
Inferior Ø65Ø
Superior Ø25V
Ventricle
Left Ø25L
Right Ø25K
Vertebra
Cervical ØP53
Lumbar ØQ5Ø
Thoracic ØP54
Vesicle
Bilateral ØV53
Left ØV52
Right ØV51
Vitreous
Left Ø8553ZZ
Right Ø8543ZZ
Vocal Cord
Left ØC5V
Right ØC5T
Vulva ØU5M
Detachment
Arm
Lower
Left ØX6FØZ
Right ØX6DØZ
Upper
Left ØX69ØZ
Right ØX68ØZ
Elbow Region
Left ØX6CØZZ
Right ØX6BØZZ
Femoral Region
Left ØY68ØZZ
Right ØY67ØZZ
Finger
Index
Left ØX6PØZ
Right ØX6NØZ
Little
Left ØX6WØZ
Right ØX6VØZ
Middle
Left ØX6RØZ
Right ØX6QØZ
Ring
Left ØX6TØZ
Right ØX6SØZ
Foot
Left ØY6NØZ
Right ØY6MØZ
Forequarter
Left ØX61ØZZ
Right ØX6ØØZZ
Hand
Left ØX6KØZ
Right ØX6JØZ
Hindquarter
Bilateral ØY64ØZZ
Left ØY63ØZZ
Right ØY62ØZZ
Knee Region
Left ØY6GØZZ
Right ØY6FØZZ
Leg
Lower
Left ØY6JØZ
Right ØY6HØZ
Upper
Left ØY6DØZ
Right ØY6CØZ
Shoulder Region
Left ØX63ØZZ
Right ØX62ØZZ
Thumb
Left ØX6MØZ
Right ØX6LØZ
Toe
1st
Left ØY6QØZ
Right ØY6PØZ
2nd
Left ØY6SØZ

Detachment — *continued*
- Toe — *continued*
  - 2nd — *continued*
    - Right ØY6RØZ
  - 3rd
    - Left ØY6UØZ
    - Right ØY6TØZ
  - 4th
    - Left ØY6WØZ
    - Right ØY6VØZ
  - 5th
    - Left ØY6YØZ
    - Right ØY6XØZ

Determination, Mental status GZ14ZZZ

Detorsion
- *see* Release
- *see* Reposition

DETOUR® System
- *use* Conduit through Femoral Vein to Popliteal Artery in New Technology
- *use* Conduit through Femoral Vein to Superficial Femoral Artery in New Technology

Detoxification Services, for substance abuse HZ2ZZZZ

Device Fitting FØDZ

Diagnostic Audiology *see* Audiology, Diagnostic

Diagnostic imaging *see* Imaging, Diagnostic

Diagnostic radiology *see* Imaging, Diagnostic

Dialysis
- Hemodialysis *see* Performance, Urinary 5A1D
- Peritoneal 3E1M39Z

Diaphragma sellae *use* Dura Mater

Diaphragmatic pacemaker generator *use* Stimulator Generator in Subcutaneous Tissue and Fascia

Diaphragmatic Pacemaker Lead
- Insertion of device in, Diaphragm ØBHT
- Removal of device from, Diaphragm ØBPT
- Revision of device in, Diaphragm ØBWT

Digital radiography, plain *see* Plain Radiography

Dilation
- Ampulla of Vater ØF7C
- Anus ØD7Q
- Aorta
  - Abdominal
  - Thoracic
    - Ascending/Arch Ø27X
    - Descending Ø27W
- Artery
  - Anterior Tibial
    - Left Ø47Q
      - Sustained Release Drug-eluting Intraluminal Device X27Q385
        - Four or More X27Q3C5
        - Three X27Q3B5
        - Two X27Q395
    - Right Ø47P
      - Sustained Release Drug-eluting Intraluminal Device X27P385
        - Four or More X27P3C5
        - Three X27P3B5
        - Two X27P395
  - Axillary
    - Left Ø376
    - Right Ø375
  - Brachial
    - Left Ø378
    - Right Ø377
  - Celiac Ø471
  - Colic
    - Left Ø477
    - Middle Ø478
    - Right Ø476
  - Common Carotid
    - Left Ø37J
    - Right Ø37H
  - Common Iliac
    - Left Ø47D
    - Right Ø47C
  - Coronary
    - Four or More Arteries Ø273
    - One Artery Ø27Ø
    - Three Arteries Ø272
    - Two Arteries Ø271
  - External Carotid
    - Left Ø37N
    - Right Ø37M

Dilation — *continued*
- Artery — *continued*
  - External Iliac
    - Left Ø47J
    - Right Ø47H
  - Face Ø37R
  - Femoral
    - Left Ø47L
      - Sustained Release Drug-eluting Intraluminal Device X27J385
        - Four or More X27J3C5
        - Three X27J3B5
        - Two X27J395
    - Right Ø47K
      - Sustained Release Drug-eluting Intraluminal Device X27H385
        - Four or More X27H3C5
        - Three X27H3B5
        - Two X27H395
  - Foot
    - Left Ø47W
    - Right Ø47V
  - Gastric Ø472
  - Hand
    - Left Ø37F
    - Right Ø37D
  - Hepatic Ø473
  - Inferior Mesenteric Ø47B
  - Innominate Ø372
  - Internal Carotid
    - Left Ø37L
    - Right Ø37K
  - Internal Iliac
    - Left Ø47F
    - Right Ø47E
  - Internal Mammary
    - Left Ø371
    - Right Ø37Ø
  - Intracranial Ø37G
  - Lower Ø47Y
  - Peroneal
    - Left Ø47U
      - Sustained Release Drug-eluting Intraluminal Device X27U385
        - Four or More X27U3C5
        - Three X27U3B5
        - Two X27U395
    - Right Ø47T
      - Sustained Release Drug-eluting Intraluminal Device X27T385
        - Four or More X27T3C5
        - Three X27T3B5
        - Two X27T395
  - Popliteal
    - Left Ø47N
    - Left Distal
      - Sustained Release Drug-eluting Intraluminal Device X27N385
        - Four or More X27N3C5
        - Three X27N3B5
        - Two X27N395
    - Left Proximal
      - Sustained Release Drug-eluting Intraluminal Device X27L385
        - Four or More X27L3C5
        - Three X27L3B5
        - Two X27L395
    - Right Ø47M
    - Right Distal
      - Sustained Release Drug-eluting Intraluminal Device X27M385
        - Four or More X27M3C5
        - Three X27M3B5
        - Two X27M395
    - Right Proximal
      - Sustained Release Drug-eluting Intraluminal Device X27K385
        - Four or More X27K3C5
        - Three X27K3B5
        - Two X27K395

Dilation — *continued*
- Artery — *continued*
  - Posterior Tibial
    - Left Ø47S
      - Sustained Release Drug-eluting Intraluminal Device X27S385
        - Four or More X27S3C5
        - Three X27S3B5
        - Two X27S395
    - Right Ø47R
      - Sustained Release Drug-eluting Intraluminal Device X27R385
        - Four or More X27R3C5
        - Three X27R3B5
        - Two X27R395
  - Pulmonary
    - Left Ø27R
    - Right Ø27Q
  - Pulmonary Trunk Ø27P
  - Radial
    - Left Ø37C
    - Right Ø37B
  - Renal
    - Left Ø47A
    - Right Ø479
  - Splenic Ø474
  - Subclavian
    - Left Ø374
    - Right Ø373
  - Superior Mesenteric Ø475
  - Temporal
    - Left Ø37T
    - Right Ø37S
  - Thyroid
    - Left Ø37V
    - Right Ø37U
  - Ulnar
    - Left Ø37A
    - Right Ø379
  - Upper Ø37Y
  - Vertebral
    - Left Ø37Q
    - Right Ø37P
- Bladder ØT7B
- Bladder Neck ØT7C
- Bronchus
  - Lingula ØB79
  - Lower Lobe
    - Left ØB7B
    - Right ØB76
  - Main
    - Left ØB77
    - Right ØB73
  - Middle Lobe, Right ØB75
  - Upper Lobe
    - Left ØB78
    - Right ØB74
- Carina ØB72
- Cecum ØD7H
- Cerebral Ventricle ØØ76
- Cervix ØU7C
- Colon
  - Ascending ØD7K
  - Descending ØD7M
  - Sigmoid ØD7N
  - Transverse ØD7L
- Duct
  - Common Bile ØF79
  - Cystic ØF78
  - Hepatic
    - Common ØF77
    - Left ØF76
    - Right ØF75
  - Lacrimal
    - Left Ø87Y
    - Right Ø87X
  - Pancreatic ØF7D
    - Accessory ØF7F
  - Parotid
    - Left ØC7C
    - Right ØC7B
- Duodenum ØD79
- Esophagogastric Junction ØD74
- Esophagus ØD75
  - Lower ØD73
  - Middle ØD72
  - Upper ØD71

Dilation — *continued*
Eustachian Tube
Left Ø97G
Right Ø97F
Fallopian Tube
Left ØU76
Right ØU75
Fallopian Tubes, Bilateral ØU77
Hymen ØU7K
Ileocecal Valve ØD7C
Ileum ØD7B
Intestine
Large ØD7E
Left ØD7G
Right ØD7F
Small ØD78
Jejunum ØD7A
Kidney Pelvis
Left ØT74
Right ØT73
Larynx ØC7S
Pharynx ØC7M
Rectum ØD7P
Stomach ØD76
Pylorus ØD77
Trachea ØB71
Ureter
Left ØT77
Right ØT76
Ureters, Bilateral ØT78
Urethra ØT7D
Uterus ØU79
Vagina ØU7G
Valve
Aortic Ø27F
Mitral Ø27G
Pulmonary Ø27H
Tricuspid Ø27J
Vas Deferens
Bilateral ØV7Q
Left ØV7P
Right ØV7N
Vein
Axillary
Left Ø578
Right Ø577
Azygos Ø57Ø
Basilic
Left Ø57C
Right Ø57B
Brachial
Left Ø57A
Right Ø579
Cephalic
Left Ø57F
Right Ø57D
Colic Ø677
Common Iliac
Left Ø67D
Right Ø67C
Esophageal Ø673
External Iliac
Left Ø67G
Right Ø67F
External Jugular
Left Ø57Q
Right Ø57P
Face
Left Ø57V
Right Ø57T
Femoral
Left Ø67N
Right Ø67M
Foot
Left Ø67V
Right Ø67T
Gastric Ø672
Hand
Left Ø57H
Right Ø57G
Hemiazygos Ø571
Hepatic Ø674
Hypogastric
Left Ø67J
Right Ø67H
Inferior Mesenteric Ø676
Innominate
Left Ø574
Right Ø573

Dilation — *continued*
Vein — *continued*
Internal Jugular
Left Ø57N
Right Ø57M
Intracranial Ø57L
Lower Ø67Y
Portal Ø678
Pulmonary
Left Ø27T
Right Ø27S
Renal
Left Ø67B
Right Ø679
Saphenous
Left Ø67Q
Right Ø67P
Splenic Ø671
Subclavian
Left Ø576
Right Ø575
Superior Mesenteric Ø675
Upper Ø57Y
Vertebral
Left Ø57S
Right Ø57R
Vena Cava
Inferior Ø67Ø
Superior Ø27V
Ventricle
Left Ø27L
Right Ø27K
Direct Lateral Interbody Fusion (DLIF) device *use* Interbody Fusion Device in Lower Joints
Disarticulation *see* Detachment
Discectomy, diskectomy
see Excision, Lower Joints ØSB
see Excision, Upper Joints ØRB
see Resection, Lower Joints ØST
see Resection, Upper Joints ØRT
Discography
see Fluoroscopy, Axial Skeleton, Except Skull and Facial Bones BR1
see Plain Radiography, Axial Skeleton, Except Skull and Facial Bones BRØ
Dismembered pyeloplasty *see* Repair, Kidney Pelvis
Distal humerus
use Humeral Shaft, Left
use Humeral Shaft, Right
Distal humerus, involving joint
use Elbow Joint, Left
use Elbow Joint, Right
Distal radioulnar joint
use Wrist Joint, Left
use Wrist Joint, Right
Diversion *see* Bypass
Diverticulectomy *see* Excision, Gastrointestinal System ØDB
Division
Acetabulum
Left ØQ85
Right ØQ84
Anal Sphincter ØD8R
Basal Ganglia ØØ88
Bladder Neck ØT8C
Bone
Ethmoid
Left ØN8G
Right ØN8F
Frontal ØN81
Hyoid ØN8X
Lacrimal
Left ØN8J
Right ØN8H
Nasal ØN8B
Occipital ØN87
Palatine
Left ØN8L
Right ØN8K
Parietal
Left ØN84
Right ØN83
Pelvic
Left ØQ83
Right ØQ82
Sphenoid ØN8C
Temporal
Left ØN86

Division — *continued*
Bone — *continued*
Temporal — *continued*
Right ØN85
Zygomatic
Left ØN8N
Right ØN8M
Brain ØØ8Ø
Bursa and Ligament
Abdomen
Left ØM8J
Right ØM8H
Ankle
Left ØM8R
Right ØM8Q
Elbow
Left ØM84
Right ØM83
Foot
Left ØM8T
Right ØM8S
Hand
Left ØM88
Right ØM87
Head and Neck ØM8Ø
Hip
Left ØM8M
Right ØM8L
Knee
Left ØM8P
Right ØM8N
Lower Extremity
Left ØM8W
Right ØM8V
Perineum ØM8K
Rib(s) ØM8G
Shoulder
Left ØM82
Right ØM81
Spine
Lower ØM8D
Upper ØM8C
Sternum ØM8F
Upper Extremity
Left ØM8B
Right ØM89
Wrist
Left ØM86
Right ØM85
Carpal
Left ØP8N
Right ØP8M
Cerebral Hemisphere ØØ87
Chordae Tendineae Ø289
Clavicle
Left ØP8B
Right ØP89
Coccyx ØQ8S
Conduction Mechanism Ø288
Esophagogastric Junction ØD84
Femoral Shaft
Left ØQ89
Right ØQ88
Femur
Lower
Left ØQ8C
Right ØQ8B
Upper
Left ØQ87
Right ØQ86
Fibula
Left ØQ8K
Right ØQ8J
Gland, Pituitary ØG8Ø
Glenoid Cavity
Left ØP88
Right ØP87
Humeral Head
Left ØP8D
Right ØP8C
Humeral Shaft
Left ØP8G
Right ØP8F
Hymen ØU8K
Kidneys, Bilateral ØT82
Liver ØF8Ø
Left Lobe ØF82
Right Lobe ØF81

Division — *continued*
Mandible
Left ØN8V
Right ØN8T
Maxilla ØN8R
Metacarpal
Left ØP8Q
Right ØP8P
Metatarsal
Left ØQ8P
Right ØQ8N
Muscle
Abdomen
Left ØK8L
Right ØK8K
Facial ØK81
Foot
Left ØK8W
Right ØK8V
Hand
Left ØK8D
Right ØK8C
Head ØK8Ø
Hip
Left ØK8P
Right ØK8N
Lower Arm and Wrist
Left ØK8B
Right ØK89
Lower Leg
Left ØK8T
Right ØK8S
Neck
Left ØK83
Right ØK82
Papillary Ø28D
Perineum ØK8M
Shoulder
Left ØK86
Right ØK85
Thorax
Left ØK8J
Right ØK8H
Tongue, Palate, Pharynx ØK84
Trunk
Left ØK8G
Right ØK8F
Upper Arm
Left ØK88
Right ØK87
Upper Leg
Left ØK8R
Right ØK8Q
Nerve
Abdominal Sympathetic Ø18M
Abducens ØØ8L
Accessory ØØ8R
Acoustic ØØ8N
Brachial Plexus Ø183
Cervical Ø181
Cervical Plexus Ø18Ø
Facial ØØ8M
Femoral Ø18D
Glossopharyngeal ØØ8P
Head and Neck Sympathetic Ø18K
Hypoglossal ØØ8S
Lumbar Ø18B
Lumbar Plexus Ø189
Lumbar Sympathetic Ø18N
Lumbosacral Plexus Ø18A
Median Ø185
Oculomotor ØØ8H
Olfactory ØØ8F
Optic ØØ8G
Peroneal Ø18H
Phrenic Ø182
Pudendal Ø18C
Radial Ø186
Sacral Ø18R
Sacral Plexus Ø18Q
Sacral Sympathetic Ø18P
Sciatic Ø18F
Thoracic Ø188
Thoracic Sympathetic Ø18L
Tibial Ø18G
Trigeminal ØØ8K
Trochlear ØØ8J
Ulnar Ø184
Vagus ØØ8Q

Division — *continued*
Orbit
Left ØN8Q
Right ØN8P
Ovary
Bilateral ØU82
Left ØU81
Right ØU8Ø
Pancreas ØF8G
Patella
Left ØQ8F
Right ØQ8D
Perineum, Female ØW8NXZZ
Phalanx
Finger
Left ØP8V
Right ØP8T
Thumb
Left ØP8S
Right ØP8R
Toe
Left ØQ8R
Right ØQ8Q
Radius
Left ØP8J
Right ØP8H
Ribs
1 to 2 ØP81
3 or More ØP82
Sacrum ØQ81
Scapula
Left ØP86
Right ØP85
Skin
Abdomen ØH87XZZ
Back ØH86XZZ
Buttock ØH88XZZ
Chest ØH85XZZ
Ear
Left ØH83XZZ
Right ØH82XZZ
Face ØH81XZZ
Foot
Left ØH8NXZZ
Right ØH8MXZZ
Hand
Left ØH8GXZZ
Right ØH8FXZZ
Inguinal ØH8AXZZ
Lower Arm
Left ØH8EXZZ
Right ØH8DXZZ
Lower Leg
Left ØH8LXZZ
Right ØH8KXZZ
Neck ØH84XZZ
Perineum ØH89XZZ
Scalp ØH8ØXZZ
Upper Arm
Left ØH8CXZZ
Right ØH8BXZZ
Upper Leg
Left ØH8JXZZ
Right ØH8HXZZ
Skull ØN8Ø
Spinal Cord
Cervical ØØ8W
Lumbar ØØ8Y
Thoracic ØØ8X
Sternum ØP8Ø
Stomach, Pylorus ØD87
Subcutaneous Tissue and Fascia
Abdomen ØJ88
Back ØJ87
Buttock ØJ89
Chest ØJ86
Face ØJ81
Foot
Left ØJ8R
Right ØJ8Q
Hand
Left ØJ8K
Right ØJ8J
Head and Neck ØJ8S
Lower Arm
Left ØJ8H
Right ØJ8G
Lower Extremity ØJ8W

Division — *continued*
Subcutaneous Tissue and Fascia — *continued*
Lower Leg
Left ØJ8P
Right ØJ8N
Neck
Left ØJ85
Right ØJ84
Pelvic Region ØJ8C
Perineum ØJ8B
Scalp ØJ8Ø
Trunk ØJ8T
Upper Arm
Left ØJ8F
Right ØJ8D
Upper Extremity ØJ8V
Upper Leg
Left ØJ8M
Right ØJ8L
Tarsal
Left ØQ8M
Right ØQ8L
Tendon
Abdomen
Left ØL8G
Right ØL8F
Ankle
Left ØL8T
Right ØL8S
Foot
Left ØL8W
Right ØL8V
Hand
Left ØL88
Right ØL87
Head and Neck ØL8Ø
Hip
Left ØL8K
Right ØL8J
Knee
Left ØL8R
Right ØL8Q
Lower Arm and Wrist
Left ØL86
Right ØL85
Lower Leg
Left ØL8P
Right ØL8N
Perineum ØL8H
Shoulder
Left ØL82
Right ØL81
Thorax
Left ØL8D
Right ØL8C
Trunk
Left ØL8B
Right ØL89
Upper Arm
Left ØL84
Right ØL83
Upper Leg
Left ØL8M
Right ØL8L
Thyroid Gland Isthmus ØG8J
Tibia
Left ØQ8H
Right ØQ8G
Turbinate, Nasal Ø98L
Ulna
Left ØP8L
Right ØP8K
Uterine Supporting Structure ØU84
Vertebra
Cervical ØP83
Lumbar ØQ8Ø
Thoracic ØP84
Doppler study *see* Ultrasonography
Dorsal digital nerve *use* Radial Nerve
Dorsal metacarpal vein
use Hand Vein, Left
use Hand Vein, Right
Dorsal metatarsal artery
use Foot Artery, Left
use Foot Artery, Right
Dorsal metatarsal vein
use Foot Vein, Left
use Foot Vein, Right

- **Dorsal root ganglion**
  - *use* Cervical Spinal Cord
  - *use* Lumbar Spinal Cord
  - *use* Spinal Cord
  - *use* Thoracic Spinal Cord
- **Dorsal scapular artery**
  - *use* Subclavian Artery, Left
  - *use* Subclavian Artery, Right
- **Dorsal scapular nerve** *use* Brachial Plexus
- **Dorsal venous arch**
  - *use* Foot Vein, Left
  - *use* Foot Vein, Right
- **Dorsalis pedis artery**
  - *use* Anterior Tibial Artery, Left
  - *use* Anterior Tibial Artery, Right
- **DownStream® System** 5AØ512C, 5AØ522C
- **Drainage**
  - Abdominal Wall ØW9F
  - Acetabulum
    - Left ØQ95
    - Right ØQ94
  - Adenoids ØC9Q
  - Ampulla of Vater ØF9C
  - Anal Sphincter ØD9R
  - Ankle Region
    - Left ØY9L
    - Right ØY9K
  - Anterior Chamber
    - Left Ø893
    - Right Ø892
  - Anus ØD9Q
  - Aorta, Abdominal Ø49Ø
  - Aortic Body ØG9D
  - Appendix ØD9J
  - Arm
    - Lower
      - Left ØX9F
      - Right ØX9D
    - Upper
      - Left ØX99
      - Right ØX98
  - Artery
    - Anterior Tibial
      - Left Ø49Q
      - Right Ø49P
    - Axillary
      - Left Ø396
      - Right Ø395
    - Brachial
      - Left Ø398
      - Right Ø397
    - Celiac Ø491
    - Colic
      - Left Ø497
      - Middle Ø498
      - Right Ø496
    - Common Carotid
      - Left Ø39J
      - Right Ø39H
    - Common Iliac
      - Left Ø49D
      - Right Ø49C
    - External Carotid
      - Left Ø39N
      - Right Ø39M
    - External Iliac
      - Left Ø49J
      - Right Ø49H
    - Face Ø39R
    - Femoral
      - Left Ø49L
      - Right Ø49K
    - Foot
      - Left Ø49W
      - Right Ø49V
    - Gastric Ø492
    - Hand
      - Left Ø39F
      - Right Ø39D
    - Hepatic Ø493
    - Inferior Mesenteric Ø49B
    - Innominate Ø392
    - Internal Carotid
      - Left Ø39L
      - Right Ø39K
    - Internal Iliac
      - Left Ø49F
      - Right Ø49E

Drainage — *continued*

- Artery — *continued*
  - Internal Mammary
    - Left Ø391
    - Right Ø39Ø
  - Intracranial Ø39G
  - Lower Ø49Y
  - Peroneal
    - Left Ø49U
    - Right Ø49T
  - Popliteal
    - Left Ø49N
    - Right Ø49M
  - Posterior Tibial
    - Left Ø49S
    - Right Ø49R
  - Radial
    - Left Ø39C
    - Right Ø39B
  - Renal
    - Left Ø49A
    - Right Ø499
  - Splenic Ø494
  - Subclavian
    - Left Ø394
    - Right Ø393
  - Superior Mesenteric Ø495
  - Temporal
    - Left Ø39T
    - Right Ø39S
  - Thyroid
    - Left Ø39V
    - Right Ø39U
  - Ulnar
    - Left Ø39A
    - Right Ø399
  - Upper Ø39Y
  - Vertebral
    - Left Ø39Q
    - Right Ø39P
- Auditory Ossicle
  - Left Ø99A
  - Right Ø999
- Axilla
  - Left ØX95
  - Right ØX94
- Back
  - Lower ØW9L
  - Upper ØW9K
- Basal Ganglia ØØ98
- Bladder ØT9B
- Bladder Neck ØT9C
- Bone
  - Ethmoid
    - Left ØN9G
    - Right ØN9F
  - Frontal ØN91
  - Hyoid ØN9X
  - Lacrimal
    - Left ØN9J
    - Right ØN9H
  - Nasal ØN9B
  - Occipital ØN97
  - Palatine
    - Left ØN9L
    - Right ØN9K
  - Parietal
    - Left ØN94
    - Right ØN93
  - Pelvic
    - Left ØQ93
    - Right ØQ92
  - Sphenoid ØN9C
  - Temporal
    - Left ØN96
    - Right ØN95
  - Zygomatic
    - Left ØN9N
    - Right ØN9M
- Bone Marrow Ø79T
- Brain ØØ9Ø
- Breast
  - Bilateral ØH9V
  - Left ØH9U
  - Right ØH9T
- Bronchus
  - Lingula ØB99
  - Lower Lobe
    - Left ØB9B

Drainage — *continued*

- Bronchus — *continued*
  - Lower Lobe — *continued*
    - Right ØB96
  - Main
    - Left ØB97
    - Right ØB93
  - Middle Lobe, Right ØB95
  - Upper Lobe
    - Left ØB98
    - Right ØB94
- Buccal Mucosa ØC94
- Bursa and Ligament
  - Abdomen
    - Left ØM9J
    - Right ØM9H
  - Ankle
    - Left ØM9R
    - Right ØM9Q
  - Elbow
    - Left ØM94
    - Right ØM93
  - Foot
    - Left ØM9T
    - Right ØM9S
  - Hand
    - Left ØM98
    - Right ØM97
  - Head and Neck ØM9Ø
  - Hip
    - Left ØM9M
    - Right ØM9L
  - Knee
    - Left ØM9P
    - Right ØM9N
  - Lower Extremity
    - Left ØM9W
    - Right ØM9V
  - Perineum ØM9K
  - Rib(s) ØM9G
  - Shoulder
    - Left ØM92
    - Right ØM91
  - Spine
    - Lower ØM9D
    - Upper ØM9C
  - Sternum ØM9F
  - Upper Extremity
    - Left ØM9B
    - Right ØM99
  - Wrist
    - Left ØM96
    - Right ØM95
- Buttock
  - Left ØY91
  - Right ØY9Ø
- Carina ØB92
- Carotid Bodies, Bilateral ØG98
- Carotid Body
  - Left ØG96
  - Right ØG97
- Carpal
  - Left ØP9N
  - Right ØP9M
- Cavity, Cranial ØW91
- Cecum ØD9H
- Cerebellum ØØ9C
- Cerebral Hemisphere ØØ97
- Cerebral Meninges ØØ91
- Cerebral Ventricle ØØ96
- Cervix ØU9C
- Chest Wall ØW98
- Choroid
  - Left Ø89B
  - Right Ø89A
- Cisterna Chyli Ø79L
- Clavicle
  - Left ØP9B
  - Right ØP99
- Clitoris ØU9J
- Coccygeal Glomus ØG9B
- Coccyx ØQ9S
- Colon
  - Ascending ØD9K
  - Descending ØD9M
  - Sigmoid ØD9N
  - Transverse ØD9L
- Conjunctiva
  - Left Ø89T

Drainage — *continued*
Conjunctiva — *continued*
Right Ø89S
Cord
Bilateral ØV9H
Left ØV9G
Right ØV9F
Cornea
Left Ø899
Right Ø898
Cul-de-sac ØU9F
Diaphragm ØB9T
Disc
Cervical Vertebral ØR93
Cervicothoracic Vertebral ØR95
Lumbar Vertebral ØS92
Lumbosacral ØS94
Thoracic Vertebral ØR99
Thoracolumbar Vertebral ØR9B
Duct
Common Bile ØF99
Cystic ØF98
Hepatic
Common ØF97
Left ØF96
Right ØF95
Lacrimal
Left Ø89Y
Right Ø89X
Pancreatic ØF9D
Accessory ØF9F
Parotid
Left ØC9C
Right ØC9B
Duodenum ØD99
Dura Mater ØØ92
Ear
External
Left Ø991
Right Ø99Ø
External Auditory Canal
Left Ø994
Right Ø993
Inner
Left Ø99E
Right Ø99D
Middle
Left Ø996
Right Ø995
Elbow Region
Left ØX9C
Right ØX9B
Epididymis
Bilateral ØV9L
Left ØV9K
Right ØV9J
Epidural Space, Intracranial ØØ93
Epiglottis ØC9R
Esophagogastric Junction ØD94
Esophagus ØD95
Lower ØD93
Middle ØD92
Upper ØD91
Eustachian Tube
Left Ø99G
Right Ø99F
Extremity
Lower
Left ØY9B
Right ØY99
Upper
Left ØX97
Right ØX96
Eye
Left Ø891
Right Ø89Ø
Eyelid
Lower
Left Ø89R
Right Ø89Q
Upper
Left Ø89P
Right Ø89N
Face ØW92
Fallopian Tube
Left ØU96
Right ØU95
Fallopian Tubes, Bilateral ØU97

Drainage — *continued*
Femoral Region
Left ØY98
Right ØY97
Femoral Shaft
Left ØQ99
Right ØQ98
Femur
Lower
Left ØQ9C
Right ØQ9B
Upper
Left ØQ97
Right ØQ96
Fibula
Left ØQ9K
Right ØQ9J
Finger Nail ØH9Q
Foot
Left ØY9N
Right ØY9M
Gallbladder ØF94
Gingiva
Lower ØC96
Upper ØC95
Gland
Adrenal
Bilateral ØG94
Left ØG92
Right ØG93
Lacrimal
Left Ø89W
Right Ø89V
Minor Salivary ØC9J
Parotid
Left ØC99
Right ØC98
Pituitary ØG9Ø
Sublingual
Left ØC9F
Right ØC9D
Submaxillary
Left ØC9H
Right ØC9G
Vestibular ØU9L
Glenoid Cavity
Left ØP98
Right ØP97
Glomus Jugulare ØG9C
Hand
Left ØX9K
Right ØX9J
Head ØW9Ø
Humeral Head
Left ØP9D
Right ØP9C
Humeral Shaft
Left ØP9G
Right ØP9F
Hymen ØU9K
Hypothalamus ØØ9A
Ileocecal Valve ØD9C
Ileum ØD9B
Inguinal Region
Left ØY96
Right ØY95
Intestine
Large ØD9E
Left ØD9G
Right ØD9F
Small ØD98
Iris
Left Ø89D
Right Ø89C
Jaw
Lower ØW95
Upper ØW94
Jejunum ØD9A
Joint
Acromioclavicular
Left ØR9H
Right ØR9G
Ankle
Left ØS9G
Right ØS9F
Carpal
Left ØR9R
Right ØR9Q

Drainage — *continued*
Joint — *continued*
Carpometacarpal
Left ØR9T
Right ØR9S
Cervical Vertebral ØR91
Cervicothoracic Vertebral ØR94
Coccygeal ØS96
Elbow
Left ØR9M
Right ØR9L
Finger Phalangeal
Left ØR9X
Right ØR9W
Hip
Left ØS9B
Right ØS99
Knee
Left ØS9D
Right ØS9C
Lumbar Vertebral ØS9Ø
Lumbosacral ØS93
Metacarpophalangeal
Left ØR9V
Right ØR9U
Metatarsal-Phalangeal
Left ØS9N
Right ØS9M
Occipital-cervical ØR9Ø
Sacrococcygeal ØS95
Sacroiliac
Left ØS98
Right ØS97
Shoulder
Left ØR9K
Right ØR9J
Sternoclavicular
Left ØR9F
Right ØR9E
Tarsal
Left ØS9J
Right ØS9H
Tarsometatarsal
Left ØS9L
Right ØS9K
Temporomandibular
Left ØR9D
Right ØR9C
Thoracic Vertebral ØR96
Thoracolumbar Vertebral ØR9A
Toe Phalangeal
Left ØS9Q
Right ØS9P
Wrist
Left ØR9P
Right ØR9N
Kidney
Left ØT91
Right ØT9Ø
Kidney Pelvis
Left ØT94
Right ØT93
Knee Region
Left ØY9G
Right ØY9F
Larynx ØC9S
Leg
Lower
Left ØY9J
Right ØY9H
Upper
Left ØY9D
Right ØY9C
Lens
Left Ø89K
Right Ø89J
Lip
Lower ØC91
Upper ØC9Ø
Liver ØF9Ø
Left Lobe ØF92
Right Lobe ØF91
Lung
Bilateral ØB9M
Left ØB9L
Lower Lobe
Left ØB9J
Right ØB9F
Middle Lobe, Right ØB9D

- **Drainage** — *continued*
  - Lung — *continued*
    - Right ØB9K
    - Upper Lobe
      - Left ØB9G
      - Right ØB9C
  - Lung Lingula ØB9H
  - Lymphatic
    - Aortic Ø79D
    - Axillary
      - Left Ø796
      - Right Ø795
    - Head Ø79Ø
    - Inguinal
      - Left Ø79J
      - Right Ø79H
    - Internal Mammary
      - Left Ø799
      - Right Ø798
    - Lower Extremity
      - Left Ø79G
      - Right Ø79F
    - Mesenteric Ø79B
    - Neck
      - Left Ø792
      - Right Ø791
    - Pelvis Ø79C
    - Thoracic Duct Ø79K
    - Thorax Ø797
    - Upper Extremity
      - Left Ø794
      - Right Ø793
  - Mandible
    - Left ØN9V
    - Right ØN9T
  - Maxilla ØN9R
  - Mediastinum ØW9C
  - Medulla Oblongata ØØ9D
  - Mesentery ØD9V
  - Metacarpal
    - Left ØP9Q
    - Right ØP9P
  - Metatarsal
    - Left ØQ9P
    - Right ØQ9N
  - Muscle
    - Abdomen
      - Left ØK9L
      - Right ØK9K
    - Extraocular
      - Left Ø89M
      - Right Ø89L
    - Facial ØK91
    - Foot
      - Left ØK9W
      - Right ØK9V
    - Hand
      - Left ØK9D
      - Right ØK9C
    - Head ØK9Ø
    - Hip
      - Left ØK9P
      - Right ØK9N
    - Lower Arm and Wrist
      - Left ØK9B
      - Right ØK99
    - Lower Leg
      - Left ØK9T
      - Right ØK9S
    - Neck
      - Left ØK93
      - Right ØK92
    - Perineum ØK9M
    - Shoulder
      - Left ØK96
      - Right ØK95
    - Thorax
      - Left ØK9J
      - Right ØK9H
    - Tongue, Palate, Pharynx ØK94
    - Trunk
      - Left ØK9G
      - Right ØK9F
    - Upper Arm
      - Left ØK98
      - Right ØK97
    - Upper Leg
      - Left ØK9R
      - Right ØK9Q
- **Drainage** — *continued*
  - Nasal Mucosa and Soft Tissue Ø99K
  - Nasopharynx Ø99N
  - Neck ØW96
  - Nerve
    - Abdominal Sympathetic Ø19M
    - Abducens ØØ9L
    - Accessory ØØ9R
    - Acoustic ØØ9N
    - Brachial Plexus Ø193
    - Cervical Ø191
    - Cervical Plexus Ø19Ø
    - Facial ØØ9M
    - Femoral Ø19D
    - Glossopharyngeal ØØ9P
    - Head and Neck Sympathetic Ø19K
    - Hypoglossal ØØ9S
    - Lumbar Ø19B
    - Lumbar Plexus Ø199
    - Lumbar Sympathetic Ø19N
    - Lumbosacral Plexus Ø19A
    - Median Ø195
    - Oculomotor ØØ9H
    - Olfactory ØØ9F
    - Optic ØØ9G
    - Peroneal Ø19H
    - Phrenic Ø192
    - Pudendal Ø19C
    - Radial Ø196
    - Sacral Ø19R
    - Sacral Plexus Ø19Q
    - Sacral Sympathetic Ø19P
    - Sciatic Ø19F
    - Thoracic Ø198
    - Thoracic Sympathetic Ø19L
    - Tibial Ø19G
    - Trigeminal ØØ9K
    - Trochlear ØØ9J
    - Ulnar Ø194
    - Vagus ØØ9Q
  - Nipple
    - Left ØH9X
    - Right ØH9W
  - Omentum ØD9U
  - Oral Cavity and Throat ØW93
  - Orbit
    - Left ØN9Q
    - Right ØN9P
  - Ovary
    - Bilateral ØU92
    - Left ØU91
    - Right ØU9Ø
  - Palate
    - Hard ØC92
    - Soft ØC93
  - Pancreas ØF9G
  - Para-aortic Body ØG99
  - Paraganglion Extremity ØG9F
  - Parathyroid Gland ØG9R
    - Inferior
      - Left ØG9P
      - Right ØG9N
    - Multiple ØG9Q
    - Superior
      - Left ØG9M
      - Right ØG9L
  - Patella
    - Left ØQ9F
    - Right ØQ9D
  - Pelvic Cavity ØW9J
  - Penis ØV9S
  - Pericardial Cavity ØW9D
  - Perineum
    - Female ØW9N
    - Male ØW9M
  - Peritoneal Cavity ØW9G
  - Peritoneum ØD9W
  - Phalanx
    - Finger
      - Left ØP9V
      - Right ØP9T
    - Thumb
      - Left ØP9S
      - Right ØP9R
    - Toe
      - Left ØQ9R
      - Right ØQ9Q
  - Pharynx ØC9M
  - Pineal Body ØG91
- **Drainage** — *continued*
  - Pleura
    - Left ØB9P
    - Right ØB9N
  - Pleural Cavity
    - Left ØW9B
    - Right ØW99
  - Pons ØØ9B
  - Prepuce ØV9T
  - Products of Conception
    - Amniotic Fluid
      - Diagnostic 1Ø9Ø
      - Therapeutic 1Ø9Ø
    - Fetal Blood 1Ø9Ø
    - Fetal Cerebrospinal Fluid 1Ø9Ø
    - Fetal Fluid, Other 1Ø9Ø
    - Fluid, Other 1Ø9Ø
  - Prostate ØV9Ø
  - Radius
    - Left ØP9J
    - Right ØP9H
  - Rectum ØD9P
  - Retina
    - Left Ø89F
    - Right Ø89E
  - Retinal Vessel
    - Left Ø89H
    - Right Ø89G
  - Retroperitoneum ØW9H
  - Ribs
    - 1 to 2 ØP91
    - 3 or More ØP92
  - Sacrum ØQ91
  - Scapula
    - Left ØP96
    - Right ØP95
  - Sclera
    - Left Ø897
    - Right Ø896
  - Scrotum ØV95
  - Septum, Nasal Ø99M
  - Shoulder Region
    - Left ØX93
    - Right ØX92
  - Sinus
    - Accessory Ø99P
    - Ethmoid
      - Left Ø99V
      - Right Ø99U
    - Frontal
      - Left Ø99T
      - Right Ø99S
    - Mastoid
      - Left Ø99C
      - Right Ø99B
    - Maxillary
      - Left Ø99R
      - Right Ø99Q
    - Sphenoid
      - Left Ø99X
      - Right Ø99W
  - Skin
    - Abdomen ØH97
    - Back ØH96
    - Buttock ØH98
    - Chest ØH95
    - Ear
      - Left ØH93
      - Right ØH92
    - Face ØH91
    - Foot
      - Left ØH9N
      - Right ØH9M
    - Hand
      - Left ØH9G
      - Right ØH9F
    - Inguinal ØH9A
    - Lower Arm
      - Left ØH9E
      - Right ØH9D
    - Lower Leg
      - Left ØH9L
      - Right ØH9K
    - Neck ØH94
    - Perineum ØH99
    - Scalp ØH9Ø
    - Upper Arm
      - Left ØH9C
      - Right ØH9B

Drainage — *continued*
Skin — *continued*
Upper Leg
Left ØH9J
Right ØH9H
Skull ØN9Ø
Spinal Canal ØØ9U
Spinal Cord
Cervical ØØ9W
Lumbar ØØ9Y
Thoracic ØØ9X
Spinal Meninges ØØ9T
Spleen Ø79P
Sternum ØP9Ø
Stomach ØD96
Pylorus ØD97
Subarachnoid Space, Intracranial ØØ95
Subcutaneous Tissue and Fascia
Abdomen ØJ98
Back ØJ97
Buttock ØJ99
Chest ØJ96
Face ØJ91
Foot
Left ØJ9R
Right ØJ9Q
Hand
Left ØJ9K
Right ØJ9J
Lower Arm
Left ØJ9H
Right ØJ9G
Lower Leg
Left ØJ9P
Right ØJ9N
Neck
Left ØJ95
Right ØJ94
Pelvic Region ØJ9C
Perineum ØJ9B
Scalp ØJ9Ø
Upper Arm
Left ØJ9F
Right ØJ9D
Upper Leg
Left ØJ9M
Right ØJ9L
Subdural Space, Intracranial ØØ94
Tarsal
Left ØQ9M
Right ØQ9L
Tendon
Abdomen
Left ØL9G
Right ØL9F
Ankle
Left ØL9T
Right ØL9S
Foot
Left ØL9W
Right ØL9V
Hand
Left ØL98
Right ØL97
Head and Neck ØL9Ø
Hip
Left ØL9K
Right ØL9J
Knee
Left ØL9R
Right ØL9Q
Lower Arm and Wrist
Left ØL96
Right ØL95
Lower Leg
Left ØL9P
Right ØL9N
Perineum ØL9H
Shoulder
Left ØL92
Right ØL91
Thorax
Left ØL9D
Right ØL9C
Trunk
Left ØL9B
Right ØL99
Upper Arm
Left ØL94

Drainage — *continued*
Tendon — *continued*
Upper Arm — *continued*
Right ØL93
Upper Leg
Left ØL9M
Right ØL9L
Testis
Bilateral ØV9C
Left ØV9B
Right ØV99
Thalamus ØØ99
Thymus Ø79M
Thyroid Gland ØG9K
Left Lobe ØG9G
Right Lobe ØG9H
Tibia
Left ØQ9H
Right ØQ9G
Toe Nail ØH9R
Tongue ØC97
Tonsils ØC9P
Tooth
Lower ØC9X
Upper ØC9W
Trachea ØB91
Tunica Vaginalis
Left ØV97
Right ØV96
Turbinate, Nasal Ø99L
Tympanic Membrane
Left Ø998
Right Ø997
Ulna
Left ØP9L
Right ØP9K
Ureter
Left ØT97
Right ØT96
Ureters, Bilateral ØT98
Urethra ØT9D
Uterine Supporting Structure ØU94
Uterus ØU99
Uvula ØC9N
Vagina ØU9G
Vas Deferens
Bilateral ØV9Q
Left ØV9P
Right ØV9N
Vein
Axillary
Left Ø598
Right Ø597
Azygos Ø59Ø
Basilic
Left Ø59C
Right Ø59B
Brachial
Left Ø59A
Right Ø599
Cephalic
Left Ø59F
Right Ø59D
Colic Ø697
Common Iliac
Left Ø69D
Right Ø69C
Esophageal Ø693
External Iliac
Left Ø69G
Right Ø69F
External Jugular
Left Ø59Q
Right Ø59P
Face
Left Ø59V
Right Ø59T
Femoral
Left Ø69N
Right Ø69M
Foot
Left Ø69V
Right Ø69T
Gastric Ø692
Hand
Left Ø59H
Right Ø59G
Hemiazygos Ø591
Hepatic Ø694

Drainage — *continued*
Vein — *continued*
Hypogastric
Left Ø69J
Right Ø69H
Inferior Mesenteric Ø696
Innominate
Left Ø594
Right Ø593
Internal Jugular
Left Ø59N
Right Ø59M
Intracranial Ø59L
Lower Ø69Y
Portal Ø698
Renal
Left Ø69B
Right Ø699
Saphenous
Left Ø69Q
Right Ø69P
Splenic Ø691
Subclavian
Left Ø596
Right Ø595
Superior Mesenteric Ø695
Upper Ø59Y
Vertebral
Left Ø59S
Right Ø59R
Vena Cava, Inferior Ø69Ø
Vertebra
Cervical ØP93
Lumbar ØQ9Ø
Thoracic ØP94
Vesicle
Bilateral ØV93
Left ØV92
Right ØV91
Vitreous
Left Ø895
Right Ø894
Vocal Cord
Left ØC9V
Right ØC9T
Vulva ØU9M
Wrist Region
Left ØX9H
Right ØX9G
Dressing
Abdominal Wall 2W23X4Z
Arm
Lower
Left 2W2DX4Z
Right 2W2CX4Z
Upper
Left 2W2BX4Z
Right 2W2AX4Z
Back 2W25X4Z
Chest Wall 2W24X4Z
Extremity
Lower
Left 2W2MX4Z
Right 2W2LX4Z
Upper
Left 2W29X4Z
Right 2W28X4Z
Face 2W21X4Z
Finger
Left 2W2KX4Z
Right 2W2JX4Z
Foot
Left 2W2TX4Z
Right 2W2SX4Z
Hand
Left 2W2FX4Z
Right 2W2EX4Z
Head 2W2ØX4Z
Inguinal Region
Left 2W27X4Z
Right 2W26X4Z
Leg
Lower
Left 2W2RX4Z
Right 2W2QX4Z
Upper
Left 2W2PX4Z
Right 2W2NX4Z
Neck 2W22X4Z

Subterms under main terms may continue to next column or page

Dressing — *continued*
Thumb
Left 2W2HX4Z
Right 2W2GX4Z
Toe
Left 2W2VX4Z
Right 2W2UX4Z
Driver stent (RX) (OTW) *use* Intraluminal Device
Drotrecogin alfa, infusion *see* Introduction of Recombinant Human-activated Protein C
Duct of Santorini *use* Pancreatic Duct, Accessory
Duct of Wirsung *use* Pancreatic Duct
Ductogram, mammary *see* Plain Radiography, Skin, Subcutaneous Tissue and Breast BHØ
Ductography, mammary *see* Plain Radiography, Skin, Subcutaneous Tissue and Breast BHØ
Ductus deferens
use Vas Deferens
use Vas Deferens, Bilateral
use Vas Deferens, Left
use Vas Deferens, Right
Duodenal ampulla *use* Ampulla of Vater
Duodenectomy
see Excision, Duodenum ØDB9
see Resection, Duodenum ØDT9
Duodenocholedochotomy *see* Drainage, Gallbladder ØF94
Duodenocystostomy
see Bypass, Gallbladder ØF14
see Drainage, Gallbladder ØF94
Duodenoenterostomy
see Bypass, Gastrointestinal System ØD1
see Drainage, Gastrointestinal System ØD9
Duodenojejunal flexure *use* Jejunum
Duodenolysis *see* Release, Duodenum ØDN9
Duodenorrhaphy *see* Repair, Duodenum ØDQ9
Duodenoscopy, single-use (aScope™ Duodeno) (EXALT™ Model D) *see* New Technology, Hepatobiliary System and Pancreas XFJ
Duodenostomy
see Bypass, Duodenum ØD19
see Drainage, Duodenum ØD99
Duodenotomy *see* Drainage, Duodenum ØD99
Dura mater, intracranial *use* Dura Mater
Dura mater, spinal *use* Spinal Meninges
DuraGraft® Endothelial Damage Inhibitor *use* Endothelial Damage Inhibitor
DuraHeart Left Ventricular Assist System *use* Implantable Heart Assist System in Heart and Great Vessels
Dural venous sinus *use* Intracranial Vein
Durata® Defibrillation Lead *use* Cardiac Lead, Defibrillator in Ø2H
Durvalumab Antineoplastic XWØ
DynaClip® (Forte)
use Internal Fixation Device, Sustained Compression in ØRG
use Internal Fixation Device, Sustained Compression in ØSG
DynaNail® (Helix)(Hybrid) (Mini)
use Internal Fixation Device, Sustained Compression in ØRG
use Internal Fixation Device, Sustained Compression in ØSG
Dynesys® Dynamic Stabilization System
use Spinal Stabilization Device, Pedicle-Based in ØRH
use Spinal Stabilization Device, Pedicle-Based in ØSH

E

Earlobe
use Ear, External, Bilateral
use Ear, External, Left
use Ear, External, Right
ECCO2R (Extracorporeal Carbon Dioxide Removal) 5AØ92ØZ
Echocardiogram *see* Ultrasonography, Heart B24
EchoGo Heart Failure 1.Ø software XXE2X19
Echography *see* Ultrasonography
EchoTip® Insight™ Portosystemic Pressure Gradient Measurement System 4AØ44B2
ECMO *see* Performance, Circulatory 5A15
ECMO, intraoperative *see* Performance, Circulatory 5A15A
Eculizumab XWØ
EDWARDS INTUITY Elite valve system (rapid deployment technique) *see* Replacement, Valve, Aortic Ø2RF
EEG (electroencephalogram) *see* Measurement, Central Nervous 4AØØ
EGD (esophagogastroduodenoscopy) ØDJØ8ZZ
Eighth cranial nerve *use* Acoustic Nerve
Ejaculatory duct
use Vas Deferens
use Vas Deferens, Bilateral
use Vas Deferens, Left
use Vas Deferens, Right
EKG (electrocardiogram) *see* Measurement, Cardiac 4AØ2
EKOS™ EkoSonic® Endovascular System *see* Fragmentation, Artery
Eladocagene exuparvovec XWØQ316
Electrical bone growth stimulator (EBGS)
use Bone Growth Stimulator in Head and Facial Bones
use Bone Growth Stimulator in Lower Bones
use Bone Growth Stimulator in Upper Bones
Electrical muscle stimulation (EMS) lead *use* Stimulator Lead in Muscles
Electrocautery
Destruction *see* Destruction
Repair *see* Repair
Electroconvulsive Therapy
Bilateral-Multiple Seizure GZB3ZZZ
Bilateral-Single Seizure GZB2ZZZ
Electroconvulsive Therapy, Other GZB4ZZZ
Unilateral-Multiple Seizure GZB1ZZZ
Unilateral-Single Seizure GZBØZZZ
Electroencephalogram (EEG) *see* Measurement, Central Nervous 4AØØ
Electromagnetic Therapy
Central Nervous 6A22
Urinary 6A21
Electronic muscle stimulator lead *use* Stimulator Lead in Muscles
Electrophysiologic stimulation (EPS) *see* Measurement, Cardiac 4AØ2
Electroshock therapy *see* Electroconvulsive Therapy
Elevation, bone fragments, skull *see* Reposition, Head and Facial Bones ØNS
Eleventh cranial nerve *use* Accessory Nerve
Ellipsys® vascular access system *see* New Technology, Cardiovascular System X2K
Elranatamab Antineoplastic XWØ13L9
E-Luminexx™ (Biliary) (Vascular) Stent *use* Intraluminal Device
Eluvia™ Drug-Eluting Vascular Stent System
use Intraluminal Device, Sustained Release Drug-eluting in New Technology
use Intraluminal Device, Sustained Release Drug-eluting, Two in New Technology
use Intraluminal Device, Sustained Release Drug-eluting, Three in New Technology
use Intraluminal Device, Sustained Release Drug-eluting, Four or More in New Technology
ELZONRIS™ *use* Tagraxofusp-erzs Antineoplastic
Embolectomy *see* Extirpation
Embolization
see Occlusion
see Restriction
Embolization coil(s) *use* Intraluminal Device
EMG (electromyogram) *see* Measurement, Musculoskeletal 4AØF
Encephalon *use* Brain
Endarterectomy
see Extirpation, Lower Arteries Ø4C
see Extirpation, Upper Arteries Ø3C
Endeavor® (III) (IV) (Sprint) Zotarolimus-eluting Coronary Stent System *use* Intraluminal Device, Drug-eluting in Heart and Great Vessels
EndoAVF procedure, using magnetic-guided radiofrequency *see* Bypass, Upper Arteries Ø31
EndoAVF procedure, using thermal resistance energy *see* New Technology, Cardiovascular System X2K
Endologix AFX® Endovascular AAA System *use* Intraluminal Device
EndoSure® sensor *use* Monitoring Device, Pressure Sensor in Ø2H
ENDOTAK RELIANCE® (G) Defibrillation Lead *use* Cardiac Lead, Defibrillator in Ø2H
Endothelial damage inhibitor, applied to vein graft XYØVX83
Endotracheal tube (cuffed) (double-lumen) *use* Intraluminal Device, Endotracheal Airway in Respiratory System
Endovascular fistula creation, using magnetic-guided radiofrequency *see* Bypass, Upper Arteries Ø31
Endovascular fistula creation, using thermal resistance energy *see* New Technology, Cardiovascular System X2K
Endurant® Endovascular Stent Graft *use* Intraluminal Device
Endurant® II AAA Stent Graft System *use* Intraluminal Device
Engineered Allogeneic Thymus Tissue XWØ2ØD8
Engineered Chimeric Antigen Receptor T-cell Immunotherapy
Allogeneic XWØ
Autologous XWØ
Enlargement
see Dilation
see Repair
EnRhythm *use* Pacemaker, Dual Chamber in ØJH
ENROUTE® Transcarotid Neuroprotection System
see New Technology, Cardiovascular System X2A
ENSPRYNG™ *use* Satralizumab-mwge
Enterorrhaphy *see* Repair, Gastrointestinal System ØDQ
Enterra gastric neurostimulator *use* Stimulator Generator, Multiple Array in ØJH
Enucleation
Eyeball *see* Resection, Eye Ø8T
Eyeball with prosthetic implant *see* Replacement, Eye Ø8R
Epcoritamab Monoclonal Antibody XWØ13S9
Ependyma *use* Cerebral Ventricle
Epicel® cultured epidermal autograft *use* Autologous Tissue Substitute
Epic™ Stented Tissue Valve (aortic) *use* Zooplastic Tissue in Heart and Great Vessels
Epidermis *use* Skin
Epididymectomy
see Excision, Male Reproductive System ØVB
see Resection, Male Reproductive System ØVT
Epididymoplasty
see Repair, Male Reproductive System ØVQ
see Supplement, Male Reproductive System ØVU
Epididymorrhaphy *see* Repair, Male Reproductive System ØVQ
Epididymotomy *see* Drainage, Male Reproductive System ØV9
Epidural space, spinal *use* Spinal Canal
Epiphysiodesis
see Insertion of device in, Lower Bones ØQH
see Insertion of device in, Upper Bones ØPH
see Repair, Lower Bones ØQQ
see Repair, Upper Bones ØPQ
Epiploic foramen *use* Peritoneum
Epiretinal Visual Prosthesis
Left Ø8H1Ø5Z
Right Ø8HØØ5Z
Episiorrhaphy *see* Repair, Perineum, Female ØWQN
Episiotomy *see* Division, Perineum, Female ØW8N
Epithalamus *use* Thalamus
Epitrochlear lymph node
use Lymphatic, Left Upper Extremity
use Lymphatic, Right Upper Extremity
EPS (electrophysiologic stimulation) *see* Measurement, Cardiac 4AØ2
Eptifibatide, infusion *see* Introduction of Platelet Inhibitor
ERCP (endoscopic retrograde cholangiopancreatography) *see* Fluoroscopy, Hepatobiliary System and Pancreas BF1
Erdafitinib Antineoplastic XWØDXL5
Erector spinae muscle
use Trunk Muscle, Left
use Trunk Muscle, Right
ERLEADA™ *use* Apalutamide Antineoplastic
Esketamine Hydrochloride XWØ97M5
Esophageal artery *use* Upper Artery
Esophageal obturator airway (EOA) *use* Intraluminal Device, Airway in Gastrointestinal System
Esophageal plexus *use* Thoracic Sympathetic Nerve
Esophagectomy
see Excision, Gastrointestinal System ØDB

Esophagectomy — *continued*
  see Resection, Gastrointestinal System ØDT
Esophagocoloplasty
  see Repair, Gastrointestinal System ØDQ
  see Supplement, Gastrointestinal System ØDU
Esophagoenterostomy
  see Bypass, Gastrointestinal System ØD1
  see Drainage, Gastrointestinal System ØD9
Esophagoesophagostomy
  see Bypass, Gastrointestinal System ØD1
  see Drainage, Gastrointestinal System ØD9
Esophagogastrectomy
  see Excision, Gastrointestinal System ØDB
  see Resection, Gastrointestinal System ØDT
Esophagogastroduodenoscopy (EGD) ØDJØ8ZZ
Esophagogastroplasty
  see Repair, Gastrointestinal System ØDQ
  see Supplement, Gastrointestinal System ØDU
Esophagogastroscopy ØDJ68ZZ
Esophagogastrostomy
  see Bypass, Gastrointestinal System ØD1
  see Drainage, Gastrointestinal System ØD9
Esophagojejunoplasty *see* Supplement, Gastrointestinal System ØDU
Esophagojejunostomy
  see Bypass, Gastrointestinal System ØD1
  see Drainage, Gastrointestinal System ØD9
Esophagomyotomy *see* Division, Esophagogastric Junction ØD84
Esophagoplasty
  see Repair, Gastrointestinal System ØDQ
  see Replacement, Esophagus ØDR5
  see Supplement, Gastrointestinal System ØDU
Esophagoplication *see* Restriction, Gastrointestinal System ØDV
Esophagorrhaphy *see* Repair, Gastrointestinal System ØDQ
Esophagoscopy ØDJØ8ZZ
Esophagotomy *see* Drainage, Gastrointestinal System ØD9
Esteem® implantable hearing system *use* Hearing Device in Ear, Nose, Sinus
ESWL (extracorporeal shock wave lithotripsy) *see* Fragmentation
Etesevimab Monoclonal Antibody XWØ
Ethmoidal air cell
  use Ethmoid Sinus, Left
  use Ethmoid Sinus, Right
Ethmoidectomy
  see Excision, Ear, Nose, Sinus Ø9B
  see Excision, Head and Facial Bones ØNB
  see Resection, Ear, Nose, Sinus Ø9T
  see Resection, Head and Facial Bones ØNT
Ethmoidotomy *see* Drainage, Ear, Nose, Sinus Ø99
EV ICD System (Extravascular implantable defibrillator lead) *use* Defibrillator Lead in Anatomical Regions, General
Evacuation
  Hematoma *see* Extirpation
  Other Fluid *see* Drainage
Evera (XT) (S) (DR/VR) *use* Defibrillator Generator in ØJH
Everolimus-eluting coronary stent *use* Intraluminal Device, Drug-eluting in Heart and Great Vessels
Evisceration
  Eyeball *see* Resection, Eye Ø8T
  Eyeball with prosthetic implant *see* Replacement, Eye Ø8R
EVUSHELD™ *use* Tixagevimab and Cilgavimab Monoclonal Antibody
Exagamglogene Autotemcel XW1
EXALT™ Model D Single-Use Duodenoscope *see* New Technology, Hepatobiliary System and Pancreas XFJ
Examination *see* Inspection
Exchange *see* Change device in
Excision
  Abdominal Wall ØWBF
  Acetabulum
    Left ØQB5
    Right ØQB4
  Adenoids ØCBQ
  Ampulla of Vater ØFBC
  Anal Sphincter ØDBR
  Ankle Region
    Left ØYBL
    Right ØYBK

Excision — *continued*
  Anus ØDBQ
  Aorta
    Abdominal
    Thoracic
      Ascending/Arch Ø2BX
      Descending Ø2BW
  Aortic Body ØGBD
  Appendix ØDBJ
  Arm
    Lower
      Left ØXBF
      Right ØXBD
    Upper
      Left ØXB9
      Right ØXB8
  Artery
    Anterior Tibial
      Left Ø4BQ
      Right Ø4BP
    Axillary
      Left Ø3B6
      Right Ø3B5
    Brachial
      Left Ø3B8
      Right Ø3B7
    Celiac Ø4B1
    Colic
      Left Ø4B7
      Middle Ø4B8
      Right Ø4B6
    Common Carotid
      Left Ø3BJ
      Right Ø3BH
    Common Iliac
      Left Ø4BD
      Right Ø4BC
    External Carotid
      Left Ø3BN
      Right Ø3BM
    External Iliac
      Left Ø4BJ
      Right Ø4BH
    Face Ø3BR
    Femoral
      Left Ø4BL
      Right Ø4BK
    Foot
      Left Ø4BW
      Right Ø4BV
    Gastric Ø4B2
    Hand
      Left Ø3BF
      Right Ø3BD
    Hepatic Ø4B3
    Inferior Mesenteric Ø4BB
    Innominate Ø3B2
    Internal Carotid
      Left Ø3BL
      Right Ø3BK
    Internal Iliac
      Left Ø4BF
      Right Ø4BE
    Internal Mammary
      Left Ø3B1
      Right Ø3BØ
    Intracranial Ø3BG
    Lower Ø4BY
    Peroneal
      Left Ø4BU
      Right Ø4BT
    Popliteal
      Left Ø4BN
      Right Ø4BM
    Posterior Tibial
      Left Ø4BS
      Right Ø4BR
    Pulmonary
      Left Ø2BR
      Right Ø2BQ
    Pulmonary Trunk Ø2BP
    Radial
      Left Ø3BC
      Right Ø3BB
    Renal
      Left Ø4BA
      Right Ø4B9
    Splenic Ø4B4

Excision — *continued*
  Artery — *continued*
    Subclavian
      Left Ø3B4
      Right Ø3B3
    Superior Mesenteric Ø4B5
    Temporal
      Left Ø3BT
      Right Ø3BS
    Thyroid
      Left Ø3BV
      Right Ø3BU
    Ulnar
      Left Ø3BA
      Right Ø3B9
    Upper Ø3BY
    Vertebral
      Left Ø3BQ
      Right Ø3BP
  Atrium
    Left Ø2B7
    Right Ø2B6
  Auditory Ossicle
    Left Ø9BA
    Right Ø9B9
  Axilla
    Left ØXB5
    Right ØXB4
  Back
    Lower ØWBL
    Upper ØWBK
  Basal Ganglia ØØB8
  Bladder ØTBB
  Bladder Neck ØTBC
  Bone
    Ethmoid
      Left ØNBG
      Right ØNBF
    Frontal ØNB1
    Hyoid ØNBX
    Lacrimal
      Left ØNBJ
      Right ØNBH
    Nasal ØNBB
    Occipital ØNB7
    Palatine
      Left ØNBL
      Right ØNBK
    Parietal
      Left ØNB4
      Right ØNB3
    Pelvic
      Left ØQB3
      Right ØQB2
    Sphenoid ØNBC
    Temporal
      Left ØNB6
      Right ØNB5
    Zygomatic
      Left ØNBN
      Right ØNBM
  Brain ØØBØ
  Breast
    Bilateral ØHBV
    Left ØHBU
    Right ØHBT
    Supernumerary ØHBY
  Bronchus
    Lingula ØBB9
    Lower Lobe
      Left ØBBB
      Right ØBB6
    Main
      Left ØBB7
      Right ØBB3
    Middle Lobe, Right ØBB5
    Upper Lobe
      Left ØBB8
      Right ØBB4
  Buccal Mucosa ØCB4
  Bursa and Ligament
    Abdomen
      Left ØMBJ
      Right ØMBH
    Ankle
      Left ØMBR
      Right ØMBQ
    Elbow
      Left ØMB4

Excision — *continued*
Bursa and Ligament — *continued*
Elbow — *continued*
Right ØMB3
Foot
Left ØMBT
Right ØMBS
Hand
Left ØMB8
Right ØMB7
Head and Neck ØMBØ
Hip
Left ØMBM
Right ØMBL
Knee
Left ØMBP
Right ØMBN
Lower Extremity
Left ØMBW
Right ØMBV
Perineum ØMBK
Rib(s) ØMBG
Shoulder
Left ØMB2
Right ØMB1
Spine
Lower ØMBD
Upper ØMBC
Sternum ØMBF
Upper Extremity
Left ØMBB
Right ØMB9
Wrist
Left ØMB6
Right ØMB5
Buttock
Left ØYB1
Right ØYBØ
Carina ØBB2
Carotid Bodies, Bilateral ØGB8
Carotid Body
Left ØGB6
Right ØGB7
Carpal
Left ØPBN
Right ØPBM
Cecum ØDBH
Cerebellum ØØBC
Cerebral Hemisphere ØØB7
Cerebral Meninges ØØB1
Cerebral Ventricle ØØB6
Cervix ØUBC
Chest Wall ØWB8
Chordae Tendineae Ø2B9
Choroid
Left Ø8BB
Right Ø8BA
Cisterna Chyli Ø7BL
Clavicle
Left ØPBB
Right ØPB9
Clitoris ØUBJ
Coccygeal Glomus ØGBB
Coccyx ØQBS
Colon
Ascending ØDBK
Descending ØDBM
Sigmoid ØDBN
Transverse ØDBL
Conduction Mechanism Ø2B8
Conjunctiva
Left Ø8BTXZ
Right Ø8BSXZ
Cord
Bilateral ØVBH
Left ØVBG
Right ØVBF
Cornea
Left Ø8B9XZ
Right Ø8B8XZ
Cul-de-sac ØUBF
Diaphragm ØBBT
Disc
Cervical Vertebral ØRB3
Cervicothoracic Vertebral ØRB5
Lumbar Vertebral ØSB2
Lumbosacral ØSB4
Thoracic Vertebral ØRB9
Thoracolumbar Vertebral ØRBB

Excision — *continued*
Duct
Common Bile ØFB9
Cystic ØFB8
Hepatic
Common ØFB7
Left ØFB6
Right ØFB5
Lacrimal
Left Ø8BY
Right Ø8BX
Pancreatic ØFBD
Accessory ØFBF
Parotid
Left ØCBC
Right ØCBB
Duodenum ØDB9
Dura Mater ØØB2
Ear
External
Left Ø9B1
Right Ø9BØ
External Auditory Canal
Left Ø9B4
Right Ø9B3
Inner
Left Ø9BE
Right Ø9BD
Middle
Left Ø9B6
Right Ø9B5
Elbow Region
Left ØXBC
Right ØXBB
Epididymis
Bilateral ØVBL
Left ØVBK
Right ØVBJ
Epiglottis ØCBR
Esophagogastric Junction ØDB4
Esophagus ØDB5
Lower ØDB3
Middle ØDB2
Upper ØDB1
Eustachian Tube
Left Ø9BG
Right Ø9BF
Extremity
Lower
Left ØYBB
Right ØYB9
Upper
Left ØXB7
Right ØXB6
Eye
Left Ø8B1
Right Ø8BØ
Eyelid
Lower
Left Ø8BR
Right Ø8BQ
Upper
Left Ø8BP
Right Ø8BN
Face ØWB2
Fallopian Tube
Left ØUB6
Right ØUB5
Fallopian Tubes, Bilateral ØUB7
Femoral Region
Left ØYB8
Right ØYB7
Femoral Shaft
Left ØQB9
Right ØQB8
Femur
Lower
Left ØQBC
Right ØQBB
Upper
Left ØQB7
Right ØQB6
Fibula
Left ØQBK
Right ØQBJ
Finger Nail ØHBQXZ
Floor of mouth *see* Excision, Oral Cavity and Throat ØWB3

Excision — *continued*
Foot
Left ØYBN
Right ØYBM
Gallbladder ØFB4
Gingiva
Lower ØCB6
Upper ØCB5
Gland
Adrenal
Bilateral ØGB4
Left ØGB2
Right ØGB3
Lacrimal
Left Ø8BW
Right Ø8BV
Minor Salivary ØCBJ
Parotid
Left ØCB9
Right ØCB8
Pituitary ØGBØ
Sublingual
Left ØCBF
Right ØCBD
Submaxillary
Left ØCBH
Right ØCBG
Vestibular ØUBL
Glenoid Cavity
Left ØPB8
Right ØPB7
Glomus Jugulare ØGBC
Hand
Left ØXBK
Right ØXBJ
Head ØWBØ
Humeral Head
Left ØPBD
Right ØPBC
Humeral Shaft
Left ØPBG
Right ØPBF
Hymen ØUBK
Hypothalamus ØØBA
Ileocecal Valve ØDBC
Ileum ØDBB
Inguinal Region
Left ØYB6
Right ØYB5
Intestine
Large ØDBE
Left ØDBG
Right ØDBF
Small ØDB8
Iris
Left Ø8BD3Z
Right Ø8BC3Z
Jaw
Lower ØWB5
Upper ØWB4
Jejunum ØDBA
Joint
Acromioclavicular
Left ØRBH
Right ØRBG
Ankle
Left ØSBG
Right ØSBF
Carpal
Left ØRBR
Right ØRBQ
Carpometacarpal
Left ØRBT
Right ØRBS
Cervical Vertebral ØRB1
Cervicothoracic Vertebral ØRB4
Coccygeal ØSB6
Elbow
Left ØRBM
Right ØRBL
Finger Phalangeal
Left ØRBX
Right ØRBW
Hip
Left ØSBB
Right ØSB9
Knee
Left ØSBD
Right ØSBC

Excision — *continued*
- Joint — *continued*
  - Lumbar Vertebral ØSBØ
  - Lumbosacral ØSB3
  - Metacarpophalangeal
    - Left ØRBV
    - Right ØRBU
  - Metatarsal-Phalangeal
    - Left ØSBN
    - Right ØSBM
  - Occipital-cervical ØRBØ
  - Sacrococcygeal ØSB5
  - Sacroiliac
    - Left ØSB8
    - Right ØSB7
  - Shoulder
    - Left ØRBK
    - Right ØRBJ
  - Sternoclavicular
    - Left ØRBF
    - Right ØRBE
  - Tarsal
    - Left ØSBJ
    - Right ØSBH
  - Tarsometatarsal
    - Left ØSBL
    - Right ØSBK
  - Temporomandibular
    - Left ØRBD
    - Right ØRBC
  - Thoracic Vertebral ØRB6
  - Thoracolumbar Vertebral ØRBA
  - Toe Phalangeal
    - Left ØSBQ
    - Right ØSBP
  - Wrist
    - Left ØRBP
    - Right ØRBN
- Kidney
  - Left ØTB1
  - Right ØTBØ
- Kidney Pelvis
  - Left ØTB4
  - Right ØTB3
- Knee Region
  - Left ØYBG
  - Right ØYBF
- Larynx ØCBS
- Leg
  - Lower
    - Left ØYBJ
    - Right ØYBH
  - Upper
    - Left ØYBD
    - Right ØYBC
- Lens
  - Left Ø8BK3Z
  - Right Ø8BJ3Z
- Lip
  - Lower ØCB1
  - Upper ØCBØ
- Liver ØFBØ
  - Left Lobe ØFB2
  - Right Lobe ØFB1
- Lung
  - Bilateral ØBBM
  - Left ØBBL
  - Lower Lobe
    - Left ØBBJ
    - Right ØBBF
  - Middle Lobe, Right ØBBD
  - Right ØBBK
  - Upper Lobe
    - Left ØBBG
    - Right ØBBC
- Lung Lingula ØBBH
- Lymphatic
  - Aortic Ø7BD
  - Axillary
    - Left Ø7B6
    - Right Ø7B5
  - Head Ø7BØ
  - Inguinal
    - Left Ø7BJ
    - Right Ø7BH
  - Internal Mammary
    - Left Ø7B9
    - Right Ø7B8

Excision — *continued*
- Lymphatic — *continued*
  - Lower Extremity
    - Left Ø7BG
    - Right Ø7BF
  - Mesenteric Ø7BB
  - Neck
    - Left Ø7B2
    - Right Ø7B1
  - Pelvis Ø7BC
  - Thoracic Duct Ø7BK
  - Thorax Ø7B7
  - Upper Extremity
    - Left Ø7B4
    - Right Ø7B3
- Mandible
  - Left ØNBV
  - Right ØNBT
- Maxilla ØNBR
- Mediastinum ØWBC
- Medulla Oblongata ØØBD
- Mesentery ØDBV
- Metacarpal
  - Left ØPBQ
  - Right ØPBP
- Metatarsal
  - Left ØQBP
  - Right ØQBN
- Muscle
  - Abdomen
    - Left ØKBL
    - Right ØKBK
  - Extraocular
    - Left Ø8BM
    - Right Ø8BL
  - Facial ØKB1
  - Foot
    - Left ØKBW
    - Right ØKBV
  - Hand
    - Left ØKBD
    - Right ØKBC
  - Head ØKBØ
  - Hip
    - Left ØKBP
    - Right ØKBN
  - Lower Arm and Wrist
    - Left ØKBB
    - Right ØKB9
  - Lower Leg
    - Left ØKBT
    - Right ØKBS
  - Neck
    - Left ØKB3
    - Right ØKB2
  - Papillary Ø2BD
  - Perineum ØKBM
  - Shoulder
    - Left ØKB6
    - Right ØKB5
  - Thorax
    - Left ØKBJ
    - Right ØKBH
  - Tongue, Palate, Pharynx ØKB4
  - Trunk
    - Left ØKBG
    - Right ØKBF
  - Upper Arm
    - Left ØKB8
    - Right ØKB7
  - Upper Leg
    - Left ØKBR
    - Right ØKBQ
- Nasal Mucosa and Soft Tissue Ø9BK
- Nasopharynx Ø9BN
- Neck ØWB6
- Nerve
  - Abdominal Sympathetic Ø1BM
  - Abducens ØØBL
  - Accessory ØØBR
  - Acoustic ØØBN
  - Brachial Plexus Ø1B3
  - Cervical Ø1B1
  - Cervical Plexus Ø1BØ
  - Facial ØØBM
  - Femoral Ø1BD
  - Glossopharyngeal ØØBP
  - Head and Neck Sympathetic Ø1BK
  - Hypoglossal ØØBS

Excision — *continued*
- Nerve — *continued*
  - Lumbar Ø1BB
  - Lumbar Plexus Ø1B9
  - Lumbar Sympathetic Ø1BN
  - Lumbosacral Plexus Ø1BA
  - Median Ø1B5
  - Oculomotor ØØBH
  - Olfactory ØØBF
  - Optic ØØBG
  - Peroneal Ø1BH
  - Phrenic Ø1B2
  - Pudendal Ø1BC
  - Radial Ø1B6
  - Sacral Ø1BR
  - Sacral Plexus Ø1BQ
  - Sacral Sympathetic Ø1BP
  - Sciatic Ø1BF
  - Thoracic Ø1B8
  - Thoracic Sympathetic Ø1BL
  - Tibial Ø1BG
  - Trigeminal ØØBK
  - Trochlear ØØBJ
  - Ulnar Ø1B4
  - Vagus ØØBQ
- Nipple
  - Left ØHBX
  - Right ØHBW
- Omentum ØDBU
- Oral Cavity and Throat ØWB3
- Orbit
  - Left ØNBQ
  - Right ØNBP
- Ovary
  - Bilateral ØUB2
  - Left ØUB1
  - Right ØUBØ
- Palate
  - Hard ØCB2
  - Soft ØCB3
- Pancreas ØFBG
- Para-aortic Body ØGB9
- Paraganglion Extremity ØGBF
- Parathyroid Gland ØGBR
  - Inferior
    - Left ØGBP
    - Right ØGBN
  - Multiple ØGBQ
  - Superior
    - Left ØGBM
    - Right ØGBL
- Patella
  - Left ØQBF
  - Right ØQBD
- Penis ØVBS
- Pericardium Ø2BN
- Perineum
  - Female ØWBN
  - Male ØWBM
- Peritoneum ØDBW
- Phalanx
  - Finger
    - Left ØPBV
    - Right ØPBT
  - Thumb
    - Left ØPBS
    - Right ØPBR
  - Toe
    - Left ØQBR
    - Right ØQBQ
- Pharynx ØCBM
- Pineal Body ØGB1
- Pleura
  - Left ØBBP
  - Right ØBBN
- Pons ØØBB
- Prepuce ØVBT
- Prostate ØVBØ
- Radius
  - Left ØPBJ
  - Right ØPBH
- Rectum ØDBP
- Retina
  - Left Ø8BF3Z
  - Right Ø8BE3Z
- Retroperitoneum ØWBH
- Ribs
  - 1 to 2 ØPB1
  - 3 or More ØPB2

Excision — *continued*
- Sacrum ØQB1
- Scapula
  - Left ØPB6
  - Right ØPB5
- Sclera
  - Left Ø8B7XZ
  - Right Ø8B6XZ
- Scrotum ØVB5
- Septum
  - Atrial Ø2B5
  - Nasal Ø9BM
  - Ventricular Ø2BM
- Shoulder Region
  - Left ØXB3
  - Right ØXB2
- Sinus
  - Accessory Ø9BP
  - Ethmoid
    - Left Ø9BV
    - Right Ø9BU
  - Frontal
    - Left Ø9BT
    - Right Ø9BS
  - Mastoid
    - Left Ø9BC
    - Right Ø9BB
  - Maxillary
    - Left Ø9BR
    - Right Ø9BQ
  - Sphenoid
    - Left Ø9BX
    - Right Ø9BW
- Skin
  - Abdomen ØHB7XZ
  - Back ØHB6XZ
  - Buttock ØHB8XZ
  - Chest ØHB5XZ
  - Ear
    - Left ØHB3XZ
    - Right ØHB2XZ
  - Face ØHB1XZ
  - Foot
    - Left ØHBNXZ
    - Right ØHBMXZ
  - Hand
    - Left ØHBGXZ
    - Right ØHBFXZ
  - Inguinal ØHBAXZ
  - Lower Arm
    - Left ØHBEXZ
    - Right ØHBDXZ
  - Lower Leg
    - Left ØHBLXZ
    - Right ØHBKXZ
  - Neck ØHB4XZ
  - Perineum ØHB9XZ
  - Scalp ØHBØXZ
  - Upper Arm
    - Left ØHBCXZ
    - Right ØHBBXZ
  - Upper Leg
    - Left ØHBJXZ
    - Right ØHBHXZ
- Skull ØNBØ
- Spinal Cord
  - Cervical ØØBW
  - Lumbar ØØBY
  - Thoracic ØØBX
- Spinal Meninges ØØBT
- Spleen Ø7BP
- Sternum ØPBØ
- Stomach ØDB6
  - Pylorus ØDB7
- Subcutaneous Tissue and Fascia
  - Abdomen ØJB8
  - Back ØJB7
  - Buttock ØJB9
  - Chest ØJB6
  - Face ØJB1
  - Foot
    - Left ØJBR
    - Right ØJBQ
  - Hand
    - Left ØJBK
    - Right ØJBJ
  - Lower Arm
    - Left ØJBH
    - Right ØJBG

Excision — *continued*
- Subcutaneous Tissue and Fascia — *continued*
  - Lower Leg
    - Left ØJBP
    - Right ØJBN
  - Neck
    - Left ØJB5
    - Right ØJB4
  - Pelvic Region ØJBC
  - Perineum ØJBB
  - Scalp ØJBØ
  - Upper Arm
    - Left ØJBF
    - Right ØJBD
  - Upper Leg
    - Left ØJBM
    - Right ØJBL
- Tarsal
  - Left ØQBM
  - Right ØQBL
- Tendon
  - Abdomen
    - Left ØLBG
    - Right ØLBF
  - Ankle
    - Left ØLBT
    - Right ØLBS
  - Foot
    - Left ØLBW
    - Right ØLBV
  - Hand
    - Left ØLB8
    - Right ØLB7
  - Head and Neck ØLBØ
  - Hip
    - Left ØLBK
    - Right ØLBJ
  - Knee
    - Left ØLBR
    - Right ØLBQ
  - Lower Arm and Wrist
    - Left ØLB6
    - Right ØLB5
  - Lower Leg
    - Left ØLBP
    - Right ØLBN
  - Perineum ØLBH
  - Shoulder
    - Left ØLB2
    - Right ØLB1
  - Thorax
    - Left ØLBD
    - Right ØLBC
  - Trunk
    - Left ØLBB
    - Right ØLB9
  - Upper Arm
    - Left ØLB4
    - Right ØLB3
  - Upper Leg
    - Left ØLBM
    - Right ØLBL
- Testis
  - Bilateral ØVBC
  - Left ØVBB
  - Right ØVB9
- Thalamus ØØB9
- Thymus Ø7BM
- Thyroid Gland
  - Left Lobe ØGBG
  - Right Lobe ØGBH
- Thyroid Gland Isthmus ØGBJ
- Tibia
  - Left ØQBH
  - Right ØQBG
- Toe Nail ØHBRXZ
- Tongue ØCB7
- Tonsils ØCBP
- Tooth
  - Lower ØCBX
  - Upper ØCBW
- Trachea ØBB1
- Tunica Vaginalis
  - Left ØVB7
  - Right ØVB6
- Turbinate, Nasal Ø9BL
- Tympanic Membrane
  - Left Ø9B8
  - Right Ø9B7

Excision — *continued*
- Ulna
  - Left ØPBL
  - Right ØPBK
- Ureter
  - Left ØTB7
  - Right ØTB6
- Urethra ØTBD
- Uterine Supporting Structure ØUB4
- Uterus ØUB9
- Uvula ØCBN
- Vagina ØUBG
- Valve
  - Aortic Ø2BF
  - Mitral Ø2BG
  - Pulmonary Ø2BH
  - Tricuspid Ø2BJ
- Vas Deferens
  - Bilateral ØVBQ
  - Left ØVBP
  - Right ØVBN
- Vein
  - Axillary
    - Left Ø5B8
    - Right Ø5B7
  - Azygos Ø5BØ
  - Basilic
    - Left Ø5BC
    - Right Ø5BB
  - Brachial
    - Left Ø5BA
    - Right Ø5B9
  - Cephalic
    - Left Ø5BF
    - Right Ø5BD
  - Colic Ø6B7
  - Common Iliac
    - Left Ø6BD
    - Right Ø6BC
  - Coronary Ø2B4
  - Esophageal Ø6B3
  - External Iliac
    - Left Ø6BG
    - Right Ø6BF
  - External Jugular
    - Left Ø5BQ
    - Right Ø5BP
  - Face
    - Left Ø5BV
    - Right Ø5BT
  - Femoral
    - Left Ø6BN
    - Right Ø6BM
  - Foot
    - Left Ø6BV
    - Right Ø6BT
  - Gastric Ø6B2
  - Hand
    - Left Ø5BH
    - Right Ø5BG
  - Hemiazygos Ø5B1
  - Hepatic Ø6B4
  - Hypogastric
    - Left Ø6BJ
    - Right Ø6BH
  - Inferior Mesenteric Ø6B6
  - Innominate
    - Left Ø5B4
    - Right Ø5B3
  - Internal Jugular
    - Left Ø5BN
    - Right Ø5BM
  - Intracranial Ø5BL
  - Lower Ø6BY
  - Portal Ø6B8
  - Pulmonary
    - Left Ø2BT
    - Right Ø2BS
  - Renal
    - Left Ø6BB
    - Right Ø6B9
  - Saphenous
    - Left Ø6BQ
    - Right Ø6BP
  - Splenic Ø6B1
  - Subclavian
    - Left Ø5B6
    - Right Ø5B5
  - Superior Mesenteric Ø6B5

Excision — *continued*
Vein — *continued*
Upper Ø5BY
Vertebral
Left Ø5BS
Right Ø5BR
Vena Cava
Inferior Ø6BØ
Superior Ø2BV
Ventricle
Left Ø2BL
Right Ø2BK
Vertebra
Cervical ØPB3
Lumbar ØQBØ
Thoracic ØPB4
Vesicle
Bilateral ØVB3
Left ØVB2
Right ØVB1
Vitreous
Left Ø8B53Z
Right Ø8B43Z
Vocal Cord
Left ØCBV
Right ØCBT
Vulva ØUBM
Wrist Region
Left ØXBH
Right ØXBG
EXCLUDER® AAA Endoprosthesis
use Intraluminal Device
use Intraluminal Device, Branched or Fenestrated, One or Two Arteries in Ø4V
use Intraluminal Device, Branched or Fenestrated, Three or More Arteries in Ø4V
EXCLUDER® IBE Endoprosthesis *use* Intraluminal Device, Branched or Fenestrated, One or Two Arteries in Ø4V
Exclusion, Left atrial appendage (LAA) *see* Occlusion, Atrium, Left Ø2L7
Exercise, rehabilitation *see* Motor Treatment, Rehabilitation FØ7
Exploration *see* Inspection
Express® Biliary SD Monorail® Premounted Stent System *use* Intraluminal Device
Express® (LD) Premounted Stent System *use* Intraluminal Device
Express® SD Renal Monorail® Premounted Stent System *use* Intraluminal Device
Ex-PRESS™ mini glaucoma shunt *use* Synthetic Substitute
Extensor carpi radialis muscle
use Lower Arm and Wrist Muscle, Left
use Lower Arm and Wrist Muscle, Right
Extensor carpi ulnaris muscle
use Lower Arm and Wrist Muscle, Left
use Lower Arm and Wrist Muscle, Right
Extensor digitorum brevis muscle
use Foot Muscle, Left
use Foot Muscle, Right
Extensor digitorum longus muscle
use Lower Leg Muscle, Left
use Lower Leg Muscle, Right
Extensor hallucis brevis muscle
use Foot Muscle, Left
use Foot Muscle, Right
Extensor hallucis longus muscle
use Lower Leg Muscle, Left
use Lower Leg Muscle, Right
External anal sphincter *use* Anal Sphincter
External auditory meatus
use External Auditory Canal, Left
use External Auditory Canal, Right
External fixator
use External Fixation Device in Head and Facial Bones
use External Fixation Device in Lower Bones
use External Fixation Device in Lower Joints
use External Fixation Device in Upper Bones
use External Fixation Device in Upper Joints
External maxillary artery *use* Face Artery
External naris *use* Nasal Mucosa and Soft Tissue
External oblique aponeurosis *use* Subcutaneous Tissue and Fascia, Trunk
External oblique muscle
use Abdomen Muscle, Left
External oblique muscle — *continued*
use Abdomen Muscle, Right
External popliteal nerve *use* Peroneal Nerve
External pudendal artery
use Femoral Artery, Left
use Femoral Artery, Right
External pudendal vein
use Saphenous Vein, Left
use Saphenous Vein, Right
External urethral sphincter *use* Urethra
Extirpation
Acetabulum
Left ØQC5
Right ØQC4
Adenoids ØCCQ
Ampulla of Vater ØFCC
Anal Sphincter ØDCR
Anterior Chamber
Left Ø8C3
Right Ø8C2
Anus ØDCQ
Aorta
Abdominal Ø4CØ
Thoracic
Ascending/Arch Ø2CX
Descending Ø2CW
Aortic Body ØGCD
Appendix ØDCJ
Artery
Anterior Tibial
Left Ø4CQ
Right Ø4CP
Axillary
Left Ø3C6
Right Ø3C5
Brachial
Left Ø3C8
Right Ø3C7
Celiac Ø4C1
Colic
Left Ø4C7
Middle Ø4C8
Right Ø4C6
Common Carotid
Left Ø3CJ
Right Ø3CH
Common Iliac
Left Ø4CD
Right Ø4CC
Coronary
Four or More Arteries Ø2C3
One Artery Ø2CØ
Three Arteries Ø2C2
Two Arteries Ø2C1
External Carotid
Left Ø3CN
Right Ø3CM
External Iliac
Left Ø4CJ
Right Ø4CH
Face Ø3CR
Femoral
Left Ø4CL
Right Ø4CK
Foot
Left Ø4CW
Right Ø4CV
Gastric Ø4C2
Hand
Left Ø3CF
Right Ø3CD
Hepatic Ø4C3
Inferior Mesenteric Ø4CB
Innominate Ø3C2
Internal Carotid
Left Ø3CL
Right Ø3CK
Internal Iliac
Left Ø4CF
Right Ø4CE
Internal Mammary
Left Ø3C1
Right Ø3CØ
Intracranial Ø3CG
Lower Ø4CY
Peroneal
Left Ø4CU
Right Ø4CT
Extirpation — *continued*
Artery — *continued*
Popliteal
Left Ø4CN
Right Ø4CM
Posterior Tibial
Left Ø4CS
Right Ø4CR
Pulmonary
Left Ø2CR
Right Ø2CQ
Pulmonary Trunk Ø2CP
Radial
Left Ø3CC
Right Ø3CB
Renal
Left Ø4CA
Right Ø4C9
Splenic Ø4C4
Subclavian
Left Ø3C4
Right Ø3C3
Superior Mesenteric Ø4C5
Temporal
Left Ø3CT
Right Ø3CS
Thyroid
Left Ø3CV
Right Ø3CU
Ulnar
Left Ø3CA
Right Ø3C9
Upper Ø3CY
Vertebral
Left Ø3CQ
Right Ø3CP
Atrium
Left Ø2C7
Right Ø2C6
Auditory Ossicle
Left Ø9CA
Right Ø9C9
Basal Ganglia ØØC8
Bladder ØTCB
Bladder Neck ØTCC
Bone
Ethmoid
Left ØNCG
Right ØNCF
Frontal ØNC1
Hyoid ØNCX
Lacrimal
Left ØNCJ
Right ØNCH
Nasal ØNCB
Occipital ØNC7
Palatine
Left ØNCL
Right ØNCK
Parietal
Left ØNC4
Right ØNC3
Pelvic
Left ØQC3
Right ØQC2
Sphenoid ØNCC
Temporal
Left ØNC6
Right ØNC5
Zygomatic
Left ØNCN
Right ØNCM
Brain ØØCØ
Breast
Bilateral ØHCV
Left ØHCU
Right ØHCT
Bronchus
Lingula ØBC9
Lower Lobe
Left ØBCB
Right ØBC6
Main
Left ØBC7
Right ØBC3
Middle Lobe, Right ØBC5
Upper Lobe
Left ØBC8
Right ØBC4

Extirpation — *continued*
Buccal Mucosa ØCC4
Bursa and Ligament
Abdomen
Left ØMCJ
Right ØMCH
Ankle
Left ØMCR
Right ØMCQ
Elbow
Left ØMC4
Right ØMC3
Foot
Left ØMCT
Right ØMCS
Hand
Left ØMC8
Right ØMC7
Head and Neck ØMCØ
Hip
Left ØMCM
Right ØMCL
Knee
Left ØMCP
Right ØMCN
Lower Extremity
Left ØMCW
Right ØMCV
Perineum ØMCK
Rib(s) ØMCG
Shoulder
Left ØMC2
Right ØMC1
Spine
Lower ØMCD
Upper ØMCC
Sternum ØMCF
Upper Extremity
Left ØMCB
Right ØMC9
Wrist
Left ØMC6
Right ØMC5
Carina ØBC2
Carotid Bodies, Bilateral ØGC8
Carotid Body
Left ØGC6
Right ØGC7
Carpal
Left ØPCN
Right ØPCM
Cavity, Cranial ØWC1
Cecum ØDCH
Cerebellum ØØCC
Cerebral Hemisphere ØØC7
Cerebral Meninges ØØC1
Cerebral Ventricle ØØC6
Cervix ØUCC
Chordae Tendineae Ø2C9
Choroid
Left Ø8CB
Right Ø8CA
Cisterna Chyli Ø7CL
Clavicle
Left ØPCB
Right ØPC9
Clitoris ØUCJ
Coccygeal Glomus ØGCB
Coccyx ØQCS
Colon
Ascending ØDCK
Descending ØDCM
Sigmoid ØDCN
Transverse ØDCL
Computer-aided Mechanical Aspiration X2C
Conduction Mechanism Ø2C8
Conjunctiva
Left Ø8CTXZZ
Right Ø8CSXZZ
Cord
Bilateral ØVCH
Left ØVCG
Right ØVCF
Cornea
Left Ø8C9XZZ
Right Ø8C8XZZ
Cul-de-sac ØUCF
Diaphragm ØBCT

Extirpation — *continued*
Disc
Cervical Vertebral ØRC3
Cervicothoracic Vertebral ØRC5
Lumbar Vertebral ØSC2
Lumbosacral ØSC4
Thoracic Vertebral ØRC9
Thoracolumbar Vertebral ØRCB
Duct
Common Bile ØFC9
Cystic ØFC8
Hepatic
Common ØFC7
Left ØFC6
Right ØFC5
Lacrimal
Left Ø8CY
Right Ø8CX
Pancreatic ØFCD
Accessory ØFCF
Parotid
Left ØCCC
Right ØCCB
Duodenum ØDC9
Dura Mater ØØC2
Ear
External
Left Ø9C1
Right Ø9CØ
External Auditory Canal
Left Ø9C4
Right Ø9C3
Inner
Left Ø9CE
Right Ø9CD
Middle
Left Ø9C6
Right Ø9C5
Endometrium ØUCB
Epididymis
Bilateral ØVCL
Left ØVCK
Right ØVCJ
Epidural Space, Intracranial ØØC3
Epiglottis ØCCR
Esophagogastric Junction ØDC4
Esophagus ØDC5
Lower ØDC3
Middle ØDC2
Upper ØDC1
Eustachian Tube
Left Ø9CG
Right Ø9CF
Eye
Left Ø8C1XZZ
Right Ø8CØXZZ
Eyelid
Lower
Left Ø8CR
Right Ø8CQ
Upper
Left Ø8CP
Right Ø8CN
Fallopian Tube
Left ØUC6
Right ØUC5
Fallopian Tubes, Bilateral ØUC7
Femoral Shaft
Left ØQC9
Right ØQC8
Femur
Lower
Left ØQCC
Right ØQCB
Upper
Left ØQC7
Right ØQC6
Fibula
Left ØQCK
Right ØQCJ
Finger Nail ØHCQXZZ
Gallbladder ØFC4
Gastrointestinal Tract ØWCP
Genitourinary Tract ØWCR
Gingiva
Lower ØCC6
Upper ØCC5

Extirpation — *continued*
Gland
Adrenal
Bilateral ØGC4
Left ØGC2
Right ØGC3
Lacrimal
Left Ø8CW
Right Ø8CV
Minor Salivary ØCCJ
Parotid
Left ØCC9
Right ØCC8
Pituitary ØGCØ
Sublingual
Left ØCCF
Right ØCCD
Submaxillary
Left ØCCH
Right ØCCG
Vestibular ØUCL
Glenoid Cavity
Left ØPC8
Right ØPC7
Glomus Jugulare ØGCC
Humeral Head
Left ØPCD
Right ØPCC
Humeral Shaft
Left ØPCG
Right ØPCF
Hymen ØUCK
Hypothalamus ØØCA
Ileocecal Valve ØDCC
Ileum ØDCB
Intestine
Large ØDCE
Left ØDCG
Right ØDCF
Small ØDC8
Iris
Left Ø8CD
Right Ø8CC
Jaw
Lower ØWC5
Upper ØWC4
Jejunum ØDCA
Joint
Acromioclavicular
Left ØRCH
Right ØRCG
Ankle
Left ØSCG
Right ØSCF
Carpal
Left ØRCR
Right ØRCQ
Carpometacarpal
Left ØRCT
Right ØRCS
Cervical Vertebral ØRC1
Cervicothoracic Vertebral ØRC4
Coccygeal ØSC6
Elbow
Left ØRCM
Right ØRCL
Finger Phalangeal
Left ØRCX
Right ØRCW
Hip
Left ØSCB
Right ØSC9
Knee
Left ØSCD
Right ØSCC
Lumbar Vertebral ØSCØ
Lumbosacral ØSC3
Metacarpophalangeal
Left ØRCV
Right ØRCU
Metatarsal-Phalangeal
Left ØSCN
Right ØSCM
Occipital-cervical ØRCØ
Sacrococcygeal ØSC5
Sacroiliac
Left ØSC8
Right ØSC7

Extirpation — *continued*
Joint — *continued*
Shoulder
Left ØRCK
Right ØRCJ
Sternoclavicular
Left ØRCF
Right ØRCE
Tarsal
Left ØSCJ
Right ØSCH
Tarsometatarsal
Left ØSCL
Right ØSCK
Temporomandibular
Left ØRCD
Right ØRCC
Thoracic Vertebral ØRC6
Thoracolumbar Vertebral ØRCA
Toe Phalangeal
Left ØSCQ
Right ØSCP
Wrist
Left ØRCP
Right ØRCN
Kidney
Left ØTC1
Right ØTCØ
Kidney Pelvis
Left ØTC4
Right ØTC3
Larynx ØCCS
Lens
Left Ø8CK
Right Ø8CJ
Lip
Lower ØCC1
Upper ØCCØ
Liver ØFCØ
Left Lobe ØFC2
Right Lobe ØFC1
Lung
Bilateral ØBCM
Left ØBCL
Lower Lobe
Left ØBCJ
Right ØBCF
Middle Lobe, Right ØBCD
Right ØBCK
Upper Lobe
Left ØBCG
Right ØBCC
Lung Lingula ØBCH
Lymphatic
Aortic Ø7CD
Axillary
Left Ø7C6
Right Ø7C5
Head Ø7CØ
Inguinal
Left Ø7CJ
Right Ø7CH
Internal Mammary
Left Ø7C9
Right Ø7C8
Lower Extremity
Left Ø7CG
Right Ø7CF
Mesenteric Ø7CB
Neck
Left Ø7C2
Right Ø7C1
Pelvis Ø7CC
Thoracic Duct Ø7CK
Thorax Ø7C7
Upper Extremity
Left Ø7C4
Right Ø7C3
Mandible
Left ØNCV
Right ØNCT
Maxilla ØNCR
Mediastinum ØWCC
Medulla Oblongata ØØCD
Mesentery ØDCV
Metacarpal
Left ØPCQ
Right ØPCP

Extirpation — *continued*
Metatarsal
Left ØQCP
Right ØQCN
Muscle
Abdomen
Left ØKCL
Right ØKCK
Extraocular
Left Ø8CM
Right Ø8CL
Facial ØKC1
Foot
Left ØKCW
Right ØKCV
Hand
Left ØKCD
Right ØKCC
Head ØKCØ
Hip
Left ØKCP
Right ØKCN
Lower Arm and Wrist
Left ØKCB
Right ØKC9
Lower Leg
Left ØKCT
Right ØKCS
Neck
Left ØKC3
Right ØKC2
Papillary Ø2CD
Perineum ØKCM
Shoulder
Left ØKC6
Right ØKC5
Thorax
Left ØKCJ
Right ØKCH
Tongue, Palate, Pharynx ØKC4
Trunk
Left ØKCG
Right ØKCF
Upper Arm
Left ØKC8
Right ØKC7
Upper Leg
Left ØKCR
Right ØKCQ
Nasal Mucosa and Soft Tissue Ø9CK
Nasopharynx Ø9CN
Nerve
Abdominal Sympathetic Ø1CM
Abducens ØØCL
Accessory ØØCR
Acoustic ØØCN
Brachial Plexus Ø1C3
Cervical Ø1C1
Cervical Plexus Ø1CØ
Facial ØØCM
Femoral Ø1CD
Glossopharyngeal ØØCP
Head and Neck Sympathetic Ø1CK
Hypoglossal ØØCS
Lumbar Ø1CB
Lumbar Plexus Ø1C9
Lumbar Sympathetic Ø1CN
Lumbosacral Plexus Ø1CA
Median Ø1C5
Oculomotor ØØCH
Olfactory ØØCF
Optic ØØCG
Peroneal Ø1CH
Phrenic Ø1C2
Pudendal Ø1CC
Radial Ø1C6
Sacral Ø1CR
Sacral Plexus Ø1CQ
Sacral Sympathetic Ø1CP
Sciatic Ø1CF
Thoracic Ø1C8
Thoracic Sympathetic Ø1CL
Tibial Ø1CG
Trigeminal ØØCK
Trochlear ØØCJ
Ulnar Ø1C4
Vagus ØØCQ
Nipple
Left ØHCX

Extirpation — *continued*
Nipple — *continued*
Right ØHCW
Omentum ØDCU
Oral Cavity and Throat ØWC3
Orbit
Left ØNCQ
Right ØNCP
Orbital Atherectomy *see* Extirpation, Heart and Great Vessels Ø2C
Ovary
Bilateral ØUC2
Left ØUC1
Right ØUCØ
Palate
Hard ØCC2
Soft ØCC3
Pancreas ØFCG
Para-aortic Body ØGC9
Paraganglion Extremity ØGCF
Parathyroid Gland ØGCR
Inferior
Left ØGCP
Right ØGCN
Multiple ØGCQ
Superior
Left ØGCM
Right ØGCL
Patella
Left ØQCF
Right ØQCD
Pelvic Cavity ØWCJ
Penis ØVCS
Pericardial Cavity ØWCD
Pericardium Ø2CN
Peritoneal Cavity ØWCG
Peritoneum ØDCW
Phalanx
Finger
Left ØPCV
Right ØPCT
Thumb
Left ØPCS
Right ØPCR
Toe
Left ØQCR
Right ØQCQ
Pharynx ØCCM
Pineal Body ØGC1
Pleura
Left ØBCP
Right ØBCN
Pleural Cavity
Left ØWCB
Right ØWC9
Pons ØØCB
Prepuce ØVCT
Prostate ØVCØ
Radius
Left ØPCJ
Right ØPCH
Rectum ØDCP
Respiratory Tract ØWCQ
Retina
Left Ø8CF
Right Ø8CE
Retinal Vessel
Left Ø8CH
Right Ø8CG
Retroperitoneum ØWCH
Ribs
1 to 2 ØPC1
3 or More ØPC2
Sacrum ØQC1
Scapula
Left ØPC6
Right ØPC5
Sclera
Left Ø8C7XZZ
Right Ø8C6XZZ
Scrotum ØVC5
Septum
Atrial Ø2C5
Nasal Ø9CM
Ventricular Ø2CM
Sinus
Accessory Ø9CP
Ethmoid
Left Ø9CV

Extirpation — *continued*
Sinus — *continued*
Ethmoid — *continued*
Right Ø9CU
Frontal
Left Ø9CT
Right Ø9CS
Mastoid
Left Ø9CC
Right Ø9CB
Maxillary
Left Ø9CR
Right Ø9CQ
Sphenoid
Left Ø9CX
Right Ø9CW
Skin
Abdomen ØHC7XZZ
Back ØHC6XZZ
Buttock ØHC8XZZ
Chest ØHC5XZZ
Ear
Left ØHC3XZZ
Right ØHC2XZZ
Face ØHC1XZZ
Foot
Left ØHCNXZZ
Right ØHCMXZZ
Hand
Left ØHCGXZZ
Right ØHCFXZZ
Inguinal ØHCAXZZ
Lower Arm
Left ØHCEXZZ
Right ØHCDXZZ
Lower Leg
Left ØHCLXZZ
Right ØHCKXZZ
Neck ØHC4XZZ
Perineum ØHC9XZZ
Scalp ØHCØXZZ
Upper Arm
Left ØHCCXZZ
Right ØHCBXZZ
Upper Leg
Left ØHCJXZZ
Right ØHCHXZZ
Spinal Canal ØØCU
Spinal Cord
Cervical ØØCW
Lumbar ØØCY
Thoracic ØØCX
Spinal Meninges ØØCT
Spleen Ø7CP
Sternum ØPCØ
Stomach ØDC6
Pylorus ØDC7
Subarachnoid Space, Intracranial ØØC5
Subcutaneous Tissue and Fascia
Abdomen ØJC8
Back ØJC7
Buttock ØJC9
Chest ØJC6
Face ØJC1
Foot
Left ØJCR
Right ØJCQ
Hand
Left ØJCK
Right ØJCJ
Lower Arm
Left ØJCH
Right ØJCG
Lower Leg
Left ØJCP
Right ØJCN
Neck
Left ØJC5
Right ØJC4
Pelvic Region ØJCC
Perineum ØJCB
Scalp ØJCØ
Upper Arm
Left ØJCF
Right ØJCD
Upper Leg
Left ØJCM
Right ØJCL
Subdural Space, Intracranial ØØC4

Extirpation — *continued*
Tarsal
Left ØQCM
Right ØQCL
Tendon
Abdomen
Left ØLCG
Right ØLCF
Ankle
Left ØLCT
Right ØLCS
Foot
Left ØLCW
Right ØLCV
Hand
Left ØLC8
Right ØLC7
Head and Neck ØLCØ
Hip
Left ØLCK
Right ØLCJ
Knee
Left ØLCR
Right ØLCQ
Lower Arm and Wrist
Left ØLC6
Right ØLC5
Lower Leg
Left ØLCP
Right ØLCN
Perineum ØLCH
Shoulder
Left ØLC2
Right ØLC1
Thorax
Left ØLCD
Right ØLCC
Trunk
Left ØLCB
Right ØLC9
Upper Arm
Left ØLC4
Right ØLC3
Upper Leg
Left ØLCM
Right ØLCL
Testis
Bilateral ØVCC
Left ØVCB
Right ØVC9
Thalamus ØØC9
Thymus Ø7CM
Thyroid Gland ØGCK
Left Lobe ØGCG
Right Lobe ØGCH
Tibia
Left ØQCH
Right ØQCG
Toe Nail ØHCRXZZ
Tongue ØCC7
Tonsils ØCCP
Tooth
Lower ØCCX
Upper ØCCW
Trachea ØBC1
Tunica Vaginalis
Left ØVC7
Right ØVC6
Turbinate, Nasal Ø9CL
Tympanic Membrane
Left Ø9C8
Right Ø9C7
Ulna
Left ØPCL
Right ØPCK
Ureter
Left ØTC7
Right ØTC6
Urethra ØTCD
Uterine Supporting Structure ØUC4
Uterus ØUC9
Uvula ØCCN
Vagina ØUCG
Valve
Aortic Ø2CF
Mitral Ø2CG
Pulmonary Ø2CH
Tricuspid Ø2CJ

Extirpation — *continued*
Vas Deferens
Bilateral ØVCQ
Left ØVCP
Right ØVCN
Vein
Axillary
Left Ø5C8
Right Ø5C7
Azygos Ø5CØ
Basilic
Left Ø5CC
Right Ø5CB
Brachial
Left Ø5CA
Right Ø5C9
Cephalic
Left Ø5CF
Right Ø5CD
Colic Ø6C7
Common Iliac
Left Ø6CD
Right Ø6CC
Coronary Ø2C4
Esophageal Ø6C3
External Iliac
Left Ø6CG
Right Ø6CF
External Jugular
Left Ø5CQ
Right Ø5CP
Face
Left Ø5CV
Right Ø5CT
Femoral
Left Ø6CN
Right Ø6CM
Foot
Left Ø6CV
Right Ø6CT
Gastric Ø6C2
Hand
Left Ø5CH
Right Ø5CG
Hemiazygos Ø5C1
Hepatic Ø6C4
Hypogastric
Left Ø6CJ
Right Ø6CH
Inferior Mesenteric Ø6C6
Innominate
Left Ø5C4
Right Ø5C3
Internal Jugular
Left Ø5CN
Right Ø5CM
Intracranial Ø5CL
Lower Ø6CY
Portal Ø6C8
Pulmonary
Left Ø2CT
Right Ø2CS
Renal
Left Ø6CB
Right Ø6C9
Saphenous
Left Ø6CQ
Right Ø6CP
Splenic Ø6C1
Subclavian
Left Ø5C6
Right Ø5C5
Superior Mesenteric Ø6C5
Upper Ø5CY
Vertebral
Left Ø5CS
Right Ø5CR
Vena Cava
Inferior Ø6CØ
Superior Ø2CV
Ventricle
Left Ø2CL
Right Ø2CK
Vertebra
Cervical ØPC3
Lumbar ØQCØ
Thoracic ØPC4
Vesicle
Bilateral ØVC3

Extirpation — *continued*
Vesicle — *continued*
Left ØVC2
Right ØVC1
Vitreous
Left Ø8C5
Right Ø8C4
Vocal Cord
Left ØCCV
Right ØCCT
Vulva ØUCM
Extracorporeal Carbon Dioxide Removal (ECCO2R) 5AØ92ØZ
Extracorporeal shock wave lithotripsy *see* Fragmentation
Extracranial-intracranial bypass (EC-IC) *see* Bypass, Upper Arteries Ø31
Extraction
Acetabulum
Left ØQD5ØZZ
Right ØQD4ØZZ
Ampulla of Vater ØFDC
Anus ØDDQ
Appendix ØDDJ
Auditory Ossicle
Left Ø9DAØZZ
Right Ø9D9ØZZ
Bone
Ethmoid
Left ØNDGØZZ
Right ØNDFØZZ
Frontal ØND1ØZZ
Hyoid ØNDXØZZ
Lacrimal
Left ØNDJØZZ
Right ØNDHØZZ
Nasal ØNDBØZZ
Occipital ØND7ØZZ
Palatine
Left ØNDLØZZ
Right ØNDKØZZ
Parietal
Left ØND4ØZZ
Right ØND3ØZZ
Pelvic
Left ØQD3ØZZ
Right ØQD2ØZZ
Sphenoid ØNDCØZZ
Temporal
Left ØND6ØZZ
Right ØND5ØZZ
Zygomatic
Left ØNDNØZZ
Right ØNDMØZZ
Bone Marrow Ø7DT
Iliac Ø7DR
Sternum Ø7DQ
Vertebral Ø7DS
Brain ØØDØ
Breast
Bilateral ØHDVØZZ
Left ØHDUØZZ
Right ØHDTØZZ
Supernumerary ØHDYØZZ
Bronchus
Lingula ØBD9
Lower Lobe
Left ØBDB
Right ØBD6
Main
Left ØBD7
Right ØBD3
Middle Lobe, Right ØBD5
Upper Lobe
Left ØBD8
Right ØBD4
Bursa and Ligament
Abdomen
Left ØMDJ
Right ØMDH
Ankle
Left ØMDR
Right ØMDQ
Elbow
Left ØMD4
Right ØMD3
Foot
Left ØMDT
Right ØMDS

Extraction — *continued*
Bursa and Ligament — *continued*
Hand
Left ØMD8
Right ØMD7
Head and Neck ØMDØ
Hip
Left ØMDM
Right ØMDL
Knee
Left ØMDP
Right ØMDN
Lower Extremity
Left ØMDW
Right ØMDV
Perineum ØMDK
Rib(s) ØMDG
Shoulder
Left ØMD2
Right ØMD1
Spine
Lower ØMDD
Upper ØMDC
Sternum ØMDF
Upper Extremity
Left ØMDB
Right ØMD9
Wrist
Left ØMD6
Right ØMD5
Carina ØBD2
Carpal
Left ØPDNØZZ
Right ØPDMØZZ
Cecum ØDDH
Cerebellum ØØDC
Cerebral Hemisphere ØØD7
Cerebral Meninges ØØD1
Cisterna Chyli Ø7DL
Clavicle
Left ØPDBØZZ
Right ØPD9ØZZ
Coccyx ØQDSØZZ
Colon
Ascending ØDDK
Descending ØDDM
Sigmoid ØDDN
Transverse ØDDL
Cornea
Left Ø8D9XZ
Right Ø8D8XZ
Duct
Common Bile ØFD9
Cystic ØFD8
Hepatic
Common ØFD7
Left ØFD6
Right ØFD5
Pancreatic ØFDD
Accessory ØFDF
Duodenum ØDD9
Dura Mater ØØD2
Endometrium ØUDB
Esophagogastric Junction ØDD4
Esophagus ØDD5
Lower ØDD3
Middle ØDD2
Upper ØDD1
Femoral Shaft
Left ØQD9ØZZ
Right ØQD8ØZZ
Femur
Lower
Left ØQDCØZZ
Right ØQDBØZZ
Upper
Left ØQD7ØZZ
Right ØQD6ØZZ
Fibula
Left ØQDKØZZ
Right ØQDJØZZ
Finger Nail ØHDQXZZ
Gallbladder ØFD4
Glenoid Cavity
Left ØPD8ØZZ
Right ØPD7ØZZ
Hair ØHDSXZZ
Humeral Head
Left ØPDDØZZ

Extraction — *continued*
Humeral Head — *continued*
Right ØPDCØZZ
Humeral Shaft
Left ØPDGØZZ
Right ØPDFØZZ
Ileocecal Valve ØDDC
Ileum ØDDB
Intestine
Large ØDDE
Left ØDDG
Right ØDDF
Small ØDD8
Jejunum ØDDA
Kidney
Left ØTD1
Right ØTDØ
Lens
Left Ø8DK3ZZ
Right Ø8DJ3ZZ
Liver ØFDØ
Left Lobe ØFD2
Right Lobe ØFD1
Lung
Bilateral ØBDM
Left ØBDL
Lower Lobe
Left ØBDJ
Right ØBDF
Middle Lobe, Right ØBDD
Right ØBDK
Upper Lobe
Left ØBDG
Right ØBDC
Lung Lingula ØBDH
Lymphatic
Aortic Ø7DD
Axillary
Left Ø7D6
Right Ø7D5
Head Ø7DØ
Inguinal
Left Ø7DJ
Right Ø7DH
Internal Mammary
Left Ø7D9
Right Ø7D8
Lower Extremity
Left Ø7DG
Right Ø7DF
Mesenteric Ø7DB
Neck
Left Ø7D2
Right Ø7D1
Pelvis Ø7DC
Thoracic Duct Ø7DK
Thorax Ø7D7
Upper Extremity
Left Ø7D4
Right Ø7D3
Mandible
Left ØNDVØZZ
Right ØNDTØZZ
Maxilla ØNDRØZZ
Metacarpal
Left ØPDQØZZ
Right ØPDPØZZ
Metatarsal
Left ØQDPØZZ
Right ØQDNØZZ
Muscle
Abdomen
Left ØKDLØZZ
Right ØKDKØZZ
Facial ØKD1ØZZ
Foot
Left ØKDWØZZ
Right ØKDVØZZ
Hand
Left ØKDDØZZ
Right ØKDCØZZ
Head ØKDØØZZ
Hip
Left ØKDPØZZ
Right ØKDNØZZ
Lower Arm and Wrist
Left ØKDBØZZ
Right ØKD9ØZZ

Extraction — *continued*
Muscle — *continued*
Lower Leg
Left ØKDTØZZ
Right ØKDSØZZ
Neck
Left ØKD3ØZZ
Right ØKD2ØZZ
Perineum ØKDMØZZ
Shoulder
Left ØKD6ØZZ
Right ØKD5ØZZ
Thorax
Left ØKDJØZZ
Right ØKDHØZZ
Tongue, Palate, Pharynx ØKD4ØZZ
Trunk
Left ØKDGØZZ
Right ØKDFØZZ
Upper Arm
Left ØKD8ØZZ
Right ØKD7ØZZ
Upper Leg
Left ØKDRØZZ
Right ØKDQØZZ
Nerve
Abdominal Sympathetic Ø1DM
Abducens ØØDL
Accessory ØØDR
Acoustic ØØDN
Brachial Plexus Ø1D3
Cervical Ø1D1
Cervical Plexus Ø1DØ
Facial ØØDM
Femoral Ø1DD
Glossopharyngeal ØØDP
Head and Neck Sympathetic Ø1DK
Hypoglossal ØØDS
Lumbar Ø1DB
Lumbar Plexus Ø1D9
Lumbar Sympathetic Ø1DN
Lumbosacral Plexus Ø1DA
Median Ø1D5
Oculomotor ØØDH
Olfactory ØØDF
Optic ØØDG
Peroneal Ø1DH
Phrenic Ø1D2
Pudendal Ø1DC
Radial Ø1D6
Sacral Ø1DR
Sacral Plexus Ø1DQ
Sacral Sympathetic Ø1DP
Sciatic Ø1DF
Thoracic Ø1D8
Thoracic Sympathetic Ø1DL
Tibial Ø1DG
Trigeminal ØØDK
Trochlear ØØDJ
Ulnar Ø1D4
Vagus ØØDQ
Orbit
Left ØNDQØZZ
Right ØNDPØZZ
Ova ØUDN
Pancreas ØFDG
Patella
Left ØQDFØZZ
Right ØQDDØZZ
Phalanx
Finger
Left ØPDVØZZ
Right ØPDTØZZ
Thumb
Left ØPDSØZZ
Right ØPDRØZZ
Toe
Left ØQDRØZZ
Right ØQDQØZZ
Pleura
Left ØBDP
Right ØBDN
Products of Conception
Ectopic 1ØD2
Extraperitoneal 1ØDØØZ2
High 1ØDØØZØ
High Forceps 1ØDØ7Z5
Internal Version 1ØDØ7Z7
Low 1ØDØØZ1

Extraction — *continued*
Products of Conception — *continued*
Low Forceps 1ØDØ7Z3
Mid Forceps 1ØDØ7Z4
Other 1ØDØ7Z8
Retained 1ØD1
Vacuum 1ØDØ7Z6
Radius
Left ØPDJØZZ
Right ØPDHØZZ
Rectum ØDDP
Ribs
1 to 2 ØPD1ØZZ
3 or More ØPD2ØZZ
Sacrum ØQD1ØZZ
Scapula
Left ØPD6ØZZ
Right ØPD5ØZZ
Septum, Nasal Ø9DM
Sinus
Accessory Ø9DP
Ethmoid
Left Ø9DV
Right Ø9DU
Frontal
Left Ø9DT
Right Ø9DS
Mastoid
Left Ø9DC
Right Ø9DB
Maxillary
Left Ø9DR
Right Ø9DQ
Sphenoid
Left Ø9DX
Right Ø9DW
Skin
Abdomen ØHD7XZZ
Back ØHD6XZZ
Buttock ØHD8XZZ
Chest ØHD5XZZ
Ear
Left ØHD3XZZ
Right ØHD2XZZ
Face ØHD1XZZ
Foot
Left ØHDNXZZ
Right ØHDMXZZ
Hand
Left ØHDGXZZ
Right ØHDFXZZ
Inguinal ØHDAXZZ
Lower Arm
Left ØHDEXZZ
Right ØHDDXZZ
Lower Leg
Left ØHDLXZZ
Right ØHDKXZZ
Neck ØHD4XZZ
Perineum ØHD9XZZ
Scalp ØHDØXZZ
Upper Arm
Left ØHDCXZZ
Right ØHDBXZZ
Upper Leg
Left ØHDJXZZ
Right ØHDHXZZ
Skull ØNDØØZZ
Spinal Meninges ØØDT
Spleen Ø7DP
Sternum ØPDØØZZ
Stomach ØDD6
Pylorus ØDD7
Subcutaneous Tissue and Fascia
Abdomen ØJD8
Back ØJD7
Buttock ØJD9
Chest ØJD6
Face ØJD1
Foot
Left ØJDR
Right ØJDQ
Hand
Left ØJDK
Right ØJDJ
Lower Arm
Left ØJDH
Right ØJDG

Extraction — *continued*
Subcutaneous Tissue and Fascia — *continued*
Lower Leg
Left ØJDP
Right ØJDN
Neck
Left ØJD5
Right ØJD4
Pelvic Region ØJDC
Perineum ØJDB
Scalp ØJDØ
Upper Arm
Left ØJDF
Right ØJDD
Upper Leg
Left ØJDM
Right ØJDL
Tarsal
Left ØQDMØZZ
Right ØQDLØZZ
Tendon
Abdomen
Left ØLDGØZZ
Right ØLDFØZZ
Ankle
Left ØLDTØZZ
Right ØLDSØZZ
Foot
Left ØLDWØZZ
Right ØLDVØZZ
Hand
Left ØLD8ØZZ
Right ØLD7ØZZ
Head and Neck ØLDØØZZ
Hip
Left ØLDKØZZ
Right ØLDJØZZ
Knee
Left ØLDRØZZ
Right ØLDQØZZ
Lower Arm and Wrist
Left ØLD6ØZZ
Right ØLD5ØZZ
Lower Leg
Left ØLDPØZZ
Right ØLDNØZZ
Perineum ØLDHØZZ
Shoulder
Left ØLD2ØZZ
Right ØLD1ØZZ
Thorax
Left ØLDDØZZ
Right ØLDCØZZ
Trunk
Left ØLDBØZZ
Right ØLD9ØZZ
Upper Arm
Left ØLD4ØZZ
Right ØLD3ØZZ
Upper Leg
Left ØLDMØZZ
Right ØDLLØZZ
Thymus Ø7DM
Tibia
Left ØQDHØZZ
Right ØQDGØZZ
Toe Nail ØHDRXZZ
Tooth
Lower ØCDXXZ
Upper ØCDWXZ
Trachea ØBD1
Turbinate, Nasal Ø9DL
Tympanic Membrane
Left Ø9D8
Right Ø9D7
Ulna
Left ØPDLØZZ
Right ØPDKØZZ
Vein
Basilic
Left Ø5DC
Right Ø5DB
Brachial
Left Ø5DA
Right Ø5D9
Cephalic
Left Ø5DF
Right Ø5DD

Extraction — *continued*
  Vein — *continued*
    Femoral
      Left Ø6DN
      Right Ø6DM
    Foot
      Left Ø6DV
      Right Ø6DT
    Hand
      Left Ø5DH
      Right Ø5DG
    Lower Ø6DY
    Saphenous
      Left Ø6DQ
      Right Ø6DP
    Upper Ø5DY
  Vertebra
    Cervical ØPD3ØZZ
    Lumbar ØQDØØZZ
    Thoracic ØPD4ØZZ
  Vocal Cord
    Left ØCDV
    Right ØCDT
Extradural space, intracranial *use* Epidural Space, Intracranial
Extradural space, spinal *use* Spinal Canal
EXtreme Lateral Interbody Fusion (XLIF) device
    use Interbody Fusion Device in Lower Joints

F

Face lift *see* Alteration, Face ØWØ2
Facet replacement spinal stabilization device
  use Spinal Stabilization Device, Facet Replacement in ØRH
  use Spinal Stabilization Device, Facet Replacement in ØSH
Facial artery *use* Face Artery
Factor Xa Inhibitor Reversal Agent, Andexanet Alfa *use* Coagulation Factor Xa, Inactivated
False vocal cord *use* Larynx
Falx cerebri *use* Dura Mater
Fascia lata
  use Subcutaneous Tissue and Fascia, Left Upper Leg
  use Subcutaneous Tissue and Fascia, Right Upper Leg
Fasciaplasty, fascioplasty
  see Repair, Subcutaneous Tissue and Fascia ØJQ
  see Replacement, Subcutaneous Tissue and Fascia ØJR
Fasciectomy *see* Excision, Subcutaneous Tissue and Fascia ØJB
Fasciorrhaphy *see* Repair, Subcutaneous Tissue and Fascia ØJQ
Fasciotomy
  see Division, Subcutaneous Tissue and Fascia ØJ8
  see Drainage, Subcutaneous Tissue and Fascia ØJ9
  see Release
Feeding Device
  Change device in
    Lower Intestinal Tract ØD2DXUZ
    Upper Intestinal Tract ØD2ØXUZ
  Insertion of device in
    Duodenum ØDH9
    Esophagus ØDH5
    Ileum ØDHB
    Intestine, Small ØDH8
    Jejunum ØDHA
    Stomach ØDH6
  Removal of device from
    Esophagus ØDP5
    Intestinal Tract
      Lower Intestinal Tract ØDPD
      Upper Intestinal Tract ØDPØ
    Stomach ØDP6
  Revision of device in
    Intestinal Tract
      Lower Intestinal Tract ØDWD
      Upper Intestinal Tract ØDWØ
    Stomach ØDW6
    Upper Intestinal Tract ØDWØ
Femoral head
  use Upper Femur, Left
  use Upper Femur, Right
Femoral lymph node
  use Lymphatic, Left Lower Extremity
Femoral lymph node — *continued*
  use Lymphatic, Right Lower Extremity
Femoropatellar joint
  use Knee Joint, Left
  use Knee Joint, Left, Tibial Surface
  use Knee Joint, Right
  use Knee Joint, Right, Femoral Surface
Femorotibial joint
  use Knee Joint, Left
  use Knee Joint, Left, Tibial Surface
  use Knee Joint, Right
  use Knee Joint, Right, Tibial Surface
FETROJA® *use* Cefiderocol Anti-infective
FGS (fluorescence-guided surgery) *see* Fluorescence Guided Procedure
Fibular artery
  use Peroneal Artery, Left
  use Peroneal Artery, Right
Fibular sesamoid
  use Metatarsal, Left
  use Metatarsal, Right
Fibularis brevis muscle
  use Lower Leg Muscle, Left
  use Lower Leg Muscle, Right
Fibularis longus muscle
  use Lower Leg Muscle, Left
  use Lower Leg Muscle, Right
Fifth cranial nerve *use* Trigeminal Nerve
Filum terminale *use* Spinal Meninges
Fimbriectomy
  see Excision, Female Reproductive System ØUB
  see Resection, Female Reproductive System ØUT
Fine needle aspiration
  Fluid or gas *see* Drainage
  Tissue biopsy
    see Excision
    see Extraction
First cranial nerve *use* Olfactory Nerve
First intercostal nerve *use* Brachial Plexus
Fistulization
  see Bypass
  see Drainage
  see Repair
Fitting
  Arch bars, for fracture reduction *see* Reposition, Mouth and Throat ØCS
  Arch bars, for immobilization *see* Immobilization, Face 2W31
  Artificial limb *see* Device Fitting, Rehabilitation FØD
  Hearing aid *see* Device Fitting, Rehabilitation FØD
  Ocular prosthesis FØDZ8UZ
  Prosthesis, limb *see* Device Fitting, Rehabilitation FØD
  Prosthesis, ocular FØDZ8UZ
Fixation, bone
  External, with fracture reduction *see* Reposition
  External, without fracture reduction *see* Insertion
  Internal, with fracture reduction *see* Reposition
  Internal, without fracture reduction *see* Insertion
FLAIR® Endovascular Stent Graft *use* Intraluminal Device
Flexible Composite Mesh *use* Synthetic Substitute
Flexor carpi radialis muscle
  use Lower Arm and Wrist Muscle, Left
  use Lower Arm and Wrist Muscle, Right
Flexor carpi ulnaris muscle
  use Lower Arm and Wrist Muscle, Left
  use Lower Arm and Wrist Muscle, Right
Flexor digitorum brevis muscle
  use Foot Muscle, Left
  use Foot Muscle, Right
Flexor digitorum longus muscle
  use Lower Leg Muscle, Left
  use Lower Leg Muscle, Right
Flexor hallucis brevis muscle
  use Foot Muscle, Left
  use Foot Muscle, Right
Flexor hallucis longus muscle
  use Lower Leg Muscle, Left
  use Lower Leg Muscle, Right
Flexor pollicis longus muscle
  use Lower Arm and Wrist Muscle, Left
  use Lower Arm and Wrist Muscle, Right
Flourish® Pediatric Esophageal Atresia Device *use* Magnetic Lengthening Device in Gastrointestinal System
Flow Diverter embolization device *use* Intraluminal Device, Flow Diverter in Ø3V
FlowSense Noninvasive Thermal Sensor 4BØØXWØ
Fluorescence Guided Procedure
  Extremity
    Lower 8EØY
    Upper 8EØX
  Head and Neck Region 8EØ9
    Aminolevulinic Acid 8EØ9ØEM
    No Qualifier 8EØ9ØEZ
  Reproductive System, Female, Pafolacianine (CYTALUX®) EØU
  Trunk Region
    No Qualifier 8EØW
    Pafolacianine (CYTALUX®) 8EØW
Fluorescent Pyrazine, Kidney XT25XE5
Fluoroscopy
  Abdomen and Pelvis BW11
  Airway, Upper BB1DZZZ
  Ankle
    Left BQ1H
    Right BQ1G
  Aorta
    Abdominal B41Ø
      Laser, Intraoperative B41Ø
    Thoracic B31Ø
      Laser, Intraoperative B31Ø
    Thoraco-Abdominal B31P
      Laser, Intraoperative B31P
  Aorta and Bilateral Lower Extremity Arteries B41D
    Laser, Intraoperative B41D
  Arm
    Left BP1FZZZ
    Right BP1EZZZ
  Artery
    Brachiocephalic-Subclavian
      Laser, Intraoperative B311
      Right B311
    Bronchial B31L
      Laser, Intraoperative B31L
    Bypass Graft, Other B21F
    Cervico-Cerebral Arch B31Q
      Laser, Intraoperative B31Q
    Common Carotid
      Bilateral B315
        Laser, Intraoperative B315
      Left B314
        Laser, Intraoperative B314
      Right B313
        Laser, Intraoperative B313
    Coronary
      Bypass Graft
        Multiple B213
          Laser, Intraoperative B213
        Single B212
          Laser, Intraoperative B212
      Multiple B211
        Laser, Intraoperative B211
      Single B21Ø
        Laser, Intraoperative B21Ø
    External Carotid
      Bilateral B31C
        Laser, Intraoperative B31C
      Left B31B
        Laser, Intraoperative B31B
      Right B319
        Laser, Intraoperative B319
    Hepatic B412
      Laser, Intraoperative B412
    Inferior Mesenteric B415
      Laser, Intraoperative B415
    Intercostal B31L
      Laser, Intraoperative B31L
    Internal Carotid
      Bilateral B318
        Laser, Intraoperative B318
      Left B317
        Laser, Intraoperative B317
      Right B316
        Laser, Intraoperative B316
    Internal Mammary Bypass Graft
      Left B218
      Right B217
    Intra-Abdominal
      Laser, Intraoperative B41B
      Other B41B

Fluoroscopy — *continued*
- Artery — *continued*
  - Intracranial B31R
    - Laser, Intraoperative B31R
  - Lower
    - Laser, Intraoperative B41J
    - Other B41J
  - Lower Extremity
    - Bilateral and Aorta B41D
      - Laser, Intraoperative B41D
    - Left B41G
      - Laser, Intraoperative B41G
    - Right B41F
      - Laser, Intraoperative B41F
  - Lumbar B419
    - Laser, Intraoperative B419
  - Pelvic B41C
    - Laser, Intraoperative B41C
  - Pulmonary
    - Left B31T
      - Laser, Intraoperative B31T
    - Right B31S
      - Laser, Intraoperative B31S
  - Pulmonary Trunk B31U
    - Laser, Intraoperative B31U
  - Renal
    - Bilateral B418
      - Laser, Intraoperative B418
    - Left B417
      - Laser, Intraoperative B417
    - Right B416
      - Laser, Intraoperative B416
  - Spinal B31M
    - Laser, Intraoperative B31M
  - Splenic B413
    - Laser, Intraoperative B413
  - Subclavian
    - Laser, Intraoperative B312
    - Left B312
  - Superior Mesenteric B414
    - Laser, Intraoperative B414
  - Upper
    - Laser, Intraoperative B31N
    - Other B31N
  - Upper Extremity
    - Bilateral B31K
      - Laser, Intraoperative B31K
    - Left B31J
      - Laser, Intraoperative B31J
    - Right B31H
      - Laser, Intraoperative B31H
  - Vertebral
    - Bilateral B31G
      - Laser, Intraoperative B31G
    - Left B31F
      - Laser, Intraoperative B31F
    - Right B31D
      - Laser, Intraoperative B31D
- Bile Duct BF1Ø
  - Pancreatic Duct and Gallbladder BF14
- Bile Duct and Gallbladder BF13
- Biliary Duct BF11
- Bladder BT1Ø
  - Kidney and Ureter BT14
    - Left BT1F
    - Right BT1D
- Bladder and Urethra BT1B
- Bowel, Small BD1
- Calcaneus
  - Left BQ1KZZZ
  - Right BQ1JZZZ
- Clavicle
  - Left BP15ZZZ
  - Right BP14ZZZ
- Coccyx BR1F
- Colon BD14
- Corpora Cavernosa BV1Ø
- Dialysis Fistula B51W
- Dialysis Shunt B51W
- Diaphragm BB16ZZZ
- Disc
  - Cervical BR11
  - Lumbar BR13
  - Thoracic BR12
- Duodenum BD19
- Elbow
  - Left BP1H
  - Right BP1G
- Epiglottis B91G

Fluoroscopy — *continued*
- Esophagus BD11
- Extremity
  - Lower BW1C
  - Upper BW1J
- Facet Joint
  - Cervical BR14
  - Lumbar BR16
  - Thoracic BR15
- Fallopian Tube
  - Bilateral BU12
  - Left BU11
  - Right BU1Ø
- Fallopian Tube and Uterus BU18
- Femur
  - Left BQ14ZZZ
  - Right BQ13ZZZ
- Finger
  - Left BP1SZZZ
  - Right BP1RZZZ
- Foot
  - Left BQ1MZZZ
  - Right BQ1LZZZ
- Forearm
  - Left BP1KZZZ
  - Right BP1JZZZ
- Gallbladder BF12
  - Bile Duct and Pancreatic Duct BF14
- Gallbladder and Bile Duct BF13
- Gastrointestinal, Upper BD1
- Hand
  - Left BP1PZZZ
  - Right BP1NZZZ
- Head and Neck BW19
- Heart
  - Left B215
  - Right B214
  - Right and Left B216
- Hip
  - Left BQ11
  - Right BQ1Ø
- Humerus
  - Left BP1BZZZ
  - Right BP1AZZZ
- Ileal Diversion Loop BT1C
- Ileal Loop, Ureters and Kidney BT1G
- Intracranial Sinus B512
- Joint
  - Acromioclavicular, Bilateral BP13ZZZ
  - Finger
    - Left BP1D
    - Right BP1C
  - Foot
    - Left BQ1Y
    - Right BQ1X
  - Hand
    - Left BP1D
    - Right BP1C
  - Lumbosacral BR1B
  - Sacroiliac BR1D
  - Sternoclavicular
    - Bilateral BP12ZZZ
    - Left BP11ZZZ
    - Right BP1ØZZZ
  - Temporomandibular
    - Bilateral BN19
    - Left BN18
    - Right BN17
  - Thoracolumbar BR18
  - Toe
    - Left BQ1Y
    - Right BQ1X
- Kidney
  - Bilateral BT13
  - Ileal Loop and Ureter BT1G
  - Left BT12
  - Right BT11
  - Ureter and Bladder BT14
    - Left BT1F
    - Right BT1D
- Knee
  - Left BQ18
  - Right BQ17
- Larynx B91J
- Leg
  - Left BQ1FZZZ
  - Right BQ1DZZZ
- Liver BF15

Fluoroscopy — *continued*
- Lung
  - Bilateral BB14ZZZ
  - Left BB13ZZZ
  - Right BB12ZZZ
- Mediastinum BB1CZZZ
- Mouth BD1B
- Neck and Head BW19
- Oropharynx BD1B
- Pancreatic Duct BF1
  - Gallbladder and Bile Buct BF14
- Patella
  - Left BQ1WZZZ
  - Right BQ1VZZZ
- Pelvis BR1C
- Pelvis and Abdomen BW11
- Pharynix B91G
- Ribs
  - Left BP1YZZZ
  - Right BP1XZZZ
- Sacrum BR1F
- Scapula
  - Left BP17ZZZ
  - Right BP16ZZZ
- Shoulder
  - Left BP19
  - Right BP18
- Sinus, Intracranial B512
- Spinal Cord BØ1B
- Spine
  - Cervical BR1Ø
  - Lumbar BR19
  - Thoracic BR17
  - Whole BR1G
- Sternum BR1H
- Stomach BD12
- Toe
  - Left BQ1QZZZ
  - Right BQ1PZZZ
- Tracheobronchial Tree
  - Bilateral BB19YZZ
  - Left BB18YZZ
  - Right BB17YZZ
- Ureter
  - Ileal Loop and Kidney BT1G
  - Kidney and Bladder BT14
    - Left BT1F
    - Right BT1D
  - Left BT17
  - Right BT16
- Urethra BT15
- Urethra and Bladder BT1B
- Uterus BU16
- Uterus and Fallopian Tube BU18
- Vagina BU19
- Vasa Vasorum BV18
- Vein
  - Cerebellar B511
  - Cerebral B511
  - Epidural B51Ø
  - Jugular
    - Bilateral B515
    - Left B514
    - Right B513
  - Lower Extremity
    - Bilateral B51D
    - Left B51C
    - Right B51B
  - Other B51V
  - Pelvic (Iliac)
    - Left B51G
    - Right B51F
  - Pelvic (Iliac) Bilateral B51H
  - Portal B51T
  - Pulmonary
    - Bilateral B51S
    - Left B51R
    - Right B51Q
  - Renal
    - Bilateral B51L
    - Left B51K
    - Right B51J
  - Spanchnic B51T
  - Subclavian
    - Left B517
    - Right B516
  - Upper Extremity
    - Bilateral B51P
    - Left B51N

Subterms under main terms may continue to next column or page

Fluoroscopy — *continued*
Vein — *continued*
Upper Extremity — *continued*
Right B51M
Vena Cava
Inferior B519
Superior B518
Wrist
Left BP1M
Right BP1L
Fluoroscopy, laser intraoperative
see Fluoroscopy, Heart B21
see Fluoroscopy, Lower Arteries B41
see Fluoroscopy, Upper Arteries B31
Flushing *see* Irrigation
Foley catheter *use* Drainage Device
Fontan completion procedure Stage II *see* Bypass, Vena Cava, Inferior Ø61Ø
Foramen magnum *use* Occipital Bone
Foramen of Monro (intraventricular) *use* Cerebral Ventricle
Foreskin *use* Prepuce
Formula™ Balloon-Expandable Renal Stent System *use* Intraluminal Device
Fosfomycin Anti-infective XWØ
Fosfomycin injection *use* Fosfomycin Anti-infective
Fossa of Rosenmuller *use* Nasopharynx
Fostamatinib XWØ
Fourth cranial nerve *use* Trochlear Nerve
Fourth ventricle *use* Cerebral Ventricle
Fovea
use Retina, Left
use Retina, Right
Fragmentation
Ampulla of Vater ØFFC
Anus ØDFQ
Appendix ØDFJ
Artery
Anterior Tibial
Left Ø4FQ3Z
Right Ø4FP3Z
Axillary
Left Ø3F63Z
Right Ø3F53Z
Brachial
Left Ø3F83Z
Right Ø3F73Z
Common Iliac
Left Ø4FD3Z
Right Ø4FC3Z
Coronary
Four or More Arteries Ø2F33ZZ
One Artery Ø2FØ3ZZ
Three Arteries Ø2F23ZZ
Two Arteries Ø2F13ZZ
External Iliac
Left Ø4FJ3Z
Right Ø4FH3Z
Femoral
Left Ø4FL3Z
Right Ø4FK3Z
Innominate Ø3F23Z
Internal Iliac
Left Ø4FF3Z
Right Ø4FE3Z
Intracranial Ø3FG3Z
Lower Ø4FY3Z
Peroneal
Left Ø4FU3Z
Right Ø4FT3Z
Popliteal
Left Ø4FN3Z
Right Ø4FM3Z
Posterior Tibial
Left Ø4FS3Z
Right Ø4FR3Z
Pulmonary
Left Ø2FR3Z
Right Ø2FQ3Z
Pulmonary Trunk Ø2FP3Z
Radial
Left Ø3FC3Z
Right Ø3FB3Z
Subclavian
Left Ø3F43Z
Right Ø3F33Z
Ulnar
Left Ø3FA3Z

Fragmentation — *continued*
Artery — *continued*
Ulnar — *continued*
Right Ø3F93Z
Upper Ø3FY3Z
Bladder ØTFB
Bladder Neck ØTFC
Bronchus
Lingula ØBF9
Lower Lobe
Left ØBFB
Right ØBF6
Main
Left ØBF7
Right ØBF3
Middle Lobe, Right ØBF5
Upper Lobe
Left ØBF8
Right ØBF4
Carina ØBF2
Cavity, Cranial ØWF1
Cecum ØDFH
Cerebral Ventricle ØØF6
Colon
Ascending ØDFK
Descending ØDFM
Sigmoid ØDFN
Transverse ØDFL
Duct
Common Bile ØFF9
Cystic ØFF8
Hepatic
Common ØFF7
Left ØFF6
Right ØFF5
Pancreatic ØFFD
Accessory ØFFF
Parotid
Left ØCFC
Right ØCFB
Duodenum ØDF9
Epidural Space, Intracranial ØØF3
Esophagus ØDF5
Fallopian Tube
Left ØUF6
Right ØUF5
Fallopian Tubes, Bilateral ØUF7
Gallbladder ØFF4
Gastrointestinal Tract ØWFP
Genitourinary Tract ØWFR
Ileum ØDFB
Intestine
Large ØDFE
Left ØDFG
Right ØDFF
Small ØDF8
Jejunum ØDFA
Kidney Pelvis
Left ØTF4
Right ØTF3
Mediastinum ØWFC
Oral Cavity and Throat ØWF3
Pelvic Cavity ØWFJ
Pericardial Cavity ØWFD
Pericardium Ø2FN
Peritoneal Cavity ØWFG
Pleural Cavity
Left ØWFB
Right ØWF9
Rectum ØDFP
Respiratory Tract ØWFQ
Spinal Canal ØØFU
Stomach ØDF6
Subarachnoid Space, Intracranial ØØF5
Subdural Space, Intracranial ØØF4
Trachea ØBF1
Ureter
Left ØTF7
Right ØTF6
Urethra ØTFD
Uterus ØUF9
Vein
Axillary
Left Ø5F83Z
Right Ø5F73Z
Basilic
Left Ø5FC3Z
Right Ø5FB3Z

Fragmentation — *continued*
Vein — *continued*
Brachial
Left Ø5FA3Z
Right Ø5F93Z
Cephalic
Left Ø5FF3Z
Right Ø5FD3Z
Common Iliac
Left Ø6FD3Z
Right Ø6FC3Z
External Iliac
Left Ø6FG3Z
Right Ø6FF3Z
Femoral
Left Ø6FN3Z
Right Ø6FM3Z
Hypogastric
Left Ø6FJ3Z
Right Ø6FH3Z
Innominate
Left Ø5F43Z
Right Ø5F33Z
Lower Ø6FY3Z
Pulmonary
Left Ø2FT3Z
Right Ø2FS3Z
Saphenous
Left Ø6FQ3Z
Right Ø6FP3Z
Subclavian
Left Ø5F63Z
Right Ø5F53Z
Upper Ø5FY3Z
Vitreous
Left Ø8F5
Right Ø8F4
Fragmentation, Ultrasonic *see* Fragmentation, Artery
Freestyle (Stentless) Aortic Root Bioprosthesis *use* Zooplastic Tissue in Heart and Great Vessels
Frenectomy
see Excision, Mouth and Throat ØCB
see Resection, Mouth and Throat ØCT
Frenoplasty, frenuloplasty
see Repair, Mouth and Throat ØCQ
see Replacement, Mouth and Throat ØCR
see Supplement, Mouth and Throat ØCU
Frenotomy
see Drainage, Mouth and Throat ØC9
see Release, Mouth and Throat ØCN
Frenulotomy
see Drainage, Mouth and Throat ØC9
see Release, Mouth and Throat ØCN
Frenulum labii inferioris *use* Lower Lip
Frenulum labii superioris *use* Upper Lip
Frenulum linguae *use* Tongue
Frenulumectomy
see Excision, Mouth and Throat ØCB
see Resection, Mouth and Throat ØCT
Frontal lobe *use* Cerebral Hemisphere
Frontal vein
use Face Vein, Left
use Face Vein, Right
Frozen elephant trunk (FET) technique, aortic arch replacement
see New Technology, Cardiovascular System X2R
see Replacement, Heart and Great Vessels Ø2R
Frozen elephant trunk (FET) technique, thoracic aorta restriction
see New Technology, Cardiovascular System X2V
see Restriction, Heart and Great Vessels Ø2V
FUJIFILM EP-7ØØØX System for Oxygen Saturation Endoscopic Imaging (OXEI) *see* New Technology, Gastrointestinal System XD2
Fulguration *see* Destruction
Fundoplication, gastroesophageal *see* Restriction, Esophagogastric Junction ØDV4
Fundus uteri *use* Uterus
Fusion
Acromioclavicular
Left ØRGH
Right ØRGG
Ankle
Left ØSGG
Open-truss Design Internal Fixation Device XRGKØB9
Right ØSGF

- **Fusion** — *continued*
  - Ankle — *continued*
    - Right — *continued*
      - Open-truss Design Internal Fixation Device XRGJØB9
  - Carpal
    - Left ØRGR
    - Right ØRGQ
  - Carpometacarpal
    - Left ØRGT
    - Right ØRGS
  - Cervical Vertebral ØRG1
    - 2 or more ØRG2
  - Cervicothoracic Vertebral ØRG4
  - Coccygeal ØSG6
  - Elbow
    - Left ØRGM
    - Right ØRGL
  - Finger Phalangeal
    - Left ØRGX
    - Right ØRGW
  - Hip
    - Left ØSGB
    - Right ØSG9
  - Knee
    - Left ØSGD
    - Right ØSGC
  - Lumbar Vertebral ØSGØ
    - 2 or more ØSG1
      - Interbody Fusion Device, Custom-Made Anatomically Designed XRGC
    - Interbody Fusion Device, Custom-Made Anatomically Designed XRGB
  - Lumbosacral ØSG3
    - Interbody Fusion Device, Custom-Made Anatomically Designed XRGD
  - Metacarpophalangeal
    - Left ØRGV
    - Right ØRGU
  - Metatarsal-Phalangeal
    - Left ØSGN
    - Right ØSGM
  - Occipital-cervical ØRGØ
  - Sacrococcygeal ØSG5
  - Sacroiliac
    - Internal Fixation Device with Tulip Connector XRG
    - Left ØSG8
    - Right ØSG7
  - Shoulder
    - Left ØRGK
    - Right ØRGJ
  - Sternoclavicular
    - Left ØRGF
    - Right ØRGE
  - Tarsal
    - Left ØSGJ
      - Open-truss Design Internal Fixation Device XRGMØB9
    - Right ØSGH
      - Open-truss Design Internal Fixation Device XRGLØB9
  - Tarsometatarsal
    - Left ØSGL
    - Right ØSGK
  - Temporomandibular
    - Left ØRGD
    - Right ØRGC
  - Thoracic Vertebral ØRG6
    - 2 to 7 ØRG7
    - 8 or more ØRG8
  - Thoracolumbar Vertebral ØRGA
    - Interbody Fusion Device, Custom-Made Anatomically Designed XRGA
  - Toe Phalangeal
    - Left ØSGQ
    - Right ØSGP
  - Wrist
    - Left ØRGP
    - Right ØRGN
- **Fusion screw (compression) (lag) (locking)**
  - *use* Internal Fixation Device in Lower Joints
  - *use* Internal Fixation Device in Upper Joints

G

- **Gait training** *see* Motor Treatment, Rehabilitation FØ7
- **Galea aponeurotica** *use* Subcutaneous Tissue and Fascia, Scalp
- **Gammaglobulin** *use* Globulin
- **GammaTile™** *use* Radioactive Element, Cesium-131 Collagen Implant in ØØH
- **GAMUNEX-C, for COVID-19 treatment** *use* High-Dose Intravenous Immune Globulin
- **Ganglion impar (ganglion of Walther)** *use* Sacral Sympathetic Nerve
- **Ganglionectomy**
  - Destruction of lesion *see* Destruction
  - Excision of lesion *see* Excision
- **Gasserian ganglion** *use* Trigeminal Nerve
- **Gastrectomy**
  - Partial *see* Excision, Stomach ØDB6
  - Total *see* Resection, Stomach ØDT6
  - Vertical (sleeve) *see* Excision, Stomach ØDB6
- **Gastric electrical stimulation (GES) lead** *use* Stimulator Lead in Gastrointestinal System
- **Gastric lymph node** *use* Lymphatic, Aortic
- **Gastric pacemaker lead** *use* Stimulator Lead in Gastrointestinal System
- **Gastric plexus** *use* Abdominal Sympathetic Nerve
- **Gastrocnemius muscle**
  - *use* Lower Leg Muscle, Left
  - *use* Lower Leg Muscle, Right
- **Gastrocolic ligament** *use* Omentum
- **Gastrocolic omentum** *use* Omentum
- **Gastrocolostomy**
  - *see* Bypass, Gastrointestinal System ØD1
  - *see* Drainage, Gastrointestinal System ØD9
- **Gastroduodenal artery** *use* Hepatic Artery
- **Gastroduodenectomy**
  - *see* Excision, Gastrointestinal System ØDB
  - *see* Resection, Gastrointestinal System ØDT
- **Gastroduodenoscopy** ØDJØ8ZZ
- **Gastroenteroplasty**
  - *see* Repair, Gastrointestinal System ØDQ
  - *see* Supplement, Gastrointestinal System ØDU
- **Gastroenterostomy**
  - *see* Bypass, Gastrointestinal System ØD1
  - *see* Drainage, Gastrointestinal System ØD9
- **Gastroesophageal (GE) junction** *use* Esophagogastric Junction
- **Gastrogastrostomy**
  - *see* Bypass, Stomach ØD16
  - *see* Drainage, Stomach ØD96
- **Gastrohepatic omentum** *use* Omentum
- **Gastrojejunostomy**
  - *see* Bypass, Stomach ØD16
  - *see* Drainage, Stomach ØD96
- **Gastrolysis** *see* Release, Stomach ØDN6
- **Gastropexy**
  - *see* Repair, Stomach ØDQ6
  - *see* Reposition, Stomach ØDS6
- **Gastrophrenic ligament** *use* Omentum
- **Gastroplasty**
  - *see* Repair, Stomach ØDQ6
  - *see* Supplement, Stomach ØDU6
- **Gastroplication** *see* Restriction, Stomach ØDV6
- **Gastropylorectomy** *see* Excision, Gastrointestinal System ØDB
- **Gastrorrhaphy** *see* Repair, Stomach ØDQ6
- **Gastroscopy** ØDJ68ZZ
- **Gastrosplenic ligament** *use* Omentum
- **Gastrostomy**
  - *see* Bypass, Stomach ØD16
  - *see* Drainage, Stomach ØD96
- **Gastrotomy** *see* Drainage, Stomach ØD96
- **Gemellus muscle**
  - *use* Hip Muscle, Left
  - *use* Hip Muscle, Right
- **Geniculate ganglion** *use* Facial Nerve
- **Geniculate nucleus** *use* Thalamus
- **Genioglossus muscle** *use* Tongue, Palate, Pharynx Muscle
- **Genioplasty** *see* Alteration, Jaw, Lower ØWØ5
- **Genitofemoral nerve** *use* Lumbar Plexus
- **GIAPREZA™** *use* Vasopressor
- **Gilteritinib Antineoplastic** XWØDXV5
- **Gingivectomy** *see* Excision, Mouth and Throat ØCB
- **Gingivoplasty**
  - *see* Repair, Mouth and Throat ØCQ
  - *see* Replacement, Mouth and Throat ØCR
  - *see* Supplement, Mouth and Throat ØCU
- **Glans penis** *use* Prepuce
- **Glenohumeral joint**
  - *use* Shoulder Joint, Left
  - *use* Shoulder Joint, Right
- **Glenohumeral ligament**
  - *use* Shoulder Bursa and Ligament, Left
  - *use* Shoulder Bursa and Ligament, Right
- **Glenoid fossa (of scapula)**
  - *use* Glenoid Cavity, Left
  - *use* Glenoid Cavity, Right
- **Glenoid ligament (labrum)**
  - *use* Shoulder Joint, Left
  - *use* Shoulder Joint, Right
- **Globus pallidus** *use* Basal Ganglia
- **Glofitamab Antineoplastic** XWØ
- **Glomectomy**
  - *see* Excision, Endocrine System ØGB
  - *see* Resection, Endocrine System ØGT
- **Glossectomy**
  - *see* Excision, Tongue ØCB7
  - *see* Resection, Tongue ØCT7
- **Glossoepiglottic fold** *use* Epiglottis
- **Glossopexy**
  - *see* Repair, Tongue ØCQ7
  - *see* Reposition, Tongue ØCS7
- **Glossoplasty**
  - *see* Repair, Tongue ØCQ7
  - *see* Replacement, Tongue ØCR7
  - *see* Supplement, Tongue ØCU7
- **Glossorrhaphy** *see* Repair, Tongue ØCQ7
- **Glossotomy** *see* Drainage, Tongue ØC97
- **Glottis** *use* Larynx
- **Gluteal Artery Perforator Flap**
  - Replacement
    - Bilateral ØHRVØ79
    - Left ØHRUØ79
    - Right ØHRTØ79
  - Transfer
    - Left ØKXG
    - Right ØKXF
- **Gluteal lymph node** *use* Lymphatic, Pelvis
- **Gluteal vein**
  - *use* Hypogastric Vein, Left
  - *use* Hypogastric Vein, Right
- **Gluteus maximus muscle**
  - *use* Hip Muscle, Left
  - *use* Hip Muscle, Right
- **Gluteus medius muscle**
  - *use* Hip Muscle, Left
  - *use* Hip Muscle, Right
- **Gluteus minimus muscle**
  - *use* Hip Muscle, Left
  - *use* Hip Muscle, Right
- **GORE EXCLUDER® AAA Endoprosthesis**
  - *use* Intraluminal Device
  - *use* Intraluminal Device, Branched or Fenestrated, One or Two Arteries in Ø4V
  - *use* Intraluminal Device, Branched or Fenestrated, Three or More Arteries in Ø4V
- **GORE EXCLUDER® IBE Endoprosthesis** *use* Intraluminal Device, Branched or Fenestrated, One or Two Arteries in Ø4V
- **GORE TAG® Thoracic Endoprosthesis** *use* Intraluminal Device
- **GORE® DUALMESH®** *use* Synthetic Substitute
- **Gracilis muscle**
  - *use* Upper Leg Muscle, Left
  - *use* Upper Leg Muscle, Right
- **Graft**
  - *see* Replacement
  - *see* Supplement
- **Great auricular nerve** *use* Cervical Plexus
- **Great cerebral vein** *use* Intracranial Vein
- **Great(er) saphenous vein**
  - *use* Saphenous Vein, Left
  - *use* Saphenous Vein, Right
- **Greater alar cartilage** *use* Nasal Mucosa and Soft Tissue
- **Greater occipital nerve** *use* Cervical Nerve
- **Greater Omentum** *use* Omentum
- **Greater splanchnic nerve** *use* Thoracic Sympathetic Nerve
- **Greater superficial petrosal nerve** *use* Facial Nerve
- **Greater trochanter**
  - *use* Upper Femur, Left
  - *use* Upper Femur, Right

Greater tuberosity
use Humeral Head, Left
use Humeral Head, Right
Greater vestibular (Bartholin's) gland *use* Vestibular Gland
Greater wing *use* Sphenoid Bone
GS-5734 *use* Remdesivir Anti-infective
Guedel airway *use* Intraluminal Device, Airway in Mouth and Throat
Guidance, catheter placement
EKG *see* Measurement, Physiological Systems 4AØ
Fluoroscopy *see* Fluoroscopy, Veins B51
Ultrasound *see* Ultrasonography, Veins B54

H

Hallux
use 1st Toe, Left
use 1st Toe, Right
Hamate bone
use Carpal, Left
use Carpal, Right
Hancock Bioprosthesis (aortic) (mitral) valve *use* Zooplastic Tissue in Heart and Great Vessels
Hancock Bioprosthetic Valved Conduit *use* Zooplastic Tissue in Heart and Great Vessels
Harmony™ transcatheter pulmonary valve (TPV) placement Ø2RH38M
Harvesting, Stem Cells *see* Pheresis, Circulatory 6A55
hdIVIG (high-dose intravenous immunoglobulin), for COVID-19 treatment *use* High-Dose Intravenous Immune Globulin
Head of fibula
use Fibula, Left
use Fibula, Right
Hearing Aid Assessment F14Z
Hearing Assessment F13Z
Hearing Device
Bone Conduction
Left Ø9HE
Right Ø9HD
Insertion of device in
Left ØNH6
Right ØNH5
Multiple Channel Cochlear Prosthesis
Left Ø9HE
Right Ø9HD
Removal of device from, Skull ØNPØ
Revision of device in, Skull ØNWØ
Single Channel Cochlear Prosthesis
Left Ø9HE
Right Ø9HD
Hearing Treatment FØ9Z
Heart Assist System
Implantable
Insertion of device in, Heart Ø2HA
Removal of device from, Heart Ø2PA
Revision of device in, Heart Ø2WA
Short-term External
Insertion of device in
Aorta, Thoracic, Descending Ø2HW3RZ
Heart Ø2HA
Removal of device from
Aorta, Thoracic, Descending Ø2PW3RZ
Heart Ø2PA
Revision of device in
Aorta, Thoracic, Descending Ø2WW3RZ
Heart Ø2WA
HeartMate 3™ LVAS *use* Implantable Heart Assist System in Heart and Great Vessels
HeartMate II® Left Ventricular Assist Device (LVAD) *use* Implantable Heart Assist System in Heart and Great Vessels
HeartMate XVE® Left Ventricular Assist Device (LVAD) *use* Implantable Heart Assist System in Heart and Great Vessels
HeartMate® implantable heart assist system *see* Insertion of device in, Heart Ø2HA
Helix
use Ear, External, Bilateral
use Ear, External, Left
use Ear, External, Right
Hematopoietic cell transplant (HCT) *see* Transfusion, Circulatory 3Ø2
Hemicolectomy *see* Resection, Gastrointestinal System ØDT
Hemicystectomy *see* Excision, Urinary System ØTB
Hemigastrectomy *see* Excision, Gastrointestinal System ØDB
Hemiglossectomy *see* Excision, Mouth and Throat ØCB
Hemilaminectomy
see Excision, Lower Bones ØQB
see Excision, Upper Bones ØPB
Hemilaminotomy
see Drainage, Lower Bones ØQ9
see Drainage, Upper Bones ØP9
see Excision, Lower Bones ØQB
see Excision, Upper Bones ØPB
see Release, Central Nervous System and Cranial Nerves ØØN
see Release, Lower Bones ØQN
see Release, Peripheral Nervous System Ø1N
see Release, Upper Bones ØPN
Hemilaryngectomy *see* Excision, Larynx ØCBS
Hemimandibulectomy *see* Excision, Head and Facial Bones ØNB
Hemimaxillectomy *see* Excision, Head and Facial Bones ØNB
Hemipylorectomy *see* Excision, Gastrointestinal System ØDB
Hemispherectomy
see Excision, Central Nervous System and Cranial Nerves ØØB
see Resection, Central Nervous System and Cranial Nerves ØØT
Hemithyroidectomy
see Excision, Endocrine System ØGB
see Resection, Endocrine System ØGT
Hemodialysis *see* Performance, Urinary 5A1D
Hemolung® Respiratory Assist System (RAS) 5AØ92ØZ
Hemospray® Endoscopic Hemostat *use* Mineral-based Topical Hemostatic Agent
Hepatectomy
see Excision, Hepatobiliary System and Pancreas ØFB
see Resection, Hepatobiliary System and Pancreas ØFT
Hepatic artery proper *use* Hepatic Artery
Hepatic flexure *use* Transverse Colon
Hepatic lymph node *use* Lymphatic, Aortic
Hepatic plexus *use* Abdominal Sympathetic Nerve
Hepatic portal vein *use* Portal Vein
Hepaticoduodenostomy
see Bypass, Hepatobiliary System and Pancreas ØF1
see Drainage, Hepatobiliary System and Pancreas ØF9
Hepaticotomy *see* Drainage, Hepatobiliary System and Pancreas ØF9
Hepatocholedochostomy *see* Drainage, Duct, Common Bile ØF99
Hepatogastric ligament *use* Omentum
Hepatopancreatic ampulla *use* Ampulla of Vater
Hepatopexy
see Repair, Hepatobiliary System and Pancreas ØFQ
see Reposition, Hepatobiliary System and Pancreas ØFS
Hepatorrhaphy *see* Repair, Hepatobiliary System and Pancreas ØFQ
Hepatotomy *see* Drainage, Hepatobiliary System and Pancreas ØF9
HEPZATO™ KIT (melphalan hydrochloride Hepatic Delivery System) *use* Melphalan Hydrochloride Antineoplastic
Herculink (RX) Elite Renal Stent System *use* Intraluminal Device
Herniorrhaphy
see Repair, Anatomical Regions, General ØWQ
see Repair, Anatomical Regions, Lower Extremities ØYQ
With synthetic substitute
see Supplement, Anatomical Regions, General ØWU
see Supplement, Anatomical Regions, Lower Extremities ØYU
HIG (hyperimmune globulin), for COVID-19 treatment *use* Hyperimmune Globulin
High-Dose Intravenous Immune Globulin, for COVID-19 treatment XW1
High-dose intravenous immunoglobulin (hdIVIG), for COVID-19 treatment *use* High-Dose Intravenous Immune Globulin
Hip (joint) liner *use* Liner in Lower Joints
HIPEC (hyperthermic intraperitoneal chemotherapy) 3EØM3ØY
HistoSonics® System *see* New Technology, Hepatobiliary System and Pancreas XF5
Histotripsy, liver *see* New Technology, Hepatobiliary System and Pancreas XF5
hIVIG (hyperimmune intravenous immunoglobulin), for COVID-19 treatment *use* Hyperimmune Globulin
Holter Monitoring 4A12X45
Holter valve ventricular shunt *use* Synthetic Substitute
Human angiotensin II, synthetic *use* Vasopressor
Humeroradial joint
use Elbow Joint, Left
use Elbow Joint, Right
Humeroulnar joint
use Elbow Joint, Left
use Elbow Joint, Right
Humerus, distal
use Humeral Shaft, Left
use Humeral Shaft, Right
Hydrocelectomy *see* Excision, Male Reproductive System ØVB
Hydrotherapy
Assisted exercise in pool *see* Motor Treatment, Rehabilitation FØ7
Whirlpool *see* Activities of Daily Living Treatment, Rehabilitation FØ8
Hymenectomy
see Excision, Hymen ØUBK
see Resection, Hymen ØUTK
Hymenoplasty
see Repair, Hymen ØUQK
see Supplement, Hymen ØUUK
Hymenorrhaphy *see* Repair, Hymen ØUQK
Hymenotomy
see Division, Hymen ØU8K
see Drainage, Hymen ØU9K
Hyoglossus muscle *use* Tongue, Palate, Pharynx Muscle
Hyoid artery
use Thyroid Artery, Left
use Thyroid Artery, Right
Hyperalimentation *see* Introduction of substance in or on
Hyperbaric oxygenation
Decompression sickness treatment *see* Decompression, Circulatory 6A15
Other treatment *see* Assistance, Circulatory 5AØ5
Hyperimmune globulin *use* Globulin
Hyperimmune Globulin, for COVID-19 treatment XW1
Hyperimmune intravenous immunoglobulin (hIVIG), for COVID-19 treatment *use* Hyperimmune Globulin
Hyperthermia
Radiation Therapy
Abdomen DWY38ZZ
Adrenal Gland DGY28ZZ
Bile Ducts DFY28ZZ
Bladder DTY28ZZ
Bone Marrow D7YØ8ZZ
Bone, Other DPYC8ZZ
Brain DØYØ8ZZ
Brain Stem DØY18ZZ
Breast
Left DMYØ8ZZ
Right DMY18ZZ
Bronchus DBY18ZZ
Cervix DUY18ZZ
Chest DWY28ZZ
Chest Wall DBY78ZZ
Colon DDY58ZZ
Diaphragm DBY88ZZ
Duodenum DDY28ZZ
Ear D9YØ8ZZ
Esophagus DDYØ8ZZ
Eye D8YØ8ZZ
Femur DPY98ZZ
Fibula DPYB8ZZ
Gallbladder DFY18ZZ
Gland
Adrenal DGY28ZZ
Parathyroid DGY48ZZ
Pituitary DGYØ8ZZ
Thyroid DGY58ZZ

Hyperthermia — *continued*
Radiation Therapy — *continued*
Glands, Salivary D9Y68ZZ
Head and Neck DWY18ZZ
Hemibody DWY48ZZ
Humerus DPY68ZZ
Hypopharynx D9Y38ZZ
Ileum DDY48ZZ
Jejunum DDY38ZZ
Kidney DTY08ZZ
Larynx D9YB8ZZ
Liver DFY08ZZ
Lung DBY28ZZ
Lymphatics
Abdomen D7Y68ZZ
Axillary D7Y48ZZ
Inguinal D7Y88ZZ
Neck D7Y38ZZ
Pelvis D7Y78ZZ
Thorax D7Y58ZZ
Mandible DPY38ZZ
Maxilla DPY28ZZ
Mediastinum DBY68ZZ
Mouth D9Y48ZZ
Nasopharynx D9YD8ZZ
Neck and Head DWY18ZZ
Nerve, Peripheral D0Y78ZZ
Nose D9Y18ZZ
Oropharynx D9YF8ZZ
Ovary DUY08ZZ
Palate
Hard D9Y88ZZ
Soft D9Y98ZZ
Pancreas DFY38ZZ
Parathyroid Gland DGY48ZZ
Pelvic Bones DPY88ZZ
Pelvic Region DWY68ZZ
Pineal Body DGY18ZZ
Pituitary Gland DGY08ZZ
Pleura DBY58ZZ
Prostate DVY08ZZ
Radius DPY78ZZ
Rectum DDY78ZZ
Rib DPY58ZZ
Sinuses D9Y78ZZ
Skin
Abdomen DHY88ZZ
Arm DHY48ZZ
Back DHY78ZZ
Buttock DHY98ZZ
Chest DHY68ZZ
Face DHY28ZZ
Leg DHYB8ZZ
Neck DHY38ZZ
Skull DPY08ZZ
Spinal Cord D0Y68ZZ
Spleen D7Y28ZZ
Sternum DPY48ZZ
Stomach DDY18ZZ
Testis DVY18ZZ
Thymus D7Y18ZZ
Thyroid Gland DGY58ZZ
Tibia DPYB8ZZ
Tongue D9Y58ZZ
Trachea DBY08ZZ
Ulna DPY78ZZ
Ureter DTY18ZZ
Urethra DTY38ZZ
Uterus DUY28ZZ
Whole Body DWY58ZZ
Whole Body 6A3Z
Hyperthermic Intraperitoneal Chemotherapy (HIPEC) 3E0M30Y
Hypnosis GZFZZZZ
Hypogastric artery
use Internal Iliac Artery, Left
use Internal Iliac Artery, Right
Hypopharynx *use* Pharynx
Hypophysectomy
see Excision, Gland, Pituitary 0GB0
see Resection, Gland, Pituitary 0GT0
Hypophysis *use* Pituitary Gland
Hypothalamotomy *see* Destruction, Thalamus 0059
Hypothenar muscle
use Hand Muscle, Left
use Hand Muscle, Right
Hypothermia, Whole Body 6A4Z
Hysterectomy
Supracervical *see* Resection, Uterus 0UT9
Total *see* Resection, Uterus 0UT9
Hysterolysis *see* Release, Uterus 0UN9
Hysteropexy
see Repair, Uterus 0UQ9
see Reposition, Uterus 0US9
Hysteroplasty *see* Repair, Uterus 0UQ9
Hysterorrhaphy *see* Repair, Uterus 0UQ9
Hysteroscopy 0UJD8ZZ
Hysterotomy *see* Drainage, Uterus 0U99
Hysterotrachelectomy
see Resection, Cervix 0UTC
see Resection, Uterus 0UT9
Hysterotracheloplasty *see* Repair, Uterus 0UQ9
Hysterotrachelorrhaphy *see* Repair, Uterus 0UQ9

I

IABP (Intra-aortic balloon pump) *see* Assistance, Cardiac 5A02
IAEMT (Intraoperative anesthetic effect monitoring and titration) *see* Monitoring, Central Nervous 4A10
IASD® (InterAtrial Shunt Device), Corvia *use* Synthetic Substitute
Idarucizumab, Pradaxa® (dabigatran) reversal agent *use* Other Therapeutic Substance
Idecabtagene Vicleucel *use* Idecabtagene Vicleucel Immunotherapy
Idecabtagene Vicleucel Immunotherapy XW0
Ide-cel *use* Idecabtagene Vicleucel Immunotherapy
iFuse Bedrock™ Granite Implant System *use* Internal Fixation Device with Tulip Connector in New Technology
IGIV-C, for COVID-19 treatment *use* Hyperimmune Globulin
IHD (Intermittent hemodialysis) 5A1D70Z
Ileal artery *use* Superior Mesenteric Artery
Ileectomy
see Excision, Ileum 0DBB
see Resection, Ileum 0DTB
Ileocolic artery *use* Superior Mesenteric Artery
Ileocolic vein *use* Colic Vein
Ileopexy
see Repair, Ileum 0DQB
see Reposition, Ileum 0DSB
Ileorrhaphy *see* Repair, Ileum 0DQB
Ileoscopy 0DJD8ZZ
Ileostomy
see Bypass, Ileum 0D1B
see Drainage, Ileum 0D9B
Ileotomy *see* Drainage, Ileum 0D9B
Ileoureterostomy *see* Bypass, Urinary System 0T1
Iliac crest
use Pelvic Bone, Left
use Pelvic Bone, Right
Iliac fascia
use Subcutaneous Tissue and Fascia, Left Upper Leg
use Subcutaneous Tissue and Fascia, Right Upper Leg
Iliac lymph node *use* Lymphatic, Pelvis
Iliacus muscle
use Hip Muscle, Left
use Hip Muscle, Right
Iliofemoral ligament
use Hip Bursa and Ligament, Left
use Hip Bursa and Ligament, Right
Iliohypogastric nerve *use* Lumbar Plexus
Ilioinguinal nerve *use* Lumbar Plexus
Iliolumbar artery
use Internal Iliac Artery, Left
use Internal Iliac Artery, Right
Iliolumbar ligament *use* Lower Spine Bursa and Ligament
Iliotibial tract (band)
use Subcutaneous Tissue and Fascia, Left Upper Leg
use Subcutaneous Tissue and Fascia, Right Upper Leg
Ilium
use Pelvic Bone, Left
use Pelvic Bone, Right
Ilizarov external fixator
use External Fixation Device, Ring in 0PH
Ilizarov external fixator — *continued*
use External Fixation Device, Ring in 0PS
use External Fixation Device, Ring in 0QH
use External Fixation Device, Ring in 0QS
Ilizarov-Vecklich device
use External Fixation Device, Limb Lengthening in 0PH
use External Fixation Device, Limb Lengthening in 0QH
Imaging, diagnostic
see Computerized Tomography (CT Scan)
see Fluoroscopy
see Magnetic Resonance Imaging (MRI)
see Plain Radiography
see Ultrasonography
Imdevimab (REGN10987) and Casirivimab (REGN10933) *use* REGN-COV2 Monoclonal Antibody
IMFINZI® *use* Durvalumab Antineoplastic
Imipenem-cilastatin-relebactam Anti-infective XW0
IMI/REL *use* Imipenem-cilastatin-relebactam Anti-infective
Immobilization
Abdominal Wall 2W33X
Arm
Lower
Left 2W3DX
Right 2W3CX
Upper
Left 2W3BX
Right 2W3AX
Back 2W35X
Chest Wall 2W34X
Extremity
Lower
Left 2W3MX
Right 2W3LX
Upper
Left 2W39X
Right 2W38X
Face 2W31X
Finger
Left 2W3KX
Right 2W3JX
Foot
Left 2W3TX
Right 2W3SX
Hand
Left 2W3FX
Right 2W3EX
Head 2W30X
Inguinal Region
Left 2W37X
Right 2W36X
Leg
Lower
Left 2W3RX
Right 2W3QX
Upper
Left 2W3PX
Right 2W3NX
Neck 2W32X
Thumb
Left 2W3HX
Right 2W3GX
Toe
Left 2W3VX
Right 2W3UX
Immunization *see* Introduction of Serum, Toxoid, and Vaccine
Immunoglobulin *use* Globulin
Immunotherapy *see* Introduction of Immunotherapeutic Substance
Immunotherapy, antineoplastic
Interferon *see* Introduction of Low-dose Interleukin-2
Interleukin-2, high-dose *see* Introduction of High-dose Interleukin-2
Interleukin-2, low-dose *see* Introduction of Low-dose Interleukin-2
Monoclonal antibody *see* Introduction of Monoclonal Antibody
Proleukin, high-dose *see* Introduction of High-dose Interleukin-2
Proleukin, low-dose *see* Introduction of Low-dose Interleukin-2

Impella® 5.5 with SmartAssist® System *use* Conduit to Short-term External Heart Assist System in New Technology
Impella® heart pump *use* Short-term External Heart Assist System in Heart and Great Vessels
Impeller Pump
Continuous, Output 5A0221D
Intermittent, Output 5A0211D
Implantable cardioverter-defibrillator (ICD) *use* Defibrillator Generator in 0JH
Implantable drug infusion pump (anti-spasmodic) (chemotherapy) (pain) *use* Infusion Device, Pump in Subcutaneous Tissue and Fascia
Implantable glucose monitoring device *use* Monitoring Device
Implantable hemodynamic monitor (IHM) *use* Monitoring Device, Hemodynamic in 0JH
Implantable hemodynamic monitoring system (IHMS) *use* Monitoring Device, Hemodynamic in 0JH
Implantable Miniature Telescope™ (IMT) *use* Synthetic Substitute, Intraocular Telescope in 08R
Implantation
see Insertion
see Replacement
Implanted (venous)(access) port *use* Vascular Access Device, Totally Implantable in Subcutaneous Tissue and Fascia
IMV (intermittent mandatory ventilation) *see* Assistance, Respiratory 5A09
In Vitro Fertilization 8E0ZXY1
Incision, abscess *see* Drainage
Incudectomy
see Excision, Ear, Nose, Sinus 09B
see Resection, Ear, Nose, Sinus 09T
Incudopexy
see Repair, Ear, Nose, Sinus 09Q
see Reposition, Ear, Nose, Sinus 09S
Incus
use Auditory Ossicle, Left
use Auditory Ossicle, Right
Induction of labor
Artificial rupture of membranes *see* Drainage, Pregnancy 109
Oxytocin *see* Introduction of Hormone
InDura, intrathecal catheter (1P) (spinal) *use* Infusion Device
Inebilizumab-cdon XW0
Inferior cardiac nerve *use* Thoracic Sympathetic Nerve
Inferior cerebellar vein *use* Intracranial Vein
Inferior cerebral vein *use* Intracranial Vein
Inferior epigastric artery
use External Iliac Artery, Left
use External Iliac Artery, Right
Inferior epigastric lymph node *use* Lymphatic, Pelvis
Inferior genicular artery
use Popliteal Artery, Left
use Popliteal Artery, Right
Inferior gluteal artery
use Internal Iliac Artery, Left
use Internal Iliac Artery, Right
Inferior gluteal nerve *use* Sacral Plexus
Inferior hypogastric plexus *use* Abdominal Sympathetic Nerve
Inferior labial artery *use* Face Artery
Inferior longitudinal muscle *use* Tongue, Palate, Pharynx Muscle
Inferior mesenteric ganglion *use* Abdominal Sympathetic Nerve
Inferior mesenteric lymph node *use* Lymphatic, Mesenteric
Inferior mesenteric plexus *use* Abdominal Sympathetic Nerve
Inferior oblique muscle
use Extraocular Muscle, Left
use Extraocular Muscle, Right
Inferior pancreaticoduodenal artery *use* Superior Mesenteric Artery
Inferior phrenic artery *use* Abdominal Aorta
Inferior rectus muscle
use Extraocular Muscle, Left
use Extraocular Muscle, Right
Inferior suprarenal artery
use Renal Artery, Left
use Renal Artery, Right
Inferior tarsal plate
use Lower Eyelid, Left
Inferior tarsal plate — *continued*
use Lower Eyelid, Right
Inferior thyroid vein
use Innominate Vein, Left
use Innominate Vein, Right
Inferior tibiofibular joint
use Ankle Joint, Left
use Ankle Joint, Right
Inferior turbinate *use* Nasal Turbinate
Inferior ulnar collateral artery
use Brachial Artery, Left
use Brachial Artery, Right
Inferior vesical artery
use Internal Iliac Artery, Left
use Internal Iliac Artery, Right
Infraauricular lymph node *use* Lymphatic, Head
Infraclavicular (deltopectoral) lymph node
use Lymphatic, Left Upper Extremity
use Lymphatic, Right Upper Extremity
Infrahyoid muscle
use Neck Muscle, Left
use Neck Muscle, Right
Infraparotid lymph node *use* Lymphatic, Head
Infraspinatus fascia
use Subcutaneous Tissue and Fascia, Left Upper Arm
use Subcutaneous Tissue and Fascia, Right Upper Arm
Infraspinatus muscle
use Shoulder Muscle, Left
use Shoulder Muscle, Right
Infundibulopelvic ligament *use* Uterine Supporting Structure
Infusion *see* Introduction of substance in or on
Infusion Device, Pump
Insertion of device in
Abdomen 0JH8
Back 0JH7
Chest 0JH6
Lower Arm
Left 0JHH
Right 0JHG
Lower Leg
Left 0JHP
Right 0JHN
Trunk 0JHT
Upper Arm
Left 0JHF
Right 0JHD
Upper Leg
Left 0JHM
Right 0JHL
Removal of device from
Lower Extremity 0JPW
Trunk 0JPT
Upper Extremity 0JPV
Revision of device in
Lower Extremity 0JWW
Trunk 0JWT
Upper Extremity 0JWV
Infusion, glucarpidase
Central Vein 3E043GQ
Peripheral Vein 3E033GQ
Inguinal canal
use Inguinal Region, Bilateral
use Inguinal Region, Left
use Inguinal Region, Right
Inguinal triangle
use Inguinal Region, Bilateral
use Inguinal Region, Left
use Inguinal Region, Right
Injection *see* Introduction of substance in or on
Injection reservoir, port *use* Vascular Access Device, Totally Implantable in Subcutaneous Tissue and Fascia
Injection reservoir, pump *use* Infusion Device, Pump in Subcutaneous Tissue and Fascia
Insemination, artificial 3E0P7LZ
Insertion
Antimicrobial envelope *see* Introduction of Anti-infective
Aqueous drainage shunt
see Bypass, Eye 081
see Drainage, Eye 089
Bone, Pelvic, Internal Fixation Device with Tulip Connector XNH
Insertion — *continued*
Conduit to Short-term External Heart Assist System X2H
Intracardiac Pacemaker, Dual-Chamber X2H
Intraluminal Device, Bioprosthetic Valve X2H
Joint
Lumbar Vertebral, Posterior Spinal Motion Preservation Device XRHB018
Lumbosacral, Posterior Spinal Motion Preservation Device XRHD018
Neurostimulator Lead, Sphenopalatine Ganglion X0HK3Q8
Neurostimulator Lead with Paired Stimulation System X0HQ3R8
Products of Conception 10H0
Spinal Stabilization Device
see Insertion of device in, Lower Joints 0SH
see Insertion of device in, Upper Joints 0RH
Tibial Extension with Motion Sensors XNH
Insertion of device in
Abdominal Wall 0WHF
Acetabulum
Left 0QH5
Right 0QH4
Anal Sphincter 0DHR
Ankle Region
Left 0YHL
Right 0YHK
Anus 0DHQ
Aorta
Abdominal 04H0
Thoracic
Ascending/Arch 02HX
Descending 02HW
Arm
Lower
Left 0XHF
Right 0XHD
Upper
Left 0XH9
Right 0XH8
Artery
Anterior Tibial
Left 04HQ
Right 04HP
Axillary
Left 03H6
Right 03H5
Brachial
Left 03H8
Right 03H7
Celiac 04H1
Colic
Left 04H7
Middle 04H8
Right 04H6
Common Carotid
Left 03HJ
Right 03HH
Common Iliac
Left 04HD
Right 04HC
Coronary
Four or More Arteries 02H3
One Artery 02H0
Three Arteries 02H2
Two Arteries 02H1
External Carotid
Left 03HN
Right 03HM
External Iliac
Left 04HJ
Right 04HH
Face 03HR
Femoral
Left 04HL
Right 04HK
Foot
Left 04HW
Right 04HV
Gastric 04H2
Hand
Left 03HF
Right 03HD
Hepatic 04H3
Inferior Mesenteric 04HB
Innominate 03H2
Internal Carotid
Left 03HL

Insertion of device in — *continued*
Artery — *continued*
Internal Carotid — *continued*
Right Ø3HK
Internal Iliac
Left Ø4HF
Right Ø4HE
Internal Mammary
Left Ø3H1
Right Ø3HØ
Intracranial Ø3HG
Lower Ø4HY
Peroneal
Left Ø4HU
Right Ø4HT
Popliteal
Left Ø4HN
Right Ø4HM
Posterior Tibial
Left Ø4HS
Right Ø4HR
Pulmonary
Left Ø2HR
Right Ø2HQ
Pulmonary Trunk Ø2HP
Radial
Left Ø3HC
Right Ø3HB
Renal
Left Ø4HA
Right Ø4H9
Splenic Ø4H4
Subclavian
Left Ø3H4
Right Ø3H3
Superior Mesenteric Ø4H5
Temporal
Left Ø3HT
Right Ø3HS
Thyroid
Left Ø3HV
Right Ø3HU
Ulnar
Left Ø3HA
Right Ø3H9
Upper Ø3HY
Vertebral
Left Ø3HQ
Right Ø3HP
Atrium
Left Ø2H7
Right Ø2H6
Axilla
Left ØXH5
Right ØXH4
Back
Lower ØWHL
Upper ØWHK
Bladder ØTHB
Bladder Neck ØTHC
Bone
Ethmoid
Left ØNHG
Right ØNHF
Facial ØNHW
Frontal ØNH1
Hyoid ØNHX
Lacrimal
Left ØNHJ
Right ØNHH
Lower ØQHY
Nasal ØNHB
Occipital ØNH7
Palatine
Left ØNHL
Right ØNHK
Parietal
Left ØNH4
Right ØNH3
Pelvic
Left ØQH3
Right ØQH2
Sphenoid ØNHC
Temporal
Left ØNH6
Right ØNH5
Upper ØPHY
Zygomatic
Left ØNHN

Insertion of device in — *continued*
Bone — *continued*
Zygomatic — *continued*
Right ØNHM
Bone Marrow Ø7HT
Brain ØØHØ
Breast
Bilateral ØHHV
Left ØHHU
Right ØHHT
Bronchus
Lingula ØBH9
Lower Lobe
Left ØBHB
Right ØBH6
Main
Left ØBH7
Right ØBH3
Middle Lobe, Right ØBH5
Upper Lobe
Left ØBH8
Right ØBH4
Bursa and Ligament
Lower ØMHY
Upper ØMHX
Buttock
Left ØYH1
Right ØYHØ
Carpal
Left ØPHN
Right ØPHM
Cavity, Cranial ØWH1
Cerebral Ventricle ØØH6
Cervix ØUHC
Chest Wall ØWH8
Cisterna Chyli Ø7HL
Clavicle
Left ØPHB
Right ØPH9
Coccyx ØQHS
Cul-de-sac ØUHF
Diaphragm ØBHT
Disc
Cervical Vertebral ØRH3
Cervicothoracic Vertebral ØRH5
Lumbar Vertebral ØSH2
Lumbosacral ØSH4
Thoracic Vertebral ØRH9
Thoracolumbar Vertebral ØRHB
Duct
Hepatobiliary ØFHB
Pancreatic ØFHD
Duodenum ØDH9
Ear
Inner
Left Ø9HE
Right Ø9HD
Left Ø9HJ
Right Ø9HH
Elbow Region
Left ØXHC
Right ØXHB
Epididymis and Spermatic Cord ØVHM
Esophagus ØDH5
Lower, Magnetic Lengthening Device ØDH37JZ
Middle, Magnetic Lengthening Device ØDH27JZ
Upper, Magnetic Lengthening Device ØDH17JZ
Extremity
Lower
Left ØYHB
Right ØYH9
Upper
Left ØXH7
Right ØXH6
Eye
Left Ø8H1
Right Ø8HØ
Face ØWH2
Fallopian Tube ØUH8
Femoral Region
Left ØYH8
Right ØYH7
Femoral Shaft
Left ØQH9
Right ØQH8

Insertion of device in — *continued*
Femur
Lower
Left ØQHC
Right ØQHB
Upper
Left ØQH7
Right ØQH6
Fibula
Left ØQHK
Right ØQHJ
Foot
Left ØYHN
Right ØYHM
Gallbladder ØFH4
Gastrointestinal Tract ØWHP
Genitourinary Tract ØWHR
Gland
Endocrine ØGHS
Salivary ØCHA
Glenoid Cavity
Left ØPH8
Right ØPH7
Hand
Left ØXHK
Right ØXHJ
Head ØWHØ
Heart Ø2HA
Humeral Head
Left ØPHD
Right ØPHC
Humeral Shaft
Left ØPHG
Right ØPHF
Ileum ØDHB
Inguinal Region
Left ØYH6
Right ØYH5
Intestinal Tract
Lower Intestinal Tract ØDHD
Upper Intestinal Tract ØDHØ
Intestine
Large ØDHE
Small ØDH8
Jaw
Lower ØWH5
Upper ØWH4
Jejunum ØDHA
Joint
Acromioclavicular
Left ØRHH
Right ØRHG
Ankle
Left ØSHG
Right ØSHF
Carpal
Left ØRHR
Right ØRHQ
Carpometacarpal
Left ØRHT
Right ØRHS
Cervical Vertebral ØRH1
Cervicothoracic Vertebral ØRH4
Coccygeal ØSH6
Elbow
Left ØRHM
Right ØRHL
Finger Phalangeal
Left ØRHX
Right ØRHW
Hip
Left ØSHB
Right ØSH9
Knee
Left ØSHD
Right ØSHC
Lumbar Vertebral ØSHØ
Lumbosacral ØSH3
Metacarpophalangeal
Left ØRHV
Right ØRHU
Metatarsal-Phalangeal
Left ØSHN
Right ØSHM
Occipital-cervical ØRHØ
Sacrococcygeal ØSH5
Sacroiliac
Left ØSH8
Right ØSH7

Insertion of device in — *continued*
Joint — *continued*
Shoulder
Left ØRHK
Right ØRHJ
Sternoclavicular
Left ØRHF
Right ØRHE
Tarsal
Left ØSHJ
Right ØSHH
Tarsometatarsal
Left ØSHL
Right ØSHK
Temporomandibular
Left ØRHD
Right ØRHC
Thoracic Vertebral ØRH6
Thoracolumbar Vertebral ØRHA
Toe Phalangeal
Left ØSHQ
Right ØSHP
Wrist
Left ØRHP
Right ØRHN
Kidney ØTH5
Knee Region
Left ØYHG
Right ØYHF
Larynx ØCHS
Leg
Lower
Left ØYHJ
Right ØYHH
Upper
Left ØYHD
Right ØYHC
Liver ØFHØ
Left Lobe ØFH2
Right Lobe ØFH1
Lung
Left ØBHL
Right ØBHK
Lymphatic Ø7HN
Thoracic Duct Ø7HK
Mandible
Left ØNHV
Right ØNHT
Maxilla ØNHR
Mediastinum ØWHC
Metacarpal
Left ØPHQ
Right ØPHP
Metatarsal
Left ØQHP
Right ØQHN
Mouth and Throat ØCHY
Muscle
Lower ØKHY
Upper ØKHX
Nasal Mucosa and Soft Tissue Ø9HK
Nasopharynx Ø9HN
Neck ØWH6
Nerve
Cranial ØØHE
Peripheral Ø1HY
Nipple
Left ØHHX
Right ØHHW
Oral Cavity and Throat ØWH3
Orbit
Left ØNHQ
Right ØNHP
Ovary ØUH3
Pancreas ØFHG
Patella
Left ØQHF
Right ØQHD
Pelvic Cavity ØWHJ
Penis ØVHS
Pericardial Cavity ØWHD
Pericardium Ø2HN
Perineum
Female ØWHN
Male ØWHM
Peritoneal Cavity ØWHG
Phalanx
Finger
Left ØPHV

Insertion of device in — *continued*
Phalanx — *continued*
Finger — *continued*
Right ØPHT
Thumb
Left ØPHS
Right ØPHR
Toe
Left ØQHR
Right ØQHQ
Pleura ØBHQ
Pleural Cavity
Left ØWHB
Right ØWH9
Prostate ØVHØ
Prostate and Seminal Vesicles ØVH4
Radius
Left ØPHJ
Right ØPHH
Rectum ØDHP
Respiratory Tract ØWHQ
Retroperitoneum ØWHH
Ribs
1 to 2 ØPH1
3 or More ØPH2
Sacrum ØQH1
Scapula
Left ØPH6
Right ØPH5
Scrotum and Tunica Vaginalis ØVH8
Shoulder Region
Left ØXH3
Right ØXH2
Sinus Ø9HY
Skin ØHHPXYZ
Skull ØNHØ
Spinal Canal ØØHU
Spinal Cord ØØHV
Spleen Ø7HP
Sternum ØPHØ
Stomach ØDH6
Subcutaneous Tissue and Fascia
Abdomen ØJH8
Back ØJH7
Buttock ØJH9
Chest ØJH6
Face ØJH1
Foot
Left ØJHR
Right ØJHQ
Hand
Left ØJHK
Right ØJHJ
Head and Neck ØJHS
Lower Arm
Left ØJHH
Right ØJHG
Lower Extremity ØJHW
Lower Leg
Left ØJHP
Right ØJHN
Neck
Left ØJH5
Right ØJH4
Pelvic Region ØJHC
Perineum ØJHB
Scalp ØJHØ
Trunk ØJHT
Upper Arm
Left ØJHF
Right ØJHD
Upper Extremity ØJHV
Upper Leg
Left ØJHM
Right ØJHL
Tarsal
Left ØQHM
Right ØQHL
Tendon
Lower ØLHY
Upper ØLHX
Testis ØVHD
Thymus Ø7HM
Tibia
Left ØQHH
Right ØQHG
Tongue ØCH7
Trachea ØBH1
Tracheobronchial Tree ØBHØ

Insertion of device in — *continued*
Ulna
Left ØPHL
Right ØPHK
Ureter ØTH9
Urethra ØTHD
Uterus ØUH9
Uterus and Cervix ØUHD
Vagina ØUHG
Vagina and Cul-de-sac ØUHH
Vas Deferens ØVHR
Vein
Axillary
Left Ø5H8
Right Ø5H7
Azygos Ø5HØ
Basilic
Left Ø5HC
Right Ø5HB
Brachial
Left Ø5HA
Right Ø5H9
Cephalic
Left Ø5HF
Right Ø5HD
Colic Ø6H7
Common Iliac
Left Ø6HD
Right Ø6HC
Coronary Ø2H4
Esophageal Ø6H3
External Iliac
Left Ø6HG
Right Ø6HF
External Jugular
Left Ø5HQ
Right Ø5HP
Face
Left Ø5HV
Right Ø5HT
Femoral
Left Ø6HN
Right Ø6HM
Foot
Left Ø6HV
Right Ø6HT
Gastric Ø6H2
Hand
Left Ø5HH
Right Ø5HG
Hemiazygos Ø5H1
Hepatic Ø6H4
Hypogastric
Left Ø6HJ
Right Ø6HH
Inferior Mesenteric Ø6H6
Innominate
Left Ø5H4
Right Ø5H3
Internal Jugular
Left Ø5HN
Right Ø5HM
Intracranial Ø5HL
Lower Ø6HY
Portal Ø6H8
Pulmonary
Left Ø2HT
Right Ø2HS
Renal
Left Ø6HB
Right Ø6H9
Saphenous
Left Ø6HQ
Right Ø6HP
Splenic Ø6H1
Subclavian
Left Ø5H6
Right Ø5H5
Superior Mesenteric Ø6H5
Upper Ø5HY
Vertebral
Left Ø5HS
Right Ø5HR
Vena Cava
Inferior Ø6HØ
Superior Ø2HV
Ventricle
Left Ø2HL
Right Ø2HK

Insertion of device in — *continued*
Vertebra
Cervical ØPH3
Lumbar ØQHØ
Thoracic ØPH4
Wrist Region
Left ØXHH
Right ØXHG
Inspection
Abdominal Wall ØWJF
Ankle Region
Left ØYJL
Right ØYJK
Arm
Lower
Left ØXJF
Right ØXJD
Upper
Left ØXJ9
Right ØXJ8
Artery
Lower Ø4JY
Upper Ø3JY
Axilla
Left ØXJ5
Right ØXJ4
Back
Lower ØWJL
Upper ØWJK
Bladder ØTJB
Bone
Facial ØNJW
Lower ØQJY
Nasal ØNJB
Upper ØPJY
Bone Marrow Ø7JT
Brain ØØJØ
Breast
Left ØHJU
Right ØHJT
Bursa and Ligament
Lower ØMJY
Upper ØMJX
Buttock
Left ØYJ1
Right ØYJØ
Cavity, Cranial ØWJ1
Chest Wall ØWJ8
Cisterna Chyli Ø7JL
Diaphragm ØBJT
Disc
Cervical Vertebral ØRJ3
Cervicothoracic Vertebral ØRJ5
Lumbar Vertebral ØSJ2
Lumbosacral ØSJ4
Thoracic Vertebral ØRJ9
Thoracolumbar Vertebral ØRJB
Duct
Hepatobiliary ØFJB
Pancreatic ØFJD
Ear
Inner
Left Ø9JE
Right Ø9JD
Left Ø9JJ
Right Ø9JH
Elbow Region
Left ØXJC
Right ØXJB
Epididymis and Spermatic Cord ØVJM
Extremity
Lower
Left ØYJB
Right ØYJ9
Upper
Left ØXJ7
Right ØXJ6
Eye
Left Ø8J1XZZ
Right Ø8JØXZZ
Face ØWJ2
Fallopian Tube ØUJ8
Femoral Region
Bilateral ØYJE
Left ØYJ8
Right ØYJ7
Finger Nail ØHJQXZZ
Foot
Left ØYJN

Inspection — *continued*
Foot — *continued*
Right ØYJM
Gallbladder ØFJ4
Gastrointestinal Tract ØWJP
Genitourinary Tract ØWJR
Gland
Adrenal ØGJ5
Endocrine ØGJS
Pituitary ØGJØ
Salivary ØCJA
Great Vessel Ø2JY
Hand
Left ØXJK
Right ØXJJ
Head ØWJØ
Heart Ø2JA
Inguinal Region
Bilateral ØYJA
Left ØYJ6
Right ØYJ5
Intestinal Tract
Lower Intestinal Tract ØDJD
Upper Intestinal Tract ØDJØ
Jaw
Lower ØWJ5
Upper ØWJ4
Joint
Acromioclavicular
Left ØRJH
Right ØRJG
Ankle
Left ØSJG
Right ØSJF
Carpal
Left ØRJR
Right ØRJQ
Carpometacarpal
Left ØRJT
Right ØRJS
Cervical Vertebral ØRJ1
Cervicothoracic Vertebral ØRJ4
Coccygeal ØSJ6
Elbow
Left ØRJM
Right ØRJL
Finger Phalangeal
Left ØRJX
Right ØRJW
Hip
Left ØSJB
Right ØSJ9
Knee
Left ØSJD
Right ØSJC
Lumbar Vertebral ØSJØ
Lumbosacral ØSJ3
Metacarpophalangeal
Left ØRJV
Right ØRJU
Metatarsal-Phalangeal
Left ØSJN
Right ØSJM
Occipital-cervical ØRJØ
Sacrococcygeal ØSJ5
Sacroiliac
Left ØSJ8
Right ØSJ7
Shoulder
Left ØRJK
Right ØRJJ
Sternoclavicular
Left ØRJF
Right ØRJE
Tarsal
Left ØSJJ
Right ØSJH
Tarsometatarsal
Left ØSJL
Right ØSJK
Temporomandibular
Left ØRJD
Right ØRJC
Thoracic Vertebral ØRJ6
Thoracolumbar Vertebral ØRJA
Toe Phalangeal
Left ØSJQ
Right ØSJP

Inspection — *continued*
Joint — *continued*
Wrist
Left ØRJP
Right ØRJN
Kidney ØTJ5
Knee Region
Left ØYJG
Right ØYJF
Larynx ØCJS
Leg
Lower
Left ØYJJ
Right ØYJH
Upper
Left ØYJD
Right ØYJC
Lens
Left Ø8JKXZZ
Right Ø8JJXZZ
Liver ØFJØ
Lung
Left ØBJL
Right ØBJK
Lymphatic Ø7JN
Thoracic Duct Ø7JK
Mediastinum ØWJC
Mesentery ØDJV
Mouth and Throat ØCJY
Muscle
Extraocular
Left Ø8JM
Right Ø8JL
Lower ØKJY
Upper ØKJX
Nasal Mucosa and Soft Tissue Ø9JK
Neck ØWJ6
Nerve
Cranial ØØJE
Peripheral Ø1JY
Omentum ØDJU
Oral Cavity and Throat ØWJ3
Ovary ØUJ3
Pancreas ØFJG
Parathyroid Gland ØGJR
Pelvic Cavity ØWJJ
Penis ØVJS
Pericardial Cavity ØWJD
Perineum
Female ØWJN
Male ØWJM
Peritoneal Cavity ØWJG
Peritoneum ØDJW
Pineal Body ØGJ1
Pleura ØBJQ
Pleural Cavity
Left ØWJB
Right ØWJ9
Products of Conception 1ØJØ
Ectopic 1ØJ2
Retained 1ØJ1
Prostate and Seminal Vesicles ØVJ4
Respiratory Tract ØWJQ
Retroperitoneum ØWJH
Scrotum and Tunica Vaginalis ØVJ8
Shoulder Region
Left ØXJ3
Right ØXJ2
Sinus Ø9JY
Skin ØHJPXZZ
Skull ØNJØ
Spinal Canal ØØJU
Spinal Cord ØØJV
Spleen Ø7JP
Stomach ØDJ6
Subcutaneous Tissue and Fascia
Head and Neck ØJJS
Lower Extremity ØJJW
Trunk ØJJT
Upper Extremity ØJJV
Tendon
Lower ØLJY
Upper ØLJX
Testis ØVJD
Thymus Ø7JM
Thyroid Gland ØGJK
Toe Nail ØHJRXZZ
Trachea ØBJ1
Tracheobronchial Tree ØBJØ

Inspection — *continued*
Tympanic Membrane
Left Ø9J8
Right Ø9J7
Ureter ØTJ9
Urethra ØTJD
Uterus and Cervix ØUJD
Vagina and Cul-de-sac ØUJH
Vas Deferens ØVJR
Vein
Lower Ø6JY
Upper Ø5JY
Vulva ØUJM
Wrist Region
Left ØXJH
Right ØXJG
Instillation *see* Introduction of substance in or on
Insufflation *see* Introduction of substance in or on
Intellis™ neurostimulator *use* Stimulator Generator, Multiple Array Rechargeable in ØJH
Interatrial septum *use* Atrial Septum
InterAtrial Shunt Device IASD®, Corvia *use* Synthetic Substitute
Interbody fusion (spine) cage
use Interbody Fusion Device in Lower Joints
use Interbody Fusion Device in Upper Joints
Interbody Fusion Device, Custom-Made Anatomically Designed
Lumbar Vertebral XRGB
2 or more XRGC
Lumbosacral XRGD
Thoracolumbar Vertebral XRGA
Intercarpal joint
use Carpal Joint, Left
use Carpal Joint, Right
Intercarpal ligament
use Hand Bursa and Ligament, Left
use Hand Bursa and Ligament, Right
INTERCEPT Blood System for Plasma Pathogen Reduced Cryoprecipitated Fibrinogen Complex *use* Pathogen Reduced Cryoprecipitated Fibrinogen Complex
INTERCEPT Fibrinogen Complex *use* Pathogen Reduced Cryoprecipitated Fibrinogen Complex
Interclavicular ligament
use Shoulder Bursa and Ligament, Left
use Shoulder Bursa and Ligament, Right
Intercostal lymph node *use* Lymphatic, Thorax
Intercostal muscle
use Thorax Muscle, Left
use Thorax Muscle, Right
Intercostal nerve *use* Thoracic Nerve
Intercostobrachial nerve *use* Thoracic Nerve
Intercuneiform joint
use Tarsal Joint, Left
use Tarsal Joint, Right
Intercuneiform ligament
use Foot Bursa and Ligament, Left
use Foot Bursa and Ligament, Right
Intermediate bronchus *use* Main Bronchus, Right
Intermediate cuneiform bone
use Tarsal, Left
use Tarsal, Right
Intermittent Coronary Sinus Occlusion X2A7358
Intermittent hemodialysis (IHD) 5A1D70Z
Intermittent mandatory ventilation *see* Assistance, Respiratory 5A09
Intermittent Negative Airway Pressure
24-96 Consecutive Hours, Ventilation 5A0945B
Greater than 96 Consecutive Hours, Ventilation 5A0955B
Less than 24 Consecutive Hours, Ventilation 5A0935B
Intermittent Positive Airway Pressure
24-96 Consecutive Hours, Ventilation 5A09458
Greater than 96 Consecutive Hours, Ventilation 5A09558
Less than 24 Consecutive Hours, Ventilation 5A09358
Intermittent positive pressure breathing *see* Assistance, Respiratory 5A09
Internal anal sphincter *use* Anal Sphincter
Internal carotid artery, intracranial portion *use* Intracranial Artery
Internal carotid plexus *use* Head and Neck Sympathetic Nerve
Internal (basal) cerebral vein *use* Intracranial Vein
Internal Fixation Device with Tulip Connector
Fusion, Joint, Sacroiliac XRG
Insertion, Bone, Pelvic XNH
Internal iliac vein
use Hypogastric Vein, Left
use Hypogastric Vein, Right
Internal maxillary artery
use External Carotid Artery, Left
use External Carotid Artery, Right
Internal naris *use* Nasal Mucosa and Soft Tissue
Internal oblique muscle
use Abdomen Muscle, Left
use Abdomen Muscle, Right
Internal pudendal artery
use Internal Iliac Artery, Left
use Internal Iliac Artery, Right
Internal pudendal vein
use Hypogastric Vein, Left
use Hypogastric Vein, Right
Internal thoracic artery
use Internal Mammary Artery, Left
use Internal Mammary Artery, Right
use Subclavian Artery, Left
use Subclavian Artery, Right
Internal urethral sphincter *use* Urethra
Interphalangeal (IP) joint
use Finger Phalangeal Joint, Left
use Finger Phalangeal Joint, Right
use Toe Phalangeal Joint, Left
use Toe Phalangeal Joint, Right
Interphalangeal ligament
use Foot Bursa and Ligament, Left
use Foot Bursa and Ligament, Right
use Hand Bursa and Ligament, Left
use Hand Bursa and Ligament, Right
Interrogation, cardiac rhythm related device
Interrogation only *see* Measurement, Cardiac 4B02
With cardiac function testing *see* Measurement, Cardiac 4A02
Interruption *see* Occlusion
Interspinalis muscle
use Trunk Muscle, Left
use Trunk Muscle, Right
Interspinous ligament, cervical *use* Head and Neck Bursa and Ligament
Interspinous ligament, lumbar *use* Lower Spine Bursa and Ligament
Interspinous ligament, thoracic *use* Upper Spine Bursa and Ligament
Interspinous process spinal stabilization device
use Spinal Stabilization Device, Interspinous Process in ØRH
use Spinal Stabilization Device, Interspinous Process in ØSH
InterStim® Therapy lead *use* Neurostimulator Lead in Peripheral Nervous System
InterStim™ II Therapy neurostimulator *use* Stimulator Generator, Single Array in ØJH
InterStim™ Micro Therapy neurostimulator *use* Stimulator Generator, Single Array Rechargeable in ØJH
Intertransversarius muscle
use Trunk Muscle, Left
use Trunk Muscle, Right
Intertransverse ligament, cervical *use* Head and Neck Bursa and Ligament
Intertransverse ligament, lumbar *use* Lower Spine Bursa and Ligament
Intertransverse ligament, thoracic *use* Upper Spine Bursa and Ligament
Interventricular foramen (Monro) *use* Cerebral Ventricle
Interventricular septum *use* Ventricular Septum
Intestinal lymphatic trunk *use* Cisterna Chyli
Intracardiac Pacemaker, Dual-Chamber, Insertion X2H
Intracranial Arterial Flow, Whole Blood mRNA XXE5XT7
Intraluminal Device
Airway
Esophagus ØDH5
Mouth and Throat ØCHY
Nasopharynx Ø9HN
Bioactive
Occlusion
Common Carotid
Left Ø3LJ
Intraluminal Device — *continued*
Bioactive — *continued*
Occlusion — *continued*
Common Carotid — *continued*
Right Ø3LH
External Carotid
Left Ø3LN
Right Ø3LM
Internal Carotid
Left Ø3LL
Right Ø3LK
Intracranial Ø3LG
Vertebral
Left Ø3LQ
Right Ø3LP
Restriction
Common Carotid
Left Ø3VJ
Right Ø3VH
External Carotid
Left Ø3VN
Right Ø3VM
Internal Carotid
Left Ø3VL
Right Ø3VK
Intracranial Ø3VG
Vertebral
Left Ø3VQ
Right Ø3VP
Bioprosthetic Valve, Insertion X2H
Endobronchial Valve
Lingula ØBH9
Lower Lobe
Left ØBHB
Right ØBH6
Main
Left ØBH7
Right ØBH3
Middle Lobe, Right ØBH5
Upper Lobe
Left ØBH8
Right ØBH4
Endotracheal Airway
Change device in, Trachea ØB21XEZ
Insertion of device in, Trachea ØBH1
Pessary
Change device in, Vagina and Cul-de-sac ØU2HXGZ
Insertion of device in
Cul-de-sac ØUHF
Vagina ØUHG
Intramedullary (IM) rod (nail)
use Internal Fixation Device, Intramedullary in Lower Bones
use Internal Fixation Device, Intramedullary in Upper Bones
Intramedullary skeletal kinetic distractor (ISKD)
use Internal Fixation Device, Intramedullary in Lower Bones
use Internal Fixation Device, Intramedullary in Upper Bones
Intraocular Telescope
Left Ø8RK3ØZ
Right Ø8RJ3ØZ
Intraoperative Radiation Therapy (IORT)
Anus DDY8CZZ
Bile Ducts DFY2CZZ
Bladder DTY2CZZ
Brain DØYØCZZ
Brain Stem DØY1CZZ
Cervix DUY1CZZ
Colon DDY5CZZ
Duodenum DDY2CZZ
Gallbladder DFY1CZZ
Ileum DDY4CZZ
Jejunum DDY3CZZ
Kidney DTYØCZZ
Larynx D9YBCZZ
Liver DFYØCZZ
Mouth D9Y4CZZ
Nasopharynx D9YDCZZ
Nerve, Peripheral DØY7CZZ
Ovary DUYØCZZ
Pancreas DFY3CZZ
Pharynx D9YCCZZ
Prostate DVYØCZZ
Rectum DDY7CZZ
Spinal Cord DØY6CZZ

Intraoperative Radiation Therapy (IORT) — *continued*
Stomach DDY1CZZ
Ureter DTY1CZZ
Urethra DTY3CZZ
Uterus DUY2CZZ
Intra.OX 8E02XDZ
Intrauterine Device (IUD) *use* Contraceptive Device in Female Reproductive System
Intravascular fluorescence angiography (IFA) *see* Monitoring, Physiological Systems 4A1
Intravascular Lithotripsy (IVL) *see* Fragmentation
Intravascular ultrasound assisted thrombolysis *see* Fragmentation, Artery
Introduction of substance in or on
Artery
Central 3E06
Analgesics 3E06
Anesthetic, Intracirculatory 3E06
Antiarrhythmic 3E06
Anti-infective 3E06
Anti-inflammatory 3E06
Antineoplastic 3E06
Destructive Agent 3E06
Diagnostic Substance, Other 3E06
Electrolytic Substance 3E06
Hormone 3E06
Hypnotics 3E06
Immunotherapeutic 3E06
Nutritional Substance 3E06
Platelet Inhibitor 3E06
Radioactive Substance 3E06
Sedatives 3E06
Serum 3E06
Thrombolytic 3E06
Toxoid 3E06
Vaccine 3E06
Vasopressor 3E06
Water Balance Substance 3E06
Coronary 3E07
Diagnostic Substance, Other 3E07
Platelet Inhibitor 3E07
Thrombolytic 3E07
Peripheral 3E05
Analgesics 3E05
Anesthetic, Intracirculatory 3E05
Antiarrhythmic 3E05
Anti-infective 3E05
Anti-inflammatory 3E05
Antineoplastic 3E05
Destructive Agent 3E05
Diagnostic Substance, Other 3E05
Electrolytic Substance 3E05
Hormone 3E05
Hypnotics 3E05
Immunotherapeutic 3E05
Nutritional Substance 3E05
Platelet Inhibitor 3E05
Radioactive Substance 3E05
Sedatives 3E05
Serum 3E05
Thrombolytic 3E05
Toxoid 3E05
Vaccine 3E05
Vasopressor 3E05
Water Balance Substance 3E05
Biliary Tract 3E0J
Analgesics 3E0J
Anesthetic Agent 3E0J
Anti-infective 3E0J
Anti-inflammatory 3E0J
Antineoplastic 3E0J
Destructive Agent 3E0J
Diagnostic Substance, Other 3E0J
Electrolytic Substance 3E0J
Gas 3E0J
Hypnotics 3E0J
Islet Cells, Pancreatic 3E0J
Nutritional Substance 3E0J
Radioactive Substance 3E0J
Sedatives 3E0J
Water Balance Substance 3E0J
Bone 3E0V
Analgesics 3E0V3NZ
Anesthetic Agent 3E0V3BZ
Anti-infective 3E0V32
Anti-inflammatory 3E0V33Z
Antineoplastic 3E0V30
Introduction of substance in or on — *continued*
Bone — *continued*
Destructive Agent 3E0V3TZ
Diagnostic Substance, Other 3E0V3KZ
Electrolytic Substance 3E0V37Z
Hypnotics 3E0V3NZ
Nutritional Substance 3E0V36Z
Radioactive Substance 3E0V3HZ
Sedatives 3E0V3NZ
Water Balance Substance 3E0V37Z
Bone Marrow 3E0A3GC
Antineoplastic 3E0A30
Brain 3E0Q
Analgesics 3E0Q
Anesthetic Agent 3E0Q
Anti-infective 3E0Q
Anti-inflammatory 3E0Q
Antineoplastic 3E0Q
Destructive Agent 3E0Q
Diagnostic Substance, Other 3E0Q
Electrolytic Substance 3E0Q
Gas 3E0Q
Hypnotics 3E0Q
Nutritional Substance 3E0Q
Radioactive Substance 3E0Q
Sedatives 3E0Q
Stem Cells
Embryonic 3E0Q
Somatic 3E0Q
Water Balance Substance 3E0Q
Cranial Cavity 3E0Q
Analgesics 3E0Q
Anesthetic Agent 3E0Q
Anti-infective 3E0Q
Anti-inflammatory 3E0Q
Antineoplastic 3E0Q
Destructive Agent 3E0Q
Diagnostic Substance, Other 3E0Q
Electrolytic Substance 3E0Q
Gas 3E0Q
Hypnotics 3E0Q
Nutritional Substance 3E0Q
Radioactive Substance 3E0Q
Sedatives 3E0Q
Stem Cells
Embryonic 3E0Q
Somatic 3E0Q
Water Balance Substance 3E0Q
Ear 3E0B
Analgesics 3E0B
Anesthetic Agent 3E0B
Anti-infective 3E0B
Anti-inflammatory 3E0B
Antineoplastic 3E0B
Destructive Agent 3E0B
Diagnostic Substance, Other 3E0B
Hypnotics 3E0B
Radioactive Substance 3E0B
Sedatives 3E0B
Epidural Space 3E0S3GC
Analgesics 3E0S3NZ
Anesthetic Agent 3E0S3BZ
Anti-infective 3E0S32
Anti-inflammatory 3E0S33Z
Antineoplastic 3E0S30
Destructive Agent 3E0S3TZ
Diagnostic Substance, Other 3E0S3KZ
Electrolytic Substance 3E0S37Z
Gas 3E0S
Hypnotics 3E0S3NZ
Nutritional Substance 3E0S36Z
Radioactive Substance 3E0S3HZ
Sedatives 3E0S3NZ
Water Balance Substance 3E0S37Z
Eye 3E0C
Analgesics 3E0C
Anesthetic Agent 3E0C
Anti-infective 3E0C
Anti-inflammatory 3E0C
Antineoplastic 3E0C
Destructive Agent 3E0C
Diagnostic Substance, Other 3E0C
Gas 3E0C
Hypnotics 3E0C
Pigment 3E0C
Radioactive Substance 3E0C
Sedatives 3E0C
Gastrointestinal Tract
Lower 3E0H
Introduction of substance in or on — *continued*
Gastrointestinal Tract — *continued*
Lower — *continued*
Analgesics 3E0H
Anesthetic Agent 3E0H
Anti-infective 3E0H
Anti-inflammatory 3E0H
Antineoplastic 3E0H
Destructive Agent 3E0H
Diagnostic Substance, Other 3E0H
Electrolytic Substance 3E0H
Gas 3E0H
Hypnotics 3E0H
Nutritional Substance 3E0H
Radioactive Substance 3E0H
Sedatives 3E0H
Water Balance Substance 3E0H
Upper 3E0G
Analgesics 3E0G
Anesthetic Agent 3E0G
Anti-infective 3E0G
Anti-inflammatory 3E0G
Antineoplastic 3E0G
Destructive Agent 3E0G
Diagnostic Substance, Other 3E0G
Electrolytic Substance 3E0G
Gas 3E0G
Hypnotics 3E0G
Nutritional Substance 3E0G
Radioactive Substance 3E0G
Sedatives 3E0G
Water Balance Substance 3E0G
Genitourinary Tract 3E0K
Analgesics 3E0K
Anesthetic Agent 3E0K
Anti-infective 3E0K
Anti-inflammatory 3E0K
Antineoplastic 3E0K
Destructive Agent 3E0K
Diagnostic Substance, Other 3E0K
Electrolytic Substance 3E0K
Gas 3E0K
Hypnotics 3E0K
Nutritional Substance 3E0K
Radioactive Substance 3E0K
Sedatives 3E0K
Water Balance Substance 3E0K
Heart 3E08
Diagnostic Substance, Other 3E08
Platelet Inhibitor 3E08
Thrombolytic 3E08
Joint 3E0U
Analgesics 3E0U3NZ
Anesthetic Agent 3E0U3BZ
Anti-infective 3E0U
Anti-inflammatory 3E0U33Z
Antineoplastic 3E0U30
Destructive Agent 3E0U3TZ
Diagnostic Substance, Other 3E0U3KZ
Electrolytic Substance 3E0U37Z
Gas 3E0U3SF
Hypnotics 3E0U3NZ
Nutritional Substance 3E0U36Z
Radioactive Substance 3E0U3HZ
Sedatives 3E0U3NZ
Water Balance Substance 3E0U37Z
Lymphatic 3E0W3GC
Analgesics 3E0W3NZ
Anesthetic Agent 3E0W3BZ
Anti-infective 3E0W32
Anti-inflammatory 3E0W33Z
Antineoplastic 3E0W30
Destructive Agent 3E0W3TZ
Diagnostic Substance, Other 3E0W3KZ
Electrolytic Substance 3E0W37Z
Hypnotics 3E0W3NZ
Nutritional Substance 3E0W36Z
Radioactive Substance 3E0W3HZ
Sedatives 3E0W3NZ
Water Balance Substance 3E0W37Z
Mouth 3E0D
Analgesics 3E0D
Anesthetic Agent 3E0D
Antiarrhythmic 3E0D
Anti-infective 3E0D
Anti-inflammatory 3E0D
Antineoplastic 3E0D
Destructive Agent 3E0D
Diagnostic Substance, Other 3E0D

Introduction of substance in or on — *continued*
Mouth — *continued*
Electrolytic Substance 3EØD
Hypnotics 3EØD
Nutritional Substance 3EØD
Radioactive Substance 3EØD
Sedatives 3EØD
Serum 3EØD
Toxoid 3EØD
Vaccine 3EØD
Water Balance Substance 3EØD
Mucous Membrane 3EØØXGC
Analgesics 3EØØXNZ
Anesthetic Agent 3EØØXBZ
Anti-infective 3EØØX2
Anti-inflammatory 3EØØX3Z
Antineoplastic 3EØØXØ
Destructive Agent 3EØØXTZ
Diagnostic Substance, Other 3EØØXKZ
Hypnotics 3EØØXNZ
Pigment 3EØØXMZ
Sedatives 3EØØXNZ
Serum 3EØØX4Z
Toxoid 3EØØX4Z
Vaccine 3EØØX4Z
Muscle 3EØ23GC
Analgesics 3EØ23NZ
Anesthetic Agent 3EØ23BZ
Anti-infective 3EØ232
Anti-inflammatory 3EØ233Z
Antineoplastic 3EØ23Ø
Destructive Agent 3EØ23TZ
Diagnostic Substance, Other 3EØ23KZ
Electrolytic Substance 3EØ237Z
Hypnotics 3EØ23NZ
Nutritional Substance 3EØ236Z
Radioactive Substance 3EØ23HZ
Sedatives 3EØ23NZ
Serum 3EØ234Z
Toxoid 3EØ234Z
Vaccine 3EØ234Z
Water Balance Substance 3EØ237Z
Nerve
Cranial 3EØX3GC
Anesthetic Agent 3EØX3BZ
Anti-inflammatory 3EØX33Z
Destructive Agent 3EØX3TZ
Peripheral 3EØT3GC
Anesthetic Agent 3EØT3BZ
Anti-inflammatory 3EØT33Z
Destructive Agent 3EØT3TZ
Plexus 3EØT3GC
Anesthetic Agent 3EØT3BZ
Anti-inflammatory 3EØT33Z
Destructive Agent 3EØT3TZ
Nose 3EØ9
Analgesics 3EØ9
Anesthetic Agent 3EØ9
Anti-infective 3EØ9
Anti-inflammatory 3EØ9
Antineoplastic 3EØ9
Destructive Agent 3EØ9
Diagnostic Substance, Other 3EØ9
Hypnotics 3EØ9
Radioactive Substance 3EØ9
Sedatives 3EØ9
Serum 3EØ9
Toxoid 3EØ9
Vaccine 3EØ9
Pancreatic Tract 3EØJ
Analgesics 3EØJ
Anesthetic Agent 3EØJ
Anti-infective 3EØJ
Anti-inflammatory 3EØJ
Antineoplastic 3EØJ
Destructive Agent 3EØJ
Diagnostic Substance, Other 3EØJ
Electrolytic Substance 3EØJ
Gas 3EØJ
Hypnotics 3EØJ
Islet Cells, Pancreatic 3EØJ
Nutritional Substance 3EØJ
Radioactive Substance 3EØJ
Sedatives 3EØJ
Water Balance Substance 3EØJ
Pericardial Cavity 3EØY
Analgesics 3EØY3NZ
Anesthetic Agent 3EØY3BZ
Anti-infective 3EØY32

Introduction of substance in or on — *continued*
Pericardial Cavity — *continued*
Anti-inflammatory 3EØY33Z
Antineoplastic 3EØY
Destructive Agent 3EØY3TZ
Diagnostic Substance, Other 3EØY3KZ
Electrolytic Substance 3EØY37Z
Gas 3EØY
Hypnotics 3EØY3NZ
Nutritional Substance 3EØY36Z
Radioactive Substance 3EØY3HZ
Sedatives 3EØY3NZ
Water Balance Substance 3EØY37Z
Peritoneal Cavity 3EØM
Adhesion Barrier 3EØM
Analgesics 3EØM3NZ
Anesthetic Agent 3EØM3BZ
Anti-infective 3EØM32
Anti-inflammatory 3EØM33Z
Antineoplastic 3EØM
Destructive Agent 3EØM3TZ
Diagnostic Substance, Other 3EØM3KZ
Electrolytic Substance 3EØM37Z
Gas 3EØM
Hypnotics 3EØM3NZ
Nutritional Substance 3EØM36Z
Radioactive Substance 3EØM3HZ
Sedatives 3EØM3NZ
Water Balance Substance 3EØM37Z
Pharynx 3EØD
Analgesics 3EØD
Anesthetic Agent 3EØD
Antiarrhythmic 3EØD
Anti-infective 3EØD
Anti-inflammatory 3EØD
Antineoplastic 3EØD
Destructive Agent 3EØD
Diagnostic Substance, Other 3EØD
Electrolytic Substance 3EØD
Hypnotics 3EØD
Nutritional Substance 3EØD
Radioactive Substance 3EØD
Sedatives 3EØD
Serum 3EØD
Toxoid 3EØD
Vaccine 3EØD
Water Balance Substance 3EØD
Pleural Cavity 3EØL
Adhesion Barrier 3EØL
Analgesics 3EØL3NZ
Anesthetic Agent 3EØL3BZ
Anti-infective 3EØL32
Anti-inflammatory 3EØL33Z
Antineoplastic 3EØL
Destructive Agent 3EØL3TZ
Diagnostic Substance, Other 3EØL3KZ
Electrolytic Substance 3EØL37Z
Gas 3EØL
Hypnotics 3EØL3NZ
Nutritional Substance 3EØL36Z
Radioactive Substance 3EØL3HZ
Sedatives 3EØL3NZ
Water Balance Substance 3EØL37Z
Products of Conception 3EØE
Analgesics 3EØE
Anesthetic Agent 3EØE
Anti-infective 3EØE
Anti-inflammatory 3EØE
Antineoplastic 3EØE
Destructive Agent 3EØE
Diagnostic Substance, Other 3EØE
Electrolytic Substance 3EØE
Gas 3EØE
Hypnotics 3EØE
Nutritional Substance 3EØE
Radioactive Substance 3EØE
Sedatives 3EØE
Water Balance Substance 3EØE
Reproductive
Female 3EØP
Adhesion Barrier 3EØP
Analgesics 3EØP
Anesthetic Agent 3EØP
Anti-infective 3EØP
Anti-inflammatory 3EØP
Antineoplastic 3EØP
Destructive Agent 3EØP
Diagnostic Substance, Other 3EØP
Electrolytic Substance 3EØP

Introduction of substance in or on — *continued*
Reproductive — *continued*
Female — *continued*
Gas 3EØP
Hormone 3EØP
Hypnotics 3EØP
Nutritional Substance 3EØP
Ovum, Fertilized 3EØP
Radioactive Substance 3EØP
Sedatives 3EØP
Sperm 3EØP
Water Balance Substance 3EØP
Male 3EØN
Analgesics 3EØN
Anesthetic Agent 3EØN
Anti-infective 3EØN
Anti-inflammatory 3EØN
Antineoplastic 3EØN
Destructive Agent 3EØN
Diagnostic Substance, Other 3EØN
Electrolytic Substance 3EØN
Gas 3EØN
Hypnotics 3EØN
Nutritional Substance 3EØN
Radioactive Substance 3EØN
Sedatives 3EØN
Water Balance Substance 3EØN
Respiratory Tract 3EØF
Analgesics 3EØF
Anesthetic Agent 3EØF
Anti-infective 3EØF
Anti-inflammatory 3EØF
Antineoplastic 3EØF
Destructive Agent 3EØF
Diagnostic Substance, Other 3EØF
Electrolytic Substance 3EØF
Gas 3EØF
Hypnotics 3EØF
Nutritional Substance 3EØF
Radioactive Substance 3EØF
Sedatives 3EØF
Water Balance Substance 3EØF
Skin 3EØØXGC
Analgesics 3EØØXNZ
Anesthetic Agent 3EØØXBZ
Anti-infective 3EØØX2
Anti-inflammatory 3EØØX3Z
Antineoplastic 3EØØXØ
Destructive Agent 3EØØXTZ
Diagnostic Substance, Other 3EØØXKZ
Hypnotics 3EØØXNZ
Pigment 3EØØXMZ
Sedatives 3EØØXNZ
Serum 3EØØX4Z
Toxoid 3EØØX4Z
Vaccine 3EØØX4Z
Spinal Canal 3EØR3GC
Analgesics 3EØR3NZ
Anesthetic Agent 3EØR3BZ
Anti-infective 3EØR32
Anti-inflammatory 3EØR33Z
Antineoplastic 3EØR3Ø
Destructive Agent 3EØR3TZ
Diagnostic Substance, Other 3EØR3KZ
Electrolytic Substance 3EØR37Z
Gas 3EØR
Hypnotics 3EØR3NZ
Nutritional Substance 3EØR36Z
Radioactive Substance 3EØR3HZ
Sedatives 3EØR3NZ
Stem Cells
Embryonic 3EØR
Somatic 3EØR
Water Balance Substance 3EØR37Z
Subcutaneous Tissue 3EØ13GC
Analgesics 3EØ13NZ
Anesthetic Agent 3EØ13BZ
Anti-infective 3EØ1
Anti-inflammatory 3EØ133Z
Antineoplastic 3EØ13Ø
Destructive Agent 3EØ13TZ
Diagnostic Substance, Other 3EØ13KZ
Electrolytic Substance 3EØ137Z
Hormone 3EØ13V
Hypnotics 3EØ13NZ
Nutritional Substance 3EØ136Z
Radioactive Substance 3EØ13HZ
Sedatives 3EØ13NZ
Serum 3EØ134Z

Subterms under main terms may continue to next column or page

Introduction of substance in or on — *continued*
Subcutaneous Tissue — *continued*
Toxoid 3E0134Z
Vaccine 3E0134Z
Water Balance Substance 3E0137Z
Vein
Central 3E04
Analgesics 3E04
Anesthetic, Intracirculatory 3E04
Antiarrhythmic 3E04
Anti-infective 3E04
Anti-inflammatory 3E04
Antineoplastic 3E04
Destructive Agent 3E04
Diagnostic Substance, Other 3E04
Electrolytic Substance 3E04
Hormone 3E04
Hypnotics 3E04
Immunotherapeutic 3E04
Nutritional Substance 3E04
Platelet Inhibitor 3E04
Radioactive Substance 3E04
Sedatives 3E04
Serum 3E04
Thrombolytic 3E04
Toxoid 3E04
Vaccine 3E04
Vasopressor 3E04
Water Balance Substance 3E04
Peripheral 3E03
Analgesics 3E03
Anesthetic, Intracirculatory 3E03
Antiarrhythmic 3E03
Anti-infective 3E03
Anti-inflammatory 3E03
Antineoplastic 3E03
Destructive Agent 3E03
Diagnostic Substance, Other 3E03
Electrolytic Substance 3E03
Hormone 3E03
Hypnotics 3E03
Immunotherapeutic 3E03
Islet Cells, Pancreatic 3E03
Nutritional Substance 3E03
Platelet Inhibitor 3E03
Radioactive Substance 3E03
Sedatives 3E03
Serum 3E03
Thrombolytic 3E03
Toxoid 3E03
Vaccine 3E03
Vasopressor 3E03
Water Balance Substance 3E03
Intubated prone positioning *see* Assistance, Respiratory 5A09
Intubation
Airway
see Insertion of device in, Esophagus 0DH5
see Insertion of device in, Mouth and Throat 0CHY
see Insertion of device in, Trachea 0BH1
Drainage device *see* Drainage
Feeding Device *see* Insertion of device in, Gastrointestinal System 0DH
INTUITY Elite valve system, EDWARDS (rapid deployment technique) *see* Replacement, Valve, Aortic 02RF
Iobenguane I-131 Antineoplastic XW0
Iobenguane I-131, High Specific Activity (HSA) *use* Iobenguane I-131 Antineoplastic
IPPB (intermittent positive pressure breathing) *see* Assistance, Respiratory 5A09
IRE (Irreversible Electroporation) *see* Destruction, Hepatobiliary System and Pancreas 0F5
Iridectomy
see Excision, Eye 08B
see Resection, Eye 08T
Iridoplasty
see Repair, Eye 08Q
see Replacement, Eye 08R
see Supplement, Eye 08U
Iridotomy *see* Drainage, Eye 089
Irreversible Electroporation (IRE) *see* Destruction, Hepatobiliary System and Pancreas 0F5
Irrigation
Biliary Tract, Irrigating Substance 3E1J
Brain, Irrigating Substance 3E1Q38Z
Cranial Cavity, Irrigating Substance 3E1Q38Z
Irrigation — *continued*
Ear, Irrigating Substance 3E1B
Epidural Space, Irrigating Substance 3E1S38Z
Eye, Irrigating Substance 3E1C
Gastrointestinal Tract
Lower, Irrigating Substance 3E1H
Upper, Irrigating Substance 3E1G
Genitourinary Tract, Irrigating Substance 3E1K
Irrigating Substance 3C1ZX8Z
Joint, Irrigating Substance 3E1U
Mucous Membrane, Irrigating Substance 3E10
Nose, Irrigating Substance 3E19
Pancreatic Tract, Irrigating Substance 3E1J
Pericardial Cavity, Irrigating Substance 3E1Y38Z
Peritoneal Cavity
Dialysate 3E1M39Z
Irrigating Substance 3E1M
Pleural Cavity, Irrigating Substance 3E1L38Z
Reproductive
Female, Irrigating Substance 3E1P
Male, Irrigating Substance 3E1N
Respiratory Tract, Irrigating Substance 3E1F
Skin, Irrigating Substance 3E10
Spinal Canal, Irrigating Substance 3E1R38Z
Isavuconazole (isavuconazonium sulfate) *use* Other Anti-infective
Ischemic Stroke System (ISS500) *use* Neurostimulator Lead in New Technology
Ischiatic nerve *use* Sciatic Nerve
Ischiocavernosus muscle *use* Perineum Muscle
Ischiofemoral ligament
use Hip Bursa and Ligament, Left
use Hip Bursa and Ligament, Right
Ischium
use Pelvic Bone, Left
use Pelvic Bone, Right
ISC-REST kit
ISCDx XXE5XT7
QIAGEN Access Anti-SARS-CoV-2 Total Test XXE5XV7
QIAstat-Dx Respiratory SARS-CoV-2 Panel XXE97U7
Isolation 8E0ZXY6
Isotope Administration, Other Radiation, Whole Body DWY5G
ISS500 (Ischemic Stroke System) *use* Neurostimulator Lead in New Technology
Itrel (3) (4) neurostimulator *use* Stimulator Generator, Single Array in 0JH

J

Jakafi® *use* Ruxolitinib
Jejunal artery *use* Superior Mesenteric Artery
Jejunectomy
see Excision, Jejunum 0DBA
see Resection, Jejunum 0DTA
Jejunocolostomy
see Bypass, Gastrointestinal System 0D1
see Drainage, Gastrointestinal System 0D9
Jejunopexy
see Repair, Jejunum 0DQA
see Reposition, Jejunum 0DSA
Jejunostomy
see Bypass, Jejunum 0D1A
see Drainage, Jejunum 0D9A
Jejunotomy *see* Drainage, Jejunum 0D9A
Joint fixation plate
use Internal Fixation Device in Lower Joints
use Internal Fixation Device in Upper Joints
Joint liner (insert) *use* Liner in Lower Joints
Joint spacer (antibiotic)
use Spacer in Lower Joints
use Spacer in Upper Joints
Jugular body *use* Glomus Jugulare
Jugular lymph node
use Lymphatic, Left Neck
use Lymphatic, Right Neck

K

Kappa *use* Pacemaker, Dual Chamber in 0JH
Kcentra *use* 4-Factor Prothrombin Complex Concentrate
Keratectomy, kerectomy
see Excision, Eye 08B
see Resection, Eye 08T
Keratocentesis *see* Drainage, Eye 089
Keratoplasty
see Repair, Eye 08Q
see Replacement, Eye 08R
see Supplement, Eye 08U
Keratotomy
see Drainage, Eye 089
see Repair, Eye 08Q
KEVZARA® *use* Sarilumab
Keystone Heart TriGuard 3™ CEPD (cerebral embolic protection device) X2A6325
Kirschner wire (K-wire)
use Internal Fixation Device in Head and Facial Bones
use Internal Fixation Device in Lower Bones
use Internal Fixation Device in Lower Joints
use Internal Fixation Device in Upper Bones
use Internal Fixation Device in Upper Joints
Knee (implant) insert *use* Liner in Lower Joints
KUB x-ray *see* Plain Radiography, Kidney, Ureter and Bladder BT04
Kuntscher nail
use Internal Fixation Device, Intramedullary in Lower Bones
use Internal Fixation Device, Intramedullary in Upper Bones
KYMRIAH® *use* Tisagenlecleucel Immunotherapy

L

Labia majora *use* Vulva
Labia minora *use* Vulva
Labial gland
use Lower Lip
use Upper Lip
Labiectomy
see Excision, Female Reproductive System 0UB
see Resection, Female Reproductive System 0UT
Lacrimal canaliculus
use Lacrimal Duct, Left
use Lacrimal Duct, Right
Lacrimal punctum
use Lacrimal Duct, Left
use Lacrimal Duct, Right
Lacrimal sac
use Lacrimal Duct, Left
use Lacrimal Duct, Right
LAGB (laparoscopic adjustable gastric banding)
Initial procedure 0DV64CZ
Surgical correction *see* Revision of device in, Stomach 0DW6
Laminectomy
see Excision, Lower Bones 0QB
see Excision, Upper Bones 0PB
see Release, Central Nervous System and Cranial Nerves 00N
see Release, Peripheral Nervous System 01N
Laminotomy
see Drainage, Lower Bones 0Q9
see Drainage, Upper Bones 0P9
see Excision, Lower Bones 0QB
see Excision, Upper Bones 0PB
see Release, Central Nervous System and Cranial Nerves 00N
see Release, Lower Bones 0QN
see Release, Peripheral Nervous System 01N
see Release, Upper Bones 0PN
Laparoscopic-assisted transanal pull-through
see Excision, Gastrointestinal System 0DB
see Resection, Gastrointestinal System 0DT
Laparoscopy *see* Inspection
Laparotomy
Drainage *see* Drainage, Peritoneal Cavity 0W9G
Exploratory *see* Inspection, Peritoneal Cavity 0WJG
LAP-BAND® adjustable gastric banding system *use* Extraluminal Device
Laryngectomy
see Excision, Larynx 0CBS
see Resection, Larynx 0CTS
Laryngocentesis *see* Drainage, Larynx 0C9S
Laryngogram *see* Fluoroscopy, Larynx B91J
Laryngopexy *see* Repair, Larynx 0CQS
Laryngopharynx *use* Pharynx
Laryngoplasty
see Repair, Larynx 0CQS
see Replacement, Larynx 0CRS

Subterms under main terms may continue to next column or page

Laryngoplasty — *continued*
see Supplement, Larynx ØCUS
Laryngorrhaphy *see* Repair, Larynx ØCQS
Laryngoscopy ØCJS8ZZ
Laryngotomy *see* Drainage, Larynx ØC9S
Laser Interstitial Thermal Therapy
Ampulla of Vater ØF5C
Anus ØD5Q
Aortic Body ØG5D
Appendix ØD5J
Brain ØØ5Ø
Breast
Bilateral ØH5V
Left ØH5U
Right ØH5T
Carotid Bodies, Bilateral ØG58
Carotid Body
Left ØG56
Right ØG57
Cecum ØD5H
Coccygeal Glomus ØG5B
Colon
Ascending ØD5K
Descending ØD5M
Sigmoid ØD5N
Transverse ØD5L
Duct
Common Bile ØF59
Cystic ØF58
Hepatic
Common ØF57
Left ØF56
Right ØF55
Pancreatic ØF5D
Accessory ØF5F
Duodenum ØD59
Esophagogastric Junction ØD54
Esophagus ØD55
Lower ØD53
Middle ØD52
Upper ØD51
Gallbladder ØF54
Gland
Adrenal
Bilateral ØG54
Left ØG52
Right ØG53
Pituitary ØG5Ø
Glomus Jugulare ØG5C
Ileocecal Valve ØD5C
Ileum ØD5B
Intestine
Large ØD5E
Left ØD5G
Right ØD5F
Small ØD58
Jejunum ØD5A
Liver ØF5Ø
Left Lobe ØF52
Right Lobe ØF51
Lung
Bilateral ØB5M
Left ØB5L
Lower Lobe
Left ØB5J
Right ØB5F
Middle Lobe, Right ØB5D
Right ØB5K
Upper Lobe
Left ØB5G
Right ØB5C
Lung Lingula ØB5H
Pancreas ØF5G
Para-aortic Body ØG59
Paraganglion Extremity ØG5F
Parathyroid Gland ØG5R
Inferior
Left ØG5P
Right ØG5N
Multiple ØG5Q
Superior
Left ØG5M
Right ØG5L
Pineal Body ØG51
Prostate ØV5Ø
Rectum ØD5P
Sacrum ØQ51
Spinal Cord
Cervical ØØ5W

Laser Interstitial Thermal Therapy — *continued*
Spinal Cord — *continued*
Lumbar ØØ5Y
Thoracic ØØ5X
Stomach ØD56
Pylorus ØD57
Thyroid Gland ØG5K
Left Lobe ØG5G
Right Lobe ØG5H
Vertebra
Cervical ØP53
Lumbar ØQ5Ø
Thoracic ØP54
Lateral canthus
use Upper Eyelid, Left
use Upper Eyelid, Right
Lateral collateral ligament (LCL)
use Knee Bursa and Ligament, Left
use Knee Bursa and Ligament, Right
Lateral condyle of femur
use Lower Femur, Left
use Lower Femur, Right
Lateral condyle of tibia
use Tibia, Left
use Tibia, Right
Lateral cuneiform bone
use Tarsal, Left
use Tarsal, Right
Lateral epicondyle of femur
use Lower Femur, Left
use Lower Femur, Right
Lateral epicondyle of humerus
use Humeral Shaft, Left
use Humeral Shaft, Right
Lateral femoral cutaneous nerve *use* Lumbar Plexus
Lateral (brachial) lymph node
use Lymphatic, Left Axillary
use Lymphatic, Right Axillary
Lateral malleolus
use Fibula, Left
use Fibula, Right
Lateral meniscus
use Knee Joint, Left
use Knee Joint, Right
Lateral nasal cartilage *use* Nasal Mucosa and Soft Tissue
Lateral plantar artery
use Foot Artery, Left
use Foot Artery, Right
Lateral plantar nerve *use* Tibial Nerve
Lateral rectus muscle
use Extraocular Muscle, Left
use Extraocular Muscle, Right
Lateral sacral artery
use Internal Iliac Artery, Left
use Internal Iliac Artery, Right
Lateral sacral vein
use Hypogastric Vein, Left
use Hypogastric Vein, Right
Lateral sural cutaneous nerve *use* Peroneal Nerve
Lateral tarsal artery
use Foot Artery, Left
use Foot Artery, Right
Lateral temporomandibular ligament *use* Head and Neck Bursa and Ligament
Lateral thoracic artery
use Axillary Artery, Left
use Axillary Artery, Right
Latissimus dorsi muscle
use Trunk Muscle, Left
use Trunk Muscle, Right
Latissimus Dorsi Myocutaneous Flap
Replacement
Bilateral ØHRVØ75
Left ØHRUØ75
Right ØHRTØ75
Transfer
Left ØKXG
Right ØKXF
Lavage
see Irrigation
Bronchial alveolar, diagnostic *see* Drainage, Respiratory System ØB9
Least splanchnic nerve *use* Thoracic Sympathetic Nerve
Lefamulin Anti-infective XWØ
Left ascending lumbar vein *use* Hemiazygos Vein

Left atrioventricular valve *use* Mitral Valve
Left auricular appendix *use* Atrium, Left
Left colic vein *use* Colic Vein
Left coronary sulcus *use* Heart, Left
Left gastric artery *use* Gastric Artery
Left gastroepiploic artery *use* Splenic Artery
Left gastroepiploic vein *use* Splenic Vein
Left inferior phrenic vein *use* Renal Vein, Left
Left inferior pulmonary vein *use* Pulmonary Vein, Left
Left jugular trunk *use* Thoracic Duct
Left lateral ventricle *use* Cerebral Ventricle
Left ovarian vein *use* Renal Vein, Left
Left second lumbar vein *use* Renal Vein, Left
Left subclavian trunk *use* Thoracic Duct
Left subcostal vein *use* Hemiazygos Vein
Left superior pulmonary vein *use* Pulmonary Vein, Left
Left suprarenal vein *use* Renal Vein, Left
Left testicular vein *use* Renal Vein, Left
Lengthening
Bone, with device *see* Insertion of Limb Lengthening Device
Muscle, by incision *see* Division, Muscles ØK8
Tendon, by incision *see* Division, Tendons ØL8
Leptomeninges, intracranial *use* Cerebral Meninges
Leptomeninges, spinal *use* Spinal Meninges
Leronlimab Monoclonal Antibody XWØ13K6
Lesser alar cartilage *use* Nasal Mucosa and Soft Tissue
Lesser occipital nerve *use* Cervical Plexus
Lesser Omentum *use* Omentum
Lesser saphenous vein
use Saphenous Vein, Left
use Saphenous Vein, Right
Lesser splanchnic nerve *use* Thoracic Sympathetic Nerve
Lesser trochanter
use Upper Femur, Left
use Upper Femur, Right
Lesser tuberosity
use Humeral Head, Left
use Humeral Head, Right
Lesser wing *use* Sphenoid Bone
Leukopheresis, therapeutic *see* Pheresis, Circulatory 6A55
Levator anguli oris muscle *use* Facial Muscle
Levator ani muscle *use* Perineum Muscle
Levator labii superioris alaeque nasi muscle *use* Facial Muscle
Levator labii superioris muscle *use* Facial Muscle
Levator palpebrae superioris muscle
use Upper Eyelid, Left
use Upper Eyelid, Right
Levator scapulae muscle
use Neck Muscle, Left
use Neck Muscle, Right
Levator veli palatini muscle *use* Tongue, Palate, Pharynx Muscle
Levatores costarum muscle
use Thorax Muscle, Left
use Thorax Muscle, Right
Lifeline ARM Automated Chest Compression (ACC) device 5A1221J
LifeStent® (Flexstar) (XL) Vascular Stent System *use* Intraluminal Device
Lifileucel *use* Lifileucel Immunotherapy
Lifileucel Immunotherapy XWØ
Ligament of head of fibula
use Knee Bursa and Ligament, Left
use Knee Bursa and Ligament, Right
Ligament of the lateral malleolus
use Ankle Bursa and Ligament, Left
use Ankle Bursa and Ligament, Right
Ligamentum flavum, cervical *use* Head and Neck Bursa and Ligament
Ligamentum flavum, lumbar *use* Lower Spine Bursa and Ligament
Ligamentum flavum, thoracic *use* Upper Spine Bursa and Ligament
LigaPASS 2.Ø™ PJK Prevention System *use* Posterior Vertebral Tether in New Technology
Ligation *see* Occlusion
Ligation, hemorrhoid *see* Occlusion, Lower Veins, Hemorrhoidal Plexus
Light Therapy GZJZZZZ

Liner
Removal of device from
Hip
Left ØSPBØ9Z
Right ØSP9Ø9Z
Knee
Left ØSPDØ9Z
Right ØSPCØ9Z
Revision of device in
Hip
Left ØSWBØ9Z
Right ØSW9Ø9Z
Knee
Left ØSWDØ9Z
Right ØSWCØ9Z
Supplement
Hip
Left ØSUBØ9Z
Acetabular Surface ØSUEØ9Z
Femoral Surface ØSUSØ9Z
Right ØSU9Ø9Z
Acetabular Surface ØSUAØ9Z
Femoral Surface ØSURØ9Z
Knee
Left ØSUDØ9
Femoral Surface ØSUUØ9Z
Tibial Surface ØSUWØ9Z
Right ØSUCØ9
Femoral Surface ØSUTØ9Z
Tibial Surface ØSUVØ9Z
Lingual artery
use External Carotid Artery, Left
use External Carotid Artery, Right
Lingual tonsil *use* Pharynx
Lingulectomy, lung
see Excision, Lung Lingula ØBBH
see Resection, Lung Lingula ØBTH
Lisocabtagene Maraleucel *use* Lisocabtagene Maraleucel Immunotherapy
Lisocabtagene Maraleucel Immunotherapy XWØ
Lithoplasty *see* Fragmentation
Lithotripsy
see Fragmentation
With removal of fragments *see* Extirpation
LITT (laser interstitial thermal therapy)
see Destruction
see Laser Interstitial Thermal Therapy
LIVIAN™ CRT-D *use* Cardiac Resynchronization Defibrillator Pulse Generator in ØJH
LIVTENCITY™ *use* Maribavir Anti-infective
Lobectomy
see Excision, Central Nervous System and Cranial Nerves ØØB
see Excision, Endocrine System ØGB
see Excision, Hepatobiliary System and Pancreas ØFB
see Excision, Respiratory System ØBB
see Resection, Endocrine System ØGT
see Resection, Hepatobiliary System and Pancreas ØFT
see Resection, Respiratory System ØBT
Lobotomy *see* Division, Brain ØØ8Ø
Localization
see Imaging
see Map
Locus ceruleus *use* Pons
Long thoracic nerve *use* Brachial Plexus
Longeviti ClearFit® Cranial Implant *use* Synthetic Substitute, Ultrasound Penetrable in New Technology
Longeviti ClearFit® OTS Cranial Implant *use* Synthetic Substitute, Ultrasound Penetrable in New Technology
Loop ileostomy *see* Bypass, Ileum ØD1B
Loop recorder, implantable *use* Monitoring Device
Lovotibeglogene Autotemcel XW1
Lower GI series *see* Fluoroscopy, Colon BD14
Lower Respiratory Fluid Nucleic Acid-base Microbial Detection XXEBXQ6
LTX Regional Anticoagulant *use* Nafamostat Anticoagulant
LUCAS® Chest Compression System 5A1221J
Lumbar artery *use* Abdominal Aorta
Lumbar facet joint *use* Lumbar Vertebral Joint
Lumbar ganglion *use* Lumbar Sympathetic Nerve
Lumbar lymph node *use* Lymphatic, Aortic
Lumbar lymphatic trunk *use* Cisterna Chyli
Lumbar splanchnic nerve *use* Lumbar Sympathetic Nerve
Lumbosacral facet joint *use* Lumbosacral Joint
Lumbosacral trunk *use* Lumbar Nerve
Lumpectomy *see* Excision
Lunate bone
use Carpal, Left
use Carpal, Right
Lunotriquetral ligament
use Hand Bursa and Ligament, Left
use Hand Bursa and Ligament, Right
LUNSUMIO™ *use* Mosunetuzumab Antineoplastic
Lurbinectedin XWØ
Lymphadenectomy
see Excision, Lymphatic and Hemic Systems Ø7B
see Resection, Lymphatic and Hemic Systems Ø7T
Lymphadenotomy *see* Drainage, Lymphatic and Hemic Systems Ø79
Lymphangiectomy
see Excision, Lymphatic and Hemic Systems Ø7B
see Resection, Lymphatic and Hemic Systems Ø7T
Lymphangiogram *see* Plain Radiography, Lymphatic System B7Ø
Lymphangioplasty
see Repair, Lymphatic and Hemic Systems Ø7Q
see Supplement, Lymphatic and Hemic Systems Ø7U
Lymphangiorrhaphy *see* Repair, Lymphatic and Hemic Systems Ø7Q
Lymphangiotomy *see* Drainage, Lymphatic and Hemic Systems Ø79
Lysis *see* Release

M

Macula XXE5XR7
use Retina, Left
use Retina, Right
MAGEC® Spinal Bracing and Distraction System
use Magnetically Controlled Growth Rod(s) in New Technology
Magnet extraction, ocular foreign body *see* Extirpation, Eye Ø8C
Magnetic Resonance Imaging (MRI)
Abdomen BW3Ø
Ankle
Left BQ3H
Right BQ3G
Aorta
Abdominal B43Ø
Thoracic B33Ø
Arm
Left BP3F
Right BP3E
Artery
Celiac B431
Cervico-Cerebral Arch B33Q
Common Carotid, Bilateral B335
Coronary
Bypass Graft, Multiple B233
Multiple B231
Internal Carotid, Bilateral B338
Intracranial B33R
Lower Extremity
Bilateral B43H
Left B43G
Right B43F
Pelvic B43C
Renal, Bilateral B438
Spinal B33M
Superior Mesenteric B434
Upper Extremity
Bilateral B33K
Left B33J
Right B33H
Vertebral, Bilateral B33G
Bladder BT3Ø
Brachial Plexus BW3P
Brain BØ3Ø
Breast
Bilateral BH32
Left BH31
Right BH3Ø
Calcaneus
Left BQ3K
Right BQ3J
Chest BW33Y
Magnetic Resonance Imaging (MRI) — *continued*
Coccyx BR3F
Connective Tissue
Lower Extremity BL31
Upper Extremity BL3Ø
Corpora Cavernosa BV3Ø
Disc
Cervical BR31
Lumbar BR33
Thoracic BR32
Ear B93Ø
Elbow
Left BP3H
Right BP3G
Eye
Bilateral B837
Left B836
Right B835
Femur
Left BQ34
Right BQ33
Fetal Abdomen BY33
Fetal Extremity BY35
Fetal Head BY3Ø
Fetal Heart BY31
Fetal Spine BY34
Fetal Thorax BY32
Fetus, Whole BY36
Foot
Left BQ3M
Right BQ3L
Forearm
Left BP3K
Right BP3J
Gland
Adrenal, Bilateral BG32
Parathyroid BG33
Parotid, Bilateral B936
Salivary, Bilateral B93D
Submandibular, Bilateral B939
Thyroid BG34
Head BW38
Heart, Right and Left B236
Hip
Left BQ31
Right BQ3Ø
Intracranial Sinus B532
Joint
Finger
Left BP3D
Right BP3C
Hand
Left BP3D
Right BP3C
Temporomandibular, Bilateral BN39
Kidney
Bilateral BT33
Left BT32
Right BT31
Transplant BT39
Knee
Left BQ38
Right BQ37
Larynx B93J
Leg
Left BQ3F
Right BQ3D
Liver BF35
Liver and Spleen BF36
Lung Apices BB3G
Lung, Bilateral, Hyperpolarized Xenon 129 (Xe-129) BB34Z3Z
Nasopharynx B93F
Neck BW3F
Nerve
Acoustic BØ3C
Brachial Plexus BW3P
Oropharynx B93F
Ovary
Bilateral BU35
Left BU34
Right BU33
Ovary and Uterus BU3C
Pancreas BF37
Patella
Left BQ3W
Right BQ3V
Pelvic Region BW3G
Pelvis BR3C

Magnetic Resonance Imaging (MRI) — *continued*
- Pituitary Gland BØ39
- Plexus, Brachial BW3P
- Prostate BV33
- Retroperitoneum BW3H
- Sacrum BR3F
- Scrotum BV34
- Sella Turcica BØ39
- Shoulder
  - Left BP39
  - Right BP38
- Sinus
  - Intracranial B532
  - Paranasal B932
- Spinal Cord BØ3B
- Spine
  - Cervical BR3Ø
  - Lumbar BR39
  - Thoracic BR37
- Spleen and Liver BF36
- Subcutaneous Tissue
  - Abdomen BH3H
  - Extremity
    - Lower BH3J
    - Upper BH3F
  - Head BH3D
  - Neck BH3D
  - Pelvis BH3H
  - Thorax BH3G
- Tendon
  - Lower Extremity BL33
  - Upper Extremity BL32
- Testicle
  - Bilateral BV37
  - Left BV36
  - Right BV35
- Toe
  - Left BQ3Q
  - Right BQ3P
- Uterus BU36
  - Pregnant BU3B
- Uterus and Ovary BU3C
- Vagina BU39
- Vein
  - Cerebellar B531
  - Cerebral B531
  - Jugular, Bilateral B535
  - Lower Extremity
    - Bilateral B53D
    - Left B53C
    - Right B53B
  - Other B53V
  - Pelvic (Iliac) Bilateral B53H
  - Portal B53T
  - Pulmonary, Bilateral B53S
  - Renal, Bilateral B53L
  - Spanchnic B53T
  - Upper Extremity
    - Bilateral B53P
    - Left B53N
    - Right B53M
- Vena Cava
  - Inferior B539
  - Superior B538
- Wrist
  - Left BP3M
  - Right BP3L

Magnetically Controlled Growth Rod(s)
- Cervical XNS3
- Lumbar XNSØ
- Thoracic XNS4

Magnetic-guided radiofrequency endovascular fistula
- Radial Artery, Left Ø31C3ZF
- Radial Artery, Right Ø31B3ZF
- Ulnar Artery, Left Ø31A3ZF
- Ulnar Artery, Right Ø3193ZF

Magnus Neuromodulation System (MNS) XØZØX18

Malleotomy *see* Drainage, Ear, Nose, Sinus Ø99

Malleus
- *use* Auditory Ossicle, Left
- *use* Auditory Ossicle, Right

Mammaplasty, mammoplasty
- *see* Alteration, Skin and Breast ØHØ
- *see* Repair, Skin and Breast ØHQ
- *see* Replacement, Skin and Breast ØHR
- *see* Supplement, Skin and Breast ØHU

Mammary duct
- *use* Breast, Bilateral
- *use* Breast, Left
- *use* Breast, Right

Mammary gland
- *use* Breast, Bilateral
- *use* Breast, Left
- *use* Breast, Right

Mammectomy
- *see* Excision, Skin and Breast ØHB
- *see* Resection, Skin and Breast ØHT

Mammillary body *use* Hypothalamus

Mammography *see* Plain Radiography, Skin, Subcutaneous Tissue and Breast BHØ

Mammotomy *see* Drainage, Skin and Breast ØH9

Mandibular nerve *use* Trigeminal Nerve

Mandibular notch
- *use* Mandible, Left
- *use* Mandible, Right

Mandibulectomy
- *see* Excision, Head and Facial Bones ØNB
- *see* Resection, Head and Facial Bones ØNT

Manipulation
- Adhesions *see* Release
- Chiropractic *see* Chiropractic Manipulation

Manual removal, retained placenta *see* Extraction, Products of Conception, Retained 1ØD1

Manubrium *use* Sternum

Map
- Basal Ganglia ØØK8
- Brain ØØKØ
- Cerebellum ØØKC
- Cerebral Hemisphere ØØK7
- Conduction Mechanism Ø2K8
- Hypothalamus ØØKA
- Medulla Oblongata ØØKD
- Pons ØØKB
- Thalamus ØØK9

Mapping
- Doppler ultrasound *see* Ultrasonography
- Electrocardiogram only *see* Measurement, Cardiac 4AØ2

Maribavir Anti-infective XWØ

Mark IV Breathing Pacemaker System *use* Stimulator Generator in Subcutaneous Tissue and Fascia

MarrowStim™ PAD Kit for CBMA (Concentrated Bone Marrow Aspirate) *use* Other Substance

MarrowStim™ PAD Kit, for injection of concentrated bone marrow aspirate *see* Introduction of substance in or on, Muscle 3EØ2

Marsupialization
- *see* Drainage
- *see* Excision

Massage, cardiac
- External 5A12Ø12
- Open Ø2QAØZZ

Masseter muscle *use* Head Muscle

Masseteric fascia *use* Subcutaneous Tissue and Fascia, Face

Mastectomy
- *see* Excision, Skin and Breast ØHB
- *see* Resection, Skin and Breast ØHT

Mastoid air cells
- *use* Mastoid Sinus, Left
- *use* Mastoid Sinus, Right

Mastoid (postauricular) lymph node
- *use* Lymphatic, Left Neck
- *use* Lymphatic, Right Neck

Mastoid process
- *use* Temporal Bone, Left
- *use* Temporal Bone, Right

Mastoidectomy
- *see* Excision, Ear, Nose, Sinus Ø9B
- *see* Resection, Ear, Nose, Sinus Ø9T

Mastoidotomy *see* Drainage, Ear, Nose, Sinus Ø99

Mastopexy
- *see* Repair, Skin and Breast ØHQ
- *see* Reposition, Skin and Breast ØHS

Mastorrhaphy *see* Repair, Skin and Breast ØHQ

Mastotomy *see* Drainage, Skin and Breast ØH9

Maxillary artery
- *use* External Carotid Artery, Left
- *use* External Carotid Artery, Right

Maxillary nerve *use* Trigeminal Nerve

Maximo II DR (VR) *use* Defibrillator Generator in ØJH

Maximo II DR CRT-D *use* Cardiac Resynchronization Defibrillator Pulse Generator in ØJH

Measurement
- Arterial
  - Flow
    - Coronary 4AØ3
    - Intracranial 4AØ3X5D
    - Peripheral 4AØ3
    - Pulmonary 4AØ3
  - Pressure
    - Coronary 4AØ3
    - Peripheral 4AØ3
    - Pulmonary 4AØ3
    - Thoracic, Other 4AØ3
  - Pulse
    - Coronary 4AØ3
    - Peripheral 4AØ3
    - Pulmonary 4AØ3
  - Saturation, Peripheral 4AØ3
  - Sound, Peripheral 4AØ3
- Biliary
  - Flow 4AØC
  - Pressure 4AØC
- Cardiac
  - Action Currents 4AØ2
  - Defibrillator 4BØ2XTZ
  - Electrical Activity 4AØ2
    - Guidance 4AØ2X4A
    - No Qualifier 4AØ2X4Z
  - Output 4AØ2
  - Pacemaker 4BØ2XSZ
  - Rate 4AØ2
  - Rhythm 4AØ2
  - Sampling and Pressure
    - Bilateral 4AØ2
    - Left Heart 4AØ2
    - Right Heart 4AØ2
  - Sound 4AØ2
  - Total Activity, Stress 4AØ2XM4
- Central Nervous
  - Cerebrospinal Fluid Shunt, Wireless Sensor 4BØØXWØ
  - Conductivity 4AØØ
  - Electrical Activity 4AØØ
  - Pressure 4AØØØBZ
    - Intracranial 4AØØ
  - Saturation, Intracranial 4AØØ
  - Stimulator 4BØØXVZ
  - Temperature, Intracranial 4AØØ
- Circulatory, Volume 4AØ5XLZ
- Gastrointestinal
  - Motility 4AØB
  - Pressure 4AØB
  - Secretion 4AØB
- Lower Respiratory Fluid Nucleic Acid-base Microbial Detection XXEBXQ6
- Lymphatic
  - Flow 4AØ6
  - Pressure 4AØ6
- Metabolism 4AØZ
- Musculoskeletal
  - Contractility 4AØF
  - Pressure 4AØF3BE
  - Stimulator 4BØFXVZ
- Olfactory, Acuity 4AØ8XØZ
- Peripheral Nervous
  - Conductivity
    - Motor 4AØ1
    - Sensory 4AØ1
  - Electrical Activity 4AØ1
  - Stimulator 4BØ1XVZ
- Positive Blood Culture Fluorescence Hybridization for Organism Identification, Concentration and Susceptibility XXE5XN6
- Products of Conception
  - Cardiac
    - Electrical Activity 4AØH
    - Rate 4AØH
    - Rhythm 4AØH
    - Sound 4AØH
  - Nervous
    - Conductivity 4AØJ
    - Electrical Activity 4AØJ
    - Pressure 4AØJ
- Respiratory
  - Capacity 4AØ9
  - Flow 4AØ9
  - Pacemaker 4BØ9XSZ
  - Rate 4AØ9
  - Resistance 4AØ9
  - Total Activity 4AØ9

Measurement — *continued*
Respiratory — *continued*
Volume 4A09
Sleep 4A0ZXQZ
Temperature 4A0Z
Urinary
Contractility 4A0D
Flow 4A0D
Pressure 4A0D
Resistance 4A0D
Volume 4A0D
Venous
Flow
Central 4A04
Peripheral 4A04
Portal 4A04
Pulmonary 4A04
Pressure
Central 4A04
Peripheral 4A04
Portal 4A04
Pulmonary 4A04
Pulse
Central 4A04
Peripheral 4A04
Portal 4A04
Pulmonary 4A04
Saturation, Peripheral 4A04
Visual
Acuity 4A07X0Z
Mobility 4A07X7Z
Pressure 4A07XBZ
Whole Blood Nucleic Acid-base Microbial Detection XXE5XM5
Meatoplasty, urethra *see* Repair, Urethra 0TQD
Meatotomy *see* Drainage, Urinary System 0T9
Mechanical chest compression (mCPR) 5A1221J
Mechanical Initial Specimen Diversion Technique Using Active Negative Pressure (blood collection) XXE5XR7
Mechanical ventilation *see* Performance, Respiratory 5A19
Medial canthus
use Lower Eyelid, Left
use Lower Eyelid, Right
Medial collateral ligament (MCL)
use Knee Bursa and Ligament, Left
use Knee Bursa and Ligament, Right
Medial condyle of femur
use Lower Femur, Left
use Lower Femur, Right
Medial condyle of tibia
use Tibia, Left
use Tibia, Right
Medial cuneiform bone
use Tarsal, Left
use Tarsal, Right
Medial epicondyle of femur
use Lower Femur, Left
use Lower Femur, Right
Medial epicondyle of humerus
use Humeral Shaft, Left
use Humeral Shaft, Right
Medial malleolus
use Tibia, Left
use Tibia, Right
Medial meniscus
use Knee Joint, Left
use Knee Joint, Right
Medial plantar artery
use Foot Artery, Left
use Foot Artery, Right
Medial plantar nerve *use* Tibial Nerve
Medial popliteal nerve *use* Tibial Nerve
Medial rectus muscle
use Extraocular Muscle, Left
use Extraocular Muscle, Right
Medial sural cutaneous nerve *use* Tibial Nerve
Median antebrachial vein
use Basilic Vein, Left
use Basilic Vein, Right
Median cubital vein
use Basilic Vein, Left
use Basilic Vein, Right
Median sacral artery *use* Abdominal Aorta
Mediastinal cavity *use* Mediastinum
Mediastinal lymph node *use* Lymphatic, Thorax
Mediastinal space *use* Mediastinum
Mediastinoscopy 0WJC4ZZ
Medication Management GZ3ZZZZ
for substance abuse
Antabuse HZ83ZZZ
Bupropion HZ87ZZZ
Clonidine HZ86ZZZ
Levo-alpha-acetyl-methadol (LAAM) HZ82ZZZ
Methadone Maintenance HZ81ZZZ
Naloxone HZ85ZZZ
Naltrexone HZ84ZZZ
Nicotine Replacement HZ80ZZZ
Other Replacement Medication HZ89ZZZ
Psychiatric Medication HZ88ZZZ
Meditation 8E0ZXY5
Medtronic Endurant® II AAA stent graft system *use* Intraluminal Device
Meissner's (submucous) plexus *use* Abdominal Sympathetic Nerve
Melody® transcatheter pulmonary valve *use* Zooplastic Tissue in Heart and Great Vessels
Melphalan Hydrochloride Antineoplastic XW053T9
Membranous urethra *use* Urethra
Meningeorrhaphy
see Repair, Cerebral Meninges 00Q1
see Repair, Spinal Meninges 00QT
Meniscectomy, knee
see Excision, Joint, Knee, Left 0SBD
see Excision, Joint, Knee, Right 0SBC
Mental foramen
use Mandible, Left
use Mandible, Right
Mentalis muscle *use* Facial Muscle
Mentoplasty *see* Alteration, Jaw, Lower 0W05
Meropenem-vaborbactam Anti-infective XW0
Mesenterectomy *see* Excision, Mesentery 0DBV
Mesenteriorrhaphy, mesenterorrhaphy *see* Repair, Mesentery 0DQV
Mesenteriplication *see* Repair, Mesentery 0DQV
Mesoappendix *use* Mesentery
Mesocolon *use* Mesentery
Metacarpal ligament
use Hand Bursa and Ligament, Left
use Hand Bursa and Ligament, Right
Metacarpophalangeal ligament
use Hand Bursa and Ligament, Left
use Hand Bursa and Ligament, Right
Metal on metal bearing surface *use* Synthetic Substitute, Metal in 0SR
Metatarsal Ligament
use Foot Bursa and Ligament, Left
use Foot Bursa and Ligament, Right
Metatarsectomy
see Excision, Lower Bones 0QB
see Resection, Lower Bones 0QT
Metatarsophalangeal (MTP) joint
use Metatarsal-Phalangeal Joint, Left
use Metatarsal-Phalangeal Joint, Right
Metatarsophalangeal Ligament
use Foot Bursa and Ligament, Left
use Foot Bursa and Ligament, Right
Metathalamus *use* Thalamus
Micro-Driver stent (RX) (OTW) *use* Intraluminal Device
MicroMed HeartAssist *use* Implantable Heart Assist System in Heart and Great Vessels
Micrus CERECYTE Microcoil *use* Intraluminal Device, Bioactive in Upper Arteries
Midcarpal joint
use Carpal Joint, Left
use Carpal Joint, Right
Middle cardiac nerve *use* Thoracic Sympathetic Nerve
Middle cerebral artery *use* Intracranial Artery
Middle cerebral vein *use* Intracranial Vein
Middle colic vein *use* Colic Vein
Middle genicular artery
use Popliteal Artery, Left
use Popliteal Artery, Right
Middle hemorrhoidal vein
use Hypogastric Vein, Left
use Hypogastric Vein, Right
Middle meningeal artery, intracranial portion *use* Intracranial Artery
Middle rectal artery
use Internal Iliac Artery, Left
use Internal Iliac Artery, Right
Middle suprarenal artery *use* Abdominal Aorta
Middle temporal artery
use Temporal Artery, Left
use Temporal Artery, Right
Middle turbinate *use* Nasal Turbinate
Mineral-based Topical Hemostatic Agent XW0
MIRODERM™ Biologic Wound Matrix *use* Nonautologous Tissue Substitute
MIRODERM™ skin graft *see* Replacement, Skin and Breast 0HR
MitraClip valve repair system *use* Synthetic Substitute
Mitral annulus *use* Mitral Valve
Mitroflow® Aortic Pericardial Heart Valve *use* Zooplastic Tissue in Heart and Great Vessels
MNS (Magnus Neuromodulation System) X0Z0X18
Mobilization, adhesions *see* Release
Molar gland *use* Buccal Mucosa
MolecuLight i:X® wound imaging *see* Other Imaging, Anatomical Regions BW5
Monitoring
Arterial
Flow
Coronary 4A13
Peripheral 4A13
Pulmonary 4A13
Pressure
Coronary 4A13
Peripheral 4A13
Pulmonary 4A13
Pulse
Coronary 4A13
Peripheral 4A13
Pulmonary 4A13
Saturation, Peripheral 4A13
Sound, Peripheral 4A13
Brain Electrical Activity, Computer-aided Detection and Notification XX20X89
Cardiac
Electrical Activity 4A12
Ambulatory 4A12X45
No Qualifier 4A12X4Z
Output 4A12
Rate 4A12
Rhythm 4A12
Sound 4A12
Total Activity, Stress 4A12XM4
Vascular Perfusion, Indocyanine Green Dye 4A12XSH
Central Nervous
Conductivity 4A10
Electrical Activity
Intraoperative 4A10
No Qualifier 4A10
Pressure 4A100BZ
Intracranial 4A10
Saturation, Intracranial 4A10
Temperature, Intracranial 4A10
Gastrointestinal
Motility 4A1B
Pressure 4A1B
Secretion 4A1B
Vascular Perfusion, Indocyanine Green Dye 4A1BXSH
Kidney, Fluorescent Pyrazine XT25XE5
Lymphatic
Flow
Indocyanine Green Dye 4A16
No Qualifier 4A16
Pressure 4A16
Muscle Compartment Pressure, Micro-Electro-Mechanical System XX2F3W9
Oxygen Saturation Endoscopic Imaging (OXEI) XD2
Peripheral Nervous
Conductivity
Motor 4A11
Sensory 4A11
Electrical Activity
Intraoperative 4A11
No Qualifier 4A11
Products of Conception
Cardiac
Electrical Activity 4A1H
Rate 4A1H
Rhythm 4A1H
Sound 4A1H
Nervous
Conductivity 4A1J
Electrical Activity 4A1J

Monitoring — *continued*
Products of Conception — *continued*
Nervous — *continued*
Pressure 4A1J
Respiratory
Capacity 4A19
Flow 4A19
Rate 4A19
Resistance 4A19
Volume 4A19
Skin and Breast, Vascular Perfusion, Indocyanine Green Dye 4A1GXSH
Sleep 4A1ZXQZ
Temperature 4A1Z
Urinary
Contractility 4A1D
Flow 4A1D
Pressure 4A1D
Resistance 4A1D
Volume 4A1D
Venous
Flow
Central 4A14
Peripheral 4A14
Portal 4A14
Pulmonary 4A14
Pressure
Central 4A14
Peripheral 4A14
Portal 4A14
Pulmonary 4A14
Pulse
Central 4A14
Peripheral 4A14
Portal 4A14
Pulmonary 4A14
Saturation
Central 4A14
Portal 4A14
Pulmonary 4A14
Monitoring Device, Hemodynamic
Abdomen ØJH8
Chest ØJH6
Mosaic Bioprosthesis (aortic) (mitral) valve *use* Zooplastic Tissue in Heart and Great Vessels
Mosunetuzumab Antineoplastic XWØ
Motor Function Assessment FØ1
Motor Treatment FØ7
MR Angiography
see Magnetic Resonance Imaging (MRI), Heart B23
see Magnetic Resonance Imaging (MRI), Lower Arteries B43
see Magnetic Resonance Imaging (MRI), Upper Arteries B33
MULTI-LINK (VISION) (MINI-VISION) (ULTRA) Coronary Stent System *use* Intraluminal Device
Multiple sleep latency test 4AØZXQZ
Muscle Compartment Pressure, Micro-Electro-Mechanical System XX2F3W9
Musculocutaneous nerve *use* Brachial Plexus
Musculopexy
see Repair, Muscles ØKQ
see Reposition, Muscles ØKS
Musculophrenic artery
use Internal Mammary Artery, Left
use Internal Mammary Artery, Right
Musculoplasty
see Repair, Muscles ØKQ
see Supplement, Muscles ØKU
Musculorrhaphy *see* Repair, Muscles ØKQ
Musculospiral nerve *use* Radial Nerve
MYØ1 Continuous Compartmental Pressure Monitor XX2F3W9
Myectomy
see Excision, Muscles ØKB
see Resection, Muscles ØKT
Myelencephalon *use* Medulla Oblongata
Myelogram
CT *see* Computerized Tomography (CT Scan), Central Nervous System BØ2
MRI *see* Magnetic Resonance Imaging (MRI), Central Nervous System BØ3
Myenteric (Auerbach's) plexus *use* Abdominal Sympathetic Nerve
Myocardial Bridge Release *see* Release, Artery, Coronary
Myomectomy *see* Excision, Female Reproductive System ØUB
Myometrium *use* Uterus
Myopexy
see Repair, Muscles ØKQ
see Reposition, Muscles ØKS
Myoplasty
see Repair, Muscles ØKQ
see Supplement, Muscles ØKU
Myorrhaphy *see* Repair, Muscles ØKQ
Myoscopy *see* Inspection, Muscles ØKJ
Myotomy
see Division, Muscles ØK8
see Drainage, Muscles ØK9
Myringectomy
see Excision, Ear, Nose, Sinus Ø9B
see Resection, Ear, Nose, Sinus Ø9T
Myringoplasty
see Repair, Ear, Nose, Sinus Ø9Q
see Replacement, Ear, Nose, Sinus Ø9R
see Supplement, Ear, Nose, Sinus Ø9U
Myringostomy *see* Drainage, Ear, Nose, Sinus Ø99
Myringotomy *see* Drainage, Ear, Nose, Sinus Ø99

N

NA-1 (Nerinitide) *use* Nerinitide
Nafamostat Anticoagulant XYØYX37
Nail bed
use Finger Nail
use Toe Nail
Nail plate
use Finger Nail
use Toe Nail
nanoLOCK™ interbody fusion device
use Interbody Fusion Device in Lower Joints
use Interbody Fusion Device in Upper Joints
Narcosynthesis GZGZZZZ
Narsoplimab Monoclonal Antibody XWØ
Nasal cavity *use* Nasal Mucosa and Soft Tissue
Nasal concha *use* Nasal Turbinate
Nasalis muscle *use* Facial Muscle
Nasolacrimal duct
use Lacrimal Duct, Left
use Lacrimal Duct, Right
Nasopharyngeal airway (NPA) *use* Intraluminal Device, Airway in Ear, Nose, Sinus
Navicular bone
use Tarsal, Left
use Tarsal, Right
Near Infrared Spectroscopy, Circulatory System 8EØ2
Neck of femur
use Upper Femur, Left
use Upper Femur, Right
Neck of humerus (anatomical) (surgical)
use Humeral Head, Left
use Humeral Head, Right
Nelli® Seizure Monitoring System XXEØX48
Neovasc Reducer™ *use* Reduction Device in New Technology
Nephrectomy
see Excision, Urinary System ØTB
see Resection, Urinary System ØTT
Nephrolithotomy *see* Extirpation, Urinary System ØTC
Nephrolysis *see* Release, Urinary System ØTN
Nephropexy
see Repair, Urinary System ØTQ
see Reposition, Urinary System ØTS
Nephroplasty
see Repair, Urinary System ØTQ
see Supplement, Urinary System ØTU
Nephropyeloureterostomy
see Bypass, Urinary System ØT1
see Drainage, Urinary System ØT9
Nephrorrhaphy *see* Repair, Urinary System ØTQ
Nephroscopy, transurethral ØTJ58ZZ
Nephrostomy
see Bypass, Urinary System ØT1
see Drainage, Urinary System ØT9
Nephrotomography
see Fluoroscopy, Urinary System BT1
see Plain Radiography, Urinary System BTØ
Nephrotomy
see Division, Urinary System ØT8
see Drainage, Urinary System ØT9
Nerinitide XWØ
Nerve conduction study
see Measurement, Central Nervous 4AØØ
see Measurement, Peripheral Nervous 4AØ1
Nerve Function Assessment FØ1
Nerve to the stapedius *use* Facial Nerve
Nesiritide *use* Human B-Type Natriuretic Peptide
Neurectomy
see Excision, Central Nervous System and Cranial Nerves ØØB
see Excision, Peripheral Nervous System Ø1B
Neurexeresis
see Extraction, Central Nervous System and Cranial Nerves ØØD
see Extraction, Peripheral Nervous System Ø1D
NeuroBlate™ System *see* Destruction
Neurohypophysis *use* Pituitary Gland
Neurolysis
see Release, Central Nervous System and Cranial Nerves ØØN
see Release, Peripheral Nervous System Ø1N
Neuromuscular electrical stimulation (NEMS) lead *use* Stimulator Lead in Muscles
Neurophysiologic monitoring *see* Monitoring, Central Nervous 4A1Ø
Neuroplasty
see Repair, Central Nervous System and Cranial Nerves ØØQ
see Repair, Peripheral Nervous System Ø1Q
see Supplement, Central Nervous System and Cranial Nerves ØØU
see Supplement, Peripheral Nervous System Ø1U
Neurorrhaphy
see Repair, Central Nervous System and Cranial Nerves ØØQ
see Repair, Peripheral Nervous System Ø1Q
Neurostimulator Generator
Insertion of device in, Skull ØNHØØNZ
Removal of device from, Skull ØNPØØNZ
Revision of device in, Skull ØNWØØNZ
Neurostimulator generator, multiple channel *use* Stimulator Generator, Multiple Array in ØJH
Neurostimulator generator, multiple channel rechargeable *use* Stimulator Generator, Multiple Array Rechargeable in ØJH
Neurostimulator generator, single channel *use* Stimulator Generator, Single Array in ØJH
Neurostimulator generator, single channel rechargeable *use* Stimulator Generator, Single Array Rechargeable in ØJH
Neurostimulator Lead
Insertion of device in
Brain ØØHØ
Cerebral Ventricle ØØH6
Nerve
Cranial ØØHE
Peripheral Ø1HY
Spinal Canal ØØHU
Spinal Cord ØØHV
Vein
Azygos Ø5HØ
Innominate
Left Ø5H4
Right Ø5H3
Removal of device from
Brain ØØPØ
Cerebral Ventricle ØØP6
Nerve
Cranial ØØPE
Peripheral Ø1PY
Spinal Canal ØØPU
Spinal Cord ØØPV
Vein
Azygos Ø5PØ
Innominate
Left Ø5P4
Right Ø5P3
Revision of device in
Brain ØØWØ
Cerebral Ventricle ØØW6
Nerve
Cranial ØØWE
Peripheral Ø1WY
Spinal Canal ØØWU
Spinal Cord ØØWV
Vein
Azygos Ø5WØ
Innominate
Left Ø5W4

Neurostimulator Lead — *continued*
Revision of device in — *continued*
Vein — *continued*
Innominate — *continued*
Right Ø5W3
Sphenopalatine Ganglion, Insertion XØHK3Q8
Neurostimulator Lead in Oropharynx XWHD7Q7
Neurostimulator Lead with Paired Stimulation System, Insertion XØHQ3R8
Neurotomy
see Division, Central Nervous System and Cranial Nerves ØØ8
see Division, Peripheral Nervous System Ø18
Neurotripsy
see Destruction, Central Nervous System and Cranial Nerves ØØ5
see Destruction, Peripheral Nervous System Ø15
Neutralization plate
use Internal Fixation Device in Head and Facial Bones
use Internal Fixation Device in Lower Bones
use Internal Fixation Device in Upper Bones
New Technology
Afamitresgene Autoleucel Immunotherapy XWØ
Amivantamab Monoclonal Antibody XWØ
Anacaulase-bcdb XWØ
Antibiotic-eluting Bone Void Filler XWØVØP7
Aorta
Thoracic Arch using Branched Synthetic Substitute with Intraluminal Device X2RXØN7
Thoracic Descending using Branched Synthetic Substitute with Intraluminal Device X2VWØN7
Apalutamide Antineoplastic XWØDXJ5
Atezolizumab Antineoplastic XWØ
Axicabtagene Ciloleucel Immunotherapy XWØ
Bamlanivimab Monoclonal Antibody XWØ
Baricitinib XWØ
Betibeglogene Autotemcel XW1
Bioengineered Allogeneic Construct, Skin XHRPXF7
Brain Electrical Activity
Computer-aided Detection and Notification XX2ØX89
Computer-aided Semiologic Analysis XXEØX48
Brexanolone XWØ
Brexucabtagene Autoleucel Immunotherapy XWØ
Broad Consortium Microbiota-based Live Biotherapeutic Suspension XWØH7X8
Bypass
Conduit through Femoral Vein to Popliteal Artery X2K
Conduit through Femoral Vein to Superficial Femoral Artery X2K
Caplacizumab XWØ
CD24Fc Immunomodulator XWØ
Cefiderocol Anti-infective XWØ
Ceftolozane/Tazobactam Anti-infective XWØ
Cerebral Embolic Filtration
Dual Filter X2A5312
Extracorporeal Flow Reversal Circuit X2A
Single Deflection Filter X2A6325
Ciltacabtagene Autoleucel XWØ
Coagulation Factor Xa, Inactivated XWØ
Computer-aided Assessment
Cardiac Output XXE2X19
Intracranial Vascular Activity XXEØXØ7
Computer-aided Guidance, Transthoracic Echocardiography X2JAX47
Computer-aided Mechanical Aspiration X2C
Computer-aided Triage and Notification, Pulmonary Artery Flow XXE3X27
Computer-aided Valve Modeling and Notification, Coronary Artery Flow XXE3X68
Computer-assisted Transcranial Magnetic Stimulation XØZØX18
Coronary Sinus, Reduction Device X2V73Q7
COVID-19 Vaccine XWØ
COVID-19 Vaccine Booster XWØ
COVID-19 Vaccine Dose 1 XWØ
COVID-19 Vaccine Dose 2 XWØ
COVID-19 Vaccine Dose 3 XWØ
Cytarabine and Daunorubicin Liposome Antineoplastic XWØ
Daratumumab and Hyaluronidase-fihj XWØ1318
Destruction
Liver, Ultrasound-guided Cavitation XF5

New Technology — *continued*
Destruction — *continued*
Renal Sympathetic Nerve(s), Ultrasound Ablation XØ51329
Dilation
Anterior Tibial
Left
Sustained Release Drug-eluting Intraluminal Device X27Q385
Four or More X27Q3C5
Three X27Q3B5
Two X27Q395
Right
Sustained Release Drug-eluting Intraluminal Device X27P385
Four or More X27P3C5
Three X27P3B5
Two X27P395
Femoral
Left
Sustained Release Drug-eluting Intraluminal Device X27J385
Four or More X27J3C5
Three X27J3B5
Two X27J395
Right
Sustained Release Drug-eluting Intraluminal Device X27H385
Four or More X27H3C5
Three X27H3B5
Two X27H395
Peroneal
Left
Sustained Release Drug-eluting Intraluminal Device X27U385
Four or More X27U3C5
Three X27U3B5
Two X27U395
Right
Sustained Release Drug-eluting Intraluminal Device X27T385
Four or More X27T3C5
Three X27T3B5
Two X27T395
Popliteal
Left Distal
Sustained Release Drug-eluting Intraluminal Device X27N385
Four or More X27N3C5
Three X27N3B5
Two X27N395
Left Proximal
Sustained Release Drug-eluting Intraluminal Device X27L385
Four or More X27L3C5
Three X27L3B5
Two X27L395
Right Distal
Sustained Release Drug-eluting Intraluminal Device X27M385
Four or More X27M3C5
Three X27M3B5
Two X27M395
Right Proximal
Sustained Release Drug-eluting Intraluminal Device X27K385
Four or More X27K3C5
Three X27K3B5
Two X27K395
Posterior Tibial
Left
Sustained Release Drug-eluting Intraluminal Device X27S385
Four or More X27S3C5
Three X27S3B5
Two X27S395

New Technology — *continued*
Dilation — *continued*
Posterior Tibial — *continued*
Right
Sustained Release Drug-eluting Intraluminal Device X27R385
Four or More X27R3C5
Three X27R3B5
Two X27R395
Durvalumab Antineoplastic XWØ
Eculizumab XWØ
Eladocagene exuparvovec XWØQ316
Elranatamab Antineoplastic XWØ13L9
Endothelial Damage Inhibitor XYØVX83
Engineered Allogeneic Thymus Tissue XWØ2ØD8
Engineered Chimeric Antigen Receptor T-cell Immunotherapy
Allogeneic XWØ
Autologous XWØ
Epcoritamab Monoclonal Antibody XWØ13S9
Erdafitinib Antineoplastic XWØDXL5
Esketamine Hydrochloride XWØ97M5
Etesevimab Monoclonal Antibody XWØ
Exagamglogene Autotemcel XW1
Fosfomycin Anti-infective XWØ
Fostamatinib XWØ
Fusion
Ankle
Left, Open-truss Design Internal Fixation Device XRGKØB9
Right, Open-truss Design Internal Fixation Device XRGJØB9
Lumbar Vertebral
2 or more, Interbody Fusion Device, Custom-Made Anatomically Designed XRGC
Interbody Fusion Device, Custom-Made Anatomically Designed XRGB
Lumbosacral, Interbody Fusion Device, Custom-Made Anatomically Designed XRGD
Sacroiliac, Internal Fixation Device with Tulip Connector XRG
Tarsal
Left, Open-truss Design Internal Fixation Device XRGMØB9
Right, Open-truss Design Internal Fixation Device XRGLØB9
Thoracolumbar Vertebral, Interbody Fusion Device, Custom-Made Anatomically Designed XRGA
Gilteritinib Antineoplastic XWØDXV5
Glofitamab Antineoplastic XWØ
High-Dose Intravenous Immune Globulin, for COVID-19 treatment XW1
Hyperimmune Globulin, for COVID-19 treatment XW1
Idecabtagene Vicleucel Immunotherapy XWØ
Imipenem-cilastatin-relebactam Anti-infective XWØ
Inebilizumab-cdon XWØ
Insertion
Bone, Pelvic, Internal Fixation Device with Tulip Connector XNH
Conduit to Short-term External Heart Assist System X2H
Intracardiac Pacemaker, Dual-Chamber X2H
Intraluminal Device, Bioprosthetic Valve X2H
Joint
Lumbar Vertebral, Posterior Spinal Motion Preservation Device XRHBØ18
Lumbosacral, Posterior Spinal Motion Preservation Device XRHDØ18
Neurostimulator Lead, Sphenopalatine Ganglion XØHK3Q8
Neurostimulator Lead with Paired Stimulation System XØHQ3R8
Tibial Extension with Motion Sensors XNH
Intermittent Coronary Sinus Occlusion X2A7358
Intracranial Arterial Flow, Whole Blood mRNA XXE5XT7
Iobenguane I-131 Antineoplastic XWØ
Kidney, Fluorescent Pyrazine XT25XE5
Lefamulin Anti-infective XWØ
Leronlimab Monoclonal Antibody XWØ13K6
Lifileucel Immunotherapy XWØ
Lisocabtagene Maraleucel Immunotherapy XWØ

New Technology — *continued*
Lovotibeglogene Autotemcel XW1
Lower Respiratory Fluid Nucleic Acid-base Microbial Detection XXEBXQ6
Lurbinectedin XWØ
Maribavir Anti-infective XWØ
Mechanical Initial Specimen Diversion Technique Using Active Negative Pressure (blood collection) XXE5XR7
Melphalan Hydrochloride Antineoplastic XWØ53T9
Meropenem-vaborbactam Anti-infective XWØ
Mineral-based Topical Hemostatic Agent XWØ
Mosunetuzumab Antineoplastic XWØ
Muscle Compartment Pressure, Micro-Electro-Mechanical System XX2F3W9
Nafamostat Anticoagulant XYØYX37
Narsoplimab Monoclonal Antibody XWØ
Nerinitide XWØ
Neurostimulator Lead in Oropharynx XWHD7Q7
Omadacycline Anti-infective XWØ
Omidubicel XW1
Other New Technology Monoclonal Antibody XWØ
Other New Technology Therapeutic Substance XWØ
Other Positive Blood/Isolated Colonies Bimodal Phenotypic Susceptibility Technology XXE5XY9
OTL-1Ø3 XW1
OTL-2ØØ XW1
Oxygen Saturation Endoscopic Imaging (OXEI) XD2
Plasma, Convalescent (Nonautologous) XW1
Positive Blood Culture Fluorescence Hybridization for Organism Identification, Concentration and Susceptibility XXE5XN6
Posoleucel XWØ
Quantitative Flow Ratio Analysis, Coronary Artery Flow XXE3X58
Quizartinib Antineoplastic XWØDXJ9
Radial artery arteriovenous fistula, using Thermal Resistance Energy X2K
REGN-COV2 Monoclonal Antibody XWØ
Remdesivir Anti-infective XWØ
Replacement
Lateral Meniscus Synthetic Substitute XRR
Medial Meniscus Synthetic Substitute XRR
Reposition
Cervical, Magnetically Controlled Growth Rod(s) XNS3
Lumbar
Magnetically Controlled Growth Rod(s) XNSØ
Posterior (Dynamic) Distraction Device XNSØ
Thoracic
Magnetically Controlled Growth Rod(s) XNS4
Posterior (Dynamic) Distraction Device XNS4
Rezafungin XWØ
Ruxolitinib XWØDXT5
Sabizabulin XWØ
Sarilumab XWØ
SARS-CoV-2 Antibody Detection, Serum/Plasma Nanoparticle Fluorescence XXE5XV7
SARS-CoV-2 Polymerase Chain Reaction, Nasopharyngeal Fluid XXE97U7
Satralizumab-mwge XWØ1397
SER-1Ø9 XWØDXN9
Single-use Duodenoscope XFJ
Single-use Oversleeve with Intraoperative Colonic Irrigation XDPH8K7
Spesolimab Monoclonal Antibody XWØ
Sulbactam-Durlobactam XWØ
Supplement
Arteriovenous Fistula, Extraluminal Support Device X2U
Bursa and Ligament, Spine, Posterior Vertebral Tether XKU
Coronary Artery/Arteries, Vein Graft Extraluminal Support Device(s) X2U4079
Vertebra
Lumbar, Mechanically Expandable (Paired) Synthetic Substitute XNUØ356
Thoracic, Mechanically Expandable (Paired) Synthetic Substitute XNU4356
Tabelecleucel Immunotherapy XWØ
Tagraxofusp-erzs Antineoplastic XWØ

New Technology — *continued*
Talar Prosthesis Synthetic Substitute XNR
Taurolidine Anti-infective and Heparin Anticoagulant XYØYX28
Teclistamab Antineoplastic XWØ1348
Terlipressin XWØ
Tisagenlecleucel Immunotherapy XWØ
Tixagevimab and Cilgavimab Monoclonal Antibody XWØ23X7
Tocilizumab XWØ
Treosulfan XWØ
Trilaciclib XWØ
Ultrasound Penetrable Synthetic Substitute, Skull XNR8ØD9
Uridine Triacetate XWØDX82
Venetoclax Antineoplastic XWØDXR5
Whole Blood Nucleic Acid-base Microbial Detection XXE5XM5
Whole Blood Reverse Transcription and Quantitative Real-time Polymerase Chain Reaction XXE5X38
NexoBrid™ *use* Anacaulase-bcdb
Ninth cranial nerve *use* Glossopharyngeal Nerve
NIRS (Near Infrared Spectroscopy) *see* Physiological Systems and Anatomical Regions 8EØ
Nitinol framed polymer mesh *use* Synthetic Substitute
Niyad™ *use* Nafamostat Anticoagulant
Nonimaging Nuclear Medicine Assay
Bladder, Kidneys and Ureters CT63
Blood C763
Kidneys, Ureters and Bladder CT63
Lymphatics and Hematologic System C76YYZZ
Ureters, Kidneys and Bladder CT63
Urinary System CT6YYZZ
Nonimaging Nuclear Medicine Probe
Abdomen CW5Ø
Abdomen and Chest CW54
Abdomen and Pelvis CW51
Brain CØ5Ø
Central Nervous System CØ5YYZZ
Chest CW53
Chest and Abdomen CW54
Chest and Neck CW56
Extremity
Lower CP5PZZZ
Upper CP5NZZZ
Head and Neck CW5B
Heart C25YYZZ
Right and Left C256
Lymphatics
Head C75J
Head and Neck C755
Lower Extremity C75P
Neck C75K
Pelvic C75D
Trunk C75M
Upper Chest C75L
Upper Extremity C75N
Lymphatics and Hematologic System C75YYZZ
Musculoskeletal System, Other CP5YYZZ
Neck and Chest CW56
Neck and Head CW5B
Pelvic Region CW5J
Pelvis and Abdomen CW51
Spine CP55ZZZ
Nonimaging Nuclear Medicine Uptake
Endocrine System CG4YYZZ
Gland, Thyroid CG42
Non-tunneled central venous catheter *use* Infusion Device
Nostril *use* Nasal Mucosa and Soft Tissue
Novacor Left Ventricular Assist Device *use* Implantable Heart Assist System in Heart and Great Vessels
Novation® Ceramic AHS® (Articulation Hip System) *use* Synthetic Substitute, Ceramic in ØSR
Nuclear medicine
see Nonimaging Nuclear Medicine Assay
see Nonimaging Nuclear Medicine Probe
see Nonimaging Nuclear Medicine Uptake
see Planar Nuclear Medicine Imaging
see Positron Emission Tomographic (PET) Imaging
see Systemic Nuclear Medicine Therapy
see Tomographic (Tomo) Nuclear Medicine Imaging
Nuclear scintigraphy *see* Nuclear Medicine

NUsurface® Meniscus Implant
use Synthetic Substitute, Lateral Meniscus in New Technology
use Synthetic Substitute, Medial Meniscus in New Technology
Nutrition, concentrated substances
Enteral infusion 3EØG36Z
Parenteral (peripheral) infusion *see* Introduction of Nutritional Substance
NUZYRA™ *use* Omadacycline Anti-infective

O

Obliteration *see* Destruction
Obturator artery
use Internal Iliac Artery, Left
use Internal Iliac Artery, Right
Obturator lymph node *use* Lymphatic, Pelvis
Obturator muscle
use Hip Muscle, Left
use Hip Muscle, Right
Obturator nerve *use* Lumbar Plexus
Obturator vein
use Hypogastric Vein, Left
use Hypogastric Vein, Right
Obtuse margin *use* Heart, Left
Occipital artery
use External Carotid Artery, Left
use External Carotid Artery, Right
Occipital lobe *use* Cerebral Hemisphere
Occipital lymph node
use Lymphatic, Left Neck
use Lymphatic, Right Neck
Occipitofrontalis muscle *use* Facial Muscle
Occlusion
Ampulla of Vater ØFLC
Anus ØDLQ
Aorta
Abdominal Ø4LØ
Thoracic, Descending Ø2LW
Artery
Anterior Tibial
Left Ø4LQ
Right Ø4LP
Axillary
Left Ø3L6
Right Ø3L5
Brachial
Left Ø3L8
Right Ø3L7
Celiac Ø4L1
Colic
Left Ø4L7
Middle Ø4L8
Right Ø4L6
Common Carotid
Left Ø3LJ
Right Ø3LH
Common Iliac
Left Ø4LD
Right Ø4LC
External Carotid
Left Ø3LN
Right Ø3LM
External Iliac
Left Ø4LJ
Right Ø4LH
Face Ø3LR
Femoral
Left Ø4LL
Right Ø4LK
Foot
Left Ø4LW
Right Ø4LV
Gastric Ø4L2
Hand
Left Ø3LF
Right Ø3LD
Hepatic Ø4L3
Inferior Mesenteric Ø4LB
Innominate Ø3L2
Internal Carotid
Left Ø3LL
Right Ø3LK
Internal Iliac
Left Ø4LF
Right Ø4LE

- **Occlusion** — *continued*
  - Artery — *continued*
    - Internal Mammary
      - Left Ø3L1
      - Right Ø3LØ
    - Intracranial Ø3LG
    - Lower Ø4LY
    - Peroneal
      - Left Ø4LU
      - Right Ø4LT
    - Popliteal
      - Left Ø4LN
      - Right Ø4LM
    - Posterior Tibial
      - Left Ø4LS
      - Right Ø4LR
    - Pulmonary
      - Left Ø2LR
      - Right Ø2LQ
    - Pulmonary Trunk Ø2LP
    - Radial
      - Left Ø3LC
      - Right Ø3LB
    - Renal
      - Left Ø4LA
      - Right Ø4L9
    - Splenic Ø4L4
    - Subclavian
      - Left Ø3L4
      - Right Ø3L3
    - Superior Mesenteric Ø4L5
    - Temporal
      - Left Ø3LT
      - Right Ø3LS
    - Thyroid
      - Left Ø3LV
      - Right Ø3LU
    - Ulnar
      - Left Ø3LA
      - Right Ø3L9
    - Upper Ø3LY
    - Vertebral
      - Left Ø3LQ
      - Right Ø3LP
  - Atrium, Left Ø2L7
  - Bladder ØTLB
  - Bladder Neck ØTLC
  - Bronchus
    - Lingula ØBL9
    - Lower Lobe
      - Left ØBLB
      - Right ØBL6
    - Main
      - Left ØBL7
      - Right ØBL3
    - Middle Lobe, Right ØBL5
    - Upper Lobe
      - Left ØBL8
      - Right ØBL4
  - Carina ØBL2
  - Cecum ØDLH
  - Cisterna Chyli Ø7LL
  - Colon
    - Ascending ØDLK
    - Descending ØDLM
    - Sigmoid ØDLN
    - Transverse ØDLL
  - Cord
    - Bilateral ØVLH
    - Left ØVLG
    - Right ØVLF
  - Cul-de-sac ØULF
  - Duct
    - Common Bile ØFL9
    - Cystic ØFL8
    - Hepatic
      - Common ØFL7
      - Left ØFL6
      - Right ØFL5
    - Lacrimal
      - Left Ø8LY
      - Right Ø8LX
    - Pancreatic ØFLD
      - Accessory ØFLF
    - Parotid
      - Left ØCLC
      - Right ØCLB
  - Duodenum ØDL9
  - Esophagogastric Junction ØDL4

- **Occlusion** — *continued*
  - Esophagus ØDL5
    - Lower ØDL3
    - Middle ØDL2
    - Upper ØDL1
  - Fallopian Tube
    - Left ØUL6
    - Right ØUL5
  - Fallopian Tubes, Bilateral ØUL7
  - Ileocecal Valve ØDLC
  - Ileum ØDLB
  - Intestine
    - Large ØDLE
      - Left ØDLG
      - Right ØDLF
    - Small ØDL8
  - Jejunum ØDLA
  - Kidney Pelvis
    - Left ØTL4
    - Right ØTL3
  - Left atrial appendage (LAA) *see* Occlusion, Atrium, Left Ø2L7
  - Lymphatic
    - Aortic Ø7LD
    - Axillary
      - Left Ø7L6
      - Right Ø7L5
    - Head Ø7LØ
    - Inguinal
      - Left Ø7LJ
      - Right Ø7LH
    - Internal Mammary
      - Left Ø7L9
      - Right Ø7L8
    - Lower Extremity
      - Left Ø7LG
      - Right Ø7LF
    - Mesenteric Ø7LB
    - Neck
      - Left Ø7L2
      - Right Ø7L1
    - Pelvis Ø7LC
    - Thoracic Duct Ø7LK
    - Thorax Ø7L7
    - Upper Extremity
      - Left Ø7L4
      - Right Ø7L3
  - Rectum ØDLP
  - Stomach ØDL6
    - Pylorus ØDL7
  - Trachea ØBL1
  - Ureter
    - Left ØTL7
    - Right ØTL6
  - Urethra ØTLD
  - Vagina ØULG
  - Valve, Pulmonary Ø2LH
  - Vas Deferens
    - Bilateral ØVLQ
    - Left ØVLP
    - Right ØVLN
  - Vein
    - Axillary
      - Left Ø5L8
      - Right Ø5L7
    - Azygos Ø5LØ
    - Basilic
      - Left Ø5LC
      - Right Ø5LB
    - Brachial
      - Left Ø5LA
      - Right Ø5L9
    - Cephalic
      - Left Ø5LF
      - Right Ø5LD
    - Colic Ø6L7
    - Common Iliac
      - Left Ø6LD
      - Right Ø6LC
    - Esophageal Ø6L3
    - External Iliac
      - Left Ø6LG
      - Right Ø6LF
    - External Jugular
      - Left Ø5LQ
      - Right Ø5LP
    - Face
      - Left Ø5LV
      - Right Ø5LT

- **Occlusion** — *continued*
  - Vein — *continued*
    - Femoral
      - Left Ø6LN
      - Right Ø6LM
    - Foot
      - Left Ø6LV
      - Right Ø6LT
    - Gastric Ø6L2
    - Hand
      - Left Ø5LH
      - Right Ø5LG
    - Hemiazygos Ø5L1
    - Hepatic Ø6L4
    - Hypogastric
      - Left Ø6LJ
      - Right Ø6LH
    - Inferior Mesenteric Ø6L6
    - Innominate
      - Left Ø5L4
      - Right Ø5L3
    - Internal Jugular
      - Left Ø5LN
      - Right Ø5LM
    - Intracranial Ø5LL
    - Lower Ø6LY
    - Portal Ø6L8
    - Pulmonary
      - Left Ø2LT
      - Right Ø2LS
    - Renal
      - Left Ø6LB
      - Right Ø6L9
    - Saphenous
      - Left Ø6LQ
      - Right Ø6LP
    - Splenic Ø6L1
    - Subclavian
      - Left Ø5L6
      - Right Ø5L5
    - Superior Mesenteric Ø6L5
    - Upper Ø5LY
    - Vertebral
      - Left Ø5LS
      - Right Ø5LR
  - Vena Cava
    - Inferior Ø6LØ
    - Superior Ø2LV
- **Occlusion, REBOA (resuscitative endovascular balloon occlusion of the aorta)**
  - Ø2LW3DJ
  - Ø4LØ3DJ
- **Occupational therapy** *see* Activities of Daily Living Treatment, Rehabilitation FØ8
- **Octagam 1Ø%, for COVID-19 treatment** *use* High-Dose Intravenous Immune Globulin
- **Odentectomy**
  - *see* Excision, Mouth and Throat ØCB
  - *see* Resection, Mouth and Throat ØCT
- **Odontoid process** *use* Cervical Vertebra
- **Olecranon bursa**
  - *use* Elbow Bursa and Ligament, Left
  - *use* Elbow Bursa and Ligament, Right
- **Olecranon process**
  - *use* Ulna, Left
  - *use* Ulna, Right
- **Olfactory bulb** *use* Olfactory Nerve
- **Olumiant®** *use* Baricitinib
- **Omadacycline Anti-infective** XWØ
- **Omentectomy, omentumectomy**
  - *see* Excision, Gastrointestinal System ØDB
  - *see* Resection, Gastrointestinal System ØDT
- **Omentofixation** *see* Repair, Gastrointestinal System ØDQ
- **Omentoplasty**
  - *see* Repair, Gastrointestinal System ØDQ
  - *see* Replacement, Gastrointestinal System ØDR
  - *see* Supplement, Gastrointestinal System ØDU
- **Omentorrhaphy** *see* Repair, Gastrointestinal System ØDQ
- **Omentotomy** *see* Drainage, Gastrointestinal System ØD9
- **Omidubicel** XW1
- **Omnilink Elite Vascular Balloon Expandable Stent System** *use* Intraluminal Device
- **Onychectomy**
  - *see* Excision, Skin and Breast ØHB
  - *see* Resection, Skin and Breast ØHT

Onychoplasty
see Repair, Skin and Breast ØHQ
see Replacement, Skin and Breast ØHR
Onychotomy *see* Drainage, Skin and Breast ØH9
Oophorectomy
see Excision, Female Reproductive System ØUB
see Resection, Female Reproductive System ØUT
Oophoropexy
see Repair, Female Reproductive System ØUQ
see Reposition, Female Reproductive System ØUS
Oophoroplasty
see Repair, Female Reproductive System ØUQ
see Supplement, Female Reproductive System ØUU
Oophororrhaphy *see* Repair, Female Reproductive System ØUQ
Oophorostomy *see* Drainage, Female Reproductive System ØU9
Oophorotomy
see Division, Female Reproductive System ØU8
see Drainage, Female Reproductive System ØU9
Oophorrhaphy *see* Repair, Female Reproductive System ØUQ
Open Pivot Aortic Valve Graft (AVG) *use* Synthetic Substitute
Open Pivot (mechanical) Valve *use* Synthetic Substitute
Open-truss Design Internal Fixation Device
Ankle
Left XRGKØB9
Right XRGJØB9
Tarsal
Left XRGMØB9
Right XRGLØB9
Ophthalmic artery *use* Intracranial Artery
Ophthalmic nerve *use* Trigeminal Nerve
Ophthalmic vein *use* Intracranial Vein
Opponensplasty
Tendon replacement *see* Replacement, Tendons ØLR
Tendon transfer *see* Transfer, Tendons ØLX
Optic chiasma *use* Optic Nerve
Optic disc
use Retina, Left
use Retina, Right
Optic foramen *use* Sphenoid Bone
Optical coherence tomography, intravascular *see* Computerized Tomography (CT Scan)
Optimizer™ III implantable pulse generator *use* Contractility Modulation Device in ØJH
Orbicularis oculi muscle
use Upper Eyelid, Left
use Upper Eyelid, Right
Orbicularis oris muscle *use* Facial Muscle
Orbital Atherectomy *see* Extirpation, Heart and Great Vessels Ø2C
Orbital fascia *use* Subcutaneous Tissue and Fascia, Face
Orbital portion of ethmoid bone
use Orbit, Left
use Orbit, Right
Orbital portion of frontal bone
use Orbit, Left
use Orbit, Right
Orbital portion of lacrimal bone
use Orbit, Left
use Orbit, Right
Orbital portion of maxilla
use Orbit, Left
use Orbit, Right
Orbital portion of palatine bone
use Orbit, Left
use Orbit, Right
Orbital portion of sphenoid bone
use Orbit, Left
use Orbit, Right
Orbital portion of zygomatic bone
use Orbit, Left
use Orbit, Right
Orchectomy, orchidectomy, orchiectomy
see Excision, Male Reproductive System ØVB
see Resection, Male Reproductive System ØVT
Orchidoplasty, orchioplasty
see Repair, Male Reproductive System ØVQ
see Replacement, Male Reproductive System ØVR
see Supplement, Male Reproductive System ØVU
Orchidorrhaphy, orchiorrhaphy *see* Repair, Male Reproductive System ØVQ
Orchidotomy, orchiotomy, orchotomy *see* Drainage, Male Reproductive System ØV9
Orchiopexy
see Repair, Male Reproductive System ØVQ
see Reposition, Male Reproductive System ØVS
Oropharyngeal airway (OPA) *use* Intraluminal Device, Airway in Mouth and Throat
Oropharynx *use* Pharynx
Ossiculectomy
see Excision, Ear, Nose, Sinus Ø9B
see Resection, Ear, Nose, Sinus Ø9T
Ossiculotomy *see* Drainage, Ear, Nose, Sinus Ø99
Ostectomy
see Excision, Head and Facial Bones ØNB
see Excision, Lower Bones ØQB
see Excision, Upper Bones ØPB
see Resection, Head and Facial Bones ØNT
see Resection, Lower Bones ØQT
see Resection, Upper Bones ØPT
Osteoclasis
see Division, Head and Facial Bones ØN8
see Division, Lower Bones ØQ8
see Division, Upper Bones ØP8
Osteolysis
see Release, Head and Facial Bones ØNN
see Release, Lower Bones ØQN
see Release, Upper Bones ØPN
Osteopathic Treatment
Abdomen 7WØ9X
Cervical 7WØ1X
Extremity
Lower 7WØ6X
Upper 7WØ7X
Head 7WØØX
Lumbar 7WØ3X
Pelvis 7WØ5X
Rib Cage 7WØ8X
Sacrum 7WØ4X
Thoracic 7WØ2X
Osteopexy
see Repair, Head and Facial Bones ØNQ
see Repair, Lower Bones ØQQ
see Repair, Upper Bones ØPQ
see Reposition, Head and Facial Bones ØNS
see Reposition, Lower Bones ØQS
see Reposition, Upper Bones ØPS
Osteoplasty
see Repair, Head and Facial Bones ØNQ
see Repair, Lower Bones ØQQ
see Repair, Upper Bones ØPQ
see Replacement, Head and Facial Bones ØNR
see Replacement, Lower Bones ØQR
see Replacement, Upper Bones ØPR
see Supplement, Head and Facial Bones ØNU
see Supplement, Lower Bones ØQU
see Supplement, Upper Bones ØPU
Osteorrhaphy
see Repair, Head and Facial Bones ØNQ
see Repair, Lower Bones ØQQ
see Repair, Upper Bones ØPQ
Osteotomy, ostotomy
see Division, Head and Facial Bones ØN8
see Division, Lower Bones ØQ8
see Division, Upper Bones ØP8
see Drainage, Head and Facial Bones ØN9
see Drainage, Lower Bones ØQ9
see Drainage, Upper Bones ØP9
Other Imaging
Bile Duct and Gallbladder, Indocyanine Green Dye, Intraoperative BF532ØØ
Bile Duct, Indocyanine Green Dye, Intraoperative BF5Ø2ØØ
Extremity
Lower BW5CZ1Z
Upper BW5JZ1Z
Gallbladder and Bile Duct, Indocyanine Green Dye, Intraoperative BF532ØØ
Gallbladder, Indocyanine Green Dye, Intraoperative BF522ØØ
Head and Neck BW59Z1Z
Hepatobiliary System, All, Indocyanine Green Dye, Intraoperative BF5C2ØØ
Liver and Spleen, Indocyanine Green Dye, Intraoperative BF562ØØ
Liver, Indocyanine Green Dye, Intraoperative BF552ØØ
Neck and Head BW59Z1Z
Other Imaging — *continued*
Pancreas, Indocyanine Green Dye, Intraoperative BF572ØØ
Spleen and Liver, Indocyanine Green Dye, Intraoperative BF562ØØ
Trunk BW52Z1Z
Other New Technology Monoclonal Antibody XWØ
Other New Technology Therapeutic Substance XWØ
Other Positive Blood/Isolated Colonies Bimodal Phenotypic Susceptibility Technology XXE5XY9
Otic ganglion *use* Head and Neck Sympathetic Nerve
OTL-1Ø1 *use* Hematopoietic Stem/Progenitor Cells, Genetically Modified
OTL-1Ø3 XW1
OTL-2ØØ XW1
Otoplasty
see Repair, Ear, Nose, Sinus Ø9Q
see Replacement, Ear, Nose, Sinus Ø9R
see Supplement, Ear, Nose, Sinus Ø9U
Otoscopy *see* Inspection, Ear, Nose, Sinus Ø9J
Oval window
use Middle Ear, Left
use Middle Ear, Right
Ovarian artery *use* Abdominal Aorta
Ovarian ligament *use* Uterine Supporting Structure
Ovariectomy
see Excision, Female Reproductive System ØUB
see Resection, Female Reproductive System ØUT
Ovariocentesis *see* Drainage, Female Reproductive System ØU9
Ovariopexy
see Repair, Female Reproductive System ØUQ
see Reposition, Female Reproductive System ØUS
Ovariotomy
see Division, Female Reproductive System ØU8
see Drainage, Female Reproductive System ØU9
Ovatio™ CRT-D *use* Cardiac Resynchronization Defibrillator Pulse Generator in ØJH
Oversewing
Gastrointestinal ulcer *see* Repair, Gastrointestinal System ØDQ
Pleural bleb *see* Repair, Respiratory System ØBQ
Oviduct
use Fallopian Tube, Left
use Fallopian Tube, Right
Oximetry, Fetal pulse 1ØHØ73Z
OXINIUM *use* Synthetic Substitute, Oxidized Zirconium on Polyethylene in ØSR
Oxygen Saturation Endoscopic Imaging (OXEI) XD2
Oxygenation
Extracorporeal membrane (ECMO) *see* Performance, Circulatory 5A15
Hyperbaric *see* Assistance, Circulatory 5AØ5
Supersaturated *see* Assistance, Cardiac 5AØ2

P

Pacemaker
Dual Chamber
Abdomen ØJH8
Chest ØJH6
Intracardiac
Insertion of device in
Atrium
Left Ø2H7
Right Ø2H6
Vein, Coronary Ø2H4
Ventricle
Left Ø2HL
Right Ø2HK
Removal of device from, Heart Ø2PA
Revision of device in, Heart Ø2WA
Single Chamber
Abdomen ØJH8
Chest ØJH6
Single Chamber Rate Responsive
Abdomen ØJH8
Chest ØJH6
Packing
Abdominal Wall 2W43X5Z
Anorectal 2Y43X5Z
Arm
Lower
Left 2W4DX5Z
Right 2W4CX5Z

Packing — *continued*
Arm — *continued*
Upper
Left 2W4BX5Z
Right 2W4AX5Z
Back 2W45X5Z
Chest Wall 2W44X5Z
Ear 2Y42X5Z
Extremity
Lower
Left 2W4MX5Z
Right 2W4LX5Z
Upper
Left 2W49X5Z
Right 2W48X5Z
Face 2W41X5Z
Finger
Left 2W4KX5Z
Right 2W4JX5Z
Foot
Left 2W4TX5Z
Right 2W4SX5Z
Genital Tract, Female 2Y44X5Z
Hand
Left 2W4FX5Z
Right 2W4EX5Z
Head 2W40X5Z
Inguinal Region
Left 2W47X5Z
Right 2W46X5Z
Leg
Lower
Left 2W4RX5Z
Right 2W4QX5Z
Upper
Left 2W4PX5Z
Right 2W4NX5Z
Mouth and Pharynx 2Y40X5Z
Nasal 2Y41X5Z
Neck 2W42X5Z
Thumb
Left 2W4HX5Z
Right 2W4GX5Z
Toe
Left 2W4VX5Z
Right 2W4UX5Z
Urethra 2Y45X5Z
Paclitaxel-eluting coronary stent *use* Intraluminal Device, Drug-eluting in Heart and Great Vessels
Paclitaxel-eluting peripheral stent
use Intraluminal Device, Drug-eluting in Lower Arteries
use Intraluminal Device, Drug-eluting in Upper Arteries
Palatine gland *use* Buccal Mucosa
Palatine tonsil *use* Tonsils
Palatine uvula *use* Uvula
Palatoglossal muscle *use* Tongue, Palate, Pharynx Muscle
Palatopharyngeal muscle *use* Tongue, Palate, Pharynx Muscle
Palatoplasty
see Repair, Mouth and Throat 0CQ
see Replacement, Mouth and Throat 0CR
see Supplement, Mouth and Throat 0CU
Palatorrhaphy *see* Repair, Mouth and Throat 0CQ
Palmar cutaneous nerve
use Median Nerve
use Radial Nerve
Palmar (volar) digital vein
use Hand Vein, Left
use Hand Vein, Right
Palmar fascia (aponeurosis)
use Subcutaneous Tissue and Fascia, Left Hand
use Subcutaneous Tissue and Fascia, Right Hand
Palmar interosseous muscle
use Hand Muscle, Left
use Hand Muscle, Right
Palmar (volar) metacarpal vein
use Hand Vein, Left
use Hand Vein, Right
Palmar ulnocarpal ligament
use Wrist Bursa and Ligament, Left
use Wrist Bursa and Ligament, Right
Palmaris longus muscle
use Lower Arm and Wrist Muscle, Left
use Lower Arm and Wrist Muscle, Right
Pancreatectomy
see Excision, Pancreas 0FBG
see Resection, Pancreas 0FTG
Pancreatic artery *use* Splenic Artery
Pancreatic plexus *use* Abdominal Sympathetic Nerve
Pancreatic vein *use* Splenic Vein
Pancreaticoduodenostomy *see* Bypass, Hepatobiliary System and Pancreas 0F1
Pancreaticosplenic lymph node *use* Lymphatic, Aortic
Pancreatogram, endoscopic retrograde *see* Fluoroscopy, Pancreatic Duct BF18
Pancreatolithotomy *see* Extirpation, Pancreas 0FCG
Pancreatotomy
see Division, Pancreas 0F8G
see Drainage, Pancreas 0F9G
Panniculectomy
see Excision, Skin, Abdomen 0HB7
see Excision, Subcutaneous Tissue and Fascia, Abdomen 0JB8
Paraaortic lymph node *use* Lymphatic, Aortic
Paracentesis
Eye *see* Drainage, Eye 089
Peritoneal Cavity *see* Drainage, Peritoneal Cavity 0W9G
Tympanum *see* Drainage, Ear, Nose, Sinus 099
Paradise™ Ultrasound Renal Denervation System X051329
Parapharyngeal space *use* Neck
Pararectal lymph node *use* Lymphatic, Mesenteric
Parasternal lymph node *use* Lymphatic, Thorax
Parathyroidectomy
see Excision, Endocrine System 0GB
see Resection, Endocrine System 0GT
Paratracheal lymph node *use* Lymphatic, Thorax
Paraurethral (Skene's) gland *use* Vestibular Gland
Parenteral nutrition, total *see* Introduction of Nutritional Substance
Parietal lobe *use* Cerebral Hemisphere
Parotid lymph node *use* Lymphatic, Head
Parotid plexus *use* Facial Nerve
Parotidectomy
see Excision, Mouth and Throat 0CB
see Resection, Mouth and Throat 0CT
Pars flaccida
use Tympanic Membrane, Left
use Tympanic Membrane, Right
Partial joint replacement
Hip *see* Replacement, Lower Joints 0SR
Knee *see* Replacement, Lower Joints 0SR
Shoulder *see* Replacement, Upper Joints 0RR
Partially absorbable mesh *use* Synthetic Substitute
Patch, blood, spinal 3E0R3GC
Patellapexy
see Repair, Lower Bones 0QQ
see Reposition, Lower Bones 0QS
Patellaplasty
see Repair, Lower Bones 0QQ
see Replacement, Lower Bones 0QR
see Supplement, Lower Bones 0QU
Patellar ligament
use Knee Bursa and Ligament, Left
use Knee Bursa and Ligament, Right
Patellar tendon
use Knee Tendon, Left
use Knee Tendon, Right
Patellectomy
see Excision, Lower Bones 0QB
see Resection, Lower Bones 0QT
Patellofemoral joint
use Knee Joint, Left
use Knee Joint, Left, Femoral Surface
use Knee Joint, Right
use Knee Joint, Right, Femoral Surface
pAVF (percutaneous arteriovenous fistula), using magnetic-guided radiofrequency *see* Bypass, Upper Arteries 031
pAVF (percutaneous arteriovenous fistula), using thermal resistance energy *see* New Technology, Cardiovascular System X2K
Pectineus muscle
use Upper Leg Muscle, Left
use Upper Leg Muscle, Right
Pectoral fascia *use* Subcutaneous Tissue and Fascia, Chest
Pectoral (anterior) lymph node
use Lymphatic Left, Axillary
use Lymphatic Right, Axillary
Pectoralis major muscle
use Thorax Muscle, Left
use Thorax Muscle, Right
Pectoralis minor muscle
use Thorax Muscle, Left
use Thorax Muscle, Right
Pedicle-based dynamic stabilization device
use Spinal Stabilization Device, Pedicle-Based in 0SH
use Spinal Stabilization Device, Pedicle-Based in 0RH
PEEP (positive end expiratory pressure) *see* Assistance, Respiratory 5A09
PEG (percutaneous endoscopic gastrostomy) 0DH63UZ
PEJ (percutaneous endoscopic jejunostomy) 0DHA3UZ
Pelvic splanchnic nerve
use Abdominal Sympathetic Nerve
use Sacral Sympathetic Nerve
Penectomy
see Excision, Male Reproductive System 0VB
see Resection, Male Reproductive System 0VT
Penile urethra *use* Urethra
Penumbra Indigo® Aspiration System *see* New Technology, Cardiovascular System X2C
PERCEPT™ PC neurostimulator *use* Stimulator Generator, Multiple Array in 0JH
Perceval sutureless valve (rapid deployment technique) *see* Replacement, Valve, Aortic 02RF
Percutaneous endoscopic gastrojejunostomy (PEG/J) tube *use* Feeding Device in Gastrointestinal System
Percutaneous endoscopic gastrostomy (PEG) tube *use* Feeding Device in Gastrointestinal System
Percutaneous nephrostomy catheter *use* Drainage Device
Percutaneous transluminal coronary angioplasty (PTCA) *see* Dilation, Heart and Great Vessels 027
Performance
Biliary
Multiple, Filtration 5A1C60Z
Single, Filtration 5A1C00Z
Cardiac
Continuous
Output 5A1221Z
Pacing 5A1223Z
Intermittent, Pacing 5A1213Z
Single, Output, Manual 5A12012
Circulatory
Continuous
Central Membrane 5A1522F
Peripheral Veno-arterial Membrane 5A1522G
Peripheral Veno-venous Membrane 5A1522H
Intraoperative
Central Membrane 5A15A2F
Peripheral Veno-arterial Membrane 5A15A2G
Peripheral Veno-venous Membrane 5A15A2H
Respiratory
24-96 Consecutive Hours, Ventilation 5A1945Z
Greater than 96 Consecutive Hours, Ventilation 5A1955Z
Less than 24 Consecutive Hours, Ventilation 5A1935Z
Single, Ventilation, Nonmechanical 5A19054
Urinary
Continuous, Greater than 18 hours per day, Filtration 5A1D90Z
Intermittent, Less than 6 Hours Per Day, Filtration 5A1D70Z
Prolonged Intermittent, 6-18 hours per day, Filtration 5A1D80Z
Perfusion *see* Introduction of substance in or on
Perfusion, donor organ
Heart 6AB50BZ
Kidney(s) 6ABT0BZ
Liver 6ABF0BZ
Lung(s) 6ABB0BZ
Perianal skin *use* Skin, Perineum

Pericardiectomy
see Excision, Pericardium Ø2BN
see Resection, Pericardium Ø2TN
Pericardiocentesis see Drainage, Pericardial Cavity ØW9D
Pericardiolysis see Release, Pericardium Ø2NN
Pericardiophrenic artery
use Internal Mammary Artery, Left
use Internal Mammary Artery, Right
Pericardioplasty
see Repair, Pericardium Ø2QN
see Replacement, Pericardium Ø2RN
see Supplement, Pericardium Ø2UN
Pericardiorrhaphy see Repair, Pericardium Ø2QN
Pericardiostomy see Drainage, Pericardial Cavity ØW9D
Pericardiotomy see Drainage, Pericardial Cavity ØW9D
Perimetrium use Uterus
Peripheral Intravascular Lithotripsy (Peripheral IVL) see Fragmentation
Peripheral parenteral nutrition see Introduction of Nutritional Substance
Peripherally inserted central catheter (PICC) use Infusion Device
Peritoneal dialysis 3E1M39Z
Peritoneocentesis
see Drainage, Peritoneal Cavity ØW9G
see Drainage, Peritoneum ØD9W
Peritoneoplasty
see Repair, Peritoneum ØDQW
see Replacement, Peritoneum ØDRW
see Supplement, Peritoneum ØDUW
Peritoneoscopy ØDJW4ZZ
Peritoneotomy see Drainage, Peritoneum ØD9W
Peritoneumectomy see Excision, Peritoneum ØDBW
Peroneus brevis muscle
use Lower Leg Muscle, Left
use Lower Leg Muscle, Right
Peroneus longus muscle
use Lower Leg Muscle, Left
use Lower Leg Muscle, Right
Pessary ring use Intraluminal Device, Pessary in Female Reproductive System
PET scan see Positron Emission Tomographic (PET) Imaging
Petrous part of temoporal bone
use Temporal Bone, Left
use Temporal Bone, Right
Phacoemulsification, lens
With IOL implant see Replacement, Eye Ø8R
Without IOL implant see Extraction, Eye Ø8D
Phagenyx® System XWHD7Q7
Phalangectomy
see Excision, Lower Bones ØQB
see Excision, Upper Bones ØPB
see Resection, Lower Bones ØQT
see Resection, Upper Bones ØPT
Phallectomy
see Excision, Penis ØVBS
see Resection, Penis ØVTS
Phalloplasty
see Repair, Penis ØVQS
see Supplement, Penis ØVUS
Phallotomy see Drainage, Penis ØV9S
Pharmacotherapy, for substance abuse
Antabuse HZ93ZZZ
Bupropion HZ97ZZZ
Clonidine HZ96ZZZ
Levo-alpha-acetyl-methadol (LAAM) HZ92ZZZ
Methadone Maintenance HZ91ZZZ
Naloxone HZ95ZZZ
Naltrexone HZ94ZZZ
Nicotine Replacement HZ9ØZZZ
Psychiatric Medication HZ98ZZZ
Replacement Medication, Other HZ99ZZZ
Pharyngeal constrictor muscle use Tongue, Palate, Pharynx Muscle
Pharyngeal plexus use Vagus Nerve
Pharyngeal recess use Nasopharynx
Pharyngeal tonsil use Adenoids
Pharyngogram see Fluoroscopy, Pharynix B91G
Pharyngoplasty
see Repair, Mouth and Throat ØCQ
see Replacement, Mouth and Throat ØCR
see Supplement, Mouth and Throat ØCU
Pharyngorrhaphy see Repair, Mouth and Throat ØCQ
Pharyngotomy see Drainage, Mouth and Throat ØC9
Pharyngotympanic tube
use Eustachian Tube, Left
use Eustachian Tube, Right
Pheresis
Erythrocytes 6A55
Leukocytes 6A55
Plasma 6A55
Platelets 6A55
Stem Cells
Cord Blood 6A55
Hematopoietic 6A55
Phlebectomy
see Excision, Lower Veins Ø6B
see Excision, Upper Veins Ø5B
see Extraction, Lower Veins Ø6D
see Extraction, Upper Veins Ø5D
Phlebography
see Plain Radiography, Veins B5Ø
Impedance 4AØ4X51
Phleborrhaphy
see Repair, Lower Veins Ø6Q
see Repair, Upper Veins Ø5Q
Phlebotomy
see Drainage, Lower Veins Ø69
see Drainage, Upper Veins Ø59
Photocoagulation
For Destruction see Destruction
For Repair see Repair
Photopheresis, therapeutic see Phototherapy, Circulatory 6A65
Phototherapy
Circulatory 6A65
Skin 6A6Ø
Ultraviolet light see Ultraviolet Light Therapy, Physiological Systems 6A8
Phrenectomy, phrenoneurectomy see Excision, Nerve, Phrenic Ø1B2
Phrenemphraxis see Destruction, Nerve, Phrenic Ø152
Phrenic nerve stimulator generator use Stimulator Generator in Subcutaneous Tissue and Fascia
Phrenic nerve stimulator lead use Diaphragmatic Pacemaker Lead in Respiratory System
Phreniclasis see Destruction, Nerve, Phrenic Ø152
Phrenicoexeresis see Extraction, Nerve, Phrenic Ø1D2
Phrenicotomy see Division, Nerve, Phrenic Ø182
Phrenicotripsy see Destruction, Nerve, Phrenic Ø152
Phrenoplasty
see Repair, Respiratory System ØBQ
see Supplement, Respiratory System ØBU
Phrenotomy see Drainage, Respiratory System ØB9
Physiatry see Motor Treatment, Rehabilitation FØ7
Physical medicine see Motor Treatment, Rehabilitation FØ7
Physical therapy see Motor Treatment, Rehabilitation FØ7
PHYSIOMESH™ Flexible Composite Mesh use Synthetic Substitute
Pia mater, intracranial use Cerebral Meninges
Pia mater, spinal use Spinal Meninges
PiCSO® Impulse System X2A7358
Pinealectomy
see Excision, Pineal Body ØGB1
see Resection, Pineal Body ØGT1
Pinealoscopy ØGJ14ZZ
Pinealotomy see Drainage, Pineal Body ØG91
Pinna
use External Ear, Bilateral
use External Ear, Left
use External Ear, Right
Pipeline™ (Flex) embolization device use Intraluminal Device, Flow Diverter in Ø3V
Piriform recess (sinus) use Pharynx
Piriformis muscle
use Hip Muscle, Left
use Hip Muscle, Right
PIRRT (Prolonged intermittent renal replacement therapy) 5A1D8ØZ
Pisiform bone
use Carpal, Left
use Carpal, Right
Pisohamate ligament
use Hand Bursa and Ligament, Left
use Hand Bursa and Ligament, Right
Pisometacarpal ligament
use Hand Bursa and Ligament, Left
use Hand Bursa and Ligament, Right
Pituitectomy
see Excision, Gland, Pituitary ØGBØ
see Resection, Gland, Pituitary ØGTØ
Plain film radiology see Plain Radiography
Plain Radiography
Abdomen BWØØZZZ
Abdomen and Pelvis BWØ1ZZZ
Abdominal Lymphatic
Bilateral B7Ø1
Unilateral B7ØØ
Airway, Upper BBØDZZZ
Ankle
Left BQØH
Right BQØG
Aorta
Abdominal B4ØØ
Thoracic B3ØØ
Thoraco-Abdominal B3ØP
Aorta and Bilateral Lower Extremity Arteries B4ØD
Arch
Bilateral BNØDZZZ
Left BNØCZZZ
Right BNØBZZZ
Arm
Left BPØFZZZ
Right BPØEZZZ
Artery
Brachiocephalic-Subclavian, Right B3Ø1
Bronchial B3ØL
Bypass Graft, Other B2ØF
Cervico-Cerebral Arch B3ØQ
Common Carotid
Bilateral B3Ø5
Left B3Ø4
Right B3Ø3
Coronary
Bypass Graft
Multiple B2Ø3
Single B2Ø2
Multiple B2Ø1
Single B2ØØ
External Carotid
Bilateral B3ØC
Left B3ØB
Right B3Ø9
Hepatic B4Ø2
Inferior Mesenteric B4Ø5
Intercostal B3ØL
Internal Carotid
Bilateral B3Ø8
Left B3Ø7
Right B3Ø6
Internal Mammary Bypass Graft
Left B2Ø8
Right B2Ø7
Intra-Abdominal, Other B4ØB
Intracranial B3ØR
Lower Extremity
Bilateral and Aorta B4ØD
Left B4ØG
Right B4ØF
Lower, Other B4ØJ
Lumbar B4Ø9
Pelvic B4ØC
Pulmonary
Left B3ØT
Right B3ØS
Renal
Bilateral B4Ø8
Left B4Ø7
Right B4Ø6
Transplant B4ØM
Spinal B3ØM
Splenic B4Ø3
Subclavian, Left B3Ø2
Superior Mesenteric B4Ø4
Upper Extremity
Bilateral B3ØK
Left B3ØJ
Right B3ØH
Upper, Other B3ØN
Vertebral
Bilateral B3ØG
Left B3ØF
Right B3ØD
Bile Duct BFØØ
Bile Duct and Gallbladder BFØ3
Bladder BTØØ
Kidney and Ureter BTØ4

Plain Radiography — *continued*
- Bladder and Urethra BTØB
- Bone
  - Facial BNØ5ZZZ
  - Nasal BNØ4ZZZ
- Bones, Long, All BWØBZZZ
- Breast
  - Bilateral BHØ2ZZZ
  - Left BHØ1ZZZ
  - Right BHØØZZZ
- Calcaneus
  - Left BQØKZZZ
  - Right BQØJZZZ
- Chest BWØ3ZZZ
- Clavicle
  - Left BPØ5ZZZ
  - Right BPØ4ZZZ
- Coccyx BRØFZZZ
- Corpora Cavernosa BVØØ
- Dialysis Fistula B5ØW
- Dialysis Shunt B5ØW
- Disc
  - Cervical BRØ1
  - Lumbar BRØ3
  - Thoracic BRØ2
- Duct
  - Lacrimal
    - Bilateral B8Ø2
    - Left B8Ø1
    - Right B8ØØ
  - Mammary
    - Multiple
      - Left BHØ6
      - Right BHØ5
    - Single
      - Left BHØ4
      - Right BHØ3
- Elbow
  - Left BPØH
  - Right BPØG
- Epididymis
  - Left BVØ2
  - Right BVØ1
- Extremity
  - Lower BWØCZZZ
  - Upper BWØJZZZ
- Eye
  - Bilateral B8Ø7ZZZ
  - Left B8Ø6ZZZ
  - Right B8Ø5ZZZ
- Facet Joint
  - Cervical BRØ4
  - Lumbar BRØ6
  - Thoracic BRØ5
- Fallopian Tube
  - Bilateral BUØ2
  - Left BUØ1
  - Right BUØØ
- Fallopian Tube and Uterus BUØ8
- Femur
  - Left, Densitometry BQØ4ZZ1
  - Right, Densitometry BQØ3ZZ1
- Finger
  - Left BPØSZZZ
  - Right BPØRZZZ
- Foot
  - Left BQØMZZZ
  - Right BQØLZZZ
- Forearm
  - Left BPØKZZZ
  - Right BPØJZZZ
- Gallbladder and Bile Duct BFØ3
- Gland
  - Parotid
    - Bilateral B9Ø6
    - Left B9Ø5
    - Right B9Ø4
  - Salivary
    - Bilateral B9ØD
    - Left B9ØC
    - Right B9ØB
  - Submandibular
    - Bilateral B9Ø9
    - Left B9Ø8
    - Right B9Ø7
- Hand
  - Left BPØPZZZ
  - Right BPØNZZZ

Plain Radiography — *continued*
- Heart
  - Left B2Ø5
  - Right B2Ø4
  - Right and Left B2Ø6
- Hepatobiliary System, All BFØC
- Hip
  - Left BQØ1
    - Densitometry BQØ1ZZ1
  - Right BQØØ
    - Densitometry BQØØZZ1
- Humerus
  - Left BPØBZZZ
  - Right BPØAZZZ
- Ileal Diversion Loop BTØC
- Intracranial Sinus B5Ø2
- Joint
  - Acromioclavicular, Bilateral BPØ3ZZZ
  - Finger
    - Left BPØD
    - Right BPØC
  - Foot
    - Left BQØY
    - Right BQØX
  - Hand
    - Left BPØD
    - Right BPØC
  - Lumbosacral BRØBZZZ
  - Sacroiliac BRØD
  - Sternoclavicular
    - Bilateral BPØ2ZZZ
    - Left BPØ1ZZZ
    - Right BPØØZZZ
  - Temporomandibular
    - Bilateral BNØ9
    - Left BNØ8
    - Right BNØ7
  - Thoracolumbar BRØ8ZZZ
  - Toe
    - Left BQØY
    - Right BQØX
- Kidney
  - Bilateral BTØ3
  - Left BTØ2
  - Right BTØ1
  - Ureter and Bladder BTØ4
- Knee
  - Left BQØ8
  - Right BQØ7
- Leg
  - Left BQØFZZZ
  - Right BQØDZZZ
- Lymphatic
  - Head B7Ø4
  - Lower Extremity
    - Bilateral B7ØB
    - Left B7Ø9
    - Right B7Ø8
  - Neck B7Ø4
  - Pelvic B7ØC
  - Upper Extremity
    - Bilateral B7Ø7
    - Left B7Ø6
    - Right B7Ø5
- Mandible BNØ6ZZZ
- Mastoid B9ØHZZZ
- Nasopharynx B9ØFZZZ
- Optic Foramina
  - Left B8Ø4ZZZ
  - Right B8Ø3ZZZ
- Orbit
  - Bilateral BNØ3ZZZ
  - Left BNØ2ZZZ
  - Right BNØ1ZZZ
- Oropharynx B9ØFZZZ
- Patella
  - Left BQØWZZZ
  - Right BQØVZZZ
- Pelvis BRØCZZZ
- Pelvis and Abdomen BWØ1ZZZ
- Prostate BVØ3
- Retroperitoneal Lymphatic
  - Bilateral B7Ø1
  - Unilateral B7ØØ
- Ribs
  - Left BPØYZZZ
  - Right BPØXZZZ
- Sacrum BRØFZZZ

Plain Radiography — *continued*
- Scapula
  - Left BPØ7ZZZ
  - Right BPØ6ZZZ
- Shoulder
  - Left BPØ9
  - Right BPØ8
- Sinus
  - Intracranial B5Ø2
  - Paranasal B9Ø2ZZZ
- Skull BNØØZZZ
- Spinal Cord BØØB
- Spine
  - Cervical, Densitometry BRØØZZ1
  - Lumbar, Densitometry BRØ9ZZ1
  - Thoracic, Densitometry BRØ7ZZ1
  - Whole, Densitometry BRØGZZ1
- Sternum BRØHZZZ
- Teeth
  - All BNØJZZZ
  - Multiple BNØHZZZ
- Testicle
  - Left BVØ6
  - Right BVØ5
- Toe
  - Left BQØQZZZ
  - Right BQØPZZZ
- Tooth, Single BNØGZZZ
- Tracheobronchial Tree
  - Bilateral BBØ9YZZ
  - Left BBØ8YZZ
  - Right BBØ7YZZ
- Ureter
  - Bilateral BTØ8
  - Kidney and Bladder BTØ4
  - Left BTØ7
  - Right BTØ6
- Urethra BTØ5
- Urethra and Bladder BTØB
- Uterus BUØ6
- Uterus and Fallopian Tube BUØ8
- Vagina BUØ9
- Vasa Vasorum BVØ8
- Vein
  - Cerebellar B5Ø1
  - Cerebral B5Ø1
  - Epidural B5ØØ
  - Jugular
    - Bilateral B5Ø5
    - Left B5Ø4
    - Right B5Ø3
  - Lower Extremity
    - Bilateral B5ØD
    - Left B5ØC
    - Right B5ØB
  - Other B5ØV
  - Pelvic (Iliac)
    - Left B5ØG
    - Right B5ØF
  - Pelvic (Iliac) Bilateral B5ØH
  - Portal B5ØT
  - Pulmonary
    - Bilateral B5ØS
    - Left B5ØR
    - Right B5ØQ
  - Renal
    - Bilateral B5ØL
    - Left B5ØK
    - Right B5ØJ
  - Spanchnic B5ØT
  - Subclavian
    - Left B5Ø7
    - Right B5Ø6
  - Upper Extremity
    - Bilateral B5ØP
    - Left B5ØN
    - Right B5ØM
- Vena Cava
  - Inferior B5Ø9
  - Superior B5Ø8
- Whole Body BWØKZZZ
  - Infant BWØMZZZ
- Whole Skeleton BWØLZZZ
- Wrist
  - Left BPØM
  - Right BPØL

Planar Nuclear Medicine Imaging
- Abdomen CW1Ø
- Abdomen and Chest CW14

Planar Nuclear Medicine Imaging — *continued*
Abdomen and Pelvis CW11
Anatomical Region, Other CW1ZZZZ
Anatomical Regions, Multiple CW1YYZZ
Bladder and Ureters CT1H
Bladder, Kidneys and Ureters CT13
Blood C713
Bone Marrow C71Ø
Brain CØ1Ø
Breast CH1YYZZ
Bilateral CH12
Left CH11
Right CH1Ø
Bronchi and Lungs CB12
Central Nervous System CØ1YYZZ
Cerebrospinal Fluid CØ15
Chest CW13
Chest and Abdomen CW14
Chest and Neck CW16
Digestive System CD1YYZZ
Ducts, Lacrimal, Bilateral C819
Ear, Nose, Mouth and Throat C91YYZZ
Endocrine System CG1YYZZ
Extremity
Lower CW1D
Bilateral CP1F
Left CP1D
Right CP1C
Upper CW1M
Bilateral CP1B
Left CP19
Right CP18
Eye C81YYZZ
Gallbladder CF14
Gastrointestinal Tract CD17
Upper CD15
Gland
Adrenal, Bilateral CG14
Parathyroid CG11
Thyroid CG12
Glands, Salivary, Bilateral C91B
Head and Neck CW1B
Heart C21YYZZ
Right and Left C216
Hepatobiliary System, All CF1C
Hepatobiliary System and Pancreas CF1YYZZ
Kidneys, Ureters and Bladder CT13
Liver CF15
Liver and Spleen CF16
Lungs and Bronchi CB12
Lymphatics
Head C71J
Head and Neck C715
Lower Extremity C71P
Neck C71K
Pelvic C71D
Trunk C71M
Upper Chest C71L
Upper Extremity C71N
Lymphatics and Hematologic System C71YYZZ
Musculoskeletal System
All CP1Z
Other CP1YYZZ
Myocardium C21G
Neck and Chest CW16
Neck and Head CW1B
Pancreas and Hepatobiliary System CF1YYZZ
Pelvic Region CW1J
Pelvis CP16
Pelvis and Abdomen CW11
Pelvis and Spine CP17
Reproductive System, Male CV1YYZZ
Respiratory System CB1YYZZ
Skin CH1YYZZ
Skull CP11
Spine CP15
Spine and Pelvis CP17
Spleen C712
Spleen and Liver CF16
Subcutaneous Tissue CH1YYZZ
Testicles, Bilateral CV19
Thorax CP14
Ureters and Bladder CT1H
Ureters, Kidneys and Bladder CT13
Urinary System CT1YYZZ
Veins C51YYZZ
Central C51R
Lower Extremity
Bilateral C51D

Planar Nuclear Medicine Imaging — *continued*
Veins — *continued*
Lower Extremity — *continued*
Left C51C
Right C51B
Upper Extremity
Bilateral C51Q
Left C51P
Right C51N
Whole Body CW1N
Plantar digital vein
use Foot Vein, Left
use Foot Vein, Right
Plantar fascia (aponeurosis)
use Subcutaneous Tissue and Fascia, Left Foot
use Subcutaneous Tissue and Fascia, Right Foot
Plantar metatarsal vein
use Foot Vein, Left
use Foot Vein, Right
Plantar venous arch
use Foot Vein, Left
use Foot Vein, Right
Plaque Radiation
Abdomen DWY3FZZ
Adrenal Gland DGY2FZZ
Anus DDY8FZZ
Bile Ducts DFY2FZZ
Bladder DTY2FZZ
Bone Marrow D7YØFZZ
Bone, Other DPYCFZZ
Brain DØYØFZZ
Brain Stem DØY1FZZ
Breast
Left DMYØFZZ
Right DMY1FZZ
Bronchus DBY1FZZ
Cervix DUY1FZZ
Chest DWY2FZZ
Chest Wall DBY7FZZ
Colon DDY5FZZ
Diaphragm DBY8FZZ
Duodenum DDY2FZZ
Ear D9YØFZZ
Esophagus DDYØFZZ
Eye D8YØFZZ
Femur DPY9FZZ
Fibula DPYBFZZ
Gallbladder DFY1FZZ
Gland
Adrenal DGY2FZZ
Parathyroid DGY4FZZ
Pituitary DGYØFZZ
Thyroid DGY5FZZ
Glands, Salivary D9Y6FZZ
Head and Neck DWY1FZZ
Hemibody DWY4FZZ
Humerus DPY6FZZ
Ileum DDY4FZZ
Jejunum DDY3FZZ
Kidney DTYØFZZ
Larynx D9YBFZZ
Liver DFYØFZZ
Lung DBY2FZZ
Lymphatics
Abdomen D7Y6FZZ
Axillary D7Y4FZZ
Inguinal D7Y8FZZ
Neck D7Y3FZZ
Pelvis D7Y7FZZ
Thorax D7Y5FZZ
Mandible DPY3FZZ
Maxilla DPY2FZZ
Mediastinum DBY6FZZ
Mouth D9Y4FZZ
Nasopharynx D9YDFZZ
Neck and Head DWY1FZZ
Nerve, Peripheral DØY7FZZ
Nose D9Y1FZZ
Ovary DUYØFZZ
Palate
Hard D9Y8FZZ
Soft D9Y9FZZ
Pancreas DFY3FZZ
Parathyroid Gland DGY4FZZ
Pelvic Bones DPY8FZZ
Pelvic Region DWY6FZZ
Pharynx D9YCFZZ
Pineal Body DGY1FZZ

Plaque Radiation — *continued*
Pituitary Gland DGYØFZZ
Pleura DBY5FZZ
Prostate DVYØFZZ
Radius DPY7FZZ
Rectum DDY7FZZ
Rib DPY5FZZ
Sinuses D9Y7FZZ
Skin
Abdomen DHY8FZZ
Arm DHY4FZZ
Back DHY7FZZ
Buttock DHY9FZZ
Chest DHY6FZZ
Face DHY2FZZ
Foot DHYCFZZ
Hand DHY5FZZ
Leg DHYBFZZ
Neck DHY3FZZ
Skull DPYØFZZ
Spinal Cord DØY6FZZ
Spleen D7Y2FZZ
Sternum DPY4FZZ
Stomach DDY1FZZ
Testis DVY1FZZ
Thymus D7Y1FZZ
Thyroid Gland DGY5FZZ
Tibia DPYBFZZ
Tongue D9Y5FZZ
Trachea DBYØFZZ
Ulna DPY7FZZ
Ureter DTY1FZZ
Urethra DTY3FZZ
Uterus DUY2FZZ
Whole Body DWY5FZZ
Plasma, Convalescent (Nonautologous) XW1
Plasmapheresis, therapeutic *see* Pheresis, Physiological Systems 6A5
Plateletpheresis, therapeutic *see* Pheresis, Physiological Systems 6A5
Platysma muscle
use Neck Muscle, Left
use Neck Muscle, Right
Plazomicin *use* Other Anti-infective
Pleurectomy
see Excision, Respiratory System ØBB
see Resection, Respiratory System ØBT
Pleurocentesis *see* Drainage, Anatomical Regions, General ØW9
Pleurodesis, pleurosclerosis
Chemical injection *see* Introduction of Substance in or on, Pleural Cavity 3EØL
Surgical *see* Destruction, Respiratory System ØB5
Pleurolysis *see* Release, Respiratory System ØBN
Pleuroscopy ØBJQ4ZZ
Pleurotomy *see* Drainage, Respiratory System ØB9
Plica semilunaris
use Conjunctiva, Left
use Conjunctiva, Right
Plication *see* Restriction
Pneumectomy
see Excision, Respiratory System ØBB
see Resection, Respiratory System ØBT
Pneumocentesis *see* Drainage, Respiratory System ØB9
Pneumogastric nerve *use* Vagus Nerve
Pneumolysis *see* Release, Respiratory System ØBN
Pneumonectomy *see* Resection, Respiratory System ØBT
Pneumonolysis *see* Release, Respiratory System ØBN
Pneumonopexy
see Repair, Respiratory System ØBQ
see Reposition, Respiratory System ØBS
Pneumonorrhaphy *see* Repair, Respiratory System ØBQ
Pneumonotomy *see* Drainage, Respiratory System ØB9
Pneumotaxic center *use* Pons
Pneumotomy *see* Drainage, Respiratory System ØB9
Pollicization *see* Transfer, Anatomical Regions, Upper Extremities ØXX
Polyclonal hyperimmune globulin *use* Globulin
Polyethylene socket *use* Synthetic Substitute, Polyethylene in ØSR
Polymethylmethacrylate (PMMA) *use* Synthetic Substitute
Polypectomy, gastrointestinal *see* Excision, Gastrointestinal System ØDB

Polypropylene mesh *use* Synthetic Substitute
Polysomnogram 4A1ZXQZ
Pontine tegmentum *use* Pons
Popliteal ligament
use Knee Bursa and Ligament, Left
use Knee Bursa and Ligament, Right
Popliteal lymph node
use Lymphatic, Left Lower Extremity
use Lymphatic, Right Lower Extremity
Popliteal vein
use Femoral Vein, Left
use Femoral Vein, Right
Popliteus muscle
use Lower Leg Muscle, Left
use Lower Leg Muscle, Right
Porcine (bioprosthetic) valve *use* Zooplastic Tissue in Heart and Great Vessels
Positive Blood Culture Fluorescence Hybridization for Organism Identification, Concentration and Susceptibility XXE5XN6
Positive end expiratory pressure *see* Performance, Respiratory 5A19
Positron Emission Tomographic (PET) Imaging
Brain CØ3Ø
Bronchi and Lungs CB32
Central Nervous System CØ3YYZZ
Heart C23YYZZ
Lungs and Bronchi CB32
Myocardium C23G
Respiratory System CB3YYZZ
Whole Body CW3NYZZ
Positron emission tomography *see* Positron Emission Tomographic (PET) Imaging
Posoleucel XWØ
Postauricular (mastoid) lymph node
use Lymphatic, Left Neck
use Lymphatic, Right Neck
Postcava *use* Inferior Vena Cava
Posterior auricular artery
use External Carotid Artery, Left
use External Carotid Artery, Right
Posterior auricular nerve *use* Facial Nerve
Posterior auricular vein
use External Jugular Vein, Left
use External Jugular Vein, Right
Posterior cerebral artery *use* Intracranial Artery
Posterior chamber
use Eye, Left
use Eye, Right
Posterior circumflex humeral artery
use Axillary Artery, Left
use Axillary Artery, Right
Posterior communicating artery *use* Intracranial Artery
Posterior cruciate ligament (PCL)
use Knee Bursa and Ligament, Left
use Knee Bursa and Ligament, Right
Posterior (Dynamic) Distraction Device
Lumbar XNSØ
Thoracic XNS4
Posterior facial (retromandibular) vein
use Face Vein, Left
use Face Vein, Right
Posterior femoral cutaneous nerve *use* Sacral Plexus
Posterior inferior cerebellar artery (PICA) *use* Intracranial Artery
Posterior interosseous nerve *use* Radial Nerve
Posterior labial nerve *use* Pudendal Nerve
Posterior (subscapular) lymph node
use Lymphatic, Left Axillary
use Lymphatic, Right Axillary
Posterior scrotal nerve *use* Pudendal Nerve
Posterior spinal artery
use Vertebral Artery, Left
use Vertebral Artery, Right
Posterior tibial recurrent artery
use Anterior Tibial Artery, Left
use Anterior Tibial Artery, Right
Posterior ulnar recurrent artery
use Ulnar Artery, Left
use Ulnar Artery, Right
Posterior vagal trunk *use* Vagus Nerve
PPN (peripheral parenteral nutrition) *see* Introduction of Nutritional Substance
Praxbind® (idarucizumab), Pradaxa® (dabigatran) reversal agent *use* Other Therapeutic Substance
Preauricular lymph node *use* Lymphatic, Head
Precava *use* Superior Vena Cava
PRECICE intramedullary limb lengthening system
use Internal Fixation Device, Intramedullary Limb Lengthening in ØPH
use Internal Fixation Device, Intramedullary Limb Lengthening in ØQH
Precision TAVI™ Coronary Obstruction Module XXE3X68
Prepatellar bursa
use Knee Bursa and Ligament, Left
use Knee Bursa and Ligament, Right
Preputiotomy *see* Drainage, Male Reproductive System ØV9
Pressure support ventilation *see* Performance, Respiratory 5A19
PRESTIGE® Cervical Disc *use* Synthetic Substitute
Pretracheal fascia
use Subcutaneous Tissue and Fascia, Left Neck
use Subcutaneous Tissue and Fascia, Right Neck
Prevertebral fascia
use Subcutaneous Tissue and Fascia, Left Neck
use Subcutaneous Tissue and Fascia, Right Neck
PrimeAdvanced neurostimulator (SureScan) (MRI Safe) *use* Stimulator Generator, Multiple Array in ØJH
Princeps pollicis artery
use Hand Artery, Left
use Hand Artery, Right
Probing, duct
Diagnostic *see* Inspection
Dilation *see* Dilation
PROCEED™ Ventral Patch *use* Synthetic Substitute
Procerus muscle *use* Facial Muscle
Proctectomy
see Excision, Rectum ØDBP
see Resection, Rectum ØDTP
Proctoclysis *see* Introduction of substance in or on, Gastrointestinal Tract, Lower 3EØH
Proctocolectomy
see Excision, Gastrointestinal System ØDB
see Resection, Gastrointestinal System ØDT
Proctocolpoplasty
see Repair, Gastrointestinal System ØDQ
see Supplement, Gastrointestinal System ØDU
Proctoperineoplasty
see Repair, Gastrointestinal System ØDQ
see Supplement, Gastrointestinal System ØDU
Proctoperineorrhaphy *see* Repair, Gastrointestinal System ØDQ
Proctopexy
see Repair, Rectum ØDQP
see Reposition, Rectum ØDSP
Proctoplasty
see Repair, Rectum ØDQP
see Supplement, Rectum ØDUP
Proctorrhaphy *see* Repair, Rectum ØDQP
Proctoscopy ØDJD8ZZ
Proctosigmoidectomy
see Excision, Gastrointestinal System ØDB
see Resection, Gastrointestinal System ØDT
Proctosigmoidoscopy ØDJD8ZZ
Proctostomy *see* Drainage, Rectum ØD9P
Proctotomy *see* Drainage, Rectum ØD9P
Prodisc-C *use* Synthetic Substitute
Prodisc-L *use* Synthetic Substitute
Production, atrial septal defect *see* Excision, Septum, Atrial Ø2B5
Profunda brachii
use Brachial Artery, Left
use Brachial Artery, Right
Profunda femoris (deep femoral) vein
use Femoral Vein, Left
use Femoral Vein, Right
PROLENE Polypropylene Hernia System (PHS) *use* Synthetic Substitute
Prolonged intermittent renal replacement therapy (PIRRT) 5A1D8ØZ
Pronator quadratus muscle
use Lower Arm and Wrist Muscle, Left
use Lower Arm and Wrist Muscle, Right
Pronator teres muscle
use Lower Arm and Wrist Muscle, Left
use Lower Arm and Wrist Muscle, Right
Prone positioning, intubated *see* Assistance, Respiratory 5AØ9
Prostatectomy
see Excision, Prostate ØVBØ
see Resection, Prostate ØVTØ
Prostatic artery
use Internal Iliac Artery, Left
use Internal Iliac Artery, Right
Prostatic urethra *use* Urethra
Prostatomy, prostatotomy *see* Drainage, Prostate ØV9Ø
Protecta XT CRT-D *use* Cardiac Resynchronization Defibrillator Pulse Generator in ØJH
Protecta XT DR (XT VR) *use* Defibrillator Generator in ØJH
Protege® RX Carotid Stent System *use* Intraluminal Device
Proximal radioulnar joint
use Elbow Joint, Left
use Elbow Joint, Right
Psoas muscle
use Hip Muscle, Left
use Hip Muscle, Right
PSV (pressure support ventilation) *see* Performance, Respiratory 5A19
Psychoanalysis GZ54ZZZ
Psychological Tests
Cognitive Status GZ14ZZZ
Developmental GZ1ØZZZ
Intellectual and Psychoeducational GZ12ZZZ
Neurobehavioral Status GZ14ZZZ
Neuropsychological GZ13ZZZ
Personality and Behavioral GZ11ZZZ
Psychotherapy
Family, Mental Health Services GZ72ZZZ
Group GZHZZZZ
Mental Health Services GZHZZZZ
Individual
see Psychotherapy, Individual, Mental Health Services
for substance abuse
12-Step HZ53ZZZ
Behavioral HZ51ZZZ
Cognitive HZ5ØZZZ
Cognitive-Behavioral HZ52ZZZ
Confrontational HZ58ZZZ
Interactive HZ55ZZZ
Interpersonal HZ54ZZZ
Motivational Enhancement HZ57ZZZ
Psychoanalysis HZ5BZZZ
Psychodynamic HZ5CZZZ
Psychoeducation HZ56ZZZ
Psychophysiological HZ5DZZZ
Supportive HZ59ZZZ
Mental Health Services
Behavioral GZ51ZZZ
Cognitive GZ52ZZZ
Cognitive-Behavioral GZ58ZZZ
Interactive GZ5ØZZZ
Interpersonal GZ53ZZZ
Psychoanalysis GZ54ZZZ
Psychodynamic GZ55ZZZ
Psychophysiological GZ59ZZZ
Supportive GZ56ZZZ
PTCA (percutaneous transluminal coronary angioplasty) *see* Dilation, Heart and Great Vessels Ø27
Pterygoid muscle *use* Head Muscle
Pterygoid process *use* Sphenoid Bone
Pterygopalatine (sphenopalatine) ganglion *use* Head and Neck Sympathetic Nerve
Pubis
use Pelvic Bone, Left
use Pelvic Bone, Right
Pubofemoral ligament
use Hip Bursa and Ligament, Left
use Hip Bursa and Ligament, Right
Pudendal nerve *use* Sacral Plexus
Pull-through, laparoscopic-assisted transanal
see Excision, Gastrointestinal System ØDB
see Resection, Gastrointestinal System ØDT
Pull-through, rectal *see* Resection, Rectum ØDTP
Pulmoaortic canal *use* Pulmonary Artery, Left
Pulmonary annulus *use* Pulmonary Valve
Pulmonary artery wedge monitoring *see* Monitoring, Arterial 4A13
Pulmonary plexus
use Thoracic Sympathetic Nerve
use Vagus Nerve
Pulmonic valve *use* Pulmonary Valve

Pulpectomy *see* Excision, Mouth and Throat ØCB
Pulverization *see* Fragmentation
Pulvinar *use* Thalamus
Pump reservoir *use* Infusion Device, Pump in Subcutaneous Tissue and Fascia
Punch biopsy *see* Excision with qualifier Diagnostic
Puncture *see* Drainage
Puncture, lumbar *see* Drainage, Spinal Canal ØØ9U
Pure-Vu® System XDPH8K7
Pyelography
see Fluoroscopy, Urinary System BT1
see Plain Radiography, Urinary System BTØ
Pyeloileostomy, urinary diversion *see* Bypass, Urinary System ØT1
Pyeloplasty
see Repair, Urinary System ØTQ
see Replacement, Urinary System ØTR
see Supplement, Urinary System ØTU
Pyeloplasty, dismembered *see* Repair, Kidney Pelvis
Pyelorrhaphy *see* Repair, Urinary System ØTQ
Pyeloscopy ØTJ58ZZ
Pyelostomy
see Bypass, Urinary System ØT1
see Drainage, Urinary System ØT9
Pyelotomy *see* Drainage, Urinary System ØT9
Pylorectomy
see Excision, Stomach, Pylorus ØDB7
see Resection, Stomach, Pylorus ØDT7
Pyloric antrum *use* Stomach, Pylorus
Pyloric canal *use* Stomach, Pylorus
Pyloric sphincter *use* Stomach, Pylorus
Pylorodiosis *see* Dilation, Stomach, Pylorus ØD77
Pylorogastrectomy
see Excision, Gastrointestinal System ØDB
see Resection, Gastrointestinal System ØDT
Pyloroplasty
see Repair, Stomach, Pylorus ØDQ7
see Supplement, Stomach, Pylorus ØDU7
Pyloroscopy ØDJ68ZZ
Pylorotomy *see* Drainage, Stomach, Pylorus ØD97
Pyramidalis muscle
use Abdomen Muscle, Left
use Abdomen Muscle, Right

Q

QAngio XA® 3D XXE3X58
QFR® (Quantitative Flow Ratio) analysis of coronary angiography XXE3X58
Quadrangular cartilage *use* Nasal Septum
Quadrant resection of breast *see* Excision, Skin and Breast ØHB
Quadrate lobe *use* Liver
Quadratus femoris muscle
use Hip Muscle, Left
use Hip Muscle, Right
Quadratus lumborum muscle
use Trunk Muscle, Left
use Trunk Muscle, Right
Quadratus plantae muscle
use Foot Muscle, Left
use Foot Muscle, Right
Quadriceps (femoris)
use Upper Leg Muscle, Left
use Upper Leg Muscle, Right
Quantitative Flow Ratio Analysis, Coronary Artery Flow XXE3X58
Quarantine 8EØZXY6
Quizartinib Antineoplastic XWØDXJ9

R

Radial artery arteriovenous fistula, using Thermal Resistance Energy X2K
Radial collateral carpal ligament
use Wrist Bursa and Ligament, Left
use Wrist Bursa and Ligament, Right
Radial collateral ligament
use Elbow Bursa and Ligament, Left
use Elbow Bursa and Ligament, Right
Radial notch
use Ulna, Left
use Ulna, Right
Radial recurrent artery
use Radial Artery, Left
Radial recurrent artery — *continued*
use Radial Artery, Right
Radial vein
use Brachial Vein, Left
use Brachial Vein, Right
Radialis indicis
use Hand Artery, Left
use Hand Artery, Right
Radiation Therapy
see Beam Radiation
see Brachytherapy
see Other Radiation
see Stereotactic Radiosurgery
Radiation treatment *see* Radiation Therapy
Radiocarpal joint
use Wrist Joint, Left
use Wrist Joint, Right
Radiocarpal ligament
use Wrist Bursa and Ligament, Left
use Wrist Bursa and Ligament, Right
Radiography *see* Plain Radiography
Radiology, analog *see* Plain Radiography
Radiology, diagnostic *see* Imaging, Diagnostic
Radioulnar ligament
use Wrist Bursa and Ligament, Left
use Wrist Bursa and Ligament, Right
Range of motion testing *see* Motor Function Assessment, Rehabilitation FØ1
Rapid ASPECTS XXEØXØ7
REALIZE® Adjustable Gastric Band *use* Extraluminal Device
Reattachment
Abdominal Wall ØWMFØZZ
Ampulla of Vater ØFMC
Ankle Region
Left ØYMLØZZ
Right ØYMKØZZ
Arm
Lower
Left ØXMFØZZ
Right ØXMDØZZ
Upper
Left ØXM9ØZZ
Right ØXM8ØZZ
Axilla
Left ØXM5ØZZ
Right ØXM4ØZZ
Back
Lower ØWMLØZZ
Upper ØWMKØZZ
Bladder ØTMB
Bladder Neck ØTMC
Breast
Bilateral ØHMVXZZ
Left ØHMUXZZ
Right ØHMTXZZ
Bronchus
Lingula ØBM9ØZZ
Lower Lobe
Left ØBMBØZZ
Right ØBM6ØZZ
Main
Left ØBM7ØZZ
Right ØBM3ØZZ
Middle Lobe, Right ØBM5ØZZ
Upper Lobe
Left ØBM8ØZZ
Right ØBM4ØZZ
Bursa and Ligament
Abdomen
Left ØMMJ
Right ØMMH
Ankle
Left ØMMR
Right ØMMQ
Elbow
Left ØMM4
Right ØMM3
Foot
Left ØMMT
Right ØMMS
Hand
Left ØMM8
Right ØMM7
Head and Neck ØMMØ
Hip
Left ØMMM
Right ØMML
Reattachment — *continued*
Bursa and Ligament — *continued*
Knee
Left ØMMP
Right ØMMN
Lower Extremity
Left ØMMW
Right ØMMV
Perineum ØMMK
Rib(s) ØMMG
Shoulder
Left ØMM2
Right ØMM1
Spine
Lower ØMMD
Upper ØMMC
Sternum ØMMF
Upper Extremity
Left ØMMB
Right ØMM9
Wrist
Left ØMM6
Right ØMM5
Buttock
Left ØYM1ØZZ
Right ØYMØØZZ
Carina ØBM2ØZZ
Cecum ØDMH
Cervix ØUMC
Chest Wall ØWM8ØZZ
Clitoris ØUMJXZZ
Colon
Ascending ØDMK
Descending ØDMM
Sigmoid ØDMN
Transverse ØDML
Cord
Bilateral ØVMH
Left ØVMG
Right ØVMF
Cul-de-sac ØUMF
Diaphragm ØBMTØZZ
Duct
Common Bile ØFM9
Cystic ØFM8
Hepatic
Common ØFM7
Left ØFM6
Right ØFM5
Pancreatic ØFMD
Accessory ØFMF
Duodenum ØDM9
Ear
Left Ø9M1XZZ
Right Ø9MØXZZ
Elbow Region
Left ØXMCØZZ
Right ØXMBØZZ
Esophagus ØDM5
Extremity
Lower
Left ØYMBØZZ
Right ØYM9ØZZ
Upper
Left ØXM7ØZZ
Right ØXM6ØZZ
Eyelid
Lower
Left Ø8MRXZZ
Right Ø8MQXZZ
Upper
Left Ø8MPXZZ
Right Ø8MNXZZ
Face ØWM2ØZZ
Fallopian Tube
Left ØUM6
Right ØUM5
Fallopian Tubes, Bilateral ØUM7
Femoral Region
Left ØYM8ØZZ
Right ØYM7ØZZ
Finger
Index
Left ØXMPØZZ
Right ØXMNØZZ
Little
Left ØXMWØZZ
Right ØXMVØZZ

Reattachment — *continued*
Finger — *continued*
Middle
Left ØXMRØZZ
Right ØXMQØZZ
Ring
Left ØXMTØZZ
Right ØXMSØZZ
Foot
Left ØYMNØZZ
Right ØYMMØZZ
Forequarter
Left ØXM1ØZZ
Right ØXMØØZZ
Gallbladder ØFM4
Gland
Left ØGM2
Right ØGM3
Hand
Left ØXMKØZZ
Right ØXMJØZZ
Hindquarter
Bilateral ØYM4ØZZ
Left ØYM3ØZZ
Right ØYM2ØZZ
Hymen ØUMK
Ileum ØDMB
Inguinal Region
Left ØYM6ØZZ
Right ØYM5ØZZ
Intestine
Large ØDME
Left ØDMG
Right ØDMF
Small ØDM8
Jaw
Lower ØWM5ØZZ
Upper ØWM4ØZZ
Jejunum ØDMA
Kidney
Left ØTM1
Right ØTMØ
Kidney Pelvis
Left ØTM4
Right ØTM3
Kidneys, Bilateral ØTM2
Knee Region
Left ØYMGØZZ
Right ØYMFØZZ
Leg
Lower
Left ØYMJØZZ
Right ØYMHØZZ
Upper
Left ØYMDØZZ
Right ØYMCØZZ
Lip
Lower ØCM1ØZZ
Upper ØCMØØZZ
Liver ØFMØ
Left Lobe ØFM2
Right Lobe ØFM1
Lung
Left ØBMLØZZ
Lower Lobe
Left ØBMJØZZ
Right ØBMFØZZ
Middle Lobe, Right ØBMDØZZ
Right ØBMKØZZ
Upper Lobe
Left ØBMGØZZ
Right ØBMCØZZ
Lung Lingula ØBMHØZZ
Muscle
Abdomen
Left ØKML
Right ØKMK
Facial ØKM1
Foot
Left ØKMW
Right ØKMV
Hand
Left ØKMD
Right ØKMC
Head ØKMØ
Hip
Left ØKMP
Right ØKMN

Reattachment — *continued*
Muscle — *continued*
Lower Arm and Wrist
Left ØKMB
Right ØKM9
Lower Leg
Left ØKMT
Right ØKMS
Neck
Left ØKM3
Right ØKM2
Perineum ØKMM
Shoulder
Left ØKM6
Right ØKM5
Thorax
Left ØKMJ
Right ØKMH
Tongue, Palate, Pharynx ØKM4
Trunk
Left ØKMG
Right ØKMF
Upper Arm
Left ØKM8
Right ØKM7
Upper Leg
Left ØKMR
Right ØKMQ
Nasal Mucosa and Soft Tissue Ø9MKXZZ
Neck ØWM6ØZZ
Nipple
Left ØHMXXZZ
Right ØHMWXZZ
Ovary
Bilateral ØUM2
Left ØUM1
Right ØUMØ
Palate, Soft ØCM3ØZZ
Pancreas ØFMG
Parathyroid Gland ØGMR
Inferior
Left ØGMP
Right ØGMN
Multiple ØGMQ
Superior
Left ØGMM
Right ØGML
Penis ØVMSXZZ
Perineum
Female ØWMNØZZ
Male ØWMMØZZ
Rectum ØDMP
Scrotum ØVM5XZZ
Shoulder Region
Left ØXM3ØZZ
Right ØXM2ØZZ
Skin
Abdomen ØHM7XZZ
Back ØHM6XZZ
Buttock ØHM8XZZ
Chest ØHM5XZZ
Ear
Left ØHM3XZZ
Right ØHM2XZZ
Face ØHM1XZZ
Foot
Left ØHMNXZZ
Right ØHMMXZZ
Hand
Left ØHMGXZZ
Right ØHMFXZZ
Inguinal ØHMAXZZ
Lower Arm
Left ØHMEXZZ
Right ØHMDXZZ
Lower Leg
Left ØHMLXZZ
Right ØHMKXZZ
Neck ØHM4XZZ
Perineum ØHM9XZZ
Scalp ØHMØXZZ
Upper Arm
Left ØHMCXZZ
Right ØHMBXZZ
Upper Leg
Left ØHMJXZZ
Right ØHMHXZZ
Stomach ØDM6

Reattachment — *continued*
Tendon
Abdomen
Left ØLMG
Right ØLMF
Ankle
Left ØLMT
Right ØLMS
Foot
Left ØLMW
Right ØLMV
Hand
Left ØLM8
Right ØLM7
Head and Neck ØLMØ
Hip
Left ØLMK
Right ØLMJ
Knee
Left ØLMR
Right ØLMQ
Lower Arm and Wrist
Left ØLM6
Right ØLM5
Lower Leg
Left ØLMP
Right ØLMN
Perineum ØLMH
Shoulder
Left ØLM2
Right ØLM1
Thorax
Left ØLMD
Right ØLMC
Trunk
Left ØLMB
Right ØLM9
Upper Arm
Left ØLM4
Right ØLM3
Upper Leg
Left ØLMM
Right ØLML
Testis
Bilateral ØVMC
Left ØVMB
Right ØVM9
Thumb
Left ØXMMØZZ
Right ØXMLØZZ
Thyroid Gland
Left Lobe ØGMG
Right Lobe ØGMH
Toe
1st
Left ØYMQØZZ
Right ØYMPØZZ
2nd
Left ØYMSØZZ
Right ØYMRØZZ
3rd
Left ØYMUØZZ
Right ØYMTØZZ
4th
Left ØYMWØZZ
Right ØYMVØZZ
5th
Left ØYMYØZZ
Right ØYMXØZZ
Tongue ØCM7ØZZ
Tooth
Lower ØCMX
Upper ØCMW
Trachea ØBM1ØZZ
Tunica Vaginalis
Left ØVM7
Right ØVM6
Ureter
Left ØTM7
Right ØTM6
Ureters, Bilateral ØTM8
Urethra ØTMD
Uterine Supporting Structure ØUM4
Uterus ØUM9
Uvula ØCMNØZZ
Vagina ØUMG
Vulva ØUMMXZZ
Wrist Region
Left ØXMHØZZ

Reattachment — *continued*
  Wrist Region — *continued*
    Right ØXMGØZZ
REBOA (resuscitative endovascular balloon occlusion of the aorta)
  Ø2LW3DJ
  Ø4LØ3DJ
Rebound HRD® (Hernia Repair Device) *use* Synthetic Substitute
REBYOTA® *use* Broad Consortium Microbiota-based Live Biotherapeutic Suspension
RECELL® cell suspension autograft *see* Replacement, Skin and Breast ØHR
Recession
  see Repair
  see Reposition
Reclosure, disrupted abdominal wall ØWQFXZZ
Reconstruction
  see Repair
  see Replacement
  see Supplement
Rectectomy
  see Excision, Rectum ØDBP
  see Resection, Rectum ØDTP
Rectocele repair *see* Repair, Subcutaneous Tissue and Fascia, Pelvic Region ØJQC
Rectopexy
  see Repair, Gastrointestinal System ØDQ
  see Reposition, Gastrointestinal System ØDS
Rectoplasty
  see Repair, Gastrointestinal System ØDQ
  see Supplement, Gastrointestinal System ØDU
Rectorrhaphy *see* Repair, Gastrointestinal System ØDQ
Rectoscopy ØDJD8ZZ
Rectosigmoid junction *use* Sigmoid Colon
Rectosigmoidectomy
  see Excision, Gastrointestinal System ØDB
  see Resection, Gastrointestinal System ØDT
Rectostomy *see* Drainage, Rectum ØD9P
Rectotomy *see* Drainage, Rectum ØD9P
Rectus abdominis muscle
  use Abdomen Muscle, Left
  use Abdomen Muscle, Right
Rectus femoris muscle
  use Upper Leg Muscle, Left
  use Upper Leg Muscle, Right
Recurrent laryngeal nerve *use* Vagus Nerve
Reducer™ System *use* Reduction Device in New Technology
Reduction
  Dislocation *see* Reposition
  Fracture *see* Reposition
  Intussusception, intestinal *see* Reposition, Gastrointestinal System ØDS
  Mammoplasty *see* Excision, Skin and Breast ØHB
  Prolapse *see* Reposition
  Torsion *see* Reposition
  Volvulus, gastrointestinal *see* Reposition, Gastrointestinal System ØDS
Reduction Device, Coronary Sinus X2V73Q7
Refusion *see* Fusion
REGN-COV2 Monoclonal Antibody XWØ
Rehabilitation
  see Activities of Daily Living Assessment, Rehabilitation FØ2
  see Activities of Daily Living Treatment, Rehabilitation FØ8
  see Caregiver Training, Rehabilitation FØF
  see Cochlear Implant Treatment, Rehabilitation FØB
  see Device Fitting, Rehabilitation FØD
  see Hearing Treatment, Rehabilitation FØ9
  see Motor Function Assessment, Rehabilitation FØ1
  see Motor Treatment, Rehabilitation FØ7
  see Speech Assessment, Rehabilitation FØØ
  see Speech Treatment, Rehabilitation FØ6
  see Vestibular Treatment, Rehabilitation FØC
Reimplantation
  see Reattachment
  see Reposition
  see Transfer
Reinforcement
  see Repair
  see Supplement
Relaxation, scar tissue *see* Release
Release
  Acetabulum
    Left ØQN5
    Right ØQN4
  Adenoids ØCNQ
  Ampulla of Vater ØFNC
  Anal Sphincter ØDNR
  Anterior Chamber
    Left Ø8N33ZZ
    Right Ø8N23ZZ
  Anus ØDNQ
  Aorta
    Abdominal Ø4NØ
    Thoracic
      Ascending/Arch Ø2NX
      Descending Ø2NW
  Aortic Body ØGND
  Appendix ØDNJ
  Artery
    Anterior Tibial
      Left Ø4NQ
      Right Ø4NP
    Axillary
      Left Ø3N6
      Right Ø3N5
    Brachial
      Left Ø3N8
      Right Ø3N7
    Celiac Ø4N1
    Colic
      Left Ø4N7
      Middle Ø4N8
      Right Ø4N6
    Common Carotid
      Left Ø3NJ
      Right Ø3NH
    Common Iliac
      Left Ø4ND
      Right Ø4NC
    Coronary
      Four or More Arteries Ø2N3
      One Artery Ø2NØ
      Three Arteries Ø2N2
      Two Arteries Ø2N1
    External Carotid
      Left Ø3NN
      Right Ø3NM
    External Iliac
      Left Ø4NJ
      Right Ø4NH
    Face Ø3NR
    Femoral
      Left Ø4NL
      Right Ø4NK
    Foot
      Left Ø4NW
      Right Ø4NV
    Gastric Ø4N2
    Hand
      Left Ø3NF
      Right Ø3ND
    Hepatic Ø4N3
    Inferior Mesenteric Ø4NB
    Innominate Ø3N2
    Internal Carotid
      Left Ø3NL
      Right Ø3NK
    Internal Iliac
      Left Ø4NF
      Right Ø4NE
    Internal Mammary
      Left Ø3N1
      Right Ø3NØ
    Intracranial Ø3NG
    Lower Ø4NY
    Peroneal
      Left Ø4NU
      Right Ø4NT
    Popliteal
      Left Ø4NN
      Right Ø4NM
    Posterior Tibial
      Left Ø4NS
      Right Ø4NR
    Pulmonary
      Left Ø2NR
      Right Ø2NQ
    Pulmonary Trunk Ø2NP
Release — *continued*
  Artery — *continued*
    Radial
      Left Ø3NC
      Right Ø3NB
    Renal
      Left Ø4NA
      Right Ø4N9
    Splenic Ø4N4
    Subclavian
      Left Ø3N4
      Right Ø3N3
    Superior Mesenteric Ø4N5
    Temporal
      Left Ø3NT
      Right Ø3NS
    Thyroid
      Left Ø3NV
      Right Ø3NU
    Ulnar
      Left Ø3NA
      Right Ø3N9
    Upper Ø3NY
    Vertebral
      Left Ø3NQ
      Right Ø3NP
  Atrium
    Left Ø2N7
    Right Ø2N6
  Auditory Ossicle
    Left Ø9NA
    Right Ø9N9
  Basal Ganglia ØØN8
  Bladder ØTNB
  Bladder Neck ØTNC
  Bone
    Ethmoid
      Left ØNNG
      Right ØNNF
    Frontal ØNN1
    Hyoid ØNNX
    Lacrimal
      Left ØNNJ
      Right ØNNH
    Nasal ØNNB
    Occipital ØNN7
    Palatine
      Left ØNNL
      Right ØNNK
    Parietal
      Left ØNN4
      Right ØNN3
    Pelvic
      Left ØQN3
      Right ØQN2
    Sphenoid ØNNC
    Temporal
      Left ØNN6
      Right ØNN5
    Zygomatic
      Left ØNNN
      Right ØNNM
  Brain ØØNØ
  Breast
    Bilateral ØHNV
    Left ØHNU
    Right ØHNT
  Bronchus
    Lingula ØBN9
    Lower Lobe
      Left ØBNB
      Right ØBN6
    Main
      Left ØBN7
      Right ØBN3
    Middle Lobe, Right ØBN5
    Upper Lobe
      Left ØBN8
      Right ØBN4
  Buccal Mucosa ØCN4
  Bursa and Ligament
    Abdomen
      Left ØMNJ
      Right ØMNH
    Ankle
      Left ØMNR
      Right ØMNQ
    Elbow
      Left ØMN4

Release — *continued*
Bursa and Ligament — *continued*
Elbow — *continued*
Right ØMN3
Foot
Left ØMNT
Right ØMNS
Hand
Left ØMN8
Right ØMN7
Head and Neck ØMNØ
Hip
Left ØMNM
Right ØMNL
Knee
Left ØMNP
Right ØMNN
Lower Extremity
Left ØMNW
Right ØMNV
Perineum ØMNK
Rib(s) ØMNG
Shoulder
Left ØMN2
Right ØMN1
Spine
Lower ØMND
Upper ØMNC
Sternum ØMNF
Upper Extremity
Left ØMNB
Right ØMN9
Wrist
Left ØMN6
Right ØMN5
Carina ØBN2
Carotid Bodies, Bilateral ØGN8
Carotid Body
Left ØGN6
Right ØGN7
Carpal
Left ØPNN
Right ØPNM
Cecum ØDNH
Cerebellum ØØNC
Cerebral Hemisphere ØØN7
Cerebral Meninges ØØN1
Cerebral Ventricle ØØN6
Cervix ØUNC
Chordae Tendineae Ø2N9
Choroid
Left Ø8NB
Right Ø8NA
Cisterna Chyli Ø7NL
Clavicle
Left ØPNB
Right ØPN9
Clitoris ØUNJ
Coccygeal Glomus ØGNB
Coccyx ØQNS
Colon
Ascending ØDNK
Descending ØDNM
Sigmoid ØDNN
Transverse ØDNL
Conduction Mechanism Ø2N8
Conjunctiva
Left Ø8NTXZZ
Right Ø8NSXZZ
Cord
Bilateral ØVNH
Left ØVNG
Right ØVNF
Cornea
Left Ø8N9XZZ
Right Ø8N8XZZ
Cul-de-sac ØUNF
Diaphragm ØBNT
Disc
Cervical Vertebral ØRN3
Cervicothoracic Vertebral ØRN5
Lumbar Vertebral ØSN2
Lumbosacral ØSN4
Thoracic Vertebral ØRN9
Thoracolumbar Vertebral ØRNB
Duct
Common Bile ØFN9
Cystic ØFN8

Release — *continued*
Duct — *continued*
Hepatic
Common ØFN7
Left ØFN6
Right ØFN5
Lacrimal
Left Ø8NY
Right Ø8NX
Pancreatic ØFND
Accessory ØFNF
Parotid
Left ØCNC
Right ØCNB
Duodenum ØDN9
Dura Mater ØØN2
Ear
External
Left Ø9N1
Right Ø9NØ
External Auditory Canal
Left Ø9N4
Right Ø9N3
Inner
Left Ø9NE
Right Ø9ND
Middle
Left Ø9N6
Right Ø9N5
Epididymis
Bilateral ØVNL
Left ØVNK
Right ØVNJ
Epiglottis ØCNR
Esophagogastric Junction ØDN4
Esophagus ØDN5
Lower ØDN3
Middle ØDN2
Upper ØDN1
Eustachian Tube
Left Ø9NG
Right Ø9NF
Eye
Left Ø8N1XZZ
Right Ø8NØXZZ
Eyelid
Lower
Left Ø8NR
Right Ø8NQ
Upper
Left Ø8NP
Right Ø8NN
Fallopian Tube
Left ØUN6
Right ØUN5
Fallopian Tubes, Bilateral ØUN7
Femoral Shaft
Left ØQN9
Right ØQN8
Femur
Lower
Left ØQNC
Right ØQNB
Upper
Left ØQN7
Right ØQN6
Fibula
Left ØQNK
Right ØQNJ
Finger Nail ØHNQXZZ
Gallbladder ØFN4
Gingiva
Lower ØCN6
Upper ØCN5
Gland
Adrenal
Bilateral ØGN4
Left ØGN2
Right ØGN3
Lacrimal
Left Ø8NW
Right Ø8NV
Minor Salivary ØCNJ
Parotid
Left ØCN9
Right ØCN8
Pituitary ØGNØ
Sublingual
Left ØCNF

Release — *continued*
Gland — *continued*
Sublingual — *continued*
Right ØCND
Submaxillary
Left ØCNH
Right ØCNG
Vestibular ØUNL
Glenoid Cavity
Left ØPN8
Right ØPN7
Glomus Jugulare ØGNC
Humeral Head
Left ØPND
Right ØPNC
Humeral Shaft
Left ØPNG
Right ØPNF
Hymen ØUNK
Hypothalamus ØØNA
Ileocecal Valve ØDNC
Ileum ØDNB
Intestine
Large ØDNE
Left ØDNG
Right ØDNF
Small ØDN8
Iris
Left Ø8ND3ZZ
Right Ø8NC3ZZ
Jejunum ØDNA
Joint
Acromioclavicular
Left ØRNH
Right ØRNG
Ankle
Left ØSNG
Right ØSNF
Carpal
Left ØRNR
Right ØRNQ
Carpometacarpal
Left ØRNT
Right ØRNS
Cervical Vertebral ØRN1
Cervicothoracic Vertebral ØRN4
Coccygeal ØSN6
Elbow
Left ØRNM
Right ØRNL
Finger Phalangeal
Left ØRNX
Right ØRNW
Hip
Left ØSNB
Right ØSN9
Knee
Left ØSND
Right ØSNC
Lumbar Vertebral ØSNØ
Lumbosacral ØSN3
Metacarpophalangeal
Left ØRNV
Right ØRNU
Metatarsal-Phalangeal
Left ØSNN
Right ØSNM
Occipital-cervical ØRNØ
Sacrococcygeal ØSN5
Sacroiliac
Left ØSN8
Right ØSN7
Shoulder
Left ØRNK
Right ØRNJ
Sternoclavicular
Left ØRNF
Right ØRNE
Tarsal
Left ØSNJ
Right ØSNH
Tarsometatarsal
Left ØSNL
Right ØSNK
Temporomandibular
Left ØRND
Right ØRNC
Thoracic Vertebral ØRN6
Thoracolumbar Vertebral ØRNA

Release — *continued*
Joint — *continued*
Toe Phalangeal
Left ØSNQ
Right ØSNP
Wrist
Left ØRNP
Right ØRNN
Kidney
Left ØTN1
Right ØTNØ
Kidney Pelvis
Left ØTN4
Right ØTN3
Larynx ØCNS
Lens
Left Ø8NK3ZZ
Right Ø8NJ3ZZ
Lip
Lower ØCN1
Upper ØCNØ
Liver ØFNØ
Left Lobe ØFN2
Right Lobe ØFN1
Lung
Bilateral ØBNM
Left ØBNL
Lower Lobe
Left ØBNJ
Right ØBNF
Middle Lobe, Right ØBND
Right ØBNK
Upper Lobe
Left ØBNG
Right ØBNC
Lung Lingula ØBNH
Lymphatic
Aortic Ø7ND
Axillary
Left Ø7N6
Right Ø7N5
Head Ø7NØ
Inguinal
Left Ø7NJ
Right Ø7NH
Internal Mammary
Left Ø7N9
Right Ø7N8
Lower Extremity
Left Ø7NG
Right Ø7NF
Mesenteric Ø7NB
Neck
Left Ø7N2
Right Ø7N1
Pelvis Ø7NC
Thoracic Duct Ø7NK
Thorax Ø7N7
Upper Extremity
Left Ø7N4
Right Ø7N3
Mandible
Left ØNNV
Right ØNNT
Maxilla ØNNR
Medulla Oblongata ØØND
Mesentery ØDNV
Metacarpal
Left ØPNQ
Right ØPNP
Metatarsal
Left ØQNP
Right ØQNN
Muscle
Abdomen
Left ØKNL
Right ØKNK
Extraocular
Left Ø8NM
Right Ø8NL
Facial ØKN1
Foot
Left ØKNW
Right ØKNV
Hand
Left ØKND
Right ØKNC
Head ØKNØ

Release — *continued*
Muscle — *continued*
Hip
Left ØKNP
Right ØKNN
Lower Arm and Wrist
Left ØKNB
Right ØKN9
Lower Leg
Left ØKNT
Right ØKNS
Neck
Left ØKN3
Right ØKN2
Papillary Ø2ND
Perineum ØKNM
Shoulder
Left ØKN6
Right ØKN5
Thorax
Left ØKNJ
Right ØKNH
Tongue, Palate, Pharynx ØKN4
Trunk
Left ØKNG
Right ØKNF
Upper Arm
Left ØKN8
Right ØKN7
Upper Leg
Left ØKNR
Right ØKNQ
Myocardial Bridge *see* Release, Artery, Coronary
Nasal Mucosa and Soft Tissue Ø9NK
Nasopharynx Ø9NN
Nerve
Abdominal Sympathetic Ø1NM
Abducens ØØNL
Accessory ØØNR
Acoustic ØØNN
Brachial Plexus Ø1N3
Cervical Ø1N1
Cervical Plexus Ø1NØ
Facial ØØNM
Femoral Ø1ND
Glossopharyngeal ØØNP
Head and Neck Sympathetic Ø1NK
Hypoglossal ØØNS
Lumbar Ø1NB
Lumbar Plexus Ø1N9
Lumbar Sympathetic Ø1NN
Lumbosacral Plexus Ø1NA
Median Ø1N5
Oculomotor ØØNH
Olfactory ØØNF
Optic ØØNG
Peroneal Ø1NH
Phrenic Ø1N2
Pudendal Ø1NC
Radial Ø1N6
Sacral Ø1NR
Sacral Plexus Ø1NQ
Sacral Sympathetic Ø1NP
Sciatic Ø1NF
Thoracic Ø1N8
Thoracic Sympathetic Ø1NL
Tibial Ø1NG
Trigeminal ØØNK
Trochlear ØØNJ
Ulnar Ø1N4
Vagus ØØNQ
Nipple
Left ØHNX
Right ØHNW
Omentum ØDNU
Orbit
Left ØNNQ
Right ØNNP
Ovary
Bilateral ØUN2
Left ØUN1
Right ØUNØ
Palate
Hard ØCN2
Soft ØCN3
Pancreas ØFNG
Para-aortic Body ØGN9
Paraganglion Extremity ØGNF
Parathyroid Gland ØGNR

Release — *continued*
Parathyroid Gland — *continued*
Inferior
Left ØGNP
Right ØGNN
Multiple ØGNQ
Superior
Left ØGNM
Right ØGNL
Patella
Left ØQNF
Right ØQND
Penis ØVNS
Pericardium Ø2NN
Peritoneum ØDNW
Phalanx
Finger
Left ØPNV
Right ØPNT
Thumb
Left ØPNS
Right ØPNR
Toe
Left ØQNR
Right ØQNQ
Pharynx ØCNM
Pineal Body ØGN1
Pleura
Left ØBNP
Right ØBNN
Pons ØØNB
Prepuce ØVNT
Prostate ØVNØ
Radius
Left ØPNJ
Right ØPNH
Rectum ØDNP
Retina
Left Ø8NF3ZZ
Right Ø8NE3ZZ
Retinal Vessel
Left Ø8NH3ZZ
Right Ø8NG3ZZ
Ribs
1 to 2 ØPN1
3 or More ØPN2
Sacrum ØQN1
Scapula
Left ØPN6
Right ØPN5
Sclera
Left Ø8N7XZZ
Right Ø8N6XZZ
Scrotum ØVN5
Septum
Atrial Ø2N5
Nasal Ø9NM
Ventricular Ø2NM
Sinus
Accessory Ø9NP
Ethmoid
Left Ø9NV
Right Ø9NU
Frontal
Left Ø9NT
Right Ø9NS
Mastoid
Left Ø9NC
Right Ø9NB
Maxillary
Left Ø9NR
Right Ø9NQ
Sphenoid
Left Ø9NX
Right Ø9NW
Skin
Abdomen ØHN7XZZ
Back ØHN6XZZ
Buttock ØHN8XZZ
Chest ØHN5XZZ
Ear
Left ØHN3XZZ
Right ØHN2XZZ
Face ØHN1XZZ
Foot
Left ØHNNXZZ
Right ØHNMXZZ
Hand
Left ØHNGXZZ

- **Release** — *continued*
  - Skin — *continued*
    - Hand — *continued*
      - Right ØHNFXZZ
    - Inguinal ØHNAXZZ
    - Lower Arm
      - Left ØHNEXZZ
      - Right ØHNDXZZ
    - Lower Leg
      - Left ØHNLXZZ
      - Right ØHNKXZZ
    - Neck ØHN4XZZ
    - Perineum ØHN9XZZ
    - Scalp ØHNØXZZ
    - Upper Arm
      - Left ØHNCXZZ
      - Right ØHNBXZZ
    - Upper Leg
      - Left ØHNJXZZ
      - Right ØHNHXZZ
  - Spinal Cord
    - Cervical ØØNW
    - Lumbar ØØNY
    - Thoracic ØØNX
  - Spinal Meninges ØØNT
  - Spleen Ø7NP
  - Sternum ØPNØ
  - Stomach ØDN6
    - Pylorus ØDN7
  - Subcutaneous Tissue and Fascia
    - Abdomen ØJN8
    - Back ØJN7
    - Buttock ØJN9
    - Chest ØJN6
    - Face ØJN1
    - Foot
      - Left ØJNR
      - Right ØJNQ
    - Hand
      - Left ØJNK
      - Right ØJNJ
    - Lower Arm
      - Left ØJNH
      - Right ØJNG
    - Lower Leg
      - Left ØJNP
      - Right ØJNN
    - Neck
      - Left ØJN5
      - Right ØJN4
    - Pelvic Region ØJNC
    - Perineum ØJNB
    - Scalp ØJNØ
    - Upper Arm
      - Left ØJNF
      - Right ØJND
    - Upper Leg
      - Left ØJNM
      - Right ØJNL
  - Tarsal
    - Left ØQNM
    - Right ØQNL
  - Tendon
    - Abdomen
      - Left ØLNG
      - Right ØLNF
    - Ankle
      - Left ØLNT
      - Right ØLNS
    - Foot
      - Left ØLNW
      - Right ØLNV
    - Hand
      - Left ØLN8
      - Right ØLN7
    - Head and Neck ØLNØ
    - Hip
      - Left ØLNK
      - Right ØLNJ
    - Knee
      - Left ØLNR
      - Right ØLNQ
    - Lower Arm and Wrist
      - Left ØLN6
      - Right ØLN5
    - Lower Leg
      - Left ØLNP
      - Right ØLNN
    - Perineum ØLNH

- **Release** — *continued*
  - Tendon — *continued*
    - Shoulder
      - Left ØLN2
      - Right ØLN1
    - Thorax
      - Left ØLND
      - Right ØLNC
    - Trunk
      - Left ØLNB
      - Right ØLN9
    - Upper Arm
      - Left ØLN4
      - Right ØLN3
    - Upper Leg
      - Left ØLNM
      - Right ØLNL
  - Testis
    - Bilateral ØVNC
    - Left ØVNB
    - Right ØVN9
  - Thalamus ØØN9
  - Thymus Ø7NM
  - Thyroid Gland ØGNK
    - Left Lobe ØGNG
    - Right Lobe ØGNH
  - Tibia
    - Left ØQNH
    - Right ØQNG
  - Toe Nail ØHNRXZZ
  - Tongue ØCN7
  - Tonsils ØCNP
  - Tooth
    - Lower ØCNX
    - Upper ØCNW
  - Trachea ØBN1
  - Tunica Vaginalis
    - Left ØVN7
    - Right ØVN6
  - Turbinate, Nasal Ø9NL
  - Tympanic Membrane
    - Left Ø9N8
    - Right Ø9N7
  - Ulna
    - Left ØPNL
    - Right ØPNK
  - Ureter
    - Left ØTN7
    - Right ØTN6
  - Urethra ØTND
  - Uterine Supporting Structure ØUN4
  - Uterus ØUN9
  - Uvula ØCNN
  - Vagina ØUNG
  - Valve
    - Aortic Ø2NF
    - Mitral Ø2NG
    - Pulmonary Ø2NH
    - Tricuspid Ø2NJ
  - Vas Deferens
    - Bilateral ØVNQ
    - Left ØVNP
    - Right ØVNN
  - Vein
    - Axillary
      - Left Ø5N8
      - Right Ø5N7
    - Azygos Ø5NØ
    - Basilic
      - Left Ø5NC
      - Right Ø5NB
    - Brachial
      - Left Ø5NA
      - Right Ø5N9
    - Cephalic
      - Left Ø5NF
      - Right Ø5ND
    - Colic Ø6N7
    - Common Iliac
      - Left Ø6ND
      - Right Ø6NC
    - Coronary Ø2N4
    - Esophageal Ø6N3
    - External Iliac
      - Left Ø6NG
      - Right Ø6NF
    - External Jugular
      - Left Ø5NQ
      - Right Ø5NP

- **Release** — *continued*
  - Vein — *continued*
    - Face
      - Left Ø5NV
      - Right Ø5NT
    - Femoral
      - Left Ø6NN
      - Right Ø6NM
    - Foot
      - Left Ø6NV
      - Right Ø6NT
    - Gastric Ø6N2
    - Hand
      - Left Ø5NH
      - Right Ø5NG
    - Hemiazygos Ø5N1
    - Hepatic Ø6N4
    - Hypogastric
      - Left Ø6NJ
      - Right Ø6NH
    - Inferior Mesenteric Ø6N6
    - Innominate
      - Left Ø5N4
      - Right Ø5N3
    - Internal Jugular
      - Left Ø5NN
      - Right Ø5NM
    - Intracranial Ø5NL
    - Lower Ø6NY
    - Portal Ø6N8
    - Pulmonary
      - Left Ø2NT
      - Right Ø2NS
    - Renal
      - Left Ø6NB
      - Right Ø6N9
    - Saphenous
      - Left Ø6NQ
      - Right Ø6NP
    - Splenic Ø6N1
    - Subclavian
      - Left Ø5N6
      - Right Ø5N5
    - Superior Mesenteric Ø6N5
    - Upper Ø5NY
    - Vertebral
      - Left Ø5NS
      - Right Ø5NR
  - Vena Cava
    - Inferior Ø6NØ
    - Superior Ø2NV
  - Ventricle
    - Left Ø2NL
    - Right Ø2NK
  - Vertebra
    - Cervical ØPN3
    - Lumbar ØQNØ
    - Thoracic ØPN4
  - Vesicle
    - Bilateral ØVN3
    - Left ØVN2
    - Right ØVN1
  - Vitreous
    - Left Ø8N53ZZ
    - Right Ø8N43ZZ
  - Vocal Cord
    - Left ØCNV
    - Right ØCNT
  - Vulva ØUNM
- **Relocation** *see* Reposition
- **Remdesivir Anti-infective** XWØ
- **Removal**
  - Abdominal Wall 2W53X
  - Anorectal 2Y53X5Z
  - Arm
    - Lower
      - Left 2W5DX
      - Right 2W5CX
    - Upper
      - Left 2W5BX
      - Right 2W5AX
  - Back 2W55X
  - Chest Wall 2W54X
  - Ear 2Y52X5Z
  - Extremity
    - Lower
      - Left 2W5MX
      - Right 2W5LX

Removal — *continued*
Extremity — *continued*
Upper
Left 2W59X
Right 2W58X
Face 2W51X
Finger
Left 2W5KX
Right 2W5JX
Foot
Left 2W5TX
Right 2W5SX
Genital Tract, Female 2Y54X5Z
Hand
Left 2W5FX
Right 2W5EX
Head 2W50X
Inguinal Region
Left 2W57X
Right 2W56X
Leg
Lower
Left 2W5RX
Right 2W5QX
Upper
Left 2W5PX
Right 2W5NX
Mouth and Pharynx 2Y50X5Z
Nasal 2Y51X5Z
Neck 2W52X
Thumb
Left 2W5HX
Right 2W5GX
Toe
Left 2W5VX
Right 2W5UX
Urethra 2Y55X5Z
Removal of device from
Abdominal Wall 0WPF
Acetabulum
Left 0QP5
Right 0QP4
Anal Sphincter 0DPR
Anus 0DPQ
Aorta, Thoracic, Descending 02PW3RZ
Artery
Lower 04PY
Upper 03PY
Back
Lower 0WPL
Upper 0WPK
Bladder 0TPB
Bone
Facial 0NPW
Lower 0QPY
Nasal 0NPB
Pelvic
Left 0QP3
Right 0QP2
Upper 0PPY
Bone Marrow 07PT
Brain 00P0
Breast
Left 0HPU
Right 0HPT
Bursa and Ligament
Lower 0MPY
Upper 0MPX
Carpal
Left 0PPN
Right 0PPM
Cavity, Cranial 0WP1
Cerebral Ventricle 00P6
Chest Wall 0WP8
Cisterna Chyli 07PL
Clavicle
Left 0PPB
Right 0PP9
Coccyx 0QPS
Diaphragm 0BPT
Disc
Cervical Vertebral 0RP3
Cervicothoracic Vertebral 0RP5
Lumbar Vertebral 0SP2
Lumbosacral 0SP4
Thoracic Vertebral 0RP9
Thoracolumbar Vertebral 0RPB
Duct
Hepatobiliary 0FPB

Removal of device from — *continued*
Duct — *continued*
Pancreatic 0FPD
Ear
Inner
Left 09PJ
Right 09PD
Left 09PJ
Right 09PH
Epididymis and Spermatic Cord 0VPM
Esophagus 0DP5
Extremity
Lower
Left 0YPB
Right 0YP9
Upper
Left 0XP7
Right 0XP6
Eye
Left 08P1
Right 08P0
Face 0WP2
Fallopian Tube 0UP8
Femoral Shaft
Left 0QP9
Right 0QP8
Femur
Lower
Left 0QPC
Right 0QPB
Upper
Left 0QP7
Right 0QP6
Fibula
Left 0QPK
Right 0QPJ
Finger Nail 0HPQX
Gallbladder 0FP4
Gastrointestinal Tract 0WPP
Genitourinary Tract 0WPR
Gland
Adrenal 0GP5
Endocrine 0GPS
Pituitary 0GP0
Salivary 0CPA
Glenoid Cavity
Left 0PP8
Right 0PP7
Great Vessel 02PY
Hair 0HPSX
Head 0WP0
Heart 02PA
Humeral Head
Left 0PPD
Right 0PPC
Humeral Shaft
Left 0PPG
Right 0PPF
Intestinal Tract
Lower Intestinal Tract 0DPD
Upper Intestinal Tract 0DP0
Jaw
Lower 0WP5
Upper 0WP4
Joint
Acromioclavicular
Left 0RPH
Right 0RPG
Ankle
Left 0SPG
Right 0SPF
Carpal
Left 0RPR
Right 0RPQ
Carpometacarpal
Left 0RPT
Right 0RPS
Cervical Vertebral 0RP1
Cervicothoracic Vertebral 0RP4
Coccygeal 0SP6
Elbow
Left 0RPM
Right 0RPL
Finger Phalangeal
Left 0RPX
Right 0RPW
Hip
Left 0SPB
Acetabular Surface 0SPE

Removal of device from — *continued*
Joint — *continued*
Hip — *continued*
Left — *continued*
Femoral Surface 0SPS
Right 0SP9
Acetabular Surface 0SPA
Femoral Surface 0SPR
Knee
Left 0SPD
Femoral Surface 0SPU
Tibial Surface 0SPW
Right 0SPC
Femoral Surface 0SPT
Tibial Surface 0SPV
Lumbar Vertebral 0SP0
Lumbosacral 0SP3
Metacarpophalangeal
Left 0RPV
Right 0RPU
Metatarsal-Phalangeal
Left 0SPN
Right 0SPM
Occipital-cervical 0RP0
Sacrococcygeal 0SP5
Sacroiliac
Left 0SP8
Right 0SP7
Shoulder
Left 0RPK
Right 0RPJ
Sternoclavicular
Left 0RPF
Right 0RPE
Tarsal
Left 0SPJ
Right 0SPH
Tarsometatarsal
Left 0SPL
Right 0SPK
Temporomandibular
Left 0RPD
Right 0RPC
Thoracic Vertebral 0RP6
Thoracolumbar Vertebral 0RPA
Toe Phalangeal
Left 0SPQ
Right 0SPP
Wrist
Left 0RPP
Right 0RPN
Kidney 0TP5
Larynx 0CPS
Lens
Left 08PK3
Right 08PJ3
Liver 0FP0
Lung
Left 0BPL
Right 0BPK
Lymphatic 07PN
Thoracic Duct 07PK
Mediastinum 0WPC
Mesentery 0DPV
Metacarpal
Left 0PPQ
Right 0PPP
Metatarsal
Left 0QPP
Right 0QPN
Mouth and Throat 0CPY
Muscle
Extraocular
Left 08PM
Right 08PL
Lower 0KPY
Upper 0KPX
Nasal Mucosa and Soft Tissue 09PK
Neck 0WP6
Nerve
Cranial 00PE
Peripheral 01PY
Omentum 0DPU
Ovary 0UP3
Pancreas 0FPG
Parathyroid Gland 0GPR
Patella
Left 0QPF
Right 0QPD

Subterms under main terms may continue to next column or page

Removal of device from — *continued*
- Pelvic Cavity ØWPJ
- Penis ØVPS
- Pericardial Cavity ØWPD
- Perineum
  - Female ØWPN
  - Male ØWPM
- Peritoneal Cavity ØWPG
- Peritoneum ØDPW
- Phalanx
  - Finger
    - Left ØPPV
    - Right ØPPT
  - Thumb
    - Left ØPPS
    - Right ØPPR
  - Toe
    - Left ØQPR
    - Right ØQPQ
- Pineal Body ØGP1
- Pleura ØBPQ
- Pleural Cavity
  - Left ØWPB
  - Right ØWP9
- Products of Conception 1ØPØ
- Prostate and Seminal Vesicles ØVP4
- Radius
  - Left ØPPJ
  - Right ØPPH
- Rectum ØDPP
- Respiratory Tract ØWPQ
- Retroperitoneum ØWPH
- Ribs
  - 1 to 2 ØPP1
  - 3 or More ØPP2
- Sacrum ØQP1
- Scapula
  - Left ØPP6
  - Right ØPP5
- Scrotum and Tunica Vaginalis ØVP8
- Sinus Ø9PY
- Skin ØHPPX
- Skull ØNPØ
- Spinal Canal ØØPU
- Spinal Cord ØØPV
- Spleen Ø7PP
- Sternum ØPPØ
- Stomach ØDP6
- Subcutaneous Tissue and Fascia
  - Head and Neck ØJPS
  - Lower Extremity ØJPW
  - Trunk ØJPT
  - Upper Extremity ØJPV
- Tarsal
  - Left ØQPM
  - Right ØQPL
- Tendon
  - Lower ØLPY
  - Upper ØLPX
- Testis ØVPD
- Thymus Ø7PM
- Thyroid Gland ØGPK
- Tibia
  - Left ØQPH
  - Right ØQPG
- Toe Nail ØHPRX
- Trachea ØBP1
- Tracheobronchial Tree ØBPØ
- Tympanic Membrane
  - Left Ø9P8
  - Right Ø9P7
- Ulna
  - Left ØPPL
  - Right ØPPK
- Ureter ØTP9
- Urethra ØTPD
- Uterus and Cervix ØUPD
- Vagina and Cul-de-sac ØUPH
- Vas Deferens ØVPR
- Vein
  - Azygos Ø5PØ
  - Innominate
    - Left Ø5P4
    - Right Ø5P3
  - Lower Ø6PY
  - Upper Ø5PY
- Vertebra
  - Cervical ØPP3
  - Lumbar ØQPØ

Removal of device from — *continued*
- Vertebra — *continued*
  - Thoracic ØPP4
- Vulva ØUPM

Renal calyx
- *use* Kidney
- *use* Kidney, Left
- *use* Kidney, Right
- *use* Kidneys, Bilateral

Renal capsule
- *use* Kidney
- *use* Kidney, Left
- *use* Kidney, Right
- *use* Kidneys, Bilateral

Renal cortex
- *use* Kidney
- *use* Kidney, Left
- *use* Kidney, Right
- *use* Kidneys, Bilateral

Renal dialysis *see* Performance, Urinary 5A1D

Renal nerve *use* Abdominal Sympathetic Nerve

Renal plexus *use* Abdominal Sympathetic Nerve

Renal segment
- *use* Kidney
- *use* Kidney, Left
- *use* Kidney, Right
- *use* Kidneys, Bilateral

Renal segmental artery
- *use* Renal Artery, Left
- *use* Renal Artery, Right

Reopening, operative site
- Control of bleeding *see* Control bleeding in
- Inspection only *see* Inspection

Repair
- Abdominal Wall ØWQF
- Acetabulum
  - Left ØQQ5
  - Right ØQQ4
- Adenoids ØCQQ
- Ampulla of Vater ØFQC
- Anal Sphincter ØDQR
- Ankle Region
  - Left ØYQL
  - Right ØYQK
- Anterior Chamber
  - Left Ø8Q33ZZ
  - Right Ø8Q23ZZ
- Anus ØDQQ
- Aorta
  - Abdominal Ø4QØ
  - Thoracic
    - Ascending/Arch Ø2QX
    - Descending Ø2QW
- Aortic Body ØGQD
- Appendix ØDQJ
- Arm
  - Lower
    - Left ØXQF
    - Right ØXQD
  - Upper
    - Left ØXQ9
    - Right ØXQ8
- Artery
  - Anterior Tibial
    - Left Ø4QQ
    - Right Ø4QP
  - Axillary
    - Left Ø3Q6
    - Right Ø3Q5
  - Brachial
    - Left Ø3Q8
    - Right Ø3Q7
  - Celiac Ø4Q1
  - Colic
    - Left Ø4Q7
    - Middle Ø4Q8
    - Right Ø4Q6
  - Common Carotid
    - Left Ø3QJ
    - Right Ø3QH
  - Common Iliac
    - Left Ø4QD
    - Right Ø4QC
  - Coronary
    - Four or More Arteries Ø2Q3
    - One Artery Ø2QØ
    - Three Arteries Ø2Q2
    - Two Arteries Ø2Q1

Repair — *continued*
- Artery — *continued*
  - External Carotid
    - Left Ø3QN
    - Right Ø3QM
  - External Iliac
    - Left Ø4QJ
    - Right Ø4QH
  - Face Ø3QR
  - Femoral
    - Left Ø4QL
    - Right Ø4QK
  - Foot
    - Left Ø4QW
    - Right Ø4QV
  - Gastric Ø4Q2
  - Hand
    - Left Ø3QF
    - Right Ø3QD
  - Hepatic Ø4Q3
  - Inferior Mesenteric Ø4QB
  - Innominate Ø3Q2
  - Internal Carotid
    - Left Ø3QL
    - Right Ø3QK
  - Internal Iliac
    - Left Ø4QF
    - Right Ø4QE
  - Internal Mammary
    - Left Ø3Q1
    - Right Ø3QØ
  - Intracranial Ø3QG
  - Lower Ø4QY
  - Peroneal
    - Left Ø4QU
    - Right Ø4QT
  - Popliteal
    - Left Ø4QN
    - Right Ø4QM
  - Posterior Tibial
    - Left Ø4QS
    - Right Ø4QR
  - Pulmonary
    - Left Ø2QR
    - Right Ø2QQ
  - Pulmonary Trunk Ø2QP
  - Radial
    - Left Ø3QC
    - Right Ø3QB
  - Renal
    - Left Ø4QA
    - Right Ø4Q9
  - Splenic Ø4Q4
  - Subclavian
    - Left Ø3Q4
    - Right Ø3Q3
  - Superior Mesenteric Ø4Q5
  - Temporal
    - Left Ø3QT
    - Right Ø3QS
  - Thyroid
    - Left Ø3QV
    - Right Ø3QU
  - Ulnar
    - Left Ø3QA
    - Right Ø3Q9
  - Upper Ø3QY
  - Vertebral
    - Left Ø3QQ
    - Right Ø3QP
- Atrium
  - Left Ø2Q7
  - Right Ø2Q6
- Auditory Ossicle
  - Left Ø9QA
  - Right Ø9Q9
- Axilla
  - Left ØXQ5
  - Right ØXQ4
- Back
  - Lower ØWQL
  - Upper ØWQK
- Basal Ganglia ØØQ8
- Bladder ØTQB
- Bladder Neck ØTQC
- Bone
  - Ethmoid
    - Left ØNQG
    - Right ØNQF

Repair — *continued*
Bone — *continued*
Frontal ØNQ1
Hyoid ØNQX
Lacrimal
Left ØNQJ
Right ØNQH
Nasal ØNQB
Occipital ØNQ7
Palatine
Left ØNQL
Right ØNQK
Parietal
Left ØNQ4
Right ØNQ3
Pelvic
Left ØQQ3
Right ØQQ2
Sphenoid ØNQC
Temporal
Left ØNQ6
Right ØNQ5
Zygomatic
Left ØNQN
Right ØNQM
Brain ØØQØ
Breast
Bilateral ØHQV
Left ØHQU
Right ØHQT
Supernumerary ØHQY
Bronchus
Lingula ØBQ9
Lower Lobe
Left ØBQB
Right ØBQ6
Main
Left ØBQ7
Right ØBQ3
Middle Lobe, Right ØBQ5
Upper Lobe
Left ØBQ8
Right ØBQ4
Buccal Mucosa ØCQ4
Bursa and Ligament
Abdomen
Left ØMQJ
Right ØMQH
Ankle
Left ØMQR
Right ØMQQ
Elbow
Left ØMQ4
Right ØMQ3
Foot
Left ØMQT
Right ØMQS
Hand
Left ØMQ8
Right ØMQ7
Head and Neck ØMQØ
Hip
Left ØMQM
Right ØMQL
Knee
Left ØMQP
Right ØMQN
Lower Extremity
Left ØMQW
Right ØMQV
Perineum ØMQK
Rib(s) ØMQG
Shoulder
Left ØMQ2
Right ØMQ1
Spine
Lower ØMQD
Upper ØMQC
Sternum ØMQF
Upper Extremity
Left ØMQB
Right ØMQ9
Wrist
Left ØMQ6
Right ØMQ5
Buttock
Left ØYQ1
Right ØYQØ
Carina ØBQ2

Repair — *continued*
Carotid Bodies, Bilateral ØGQ8
Carotid Body
Left ØGQ6
Right ØGQ7
Carpal
Left ØPQN
Right ØPQM
Cecum ØDQH
Cerebellum ØØQC
Cerebral Hemisphere ØØQ7
Cerebral Meninges ØØQ1
Cerebral Ventricle ØØQ6
Cervix ØUQC
Chest Wall ØWQ8
Chordae Tendineae Ø2Q9
Choroid
Left Ø8QB
Right Ø8QA
Cisterna Chyli Ø7QL
Clavicle
Left ØPQB
Right ØPQ9
Clitoris ØUQJ
Coccygeal Glomus ØGQB
Coccyx ØQQS
Colon
Ascending ØDQK
Descending ØDQM
Sigmoid ØDQN
Transverse ØDQL
Conduction Mechanism Ø2Q8
Conjunctiva
Left Ø8QTXZZ
Right Ø8QSXZZ
Cord
Bilateral ØVQH
Left ØVQG
Right ØVQF
Cornea
Left Ø8Q9XZZ
Right Ø8Q8XZZ
Cul-de-sac ØUQF
Diaphragm ØBQT
Disc
Cervical Vertebral ØRQ3
Cervicothoracic Vertebral ØRQ5
Lumbar Vertebral ØSQ2
Lumbosacral ØSQ4
Thoracic Vertebral ØRQ9
Thoracolumbar Vertebral ØRQB
Duct
Common Bile ØFQ9
Cystic ØFQ8
Hepatic
Common ØFQ7
Left ØFQ6
Right ØFQ5
Lacrimal
Left Ø8QY
Right Ø8QX
Pancreatic ØFQD
Accessory ØFQF
Parotid
Left ØCQC
Right ØCQB
Duodenum ØDQ9
Dura Mater ØØQ2
Ear
External
Bilateral Ø9Q2
Left Ø9Q1
Right Ø9QØ
External Auditory Canal
Left Ø9Q4
Right Ø9Q3
Inner
Left Ø9QE
Right Ø9QD
Middle
Left Ø9Q6
Right Ø9Q5
Elbow Region
Left ØXQC
Right ØXQB
Epididymis
Bilateral ØVQL
Left ØVQK
Right ØVQJ

Repair — *continued*
Epiglottis ØCQR
Esophagogastric Junction ØDQ4
Esophagus ØDQ5
Lower ØDQ3
Middle ØDQ2
Upper ØDQ1
Eustachian Tube
Left Ø9QG
Right Ø9QF
Extremity
Lower
Left ØYQB
Right ØYQ9
Upper
Left ØXQ7
Right ØXQ6
Eye
Left Ø8Q1XZZ
Right Ø8QØXZZ
Eyelid
Lower
Left Ø8QR
Right Ø8QQ
Upper
Left Ø8QP
Right Ø8QN
Face ØWQ2
Fallopian Tube
Left ØUQ6
Right ØUQ5
Fallopian Tubes, Bilateral ØUQ7
Femoral Region
Bilateral ØYQE
Left ØYQ8
Right ØYQ7
Femoral Shaft
Left ØQQ9
Right ØQQ8
Femur
Lower
Left ØQQC
Right ØQQB
Upper
Left ØQQ7
Right ØQQ6
Fibula
Left ØQQK
Right ØQQJ
Finger
Index
Left ØXQP
Right ØXQN
Little
Left ØXQW
Right ØXQV
Middle
Left ØXQR
Right ØXQQ
Ring
Left ØXQT
Right ØXQS
Finger Nail ØHQQXZZ
Floor of mouth *see* Repair, Oral Cavity and Throat ØWQ3
Foot
Left ØYQN
Right ØYQM
Gallbladder ØFQ4
Gingiva
Lower ØCQ6
Upper ØCQ5
Gland
Adrenal
Bilateral ØGQ4
Left ØGQ2
Right ØGQ3
Lacrimal
Left Ø8QW
Right Ø8QV
Minor Salivary ØCQJ
Parotid
Left ØCQ9
Right ØCQ8
Pituitary ØGQØ
Sublingual
Left ØCQF
Right ØCQD

Subterms under main terms may continue to next column or page

Repair — *continued*
- Gland — *continued*
  - Submaxillary
    - Left ØCQH
    - Right ØCQG
  - Vestibular ØUQL
- Glenoid Cavity
  - Left ØPQ8
  - Right ØPQ7
- Glomus Jugulare ØGQC
- Hand
  - Left ØXQK
  - Right ØXQJ
- Head ØWQØ
- Heart Ø2QA
  - Left Ø2QC
  - Right Ø2QB
- Humeral Head
  - Left ØPQD
  - Right ØPQC
- Humeral Shaft
  - Left ØPQG
  - Right ØPQF
- Hymen ØUQK
- Hypothalamus ØØQA
- Ileocecal Valve ØDQC
- Ileum ØDQB
- Inguinal Region
  - Bilateral ØYQA
  - Left ØYQ6
  - Right ØYQ5
- Intestine
  - Large ØDQE
    - Left ØDQG
    - Right ØDQF
  - Small ØDQ8
- Iris
  - Left Ø8QD3ZZ
  - Right Ø8QC3ZZ
- Jaw
  - Lower ØWQ5
  - Upper ØWQ4
- Jejunum ØDQA
- Joint
  - Acromioclavicular
    - Left ØRQH
    - Right ØRQG
  - Ankle
    - Left ØSQG
    - Right ØSQF
  - Carpal
    - Left ØRQR
    - Right ØRQQ
  - Carpometacarpal
    - Left ØRQT
    - Right ØRQS
  - Cervical Vertebral ØRQ1
  - Cervicothoracic Vertebral ØRQ4
  - Coccygeal ØSQ6
  - Elbow
    - Left ØRQM
    - Right ØRQL
  - Finger Phalangeal
    - Left ØRQX
    - Right ØRQW
  - Hip
    - Left ØSQB
    - Right ØSQ9
  - Knee
    - Left ØSQD
    - Right ØSQC
  - Lumbar Vertebral ØSQØ
  - Lumbosacral ØSQ3
  - Metacarpophalangeal
    - Left ØRQV
    - Right ØRQU
  - Metatarsal-Phalangeal
    - Left ØSQN
    - Right ØSQM
  - Occipital-cervical ØRQØ
  - Sacrococcygeal ØSQ5
  - Sacroiliac
    - Left ØSQ8
    - Right ØSQ7
  - Shoulder
    - Left ØRQK
    - Right ØRQJ
  - Sternoclavicular
    - Left ØRQF

Repair — *continued*
- Joint — *continued*
  - Sternoclavicular — *continued*
    - Right ØRQE
  - Tarsal
    - Left ØSQJ
    - Right ØSQH
  - Tarsometatarsal
    - Left ØSQL
    - Right ØSQK
  - Temporomandibular
    - Left ØRQD
    - Right ØRQC
  - Thoracic Vertebral ØRQ6
  - Thoracolumbar Vertebral ØRQA
  - Toe Phalangeal
    - Left ØSQQ
    - Right ØSQP
  - Wrist
    - Left ØRQP
    - Right ØRQN
- Kidney
  - Left ØTQ1
  - Right ØTQØ
- Kidney Pelvis
  - Left ØTQ4
  - Right ØTQ3
- Knee Region
  - Left ØYQG
  - Right ØYQF
- Larynx ØCQS
- Leg
  - Lower
    - Left ØYQJ
    - Right ØYQH
  - Upper
    - Left ØYQD
    - Right ØYQC
- Lens
  - Left Ø8QK3ZZ
  - Right Ø8QJ3ZZ
- Lip
  - Lower ØCQ1
  - Upper ØCQØ
- Liver ØFQØ
  - Left Lobe ØFQ2
  - Right Lobe ØFQ1
- Lung
  - Bilateral ØBQM
  - Left ØBQL
  - Lower Lobe
    - Left ØBQJ
    - Right ØBQF
  - Middle Lobe, Right ØBQD
  - Right ØBQK
  - Upper Lobe
    - Left ØBQG
    - Right ØBQC
- Lung Lingula ØBQH
- Lymphatic
  - Aortic Ø7QD
  - Axillary
    - Left Ø7Q6
    - Right Ø7Q5
  - Head Ø7QØ
  - Inguinal
    - Left Ø7QJ
    - Right Ø7QH
  - Internal Mammary
    - Left Ø7Q9
    - Right Ø7Q8
  - Lower Extremity
    - Left Ø7QG
    - Right Ø7QF
  - Mesenteric Ø7QB
  - Neck
    - Left Ø7Q2
    - Right Ø7Q1
  - Pelvis Ø7QC
  - Thoracic Duct Ø7QK
  - Thorax Ø7Q7
  - Upper Extremity
    - Left Ø7Q4
    - Right Ø7Q3
- Mandible
  - Left ØNQV
  - Right ØNQT
- Maxilla ØNQR
- Mediastinum ØWQC

Repair — *continued*
- Medulla Oblongata ØØQD
- Mesentery ØDQV
- Metacarpal
  - Left ØPQQ
  - Right ØPQP
- Metatarsal
  - Left ØQQP
  - Right ØQQN
- Muscle
  - Abdomen
    - Left ØKQL
    - Right ØKQK
  - Extraocular
    - Left Ø8QM
    - Right Ø8QL
  - Facial ØKQ1
  - Foot
    - Left ØKQW
    - Right ØKQV
  - Hand
    - Left ØKQD
    - Right ØKQC
  - Head ØKQØ
  - Hip
    - Left ØKQP
    - Right ØKQN
  - Lower Arm and Wrist
    - Left ØKQB
    - Right ØKQ9
  - Lower Leg
    - Left ØKQT
    - Right ØKQS
  - Neck
    - Left ØKQ3
    - Right ØKQ2
  - Papillary Ø2QD
  - Perineum ØKQM
  - Shoulder
    - Left ØKQ6
    - Right ØKQ5
  - Thorax
    - Left ØKQJ
    - Right ØKQH
  - Tongue, Palate, Pharynx ØKQ4
  - Trunk
    - Left ØKQG
    - Right ØKQF
  - Upper Arm
    - Left ØKQ8
    - Right ØKQ7
  - Upper Leg
    - Left ØKQR
    - Right ØKQQ
- Nasal Mucosa and Soft Tissue Ø9QK
- Nasopharynx Ø9QN
- Neck ØWQ6
- Nerve
  - Abdominal Sympathetic Ø1QM
  - Abducens ØØQL
  - Accessory ØØQR
  - Acoustic ØØQN
  - Brachial Plexus Ø1Q3
  - Cervical Ø1Q1
  - Cervical Plexus Ø1QØ
  - Facial ØØQM
  - Femoral Ø1QD
  - Glossopharyngeal ØØQP
  - Head and Neck Sympathetic Ø1QK
  - Hypoglossal ØØQS
  - Lumbar Ø1QB
  - Lumbar Plexus Ø1Q9
  - Lumbar Sympathetic Ø1QN
  - Lumbosacral Plexus Ø1QA
  - Median Ø1Q5
  - Oculomotor ØØQH
  - Olfactory ØØQF
  - Optic ØØQG
  - Peroneal Ø1QH
  - Phrenic Ø1Q2
  - Pudendal Ø1QC
  - Radial Ø1Q6
  - Sacral Ø1QR
  - Sacral Plexus Ø1QQ
  - Sacral Sympathetic Ø1QP
  - Sciatic Ø1QF
  - Thoracic Ø1Q8
  - Thoracic Sympathetic Ø1QL
  - Tibial Ø1QG

- **Repair** — *continued*
  - Nerve — *continued*
    - Trigeminal ØØQK
    - Trochlear ØØQJ
    - Ulnar Ø1Q4
    - Vagus ØØQQ
  - Nipple
    - Left ØHQX
    - Right ØHQW
  - Omentum ØDQU
  - Oral Cavity and Throat ØWQ3
  - Orbit
    - Left ØNQQ
    - Right ØNQP
  - Ovary
    - Bilateral ØUQ2
    - Left ØUQ1
    - Right ØUQØ
  - Palate
    - Hard ØCQ2
    - Soft ØCQ3
  - Pancreas ØFQG
  - Para-aortic Body ØGQ9
  - Paraganglion Extremity ØGQF
  - Parathyroid Gland ØGQR
    - Inferior
      - Left ØGQP
      - Right ØGQN
    - Multiple ØGQQ
    - Superior
      - Left ØGQM
      - Right ØGQL
  - Patella
    - Left ØQQF
    - Right ØQQD
  - Penis ØVQS
  - Pericardium Ø2QN
  - Perineum
    - Female ØWQN
    - Male ØWQM
  - Peritoneum ØDQW
  - Phalanx
    - Finger
      - Left ØPQV
      - Right ØPQT
    - Thumb
      - Left ØPQS
      - Right ØPQR
    - Toe
      - Left ØQQR
      - Right ØQQQ
  - Pharynx ØCQM
  - Pineal Body ØGQ1
  - Pleura
    - Left ØBQP
    - Right ØBQN
  - Pons ØØQB
  - Prepuce ØVQT
  - Products of Conception 1ØQØ
  - Prostate ØVQØ
  - Radius
    - Left ØPQJ
    - Right ØPQH
  - Rectum ØDQP
  - Retina
    - Left Ø8QF3ZZ
    - Right Ø8QE3ZZ
  - Retinal Vessel
    - Left Ø8QH3ZZ
    - Right Ø8QG3ZZ
  - Ribs
    - 1 to 2 ØPQ1
    - 3 or More ØPQ2
  - Sacrum ØQQ1
  - Scapula
    - Left ØPQ6
    - Right ØPQ5
  - Sclera
    - Left Ø8Q7XZZ
    - Right Ø8Q6XZZ
  - Scrotum ØVQ5
  - Septum
    - Atrial Ø2Q5
    - Nasal Ø9QM
    - Ventricular Ø2QM
  - Shoulder Region
    - Left ØXQ3
    - Right ØXQ2

- **Repair** — *continued*
  - Sinus
    - Accessory Ø9QP
    - Ethmoid
      - Left Ø9QV
      - Right Ø9QU
    - Frontal
      - Left Ø9QT
      - Right Ø9QS
    - Mastoid
      - Left Ø9QC
      - Right Ø9QB
    - Maxillary
      - Left Ø9QR
      - Right Ø9QQ
    - Sphenoid
      - Left Ø9QX
      - Right Ø9QW
  - Skin
    - Abdomen ØHQ7XZZ
    - Back ØHQ6XZZ
    - Buttock ØHQ8XZZ
    - Chest ØHQ5XZZ
    - Ear
      - Left ØHQ3XZZ
      - Right ØHQ2XZZ
    - Face ØHQ1XZZ
    - Foot
      - Left ØHQNXZZ
      - Right ØHQMXZZ
    - Hand
      - Left ØHQGXZZ
      - Right ØHQFXZZ
    - Inguinal ØHQAXZZ
    - Lower Arm
      - Left ØHQEXZZ
      - Right ØHQDXZZ
    - Lower Leg
      - Left ØHQLXZZ
      - Right ØHQKXZZ
    - Neck ØHQ4XZZ
    - Perineum ØHQ9XZZ
    - Scalp ØHQØXZZ
    - Upper Arm
      - Left ØHQCXZZ
      - Right ØHQBXZZ
    - Upper Leg
      - Left ØHQJXZZ
      - Right ØHQHXZZ
  - Skull ØNQØ
  - Spinal Cord
    - Cervical ØØQW
    - Lumbar ØØQY
    - Thoracic ØØQX
  - Spinal Meninges ØØQT
  - Spleen Ø7QP
  - Sternum ØPQØ
  - Stomach ØDQ6
    - Pylorus ØDQ7
  - Subcutaneous Tissue and Fascia
    - Abdomen ØJQ8
    - Back ØJQ7
    - Buttock ØJQ9
    - Chest ØJQ6
    - Face ØJQ1
    - Foot
      - Left ØJQR
      - Right ØJQQ
    - Hand
      - Left ØJQK
      - Right ØJQJ
    - Lower Arm
      - Left ØJQH
      - Right ØJQG
    - Lower Leg
      - Left ØJQP
      - Right ØJQN
    - Neck
      - Left ØJQ5
      - Right ØJQ4
    - Pelvic Region ØJQC
    - Perineum ØJQB
    - Scalp ØJQØ
    - Upper Arm
      - Left ØJQF
      - Right ØJQD
    - Upper Leg
      - Left ØJQM
      - Right ØJQL

- **Repair** — *continued*
  - Tarsal
    - Left ØQQM
    - Right ØQQL
  - Tendon
    - Abdomen
      - Left ØLQG
      - Right ØLQF
    - Ankle
      - Left ØLQT
      - Right ØLQS
    - Foot
      - Left ØLQW
      - Right ØLQV
    - Hand
      - Left ØLQ8
      - Right ØLQ7
    - Head and Neck ØLQØ
    - Hip
      - Left ØLQK
      - Right ØLQJ
    - Knee
      - Left ØLQR
      - Right ØLQQ
    - Lower Arm and Wrist
      - Left ØLQ6
      - Right ØLQ5
    - Lower Leg
      - Left ØLQP
      - Right ØLQN
    - Perineum ØLQH
    - Shoulder
      - Left ØLQ2
      - Right ØLQ1
    - Thorax
      - Left ØLQD
      - Right ØLQC
    - Trunk
      - Left ØLQB
      - Right ØLQ9
    - Upper Arm
      - Left ØLQ4
      - Right ØLQ3
    - Upper Leg
      - Left ØLQM
      - Right ØLQL
  - Testis
    - Bilateral ØVQC
    - Left ØVQB
    - Right ØVQ9
  - Thalamus ØØQ9
  - Thumb
    - Left ØXQM
    - Right ØXQL
  - Thymus Ø7QM
  - Thyroid Gland ØGQK
    - Left Lobe ØGQG
    - Right Lobe ØGQH
  - Thyroid Gland Isthmus ØGQJ
  - Tibia
    - Left ØQQH
    - Right ØQQG
  - Toe
    - 1st
      - Left ØYQQ
      - Right ØYQP
    - 2nd
      - Left ØYQS
      - Right ØYQR
    - 3rd
      - Left ØYQU
      - Right ØYQT
    - 4th
      - Left ØYQW
      - Right ØYQV
    - 5th
      - Left ØYQY
      - Right ØYQX
  - Toe Nail ØHQRXZZ
  - Tongue ØCQ7
  - Tonsils ØCQP
  - Tooth
    - Lower ØCQX
    - Upper ØCQW
  - Trachea ØBQ1
  - Tunica Vaginalis
    - Left ØVQ7
    - Right ØVQ6
  - Turbinate, Nasal Ø9QL

Repair — *continued*
  Tympanic Membrane
    Left Ø9Q8
    Right Ø9Q7
  Ulna
    Left ØPQL
    Right ØPQK
  Ureter
    Left ØTQ7
    Right ØTQ6
  Urethra ØTQD
  Uterine Supporting Structure ØUQ4
  Uterus ØUQ9
  Uvula ØCQN
  Vagina ØUQG
  Valve
    Aortic Ø2QF
    Mitral Ø2QG
    Pulmonary Ø2QH
    Tricuspid Ø2QJ
  Vas Deferens
    Bilateral ØVQQ
    Left ØVQP
    Right ØVQN
  Vein
    Axillary
      Left Ø5Q8
      Right Ø5Q7
    Azygos Ø5QØ
    Basilic
      Left Ø5QC
      Right Ø5QB
    Brachial
      Left Ø5QA
      Right Ø5Q9
    Cephalic
      Left Ø5QF
      Right Ø5QD
    Colic Ø6Q7
    Common Iliac
      Left Ø6QD
      Right Ø6QC
    Coronary Ø2Q4
    Esophageal Ø6Q3
    External Iliac
      Left Ø6QG
      Right Ø6QF
    External Jugular
      Left Ø5QQ
      Right Ø5QP
    Face
      Left Ø5QV
      Right Ø5QT
    Femoral
      Left Ø6QN
      Right Ø6QM
    Foot
      Left Ø6QV
      Right Ø6QT
    Gastric Ø6Q2
    Hand
      Left Ø5QH
      Right Ø5QG
    Hemiazygos Ø5Q1
    Hepatic Ø6Q4
    Hypogastric
      Left Ø6QJ
      Right Ø6QH
    Inferior Mesenteric Ø6Q6
    Innominate
      Left Ø5Q4
      Right Ø5Q3
    Internal Jugular
      Left Ø5QN
      Right Ø5QM
    Intracranial Ø5QL
    Lower Ø6QY
    Portal Ø6Q8
    Pulmonary
      Left Ø2QT
      Right Ø2QS
    Renal
      Left Ø6QB
      Right Ø6Q9
    Saphenous
      Left Ø6QQ
      Right Ø6QP
    Splenic Ø6Q1

Repair — *continued*
  Vein — *continued*
    Subclavian
      Left Ø5Q6
      Right Ø5Q5
    Superior Mesenteric Ø6Q5
    Upper Ø5QY
    Vertebral
      Left Ø5QS
      Right Ø5QR
  Vena Cava
    Inferior Ø6QØ
    Superior Ø2QV
  Ventricle
    Left Ø2QL
    Right Ø2QK
  Vertebra
    Cervical ØPQ3
    Lumbar ØQQØ
    Thoracic ØPQ4
  Vesicle
    Bilateral ØVQ3
    Left ØVQ2
    Right ØVQ1
  Vitreous
    Left Ø8Q53ZZ
    Right Ø8Q43ZZ
  Vocal Cord
    Left ØCQV
    Right ØCQT
  Vulva ØUQM
  Wrist Region
    Left ØXQH
    Right ØXQG
Repair, obstetric laceration, periurethral ØUQMXZZ
Replacement
  Acetabulum
    Left ØQR5
    Right ØQR4
  Ampulla of Vater ØFRC
  Anal Sphincter ØDRR
  Aorta
    Abdominal Ø4RØ
    Thoracic
      Ascending/Arch Ø2RX
      Descending Ø2RW
  Artery
    Anterior Tibial
      Left Ø4RQ
      Right Ø4RP
    Axillary
      Left Ø3R6
      Right Ø3R5
    Brachial
      Left Ø3R8
      Right Ø3R7
    Celiac Ø4R1
    Colic
      Left Ø4R7
      Middle Ø4R8
      Right Ø4R6
    Common Carotid
      Left Ø3RJ
      Right Ø3RH
    Common Iliac
      Left Ø4RD
      Right Ø4RC
    External Carotid
      Left Ø3RN
      Right Ø3RM
    External Iliac
      Left Ø4RJ
      Right Ø4RH
    Face Ø3RR
    Femoral
      Left Ø4RL
      Right Ø4RK
    Foot
      Left Ø4RW
      Right Ø4RV
    Gastric Ø4R2
    Hand
      Left Ø3RF
      Right Ø3RD
    Hepatic Ø4R3
    Inferior Mesenteric Ø4RB
    Innominate Ø3R2
    Internal Carotid
      Left Ø3RL

Replacement — *continued*
  Artery — *continued*
    Internal Carotid — *continued*
      Right Ø3RK
    Internal Iliac
      Left Ø4RF
      Right Ø4RE
    Internal Mammary
      Left Ø3R1
      Right Ø3RØ
    Intracranial Ø3RG
    Lower Ø4RY
    Peroneal
      Left Ø4RU
      Right Ø4RT
    Popliteal
      Left Ø4RN
      Right Ø4RM
    Posterior Tibial
      Left Ø4RS
      Right Ø4RR
    Pulmonary
      Left Ø2RR
      Right Ø2RQ
    Pulmonary Trunk Ø2RP
    Radial
      Left Ø3RC
      Right Ø3RB
    Renal
      Left Ø4RA
      Right Ø4R9
    Splenic Ø4R4
    Subclavian
      Left Ø3R4
      Right Ø3R3
    Superior Mesenteric Ø4R5
    Temporal
      Left Ø3RT
      Right Ø3RS
    Thyroid
      Left Ø3RV
      Right Ø3RU
    Ulnar
      Left Ø3RA
      Right Ø3R9
    Upper Ø3RY
    Vertebral
      Left Ø3RQ
      Right Ø3RP
  Atrium
    Left Ø2R7
    Right Ø2R6
  Auditory Ossicle
    Left Ø9RAØ
    Right Ø9R9Ø
  Bladder ØTRB
  Bladder Neck ØTRC
  Bone
    Ethmoid
      Left ØNRG
      Right ØNRF
    Frontal ØNR1
    Hyoid ØNRX
    Lacrimal
      Left ØNRJ
      Right ØNRH
    Nasal ØNRB
    Occipital ØNR7
    Palatine
      Left ØNRL
      Right ØNRK
    Parietal
      Left ØNR4
      Right ØNR3
    Pelvic
      Left ØQR3
      Right ØQR2
    Sphenoid ØNRC
    Temporal
      Left ØNR6
      Right ØNR5
    Zygomatic
      Left ØNRN
      Right ØNRM
  Breast
    Bilateral ØHRV
    Left ØHRU
    Right ØHRT

Replacement — *continued*
Bronchus
Lingula ØBR9
Lower Lobe
Left ØBRB
Right ØBR6
Main
Left ØBR7
Right ØBR3
Middle Lobe, Right ØBR5
Upper Lobe
Left ØBR8
Right ØBR4
Buccal Mucosa ØCR4
Bursa and Ligament
Abdomen
Left ØMRJ
Right ØMRH
Ankle
Left ØMRR
Right ØMRQ
Elbow
Left ØMR4
Right ØMR3
Foot
Left ØMRT
Right ØMRS
Hand
Left ØMR8
Right ØMR7
Head and Neck ØMRØ
Hip
Left ØMRM
Right ØMRL
Knee
Left ØMRP
Right ØMRN
Lower Extremity
Left ØMRW
Right ØMRV
Perineum ØMRK
Rib(s) ØMRG
Shoulder
Left ØMR2
Right ØMR1
Spine
Lower ØMRD
Upper ØMRC
Sternum ØMRF
Upper Extremity
Left ØMRB
Right ØMR9
Wrist
Left ØMR6
Right ØMR5
Carina ØBR2
Carpal
Left ØPRN
Right ØPRM
Cerebral Meninges ØØR1
Cerebral Ventricle ØØR6
Chordae Tendineae Ø2R9
Choroid
Left Ø8RB
Right Ø8RA
Clavicle
Left ØPRB
Right ØPR9
Coccyx ØQRS
Conjunctiva
Left Ø8RTX
Right Ø8RSX
Cornea
Left Ø8R9
Right Ø8R8
Diaphragm ØBRT
Disc
Cervical Vertebral ØRR3Ø
Cervicothoracic Vertebral ØRR5Ø
Lumbar Vertebral ØSR2Ø
Lumbosacral ØSR4Ø
Thoracic Vertebral ØRR9Ø
Thoracolumbar Vertebral ØRRBØ
Duct
Common Bile ØFR9
Cystic ØFR8
Hepatic
Common ØFR7
Left ØFR6

Replacement — *continued*
Duct — *continued*
Hepatic — *continued*
Right ØFR5
Lacrimal
Left Ø8RY
Right Ø8RX
Pancreatic ØFRD
Accessory ØFRF
Parotid
Left ØCRC
Right ØCRB
Dura Mater ØØR2
Ear
External
Bilateral Ø9R2
Left Ø9R1
Right Ø9RØ
Inner
Left Ø9REØ
Right Ø9RDØ
Middle
Left Ø9R6Ø
Right Ø9R5Ø
Epiglottis ØCRR
Esophagus ØDR5
Eye
Left Ø8R1
Right Ø8RØ
Eyelid
Lower
Left Ø8RR
Right Ø8RQ
Upper
Left Ø8RP
Right Ø8RN
Femoral Shaft
Left ØQR9
Right ØQR8
Femur
Lower
Left ØQRC
Right ØQRB
Upper
Left ØQR7
Right ØQR6
Fibula
Left ØQRK
Right ØQRJ
Finger Nail ØHRQX
Gingiva
Lower ØCR6
Upper ØCR5
Glenoid Cavity
Left ØPR8
Right ØPR7
Hair ØHRSX
Heart Ø2RAØ
Humeral Head
Left ØPRD
Right ØPRC
Humeral Shaft
Left ØPRG
Right ØPRF
Iris
Left Ø8RD3
Right Ø8RC3
Joint
Acromioclavicular
Left ØRRHØ
Right ØRRGØ
Ankle
Left ØSRG
Right ØSRF
Carpal
Left ØRRRØ
Right ØRRQØ
Carpometacarpal
Left ØRRTØ
Right ØRRSØ
Cervical Vertebral ØRR1Ø
Cervicothoracic Vertebral ØRR4Ø
Coccygeal ØSR6Ø
Elbow
Left ØRRMØ
Right ØRRLØ
Finger Phalangeal
Left ØRRXØ
Right ØRRWØ

Replacement — *continued*
Joint — *continued*
Hip
Left ØSRB
Acetabular Surface ØSRE
Femoral Surface ØSRS
Right ØSR9
Acetabular Surface ØSRA
Femoral Surface ØSRR
Knee
Left ØSRD
Femoral Surface ØSRU
Tibial Surface ØSRW
Right ØSRC
Femoral Surface ØSRT
Tibial Surface ØSRV
Lumbar Vertebral ØSRØØ
Lumbosacral ØSR3Ø
Metacarpophalangeal
Left ØRRVØ
Right ØRRUØ
Metatarsal-Phalangeal
Left ØSRNØ
Right ØSRMØ
Occipital-cervical ØRRØØ
Sacrococcygeal ØSR5Ø
Sacroiliac
Left ØSR8Ø
Right ØSR7Ø
Shoulder
Left ØRRK
Right ØRRJ
Sternoclavicular
Left ØRRFØ
Right ØRREØ
Tarsal
Left ØSRJØ
Right ØSRHØ
Tarsometatarsal
Left ØSRLØ
Right ØSRKØ
Temporomandibular
Left ØRRDØ
Right ØRRCØ
Thoracic Vertebral ØRR6Ø
Thoracolumbar Vertebral ØRRAØ
Toe Phalangeal
Left ØSRQØ
Right ØSRPØ
Wrist
Left ØRRPØ
Right ØRRNØ
Kidney Pelvis
Left ØTR4
Right ØTR3
Larynx ØCRS
Lens
Left Ø8RK3ØZ
Right Ø8RJ3ØZ
Lip
Lower ØCR1
Upper ØCRØ
Mandible
Left ØNRV
Right ØNRT
Maxilla ØNRR
Mesentery ØDRV
Metacarpal
Left ØPRQ
Right ØPRP
Metatarsal
Left ØQRP
Right ØQRN
Muscle
Abdomen
Left ØKRL
Right ØKRK
Facial ØKR1
Foot
Left ØKRW
Right ØKRV
Hand
Left ØKRD
Right ØKRC
Head ØKRØ
Hip
Left ØKRP
Right ØKRN

Replacement — *continued*
- Muscle — *continued*
  - Lower Arm and Wrist
    - Left ØKRB
    - Right ØKR9
  - Lower Leg
    - Left ØKRT
    - Right ØKRS
  - Neck
    - Left ØKR3
    - Right ØKR2
  - Papillary Ø2RD
  - Perineum ØKRM
  - Shoulder
    - Left ØKR6
    - Right ØKR5
  - Thorax
    - Left ØKRJ
    - Right ØKRH
  - Tongue, Palate, Pharynx ØKR4
  - Trunk
    - Left ØKRG
    - Right ØKRF
  - Upper Arm
    - Left ØKR8
    - Right ØKR7
  - Upper Leg
    - Left ØKRR
    - Right ØKRQ
- Nasal Mucosa and Soft Tissue Ø9RK
- Nasopharynx Ø9RN
- Nerve
  - Abducens ØØRL
  - Accessory ØØRR
  - Acoustic ØØRN
  - Cervical Ø1R1
  - Facial ØØRM
  - Femoral Ø1RD
  - Glossopharyngeal ØØRP
  - Hypoglossal ØØRS
  - Lumbar Ø1RB
  - Median Ø1R5
  - Oculomotor ØØRH
  - Olfactory ØØRF
  - Optic ØØRG
  - Peroneal Ø1RH
  - Phrenic Ø1R2
  - Pudendal Ø1RC
  - Radial Ø1R6
  - Sacral Ø1RR
  - Sciatic Ø1RF
  - Thoracic Ø1R8
  - Tibial Ø1RG
  - Trigeminal ØØRK
  - Trochlear ØØRJ
  - Ulnar Ø1R4
  - Vagus ØØRQ
- Nipple
  - Left ØHRX
  - Right ØHRW
- Omentum ØDRU
- Orbit
  - Left ØNRQ
  - Right ØNRP
- Palate
  - Hard ØCR2
  - Soft ØCR3
- Patella
  - Left ØQRF
  - Right ØQRD
- Pericardium Ø2RN
- Peritoneum ØDRW
- Phalanx
  - Finger
    - Left ØPRV
    - Right ØPRT
  - Thumb
    - Left ØPRS
    - Right ØPRR
  - Toe
    - Left ØQRR
    - Right ØQRQ
- Pharynx ØCRM
- Radius
  - Left ØPRJ
  - Right ØPRH
- Retinal Vessel
  - Left Ø8RH3
  - Right Ø8RG3

Replacement — *continued*
- Ribs
  - 1 to 2 ØPR1
  - 3 or More ØPR2
- Sacrum ØQR1
- Scapula
  - Left ØPR6
  - Right ØPR5
- Sclera
  - Left Ø8R7X
  - Right Ø8R6X
- Septum
  - Atrial Ø2R5
  - Nasal Ø9RM
  - Ventricular Ø2RM
- Skin
  - Abdomen ØHR7
  - Back ØHR6
  - Buttock ØHR8
  - Chest ØHR5
  - Ear
    - Left ØHR3
    - Right ØHR2
  - Face ØHR1
  - Foot
    - Left ØHRN
    - Right ØHRM
  - Hand
    - Left ØHRG
    - Right ØHRF
  - Inguinal ØHRA
  - Lower Arm
    - Left ØHRE
    - Right ØHRD
  - Lower Leg
    - Left ØHRL
    - Right ØHRK
  - Neck ØHR4
  - Perineum ØHR9
  - Scalp ØHRØ
  - Upper Arm
    - Left ØHRC
    - Right ØHRB
  - Upper Leg
    - Left ØHRJ
    - Right ØHRH
- Skull ØNRØ
- Spinal Meninges ØØRT
- Sternum ØPRØ
- Subcutaneous Tissue and Fascia
  - Abdomen ØJR8
  - Back ØJR7
  - Buttock ØJR9
  - Chest ØJR6
  - Face ØJR1
  - Foot
    - Left ØJRR
    - Right ØJRQ
  - Hand
    - Left ØJRK
    - Right ØJRJ
  - Lower Arm
    - Left ØJRH
    - Right ØJRG
  - Lower Leg
    - Left ØJRP
    - Right ØJRN
  - Neck
    - Left ØJR5
    - Right ØJR4
  - Pelvic Region ØJRC
  - Perineum ØJRB
  - Scalp ØJRØ
  - Upper Arm
    - Left ØJRF
    - Right ØJRD
  - Upper Leg
    - Left ØJRM
    - Right ØJRL
- Tarsal
  - Left ØQRM
  - Right ØQRL
- Tendon
  - Abdomen
    - Left ØLRG
    - Right ØLRF
  - Ankle
    - Left ØLRT
    - Right ØLRS

Replacement — *continued*
- Tendon — *continued*
  - Foot
    - Left ØLRW
    - Right ØLRV
  - Hand
    - Left ØLR8
    - Right ØLR7
  - Head and Neck ØLRØ
  - Hip
    - Left ØLRK
    - Right ØLRJ
  - Knee
    - Left ØLRR
    - Right ØLRQ
  - Lower Arm and Wrist
    - Left ØLR6
    - Right ØLR5
  - Lower Leg
    - Left ØLRP
    - Right ØLRN
  - Perineum ØLRH
  - Shoulder
    - Left ØLR2
    - Right ØLR1
  - Thorax
    - Left ØLRD
    - Right ØLRC
  - Trunk
    - Left ØLRB
    - Right ØLR9
  - Upper Arm
    - Left ØLR4
    - Right ØLR3
  - Upper Leg
    - Left ØLRM
    - Right ØLRL
- Testis
  - Bilateral ØVRCØJZ
  - Left ØVRBØJZ
  - Right ØVR9ØJZ
- Thumb
  - Left ØXRM
  - Right ØXRL
- Tibia
  - Left ØQRH
  - Right ØQRG
- Toe Nail ØHRRX
- Tongue ØCR7
- Tooth
  - Lower ØCRX
  - Upper ØCRW
- Trachea ØBR1
- Turbinate, Nasal Ø9RL
- Tympanic Membrane
  - Left Ø9R8
  - Right Ø9R7
- Ulna
  - Left ØPRL
  - Right ØPRK
- Ureter
  - Left ØTR7
  - Right ØTR6
- Urethra ØTRD
- Uvula ØCRN
- Valve
  - Aortic Ø2RF
  - Mitral Ø2RG
  - Pulmonary Ø2RH
  - Tricuspid Ø2RJ
- Vein
  - Axillary
    - Left Ø5R8
    - Right Ø5R7
  - Azygos Ø5RØ
  - Basilic
    - Left Ø5RC
    - Right Ø5RB
  - Brachial
    - Left Ø5RA
    - Right Ø5R9
  - Cephalic
    - Left Ø5RF
    - Right Ø5RD
  - Colic Ø6R7
  - Common Iliac
    - Left Ø6RD
    - Right Ø6RC
  - Esophageal Ø6R3

Replacement — *continued*
Vein — *continued*
External Iliac
Left Ø6RG
Right Ø6RF
External Jugular
Left Ø5RQ
Right Ø5RP
Face
Left Ø5RV
Right Ø5RT
Femoral
Left Ø6RN
Right Ø6RM
Foot
Left Ø6RV
Right Ø6RT
Gastric Ø6R2
Hand
Left Ø5RH
Right Ø5RG
Hemiazygos Ø5R1
Hepatic Ø6R4
Hypogastric
Left Ø6RJ
Right Ø6RH
Inferior Mesenteric Ø6R6
Innominate
Left Ø5R4
Right Ø5R3
Internal Jugular
Left Ø5RN
Right Ø5RM
Intracranial Ø5RL
Lower Ø6RY
Portal Ø6R8
Pulmonary
Left Ø2RT
Right Ø2RS
Renal
Left Ø6RB
Right Ø6R9
Saphenous
Left Ø6RQ
Right Ø6RP
Splenic Ø6R1
Subclavian
Left Ø5R6
Right Ø5R5
Superior Mesenteric Ø6R5
Upper Ø5RY
Vertebral
Left Ø5RS
Right Ø5RR
Vena Cava
Inferior Ø6RØ
Superior Ø2RV
Ventricle
Left Ø2RL
Right Ø2RK
Vertebra
Cervical ØPR3
Lumbar ØQRØ
Thoracic ØPR4
Vitreous
Left Ø8R53
Right Ø8R43
Vocal Cord
Left ØCRV
Right ØCRT
Replacement, hip
Partial or total *see* Replacement, Lower Joints ØSR
Resurfacing only *see* Supplement, Lower Joints ØSU
Replacement, knee
Meniscus implant only *see* New Technology, Joints XRR
Partial or total *see* Replacement, Lower Joints ØSR
Replantation *see* Reposition
Replantation, scalp *see* Reattachment, Skin, Scalp ØHMØ
Reposition
Acetabulum
Left ØQS5
Right ØQS4
Ampulla of Vater ØFSC
Anus ØDSQ

Reposition — *continued*
Aorta
Abdominal Ø4SØ
Thoracic
Ascending/Arch Ø2SXØZZ
Descending Ø2SWØZZ
Artery
Anterior Tibial
Left Ø4SQ
Right Ø4SP
Axillary
Left Ø3S6
Right Ø3S5
Brachial
Left Ø3S8
Right Ø3S7
Celiac Ø4S1
Colic
Left Ø4S7
Middle Ø4S8
Right Ø4S6
Common Carotid
Left Ø3SJ
Right Ø3SH
Common Iliac
Left Ø4SD
Right Ø4SC
Coronary
One Artery Ø2SØØZZ
Two Arteries Ø2S1ØZZ
External Carotid
Left Ø3SN
Right Ø3SM
External Iliac
Left Ø4SJ
Right Ø4SH
Face Ø3SR
Femoral
Left Ø4SL
Right Ø4SK
Foot
Left Ø4SW
Right Ø4SV
Gastric Ø4S2
Hand
Left Ø3SF
Right Ø3SD
Hepatic Ø4S3
Inferior Mesenteric Ø4SB
Innominate Ø3S2
Internal Carotid
Left Ø3SL
Right Ø3SK
Internal Iliac
Left Ø4SF
Right Ø4SE
Internal Mammary
Left Ø3S1
Right Ø3SØ
Intracranial Ø3SG
Lower Ø4SY
Peroneal
Left Ø4SU
Right Ø4ST
Popliteal
Left Ø4SN
Right Ø4SM
Posterior Tibial
Left Ø4SS
Right Ø4SR
Pulmonary
Left Ø2SRØZZ
Right Ø2SQØZZ
Pulmonary Trunk Ø2SPØZZ
Radial
Left Ø3SC
Right Ø3SB
Renal
Left Ø4SA
Right Ø4S9
Splenic Ø4S4
Subclavian
Left Ø3S4
Right Ø3S3
Superior Mesenteric Ø4S5
Temporal
Left Ø3ST
Right Ø3SS

Reposition — *continued*
Artery — *continued*
Thyroid
Left Ø3SV
Right Ø3SU
Ulnar
Left Ø3SA
Right Ø3S9
Upper Ø3SY
Vertebral
Left Ø3SQ
Right Ø3SP
Auditory Ossicle
Left Ø9SA
Right Ø9S9
Bladder ØTSB
Bladder Neck ØTSC
Bone
Ethmoid
Left ØNSG
Right ØNSF
Frontal ØNS1
Hyoid ØNSX
Lacrimal
Left ØNSJ
Right ØNSH
Nasal ØNSB
Occipital ØNS7
Palatine
Left ØNSL
Right ØNSK
Parietal
Left ØNS4
Right ØNS3
Pelvic
Left ØQS3
Right ØQS2
Sphenoid ØNSC
Temporal
Left ØNS6
Right ØNS5
Zygomatic
Left ØNSN
Right ØNSM
Breast
Bilateral ØHSVØZZ
Left ØHSUØZZ
Right ØHSTØZZ
Bronchus
Lingula ØBS9ØZZ
Lower Lobe
Left ØBSBØZZ
Right ØBS6ØZZ
Main
Left ØBS7ØZZ
Right ØBS3ØZZ
Middle Lobe, Right ØBS5ØZZ
Upper Lobe
Left ØBS8ØZZ
Right ØBS4ØZZ
Bursa and Ligament
Abdomen
Left ØMSJ
Right ØMSH
Ankle
Left ØMSR
Right ØMSQ
Elbow
Left ØMS4
Right ØMS3
Foot
Left ØMST
Right ØMSS
Hand
Left ØMS8
Right ØMS7
Head and Neck ØMSØ
Hip
Left ØMSM
Right ØMSL
Knee
Left ØMSP
Right ØMSN
Lower Extremity
Left ØMSW
Right ØMSV
Perineum ØMSK
Rib(s) ØMSG

Reposition — *continued*
Bursa and Ligament — *continued*
Shoulder
Left ØMS2
Right ØMS1
Spine
Lower ØMSD
Upper ØMSC
Sternum ØMSF
Upper Extremity
Left ØMSB
Right ØMS9
Wrist
Left ØMS6
Right ØMS5
Carina ØBS2ØZZ
Carpal
Left ØPSN
Right ØPSM
Cecum ØDSH
Cervix ØUSC
Clavicle
Left ØPSB
Right ØPS9
Coccyx ØQSS
Colon
Ascending ØDSK
Descending ØDSM
Sigmoid ØDSN
Transverse ØDSL
Cord
Bilateral ØVSH
Left ØVSG
Right ØVSF
Cul-de-sac ØUSF
Diaphragm ØBSTØZZ
Duct
Common Bile ØFS9
Cystic ØFS8
Hepatic
Common ØFS7
Left ØFS6
Right ØFS5
Lacrimal
Left Ø8SY
Right Ø8SX
Pancreatic ØFSD
Accessory ØFSF
Parotid
Left ØCSC
Right ØCSB
Duodenum ØDS9
Ear
Bilateral Ø9S2
Left Ø9S1
Right Ø9SØ
Epiglottis ØCSR
Esophagus ØDS5
Eustachian Tube
Left Ø9SG
Right Ø9SF
Eyelid
Lower
Left Ø8SR
Right Ø8SQ
Upper
Left Ø8SP
Right Ø8SN
Fallopian Tube
Left ØUS6
Right ØUS5
Fallopian Tubes, Bilateral ØUS7
Femoral Shaft
Left ØQS9
Right ØQS8
Femur
Lower
Left ØQSC
Right ØQSB
Upper
Left ØQS7
Right ØQS6
Fibula
Left ØQSK
Right ØQSJ
Gallbladder ØFS4
Gland
Adrenal
Left ØGS2

Reposition — *continued*
Gland — *continued*
Adrenal — *continued*
Right ØGS3
Lacrimal
Left Ø8SW
Right Ø8SV
Glenoid Cavity
Left ØPS8
Right ØPS7
Hair ØHSSXZZ
Humeral Head
Left ØPSD
Right ØPSC
Humeral Shaft
Left ØPSG
Right ØPSF
Ileum ØDSB
Intestine
Large ØDSE
Small ØDS8
Iris
Left Ø8SD3ZZ
Right Ø8SC3ZZ
Jejunum ØDSA
Joint
Acromioclavicular
Left ØRSH
Right ØRSG
Ankle
Left ØSSG
Right ØSSF
Carpal
Left ØRSR
Right ØRSQ
Carpometacarpal
Left ØRST
Right ØRSS
Cervical Vertebral ØRS1
Cervicothoracic Vertebral ØRS4
Coccygeal ØSS6
Elbow
Left ØRSM
Right ØRSL
Finger Phalangeal
Left ØRSX
Right ØRSW
Hip
Left ØSSB
Right ØSS9
Knee
Left ØSSD
Right ØSSC
Lumbar Vertebral ØSSØ
Lumbosacral ØSS3
Metacarpophalangeal
Left ØRSV
Right ØRSU
Metatarsal-Phalangeal
Left ØSSN
Right ØSSM
Occipital-cervical ØRSØ
Sacrococcygeal ØSS5
Sacroiliac
Left ØSS8
Right ØSS7
Shoulder
Left ØRSK
Right ØRSJ
Sternoclavicular
Left ØRSF
Right ØRSE
Tarsal
Left ØSSJ
Right ØSSH
Tarsometatarsal
Left ØSSL
Right ØSSK
Temporomandibular
Left ØRSD
Right ØRSC
Thoracic Vertebral ØRS6
Thoracolumbar Vertebral ØRSA
Toe Phalangeal
Left ØSSQ
Right ØSSP
Wrist
Left ØRSP
Right ØRSN

Reposition — *continued*
Kidney
Left ØTS1
Right ØTSØ
Kidney Pelvis
Left ØTS4
Right ØTS3
Kidneys, Bilateral ØTS2
Larynx ØCSS
Lens
Left Ø8SK3ZZ
Right Ø8SJ3ZZ
Lip
Lower ØCS1
Upper ØCSØ
Liver ØFSØ
Lung
Left ØBSLØZZ
Lower Lobe
Left ØBSJØZZ
Right ØBSFØZZ
Middle Lobe, Right ØBSDØZZ
Right ØBSKØZZ
Upper Lobe
Left ØBSGØZZ
Right ØBSCØZZ
Lung Lingula ØBSHØZZ
Mandible
Left ØNSV
Right ØNST
Maxilla ØNSR
Metacarpal
Left ØPSQ
Right ØPSP
Metatarsal
Left ØQSP
Right ØQSN
Muscle
Abdomen
Left ØKSL
Right ØKSK
Extraocular
Left Ø8SM
Right Ø8SL
Facial ØKS1
Foot
Left ØKSW
Right ØKSV
Hand
Left ØKSD
Right ØKSC
Head ØKSØ
Hip
Left ØKSP
Right ØKSN
Lower Arm and Wrist
Left ØKSB
Right ØKS9
Lower Leg
Left ØKST
Right ØKSS
Neck
Left ØKS3
Right ØKS2
Perineum ØKSM
Shoulder
Left ØKS6
Right ØKS5
Thorax
Left ØKSJ
Right ØKSH
Tongue, Palate, Pharynx ØKS4
Trunk
Left ØKSG
Right ØKSF
Upper Arm
Left ØKS8
Right ØKS7
Upper Leg
Left ØKSR
Right ØKSQ
Nasal Mucosa and Soft Tissue Ø9SK
Nerve
Abducens ØØSL
Accessory ØØSR
Acoustic ØØSN
Brachial Plexus Ø1S3
Cervical Ø1S1
Cervical Plexus Ø1SØ

Reposition — *continued*
Nerve — *continued*
Facial ØØSM
Femoral Ø1SD
Glossopharyngeal ØØSP
Hypoglossal ØØSS
Lumbar Ø1SB
Lumbar Plexus Ø1S9
Lumbosacral Plexus Ø1SA
Median Ø1S5
Oculomotor ØØSH
Olfactory ØØSF
Optic ØØSG
Peroneal Ø1SH
Phrenic Ø1S2
Pudendal Ø1SC
Radial Ø1S6
Sacral Ø1SR
Sacral Plexus Ø1SQ
Sciatic Ø1SF
Thoracic Ø1S8
Tibial Ø1SG
Trigeminal ØØSK
Trochlear ØØSJ
Ulnar Ø1S4
Vagus ØØSQ
Nipple
Left ØHSXXZZ
Right ØHSWXZZ
Orbit
Left ØNSQ
Right ØNSP
Ovary
Bilateral ØUS2
Left ØUS1
Right ØUSØ
Palate
Hard ØCS2
Soft ØCS3
Pancreas ØFSG
Parathyroid Gland ØGSR
Inferior
Left ØGSP
Right ØGSN
Multiple ØGSQ
Superior
Left ØGSM
Right ØGSL
Patella
Left ØQSF
Right ØQSD
Phalanx
Finger
Left ØPSV
Right ØPST
Thumb
Left ØPSS
Right ØPSR
Toe
Left ØQSR
Right ØQSQ
Products of Conception 1ØSØ
Ectopic 1ØS2
Radius
Left ØPSJ
Right ØPSH
Rectum ØDSP
Retinal Vessel
Left Ø8SH3ZZ
Right Ø8SG3ZZ
Ribs
1 to 2 ØPS1
3 or More ØPS2
Sacrum ØQS1
Scapula
Left ØPS6
Right ØPS5
Septum, Nasal Ø9SM
Sesamoid Bone(s) 1st Toe
see Reposition, Metatarsal, Left ØQSP
see Reposition, Metatarsal, Right ØQSN
Skull ØNSØ
Spinal Cord
Cervical ØØSW
Lumbar ØØSY
Thoracic ØØSX
Spleen Ø7SPØZZ
Sternum ØPSØ
Stomach ØDS6

Reposition — *continued*
Tarsal
Left ØQSM
Right ØQSL
Tendon
Abdomen
Left ØLSG
Right ØLSF
Ankle
Left ØLST
Right ØLSS
Foot
Left ØLSW
Right ØLSV
Hand
Left ØLS8
Right ØLS7
Head and Neck ØLSØ
Hip
Left ØLSK
Right ØLSJ
Knee
Left ØLSR
Right ØLSQ
Lower Arm and Wrist
Left ØLS6
Right ØLS5
Lower Leg
Left ØLSP
Right ØLSN
Perineum ØLSH
Shoulder
Left ØLS2
Right ØLS1
Thorax
Left ØLSD
Right ØLSC
Trunk
Left ØLSB
Right ØLS9
Upper Arm
Left ØLS4
Right ØLS3
Upper Leg
Left ØLSM
Right ØLSL
Testis
Bilateral ØVSC
Left ØVSB
Right ØVS9
Thymus Ø7SMØZZ
Thyroid Gland
Left Lobe ØGSG
Right Lobe ØGSH
Tibia
Left ØQSH
Right ØQSG
Tongue ØCS7
Tooth
Lower ØCSX
Upper ØCSW
Trachea ØBS1ØZZ
Turbinate, Nasal Ø9SL
Tympanic Membrane
Left Ø9S8
Right Ø9S7
Ulna
Left ØPSL
Right ØPSK
Ureter
Left ØTS7
Right ØTS6
Ureters, Bilateral ØTS8
Urethra ØTSD
Uterine Supporting Structure ØUS4
Uterus ØUS9
Uvula ØCSN
Vagina ØUSG
Vein
Axillary
Left Ø5S8
Right Ø5S7
Azygos Ø5SØ
Basilic
Left Ø5SC
Right Ø5SB
Brachial
Left Ø5SA
Right Ø5S9

Reposition — *continued*
Vein — *continued*
Cephalic
Left Ø5SF
Right Ø5SD
Colic Ø6S7
Common Iliac
Left Ø6SD
Right Ø6SC
Esophageal Ø6S3
External Iliac
Left Ø6SG
Right Ø6SF
External Jugular
Left Ø5SQ
Right Ø5SP
Face
Left Ø5SV
Right Ø5ST
Femoral
Left Ø6SN
Right Ø6SM
Foot
Left Ø6SV
Right Ø6ST
Gastric Ø6S2
Hand
Left Ø5SH
Right Ø5SG
Hemiazygos Ø5S1
Hepatic Ø6S4
Hypogastric
Left Ø6SJ
Right Ø6SH
Inferior Mesenteric Ø6S6
Innominate
Left Ø5S4
Right Ø5S3
Internal Jugular
Left Ø5SN
Right Ø5SM
Intracranial Ø5SL
Lower Ø6SY
Portal Ø6S8
Pulmonary
Left Ø2STØZZ
Right Ø2SSØZZ
Renal
Left Ø6SB
Right Ø6S9
Saphenous
Left Ø6SQ
Right Ø6SP
Splenic Ø6S1
Subclavian
Left Ø5S6
Right Ø5S5
Superior Mesenteric Ø6S5
Upper Ø5SY
Vertebral
Left Ø5SS
Right Ø5SR
Vena Cava
Inferior Ø6SØ
Superior Ø2SVØZZ
Vertebra
Cervical ØPS3
Magnetically Controlled Growth Rod(s) XNS3
Lumbar ØQSØ
Magnetically Controlled Growth Rod(s) XNSØ
Posterior (Dynamic) Distraction Device XNSØ
Thoracic ØPS4
Magnetically Controlled Growth Rod(s) XNS4
Posterior (Dynamic) Distraction Device XNS4
Vocal Cord
Left ØCSV
Right ØCST
Resection
Acetabulum
Left ØQT5ØZZ
Right ØQT4ØZZ
Adenoids ØCTQ
Ampulla of Vater ØFTC
Anal Sphincter ØDTR

- **Resection** — *continued*
  - Anus ØDTQ
  - Aortic Body ØGTD
  - Appendix ØDTJ
  - Auditory Ossicle
    - Left Ø9TA
    - Right Ø9T9
  - Bladder ØTTB
  - Bladder Neck ØTTC
  - Bone
    - Ethmoid
      - Left ØNTGØZZ
      - Right ØNTFØZZ
    - Frontal ØNT1ØZZ
    - Hyoid ØNTXØZZ
    - Lacrimal
      - Left ØNTJØZZ
      - Right ØNTHØZZ
    - Nasal ØNTBØZZ
    - Occipital ØNT7ØZZ
    - Palatine
      - Left ØNTLØZZ
      - Right ØNTKØZZ
    - Parietal
      - Left ØNT4ØZZ
      - Right ØNT3ØZZ
    - Pelvic
      - Left ØQT3ØZZ
      - Right ØQT2ØZZ
    - Sphenoid ØNTCØZZ
    - Temporal
      - Left ØNT6ØZZ
      - Right ØNT5ØZZ
    - Zygomatic
      - Left ØNTNØZZ
      - Right ØNTMØZZ
  - Breast
    - Bilateral ØHTVØZZ
    - Left ØHTUØZZ
    - Right ØHTTØZZ
    - Supernumerary ØHTYØZZ
  - Bronchus
    - Lingula ØBT9
    - Lower Lobe
      - Left ØBTB
      - Right ØBT6
    - Main
      - Left ØBT7
      - Right ØBT3
    - Middle Lobe, Right ØBT5
    - Upper Lobe
      - Left ØBT8
      - Right ØBT4
  - Bursa and Ligament
    - Abdomen
      - Left ØMTJ
      - Right ØMTH
    - Ankle
      - Left ØMTR
      - Right ØMTQ
    - Elbow
      - Left ØMT4
      - Right ØMT3
    - Foot
      - Left ØMTT
      - Right ØMTS
    - Hand
      - Left ØMT8
      - Right ØMT7
    - Head and Neck ØMTØ
    - Hip
      - Left ØMTM
      - Right ØMTL
    - Knee
      - Left ØMTP
      - Right ØMTN
    - Lower Extremity
      - Left ØMTW
      - Right ØMTV
    - Perineum ØMTK
    - Rib(s) ØMTG
    - Shoulder
      - Left ØMT2
      - Right ØMT1
    - Spine
      - Lower ØMTD
      - Upper ØMTC
    - Sternum ØMTF

- **Resection** — *continued*
  - Bursa and Ligament — *continued*
    - Upper Extremity
      - Left ØMTB
      - Right ØMT9
    - Wrist
      - Left ØMT6
      - Right ØMT5
  - Carina ØBT2
  - Carotid Bodies, Bilateral ØGT8
  - Carotid Body
    - Left ØGT6
    - Right ØGT7
  - Carpal
    - Left ØPTNØZZ
    - Right ØPTMØZZ
  - Cecum ØDTH
  - Cerebral Hemisphere ØØT7
  - Cervix ØUTC
  - Chordae Tendineae Ø2T9
  - Cisterna Chyli Ø7TL
  - Clavicle
    - Left ØPTBØZZ
    - Right ØPT9ØZZ
  - Clitoris ØUTJ
  - Coccygeal Glomus ØGTB
  - Coccyx ØQTSØZZ
  - Colon
    - Ascending ØDTK
    - Descending ØDTM
    - Sigmoid ØDTN
    - Transverse ØDTL
  - Conduction Mechanism Ø2T8
  - Cord
    - Bilateral ØVTH
    - Left ØVTG
    - Right ØVTF
  - Cornea
    - Left Ø8T9XZZ
    - Right Ø8T8XZZ
  - Cul-de-sac ØUTF
  - Diaphragm ØBTT
  - Disc
    - Cervical Vertebral ØRT3ØZZ
    - Cervicothoracic Vertebral ØRT5ØZZ
    - Lumbar Vertebral ØST2ØZZ
    - Lumbosacral ØST4ØZZ
    - Thoracic Vertebral ØRT9ØZZ
    - Thoracolumbar Vertebral ØRTBØZZ
  - Duct
    - Common Bile ØFT9
    - Cystic ØFT8
    - Hepatic
      - Common ØFT7
      - Left ØFT6
      - Right ØFT5
    - Lacrimal
      - Left Ø8TY
      - Right Ø8TX
    - Pancreatic ØFTD
      - Accessory ØFTF
    - Parotid
      - Left ØCTCØZZ
      - Right ØCTBØZZ
  - Duodenum ØDT9
  - Ear
    - External
      - Left Ø9T1
      - Right Ø9TØ
    - Inner
      - Left Ø9TE
      - Right Ø9TD
    - Middle
      - Left Ø9T6
      - Right Ø9T5
  - Epididymis
    - Bilateral ØVTL
    - Left ØVTK
    - Right ØVTJ
  - Epiglottis ØCTR
  - Esophagogastric Junction ØDT4
  - Esophagus ØDT5
    - Lower ØDT3
    - Middle ØDT2
    - Upper ØDT1
  - Eustachian Tube
    - Left Ø9TG
    - Right Ø9TF

- **Resection** — *continued*
  - Eye
    - Left Ø8T1XZZ
    - Right Ø8TØXZZ
  - Eyelid
    - Lower
      - Left Ø8TR
      - Right Ø8TQ
    - Upper
      - Left Ø8TP
      - Right Ø8TN
  - Fallopian Tube
    - Left ØUT6
    - Right ØUT5
  - Fallopian Tubes, Bilateral ØUT7
  - Femoral Shaft
    - Left ØQT9ØZZ
    - Right ØQT8ØZZ
  - Femur
    - Lower
      - Left ØQTCØZZ
      - Right ØQTBØZZ
    - Upper
      - Left ØQT7ØZZ
      - Right ØQT6ØZZ
  - Fibula
    - Left ØQTKØZZ
    - Right ØQTJØZZ
  - Finger Nail ØHTQXZZ
  - Gallbladder ØFT4
  - Gland
    - Adrenal
      - Bilateral ØGT4
      - Left ØGT2
      - Right ØGT3
    - Lacrimal
      - Left Ø8TW
      - Right Ø8TV
    - Minor Salivary ØCTJØZZ
    - Parotid
      - Left ØCT9ØZZ
      - Right ØCT8ØZZ
    - Pituitary ØGTØ
    - Sublingual
      - Left ØCTFØZZ
      - Right ØCTDØZZ
    - Submaxillary
      - Left ØCTHØZZ
      - Right ØCTGØZZ
    - Vestibular ØUTL
  - Glenoid Cavity
    - Left ØPT8ØZZ
    - Right ØPT7ØZZ
  - Glomus Jugulare ØGTC
  - Humeral Head
    - Left ØPTDØZZ
    - Right ØPTCØZZ
  - Humeral Shaft
    - Left ØPTGØZZ
    - Right ØPTFØZZ
  - Hymen ØUTK
  - Ileocecal Valve ØDTC
  - Ileum ØDTB
  - Intestine
    - Large ØDTE
      - Left ØDTG
      - Right ØDTF
    - Small ØDT8
  - Iris
    - Left Ø8TD3ZZ
    - Right Ø8TC3ZZ
  - Jejunum ØDTA
  - Joint
    - Acromioclavicular
      - Left ØRTHØZZ
      - Right ØRTGØZZ
    - Ankle
      - Left ØSTGØZZ
      - Right ØSTFØZZ
    - Carpal
      - Left ØRTRØZZ
      - Right ØRTQØZZ
    - Carpometacarpal
      - Left ØRTTØZZ
      - Right ØRTSØZZ
    - Cervicothoracic Vertebral ØRT4ØZZ
    - Coccygeal ØST6ØZZ
    - Elbow
      - Left ØRTMØZZ

Resection — *continued*
Joint — *continued*
Elbow — *continued*
Right ØRTLØZZ
Finger Phalangeal
Left ØRTXØZZ
Right ØRTWØZZ
Hip
Left ØSTBØZZ
Right ØST9ØZZ
Knee
Left ØSTDØZZ
Right ØSTCØZZ
Metacarpophalangeal
Left ØRTVØZZ
Right ØRTUØZZ
Metatarsal-Phalangeal
Left ØSTNØZZ
Right ØSTMØZZ
Sacrococcygeal ØST5ØZZ
Sacroiliac
Left ØST8ØZZ
Right ØST7ØZZ
Shoulder
Left ØRTKØZZ
Right ØRTJØZZ
Sternoclavicular
Left ØRTFØZZ
Right ØRTEØZZ
Tarsal
Left ØSTJØZZ
Right ØSTHØZZ
Tarsometatarsal
Left ØSTLØZZ
Right ØSTKØZZ
Temporomandibular
Left ØRTDØZZ
Right ØRTCØZZ
Toe Phalangeal
Left ØSTQØZZ
Right ØSTPØZZ
Wrist
Left ØRTPØZZ
Right ØRTNØZZ
Kidney
Left ØTT1
Right ØTTØ
Kidney Pelvis
Left ØTT4
Right ØTT3
Kidneys, Bilateral ØTT2
Larynx ØCTS
Lens
Left Ø8TK3ZZ
Right Ø8TJ3ZZ
Lip
Lower ØCT1
Upper ØCTØ
Liver ØFTØ
Left Lobe ØFT2
Right Lobe ØFT1
Lung
Bilateral ØBTM
Left ØBTL
Lower Lobe
Left ØBTJ
Right ØBTF
Middle Lobe, Right ØBTD
Right ØBTK
Upper Lobe
Left ØBTG
Right ØBTC
Lung Lingula ØBTH
Lymphatic
Aortic Ø7TD
Axillary
Left Ø7T6
Right Ø7T5
Head Ø7TØ
Inguinal
Left Ø7TJ
Right Ø7TH
Internal Mammary
Left Ø7T9
Right Ø7T8
Lower Extremity
Left Ø7TG
Right Ø7TF
Mesenteric Ø7TB

Resection — *continued*
Lymphatic — *continued*
Neck
Left Ø7T2
Right Ø7T1
Pelvis Ø7TC
Thoracic Duct Ø7TK
Thorax Ø7T7
Upper Extremity
Left Ø7T4
Right Ø7T3
Mandible
Left ØNTVØZZ
Right ØNTTØZZ
Maxilla ØNTRØZZ
Metacarpal
Left ØPTQØZZ
Right ØPTPØZZ
Metatarsal
Left ØQTPØZZ
Right ØQTNØZZ
Muscle
Abdomen
Left ØKTL
Right ØKTK
Extraocular
Left Ø8TM
Right Ø8TL
Facial ØKT1
Foot
Left ØKTW
Right ØKTV
Hand
Left ØKTD
Right ØKTC
Head ØKTØ
Hip
Left ØKTP
Right ØKTN
Lower Arm and Wrist
Left ØKTB
Right ØKT9
Lower Leg
Left ØKTT
Right ØKTS
Neck
Left ØKT3
Right ØKT2
Papillary Ø2TD
Perineum ØKTM
Shoulder
Left ØKT6
Right ØKT5
Thorax
Left ØKTJ
Right ØKTH
Tongue, Palate, Pharynx ØKT4
Trunk
Left ØKTG
Right ØKTF
Upper Arm
Left ØKT8
Right ØKT7
Upper Leg
Left ØKTR
Right ØKTQ
Nasal Mucosa and Soft Tissue Ø9TK
Nasopharynx Ø9TN
Nipple
Left ØHTXXZZ
Right ØHTWXZZ
Omentum ØDTU
Orbit
Left ØNTQØZZ
Right ØNTPØZZ
Ovary
Bilateral ØUT2
Left ØUT1
Right ØUTØ
Palate
Hard ØCT2
Soft ØCT3
Pancreas ØFTG
Para-aortic Body ØGT9
Paraganglion Extremity ØGTF
Parathyroid Gland ØGTR
Inferior
Left ØGTP
Right ØGTN

Resection — *continued*
Parathyroid Gland — *continued*
Multiple ØGTQ
Superior
Left ØGTM
Right ØGTL
Patella
Left ØQTFØZZ
Right ØQTDØZZ
Penis ØVTS
Pericardium Ø2TN
Phalanx
Finger
Left ØPTVØZZ
Right ØPTTØZZ
Thumb
Left ØPTSØZZ
Right ØPTRØZZ
Toe
Left ØQTRØZZ
Right ØQTQØZZ
Pharynx ØCTM
Pineal Body ØGT1
Prepuce ØVTT
Products of Conception, Ectopic 1ØT2
Prostate ØVTØ
Radius
Left ØPTJØZZ
Right ØPTHØZZ
Rectum ØDTP
Ribs
1 to 2 ØPT1ØZZ
3 or More ØPT2ØZZ
Scapula
Left ØPT6ØZZ
Right ØPT5ØZZ
Scrotum ØVT5
Septum
Atrial Ø2T5
Nasal Ø9TM
Ventricular Ø2TM
Sinus
Accessory Ø9TP
Ethmoid
Left Ø9TV
Right Ø9TU
Frontal
Left Ø9TT
Right Ø9TS
Mastoid
Left Ø9TC
Right Ø9TB
Maxillary
Left Ø9TR
Right Ø9TQ
Sphenoid
Left Ø9TX
Right Ø9TW
Spleen Ø7TP
Sternum ØPTØØZZ
Stomach ØDT6
Pylorus ØDT7
Tarsal
Left ØQTMØZZ
Right ØQTLØZZ
Tendon
Abdomen
Left ØLTG
Right ØLTF
Ankle
Left ØLTT
Right ØLTS
Foot
Left ØLTW
Right ØLTV
Hand
Left ØLT8
Right ØLT7
Head and Neck ØLTØ
Hip
Left ØLTK
Right ØLTJ
Knee
Left ØLTR
Right ØLTQ
Lower Arm and Wrist
Left ØLT6
Right ØLT5

Resection — *continued*
Tendon — *continued*
Lower Leg
Left ØLTP
Right ØLTN
Perineum ØLTH
Shoulder
Left ØLT2
Right ØLT1
Thorax
Left ØLTD
Right ØLTC
Trunk
Left ØLTB
Right ØLT9
Upper Arm
Left ØLT4
Right ØLT3
Upper Leg
Left ØLTM
Right ØLTL
Testis
Bilateral ØVTC
Left ØVTB
Right ØVT9
Thymus Ø7TM
Thyroid Gland ØGTK
Left Lobe ØGTG
Right Lobe ØGTH
Thyroid Gland Isthmus ØGTJ
Tibia
Left ØQTHØZZ
Right ØQTGØZZ
Toe Nail ØHTRXZZ
Tongue ØCT7
Tonsils ØCTP
Tooth
Lower ØCTXØZ
Upper ØCTWØZ
Trachea ØBT1
Tunica Vaginalis
Left ØVT7
Right ØVT6
Turbinate, Nasal Ø9TL
Tympanic Membrane
Left Ø9T8
Right Ø9T7
Ulna
Left ØPTLØZZ
Right ØPTKØZZ
Ureter
Left ØTT7
Right ØTT6
Urethra ØTTD
Uterine Supporting Structure ØUT4
Uterus ØUT9
Uvula ØCTN
Vagina ØUTG
Valve, Pulmonary Ø2TH
Vas Deferens
Bilateral ØVTQ
Left ØVTP
Right ØVTN
Vesicle
Bilateral ØVT3
Left ØVT2
Right ØVT1
Vitreous
Left Ø8T53ZZ
Right Ø8T43ZZ
Vocal Cord
Left ØCTV
Right ØCTT
Vulva ØUTM
Resection, Left ventricular outflow tract obstruction (LVOT) *see* Dilation, Ventricle, Left Ø27L
Resection, Subaortic membrane (Left ventricular outflow tract obstruction) *see* Dilation, Ventricle, Left Ø27L
Restoration, Cardiac, Single, Rhythm 5A22Ø4Z
RestoreAdvanced neurostimulator (SureScan) (MRI Safe) *use* Stimulator Generator, Multiple Array Rechargeable in ØJH
RestoreSensor neurostimulator (SureScan) (MRI Safe) *use* Stimulator Generator, Multiple Array Rechargeable in ØJH
RestoreUltra neurostimulator (SureScan) (MRI Safe) *use* Stimulator Generator, Multiple Array Rechargeable in ØJH
Restriction
Ampulla of Vater ØFVC
Anus ØDVQ
Aorta
Abdominal Ø4VØ
Intraluminal Device, Branched or Fenestrated Ø4VØ
Thoracic
Ascending/Arch, Intraluminal Device, Branched or Fenestrated Ø2VX
Descending, Intraluminal Device, Branched or Fenestrated Ø2VW
Artery
Anterior Tibial
Left Ø4VQ
Right Ø4VP
Axillary
Left Ø3V6
Right Ø3V5
Brachial
Left Ø3V8
Right Ø3V7
Celiac Ø4V1
Colic
Left Ø4V7
Middle Ø4V8
Right Ø4V6
Common Carotid
Left Ø3VJ
Right Ø3VH
Common Iliac
Left Ø4VD
Right Ø4VC
External Carotid
Left Ø3VN
Right Ø3VM
External Iliac
Left Ø4VJ
Right Ø4VH
Face Ø3VR
Femoral
Left Ø4VL
Right Ø4VK
Foot
Left Ø4VW
Right Ø4VV
Gastric Ø4V2
Hand
Left Ø3VF
Right Ø3VD
Hepatic Ø4V3
Inferior Mesenteric Ø4VB
Innominate Ø3V2
Internal Carotid
Left Ø3VL
Right Ø3VK
Internal Iliac
Left Ø4VF
Right Ø4VE
Internal Mammary
Left Ø3V1
Right Ø3VØ
Intracranial Ø3VG
Lower Ø4VY
Peroneal
Left Ø4VU
Right Ø4VT
Popliteal
Left Ø4VN
Right Ø4VM
Posterior Tibial
Left Ø4VS
Right Ø4VR
Pulmonary
Left Ø2VR
Right Ø2VQ
Pulmonary Trunk Ø2VP
Radial
Left Ø3VC
Right Ø3VB
Renal
Left Ø4VA
Right Ø4V9
Splenic Ø4V4
Subclavian
Left Ø3V4
Restriction — *continued*
Artery — *continued*
Subclavian — *continued*
Right Ø3V3
Superior Mesenteric Ø4V5
Temporal
Left Ø3VT
Right Ø3VS
Thyroid
Left Ø3VV
Right Ø3VU
Ulnar
Left Ø3VA
Right Ø3V9
Upper Ø3VY
Vertebral
Left Ø3VQ
Right Ø3VP
Bladder ØTVB
Bladder Neck ØTVC
Bronchus
Lingula ØBV9
Lower Lobe
Left ØBVB
Right ØBV6
Main
Left ØBV7
Right ØBV3
Middle Lobe, Right ØBV5
Upper Lobe
Left ØBV8
Right ØBV4
Carina ØBV2
Cecum ØDVH
Cervix ØUVC
Cisterna Chyli Ø7VL
Colon
Ascending ØDVK
Descending ØDVM
Sigmoid ØDVN
Transverse ØDVL
Duct
Common Bile ØFV9
Cystic ØFV8
Hepatic
Common ØFV7
Left ØFV6
Right ØFV5
Lacrimal
Left Ø8VY
Right Ø8VX
Pancreatic ØFVD
Accessory ØFVF
Parotid
Left ØCVC
Right ØCVB
Duodenum ØDV9
Esophagogastric Junction ØDV4
Esophagus ØDV5
Lower ØDV3
Middle ØDV2
Upper ØDV1
Heart Ø2VA
Ileocecal Valve ØDVC
Ileum ØDVB
Intestine
Large ØDVE
Left ØDVG
Right ØDVF
Small ØDV8
Jejunum ØDVA
Kidney Pelvis
Left ØTV4
Right ØTV3
Lymphatic
Aortic Ø7VD
Axillary
Left Ø7V6
Right Ø7V5
Head Ø7VØ
Inguinal
Left Ø7VJ
Right Ø7VH
Internal Mammary
Left Ø7V9
Right Ø7V8
Lower Extremity
Left Ø7VG
Right Ø7VF

Restriction — *continued*
Lymphatic — *continued*
Mesenteric Ø7VB
Neck
Left Ø7V2
Right Ø7V1
Pelvis Ø7VC
Thoracic Duct Ø7VK
Thorax Ø7V7
Upper Extremity
Left Ø7V4
Right Ø7V3
Rectum ØDVP
Stomach ØDV6
Pylorus ØDV7
Trachea ØBV1
Ureter
Left ØTV7
Right ØTV6
Urethra ØTVD
Valve, Mitral Ø2VG
Vein
Axillary
Left Ø5V8
Right Ø5V7
Azygos Ø5VØ
Basilic
Left Ø5VC
Right Ø5VB
Brachial
Left Ø5VA
Right Ø5V9
Cephalic
Left Ø5VF
Right Ø5VD
Colic Ø6V7
Common Iliac
Left Ø6VD
Right Ø6VC
Esophageal Ø6V3
External Iliac
Left Ø6VG
Right Ø6VF
External Jugular
Left Ø5VQ
Right Ø5VP
Face
Left Ø5VV
Right Ø5VT
Femoral
Left Ø6VN
Right Ø6VM
Foot
Left Ø6VV
Right Ø6VT
Gastric Ø6V2
Hand
Left Ø5VH
Right Ø5VG
Hemiazygos Ø5V1
Hepatic Ø6V4
Hypogastric
Left Ø6VJ
Right Ø6VH
Inferior Mesenteric Ø6V6
Innominate
Left Ø5V4
Right Ø5V3
Internal Jugular
Left Ø5VN
Right Ø5VM
Intracranial Ø5VL
Lower Ø6VY
Portal Ø6V8
Pulmonary
Left Ø2VT
Right Ø2VS
Renal
Left Ø6VB
Right Ø6V9
Saphenous
Left Ø6VQ
Right Ø6VP
Splenic Ø6V1
Subclavian
Left Ø5V6
Right Ø5V5
Superior Mesenteric Ø6V5
Upper Ø5VY

Restriction — *continued*
Vein — *continued*
Vertebral
Left Ø5VS
Right Ø5VR
Vena Cava
Inferior Ø6VØ
Superior Ø2VV
Ventricle, Left Ø2VL
Resurfacing Device
Removal of device from
Left ØSPBØBZ
Right ØSP9ØBZ
Revision of device in
Left ØSWBØBZ
Right ØSW9ØBZ
Supplement
Left ØSUBØBZ
Acetabular Surface ØSUEØBZ
Femoral Surface ØSUSØBZ
Right ØSU9ØBZ
Acetabular Surface ØSUAØBZ
Femoral Surface ØSURØBZ
Resuscitation
Cardiopulmonary *see* Assistance, Cardiac 5AØ2
Cardioversion 5A22Ø4Z
Defibrillation 5A22Ø4Z
Endotracheal intubation *see* Insertion of device in, Trachea ØBH1
External chest compression, manual 5A12Ø12
External chest compression, mechanical 5A1221J
Pulmonary 5A19Ø54
Resuscitative endovascular balloon occlusion of the aorta (REBOA)
Ø2LW3DJ
Ø4LØ3DJ
Resuture, Heart valve prosthesis *see* Revision of device in, Heart and Great Vessels Ø2W
Retained placenta, manual removal *see* Extraction, Products of Conception, Retained 1ØD1
RETHYMIC® *use* Engineered Allogeneic Thymus Tissue
Retraining
Cardiac *see* Motor Treatment, Rehabilitation FØ7
Vocational *see* Activities of Daily Living Treatment, Rehabilitation FØ8
Retrogasserian rhizotomy *see* Division, Nerve, Trigeminal ØØ8K
Retroperitoneal cavity *use* Retroperitoneum
Retroperitoneal lymph node *use* Lymphatic, Aortic
Retroperitoneal space *use* Retroperitoneum
Retropharyngeal lymph node
use Lymphatic, Left Neck
use Lymphatic, Right Neck
Retropharyngeal space *use* Neck
Retropubic space *use* Pelvic Cavity
Reveal (LINQ) (DX) (XT) *use* Monitoring Device
Reverse total shoulder replacement *see* Replacement, Upper Joints ØRR
Reverse® Shoulder Prosthesis *use* Synthetic Substitute, Reverse Ball and Socket in ØRR
Revision
Correcting a portion of existing device *see* Revision of device in
Removal of device without replacement *see* Removal of device from
Replacement of existing device
see Removal of device from
see Root operation to place new device, e.g., Insertion, Replacement, Supplement
Revision of device in
Abdominal Wall ØWWF
Acetabulum
Left ØQW5
Right ØQW4
Anal Sphincter ØDWR
Anus ØDWQ
Aorta, Thoracic, Descending Ø2WW3RZ
Artery
Lower Ø4WY
Upper Ø3WY
Auditory Ossicle
Left Ø9WA
Right Ø9W9
Back
Lower ØWWL
Upper ØWWK
Bladder ØTWB

Revision of device in — *continued*
Bone
Facial ØNWW
Lower ØQWY
Nasal ØNWB
Pelvic
Left ØQW3
Right ØQW2
Upper ØPWY
Bone Marrow Ø7WT
Brain ØØWØ
Breast
Left ØHWU
Right ØHWT
Bursa and Ligament
Lower ØMWY
Upper ØMWX
Carpal
Left ØPWN
Right ØPWM
Cavity, Cranial ØWW1
Cerebral Ventricle ØØW6
Chest Wall ØWW8
Cisterna Chyli Ø7WL
Clavicle
Left ØPWB
Right ØPW9
Coccyx ØQWS
Diaphragm ØBWT
Disc
Cervical Vertebral ØRW3
Cervicothoracic Vertebral ØRW5
Lumbar Vertebral ØSW2
Lumbosacral ØSW4
Thoracic Vertebral ØRW9
Thoracolumbar Vertebral ØRWB
Duct
Hepatobiliary ØFWB
Pancreatic ØFWD
Ear
Inner
Left Ø9WE
Right Ø9WD
Left Ø9WJ
Right Ø9WH
Epididymis and Spermatic Cord ØVWM
Esophagus ØDW5
Extremity
Lower
Left ØYWB
Right ØYW9
Upper
Left ØXW7
Right ØXW6
Eye
Left Ø8W1
Right Ø8WØ
Face ØWW2
Fallopian Tube ØUW8
Femoral Shaft
Left ØQW9
Right ØQW8
Femur
Lower
Left ØQWC
Right ØQWB
Upper
Left ØQW7
Right ØQW6
Fibula
Left ØQWK
Right ØQWJ
Finger Nail ØHWQX
Gallbladder ØFW4
Gastrointestinal Tract ØWWP
Genitourinary Tract ØWWR
Gland
Adrenal ØGW5
Endocrine ØGWS
Pituitary ØGWØ
Salivary ØCWA
Glenoid Cavity
Left ØPW8
Right ØPW7
Great Vessel Ø2WY
Hair ØHWSX
Head ØWWØ
Heart Ø2WA

Revision of device in — *continued*
- Humeral Head
  - Left ØPWD
  - Right ØPWC
- Humeral Shaft
  - Left ØPWG
  - Right ØPWF
- Intestinal Tract
  - Lower Intestinal Tract ØDWD
  - Upper Intestinal Tract ØDWØ
- Intestine
  - Large ØDWE
  - Small ØDW8
- Jaw
  - Lower ØWW5
  - Upper ØWW4
- Joint
  - Acromioclavicular
    - Left ØRWH
    - Right ØRWG
  - Ankle
    - Left ØSWG
    - Right ØSWF
  - Carpal
    - Left ØRWR
    - Right ØRWQ
  - Carpometacarpal
    - Left ØRWT
    - Right ØRWS
  - Cervical Vertebral ØRW1
  - Cervicothoracic Vertebral ØRW4
  - Coccygeal ØSW6
  - Elbow
    - Left ØRWM
    - Right ØRWL
  - Finger Phalangeal
    - Left ØRWX
    - Right ØRWW
  - Hip
    - Left ØSWB
      - Acetabular Surface ØSWE
      - Femoral Surface ØSWS
    - Right ØSW9
      - Acetabular Surface ØSWA
      - Femoral Surface ØSWR
  - Knee
    - Left ØSWD
      - Femoral Surface ØSWU
      - Tibial Surface ØSWW
    - Right ØSWC
      - Femoral Surface ØSWT
      - Tibial Surface ØSWV
  - Lumbar Vertebral ØSWØ
  - Lumbosacral ØSW3
  - Metacarpophalangeal
    - Left ØRWV
    - Right ØRWU
  - Metatarsal-Phalangeal
    - Left ØSWN
    - Right ØSWM
  - Occipital-cervical ØRWØ
  - Sacrococcygeal ØSW5
  - Sacroiliac
    - Left ØSW8
    - Right ØSW7
  - Shoulder
    - Left ØRWK
    - Right ØRWJ
  - Sternoclavicular
    - Left ØRWF
    - Right ØRWE
  - Tarsal
    - Left ØSWJ
    - Right ØSWH
  - Tarsometatarsal
    - Left ØSWL
    - Right ØSWK
  - Temporomandibular
    - Left ØRWD
    - Right ØRWC
  - Thoracic Vertebral ØRW6
  - Thoracolumbar Vertebral ØRWA
  - Toe Phalangeal
    - Left ØSWQ
    - Right ØSWP
  - Wrist
    - Left ØRWP
    - Right ØRWN
- Kidney ØTW5

Revision of device in — *continued*
- Larynx ØCWS
- Lens
  - Left Ø8WK
  - Right Ø8WJ
- Liver ØFWØ
- Lung
  - Left ØBWL
  - Right ØBWK
- Lymphatic Ø7WN
  - Thoracic Duct Ø7WK
- Mediastinum ØWWC
- Mesentery ØDWV
- Metacarpal
  - Left ØPWQ
  - Right ØPWP
- Metatarsal
  - Left ØQWP
  - Right ØQWN
- Mouth and Throat ØCWY
- Muscle
  - Extraocular
    - Left Ø8WM
    - Right Ø8WL
  - Lower ØKWY
  - Upper ØKWX
- Nasal Mucosa and Soft Tissue Ø9WK
- Neck ØWW6
- Nerve
  - Cranial ØØWE
  - Peripheral Ø1WY
- Omentum ØDWU
- Ovary ØUW3
- Pancreas ØFWG
- Parathyroid Gland ØGWR
- Patella
  - Left ØQWF
  - Right ØQWD
- Pelvic Cavity ØWWJ
- Penis ØVWS
- Pericardial Cavity ØWWD
- Perineum
  - Female ØWWN
  - Male ØWWM
- Peritoneal Cavity ØWWG
- Peritoneum ØDWW
- Phalanx
  - Finger
    - Left ØPWV
    - Right ØPWT
  - Thumb
    - Left ØPWS
    - Right ØPWR
  - Toe
    - Left ØQWR
    - Right ØQWQ
- Pineal Body ØGW1
- Pleura ØBWQ
- Pleural Cavity
  - Left ØWWB
  - Right ØWW9
- Prostate and Seminal Vesicles ØVW4
- Radius
  - Left ØPWJ
  - Right ØPWH
- Respiratory Tract ØWWQ
- Retroperitoneum ØWWH
- Ribs
  - 1 to 2 ØPW1
  - 3 or More ØPW2
- Sacrum ØQW1
- Scapula
  - Left ØPW6
  - Right ØPW5
- Scrotum and Tunica Vaginalis ØVW8
- Septum
  - Atrial Ø2W5
  - Ventricular Ø2WM
- Sinus Ø9WY
- Skin ØHWPX
- Skull ØNWØ
- Spinal Canal ØØWU
- Spinal Cord ØØWV
- Spleen Ø7WP
- Sternum ØPWØ
- Stomach ØDW6
- Subcutaneous Tissue and Fascia
  - Head and Neck ØJWS
  - Lower Extremity ØJWW

Revision of device in — *continued*
- Subcutaneous Tissue and Fascia — *continued*
  - Trunk ØJWT
  - Upper Extremity ØJWV
- Tarsal
  - Left ØQWM
  - Right ØQWL
- Tendon
  - Lower ØLWY
  - Upper ØLWX
- Testis ØVWD
- Thymus Ø7WM
- Thyroid Gland ØGWK
- Tibia
  - Left ØQWH
  - Right ØQWG
- Toe Nail ØHWRX
- Trachea ØBW1
- Tracheobronchial Tree ØBWØ
- Tympanic Membrane
  - Left Ø9W8
  - Right Ø9W7
- Ulna
  - Left ØPWL
  - Right ØPWK
- Ureter ØTW9
- Urethra ØTWD
- Uterus and Cervix ØUWD
- Vagina and Cul-de-sac ØUWH
- Valve
  - Aortic Ø2WF
  - Mitral Ø2WG
  - Pulmonary Ø2WH
  - Tricuspid Ø2WJ
- Vas Deferens ØVWR
- Vein
  - Azygos Ø5WØ
  - Innominate
    - Left Ø5W4
    - Right Ø5W3
  - Lower Ø6WY
  - Upper Ø5WY
- Vertebra
  - Cervical ØPW3
  - Lumbar ØQWØ
  - Thoracic ØPW4
- Vulva ØUWM

Revo MRI™ SureScan® pacemaker *use* Pacemaker, Dual Chamber in ØJH

Rezafungin XWØ

rhBMP-2 *use* Recombinant Bone Morphogenetic Protein

Rheos® System device *use* Stimulator Generator in Subcutaneous Tissue and Fascia

Rheos® System lead *use* Stimulator Lead in Upper Arteries

Rhinopharynx *use* Nasopharynx

Rhinoplasty
- *see* Alteration, Nasal Mucosa and Soft Tissue Ø9ØK
- *see* Repair, Nasal Mucosa and Soft Tissue Ø9QK
- *see* Replacement, Nasal Mucosa and Soft Tissue Ø9RK
- *see* Supplement, Nasal Mucosa and Soft Tissue Ø9UK

Rhinorrhaphy *see* Repair, Nasal Mucosa and Soft Tissue Ø9QK

Rhinoscopy Ø9JKXZZ

Rhizotomy
- *see* Division, Central Nervous System and Cranial Nerves ØØ8
- *see* Division, Peripheral Nervous System Ø18

Rhomboid major muscle
- *use* Trunk Muscle, Left
- *use* Trunk Muscle, Right

Rhomboid minor muscle
- *use* Trunk Muscle, Left
- *use* Trunk Muscle, Right

Rhythm electrocardiogram *see* Measurement, Cardiac 4AØ2

Rhytidectomy *see* Alteration, Face ØWØ2

Right ascending lumbar vein *use* Azygos Vein

Right atrioventricular valve *use* Tricuspid Valve

Right auricular appendix *use* Atrium, Right

Right colic vein *use* Colic Vein

Right coronary sulcus *use* Heart, Right

Right gastric artery *use* Gastric Artery

Right gastroepiploic vein *use* Superior Mesenteric Vein

Right inferior phrenic vein *use* Inferior Vena Cava
Right inferior pulmonary vein *use* Pulmonary Vein, Right
Right jugular trunk *use* Lymphatic, Right Neck
Right lateral ventricle *use* Cerebral Ventricle
Right lymphatic duct *use* Lymphatic, Right Neck
Right ovarian vein *use* Inferior Vena Cava
Right second lumbar vein *use* Inferior Vena Cava
Right subclavian trunk *use* Lymphatic, Right Neck
Right subcostal vein *use* Azygos Vein
Right superior pulmonary vein *use* Pulmonary Vein, Right
Right suprarenal vein *use* Inferior Vena Cava
Right testicular vein *use* Inferior Vena Cava
Rima glottidis *use* Larynx
Risorius muscle *use* Facial Muscle
RNS System lead *use* Neurostimulator Lead in Central Nervous System and Cranial Nerves
RNS system neurostimulator generator *use* Neurostimulator Generator in Head and Facial Bones
Robotic Assisted Procedure
  Extremity
    Lower 8EØY
    Upper 8EØX
  Head and Neck Region 8EØ9
  Trunk Region 8EØW
Rotation of fetal head
  Forceps 1ØSØ7ZZ
  Manual 1ØSØXZZ
Round ligament of uterus *use* Uterine Supporting Structure
Round window
  use Inner Ear, Left
  use Inner Ear, Right
Roux-en-Y operation
  see Bypass, Gastrointestinal System ØD1
  see Bypass, Hepatobiliary System and Pancreas ØF1
Rupture
  Adhesions *see* Release
  Fluid collection *see* Drainage
Ruxolitinib XWØDXT5
RYBREVANT™ *use* Amivantamab Monoclonal Antibody

S

Sabizabulin XWØ
Sacral ganglion *use* Sacral Sympathetic Nerve
Sacral lymph node *use* Lymphatic, Pelvis
Sacral nerve modulation (SNM) lead *use* Stimulator Lead in Urinary System
Sacral neuromodulation lead *use* Stimulator Lead in Urinary System
Sacral splanchnic nerve *use* Sacral Sympathetic Nerve
Sacrectomy *see* Excision, Lower Bones ØQB
Sacrococcygeal ligament *use* Lower Spine Bursa and Ligament
Sacrococcygeal symphysis *use* Sacrococcygeal Joint
Sacroiliac ligament *use* Lower Spine Bursa and Ligament
Sacrospinous ligament *use* Lower Spine Bursa and Ligament
Sacrotuberous ligament *use* Lower Spine Bursa and Ligament
Salpingectomy
  see Excision, Female Reproductive System ØUB
  see Resection, Female Reproductive System ØUT
Salpingolysis *see* Release, Female Reproductive System ØUN
Salpingopexy
  see Repair, Female Reproductive System ØUQ
  see Reposition, Female Reproductive System ØUS
Salpingopharyngeus muscle *use* Tongue, Palate, Pharynx Muscle
Salpingoplasty
  see Repair, Female Reproductive System ØUQ
  see Supplement, Female Reproductive System ØUU
Salpingorrhaphy *see* Repair, Female Reproductive System ØUQ
Salpingoscopy ØUJ88ZZ
Salpingostomy *see* Drainage, Female Reproductive System ØU9
Salpingotomy *see* Drainage, Female Reproductive System ØU9
Salpinx
  use Fallopian Tube, Left
Salpinx — *continued*
  use Fallopian Tube, Right
Saphenous nerve *use* Femoral Nerve
SAPIEN transcatheter aortic valve *use* Zooplastic Tissue in Heart and Great Vessels
Sarilumab XWØ
SARS-CoV-2 Antibody Detection, Serum/Plasma Nanoparticle Fluorescence XXE5XV7
SARS-CoV-2 Polymerase Chain Reaction, Nasopharyngeal Fluid XXE97U7
Sartorius muscle
  use Upper Leg Muscle, Left
  use Upper Leg Muscle, Right
Satralizumab-mwge XWØ1397
SAVAL below-the-knee (BTK) drug-eluting stent system
  use Intraluminal Device, Sustained Release Drug-eluting in New Technology
  use Intraluminal Device, Sustained Release Drug-eluting, Two in New Technology
  use Intraluminal Device, Sustained Release Drug-eluting, Three in New Technology
  use Intraluminal Device, Sustained Release Drug-eluting, Four or More in New Technology
Scalene muscle
  use Neck Muscle, Left
  use Neck Muscle, Right
Scan
  Computerized Tomography (CT) *see* Computerized Tomography (CT Scan)
  Radioisotope *see* Planar Nuclear Medicine Imaging
Scaphoid bone
  use Carpal, Left
  use Carpal, Right
Scapholunate ligament
  use Wrist Bursa and Ligament, Left
  use Wrist Bursa and Ligament, Right
Scaphotrapezium ligament
  use Hand Bursa and Ligament, Left
  use Hand Bursa and Ligament, Right
Scapulectomy
  see Excision, Upper Bones ØPB
  see Resection, Upper Bones ØPT
Scapulopexy
  see Repair, Upper Bones ØPQ
  see Reposition, Upper Bones ØPS
Scarpa's (vestibular) ganglion *use* Acoustic Nerve
Sclerectomy *see* Excision, Eye Ø8B
Sclerotherapy, mechanical *see* Destruction
Sclerotherapy, via injection of sclerosing agent
  see Introduction, Destructive Agent
Sclerotomy *see* Drainage, Eye Ø89
Scrotectomy
  see Excision, Male Reproductive System ØVB
  see Resection, Male Reproductive System ØVT
Scrotoplasty
  see Repair, Male Reproductive System ØVQ
  see Supplement, Male Reproductive System ØVU
Scrotorrhaphy *see* Repair, Male Reproductive System ØVQ
Scrototomy *see* Drainage, Male Reproductive System ØV9
Sebaceous gland *use* Skin
Second cranial nerve *use* Optic Nerve
Section, cesarean *see* Extraction, Pregnancy 1ØD
Secura (DR) (VR) *use* Defibrillator Generator in ØJH
Sella turcica *use* Sphenoid Bone
Selux Rapid AST Platform XXE5XY9
Semicircular canal
  use Inner Ear, Left
  use Inner Ear, Right
Semimembranosus muscle
  use Upper Leg Muscle, Left
  use Upper Leg Muscle, Right
Semitendinosus muscle
  use Upper Leg Muscle, Left
  use Upper Leg Muscle, Right
Sentinel™ Cerebral Protection System (CPS) X2A5312
Seprafilm *use* Adhesion Barrier
Septal cartilage *use* Nasal Septum
Septectomy
  see Excision, Ear, Nose, Sinus Ø9B
  see Excision, Heart and Great Vessels Ø2B
  see Resection, Ear, Nose, Sinus Ø9T
  see Resection, Heart and Great Vessels Ø2T
SeptiCyte® RAPID XXE5X38
Septoplasty
  see Repair, Ear, Nose, Sinus Ø9Q
  see Repair, Heart and Great Vessels Ø2Q
  see Replacement, Ear, Nose, Sinus Ø9R
  see Replacement, Heart and Great Vessels Ø2R
  see Reposition, Ear, Nose, Sinus Ø9S
  see Supplement, Ear, Nose, Sinus Ø9U
  see Supplement, Heart and Great Vessels Ø2U
Septostomy, balloon atrial Ø2163Z7
Septotomy *see* Drainage, Ear, Nose, Sinus Ø99
Sequestrectomy, bone *see* Extirpation
SER-1Ø9 XWØDXN9
Serratus anterior muscle
  use Thorax Muscle, Left
  use Thorax Muscle, Right
Serratus posterior muscle
  use Trunk Muscle, Left
  use Trunk Muscle, Right
Seventh cranial nerve *use* Facial Nerve
Shapshot_NIR 8EØ2XDZ
Sheffield hybrid external fixator
  use External Fixation Device, Hybrid in ØPH
  use External Fixation Device, Hybrid in ØPS
  use External Fixation Device, Hybrid in ØQH
  use External Fixation Device, Hybrid in ØQS
Sheffield ring external fixator
  use External Fixation Device, Ring in ØPH
  use External Fixation Device, Ring in ØPS
  use External Fixation Device, Ring in ØQH
  use External Fixation Device, Ring in ØQS
Shirodkar cervical cerclage ØUVC7ZZ
Shock Wave Therapy, Musculoskeletal 6A93
Shockwave Intravascular Lithotripsy (Shockwave IVL) *see* Fragmentation
Short gastric artery *use* Splenic Artery
Shortening
  see Excision
  see Repair
  see Reposition
Shunt creation *see* Bypass
Sialoadenectomy
  Complete *see* Resection, Mouth and Throat ØCT
  Partial *see* Excision, Mouth and Throat ØCB
Sialodochoplasty
  see Repair, Mouth and Throat ØCQ
  see Replacement, Mouth and Throat ØCR
  see Supplement, Mouth and Throat ØCU
Sialoectomy
  see Excision, Mouth and Throat ØCB
  see Resection, Mouth and Throat ØCT
Sialography *see* Plain Radiography, Ear, Nose, Mouth and Throat B9Ø
Sialolithotomy *see* Extirpation, Mouth and Throat ØCC
S-ICD™ lead *use* Subcutaneous Defibrillator Lead in Subcutaneous Tissue and Fascia
Sigmoid artery *use* Inferior Mesenteric Artery
Sigmoid flexure *use* Sigmoid Colon
Sigmoid vein *use* Inferior Mesenteric Vein
Sigmoidectomy
  see Excision, Gastrointestinal System ØDB
  see Resection, Gastrointestinal System ØDT
Sigmoidorrhaphy *see* Repair, Gastrointestinal System ØDQ
Sigmoidoscopy ØDJD8ZZ
Sigmoidotomy *see* Drainage, Gastrointestinal System ØD9
Single lead pacemaker (atrium) (ventricle) *use* Pacemaker, Single Chamber in ØJH
Single lead rate responsive pacemaker (atrium) (ventricle) *use* Pacemaker, Single Chamber Rate Responsive in ØJH
Single-use Duodenoscope XFJ
Single-use Oversleeve with Intraoperative Colonic Irrigation XDPH8K7
Sinoatrial node *use* Conduction Mechanism
Sinogram
  Abdominal Wall *see* Fluoroscopy, Abdomen and Pelvis BW11
  Chest Wall *see* Plain Radiography, Chest BWØ3
  Retroperitoneum *see* Fluoroscopy, Abdomen and Pelvis BW11
Sinus venosus *use* Atrium, Right
Sinusectomy
  see Excision, Ear, Nose, Sinus Ø9B
  see Resection, Ear, Nose, Sinus Ø9T

Sinusoscopy Ø9JY4ZZ
Sinusotomy *see* Drainage, Ear, Nose, Sinus Ø99
Sirolimus-eluting coronary stent *use* Intraluminal Device, Drug-eluting in Heart and Great Vessels
Sixth cranial nerve *use* Abducens Nerve
Size reduction, breast *see* Excision, Skin and Breast ØHB
SJM Biocor® Stented Valve System *use* Zooplastic Tissue in Heart and Great Vessels
Skene's (paraurethral) gland *use* Vestibular Gland
Sling
Fascial, orbicularis muscle (mouth) *see* Supplement, Muscle, Facial ØKU1
Levator muscle, for urethral suspension *see* Reposition, Bladder Neck ØTSC
Pubococcygeal, for urethral suspension *see* Reposition, Bladder Neck ØTSC
Rectum *see* Reposition, Rectum ØDSP
Small bowel series *see* Fluoroscopy, Bowel, Small BD13
Small saphenous vein
use Saphenous Vein, Left
use Saphenous Vein, Right
Snapshot_NIR 8EØ2XDZ
Snaring, polyp, colon *see* Excision, Gastrointestinal System ØDB
Solar (celiac) plexus *use* Abdominal Sympathetic Nerve
Soleus muscle
use Lower Leg Muscle, Left
use Lower Leg Muscle, Right
Soliris® *use* Eculizumab
Space of Retzius *use* Pelvic Cavity
Spacer
Insertion of device in
Disc
Lumbar Vertebral ØSH2
Lumbosacral ØSH4
Joint
Acromioclavicular
Left ØRHH
Right ØRHG
Ankle
Left ØSHG
Right ØSHF
Carpal
Left ØRHR
Right ØRHQ
Carpometacarpal
Left ØRHT
Right ØRHS
Cervical Vertebral ØRH1
Cervicothoracic Vertebral ØRH4
Coccygeal ØSH6
Elbow
Left ØRHM
Right ØRHL
Finger Phalangeal
Left ØRHX
Right ØRHW
Hip
Left ØSHB
Right ØSH9
Knee
Left ØSHD
Right ØSHC
Lumbar Vertebral ØSHØ
Lumbosacral ØSH3
Metacarpophalangeal
Left ØRHV
Right ØRHU
Metatarsal-Phalangeal
Left ØSHN
Right ØSHM
Occipital-cervical ØRHØ
Sacrococcygeal ØSH5
Sacroiliac
Left ØSH8
Right ØSH7
Shoulder
Left ØRHK
Right ØRHJ
Sternoclavicular
Left ØRHF
Right ØRHE
Tarsal
Left ØSHJ
Right ØSHH
Spacer — *continued*
Insertion of device in — *continued*
Joint — *continued*
Tarsometatarsal
Left ØSHL
Right ØSHK
Temporomandibular
Left ØRHD
Right ØRHC
Thoracic Vertebral ØRH6
Thoracolumbar Vertebral ØRHA
Toe Phalangeal
Left ØSHQ
Right ØSHP
Wrist
Left ØRHP
Right ØRHN
Removal of device from
Acromioclavicular
Left ØRPH
Right ØRPG
Ankle
Left ØSPG
Right ØSPF
Carpal
Left ØRPR
Right ØRPQ
Carpometacarpal
Left ØRPT
Right ØRPS
Cervical Vertebral ØRP1
Cervicothoracic Vertebral ØRP4
Coccygeal ØSP6
Elbow
Left ØRPM
Right ØRPL
Finger Phalangeal
Left ØRPX
Right ØRPW
Hip
Left ØSPB
Right ØSP9
Knee
Left ØSPD
Right ØSPC
Lumbar Vertebral ØSPØ
Lumbosacral ØSP3
Metacarpophalangeal
Left ØRPV
Right ØRPU
Metatarsal-Phalangeal
Left ØSPN
Right ØSPM
Occipital-cervical ØRPØ
Sacrococcygeal ØSP5
Sacroiliac
Left ØSP8
Right ØSP7
Shoulder
Left ØRPK
Right ØRPJ
Sternoclavicular
Left ØRPF
Right ØRPE
Tarsal
Left ØSPJ
Right ØSPH
Tarsometatarsal
Left ØSPL
Right ØSPK
Temporomandibular
Left ØRPD
Right ØRPC
Thoracic Vertebral ØRP6
Thoracolumbar Vertebral ØRPA
Toe Phalangeal
Left ØSPQ
Right ØSPP
Wrist
Left ØRPP
Right ØRPN
Revision of device in
Acromioclavicular
Left ØRWH
Right ØRWG
Ankle
Left ØSWG
Right ØSWF
Spacer — *continued*
Revision of device in — *continued*
Carpal
Left ØRWR
Right ØRWQ
Carpometacarpal
Left ØRWT
Right ØRWS
Cervical Vertebral ØRW1
Cervicothoracic Vertebral ØRW4
Coccygeal ØSW6
Elbow
Left ØRWM
Right ØRWL
Finger Phalangeal
Left ØRWX
Right ØRWW
Hip
Left ØSWB
Right ØSW9
Knee
Left ØSWD
Right ØSWC
Lumbar Vertebral ØSWØ
Lumbosacral ØSW3
Metacarpophalangeal
Left ØRWV
Right ØRWU
Metatarsal-Phalangeal
Left ØSWN
Right ØSWM
Occipital-cervical ØRWØ
Sacrococcygeal ØSW5
Sacroiliac
Left ØSW8
Right ØSW7
Shoulder
Left ØRWK
Right ØRWJ
Sternoclavicular
Left ØRWF
Right ØRWE
Tarsal
Left ØSWJ
Right ØSWH
Tarsometatarsal
Left ØSWL
Right ØSWK
Temporomandibular
Left ØRWD
Right ØRWC
Thoracic Vertebral ØRW6
Thoracolumbar Vertebral ØRWA
Toe Phalangeal
Left ØSWQ
Right ØSWP
Wrist
Left ØRWP
Right ØRWN
Spacer, Articulating (Antibiotic) *use* Articulating Spacer in Lower Joints
Spacer, Static (Antibiotic) *use* Spacer in Lower Joints
Spectroscopy
Intravascular Near Infrared 8EØ23DZ
Near Infrared *see* Physiological Systems and Anatomical Regions 8EØ
Speech Assessment FØØ
Speech therapy *see* Speech Treatment, Rehabilitation FØ6
Speech Treatment FØ6
Spesolimab Monoclonal Antibody XWØ
Sphenoidectomy
see Excision, Ear, Nose, Sinus Ø9B
see Excision, Head and Facial Bones ØNB
see Resection, Ear, Nose, Sinus Ø9T
see Resection, Head and Facial Bones ØNT
Sphenoidotomy *see* Drainage, Ear, Nose, Sinus Ø99
Sphenomandibular ligament *use* Head and Neck Bursa and Ligament
Sphenopalatine (pterygopalatine) ganglion *use* Head and Neck Sympathetic Nerve
Sphincterorrhaphy, anal *see* Repair, Anal Sphincter ØDQR
Sphincterotomy, anal
see Division, Anal Sphincter ØD8R
see Drainage, Anal Sphincter ØD9R
SPIKEVAX™
use COVID-19 Vaccine

SPIKEVAX™ — *continued*
use COVID-19 Vaccine Booster
use COVID-19 Vaccine Dose 1
use COVID-19 Vaccine Dose 2
use COVID-19 Vaccine Dose 3
Spinal cord neurostimulator lead *use* Neurostimulator Lead in Central Nervous System and Cranial Nerves
Spinal growth rods, magnetically controlled *use* Magnetically Controlled Growth Rod(s) in New Technology
Spinal nerve, cervical *use* Cervical Nerve
Spinal nerve, lumbar *use* Lumbar Nerve
Spinal nerve, sacral *use* Sacral Nerve
Spinal nerve, thoracic *use* Thoracic Nerve
Spinal Stabilization Device
Facet Replacement
Cervical Vertebral ØRH1
Cervicothoracic Vertebral ØRH4
Lumbar Vertebral ØSHØ
Lumbosacral ØSH3
Occipital-cervical ØRHØ
Thoracic Vertebral ØRH6
Thoracolumbar Vertebral ØRHA
Interspinous Process
Cervical Vertebral ØRH1
Cervicothoracic Vertebral ØRH4
Lumbar Vertebral ØSHØ
Lumbosacral ØSH3
Occipital-cervical ØRHØ
Thoracic Vertebral ØRH6
Thoracolumbar Vertebral ØRHA
Pedicle-Based
Cervical Vertebral ØRH1
Cervicothoracic Vertebral ØRH4
Lumbar Vertebral ØSHØ
Lumbosacral ØSH3
Occipital-cervical ØRHØ
Thoracic Vertebral ØRH6
Thoracolumbar Vertebral ØRHA
SpineJack® system *use* Synthetic Substitute, Mechanically Expandable (Paired) in New Technology
Spinous process
use Cervical Vertebra
use Lumbar Vertebra
use Thoracic Vertebra
Spiral ganglion *use* Acoustic Nerve
Spiration IBV™ Valve System *use* Intraluminal Device, Endobronchial Valve in Respiratory System
Splenectomy
see Excision, Lymphatic and Hemic Systems Ø7B
see Resection, Lymphatic and Hemic Systems Ø7T
Splenic flexure *use* Transverse Colon
Splenic plexus *use* Abdominal Sympathetic Nerve
Splenius capitis muscle *use* Head Muscle
Splenius cervicis muscle
use Neck Muscle, Left
use Neck Muscle, Right
Splenolysis *see* Release, Lymphatic and Hemic Systems Ø7N
Splenopexy
see Repair, Lymphatic and Hemic Systems Ø7Q
see Reposition, Lymphatic and Hemic Systems Ø7S
Splenoplasty *see* Repair, Lymphatic and Hemic Systems Ø7Q
Splenorrhaphy *see* Repair, Lymphatic and Hemic Systems Ø7Q
Splenotomy *see* Drainage, Lymphatic and Hemic Systems Ø79
Splinting, musculoskeletal *see* Immobilization, Anatomical Regions 2W3
SPRAVATO™ *use* Esketamine Hydrochloride
SPY PINPOINT fluorescence imaging system
see Monitoring, Physiological Systems 4A1
see Other Imaging, Hepatobiliary System and Pancreas BF5
SPY system intraoperative fluorescence cholangiography *see* Other Imaging, Hepatobiliary System and Pancreas BF5
SPY system intravascular fluorescence angiography *see* Monitoring, Physiological Systems 4A1
SSO2 (Supersaturated Oxygen) therapy, cardiac intra-arterial 5AØ222C
Staged hepatectomy
see Division, Hepatobiliary System and Pancreas ØF8
Staged hepatectomy — *continued*
see Resection, Hepatobiliary System and Pancreas ØFT
Stapedectomy
see Excision, Ear, Nose, Sinus Ø9B
see Resection, Ear, Nose, Sinus Ø9T
Stapediolysis *see* Release, Ear, Nose, Sinus Ø9N
Stapedioplasty
see Repair, Ear, Nose, Sinus Ø9Q
see Replacement, Ear, Nose, Sinus Ø9R
see Supplement, Ear, Nose, Sinus Ø9U
Stapedotomy *see* Drainage, Ear, Nose, Sinus Ø99
Stapes
use Auditory Ossicle, Left
use Auditory Ossicle, Right
Static Spacer (Antibiotic) *use* Spacer in Lower Joints
STELARA® *use* Other New Technology Therapeutic Substance
Stellate ganglion *use* Head and Neck Sympathetic Nerve
Stem cell transplant *see* Transfusion, Circulatory 3Ø2
Stensen's duct
use Parotid Duct, Left
use Parotid Duct, Right
Stent, intraluminal (cardiovascular) (gastrointestinal) (hepatobiliary) (urinary) *use* Intraluminal Device
Stent retriever thrombectomy *see* Extirpation, Upper Arteries Ø3C
Stented tissue valve *use* Zooplastic Tissue in Heart and Great Vessels
Stereotactic Radiosurgery
Abdomen DW23
Adrenal Gland DG22
Bile Ducts DF22
Bladder DT22
Bone Marrow D72Ø
Brain DØ2Ø
Brain Stem DØ21
Breast
Left DM2Ø
Right DM21
Bronchus DB21
Cervix DU21
Chest DW22
Chest Wall DB27
Colon DD25
Diaphragm DB28
Duodenum DD22
Ear D92Ø
Esophagus DD2Ø
Eye D82Ø
Gallbladder DF21
Gamma Beam
Abdomen DW23JZZ
Adrenal Gland DG22JZZ
Bile Ducts DF22JZZ
Bladder DT22JZZ
Bone Marrow D72ØJZZ
Brain DØ2ØJZZ
Brain Stem DØ21JZZ
Breast
Left DM2ØJZZ
Right DM21JZZ
Bronchus DB21JZZ
Cervix DU21JZZ
Chest DW22JZZ
Chest Wall DB27JZZ
Colon DD25JZZ
Diaphragm DB28JZZ
Duodenum DD22JZZ
Ear D92ØJZZ
Esophagus DD2ØJZZ
Eye D82ØJZZ
Gallbladder DF21JZZ
Gland
Adrenal DG22JZZ
Parathyroid DG24JZZ
Pituitary DG2ØJZZ
Thyroid DG25JZZ
Glands, Salivary D926JZZ
Head and Neck DW21JZZ
Ileum DD24JZZ
Jejunum DD23JZZ
Kidney DT2ØJZZ
Larynx D92BJZZ
Liver DF2ØJZZ
Lung DB22JZZ
Stereotactic Radiosurgery — *continued*
Gamma Beam — *continued*
Lymphatics
Abdomen D726JZZ
Axillary D724JZZ
Inguinal D728JZZ
Neck D723JZZ
Pelvis D727JZZ
Thorax D725JZZ
Mediastinum DB26JZZ
Mouth D924JZZ
Nasopharynx D92DJZZ
Neck and Head DW21JZZ
Nerve, Peripheral DØ27JZZ
Nose D921JZZ
Ovary DU2ØJZZ
Palate
Hard D928JZZ
Soft D929JZZ
Pancreas DF23JZZ
Parathyroid Gland DG24JZZ
Pelvic Region DW26JZZ
Pharynx D92CJZZ
Pineal Body DG21JZZ
Pituitary Gland DG2ØJZZ
Pleura DB25JZZ
Prostate DV2ØJZZ
Rectum DD27JZZ
Sinuses D927JZZ
Spinal Cord DØ26JZZ
Spleen D722JZZ
Stomach DD21JZZ
Testis DV21JZZ
Thymus D721JZZ
Thyroid Gland DG25JZZ
Tongue D925JZZ
Trachea DB2ØJZZ
Ureter DT21JZZ
Urethra DT23JZZ
Uterus DU22JZZ
Gland
Adrenal DG22
Parathyroid DG24
Pituitary DG2Ø
Thyroid DG25
Glands, Salivary D926
Head and Neck DW21
Ileum DD24
Jejunum DD23
Kidney DT2Ø
Larynx D92B
Liver DF2Ø
Lung DB22
Lymphatics
Abdomen D726
Axillary D724
Inguinal D728
Neck D723
Pelvis D727
Thorax D725
Mediastinum DB26
Mouth D924
Nasopharynx D92D
Neck and Head DW21
Nerve, Peripheral DØ27
Nose D921
Other Photon
Abdomen DW23DZZ
Adrenal Gland DG22DZZ
Bile Ducts DF22DZZ
Bladder DT22DZZ
Bone Marrow D72ØDZZ
Brain DØ2ØDZZ
Brain Stem DØ21DZZ
Breast
Left DM2ØDZZ
Right DM21DZZ
Bronchus DB21DZZ
Cervix DU21DZZ
Chest DW22DZZ
Chest Wall DB27DZZ
Colon DD25DZZ
Diaphragm DB28DZZ
Duodenum DD22DZZ
Ear D92ØDZZ
Esophagus DD2ØDZZ
Eye D82ØDZZ
Gallbladder DF21DZZ

Stereotactic Radiosurgery — *continued*
Other Photon — *continued*
Gland
Adrenal DG22DZZ
Parathyroid DG24DZZ
Pituitary DG20DZZ
Thyroid DG25DZZ
Glands, Salivary D926DZZ
Head and Neck DW21DZZ
Ileum DD24DZZ
Jejunum DD23DZZ
Kidney DT20DZZ
Larynx D92BDZZ
Liver DF20DZZ
Lung DB22DZZ
Lymphatics
Abdomen D726DZZ
Axillary D724DZZ
Inguinal D728DZZ
Neck D723DZZ
Pelvis D727DZZ
Thorax D725DZZ
Mediastinum DB26DZZ
Mouth D924DZZ
Nasopharynx D92DDZZ
Neck and Head DW21DZZ
Nerve, Peripheral D027DZZ
Nose D921DZZ
Ovary DU20DZZ
Palate
Hard D928DZZ
Soft D929DZZ
Pancreas DF23DZZ
Parathyroid Gland DG24DZZ
Pelvic Region DW26DZZ
Pharynx D92CDZZ
Pineal Body DG21DZZ
Pituitary Gland DG20DZZ
Pleura DB25DZZ
Prostate DV20DZZ
Rectum DD27DZZ
Sinuses D927DZZ
Spinal Cord D026DZZ
Spleen D722DZZ
Stomach DD21DZZ
Testis DV21DZZ
Thymus D721DZZ
Thyroid Gland DG25DZZ
Tongue D925DZZ
Trachea DB20DZZ
Ureter DT21DZZ
Urethra DT23DZZ
Uterus DU22DZZ
Ovary DU20
Palate
Hard D928
Soft D929
Pancreas DF23
Parathyroid Gland DG24
Particulate
Abdomen DW23HZZ
Adrenal Gland DG22HZZ
Bile Ducts DF22HZZ
Bladder DT22HZZ
Bone Marrow D720HZZ
Brain D020HZZ
Brain Stem D021HZZ
Breast
Left DM20HZZ
Right DM21HZZ
Bronchus DB21HZZ
Cervix DU21HZZ
Chest DW22HZZ
Chest Wall DB27HZZ
Colon DD25HZZ
Diaphragm DB28HZZ
Duodenum DD22HZZ
Ear D920HZZ
Esophagus DD20HZZ
Eye D820HZZ
Gallbladder DF21HZZ
Gland
Adrenal DG22HZZ
Parathyroid DG24HZZ
Pituitary DG20HZZ
Thyroid DG25HZZ
Glands, Salivary D926HZZ
Head and Neck DW21HZZ
Ileum DD24HZZ

Stereotactic Radiosurgery — *continued*
Particulate — *continued*
Jejunum DD23HZZ
Kidney DT20HZZ
Larynx D92BHZZ
Liver DF20HZZ
Lung DB22HZZ
Lymphatics
Abdomen D726HZZ
Axillary D724HZZ
Inguinal D728HZZ
Neck D723HZZ
Pelvis D727HZZ
Thorax D725HZZ
Mediastinum DB26HZZ
Mouth D924HZZ
Nasopharynx D92DHZZ
Neck and Head DW21HZZ
Nerve, Peripheral D027HZZ
Nose D921HZZ
Ovary DU20HZZ
Palate
Hard D928HZZ
Soft D929HZZ
Pancreas DF23HZZ
Parathyroid Gland DG24HZZ
Pelvic Region DW26HZZ
Pharynx D92CHZZ
Pineal Body DG21HZZ
Pituitary Gland DG20HZZ
Pleura DB25HZZ
Prostate DV20HZZ
Rectum DD27HZZ
Sinuses D927HZZ
Spinal Cord D026HZZ
Spleen D722HZZ
Stomach DD21HZZ
Testis DV21HZZ
Thymus D721HZZ
Thyroid Gland DG25HZZ
Tongue D925HZZ
Trachea DB20HZZ
Ureter DT21HZZ
Urethra DT23HZZ
Uterus DU22HZZ
Pelvic Region DW26
Pharynx D92C
Pineal Body DG21
Pituitary Gland DG20
Pleura DB25
Prostate DV20
Rectum DD27
Sinuses D927
Spinal Cord D026
Spleen D722
Stomach DD21
Testis DV21
Thymus D721
Thyroid Gland DG25
Tongue D925
Trachea DB20
Ureter DT21
Urethra DT23
Uterus DU22
Steripath® Micro™ Blood Collection System XXE5XR7
Sternoclavicular ligament
use Shoulder Bursa and Ligament, Left
use Shoulder Bursa and Ligament, Right
Sternocleidomastoid artery
use Thyroid Artery, Left
use Thyroid Artery, Right
Sternocleidomastoid muscle
use Neck Muscle, Left
use Neck Muscle, Right
Sternocostal ligament *use* Sternum Bursa and Ligament
Sternotomy
see Division, Sternum 0P80
see Drainage, Sternum 0P90
Stimulation, cardiac
Cardioversion 5A2204Z
Electrophysiologic testing *see* Measurement, Cardiac 4A02
Stimulator Generator
Insertion of device in
Abdomen 0JH8
Back 0JH7

Stimulator Generator — *continued*
Insertion of device in — *continued*
Chest 0JH6
Multiple Array
Abdomen 0JH8
Back 0JH7
Chest 0JH6
Multiple Array Rechargeable
Abdomen 0JH8
Back 0JH7
Chest 0JH6
Removal of device from, Subcutaneous Tissue and Fascia, Trunk 0JPT
Revision of device in, Subcutaneous Tissue and Fascia, Trunk 0JWT
Single Array
Abdomen 0JH8
Back 0JH7
Chest 0JH6
Single Array Rechargeable
Abdomen 0JH8
Back 0JH7
Chest 0JH6
Stimulator Lead
Insertion of device in
Anal Sphincter 0DHR
Artery
Left 03HL
Right 03HK
Bladder 0THB
Muscle
Lower 0KHY
Upper 0KHX
Stomach 0DH6
Ureter 0TH9
Removal of device from
Anal Sphincter 0DPR
Artery, Upper 03PY
Bladder 0TPB
Muscle
Lower 0KPY
Upper 0KPX
Stomach 0DP6
Ureter 0TP9
Revision of device in
Anal Sphincter 0DWR
Artery, Upper 03WY
Bladder 0TWB
Muscle
Lower 0KWY
Upper 0KWX
Stomach 0DW6
Ureter 0TW9
Stoma
Excision
Abdominal Wall 0WBFXZ2
Neck 0WB6XZ2
Repair
Abdominal Wall 0WQFXZ2
Neck 0WQ6XZ2
Stomatoplasty
see Repair, Mouth and Throat 0CQ
see Replacement, Mouth and Throat 0CR
see Supplement, Mouth and Throat 0CU
Stomatorrhaphy *see* Repair, Mouth and Throat 0CQ
StrataGraft® *use* Bioengineered Allogeneic Construct
Stratos LV *use* Cardiac Resynchronization Pacemaker Pulse Generator in 0JH
Stress test 4A02XM4, 4A12XM4
Stripping *see* Extraction
Study
Electrophysiologic stimulation, cardiac *see* Measurement, Cardiac 4A02
Ocular motility 4A07X7Z
Pulmonary airway flow measurement *see* Measurement, Respiratory 4A09
Visual acuity 4A07X0Z
Styloglossus muscle *use* Tongue, Palate, Pharynx Muscle
Stylomandibular ligament *use* Head and Neck Bursa and Ligament
Stylopharyngeus muscle *use* Tongue, Palate, Pharynx Muscle
Subacromial bursa
use Shoulder Bursa and Ligament, Left
use Shoulder Bursa and Ligament, Right
Subaortic (common iliac) lymph node *use* Lymphatic, Pelvis

Subarachnoid space, spinal *use* Spinal Canal
Subclavicular (apical) lymph node
use Lymphatic, Left Axillary
use Lymphatic, Right Axillary
Subclavius muscle
use Thorax Muscle, Left
use Thorax Muscle, Right
Subclavius nerve *use* Brachial Plexus
Subcostal artery *use* Upper Artery
Subcostal muscle
use Thorax Muscle, Left
use Thorax Muscle, Right
Subcostal nerve *use* Thoracic Nerve
Subcutaneous Defibrillator Lead
Insertion of device in, Subcutaneous Tissue and Fascia, Chest ØJH6
Removal of device from, Subcutaneous Tissue and Fascia, Trunk ØJPT
Revision of device in, Subcutaneous Tissue and Fascia, Trunk ØJWT
Subcutaneous injection reservoir, port *use* Vascular Access Device, Totally Implantable in Subcutaneous Tissue and Fascia
Subcutaneous injection reservoir, pump *use* Infusion Device, Pump in Subcutaneous Tissue and Fascia
Subdermal progesterone implant *use* Contraceptive Device in Subcutaneous Tissue and Fascia
Subdural space, spinal *use* Spinal Canal
Submandibular ganglion
use Facial Nerve
use Head and Neck Sympathetic Nerve
Submandibular gland
use Submaxillary Gland, Left
use Submaxillary Gland, Right
Submandibular lymph node *use* Lymphatic, Head
Submandibular space *use* Subcutaneous Tissue and Fascia, Face
Submaxillary ganglion *use* Head and Neck Sympathetic Nerve
Submaxillary lymph node *use* Lymphatic, Head
Submental artery *use* Face Artery
Submental lymph node *use* Lymphatic, Head
Submucous (Meissner's) plexus *use* Abdominal Sympathetic Nerve
Suboccipital nerve *use* Cervical Nerve
Suboccipital venous plexus
use Vertebral Vein, Left
use Vertebral Vein, Right
Subparotid lymph node *use* Lymphatic, Head
Subscapular aponeurosis
use Subcutaneous Tissue and Fascia, Left Upper Arm
use Subcutaneous Tissue and Fascia, Right Upper Arm
Subscapular artery
use Axillary Artery, Left
use Axillary Artery, Right
Subscapular (posterior) lymph node
use Lymphatic, Axillary, Left
use Lymphatic, Axillary, Right
Subscapularis muscle
use Shoulder Muscle, Left
use Shoulder Muscle, Right
Substance Abuse Treatment
Counseling
Family, for substance abuse, Other Family Counseling HZ63ZZZ
Group
12-Step HZ43ZZZ
Behavioral HZ41ZZZ
Cognitive HZ40ZZZ
Cognitive-Behavioral HZ42ZZZ
Confrontational HZ48ZZZ
Continuing Care HZ49ZZZ
Infectious Disease
Post-Test HZ4CZZZ
Pre-Test HZ4CZZZ
Interpersonal HZ44ZZZ
Motivational Enhancement HZ47ZZZ
Psychoeducation HZ46ZZZ
Spiritual HZ4BZZZ
Vocational HZ45ZZZ
Individual
12-Step HZ33ZZZ
Behavioral HZ31ZZZ
Cognitive HZ30ZZZ

Substance Abuse Treatment — *continued*
Counseling — *continued*
Individual — *continued*
Cognitive-Behavioral HZ32ZZZ
Confrontational HZ38ZZZ
Continuing Care HZ39ZZZ
Infectious Disease
Post-Test HZ3CZZZ
Pre-Test HZ3CZZZ
Interpersonal HZ34ZZZ
Motivational Enhancement HZ37ZZZ
Psychoeducation HZ36ZZZ
Spiritual HZ3BZZZ
Vocational HZ35ZZZ
Detoxification Services, for substance abuse HZ2ZZZZ
Medication Management
Antabuse HZ83ZZZ
Bupropion HZ87ZZZ
Clonidine HZ86ZZZ
Levo-alpha-acetyl-methadol (LAAM) HZ82ZZZ
Methadone Maintenance HZ81ZZZ
Naloxone HZ85ZZZ
Naltrexone HZ84ZZZ
Nicotine Replacement HZ8ØZZZ
Other Replacement Medication HZ89ZZZ
Psychiatric Medication HZ88ZZZ
Pharmacotherapy
Antabuse HZ93ZZZ
Bupropion HZ97ZZZ
Clonidine HZ96ZZZ
Levo-alpha-acetyl-methadol (LAAM) HZ92ZZZ
Methadone Maintenance HZ91ZZZ
Naloxone HZ95ZZZ
Naltrexone HZ94ZZZ
Nicotine Replacement HZ9ØZZZ
Psychiatric Medication HZ98ZZZ
Replacement Medication, Other HZ99ZZZ
Psychotherapy
12-Step HZ53ZZZ
Behavioral HZ51ZZZ
Cognitive HZ5ØZZZ
Cognitive-Behavioral HZ52ZZZ
Confrontational HZ58ZZZ
Interactive HZ55ZZZ
Interpersonal HZ54ZZZ
Motivational Enhancement HZ57ZZZ
Psychoanalysis HZ5BZZZ
Psychodynamic HZ5CZZZ
Psychoeducation HZ56ZZZ
Psychophysiological HZ5DZZZ
Supportive HZ59ZZZ
Substantia nigra *use* Basal Ganglia
Subtalar (talocalcaneal) joint
use Tarsal Joint, Left
use Tarsal Joint, Right
Subtalar ligament
use Foot Bursa and Ligament, Left
use Foot Bursa and Ligament, Right
Subthalamic nucleus *use* Basal Ganglia
Suction curettage (D&C), nonobstetric *see* Extraction, Endometrium ØUDB
Suction curettage, obstetric post-delivery *see* Extraction, Products of Conception, Retained 1ØD1
Sulbactam-Durlobactam XWØ
SUL-DUR *use* Sulbactam-Durlobactam
Superficial circumflex iliac vein
use Saphenous Vein, Left
use Saphenous Vein, Right
Superficial epigastric artery
use Femoral Artery, Left
use Femoral Artery, Right
Superficial epigastric vein
use Saphenous Vein, Left
use Saphenous Vein, Right
Superficial Inferior Epigastric Artery Flap
Replacement
Bilateral ØHRVØ78
Left ØHRUØ78
Right ØHRTØ78
Transfer
Left ØKXG
Right ØKXF
Superficial palmar arch
use Hand Artery, Left
use Hand Artery, Right

Superficial palmar venous arch
use Hand Vein, Left
use Hand Vein, Right
Superficial temporal artery
use Temporal Artery, Left
use Temporal Artery, Right
Superficial transverse perineal muscle *use* Perineum Muscle
Superior cardiac nerve *use* Thoracic Sympathetic Nerve
Superior cerebellar vein *use* Intracranial Vein
Superior cerebral vein *use* Intracranial Vein
Superior clunic (cluneal) nerve *use* Lumbar Nerve
Superior epigastric artery
use Internal Mammary Artery, Left
use Internal Mammary Artery, Right
Superior genicular artery
use Popliteal Artery, Left
use Popliteal Artery, Right
Superior gluteal artery
use Internal Iliac Artery, Left
use Internal Iliac Artery, Right
Superior gluteal nerve *use* Lumbar Plexus
Superior hypogastric plexus *use* Abdominal Sympathetic Nerve
Superior labial artery *use* Face Artery
Superior laryngeal artery
use Thyroid Artery, Left
use Thyroid Artery, Right
Superior laryngeal nerve *use* Vagus Nerve
Superior longitudinal muscle *use* Tongue, Palate, Pharynx Muscle
Superior mesenteric ganglion *use* Abdominal Sympathetic Nerve
Superior mesenteric lymph node *use* Lymphatic, Mesenteric
Superior mesenteric plexus *use* Abdominal Sympathetic Nerve
Superior oblique muscle
use Extraocular Muscle, Left
use Extraocular Muscle, Right
Superior olivary nucleus *use* Pons
Superior rectal artery *use* Inferior Mesenteric Artery
Superior rectal vein *use* Inferior Mesenteric Vein
Superior rectus muscle
use Extraocular Muscle, Left
use Extraocular Muscle, Right
Superior tarsal plate
use Upper Eyelid, Left
use Upper Eyelid, Right
Superior thoracic artery
use Axillary Artery, Left
use Axillary Artery, Right
Superior thyroid artery
use External Carotid Artery, Left
use External Carotid Artery, Right
use Thyroid Artery, Left
use Thyroid Artery, Right
Superior turbinate *use* Nasal Turbinate
Superior ulnar collateral artery
use Brachial Artery, Left
use Brachial Artery, Right
Superior vesical artery
use Internal Iliac Artery, Left
use Internal Iliac Artery, Right
Supersaturated Oxygen (SSO2) therapy, cardiac intra-arterial 5AØ222C
Supplement
Abdominal Wall ØWUF
Acetabulum
Left ØQU5
Right ØQU4
Ampulla of Vater ØFUC
Anal Sphincter ØDUR
Ankle Region
Left ØYUL
Right ØYUK
Anus ØDUQ
Aorta
Abdominal Ø4UØ
Thoracic
Ascending/Arch Ø2UX
Descending Ø2UW
Arm
Lower
Left ØXUF
Right ØXUD

Supplement — *continued*
Arm — *continued*
Upper
Left ØXU9
Right ØXU8
Arteriovenous Fistula, Extraluminal Support Device X2U
Artery
Anterior Tibial
Left Ø4UQ
Right Ø4UP
Axillary
Left Ø3U6
Right Ø3U5
Brachial
Left Ø3U8
Right Ø3U7
Celiac Ø4U1
Colic
Left Ø4U7
Middle Ø4U8
Right Ø4U6
Common Carotid
Left Ø3UJ
Right Ø3UH
Common Iliac
Left Ø4UD
Right Ø4UC
Coronary
Four or More Arteries Ø2U3
One Artery Ø2UØ
Three Arteries Ø2U2
Two Arteries Ø2U1
External Carotid
Left Ø3UN
Right Ø3UM
External Iliac
Left Ø4UJ
Right Ø4UH
Face Ø3UR
Femoral
Left Ø4UL
Right Ø4UK
Foot
Left Ø4UW
Right Ø4UV
Gastric Ø4U2
Hand
Left Ø3UF
Right Ø3UD
Hepatic Ø4U3
Inferior Mesenteric Ø4UB
Innominate Ø3U2
Internal Carotid
Left Ø3UL
Right Ø3UK
Internal Iliac
Left Ø4UF
Right Ø4UE
Internal Mammary
Left Ø3U1
Right Ø3UØ
Intracranial Ø3UG
Lower Ø4UY
Peroneal
Left Ø4UU
Right Ø4UT
Popliteal
Left Ø4UN
Right Ø4UM
Posterior Tibial
Left Ø4US
Right Ø4UR
Pulmonary
Left Ø2UR
Right Ø2UQ
Pulmonary Trunk Ø2UP
Radial
Left Ø3UC
Right Ø3UB
Renal
Left Ø4UA
Right Ø4U9
Splenic Ø4U4
Subclavian
Left Ø3U4
Right Ø3U3
Superior Mesenteric Ø4U5

Supplement — *continued*
Artery — *continued*
Temporal
Left Ø3UT
Right Ø3US
Thyroid
Left Ø3UV
Right Ø3UU
Ulnar
Left Ø3UA
Right Ø3U9
Upper Ø3UY
Vertebral
Left Ø3UQ
Right Ø3UP
Atrium
Left Ø2U7
Right Ø2U6
Auditory Ossicle
Left Ø9UA
Right Ø9U9
Axilla
Left ØXU5
Right ØXU4
Back
Lower ØWUL
Upper ØWUK
Bladder ØTUB
Bladder Neck ØTUC
Bone
Ethmoid
Left ØNUG
Right ØNUF
Frontal ØNU1
Hyoid ØNUX
Lacrimal
Left ØNUJ
Right ØNUH
Nasal ØNUB
Occipital ØNU7
Palatine
Left ØNUL
Right ØNUK
Parietal
Left ØNU4
Right ØNU3
Pelvic
Left ØQU3
Right ØQU2
Sphenoid ØNUC
Temporal
Left ØNU6
Right ØNU5
Zygomatic
Left ØNUN
Right ØNUM
Breast
Bilateral ØHUV
Left ØHUU
Right ØHUT
Bronchus
Lingula ØBU9
Lower Lobe
Left ØBUB
Right ØBU6
Main
Left ØBU7
Right ØBU3
Middle Lobe, Right ØBU5
Upper Lobe
Left ØBU8
Right ØBU4
Buccal Mucosa ØCU4
Bursa and Ligament
Abdomen
Left ØMUJ
Right ØMUH
Ankle
Left ØMUR
Right ØMUQ
Elbow
Left ØMU4
Right ØMU3
Foot
Left ØMUT
Right ØMUS
Hand
Left ØMU8
Right ØMU7

Supplement — *continued*
Bursa and Ligament — *continued*
Head and Neck ØMUØ
Hip
Left ØMUM
Right ØMUL
Knee
Left ØMUP
Right ØMUN
Lower Extremity
Left ØMUW
Right ØMUV
Perineum ØMUK
Rib(s) ØMUG
Shoulder
Left ØMU2
Right ØMU1
Spine
Lower ØMUD
Posterior Vertebral Tether XKU
Upper ØMUC
Sternum ØMUF
Upper Extremity
Left ØMUB
Right ØMU9
Wrist
Left ØMU6
Right ØMU5
Buttock
Left ØYU1
Right ØYUØ
Carina ØBU2
Carpal
Left ØPUN
Right ØPUM
Cecum ØDUH
Cerebral Meninges ØØU1
Cerebral Ventricle ØØU6
Chest Wall ØWU8
Chordae Tendineae Ø2U9
Cisterna Chyli Ø7UL
Clavicle
Left ØPUB
Right ØPU9
Clitoris ØUUJ
Coccyx ØQUS
Colon
Ascending ØDUK
Descending ØDUM
Sigmoid ØDUN
Transverse ØDUL
Cord
Bilateral ØVUH
Left ØVUG
Right ØVUF
Cornea
Left Ø8U9
Right Ø8U8
Coronary Artery/Arteries, Vein Graft Extraluminal Support Device(s) X2U4079
Cul-de-sac ØUUF
Diaphragm ØBUT
Disc
Cervical Vertebral ØRU3
Cervicothoracic Vertebral ØRU5
Lumbar Vertebral ØSU2
Lumbosacral ØSU4
Thoracic Vertebral ØRU9
Thoracolumbar Vertebral ØRUB
Duct
Common Bile ØFU9
Cystic ØFU8
Hepatic
Common ØFU7
Left ØFU6
Right ØFU5
Lacrimal
Left Ø8UY
Right Ø8UX
Pancreatic ØFUD
Accessory ØFUF
Duodenum ØDU9
Dura Mater ØØU2
Ear
External
Bilateral Ø9U2
Left Ø9U1
Right Ø9UØ

Supplement — *continued*
- Ear — *continued*
  - Inner
    - Left Ø9UE
    - Right Ø9UD
  - Middle
    - Left Ø9U6
    - Right Ø9U5
- Elbow Region
  - Left ØXUC
  - Right ØXUB
- Epididymis
  - Bilateral ØVUL
  - Left ØVUK
  - Right ØVUJ
- Epiglottis ØCUR
- Esophagogastric Junction ØDU4
- Esophagus ØDU5
  - Lower ØDU3
  - Middle ØDU2
  - Upper ØDU1
- Extremity
  - Lower
    - Left ØYUB
    - Right ØYU9
  - Upper
    - Left ØXU7
    - Right ØXU6
- Eye
  - Left Ø8U1
  - Right Ø8UØ
- Eyelid
  - Lower
    - Left Ø8UR
    - Right Ø8UQ
  - Upper
    - Left Ø8UP
    - Right Ø8UN
- Face ØWU2
- Fallopian Tube
  - Left ØUU6
  - Right ØUU5
- Fallopian Tubes, Bilateral ØUU7
- Femoral Region
  - Bilateral ØYUE
  - Left ØYU8
  - Right ØYU7
- Femoral Shaft
  - Left ØQU9
  - Right ØQU8
- Femur
  - Lower
    - Left ØQUC
    - Right ØQUB
  - Upper
    - Left ØQU7
    - Right ØQU6
- Fibula
  - Left ØQUK
  - Right ØQUJ
- Finger
  - Index
    - Left ØXUP
    - Right ØXUN
  - Little
    - Left ØXUW
    - Right ØXUV
  - Middle
    - Left ØXUR
    - Right ØXUQ
  - Ring
    - Left ØXUT
    - Right ØXUS
- Foot
  - Left ØYUN
  - Right ØYUM
- Gingiva
  - Lower ØCU6
  - Upper ØCU5
- Glenoid Cavity
  - Left ØPU8
  - Right ØPU7
- Hand
  - Left ØXUK
  - Right ØXUJ
- Head ØWUØ
- Heart Ø2UA
- Humeral Head
  - Left ØPUD

Supplement — *continued*
- Humeral Head — *continued*
  - Right ØPUC
- Humeral Shaft
  - Left ØPUG
  - Right ØPUF
- Hymen ØUUK
- Ileocecal Valve ØDUC
- Ileum ØDUB
- Inguinal Region
  - Bilateral ØYUA
  - Left ØYU6
  - Right ØYU5
- Intestine
  - Large ØDUE
    - Left ØDUG
    - Right ØDUF
  - Small ØDU8
- Iris
  - Left Ø8UD
  - Right Ø8UC
- Jaw
  - Lower ØWU5
  - Upper ØWU4
- Jejunum ØDUA
- Joint
  - Acromioclavicular
    - Left ØRUH
    - Right ØRUG
  - Ankle
    - Left ØSUG
    - Right ØSUF
  - Carpal
    - Left ØRUR
    - Right ØRUQ
  - Carpometacarpal
    - Left ØRUT
    - Right ØRUS
  - Cervical Vertebral ØRU1
  - Cervicothoracic Vertebral ØRU4
  - Coccygeal ØSU6
  - Elbow
    - Left ØRUM
    - Right ØRUL
  - Finger Phalangeal
    - Left ØRUX
    - Right ØRUW
  - Hip
    - Left ØSUB
      - Acetabular Surface ØSUE
      - Femoral Surface ØSUS
    - Right ØSU9
      - Acetabular Surface ØSUA
      - Femoral Surface ØSUR
  - Knee
    - Left ØSUD
      - Femoral Surface ØSUUØ9Z
      - Tibial Surface ØSUWØ9Z
    - Right ØSUC
      - Femoral Surface ØSUTØ9Z
      - Tibial Surface ØSUVØ9Z
  - Lumbar Vertebral ØSUØ
  - Lumbosacral ØSU3
  - Metacarpophalangeal
    - Left ØRUV
    - Right ØRUU
  - Metatarsal-Phalangeal
    - Left ØSUN
    - Right ØSUM
  - Occipital-cervical ØRUØ
  - Sacrococcygeal ØSU5
  - Sacroiliac
    - Left ØSU8
    - Right ØSU7
  - Shoulder
    - Left ØRUK
    - Right ØRUJ
  - Sternoclavicular
    - Left ØRUF
    - Right ØRUE
  - Tarsal
    - Left ØSUJ
    - Right ØSUH
  - Tarsometatarsal
    - Left ØSUL
    - Right ØSUK
  - Temporomandibular
    - Left ØRUD
    - Right ØRUC

Supplement — *continued*
- Joint — *continued*
  - Thoracic Vertebral ØRU6
  - Thoracolumbar Vertebral ØRUA
  - Toe Phalangeal
    - Left ØSUQ
    - Right ØSUP
  - Wrist
    - Left ØRUP
    - Right ØRUN
- Kidney Pelvis
  - Left ØTU4
  - Right ØTU3
- Knee Region
  - Left ØYUG
  - Right ØYUF
- Larynx ØCUS
- Leg
  - Lower
    - Left ØYUJ
    - Right ØYUH
  - Upper
    - Left ØYUD
    - Right ØYUC
- Lip
  - Lower ØCU1
  - Upper ØCUØ
- Lymphatic
  - Aortic Ø7UD
  - Axillary
    - Left Ø7U6
    - Right Ø7U5
  - Head Ø7UØ
  - Inguinal
    - Left Ø7UJ
    - Right Ø7UH
  - Internal Mammary
    - Left Ø7U9
    - Right Ø7U8
  - Lower Extremity
    - Left Ø7UG
    - Right Ø7UF
  - Mesenteric Ø7UB
  - Neck
    - Left Ø7U2
    - Right Ø7U1
  - Pelvis Ø7UC
  - Thoracic Duct Ø7UK
  - Thorax Ø7U7
  - Upper Extremity
    - Left Ø7U4
    - Right Ø7U3
- Mandible
  - Left ØNUV
  - Right ØNUT
- Maxilla ØNUR
- Mediastinum ØWUC
- Mesentery ØDUV
- Metacarpal
  - Left ØPUQ
  - Right ØPUP
- Metatarsal
  - Left ØQUP
  - Right ØQUN
- Muscle
  - Abdomen
    - Left ØKUL
    - Right ØKUK
  - Extraocular
    - Left Ø8UM
    - Right Ø8UL
  - Facial ØKU1
  - Foot
    - Left ØKUW
    - Right ØKUV
  - Hand
    - Left ØKUD
    - Right ØKUC
  - Head ØKUØ
  - Hip
    - Left ØKUP
    - Right ØKUN
  - Lower Arm and Wrist
    - Left ØKUB
    - Right ØKU9
  - Lower Leg
    - Left ØKUT
    - Right ØKUS

- **Supplement** — *continued*
  - Muscle — *continued*
    - Neck
      - Left ØKU3
      - Right ØKU2
    - Papillary Ø2UD
    - Perineum ØKUM
    - Shoulder
      - Left ØKU6
      - Right ØKU5
    - Thorax
      - Left ØKUJ
      - Right ØKUH
    - Tongue, Palate, Pharynx ØKU4
    - Trunk
      - Left ØKUG
      - Right ØKUF
    - Upper Arm
      - Left ØKU8
      - Right ØKU7
    - Upper Leg
      - Left ØKUR
      - Right ØKUQ
  - Nasal Mucosa and Soft Tissue Ø9UK
  - Nasopharynx Ø9UN
  - Neck ØWU6
  - Nerve
    - Abducens ØØUL
    - Accessory ØØUR
    - Acoustic ØØUN
    - Cervical Ø1U1
    - Facial ØØUM
    - Femoral Ø1UD
    - Glossopharyngeal ØØUP
    - Hypoglossal ØØUS
    - Lumbar Ø1UB
    - Median Ø1U5
    - Oculomotor ØØUH
    - Olfactory ØØUF
    - Optic ØØUG
    - Peroneal Ø1UH
    - Phrenic Ø1U2
    - Pudendal Ø1UC
    - Radial Ø1U6
    - Sacral Ø1UR
    - Sciatic Ø1UF
    - Thoracic Ø1U8
    - Tibial Ø1UG
    - Trigeminal ØØUK
    - Trochlear ØØUJ
    - Ulnar Ø1U4
    - Vagus ØØUQ
  - Nipple
    - Left ØHUX
    - Right ØHUW
  - Omentum ØDUU
  - Orbit
    - Left ØNUQ
    - Right ØNUP
  - Palate
    - Hard ØCU2
    - Soft ØCU3
  - Patella
    - Left ØQUF
    - Right ØQUD
  - Penis ØVUS
  - Pericardium Ø2UN
  - Perineum
    - Female ØWUN
    - Male ØWUM
  - Peritoneum ØDUW
  - Phalanx
    - Finger
      - Left ØPUV
      - Right ØPUT
    - Thumb
      - Left ØPUS
      - Right ØPUR
    - Toe
      - Left ØQUR
      - Right ØQUQ
  - Pharynx ØCUM
  - Prepuce ØVUT
  - Radius
    - Left ØPUJ
    - Right ØPUH
  - Rectum ØDUP
  - Retina
    - Left Ø8UF
- **Supplement** — *continued*
  - Retina — *continued*
    - Right Ø8UE
  - Retinal Vessel
    - Left Ø8UH
    - Right Ø8UG
  - Ribs
    - 1 to 2 ØPU1
    - 3 or More ØPU2
  - Sacrum ØQU1
  - Scapula
    - Left ØPU6
    - Right ØPU5
  - Scrotum ØVU5
  - Septum
    - Atrial Ø2U5
    - Nasal Ø9UM
    - Ventricular Ø2UM
  - Shoulder Region
    - Left ØXU3
    - Right ØXU2
  - Sinus
    - Accessory Ø9UP
    - Ethmoid
      - Left Ø9UV
      - Right Ø9UU
    - Frontal
      - Left Ø9UT
      - Right Ø9US
    - Mastoid
      - Left Ø9UC
      - Right Ø9UB
    - Maxillary
      - Left Ø9UR
      - Right Ø9UQ
    - Sphenoid
      - Left Ø9UX
      - Right Ø9UW
  - Skull ØNUØ
  - Spinal Meninges ØØUT
  - Sternum ØPUØ
  - Stomach ØDU6
    - Pylorus ØDU7
  - Subcutaneous Tissue and Fascia
    - Abdomen ØJU8
    - Back ØJU7
    - Buttock ØJU9
    - Chest ØJU6
    - Face ØJU1
    - Foot
      - Left ØJUR
      - Right ØJUQ
    - Hand
      - Left ØJUK
      - Right ØJUJ
    - Lower Arm
      - Left ØJUH
      - Right ØJUG
    - Lower Leg
      - Left ØJUP
      - Right ØJUN
    - Neck
      - Left ØJU5
      - Right ØJU4
    - Pelvic Region ØJUC
    - Perineum ØJUB
    - Scalp ØJUØ
    - Upper Arm
      - Left ØJUF
      - Right ØJUD
    - Upper Leg
      - Left ØJUM
      - Right ØJUL
  - Tarsal
    - Left ØQUM
    - Right ØQUL
  - Tendon
    - Abdomen
      - Left ØLUG
      - Right ØLUF
    - Ankle
      - Left ØLUT
      - Right ØLUS
    - Foot
      - Left ØLUW
      - Right ØLUV
    - Hand
      - Left ØLU8
      - Right ØLU7
- **Supplement** — *continued*
  - Tendon — *continued*
    - Head and Neck ØLUØ
    - Hip
      - Left ØLUK
      - Right ØLUJ
    - Knee
      - Left ØLUR
      - Right ØLUQ
    - Lower Arm and Wrist
      - Left ØLU6
      - Right ØLU5
    - Lower Leg
      - Left ØLUP
      - Right ØLUN
    - Perineum ØLUH
    - Shoulder
      - Left ØLU2
      - Right ØLU1
    - Thorax
      - Left ØLUD
      - Right ØLUC
    - Trunk
      - Left ØLUB
      - Right ØLU9
    - Upper Arm
      - Left ØLU4
      - Right ØLU3
    - Upper Leg
      - Left ØLUM
      - Right ØLUL
  - Testis
    - Bilateral ØVUCØ
    - Left ØVUBØ
    - Right ØVU9Ø
  - Thumb
    - Left ØXUM
    - Right ØXUL
  - Tibia
    - Left ØQUH
    - Right ØQUG
  - Toe
    - 1st
      - Left ØYUQ
      - Right ØYUP
    - 2nd
      - Left ØYUS
      - Right ØYUR
    - 3rd
      - Left ØYUU
      - Right ØYUT
    - 4th
      - Left ØYUW
      - Right ØYUV
    - 5th
      - Left ØYUY
      - Right ØYUX
  - Tongue ØCU7
  - Trachea ØBU1
  - Tunica Vaginalis
    - Left ØVU7
    - Right ØVU6
  - Turbinate, Nasal Ø9UL
  - Tympanic Membrane
    - Left Ø9U8
    - Right Ø9U7
  - Ulna
    - Left ØPUL
    - Right ØPUK
  - Ureter
    - Left ØTU7
    - Right ØTU6
  - Urethra ØTUD
  - Uterine Supporting Structure ØUU4
  - Uvula ØCUN
  - Vagina ØUUG
  - Valve
    - Aortic Ø2UF
    - Mitral Ø2UG
    - Pulmonary Ø2UH
    - Tricuspid Ø2UJ
  - Vas Deferens
    - Bilateral ØVUQ
    - Left ØVUP
    - Right ØVUN
  - Vein
    - Axillary
      - Left Ø5U8
      - Right Ø5U7

Subterms under main terms may continue to next column or page

Supplement — *continued*
Vein — *continued*
Azygos Ø5UØ
Basilic
Left Ø5UC
Right Ø5UB
Brachial
Left Ø5UA
Right Ø5U9
Cephalic
Left Ø5UF
Right Ø5UD
Colic Ø6U7
Common Iliac
Left Ø6UD
Right Ø6UC
Esophageal Ø6U3
External Iliac
Left Ø6UG
Right Ø6UF
External Jugular
Left Ø5UQ
Right Ø5UP
Face
Left Ø5UV
Right Ø5UT
Femoral
Left Ø6UN
Right Ø6UM
Foot
Left Ø6UV
Right Ø6UT
Gastric Ø6U2
Hand
Left Ø5UH
Right Ø5UG
Hemiazygos Ø5U1
Hepatic Ø6U4
Hypogastric
Left Ø6UJ
Right Ø6UH
Inferior Mesenteric Ø6U6
Innominate
Left Ø5U4
Right Ø5U3
Internal Jugular
Left Ø5UN
Right Ø5UM
Intracranial Ø5UL
Lower Ø6UY
Portal Ø6U8
Pulmonary
Left Ø2UT
Right Ø2US
Renal
Left Ø6UB
Right Ø6U9
Saphenous
Left Ø6UQ
Right Ø6UP
Splenic Ø6U1
Subclavian
Left Ø5U6
Right Ø5U5
Superior Mesenteric Ø6U5
Upper Ø5UY
Vertebral
Left Ø5US
Right Ø5UR
Vena Cava
Inferior Ø6UØ
Superior Ø2UV
Ventricle
Left Ø2UL
Right Ø2UK
Vertebra
Cervical ØPU3
Lumbar ØQUØ
Mechanically Expandable (Paired) Synthetic Substitute XNUØ356
Thoracic ØPU4
Mechanically Expandable (Paired) Synthetic Substitute XNU4356
Vesicle
Bilateral ØVU3
Left ØVU2
Right ØVU1
Vocal Cord
Left ØCUV

Supplement — *continued*
Vocal Cord — *continued*
Right ØCUT
Vulva ØUUM
Wrist Region
Left ØXUH
Right ØXUG
Supraclavicular (Virchow's) lymph node
use Lymphatic, Left Neck
use Lymphatic, Right Neck
Supraclavicular nerve *use* Cervical Plexus
Suprahyoid lymph node *use* Lymphatic, Head
Suprahyoid muscle
use Neck Muscle, Left
use Neck Muscle, Right
Suprainguinal lymph node *use* Lymphatic, Pelvis
Supraorbital vein
use Face Vein, Left
use Face Vein, Right
Suprarenal gland
use Adrenal Gland
use Adrenal Gland, Bilateral
use Adrenal Gland, Left
use Adrenal Gland, Right
Suprarenal plexus *use* Abdominal Sympathetic Nerve
Suprascapular nerve *use* Brachial Plexus
Supraspinatus fascia
use Subcutaneous Tissue and Fascia, Left Upper Arm
use Subcutaneous Tissue and Fascia, Right Upper Arm
Supraspinatus muscle
use Shoulder Muscle, Left
use Shoulder Muscle, Right
Supraspinous ligament
use Lower Spine Bursa and Ligament
use Upper Spine Bursa and Ligament
Suprasternal notch *use* Sternum
Supratrochlear lymph node
use Lymphatic, Left Upper Extremity
use Lymphatic, Right Upper Extremity
Sural artery
use Popliteal Artery, Left
use Popliteal Artery, Right
Surpass Streamline™ Flow Diverter *use* Intraluminal Device, Flow Diverter in Ø3V
Suspension
Bladder Neck *see* Reposition, Bladder Neck ØTSC
Kidney *see* Reposition, Urinary System ØTS
Urethra *see* Reposition, Urinary System ØTS
Urethrovesical *see* Reposition, Bladder Neck ØTSC
Uterus *see* Reposition, Uterus ØUS9
Vagina *see* Reposition, Vagina ØUSG
Sustained Release Drug-eluting Intraluminal Device
Dilation
Anterior Tibial
Left X27Q385
Right X27P385
Femoral
Left X27J385
Right X27H385
Peroneal
Left X27U385
Right X27T385
Popliteal
Left Distal X27N385
Left Proximal X27L385
Right Distal X27M385
Right Proximal X27K385
Posterior Tibial
Left X27S385
Right X27R385
Four or More
Anterior Tibial
Left X27Q3C5
Right X27P3C5
Femoral
Left X27J3C5
Right X27H3C5
Peroneal
Left X27U3C5
Right X27T3C5
Popliteal
Left Distal X27N3C5
Left Proximal X27L3C5
Right Distal X27M3C5

Sustained Release Drug-eluting Intraluminal Device — *continued*
Four or More — *continued*
Popliteal — *continued*
Right Proximal X27K3C5
Posterior Tibial
Left X27S3C5
Right X27R3C5
Three
Anterior Tibial
Left X27Q3B5
Right X27P3B5
Femoral
Left X27J3B5
Right X27H3B5
Peroneal
Left X27U3B5
Right X27T3B5
Popliteal
Left Distal X27N3B5
Left Proximal X27L3B5
Right Distal X27M3B5
Right Proximal X27K3B5
Posterior Tibial
Left X27S3B5
Right X27R3B5
Two
Anterior Tibial
Left X27Q395
Right X27P395
Femoral
Left X27J395
Right X27H395
Peroneal
Left X27U395
Right X27T395
Popliteal
Left Distal X27N395
Left Proximal X27L395
Right Distal X27M395
Right Proximal X27K395
Posterior Tibial
Left X27S395
Right X27R395
Suture
Laceration repair *see* Repair
Ligation *see* Occlusion
Suture Removal
Extremity
Lower 8EØYXY8
Upper 8EØXXY8
Head and Neck Region 8EØ9XY8
Trunk Region 8EØWXY8
Sutureless valve, Perceval (rapid deployment technique) *see* Replacement, Valve, Aortic Ø2RF
Sweat gland *use* Skin
Sympathectomy *see* Excision, Peripheral Nervous System Ø1B
SynCardia (temporary) total artificial heart (TAH) *use* Synthetic Substitute, Pneumatic in Ø2R
SynCardia Total Artificial Heart *use* Synthetic Substitute
Synchra CRT-P *use* Cardiac Resynchronization Pacemaker Pulse Generator in ØJH
SynchroMed pump *use* Infusion Device, Pump in Subcutaneous Tissue and Fascia
Synechiotomy, iris *see* Release, Eye Ø8N
Synovectomy
Lower joint *see* Excision, Lower Joints ØSB
Upper joint *see* Excision, Upper Joints ØRB
Systemic Nuclear Medicine Therapy
Abdomen CW7Ø
Anatomical Regions, Multiple CW7YYZZ
Chest CW73
Thyroid CW7G
Whole Body CW7N

T

tab-cel® *use* Tabelecleucel Immunotherapy
Tabelecleucel Immunotherapy XWØ
Tagraxofusp-erzs Antineoplastic XWØ
Takedown
Arteriovenous shunt *see* Removal of device from, Upper Arteries Ø3P
Arteriovenous shunt, with creation of new shunt *see* Bypass, Upper Arteries Ø31

Takedown — *continued*
Stoma
see Excision
see Reposition
Talent® Converter *use* Intraluminal Device
Talent® Occluder *use* Intraluminal Device
Talent® Stent Graft (abdominal) (thoracic) *use* Intraluminal Device
Talocalcaneal (subtalar) joint
use Tarsal Joint, Left
use Tarsal Joint, Right
Talocalcaneal ligament
use Foot Bursa and Ligament, Left
use Foot Bursa and Ligament, Right
Talocalcaneonavicular joint
use Tarsal Joint, Left
use Tarsal Joint, Right
Talocalcaneonavicular ligament
use Foot Bursa and Ligament, Left
use Foot Bursa and Ligament, Right
Talocrural joint
use Ankle Joint, Left
use Joint, Ankle, Right
Talofibular ligament
use Ankle Bursa and Ligament, Left
use Ankle Bursa and Ligament, Right
Talus bone
use Tarsal, Left
use Tarsal, Right
TandemHeart® System *use* Short-term External Heart Assist System in Heart and Great Vessels
Tarsectomy
see Excision, Lower Bones ØQB
see Resection, Lower Bones ØQT
Tarsometatarsal ligament
use Foot Bursa and Ligament, Left
use Foot Bursa and Ligament, Right
Tarsorrhaphy *see* Repair, Eye Ø8Q
Tattooing
Cornea 3EØCXMZ
Skin *see* Introduction of substance in or on, Skin 3EØØ
Taurolidine Anti-infective and Heparin Anticoagulant XYØYX28
TAXUS® Liberte® Paclitaxel-eluting Coronary Stent System *use* Intraluminal Device, Drug-eluting in Heart and Great Vessels
TBNA (transbronchial needle aspiration)
Fluid or gas *see* Drainage, Respiratory System ØB9
Tissue biopsy *see* Extraction, Respiratory System ØBD
Tecartus™ *use* Brexucabtagene Autoleucel Immunotherapy
TECENTRIQ® *use* Atezolizumab Antineoplastic
Teclistamab Antineoplastic XWØ1348
Telemetry 4A12X4Z
Ambulatory 4A12X45
Temperature gradient study 4AØZXKZ
Temporal lobe *use* Cerebral Hemisphere
Temporalis muscle *use* Head Muscle
Temporoparietalis muscle *use* Head Muscle
Tendolysis *see* Release, Tendons ØLN
Tendonectomy
see Excision, Tendons ØLB
see Resection, Tendons ØLT
Tendonoplasty, tenoplasty
see Repair, Tendons ØLQ
see Replacement, Tendons ØLR
see Supplement, Tendons ØLU
Tendorrhaphy *see* Repair, Tendons ØLQ
Tendototomy
see Division, Tendons ØL8
see Drainage, Tendons ØL9
Tenectomy, tenonectomy
see Excision, Tendons ØLB
see Resection, Tendons ØLT
Tenolysis *see* Release, Tendons ØLN
Tenontorrhaphy *see* Repair, Tendons ØLQ
Tenontotomy
see Division, Tendons ØL8
see Drainage, Tendons ØL9
Tenorrhaphy *see* Repair, Tendons ØLQ
Tenosynovectomy
see Excision, Tendons ØLB
see Resection, Tendons ØLT
Tenotomy
see Division, Tendons ØL8
see Drainage, Tendons ØL9
Tensor fasciae latae muscle
use Hip Muscle, Left
use Hip Muscle, Right
Tensor veli palatini muscle *use* Tongue, Palate, Pharynx Muscle
Tenth cranial nerve *use* Vagus Nerve
Tentorium cerebelli *use* Dura Mater
Teres major muscle
use Shoulder Muscle, Left
use Shoulder Muscle, Right
Teres minor muscle
use Shoulder Muscle, Left
use Shoulder Muscle, Right
Terlipressin XWØ
TERLIVAZ® *use* Terlipressin
Termination of pregnancy
Aspiration curettage 1ØAØ7ZZ
Dilation and curettage 1ØAØ7ZZ
Hysterotomy 1ØAØØZZ
Intra-amniotic injection 1ØAØ3ZZ
Laminaria 1ØAØ7ZW
Vacuum 1ØAØ7Z6
Testectomy
see Excision, Male Reproductive System ØVB
see Resection, Male Reproductive System ØVT
Testicular artery *use* Abdominal Aorta
Testing
Glaucoma 4AØ7XBZ
Hearing *see* Hearing Assessment, Diagnostic Audiology F13
Mental health *see* Psychological Tests
Muscle function, electromyography (EMG) *see* Measurement, Musculoskeletal 4AØF
Muscle function, manual *see* Motor Function Assessment, Rehabilitation FØ1
Neurophysiologic monitoring, intra-operative *see* Monitoring, Physiological Systems 4A1
Range of motion *see* Motor Function Assessment, Rehabilitation FØ1
Vestibular function *see* Vestibular Assessment, Diagnostic Audiology F15
Thalamectomy *see* Excision, Thalamus ØØB9
Thalamotomy *see* Drainage, Thalamus ØØ99
Thenar muscle
use Hand Muscle, Left
use Hand Muscle, Right
Therapeutic Massage
Musculoskeletal System 8EØKX1Z
Reproductive System
Prostate 8EØVX1C
Rectum 8EØVX1D
Therapeutic occlusion coil(s) *use* Intraluminal Device
Thermography 4AØZXKZ
Thermotherapy, prostate *see* Destruction, Prostate ØV5Ø
Third cranial nerve *use* Oculomotor Nerve
Third occipital nerve *use* Cervical Nerve
Third ventricle *use* Cerebral Ventricle
Thoracectomy *see* Excision, Anatomical Regions, General ØWB
Thoracentesis *see* Drainage, Anatomical Regions, General ØW9
Thoracic aortic plexus *use* Thoracic Sympathetic Nerve
Thoracic esophagus *use* Esophagus, Middle
Thoracic facet joint *use* Thoracic Vertebral Joint
Thoracic ganglion *use* Thoracic Sympathetic Nerve
Thoracoacromial artery
use Axillary Artery, Left
use Axillary Artery, Right
Thoracocentesis *see* Drainage, Anatomical Regions, General ØW9
Thoracolumbar facet joint *use* Thoracolumbar Vertebral Joint
Thoracoplasty
see Repair, Anatomical Regions, General ØWQ
see Supplement, Anatomical Regions, General ØWU
Thoracostomy, for lung collapse *see* Drainage, Respiratory System ØB9
Thoracostomy tube *use* Drainage Device
Thoracotomy *see* Drainage, Anatomical Regions, General ØW9
Thoraflex™ Hybrid device *use* Branched Synthetic Substitute with Intraluminal Device in New Technology
Thoratec IVAD (Implantable Ventricular Assist Device) *use* Implantable Heart Assist System in Heart and Great Vessels
Thoratec Paracorporeal Ventricular Assist Device *use* Short-term External Heart Assist System in Heart and Great Vessels
Thrombectomy *see* Extirpation
Thrombolysis, Ultrasound assisted *see* Fragmentation, Artery
Thymectomy
see Excision, Lymphatic and Hemic Systems Ø7B
see Resection, Lymphatic and Hemic Systems Ø7T
Thymopexy
see Repair, Lymphatic and Hemic Systems Ø7Q
see Reposition, Lymphatic and Hemic Systems Ø7S
Thymus gland *use* Thymus
Thyroarytenoid muscle
use Neck Muscle, Left
use Neck Muscle, Right
Thyrocervical trunk
use Thyroid Artery, Left
use Thyroid Artery, Right
Thyroid cartilage *use* Larynx
Thyroidectomy
see Excision, Endocrine System ØGB
see Resection, Endocrine System ØGT
Thyroidorrhaphy *see* Repair, Endocrine System ØGQ
Thyroidoscopy ØGJK4ZZ
Thyroidotomy *see* Drainage, Endocrine System ØG9
Tibial Extension with Motion Sensors, Insertion XNH
Tibial insert *use* Liner in Lower Joints
Tibial sesamoid
use Metatarsal, Left
use Metatarsal, Right
Tibialis anterior muscle
use Lower Leg Muscle, Left
use Lower Leg Muscle, Right
Tibialis posterior muscle
use Lower Leg Muscle, Left
use Lower Leg Muscle, Right
Tibiofemoral joint
use Knee Joint, Left
use Knee Joint, Right
use Knee Joint, Tibial Surface, Left
use Knee Joint, Tibial Surface, Right
Tibioperoneal trunk
use Popliteal Artery, Left
use Popliteal Artery, Right
Tisagenlecleucel *use* Tisagenlecleucel Immunotherapy
Tisagenlecleucel Immunotherapy XWØ
Tissue bank graft *use* Nonautologous Tissue Substitute
Tissue expander (inflatable) (injectable)
use Tissue Expander in Skin and Breast
use Tissue Expander in Subcutaneous Tissue and Fascia
Tissue Expander
Insertion of device in
Breast
Bilateral ØHHV
Left ØHHU
Right ØHHT
Nipple
Left ØHHX
Right ØHHW
Subcutaneous Tissue and Fascia
Abdomen ØJH8
Back ØJH7
Buttock ØJH9
Chest ØJH6
Face ØJH1
Foot
Left ØJHR
Right ØJHQ
Hand
Left ØJHK
Right ØJHJ
Lower Arm
Left ØJHH
Right ØJHG
Lower Leg
Left ØJHP
Right ØJHN
Neck
Left ØJH5
Right ØJH4
Pelvic Region ØJHC

Subterms under main terms may continue to next column or page

- **Tissue Expander** — *continued*
  - Insertion of device in — *continued*
    - Subcutaneous Tissue and Fascia — *continued*
      - Perineum ØJHB
      - Scalp ØJHØ
      - Upper Arm
        - Left ØJHF
        - Right ØJHD
      - Upper Leg
        - Left ØJHM
        - Right ØJHL
  - Removal of device from
    - Breast
      - Left ØHPU
      - Right ØHPT
    - Subcutaneous Tissue and Fascia
      - Head and Neck ØJPS
      - Lower Extremity ØJPW
      - Trunk ØJPT
      - Upper Extremity ØJPV
  - Revision of device in
    - Breast
      - Left ØHWU
      - Right ØHWT
    - Subcutaneous Tissue and Fascia
      - Head and Neck ØJWS
      - Lower Extremity ØJWW
      - Trunk ØJWT
      - Upper Extremity ØJWV
- **Tissue Plasminogen Activator (tPA) (r-tPA)** *use* Other Thrombolytic
- **Titan Endoskeleton™**
  - *use* Interbody Fusion Device in Lower Joints
  - *use* Interbody Fusion Device in Upper Joints
- **Titanium Sternal Fixation System (TSFS)**
  - *use* Internal Fixation Device, Rigid Plate in ØPS
  - *use* Internal Fixation Device, Rigid Plate in ØPH
- **Tixagevimab and Cilgavimab Monoclonal Antibody** XWØ23X7
- **Tocilizumab** XWØ
- **Tomographic (Tomo) Nuclear Medicine Imaging**
  - Abdomen CW2Ø
  - Abdomen and Chest CW24
  - Abdomen and Pelvis CW21
  - Anatomical Regions, Multiple CW2YYZZ
  - Bladder, Kidneys and Ureters CT23
  - Brain CØ2Ø
  - Breast CH2YYZZ
    - Bilateral CH22
    - Left CH21
    - Right CH2Ø
  - Bronchi and Lungs CB22
  - Central Nervous System CØ2YYZZ
  - Cerebrospinal Fluid CØ25
  - Chest CW23
  - Chest and Abdomen CW24
  - Chest and Neck CW26
  - Digestive System CD2YYZZ
  - Endocrine System CG2YYZZ
  - Extremity
    - Lower CW2D
      - Bilateral CP2F
      - Left CP2D
      - Right CP2C
    - Upper CW2M
      - Bilateral CP2B
      - Left CP29
      - Right CP28
  - Gallbladder CF24
  - Gastrointestinal Tract CD27
  - Gland, Parathyroid CG21
  - Head and Neck CW2B
  - Heart C22YYZZ
    - Right and Left C226
  - Hepatobiliary System and Pancreas CF2YYZZ
  - Kidneys, Ureters and Bladder CT23
  - Liver CF25
  - Liver and Spleen CF26
  - Lungs and Bronchi CB22
  - Lymphatics and Hematologic System C72YYZZ
  - Musculoskeletal System, Other CP2YYZZ
  - Myocardium C22G
  - Neck and Chest CW26
  - Neck and Head CW2B
  - Pancreas and Hepatobiliary System CF2YYZZ
  - Pelvic Region CW2J
  - Pelvis CP26
- **Tomographic (Tomo) Nuclear Medicine Imaging** — *continued*
  - Pelvis and Abdomen CW21
  - Pelvis and Spine CP27
  - Respiratory System CB2YYZZ
  - Skin CH2YYZZ
  - Skull CP21
  - Skull and Cervical Spine CP23
  - Spine
    - Cervical CP22
    - Cervical and Skull CP23
    - Lumbar CP2H
    - Thoracic CP2G
    - Thoracolumbar CP2J
  - Spine and Pelvis CP27
  - Spleen C722
  - Spleen and Liver CF26
  - Subcutaneous Tissue CH2YYZZ
  - Thorax CP24
  - Ureters, Kidneys and Bladder CT23
  - Urinary System CT2YYZZ
- **Tomography, computerized** *see* Computerized Tomography (CT Scan)
- **Tongue, base of** *use* Pharynx
- **Tonometry** 4AØ7XBZ
- **Tonsillectomy**
  - *see* Excision, Mouth and Throat ØCB
  - *see* Resection, Mouth and Throat ØCT
- **Tonsillotomy** *see* Drainage, Mouth and Throat ØC9
- **TOPS™ System** *use* Posterior Spinal Motion Preservation Device in New Technology
- **Total Ankle Talar Replacement™ (TATR)** *use* Synthetic Substitute, Talar Prosthesis in New Technology
- **Total Anomalous Pulmonary Venous Return (TAPVR) repair**
  - *see* Bypass, Atrium, Left Ø217
  - *see* Bypass, Vena Cava, Superior Ø21V
- **Total artificial (replacement) heart** *use* Synthetic Substitute
- **Total parenteral nutrition (TPN)** *see* Introduction of Nutritional Substance
- **Tourniquet, External** *see* Compression, Anatomical Regions 2W1
- **Trachectomy**
  - *see* Excision, Trachea ØBB1
  - *see* Resection, Trachea ØBT1
- **Trachelectomy**
  - *see* Excision, Cervix ØUBC
  - *see* Resection, Cervix ØUTC
- **Trachelopexy**
  - *see* Repair, Cervix ØUQC
  - *see* Reposition, Cervix ØUSC
- **Tracheloplasty** *see* Repair, Cervix ØUQC
- **Trachelorrhaphy** *see* Repair, Cervix ØUQC
- **Trachelotomy** *see* Drainage, Cervix ØU9C
- **Tracheobronchial lymph node** *use* Lymphatic, Thorax
- **Tracheoesophageal fistulization** ØB11ØD6
- **Tracheolysis** *see* Release, Respiratory System ØBN
- **Tracheoplasty**
  - *see* Repair, Respiratory System ØBQ
  - *see* Supplement, Respiratory System ØBU
- **Tracheorrhaphy** *see* Repair, Respiratory System ØBQ
- **Tracheoscopy** ØBJ18ZZ
- **Tracheostomy** *see* Bypass, Respiratory System ØB1
- **Tracheostomy Device**
  - Bypass, Trachea ØB11
  - Change device in, Trachea ØB21XFZ
  - Removal of device from, Trachea ØBP1
  - Revision of device in, Trachea ØBW1
- **Tracheostomy tube** *use* Tracheostomy Device in Respiratory System
- **Tracheotomy** *see* Drainage, Respiratory System ØB9
- **Traction**
  - Abdominal Wall 2W63X
  - Arm
    - Lower
      - Left 2W6DX
      - Right 2W6CX
    - Upper
      - Left 2W6BX
      - Right 2W6AX
  - Back 2W65X
  - Chest Wall 2W64X
  - Extremity
    - Lower
      - Left 2W6MX
      - Right 2W6LX
- **Traction** — *continued*
  - Extremity — *continued*
    - Upper
      - Left 2W69X
      - Right 2W68X
  - Face 2W61X
  - Finger
    - Left 2W6KX
    - Right 2W6JX
  - Foot
    - Left 2W6TX
    - Right 2W6SX
  - Hand
    - Left 2W6FX
    - Right 2W6EX
  - Head 2W6ØX
  - Inguinal Region
    - Left 2W67X
    - Right 2W66X
  - Leg
    - Lower
      - Left 2W6RX
      - Right 2W6QX
    - Upper
      - Left 2W6PX
      - Right 2W6NX
  - Neck 2W62X
  - Thumb
    - Left 2W6HX
    - Right 2W6GX
  - Toe
    - Left 2W6VX
    - Right 2W6UX
- **Tractotomy** *see* Division, Central Nervous System and Cranial Nerves ØØ8
- **Tragus**
  - *use* External Ear, Bilateral
  - *use* External Ear, Left
  - *use* External Ear, Right
- **Training, caregiver** *see* Caregiver Training
- **TRAM (transverse rectus abdominis myocutaneous) flap reconstruction**
  - Free *see* Replacement, Skin and Breast ØHR
  - Pedicled *see* Transfer, Muscles ØKX
- **Transcatheter Pulmonary Valve (TPV) placement**
  - In conduit Ø2RH38L
  - Native site Ø2RH38M
- **Transdermal Glomerular Filtration Rate (GFR) Measurement System** XT25XE5
- **Transection** *see* Division
- **Transfer**
  - Buccal Mucosa ØCX4
  - Bursa and Ligament
    - Abdomen
      - Left ØMXJ
      - Right ØMXH
    - Ankle
      - Left ØMXR
      - Right ØMXQ
    - Elbow
      - Left ØMX4
      - Right ØMX3
    - Foot
      - Left ØMXT
      - Right ØMXS
    - Hand
      - Left ØMX8
      - Right ØMX7
    - Head and Neck ØMXØ
    - Hip
      - Left ØMXM
      - Right ØMXL
    - Knee
      - Left ØMXP
      - Right ØMXN
    - Lower Extremity
      - Left ØMXW
      - Right ØMXV
    - Perineum ØMXK
    - Rib(s) ØMXG
    - Shoulder
      - Left ØMX2
      - Right ØMX1
    - Spine
      - Lower ØMXD
      - Upper ØMXC
    - Sternum ØMXF

Transfer — *continued*
Bursa and Ligament — *continued*
Upper Extremity
Left ØMXB
Right ØMX9
Wrist
Left ØMX6
Right ØMX5
Finger
Left ØXXPØZM
Right ØXXNØZL
Gingiva
Lower ØCX6
Upper ØCX5
Intestine
Large ØDXE
Small ØDX8
Lip
Lower ØCX1
Upper ØCXØ
Muscle
Abdomen
Left ØKXL
Right ØKXK
Extraocular
Left Ø8XM
Right Ø8XL
Facial ØKX1
Foot
Left ØKXW
Right ØKXV
Hand
Left ØKXD
Right ØKXC
Head ØKXØ
Hip
Left ØKXP
Right ØKXN
Lower Arm and Wrist
Left ØKXB
Right ØKX9
Lower Leg
Left ØKXT
Right ØKXS
Neck
Left ØKX3
Right ØKX2
Perineum ØKXM
Shoulder
Left ØKX6
Right ØKX5
Thorax
Left ØKXJ
Right ØKXH
Tongue, Palate, Pharynx ØKX4
Trunk
Left ØKXG
Right ØKXF
Upper Arm
Left ØKX8
Right ØKX7
Upper Leg
Left ØKXR
Right ØKXQ
Nerve
Abducens ØØXL
Accessory ØØXR
Acoustic ØØXN
Cervical Ø1X1
Facial ØØXM
Femoral Ø1XD
Glossopharyngeal ØØXP
Hypoglossal ØØXS
Lumbar Ø1XB
Median Ø1X5
Oculomotor ØØXH
Olfactory ØØXF
Optic ØØXG
Peroneal Ø1XH
Phrenic Ø1X2
Pudendal Ø1XC
Radial Ø1X6
Sciatic Ø1XF
Thoracic Ø1X8
Tibial Ø1XG
Trigeminal ØØXK
Trochlear ØØXJ
Ulnar Ø1X4
Vagus ØØXQ

Transfer — *continued*
Palate, Soft ØCX3
Prepuce ØVXT
Skin
Abdomen ØHX7XZZ
Back ØHX6XZZ
Buttock ØHX8XZZ
Chest ØHX5XZZ
Ear
Left ØHX3XZZ
Right ØHX2XZZ
Face ØHX1XZZ
Foot
Left ØHXNXZZ
Right ØHXMXZZ
Hand
Left ØHXGXZZ
Right ØHXFXZZ
Inguinal ØHXAXZZ
Lower Arm
Left ØHXEXZZ
Right ØHXDXZZ
Lower Leg
Left ØHXLXZZ
Right ØHXKXZZ
Neck ØHX4XZZ
Perineum ØHX9XZZ
Scalp ØHXØXZZ
Upper Arm
Left ØHXCXZZ
Right ØHXBXZZ
Upper Leg
Left ØHXJXZZ
Right ØHXHXZZ
Stomach ØDX6
Subcutaneous Tissue and Fascia
Abdomen ØJX8
Back ØJX7
Buttock ØJX9
Chest ØJX6
Face ØJX1
Foot
Left ØJXR
Right ØJXQ
Hand
Left ØJXK
Right ØJXJ
Lower Arm
Left ØJXH
Right ØJXG
Lower Leg
Left ØJXP
Right ØJXN
Neck
Left ØJX5
Right ØJX4
Pelvic Region ØJXC
Perineum ØJXB
Scalp ØJXØ
Upper Arm
Left ØJXF
Right ØJXD
Upper Leg
Left ØJXM
Right ØJXL
Tendon
Abdomen
Left ØLXG
Right ØLXF
Ankle
Left ØLXT
Right ØLXS
Foot
Left ØLXW
Right ØLXV
Hand
Left ØLX8
Right ØLX7
Head and Neck ØLXØ
Hip
Left ØLXK
Right ØLXJ
Knee
Left ØLXR
Right ØLXQ
Lower Arm and Wrist
Left ØLX6
Right ØLX5

Transfer — *continued*
Tendon — *continued*
Lower Leg
Left ØLXP
Right ØLXN
Perineum ØLXH
Shoulder
Left ØLX2
Right ØLX1
Thorax
Left ØLXD
Right ØLXC
Trunk
Left ØLXB
Right ØLX9
Upper Arm
Left ØLX4
Right ØLX3
Upper Leg
Left ØLXM
Right ØLXL
Tongue ØCX7
Transfusion
Bone Marrow
Blood
Platelets 3Ø2A3R
Red Cells 3Ø2A3N
Frozen 3Ø2A3P
Whole 3Ø2A3H
Plasma
Fresh 3Ø2A3L
Frozen 3Ø2A3K
Serum Albumin 3Ø2A3J
New Technology *see* New Technology, Anatomical Regions XW1
Products of Conception
Antihemophilic Factors 3Ø27
Blood
Platelets 3Ø27
Red Cells 3Ø27
Frozen 3Ø27
White Cells 3Ø27
Whole 3Ø27
Factor IX 3Ø27
Fibrinogen 3Ø27
Globulin 3Ø27
Plasma
Fresh 3Ø27
Frozen 3Ø27
Plasma Cryoprecipitate 3Ø27
Serum Albumin 3Ø27
Vein
4-Factor Prothrombin Complex Concentrate 3Ø283B1
Central
Antihemophilic Factors 3Ø243V
Blood
Platelets 3Ø243R
Red Cells 3Ø243N
Frozen 3Ø243P
White Cells 3Ø243Q
Whole 3Ø243H
Bone Marrow 3Ø243G
Factor IX 3Ø243W
Fibrinogen 3Ø243T
Globulin 3Ø243S
Hematopoietic Stem/Progenitor Cells (HSPC), Genetically Modified 3Ø243CØ
Pathogen Reduced Cryoprecipitated Fibrinogen Complex 3Ø243D1
Plasma
Fresh 3Ø243L
Frozen 3Ø243K
Plasma Cryoprecipitate 3Ø243M
Serum Albumin 3Ø243J
Stem Cells
Cord Blood 3Ø243X
Embryonic 3Ø243AZ
Hematopoietic 3Ø243Y
T-cell Depleted Hematopoietic 3Ø243U
Peripheral
Antihemophilic Factors 3Ø233V
Blood
Platelets 3Ø233R
Red Cells 3Ø233N
Frozen 3Ø233P
White Cells 3Ø233Q

Transfusion — *continued*
Vein — *continued*
Peripheral — *continued*
Blood — *continued*
Whole 30233H
Bone Marrow 30233G
Factor IX 30233W
Fibrinogen 30233T
Globulin 30233S
Hematopoietic Stem/Progenitor Cells (HSPC), Genetically Modified 30233C0
Pathogen Reduced Cryoprecipitated Fibrinogen Complex 30233D1
Plasma
Fresh 30233L
Frozen 30233K
Plasma Cryoprecipitate 30233M
Serum Albumin 30233J
Stem Cells
Cord Blood 30233X
Embryonic 30233AZ
Hematopoietic 30233Y
T-cell Depleted Hematopoietic 30233U
Transplant *see* Transplantation
Transplantation
Bone marrow *see* Transfusion, Circulatory 302
Esophagus 0DY50Z
Face 0WY20Z
Hand
Left 0XYK0Z
Right 0XYJ0Z
Heart 02YA0Z
Hematopoietic cell *see* Transfusion, Circulatory 302
Intestine
Large 0DYE0Z
Small 0DY80Z
Kidney
Left 0TY10Z
Right 0TY00Z
Liver 0FY00Z
Lung
Bilateral 0BYM0Z
Left 0BYL0Z
Lower Lobe
Left 0BYJ0Z
Right 0BYF0Z
Middle Lobe, Right 0BYD0Z
Right 0BYK0Z
Upper Lobe
Left 0BYG0Z
Right 0BYC0Z
Lung Lingula 0BYH0Z
Ovary
Left 0UY10Z
Right 0UY00Z
Pancreas 0FYG0Z
Penis 0VYS0Z
Products of Conception 10Y0
Scrotum 0VY50Z
Spleen 07YP0Z
Stem cell *see* Transfusion, Circulatory 302
Stomach 0DY60Z
Thymus 07YM0Z
Uterus 0UY90Z
Transposition
see Bypass
see Reposition
see Transfer
Transversalis fascia *use* Subcutaneous Tissue and Fascia, Trunk
Transverse acetabular ligament
use Hip Bursa and Ligament, Left
use Hip Bursa and Ligament, Right
Transverse (cutaneous) cervical nerve *use* Cervical Plexus
Transverse facial artery
use Temporal Artery, Left
use Temporal Artery, Right
Transverse foramen *use* Cervical Vertebra
Transverse humeral ligament
use Shoulder Bursa and Ligament, Left
use Shoulder Bursa and Ligament, Right
Transverse ligament of atlas *use* Head and Neck Bursa and Ligament
Transverse process
use Cervical Vertebra
use Lumbar Vertebra
use Thoracic Vertebra
Transverse Rectus Abdominis Myocutaneous Flap
Replacement
Bilateral 0HRV076
Left 0HRU076
Right 0HRT076
Transfer
Left 0KXL
Right 0KXK
Transverse scapular ligament
use Shoulder Bursa and Ligament, Left
use Shoulder Bursa and Ligament, Right
Transverse thoracis muscle
use Thorax Muscle, Left
use Thorax Muscle, Right
Transversospinalis muscle
use Trunk Muscle, Left
use Trunk Muscle, Right
Transversus abdominis muscle
use Abdomen Muscle, Left
use Abdomen Muscle, Right
Trapezium bone
use Carpal, Left
use Carpal, Right
Trapezius muscle
use Trunk Muscle, Left
use Trunk Muscle, Right
Trapezoid bone
use Carpal, Left
use Carpal, Right
Treosulfan XW0
Triceps brachii muscle
use Upper Arm Muscle, Left
use Upper Arm Muscle, Right
Tricuspid annulus *use* Tricuspid Valve
TricValve® Transcatheter Bicaval Valve System *use* Intraluminal Device, Bioprosthetic Valve in New Technology
Trifacial nerve *use* Trigeminal Nerve
Trifecta™ Valve (aortic) *use* Zooplastic Tissue in Heart and Great Vessels
Trigone of bladder *use* Bladder
TriGuard 3™ CEPD (cerebral embolic protection device) X2A6325
Trilaciclib XW0
Trimming, excisional *see* Excision
Triquetral bone
use Carpal, Left
use Carpal, Right
Trochanteric bursa
use Hip Bursa and Ligament, Left
use Hip Bursa and Ligament, Right
TUMT (transurethral microwave thermotherapy of prostate) 0V507ZZ
TUNA (transurethral needle ablation of prostate) 0V507ZZ
Tunneled central venous catheter *use* Vascular Access Device, Tunneled in Subcutaneous Tissue and Fascia
Tunneled spinal (intrathecal) catheter *use* Infusion Device
Turbinectomy
see Excision, Ear, Nose, Sinus 09B
see Resection, Ear, Nose, Sinus 09T
Turbinoplasty
see Repair, Ear, Nose, Sinus 09Q
see Replacement, Ear, Nose, Sinus 09R
see Supplement, Ear, Nose, Sinus 09U
Turbinotomy
see Division, Ear, Nose, Sinus 098
see Drainage, Ear, Nose, Sinus 099
TURP (transurethral resection of prostate) 0VB07ZZ
see Excision, Prostate 0VB0
see Resection, Prostate 0VT0
Twelfth cranial nerve *use* Hypoglossal Nerve
Two lead pacemaker *use* Pacemaker, Dual Chamber in 0JH
Tympanic cavity
use Middle Ear, Left
use Middle Ear, Right
Tympanic nerve *use* Glossopharyngeal Nerve
Tympanic part of temporal bone
use Temporal Bone, Left
Tympanic part of temporal bone — *continued*
use Temporal Bone, Right
Tympanogram *see* Hearing Assessment, Diagnostic Audiology F13
Tympanoplasty
see Repair, Ear, Nose, Sinus 09Q
see Replacement, Ear, Nose, Sinus 09R
see Supplement, Ear, Nose, Sinus 09U
Tympanosympathectomy *see* Excision, Nerve, Head and Neck Sympathetic 01BK
Tympanotomy *see* Drainage, Ear, Nose, Sinus 099
TYRX Antibacterial Envelope *use* Anti-Infective Envelope

U

Ulnar collateral carpal ligament
use Wrist Bursa and Ligament, Left
use Wrist Bursa and Ligament, Right
Ulnar collateral ligament
use Elbow Bursa and Ligament, Left
use Elbow Bursa and Ligament, Right
Ulnar notch
use Radius, Left
use Radius, Right
Ulnar vein
use Brachial Vein, Left
use Brachial Vein, Right
Ultrafiltration
Hemodialysis *see* Performance, Urinary 5A1D
Therapeutic plasmapheresis *see* Pheresis, Circulatory 6A55
Ultraflex™ Precision Colonic Stent System *use* Intraluminal Device
ULTRAPRO Hernia System (UHS) *use* Synthetic Substitute
ULTRAPRO Partially Absorbable Lightweight Mesh *use* Synthetic Substitute
ULTRAPRO Plug *use* Synthetic Substitute
Ultrasonic osteogenic stimulator
use Bone Growth Stimulator in Head and Facial Bones
use Bone Growth Stimulator in Lower Bones
use Bone Growth Stimulator in Upper Bones
Ultrasonography
Abdomen BW40ZZZ
Abdomen and Pelvis BW41ZZZ
Abdominal Wall BH49ZZZ
Aorta
Abdominal, Intravascular B440ZZ3
Thoracic, Intravascular B340ZZ3
Appendix BD48ZZZ
Artery
Brachiocephalic-Subclavian, Right, Intravascular B341ZZ3
Celiac and Mesenteric, Intravascular B44KZZ3
Common Carotid
Bilateral, Intravascular B345ZZ3
Left, Intravascular B344ZZ3
Right, Intravascular B343ZZ3
Coronary
Multiple B241YZZ
Intravascular B241ZZ3
Transesophageal B241ZZ4
Single B240YZZ
Intravascular B240ZZ3
Transesophageal B240ZZ4
Femoral, Intravascular B44LZZ3
Inferior Mesenteric, Intravascular B445ZZ3
Internal Carotid
Bilateral, Intravascular B348ZZ3
Left, Intravascular B347ZZ3
Right, Intravascular B346ZZ3
Intra-Abdominal, Other, Intravascular B44BZZ3
Intracranial, Intravascular B34RZZ3
Lower Extremity
Bilateral, Intravascular B44HZZ3
Left, Intravascular B44GZZ3
Right, Intravascular B44FZZ3
Mesenteric and Celiac, Intravascular B44KZZ3
Ophthalmic, Intravascular B34VZZ3
Penile, Intravascular B44NZZ3
Pulmonary
Left, Intravascular B34TZZ3
Right, Intravascular B34SZZ3

- **Ultrasonography** — *continued*
  - Artery — *continued*
    - Renal
      - Bilateral, Intravascular B448ZZ3
      - Left, Intravascular B447ZZ3
      - Right, Intravascular B446ZZ3
    - Subclavian, Left, Intravascular B342ZZ3
    - Superior Mesenteric, Intravascular B444ZZ3
    - Upper Extremity
      - Bilateral, Intravascular B34KZZ3
      - Left, Intravascular B34JZZ3
      - Right, Intravascular B34HZZ3
  - Bile Duct BF4ØZZZ
  - Bile Duct and Gallbladder BF43ZZZ
  - Bladder BT4ØZZZ
    - and Kidney BT4JZZZ
  - Brain BØ4ØZZZ
  - Breast
    - Bilateral BH42ZZZ
    - Left BH41ZZZ
    - Right BH4ØZZZ
  - Chest Wall BH4BZZZ
  - Coccyx BR4FZZZ
  - Connective Tissue
    - Lower Extremity BL41ZZZ
    - Upper Extremity BL4ØZZZ
  - Duodenum BD49ZZZ
  - Elbow
    - Left, Densitometry BP4HZZ1
    - Right, Densitometry BP4GZZ1
  - Esophagus BD41ZZZ
  - Extremity
    - Lower BH48ZZZ
    - Upper BH47ZZZ
  - Eye
    - Bilateral B847ZZZ
    - Left B846ZZZ
    - Right B845ZZZ
  - Fallopian Tube
    - Bilateral BU42
    - Left BU41
    - Right BU4Ø
  - Fetal Umbilical Cord BY47ZZZ
  - Fetus
    - First Trimester, Multiple Gestation BY4BZZZ
    - Second Trimester, Multiple Gestation BY4DZZZ
    - Single
      - First Trimester BY49ZZZ
      - Second Trimester BY4CZZZ
      - Third Trimester BY4FZZZ
    - Third Trimester, Multiple Gestation BY4GZZZ
  - Gallbladder BF42ZZZ
  - Gallbladder and Bile Duct BF43ZZZ
  - Gastrointestinal Tract BD47ZZZ
  - Gland
    - Adrenal
      - Bilateral BG42ZZZ
      - Left BG41ZZZ
      - Right BG4ØZZZ
    - Parathyroid BG43ZZZ
    - Thyroid BG44ZZZ
  - Hand
    - Left, Densitometry BP4PZZ1
    - Right, Densitometry BP4NZZ1
  - Head and Neck BH4CZZZ
  - Heart
    - Left B245YZZ
      - Intravascular B245ZZ3
      - Transesophageal B245ZZ4
    - Pediatric B24DYZZ
      - Intravascular B24DZZ3
      - Transesophageal B24DZZ4
    - Right B244YZZ
      - Intravascular B244ZZ3
      - Transesophageal B244ZZ4
    - Right and Left B246YZZ
      - Intravascular B246ZZ3
      - Transesophageal B246ZZ4
  - Heart with Aorta B24BYZZ
    - Intravascular B24BZZ3
    - Transesophageal B24BZZ4
  - Hepatobiliary System, All BF4CZZZ
  - Hip
    - Bilateral BQ42ZZZ
    - Left BQ41ZZZ
    - Right BQ4ØZZZ
  - Kidney
    - and Bladder BT4JZZZ
- **Ultrasonography** — *continued*
  - Kidney — *continued*
    - Bilateral BT43ZZZ
    - Left BT42ZZZ
    - Right BT41ZZZ
    - Transplant BT49ZZZ
  - Knee
    - Bilateral BQ49ZZZ
    - Left BQ48ZZZ
    - Right BQ47ZZZ
  - Liver BF45ZZZ
  - Liver and Spleen BF46ZZZ
  - Mediastinum BB4CZZZ
  - Neck BW4FZZZ
  - Ovary
    - Bilateral BU45
    - Left BU44
    - Right BU43
  - Ovary and Uterus BU4C
  - Pancreas BF47ZZZ
  - Pelvic Region BW4GZZZ
  - Pelvis and Abdomen BW41ZZZ
  - Penis BV4BZZZ
  - Pericardium B24CYZZ
    - Intravascular B24CZZ3
    - Transesophageal B24CZZ4
  - Placenta BY48ZZZ
  - Pleura BB4BZZZ
  - Prostate and Seminal Vesicle BV49ZZZ
  - Rectum BD4CZZZ
  - Sacrum BR4FZZZ
  - Scrotum BV44ZZZ
  - Seminal Vesicle and Prostate BV49ZZZ
  - Shoulder
    - Left, Densitometry BP49ZZ1
    - Right, Densitometry BP48ZZ1
  - Spinal Cord BØ4BZZZ
  - Spine
    - Cervical BR4ØZZZ
    - Lumbar BR49ZZZ
    - Thoracic BR47ZZZ
  - Spleen and Liver BF46ZZZ
  - Stomach BD42ZZZ
  - Tendon
    - Lower Extremity BL43ZZZ
    - Upper Extremity BL42ZZZ
  - Ureter
    - Bilateral BT48ZZZ
    - Left BT47ZZZ
    - Right BT46ZZZ
  - Urethra BT45ZZZ
  - Uterus BU46
  - Uterus and Ovary BU4C
  - Vein
    - Jugular
      - Left, Intravascular B544ZZ3
      - Right, Intravascular B543ZZ3
    - Lower Extremity
      - Bilateral, Intravascular B54DZZ3
      - Left, Intravascular B54CZZ3
      - Right, Intravascular B54BZZ3
    - Portal, Intravascular B54TZZ3
    - Renal
      - Bilateral, Intravascular B54LZZ3
      - Left, Intravascular B54KZZ3
      - Right, Intravascular B54JZZ3
    - Spanchnic, Intravascular B54TZZ3
    - Subclavian
      - Left, Intravascular B547ZZ3
      - Right, Intravascular B546ZZ3
    - Upper Extremity
      - Bilateral, Intravascular B54PZZ3
      - Left, Intravascular B54NZZ3
      - Right, Intravascular B54MZZ3
  - Vena Cava
    - Inferior, Intravascular B549ZZ3
    - Superior, Intravascular B548ZZ3
  - Wrist
    - Left, Densitometry BP4MZZ1
    - Right, Densitometry BP4LZZ1
- **Ultrasound Ablation, Destruction, Renal Sympathetic Nerve(s)** XØ51329
- **Ultrasound bone healing system**
  - *use* Bone Growth Stimulator in Head and Facial Bones
  - *use* Bone Growth Stimulator in Lower Bones
  - *use* Bone Growth Stimulator in Upper Bones
- **Ultrasound Penetrable Synthetic Substitute, Skull** XNR8ØD9
- **Ultrasound Therapy**
  - Heart 6A75
  - No Qualifier 6A75
  - Vessels
    - Head and Neck 6A75
    - Other 6A75
    - Peripheral 6A75
- **Ultraviolet Light Therapy, Skin** 6A8Ø
- **Umbilical artery**
  - *use* Internal Iliac Artery, Left
  - *use* Internal Iliac Artery, Right
  - *use* Lower Artery
- **Uniplanar external fixator**
  - *use* External Fixation Device, Monoplanar in ØPH
  - *use* External Fixation Device, Monoplanar in ØPS
  - *use* External Fixation Device, Monoplanar in ØQH
  - *use* External Fixation Device, Monoplanar in ØQS
- **UPLIZNA®** *use* Inebilizumab-cdon
- **Upper GI series** *see* Fluoroscopy, Gastrointestinal, Upper BD15
- **Ureteral orifice**
  - *use* Ureter
  - *use* Ureter, Left
  - *use* Ureter, Right
  - *use* Ureters, Bilateral
- **Ureterectomy**
  - *see* Excision, Urinary System ØTB
  - *see* Resection, Urinary System ØTT
- **Ureterocolostomy** *see* Bypass, Urinary System ØT1
- **Ureterocystostomy** *see* Bypass, Urinary System ØT1
- **Ureteroenterostomy** *see* Bypass, Urinary System ØT1
- **Ureteroileostomy** *see* Bypass, Urinary System ØT1
- **Ureterolithotomy** *see* Extirpation, Urinary System ØTC
- **Ureterolysis** *see* Release, Urinary System ØTN
- **Ureteroneocystostomy**
  - *see* Bypass, Urinary System ØT1
  - *see* Reposition, Urinary System ØTS
- **Ureteropelvic junction (UPJ)**
  - *use* Kidney Pelvis, Left
  - *use* Kidney Pelvis, Right
- **Ureteropexy**
  - *see* Repair, Urinary System ØTQ
  - *see* Reposition, Urinary System ØTS
- **Ureteroplasty**
  - *see* Repair, Urinary System ØTQ
  - *see* Replacement, Urinary System ØTR
  - *see* Supplement, Urinary System ØTU
- **Ureteroplication** *see* Restriction, Urinary System ØTV
- **Ureteropyelography** *see* Fluoroscopy, Urinary System BT1
- **Ureterorrhaphy** *see* Repair, Urinary System ØTQ
- **Ureteroscopy** ØTJ98ZZ
- **Ureterostomy**
  - *see* Bypass, Urinary System ØT1
  - *see* Drainage, Urinary System ØT9
- **Ureterotomy** *see* Drainage, Urinary System ØT9
- **Ureteroureterostomy** *see* Bypass, Urinary System ØT1
- **Ureterovesical orifice**
  - *use* Ureter
  - *use* Ureter, Left
  - *use* Ureter, Right
  - *use* Ureters, Bilateral
- **Urethral catheterization, indwelling** ØT9B7ØZ
- **Urethrectomy**
  - *see* Excision, Urethra ØTBD
  - *see* Resection, Urethra ØTTD
- **Urethrolithotomy** *see* Extirpation, Urethra ØTCD
- **Urethrolysis** *see* Release, Urethra ØTND
- **Urethropexy**
  - *see* Repair, Urethra ØTQD
  - *see* Reposition, Urethra ØTSD
- **Urethroplasty**
  - *see* Repair, Urethra ØTQD
  - *see* Replacement, Urethra ØTRD
  - *see* Supplement, Urethra ØTUD
- **Urethrorrhaphy** *see* Repair, Urethra ØTQD
- **Urethroscopy** ØTJD8ZZ
- **Urethrotomy** *see* Drainage, Urethra ØT9D
- **Uridine Triacetate** XWØDX82
- **Urinary incontinence stimulator lead** *use* Stimulator Lead in Urinary System
- **Urography** *see* Fluoroscopy, Urinary System BT1
- **Ustekinumab** *use* Other New Technology Therapeutic Substance

Uterine Artery
use Internal Iliac Artery, Left
use Internal Iliac Artery, Right
Uterine artery embolization (UAE) *see* Occlusion, Lower Arteries Ø4L
Uterine cornu *use* Uterus
Uterine tube
use Fallopian Tube, Left
use Fallopian Tube, Right
Uterine vein
use Hypogastric Vein, Left
use Hypogastric Vein, Right
Uvulectomy
see Excision, Uvula ØCBN
see Resection, Uvula ØCTN
Uvulorrhaphy *see* Repair, Uvula ØCQN
Uvulotomy *see* Drainage, Uvula ØC9N

Vabomere™ *use* Meropenem-vaborbactam Anti-infective
Vaccination *see* Introduction of Serum, Toxoid, and Vaccine
Vacuum extraction, obstetric 1ØDØ7Z6
Vaginal artery
use Internal Iliac Artery, Left
use Internal Iliac Artery, Right
Vaginal pessary *use* Intraluminal Device, Pessary in Female Reproductive System
Vaginal vein
use Hypogastric Vein, Left
use Hypogastric Vein, Right
Vaginectomy
see Excision, Vagina ØUBG
see Resection, Vagina ØUTG
Vaginofixation
see Repair, Vagina ØUQG
see Reposition, Vagina ØUSG
Vaginoplasty
see Repair, Vagina ØUQG
see Supplement, Vagina ØUUG
Vaginorrhaphy *see* Repair, Vagina ØUQG
Vaginoscopy ØUJH8ZZ
Vaginotomy *see* Drainage, Female Reproductive System ØU9
Vagotomy *see* Division, Nerve, Vagus ØØ8Q
Valiant Thoracic Stent Graft *use* Intraluminal Device
Valvotomy, valvulotomy
see Division, Heart and Great Vessels Ø28
see Release, Heart and Great Vessels Ø2N
Valvuloplasty
see Repair, Heart and Great Vessels Ø2Q
see Replacement, Heart and Great Vessels Ø2R
see Supplement, Heart and Great Vessels Ø2U
Valvuloplasty, Alfieri Stitch *see* Restriction, Valve, Mitral Ø2VG
Vanta™ PC neurostimulator *use* Stimulator Generator, Multiple Array in ØJH
Vascular Access Device
Totally Implantable
Insertion of device in
Abdomen ØJH8
Chest ØJH6
Lower Arm
Left ØJHH
Right ØJHG
Lower Leg
Left ØJHP
Right ØJHN
Upper Arm
Left ØJHF
Right ØJHD
Upper Leg
Left ØJHM
Right ØJHL
Removal of device from
Lower Extremity ØJPW
Trunk ØJPT
Upper Extremity ØJPV
Revision of device in
Lower Extremity ØJWW
Trunk ØJWT
Upper Extremity ØJWV
Vascular Access Device — *continued*
Tunneled
Insertion of device in
Abdomen ØJH8
Chest ØJH6
Lower Arm
Left ØJHH
Right ØJHG
Lower Leg
Left ØJHP
Right ØJHN
Upper Arm
Left ØJHF
Right ØJHD
Upper Leg
Left ØJHM
Right ØJHL
Removal of device from
Lower Extremity ØJPW
Trunk ØJPT
Upper Extremity ØJPV
Revision of device in
Lower Extremity ØJWW
Trunk ØJWT
Upper Extremity ØJWV
Vasectomy *see* Excision, Male Reproductive System ØVB
Vasography
see Fluoroscopy, Male Reproductive System BV1
see Plain Radiography, Male Reproductive System BVØ
Vasoligation *see* Occlusion, Male Reproductive System ØVL
Vasorrhaphy *see* Repair, Male Reproductive System ØVQ
Vasostomy *see* Bypass, Male Reproductive System ØV1
Vasotomy
Drainage *see* Drainage, Male Reproductive System ØV9
With ligation *see* Occlusion, Male Reproductive System ØVL
Vasovasostomy *see* Repair, Male Reproductive System ØVQ
VasQ™ External Support device *use* Synthetic Substitute, Extraluminal Support Device in New Technology
Vastus intermedius muscle
use Upper Leg Muscle, Left
use Upper Leg Muscle, Right
Vastus lateralis muscle
use Upper Leg Muscle, Left
use Upper Leg Muscle, Right
Vastus medialis muscle
use Upper Leg Muscle, Left
use Upper Leg Muscle, Right
VCG (vectorcardiogram) *see* Measurement, Cardiac 4AØ2
Vectra® Vascular Access Graft *use* Vascular Access Device, Tunneled in Subcutaneous Tissue and Fascia
Vein Graft Extraluminal Support Device(s), Supplement, Coronary Artery/Arteries X2U4Ø79
Veklury *use* Remdesivir Anti-infective
Venclexta® *use* Venetoclax Antineoplastic
Venectomy
see Excision, Lower Veins Ø6B
see Excision, Upper Veins Ø5B
Venetoclax Antineoplastic XWØDXR5
Venography
see Fluoroscopy, Veins B51
see Plain Radiography, Veins B5Ø
Venorrhaphy
see Repair, Lower Veins Ø6Q
see Repair, Upper Veins Ø5Q
Venotripsy
see Occlusion, Lower Veins Ø6L
see Occlusion, Upper Veins Ø5L
VenoValve® *use* Intraluminal Device, Bioprosthetic Valve in New Technology
Ventricular fold *use* Larynx
Ventriculoatriostomy *see* Bypass, Central Nervous System and Cranial Nerves ØØ1
Ventriculocisternostomy *see* Bypass, Central Nervous System and Cranial Nerves ØØ1
Ventriculogram, cardiac
Combined left and right heart *see* Fluoroscopy, Heart, Right and Left B216
Ventriculogram, cardiac — *continued*
Left ventricle *see* Fluoroscopy, Heart, Left B215
Right ventricle *see* Fluoroscopy, Heart, Right B214
Ventriculopuncture, through previously implanted catheter 8CØ1X6J
Ventriculoscopy ØØJØ4ZZ
Ventriculostomy
External drainage *see* Drainage, Cerebral Ventricle ØØ96
Internal shunt *see* Bypass, Cerebral Ventricle ØØ16
Ventriculovenostomy *see* Bypass, Cerebral Ventricle ØØ16
Ventrio™ Hernia Patch *use* Synthetic Substitute
VEP (visual evoked potential) 4AØ7XØZ
Vermiform appendix *use* Appendix
Vermilion border
use Lower Lip
use Upper Lip
Versa *use* Pacemaker, Dual Chamber in ØJH
Version, obstetric
External 1ØSØXZZ
Internal 1ØSØ7ZZ
Vertebral arch
use Cervical Vertebra
use Lumbar Vertebra
use Thoracic Vertebra
Vertebral artery, intracranial portion *use* Intracranial Artery
Vertebral body
use Cervical Vertebra
use Lumbar Vertebra
use Thoracic Vertebra
Vertebral canal *use* Spinal Canal
Vertebral foramen
use Cervical Vertebra
use Lumbar Vertebra
use Thoracic Vertebra
Vertebral lamina
use Cervical Vertebra
use Lumbar Vertebra
use Thoracic Vertebra
Vertebral pedicle
use Cervical Vertebra
use Lumbar Vertebra
use Thoracic Vertebra
Vesical vein
use Hypogastric Vein, Left
use Hypogastric Vein, Right
Vesicotomy *see* Drainage, Urinary System ØT9
Vesiculectomy
see Excision, Male Reproductive System ØVB
see Resection, Male Reproductive System ØVT
Vesiculogram, seminal *see* Plain Radiography, Male Reproductive System BVØ
Vesiculotomy *see* Drainage, Male Reproductive System ØV9
Vestibular Assessment F15Z
Vestibular (Scarpa's) ganglion *use* Acoustic Nerve
Vestibular nerve *use* Acoustic Nerve
Vestibular Treatment FØC
Vestibulocochlear nerve *use* Acoustic Nerve
VEST™ Venous External Support device *use* Vein Graft Extraluminal Support Device(s) in New Technology
VH-IVUS (virtual histology intravascular ultrasound) *see* Ultrasonography, Heart B24
Virchow's (supraclavicular) lymph node
use Lymphatic, Left Neck
use Lymphatic, Right Neck
Virtuoso (II) (DR) (VR) *use* Defibrillator Generator in ØJH
Vistogard® *use* Uridine Triacetate
Visualase™ MRI-Guided Laser Ablation System *see* Destruction
Vitrectomy
see Excision, Eye Ø8B
see Resection, Eye Ø8T
Vitreous body
use Vitreous, Left
use Vitreous, Right
Viva (XT) (S) *use* Cardiac Resynchronization Defibrillator Pulse Generator in ØJH
Vivistim® Paired VNS System Lead *use* Neurostimulator Lead with Paired Stimulation System in New Technology

Vocal fold
use Vocal Cord, Left
use Vocal Cord, Right
Vocational
Assessment *see* Activities of Daily Living Assessment, Rehabilitation FØ2
Retraining *see* Activities of Daily Living Treatment, Rehabilitation FØ8
Volar (palmar) digital vein
use Hand Vein, Left
use Hand Vein, Right
Volar (palmar) metacarpal vein
use Hand Vein, Left
use Hand Vein, Right
Vomer bone *use* Nasal Septum
Vomer of nasal septum *use* Nasal Bone
Voraxaze *use* Glucarpidase
Vulvectomy
see Excision, Female Reproductive System ØUB
see Resection, Female Reproductive System ØUT
V-Wave Interatrial Shunt System *use* Synthetic Substitute
VYXEOS™ *use* Cytarabine and Daunorubicin Liposome Antineoplastic

W

WALLSTENT® Endoprosthesis *use* Intraluminal Device
Washing *see* Irrigation
WavelinQ EndoAVF system
Radial Artery, Left Ø31C3ZF
Radial Artery, Right Ø31B3ZF
Ulnar Artery, Left Ø31A3ZF
Ulnar Artery, Right Ø3193ZF
Wedge resection, pulmonary *see* Excision, Respiratory System ØBB
Whole Blood Nucleic Acid-base Microbial Detection XXE5XM5
Whole Blood Reverse Transcription and Quantitative Real-time Polymerase Chain Reaction XXE5X38
Window *see* Drainage
Wiring, dental 2W31X9Z

X

Xact Carotid Stent System *use* Intraluminal Device
XENLETA™ *use* Lefamulin Anti-infective
Xenograft *use* Zooplastic Tissue in Heart and Great Vessels
XENOVIEW™ BB34Z3Z
XIENCE Everolimus Eluting Coronary Stent System
use Intraluminal Device, Drug-eluting in Heart and Great Vessels
Xiphoid process *use* Sternum
XLIF® System *use* Interbody Fusion Device in Lower Joints
XOSPATA® *use* Gilteritinib Antineoplastic
X-ray *see* Plain Radiography
X-Spine Axle Cage
use Spinal Stabilization Device, Interspinous Process in ØRH
use Spinal Stabilization Device, Interspinous Process in ØSH
X-STOP® Spacer
use Spinal Stabilization Device, Interspinous Process in ØRH
use Spinal Stabilization Device, Interspinous Process in ØSH

Y

Yescarta® *use* Axicabtagene Ciloleucel Immunotherapy
Yoga Therapy 8EØZXY4

Z

Zenith AAA Endovascular Graft *use* Intraluminal Device
Zenith Flex® AAA Endovascular Graft *use* Intraluminal Device
Zenith TX2® TAA Endovascular Graft *use* Intraluminal Device
Zenith® Fenestrated AAA Endovascular Graft
use Intraluminal Device, Branched or Fenestrated, One or Two Arteries in Ø4V
use Intraluminal Device, Branched or Fenestrated, Three or More Arteries in Ø4V
Zenith® Renu™ AAA Ancillary Graft *use* Intraluminal Device
ZEPZELCA™ *use* Lurbinectedin
ZERBAXA® *use* Ceftolozane/Tazobactam Anti-infective
Zilver® PTX® (paclitaxel) Drug-Eluting Peripheral Stent
use Intraluminal Device, Drug-eluting in Lower Arteries
use Intraluminal Device, Drug-eluting in Upper Arteries
Zimmer® NexGen® LPS Mobile Bearing Knee *use* Synthetic Substitute
Zimmer® NexGen® LPS-Flex Mobile Knee *use* Synthetic Substitute
Zonule of Zinn
use Lens, Left
use Lens, Right
Zotarolimus-eluting Coronary Stent *use* Intraluminal Device, Drug-eluting in Heart and Great Vessels
Z-plasty, skin for scar contracture *see* Release, Skin and Breast ØHN
ZULRESSO™ use Brexanolone
Zygomatic process of frontal bone *use* Frontal Bone
Zygomatic process of temporal bone
use Temporal Bone, Left
use Temporal Bone, Right
Zygomaticus muscle *use* Facial Muscle
ZYNTEGLO® *use* Betibeglogene Autotemcel
Zyvox *use* Oxazolidinones

ICD-10-PCS Tables

Central Nervous System and Cranial Nerves ØØ1–ØØX

Character Meanings

This Character Meaning table is provided as a guide to assist the user in the identification of character members that may be found in this section of code tables. It **SHOULD NOT** be used to build a PCS code.

Operation–Character 3		Body Part–Character 4		Approach–Character 5		Device–Character 6		Qualifier–Character 7	
1	Bypass	Ø	Brain	Ø	Open	Ø	Drainage Device	Ø	Nasopharynx
2	Change	1	Cerebral Meninges	3	Percutaneous	1	Radioactive Element	1	Mastoid Sinus
5	Destruction	2	Dura Mater	4	Percutaneous Endoscopic	2	Monitoring Device	2	Atrium
7	Dilation	3	Epidural Space, Intracranial	X	External	3	Infusion Device	3	Blood Vessel OR Laser Interstitial Thermal Therapy
8	Division	4	Subdural Space, Intracranial			4	Radioactive Element, Cesium-131 Collagen Implant	4	Pleural Cavity
9	Drainage	5	Subarachnoid Space, Intracranial			7	Autologous Tissue Substitute	5	Intestine
B	Excision	6	Cerebral Ventricle			J	Synthetic Substitute	6	Peritoneal Cavity
C	Extirpation	7	Cerebral Hemisphere			K	Nonautologous Tissue Substitute	7	Urinary Tract
D	Extraction	8	Basal Ganglia			M	Neurostimulator Lead	8	Bone Marrow
F	Fragmentation	9	Thalamus			Y	Other Device	9	Fallopian Tube
H	Insertion	A	Hypothalamus			Z	No Device	A	Subgaleal Space
J	Inspection	B	Pons					B	Cerebral Cisterns
K	Map	C	Cerebellum					F	Olfactory Nerve
N	Release	D	Medulla Oblongata					G	Optic Nerve
P	Removal	E	Cranial Nerve					H	Oculomotor Nerve
Q	Repair	F	Olfactory Nerve					J	Trochlear Nerve
R	Replacement	G	Optic Nerve					K	Trigeminal Nerve
S	Reposition	H	Oculomotor Nerve					L	Abducens Nerve
T	Resection	J	Trochlear Nerve					M	Facial Nerve
U	Supplement	K	Trigeminal Nerve					N	Acoustic Nerve
W	Revision	L	Abducens Nerve					P	Glossopharyngeal Nerve
X	Transfer	M	Facial Nerve					Q	Vagus Nerve
		N	Acoustic Nerve					R	Accessory Nerve
		P	Glossopharyngeal Nerve					S	Hypoglossal Nerve
		Q	Vagus Nerve					X	Diagnostic
		R	Accessory Nerve					Z	No Qualifier
		S	Hypoglossal Nerve						
		T	Spinal Meninges						
		U	Spinal Canal						
		V	Spinal Cord						
		W	Cervical Spinal Cord						
		X	Thoracic Spinal Cord						
		Y	Lumbar Spinal Cord						

AHA Coding Clinic for table ØØ1

2021, 2Q, 19	Electromagnetic stealth guided ventriculoperitoneal shunt insertion with endoscopy
2019, 4Q, 21-22	Cerebral ventricle bypass Qualifier
2018, 4Q, 86	Placement of lumboatrial shunt
2017, 4Q, 39-41	Dilation and bypass of cerebral ventricle
2015, 2Q, 9	Revision of ventriculoperitoneal (VP) shunt
2013, 2Q, 36	Insertion of ventriculoperitoneal shunt with laparoscopic assistance

AHA Coding Clinic for table ØØ5

2022, 4Q, 53-54	Laser interstitial thermal therapy
2022, 1Q, 50	Percutaneous ganglion balloon compression
2021, 3Q, 16	Decompression of Chiari malformation by excision
2021, 2Q, 17	Dorsal root entry zone procedure

AHA Coding Clinic for table ØØ7

2017, 4Q, 39-41	Dilation and bypass of cerebral ventricle

AHA Coding Clinic for table ØØ9

2018, 4Q, 85	Externalization of lumboatrial shunt
2017, 1Q, 50	Failed lumbar puncture
2015, 3Q, 10	Open evacuation of subdural hematoma
2015, 3Q, 11	Percutaneous drainage of subdural hematoma
2015, 3Q, 12	Subdural evacuation portal system (SEPS) placement
2015, 3Q, 12	Placement of ventriculostomy catheter via burr hole
2015, 2Q, 30	Drainage of syrinx
2015, 1Q, 31	Intrathecal chemotherapy
2014, 1Q, 8	Diagnostic lumbar tap
2014, 1Q, 8	Lumbar drainage port aspiration

AHA Coding Clinic for table ØØB

2021, 3Q, 16	Decompression of Chiari malformation by excision
2017, 3Q, 17	Resection of schwannoma and placement of DuraGen and Lorenz cranial plating system
2016, 2Q, 12	Resection of malignant neoplasm of infratemporal fossa
2016, 2Q, 18	Amygdalohippocampectomy
2014, 4Q, 34	Resection of brain malignancy with implantation of chemotherapeutic wafer
2014, 3Q, 24	Repair of lipomyelomeningocele and tethered cord

AHA Coding Clinic for table ØØC

2019, 3Q, 4	Evacuation of subdural hematoma and control of bleeding artery
2019, 2Q, 36	Evacuation of hematoma using NICO Brainpath® technology
2017, 4Q, 48	New and revised body part values - Extirpation spinal canal
2016, 2Q, 29	Decompressive craniectomy with cryopreservation and storage of bone flap
2015, 3Q, 10	Open evacuation of subdural hematoma
2015, 3Q, 11	Percutaneous drainage of subdural hematoma
2015, 3Q, 13	Evacuation of intracerebral hematoma

AHA Coding Clinic for table ØØD

2022, 4Q, 54	Ultrasonic surgical aspiration of brain
2021, 4Q, 38-40	Ultrasonic surgical aspiration of brain
2015, 3Q, 13	Nonexcisional debridement of cranial wound with removal and replacement of hardware

AHA Coding Clinic for table ØØH

2020, 4Q, 43-44	Insertion of radioactive element
2020, 2Q, 15	Ommaya reservoir with ventricular catheter placement
2020, 2Q, 16	Ommaya reservoir placement for cerebrospinal fluid infusion therapy
2017, 4Q, 30-31	Radiotherapeutic brain implant
2017, 3Q, 13	Implantation of bilateral neurostimulator electrodes
2014, 3Q, 19	End of life replacement of Baclofen pump

AHA Coding Clinic for table ØØJ

2021, 2Q, 19	Electromagnetic stealth guided ventriculoperitoneal shunt insertion with endoscopy
2019, 2Q, 36	Evacuation of hematoma using NICO Brainpath® technology
2017, 1Q, 50	Failed lumbar puncture

AHA Coding Clinic for table ØØN

2019, 2Q, 19	Cervical spinal fusion, decompression and placement of interfacet stabilization device
2019, 1Q, 28	Decompressive laminectomy of both spinal cord and nerve roots
2018, 3Q, 30	Decompressive laminectomy (release of spinal cord versus release of spinal meninges)
2017, 3Q, 10	Repair of Chiari malformation
2017, 2Q, 23	Decompression of spinal cord and placement of instrumentation
2016, 2Q, 29	Decompressive craniectomy with cryopreservation and storage of bone flap
2015, 2Q, 20	Cervical laminoplasty
2015, 2Q, 21	Multiple decompressive cervical laminectomies
2015, 2Q, 34	Decompressive laminectomy
2014, 3Q, 24	Repair of lipomyelomeningocele and tethered cord

AHA Coding Clinic for table ØØP

2014, 3Q, 19	End of life replacement of Baclofen pump

AHA Coding Clinic for table ØØQ

2014, 3Q, 7	Hemi-cranioplasty for repair of cranial defect
2013, 3Q, 25	Fracture of frontal bone with repair and coagulation for hemostasis

AHA Coding Clinic for table ØØS

2014, 4Q, 35	Reimplantation of buccal nerve

AHA Coding Clinic for table ØØU

2021, 3Q, 16	Decompression of Chiari malformation by excision
2018, 1Q, 9	Craniectomy with DuraGaurd placement
2017, 4Q, 62	Added and revised device values - Nerve substitutes
2017, 3Q, 10	Repair of Chiari malformation
2017, 3Q, 17	Resection of schwannoma and placement of DuraGen and Lorenz cranial plating system
2015, 4Q, 39	Dural patch graft
2014, 3Q, 24	Repair of lipomyelomeningocele and tethered cord

AHA Coding Clinic for table ØØW

2018, 4Q, 86	Placement of lumboatrial shunt

Brain

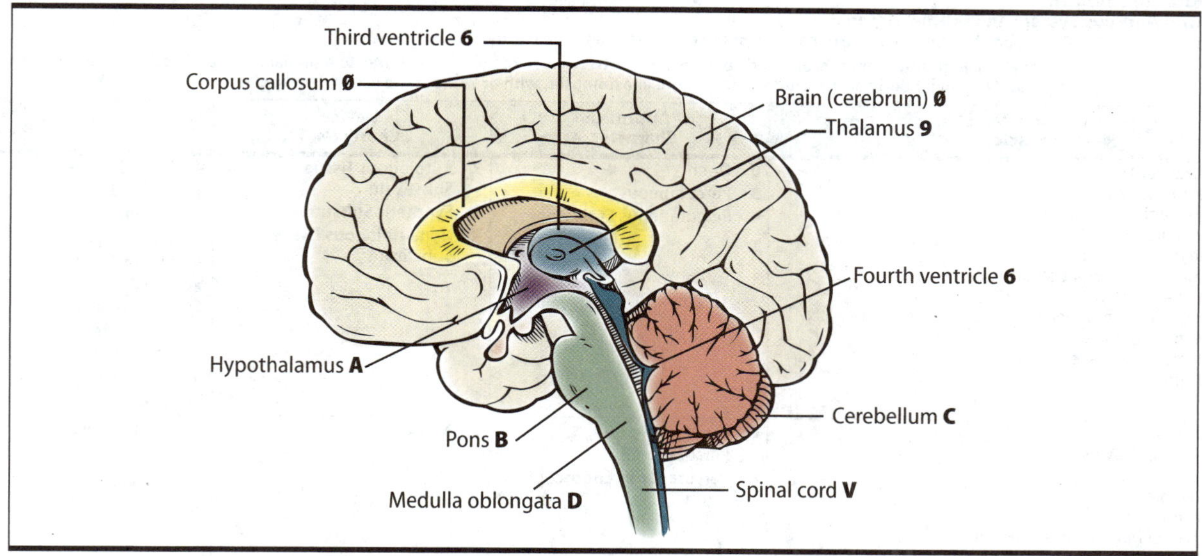

Cranial Nerves

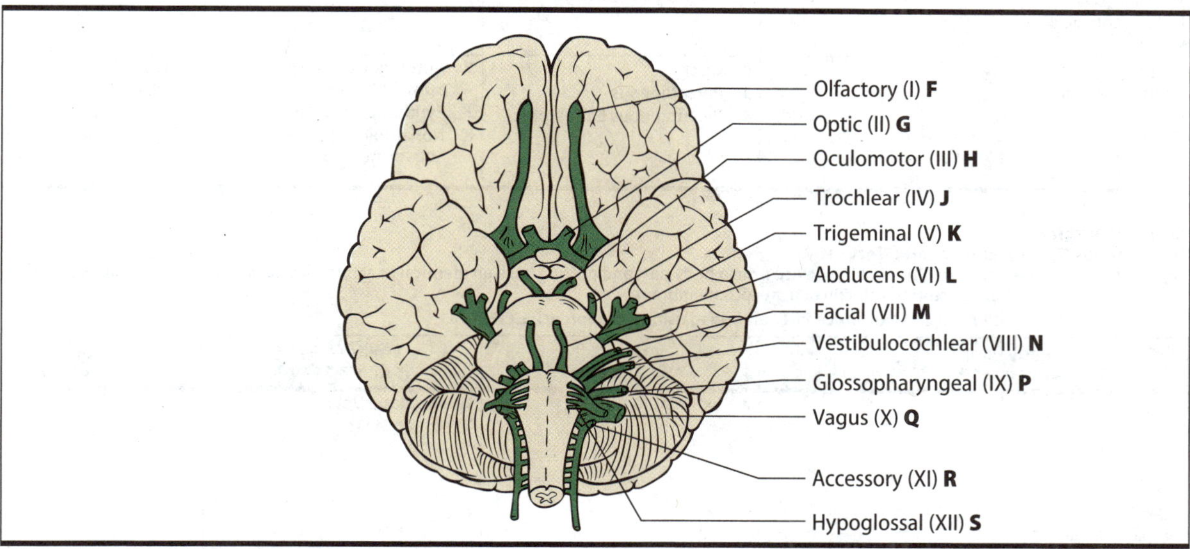

Ø Medical and Surgical
Ø Central Nervous System and Cranial Nerves
1 Bypass Definition: Altering the route of passage of the contents of a tubular body part

Explanation: Rerouting contents of a body part to a downstream area of the normal route, to a similar route and body part, or to an abnormal route and dissimilar body part. Includes one or more anastomoses, with or without the use of a device.

Body Part Character 4	Approach Character 5	Device Character 6	Qualifier Character 7
6 Cerebral Ventricle Aqueduct of Sylvius Cerebral aqueduct (Sylvius) Choroid plexus Ependyma Foramen of Monro (intraventricular) Fourth ventricle Interventricular foramen (Monro) Left lateral ventricle Right lateral ventricle Third ventricle	**Ø Open** **3 Percutaneous** **4 Percutaneous Endoscopic**	**7 Autologous Tissue Substitute** **J Synthetic Substitute** **K Nonautologous Tissue Substitute**	**Ø Nasopharynx** **1 Mastoid Sinus** **2 Atrium** **3 Blood Vessel** **4 Pleural Cavity** **5 Intestine** **6 Peritoneal Cavity** **7 Urinary Tract** **8 Bone Marrow** **A Subgaleal Space** **B Cerebral Cisterns**
6 Cerebral Ventricle Aqueduct of Sylvius Cerebral aqueduct (Sylvius) Choroid plexus Ependyma Foramen of Monro (intraventricular) Fourth ventricle Interventricular foramen (Monro) Left lateral ventricle Right lateral ventricle Third ventricle	**Ø Open** **3 Percutaneous** **4 Percutaneous Endoscopic**	**Z No Device**	**B Cerebral Cisterns**
U Spinal Canal Epidural space, spinal Extradural space, spinal Subarachnoid space, spinal Subdural space, spinal Vertebral canal	**Ø Open** **3 Percutaneous** **4 Percutaneous Endoscopic**	**7 Autologous Tissue Substitute** **J Synthetic Substitute** **K Nonautologous Tissue Substitute**	**2 Atrium** **4 Pleural Cavity** **6 Peritoneal Cavity** **7 Urinary Tract** **9 Fallopian Tube**

Ø Medical and Surgical
Ø Central Nervous System and Cranial Nerves
2 Change Definition: Taking out or off a device from a body part and putting back an identical or similar device in or on the same body part without cutting or puncturing the skin or a mucous membrane

Explanation: All CHANGE procedures are coded using the approach EXTERNAL

Body Part Character 4	Approach Character 5	Device Character 6	Qualifier Character 7
Ø Brain Cerebrum Corpus callosum Encephalon **E Cranial Nerve** **U Spinal Canal** Epidural space, spinal Extradural space, spinal Subarachnoid space, spinal Subdural space, spinal Vertebral canal	**X External**	**Ø Drainage Device** **Y Other Device**	**Z No Qualifier**

Non-OR All body part, approach, device, and qualifier values

0 Medical and Surgical
0 Central Nervous System and Cranial Nerves
5 Destruction Definition: Physical eradication of all or a portion of a body part by the direct use of energy, force, or a destructive agent
Explanation: None of the body part is physically taken out

Body Part Character 4	Approach Character 5	Device Character 6	Qualifier Character 7
0 Brain Cerebrum Corpus callosum Encephalon **W Cervical Spinal Cord** Dorsal root ganglion **X Thoracic Spinal Cord** Dorsal root ganglion **Y Lumbar Spinal Cord** Cauda equina Conus medullaris Dorsal root ganglion	**0 Open** **3 Percutaneous** **4 Percutaneous Endoscopic**	**Z No Device**	**3 Laser Interstitial Thermal Therapy** **Z No Qualifier**
1 Cerebral Meninges Arachnoid mater, intracranial Leptomeninges, intracranial Pia mater, intracranial **2 Dura Mater** Diaphragma sellae Dura mater, intracranial Falx cerebri Tentorium cerebelli **6 Cerebral Ventricle** Aqueduct of Sylvius Cerebral aqueduct (Sylvius) Choroid plexus Ependyma Foramen of Monro (intraventricular) Fourth ventricle Interventricular foramen (Monro) Left lateral ventricle Right lateral ventricle Third ventricle **7 Cerebral Hemisphere** Frontal lobe Occipital lobe Parietal lobe Temporal lobe **8 Basal Ganglia** Basal nuclei Claustrum Corpus striatum Globus pallidus Substantia nigra Subthalamic nucleus **9 Thalamus** Epithalamus Geniculate nucleus Metathalamus Pulvinar **A Hypothalamus** Mammillary body **B Pons** Apneustic center Basis pontis Locus ceruleus Pneumotaxic center Pontine tegmentum Superior olivary nucleus **C Cerebellum** Culmen **D Medulla Oblongata** Myelencephalon **F Olfactory Nerve** First cranial nerve Olfactory bulb **G Optic Nerve** Optic chiasma Second cranial nerve **H Oculomotor Nerve** Third cranial nerve **J Trochlear Nerve** Fourth cranial nerve **K Trigeminal Nerve** Fifth cranial nerve Gasserian ganglion Mandibular nerve Maxillary nerve Ophthalmic nerve Trifacial nerve **L Abducens Nerve** Sixth cranial nerve **M Facial Nerve** Chorda tympani Geniculate ganglion Greater superficial petrosal nerve Nerve to the stapedius Parotid plexus Posterior auricular nerve Seventh cranial nerve Submandibular ganglion **N Acoustic Nerve** Cochlear nerve Eighth cranial nerve Scarpa's (vestibular) ganglion Spiral ganglion Vestibular (Scarpa's) ganglion Vestibular nerve Vestibulocochlear nerve **P Glossopharyngeal Nerve** Carotid sinus nerve Ninth cranial nerve Tympanic nerve **Q Vagus Nerve** Anterior vagal trunk Pharyngeal plexus Pneumogastric nerve Posterior vagal trunk Pulmonary plexus Recurrent laryngeal nerve Superior laryngeal nerve Tenth cranial nerve **R Accessory Nerve** Eleventh cranial nerve **S Hypoglossal Nerve** Twelfth cranial nerve **T Spinal Meninges** Arachnoid mater, spinal Denticulate (dentate) ligament Dura mater, spinal Filum terminale Leptomeninges, spinal Pia mater, spinal	**0 Open** **3 Percutaneous** **4 Percutaneous Endoscopic**	**Z No Device**	**Z No Qualifier**

Non-OR 005[F,G,H,J,K,L,M,N,P,Q,R,S][0,3,4]ZZ

Ø Medical and Surgical
Ø Central Nervous System and Cranial Nerves
7 Dilation

Definition: Expanding an orifice or the lumen of a tubular body part

Explanation: The orifice can be a natural orifice or an artificially created orifice. Accomplished by stretching a tubular body part using intraluminal pressure or by cutting part of the orifice or wall of the tubular body part.

Body Part Character 4	Approach Character 5	Device Character 6	Qualifier Character 7
6 Cerebral Ventricle Aqueduct of Sylvius Cerebral aqueduct (Sylvius) Choroid plexus Ependyma Foramen of Monro (intraventricular) Fourth ventricle Interventricular foramen (Monro) Left lateral ventricle Right lateral ventricle Third ventricle	**Ø Open** **3 Percutaneous** **4 Percutaneous Endoscopic**	**Z No Device**	**Z No Qualifier**

Ø Medical and Surgical
Ø Central Nervous System and Cranial Nerves
8 Division

Definition: Cutting into a body part, without draining fluids and/or gases from the body part, in order to separate or transect a body part

Explanation: All or a portion of the body part is separated into two or more portions

Body Part Character 4	Approach Character 5	Device Character 6	Qualifier Character 7
Ø Brain Cerebrum Corpus callosum Encephalon **7 Cerebral Hemisphere** Frontal lobe Occipital lobe Parietal lobe Temporal lobe **8 Basal Ganglia** Basal nuclei Claustrum Corpus striatum Globus pallidus Substantia nigra Subthalamic nucleus **F Olfactory Nerve** First cranial nerve Olfactory bulb **G Optic Nerve** Optic chiasma Second cranial nerve **H Oculomotor Nerve** Third cranial nerve **J Trochlear Nerve** Fourth cranial nerve **K Trigeminal Nerve** Fifth cranial nerve Gasserian ganglion Mandibular nerve Maxillary nerve Ophthalmic nerve Trifacial nerve **L Abducens Nerve** Sixth cranial nerve **M Facial Nerve** Chorda tympani Geniculate ganglion Greater superficial petrosal nerve Nerve to the stapedius Parotid plexus Posterior auricular nerve Seventh cranial nerve Submandibular ganglion **N Acoustic Nerve** Cochlear nerve Eighth cranial nerve Scarpa's (vestibular) ganglion Spiral ganglion Vestibular (Scarpa's) ganglion Vestibular nerve Vestibulocochlear nerve **P Glossopharyngeal Nerve** Carotid sinus nerve Ninth cranial nerve Tympanic nerve **Q Vagus Nerve** Anterior vagal trunk Pharyngeal plexus Pneumogastric nerve Posterior vagal trunk Pulmonary plexus Recurrent laryngeal nerve Superior laryngeal nerve Tenth cranial nerve **R Accessory Nerve** Eleventh cranial nerve **S Hypoglossal Nerve** Twelfth cranial nerve **W Cervical Spinal Cord** Dorsal root ganglion **X Thoracic Spinal Cord** Dorsal root ganglion **Y Lumbar Spinal Cord** Cauda equina Conus medullaris Dorsal root ganglion	**Ø Open** **3 Percutaneous** **4 Percutaneous Endoscopic**	**Z No Device**	**Z No Qualifier**

Ø Medical and Surgical
Ø Central Nervous System and Cranial Nerves
9 Drainage Definition: Taking or letting out fluids and/or gases from a body part
Explanation: The qualifier DIAGNOSTIC is used to identify drainage procedures that are biopsies

Body Part Character 4	Approach Character 5	Device Character 6	Qualifier Character 7
Ø Brain Cerebrum Corpus callosum Encephalon **1 Cerebral Meninges** Arachnoid mater, intracranial Leptomeninges, intracranial Pia mater, intracranial **2 Dura Mater** Diaphragma sellae Dura mater, intracranial Falx cerebri Tentorium cerebelli **3 Epidural Space, Intracranial** Extradural space, intracranial **4 Subdural Space, Intracranial** **5 Subarachnoid Space, Intracranial** **6 Cerebral Ventricle** Aqueduct of Sylvius Cerebral aqueduct (Sylvius) Choroid plexus Ependyma Foramen of Monro (intraventricular) Fourth ventricle Interventricular foramen (Monro) Left lateral ventricle Right lateral ventricle Third ventricle **7 Cerebral Hemisphere** Frontal lobe Occipital lobe Parietal lobe Temporal lobe **8 Basal Ganglia** Basal nuclei Claustrum Corpus striatum Globus pallidus Substantia nigra Subthalamic nucleus **9 Thalamus** Epithalamus Geniculate nucleus Metathalamus Pulvinar **A Hypothalamus** Mammillary body **B Pons** Apneustic center Basis pontis Locus ceruleus Pneumotaxic center Pontine tegmentum Superior olivary nucleus **C Cerebellum** Culmen **D Medulla Oblongata** Myelencephalon **F Olfactory Nerve** First cranial nerve Olfactory bulb **G Optic Nerve** Optic chiasma Second cranial nerve **H Oculomotor Nerve** Third cranial nerve **J Trochlear Nerve** Fourth cranial nerve **K Trigeminal Nerve** Fifth cranial nerve Gasserian ganglion Mandibular nerve Maxillary nerve Ophthalmic nerve Trifacial nerve **L Abducens Nerve** Sixth cranial nerve **M Facial Nerve** Chorda tympani Geniculate ganglion Greater superficial petrosal nerve Nerve to the stapedius Parotid plexus Posterior auricular nerve Seventh cranial nerve Submandibular ganglion **N Acoustic Nerve** Cochlear nerve Eighth cranial nerve Scarpa's (vestibular) ganglion Spiral ganglion Vestibular (Scarpa's) ganglion Vestibular nerve Vestibulocochlear nerve **P Glossopharyngeal Nerve** Carotid sinus nerve Ninth cranial nerve Tympanic nerve **Q Vagus Nerve** Anterior vagal trunk Pharyngeal plexus Pneumogastric nerve Posterior vagal trunk Pulmonary plexus Recurrent laryngeal nerve Superior laryngeal nerve Tenth cranial nerve **R Accessory Nerve** Eleventh cranial nerve **S Hypoglossal Nerve** Twelfth cranial nerve **T Spinal Meninges** Arachnoid mater, spinal Denticulate (dentate) ligament Dura mater, spinal Filum terminale Leptomeninges, spinal Pia mater, spinal **U Spinal Canal** Epidural space, spinal Extradural space, spinal Subarachnoid space, spinal Subdural space, spinal Vertebral canal **W Cervical Spinal Cord** Dorsal root ganglion **X Thoracic Spinal Cord** Dorsal root ganglion **Y Lumbar Spinal Cord** Cauda equina Conus medullaris Dorsal root ganglion	**Ø Open** **3 Percutaneous** **4 Percutaneous Endoscopic**	**Ø Drainage Device**	**Z No Qualifier**

Non-OR ØØ9[T,W,X,Y]3ØZ
Non-OR ØØ9U[3,4]ØZ

ØØ9 Continued on next page

ØØ9 Continued

Ø Medical and Surgical
Ø Central Nervous System and Cranial Nerves
9 Drainage Definition: Taking or letting out fluids and/or gases from a body part
Explanation: The qualifier DIAGNOSTIC is used to identify drainage procedures that are biopsies

Body Part Character 4	Approach Character 5	Device Character 6	Qualifier Character 7
Ø Brain Cerebrum Corpus callosum Encephalon **1 Cerebral Meninges** Arachnoid mater, intracranial Leptomeninges, intracranial Pia mater, intracranial **2 Dura Mater** Diaphragma sellae Dura mater, intracranial Falx cerebri Tentorium cerebelli **3 Epidural Space, Intracranial** Extradural space, intracranial **4 Subdural Space, Intracranial** **5 Subarachnoid Space, Intracranial** **6 Cerebral Ventricle** Aqueduct of Sylvius Cerebral aqueduct (Sylvius) Choroid plexus Ependyma Foramen of Monro (intraventricular) Fourth ventricle Interventricular foramen (Monro) Left lateral ventricle Right lateral ventricle Third ventricle **7 Cerebral Hemisphere** Frontal lobe Occipital lobe Parietal lobe Temporal lobe **8 Basal Ganglia** Basal nuclei Claustrum Corpus striatum Globus pallidus Substantia nigra Subthalamic nucleus **9 Thalamus** Epithalamus Geniculate nucleus Metathalamus Pulvinar **A Hypothalamus** Mammillary body **B Pons** Apneustic center Basis pontis Locus ceruleus Pneumotaxic center Pontine tegmentum Superior olivary nucleus **C Cerebellum** Culmen **D Medulla Oblongata** Myelencephalon **F Olfactory Nerve** First cranial nerve Olfactory bulb **G Optic Nerve** Optic chiasma Second cranial nerve **H Oculomotor Nerve** Third cranial nerve **J Trochlear Nerve** Fourth cranial nerve **K Trigeminal Nerve** Fifth cranial nerve Gasserian ganglion Mandibular nerve Maxillary nerve Ophthalmic nerve Trifacial nerve **L Abducens Nerve** Sixth cranial nerve **M Facial Nerve** Chorda tympani Geniculate ganglion Greater superficial petrosal nerve Nerve to the stapedius Parotid plexus Posterior auricular nerve Seventh cranial nerve Submandibular ganglion **N Acoustic Nerve** Cochlear nerve Eighth cranial nerve Scarpa's (vestibular) ganglion Spiral ganglion Vestibular (Scarpa's) ganglion Vestibular nerve Vestibulocochlear nerve **P Glossopharyngeal Nerve** Carotid sinus nerve Ninth cranial nerve Tympanic nerve **Q Vagus Nerve** Anterior vagal trunk Pharyngeal plexus Pneumogastric nerve Posterior vagal trunk Pulmonary plexus Recurrent laryngeal nerve Superior laryngeal nerve Tenth cranial nerve **R Accessory Nerve** Eleventh cranial nerve **S Hypoglossal Nerve** Twelfth cranial nerve **T Spinal Meninges** Arachnoid mater, spinal Denticulate (dentate) ligament Dura mater, spinal Filum terminale Leptomeninges, spinal Pia mater, spinal **U Spinal Canal** Epidural space, spinal Extradural space, spinal Subarachnoid space, spinal Subdural space, spinal Vertebral canal **W Cervical Spinal Cord** Dorsal root ganglion **X Thoracic Spinal Cord** Dorsal root ganglion **Y Lumbar Spinal Cord** Cauda equina Conus medullaris Dorsal root ganglion	**Ø Open** **3 Percutaneous** **4 Percutaneous Endoscopic**	**Z No Device**	**X Diagnostic** **Z No Qualifier**

Non-OR ØØ9[Ø,1,2,3,4,5,6,7,8,9,A,B,C,D,F,G,H,J,K,L,M,N,P,Q,R,S][3,4]ZX
Non-OR ØØ9[T,W,X,Y]3Z[X,Z]
Non-OR ØØ9U[3,4]Z[X,Z]

Ø Medical and Surgical
Ø Central Nervous System and Cranial Nerves
B Excision Definition: Cutting out or off, without replacement, a portion of a body part
Explanation: The qualifier DIAGNOSTIC is used to identify excision procedures that are biopsies

Body Part Character 4	Approach Character 5	Device Character 6	Qualifier Character 7
Ø Brain Cerebrum Corpus callosum Encephalon 1 Cerebral Meninges Arachnoid mater, intracranial Leptomeninges, intracranial Pia mater, intracranial 2 Dura Mater Diaphragma sellae Dura mater, intracranial Falx cerebri Tentorium cerebelli 6 Cerebral Ventricle Aqueduct of Sylvius Cerebral aqueduct (Sylvius) Choroid plexus Ependyma Foramen of Monro (intraventricular) Fourth ventricle Interventricular foramen (Monro) Left lateral ventricle Right lateral ventricle Third ventricle 7 Cerebral Hemisphere Frontal lobe Occipital lobe Parietal lobe Temporal lobe 8 Basal Ganglia Basal nuclei Claustrum Corpus striatum Globus pallidus Substantia nigra Subthalamic nucleus 9 Thalamus Epithalamus Geniculate nucleus Metathalamus Pulvinar A Hypothalamus Mammillary body B Pons Apneustic center Basis pontis Locus ceruleus Pneumotaxic center Pontine tegmentum Superior olivary nucleus C Cerebellum Culmen D Medulla Oblongata Myelencephalon F Olfactory Nerve First cranial nerve Olfactory bulb G Optic Nerve Optic chiasma Second cranial nerve H Oculomotor Nerve Third cranial nerve J Trochlear Nerve Fourth cranial nerve K Trigeminal Nerve Fifth cranial nerve Gasserian ganglion Mandibular nerve Maxillary nerve Ophthalmic nerve Trifacial nerve L Abducens Nerve Sixth cranial nerve M Facial Nerve Chorda tympani Geniculate ganglion Greater superficial petrosal nerve Nerve to the stapedius Parotid plexus Posterior auricular nerve Seventh cranial nerve Submandibular ganglion N Acoustic Nerve Cochlear nerve Eighth cranial nerve Scarpa's (vestibular) ganglion Spiral ganglion Vestibular (Scarpa's) ganglion Vestibular nerve Vestibulocochlear nerve P Glossopharyngeal Nerve Carotid sinus nerve Ninth cranial nerve Tympanic nerve Q Vagus Nerve Anterior vagal trunk Pharyngeal plexus Pneumogastric nerve Posterior vagal trunk Pulmonary plexus Recurrent laryngeal nerve Superior laryngeal nerve Tenth cranial nerve R Accessory Nerve Eleventh cranial nerve S Hypoglossal Nerve Twelfth cranial nerve T Spinal Meninges Arachnoid mater, spinal Denticulate (dentate) ligament Dura mater, spinal Filum terminale Leptomeninges, spinal Pia mater, spinal W Cervical Spinal Cord Dorsal root ganglion X Thoracic Spinal Cord Dorsal root ganglion Y Lumbar Spinal Cord Cauda equina Conus medullaris Dorsal root ganglion	Ø Open 3 Percutaneous 4 Percutaneous Endoscopic	Z No Device	X Diagnostic Z No Qualifier

Non-OR ØØB[F,G,H,J,K,L,M,N,P,Q,R,S][3,4]ZX

Ø Medical and Surgical
Ø Central Nervous System and Cranial Nerves
C Extirpation Definition: Taking or cutting out solid matter from a body part

Explanation: The solid matter may be an abnormal byproduct of a biological function or a foreign body; it may be imbedded in a body part or in the lumen of a tubular body part. The solid matter may or may not have been previously broken into pieces.

Body Part Character 4		Approach Character 5	Device Character 6	Qualifier Character 7
Ø Brain Cerebrum Corpus callosum Encephalon **1 Cerebral Meninges** Arachnoid mater, intracranial Leptomeninges, intracranial Pia mater, intracranial **2 Dura Mater** Diaphragma sellae Dura mater, intracranial Falx cerebri Tentorium cerebelli **3 Epidural Space, Intracranial** Extradural space, intracranial **4 Subdural Space, Intracranial** **5 Subarachnoid Space, Intracranial** **6 Cerebral Ventricle** Aqueduct of Sylvius Cerebral aqueduct (Sylvius) Choroid plexus Ependyma Foramen of Monro (intraventricular) Fourth ventricle Interventricular foramen (Monro) Left lateral ventricle Right lateral ventricle Third ventricle **7 Cerebral Hemisphere** Frontal lobe Occipital lobe Parietal lobe Temporal lobe **8 Basal Ganglia** Basal nuclei Claustrum Corpus striatum Globus pallidus Substantia nigra Subthalamic nucleus **9 Thalamus** Epithalamus Geniculate nucleus Metathalamus Pulvinar **A Hypothalamus** Mammillary body **B Pons** Apneustic center Basis pontis Locus ceruleus Pneumotaxic center Pontine tegmentum Superior olivary nucleus **C Cerebellum** Culmen **D Medulla Oblongata** Myelencephalon **F Olfactory Nerve** First cranial nerve Olfactory bulb	**G Optic Nerve** Optic chiasma Second cranial nerve **H Oculomotor Nerve** Third cranial nerve **J Trochlear Nerve** Fourth cranial nerve **K Trigeminal Nerve** Fifth cranial nerve Gasserian ganglion Mandibular nerve Maxillary nerve Ophthalmic nerve Trifacial nerve **L Abducens Nerve** Sixth cranial nerve **M Facial Nerve** Chorda tympani Geniculate ganglion Greater superficial petrosal nerve Nerve to the stapedius Parotid plexus Posterior auricular nerve Seventh cranial nerve Submandibular ganglion **N Acoustic Nerve** Cochlear nerve Eighth cranial nerve Scarpa's (vestibular) ganglion Spiral ganglion Vestibular (Scarpa's) ganglion Vestibular nerve Vestibulocochlear nerve **P Glossopharyngeal Nerve** Carotid sinus nerve Ninth cranial nerve Tympanic nerve **Q Vagus Nerve** Anterior vagal trunk Pharyngeal plexus Pneumogastric nerve Posterior vagal trunk Pulmonary plexus Recurrent laryngeal nerve Superior laryngeal nerve Tenth cranial nerve **R Accessory Nerve** Eleventh cranial nerve **S Hypoglossal Nerve** Twelfth cranial nerve **T Spinal Meninges** Arachnoid mater, spinal Denticulate (dentate) ligament Dura mater, spinal Filum terminale Leptomeninges, spinal Pia mater, spinal **U Spinal Canal** **W Cervical Spinal Cord** Dorsal root ganglion **X Thoracic Spinal Cord** Dorsal root ganglion **Y Lumbar Spinal Cord** Cauda equina Conus medullaris Dorsal root ganglion	**Ø Open** **3 Percutaneous** **4 Percutaneous Endoscopic**	**Z No Device**	**Z No Qualifier**

0 Medical and Surgical
0 Central Nervous System and Cranial Nerves
D Extraction Definition: Pulling or stripping out or off all or a portion of a body part by the use of force
Explanation: The qualifier DIAGNOSTIC is used to identify extraction procedures that are biopsies

Body Part Character 4		Approach Character 5	Device Character 6	Qualifier Character 7
0 Brain Cerebrum Corpus callosum Encephalon **1 Cerebral Meninges** Arachnoid mater, intracranial Leptomeninges, intracranial Pia mater, intracranial **2 Dura Mater** Diaphragma sellae Dura mater, intracranial Falx cerebri Tentorium cerebelli **7 Cerebral Hemisphere** Frontal lobe Occipital lobe Parietal lobe Temporal lobe **C Cerebellum** Culmen **F Olfactory Nerve** First cranial nerve Olfactory bulb **G Optic Nerve** Optic chiasma Second cranial nerve **H Oculomotor Nerve** Third cranial nerve **J Trochlear Nerve** Fourth cranial nerve **K Trigeminal Nerve** Fifth cranial nerve Gasserian ganglion Mandibular nerve Maxillary nerve Ophthalmic nerve Trifacial nerve **L Abducens Nerve** Sixth cranial nerve	**M Facial Nerve** Chorda tympani Geniculate ganglion Greater superficial petrosal nerve Nerve to the stapedius Parotid plexus Posterior auricular nerve Seventh cranial nerve Submandibular ganglion **N Acoustic Nerve** Cochlear nerve Eighth cranial nerve Scarpa's (vestibular) ganglion Spiral ganglion Vestibular (Scarpa's) ganglion Vestibular nerve Vestibulocochlear nerve **P Glossopharyngeal Nerve** Carotid sinus nerve Ninth cranial nerve Tympanic nerve **Q Vagus Nerve** Anterior vagal trunk Pharyngeal plexus Pneumogastric nerve Posterior vagal trunk Pulmonary plexus Recurrent laryngeal nerve Superior laryngeal nerve Tenth cranial nerve **R Accessory Nerve** Eleventh cranial nerve **S Hypoglossal Nerve** Twelfth cranial nerve **T Spinal Meninges** Arachnoid mater, spinal Denticulate (dentate) ligament Dura mater, spinal Filum terminale Leptomeninges, spinal Pia mater, spinal	**0 Open** **3 Percutaneous** **4 Percutaneous Endoscopic**	**Z No Device**	**Z No Qualifier**

Ø Medical and Surgical
Ø Central Nervous System and Cranial Nerves
F Fragmentation Definition: Breaking solid matter in a body part into pieces

Explanation: Physical force (e.g., manual, ultrasonic) applied directly or indirectly is used to break the solid matter into pieces. The solid matter may be an abnormal byproduct of a biological function or a foreign body. The pieces of solid matter are not taken out.

Body Part Character 4	Approach Character 5	Device Character 6	Qualifier Character 7
3 Epidural Space, Intracranial NC Extradural space, intracranial **4** Subdural Space, Intracranial NC **5** Subarachnoid Space, Intracranial NC **6** Cerebral Ventricle NC Aqueduct of Sylvius Cerebral aqueduct (Sylvius) Choroid plexus Ependyma Foramen of Monro (intraventricular) Fourth ventricle Interventricular foramen (Monro) Left lateral ventricle Right lateral ventricle Third ventricle **U** Spinal Canal Epidural space, spinal Extradural space, spinal Subarachnoid space, spinal Subdural space, spinal Vertebral canal	**Ø** Open **3** Percutaneous **4** Percutaneous Endoscopic **X** External	**Z** No Device	**Z** No Qualifier

Non-OR ØØF[3,4,5,6]XZZ
NC ØØF[3,4,5,6]XZZ

Ø Medical and Surgical
Ø Central Nervous System and Cranial Nerves
H Insertion Definition: Putting in a nonbiological appliance that monitors, assists, performs, or prevents a physiological function but does not physically take the place of a body part

Explanation: None

Body Part Character 4	Approach Character 5	Device Character 6	Qualifier Character 7
Ø Brain ⊞ Cerebrum Corpus callosum Encephalon	**Ø** Open	**1** Radioactive Element **2** Monitoring Device **3** Infusion Device **4** Radioactive Element, Cesium-131 Collagen Implant **M** Neurostimulator Lead **Y** Other Device	**Z** No Qualifier
Ø Brain ⊞ Cerebrum Corpus callosum Encephalon	**3** Percutaneous **4** Percutaneous Endoscopic	**1** Radioactive Element **2** Monitoring Device **3** Infusion Device **M** Neurostimulator Lead **Y** Other Device	**Z** No Qualifier
6 Cerebral Ventricle ⊞ Aqueduct of Sylvius Cerebral aqueduct (Sylvius) Choroid plexus Ependyma Foramen of Monro (intraventricular) Fourth ventricle Interventricular foramen (Monro) Left lateral ventricle Right lateral ventricle Third ventricle **E** Cranial Nerve ⊞ **U** Spinal Canal ⊞ Epidural space, spinal Extradural space, spinal Subarachnoid space, spinal Subdural space, spinal Vertebral canal **V** Spinal Cord ⊞ Dorsal root ganglion	**Ø** Open **3** Percutaneous **4** Percutaneous Endoscopic	**1** Radioactive Element **2** Monitoring Device **3** Infusion Device **M** Neurostimulator Lead **Y** Other Device	**Z** No Qualifier

DRG Non-OR ØØHØØ4Z
Non-OR ØØH[E,U,V]32Z
Non-OR ØØH[E,U][3,4]YZ
Non-OR ØØH[U,V][Ø,3,4]3Z

See Appendix L for Procedure Combinations
⊞ ØØHØØMZ
⊞ ØØHØ[3,4]MZ
⊞ ØØH[6,E,U,V][Ø,3,4]MZ

Ø Medical and Surgical
Ø Central Nervous System and Cranial Nerves
J Inspection Definition: Visually and/or manually exploring a body part

Explanation: Visual exploration may be performed with or without optical instrumentation. Manual exploration may be performed directly or through intervening body layers.

Body Part Character 4	Approach Character 5	Device Character 6	Qualifier Character 7
Ø Brain Cerebrum Corpus callosum Encephalon E Cranial Nerve U Spinal Canal Epidural space, spinal Extradural space, spinal Subarachnoid space, spinal Subdural space, spinal Vertebral canal V Spinal Cord Dorsal root ganglion	Ø Open 3 Percutaneous 4 Percutaneous Endoscopic	Z No Device	Z No Qualifier

Non-OR ØØJ[Ø,E,U,V]3ZZ

Ø Medical and Surgical
Ø Central Nervous System and Cranial Nerves
K Map Definition: Locating the route of passage of electrical impulses and/or locating functional areas in a body part

Explanation: Applicable only to the cardiac conduction mechanism and the central nervous system

Body Part Character 4	Approach Character 5	Device Character 6	Qualifier Character 7
Ø Brain Cerebrum Corpus callosum Encephalon 7 Cerebral Hemisphere Frontal lobe Occipital lobe Parietal lobe Temporal lobe 8 Basal Ganglia Basal nuclei Claustrum Corpus striatum Globus pallidus Substantia nigra Subthalamic nucleus 9 Thalamus Epithalamus Geniculate nucleus Metathalamus Pulvinar A Hypothalamus Mammillary body B Pons Apneustic center Basis pontis Locus ceruleus Pneumotaxic center Pontine tegmentum Superior olivary nucleus C Cerebellum Culmen D Medulla Oblongata Myelencephalon	Ø Open 3 Percutaneous 4 Percutaneous Endoscopic	Z No Device	Z No Qualifier

Ø Medical and Surgical
Ø Central Nervous System and Cranial Nerves
N Release
Definition: Freeing a body part from an abnormal physical constraint by cutting or by the use of force
Explanation: Some of the restraining tissue may be taken out but none of the body part is taken out

Body Part Character 4		Approach Character 5	Device Character 6	Qualifier Character 7
Ø Brain Cerebrum Corpus callosum Encephalon **1 Cerebral Meninges** Arachnoid mater, intracranial Leptomeninges, intracranial Pia mater, intracranial **2 Dura Mater** Diaphragma sellae Dura mater, intracranial Falx cerebri Tentorium cerebelli **6 Cerebral Ventricle** Aqueduct of Sylvius Cerebral aqueduct (Sylvius) Choroid plexus Ependyma Foramen of Monro (intraventricular) Fourth ventricle Interventricular foramen (Monro) Left lateral ventricle Right lateral ventricle Third ventricle **7 Cerebral Hemisphere** Frontal lobe Occipital lobe Parietal lobe Temporal lobe **8 Basal Ganglia** Basal nuclei Claustrum Corpus striatum Globus pallidus Substantia nigra Subthalamic nucleus **9 Thalamus** Epithalamus Geniculate nucleus Metathalamus Pulvinar **A Hypothalamus** Mammillary body **B Pons** Apneustic center Basis pontis Locus ceruleus Pneumotaxic center Pontine tegmentum Superior olivary nucleus **C Cerebellum** Culmen **D Medulla Oblongata** Myelencephalon **F Olfactory Nerve** First cranial nerve Olfactory bulb **G Optic Nerve** Optic chiasma Second cranial nerve	**H Oculomotor Nerve** Third cranial nerve **J Trochlear Nerve** Fourth cranial nerve **K Trigeminal Nerve** Fifth cranial nerve Gasserian ganglion Mandibular nerve Maxillary nerve Ophthalmic nerve Trifacial nerve **L Abducens Nerve** Sixth cranial nerve **M Facial Nerve** Chorda tympani Geniculate ganglion Greater superficial petrosal nerve Nerve to the stapedius Parotid plexus Posterior auricular nerve Seventh cranial nerve Submandibular ganglion **N Acoustic Nerve** Cochlear nerve Eighth cranial nerve Scarpa's (vestibular) ganglion Spiral ganglion Vestibular (Scarpa's) ganglion Vestibular nerve Vestibulocochlear nerve **P Glossopharyngeal Nerve** Carotid sinus nerve Ninth cranial nerve Tympanic nerve **Q Vagus Nerve** Anterior vagal trunk Pharyngeal plexus Pneumogastric nerve Posterior vagal trunk Pulmonary plexus Recurrent laryngeal nerve Superior laryngeal nerve Tenth cranial nerve **R Accessory Nerve** Eleventh cranial nerve **S Hypoglossal Nerve** Twelfth cranial nerve **T Spinal Meninges** Arachnoid mater, spinal Denticulate (dentate) ligament Dura mater, spinal Filum terminale Leptomeninges, spinal Pia mater, spinal **W Cervical Spinal Cord** Dorsal root ganglion **X Thoracic Spinal Cord** Dorsal root ganglion **Y Lumbar Spinal Cord** Cauda equina Conus medullaris Dorsal root ganglion	**Ø Open** **3 Percutaneous** **4 Percutaneous Endoscopic**	**Z No Device**	**Z No Qualifier**

Ø Medical and Surgical
Ø Central Nervous System and Cranial Nerves
P Removal Definition: Taking out or off a device from a body part

Explanation: If a device is taken out and a similar device put in without cutting or puncturing the skin or mucous membrane, the procedure is coded to the root operation CHANGE. Otherwise, the procedure for taking out a device is coded to the root operation REMOVAL.

Body Part Character 4	Approach Character 5	Device Character 6	Qualifier Character 7
Ø Brain Cerebrum Corpus callosum Encephalon **V Spinal Cord** Dorsal root ganglion	Ø Open 3 Percutaneous 4 Percutaneous Endoscopic	Ø Drainage Device 2 Monitoring Device 3 Infusion Device 7 Autologous Tissue Substitute J Synthetic Substitute K Nonautologous Tissue Substitute M Neurostimulator Lead Y Other Device	Z No Qualifier
Ø Brain Cerebrum Corpus callosum Encephalon **V Spinal Cord** Dorsal root ganglion	X External	Ø Drainage Device 2 Monitoring Device 3 Infusion Device M Neurostimulator Lead	Z No Qualifier
6 Cerebral Ventricle Aqueduct of Sylvius Cerebral aqueduct (Sylvius) Choroid plexus Ependyma Foramen of Monro (intraventricular) Fourth ventricle Interventricular foramen (Monro) Left lateral ventricle Right lateral ventricle Third ventricle **U Spinal Canal** Epidural space, spinal Extradural space, spinal Subarachnoid space, spinal Subdural space, spinal Vertebral canal	Ø Open 3 Percutaneous 4 Percutaneous Endoscopic	Ø Drainage Device 2 Monitoring Device 3 Infusion Device J Synthetic Substitute M Neurostimulator Lead Y Other Device	Z No Qualifier
6 Cerebral Ventricle Aqueduct of Sylvius Cerebral aqueduct (Sylvius) Choroid plexus Ependyma Foramen of Monro (intraventricular) Fourth ventricle Interventricular foramen (Monro) Left lateral ventricle Right lateral ventricle Third ventricle **U Spinal Canal** Epidural space, spinal Extradural space, spinal Subarachnoid space, spinal Subdural space, spinal Vertebral canal	X External	Ø Drainage Device 2 Monitoring Device 3 Infusion Device M Neurostimulator Lead	Z No Qualifier
E Cranial Nerve	Ø Open 3 Percutaneous 4 Percutaneous Endoscopic	Ø Drainage Device 2 Monitoring Device 3 Infusion Device 7 Autologous Tissue Substitute M Neurostimulator Lead Y Other Device	Z No Qualifier
E Cranial Nerve	X External	Ø Drainage Device 2 Monitoring Device 3 Infusion Device M Neurostimulator Lead	Z No Qualifier

Non-OR ØØP[Ø,V]3[Ø,2,3]Z
Non-OR ØØP[Ø,V][3,4]YZ
Non-OR ØØP[Ø,V]X[Ø,2,3,M]Z
Non-OR ØØP[6,U]3[Ø,2,3]Z
Non-OR ØØP[6,U][3,4]YZ
Non-OR ØØP[6,U]X[Ø,2,3,M]Z
Non-OR ØØPE3[Ø,2,3]Z
Non-OR ØØPE[3,4]YZ
Non-OR ØØPEX[Ø,2,3,M]Z

Ø Medical and Surgical
Ø Central Nervous System and Cranial Nerves
Q Repair Definition: Restoring, to the extent possible, a body part to its normal anatomic structure and function
Explanation: Used only when the method to accomplish the repair is not one of the other root operations

Body Part Character 4		Approach Character 5	Device Character 6	Qualifier Character 7
Ø Brain Cerebrum Corpus callosum Encephalon **1 Cerebral Meninges** Arachnoid mater, intracranial Leptomeninges, intracranial Pia mater, intracranial **2 Dura Mater** Diaphragma sellae Dura mater, intracranial Falx cerebri Tentorium cerebelli **6 Cerebral Ventricle** Aqueduct of Sylvius Cerebral aqueduct (Sylvius) Choroid plexus Ependyma Foramen of Monro (intraventricular) Fourth ventricle Interventricular foramen (Monro) Left lateral ventricle Right lateral ventricle Third ventricle **7 Cerebral Hemisphere** Frontal lobe Occipital lobe Parietal lobe Temporal lobe **8 Basal Ganglia** Basal nuclei Claustrum Corpus striatum Globus pallidus Substantia nigra Subthalamic nucleus **9 Thalamus** Epithalamus Geniculate nucleus Metathalamus Pulvinar **A Hypothalamus** Mammillary body **B Pons** Apneustic center Basis pontis Locus ceruleus Pneumotaxic center Pontine tegmentum Superior olivary nucleus **C Cerebellum** Culmen **D Medulla Oblongata** Myelencephalon **F Olfactory Nerve** First cranial nerve Olfactory bulb **G Optic Nerve** Optic chiasma Second cranial nerve	**H Oculomotor Nerve** Third cranial nerve **J Trochlear Nerve** Fourth cranial nerve **K Trigeminal Nerve** Fifth cranial nerve Gasserian ganglion Mandibular nerve Maxillary nerve Ophthalmic nerve Trifacial nerve **L Abducens Nerve** Sixth cranial nerve **M Facial Nerve** Chorda tympani Geniculate ganglion Greater superficial petrosal nerve Nerve to the stapedius Parotid plexus Posterior auricular nerve Seventh cranial nerve Submandibular ganglion **N Acoustic Nerve** Cochlear nerve Eighth cranial nerve Scarpa's (vestibular) ganglion Spiral ganglion Vestibular (Scarpa's) ganglion Vestibular nerve Vestibulocochlear nerve **P Glossopharyngeal Nerve** Carotid sinus nerve Ninth cranial nerve Tympanic nerve **Q Vagus Nerve** Anterior vagal trunk Pharyngeal plexus Pneumogastric nerve Posterior vagal trunk Pulmonary plexus Recurrent laryngeal nerve Superior laryngeal nerve Tenth cranial nerve **R Accessory Nerve** Eleventh cranial nerve **S Hypoglossal Nerve** Twelfth cranial nerve **T Spinal Meninges** Arachnoid mater, spinal Denticulate (dentate) ligament Dura mater, spinal Filum terminale Leptomeninges, spinal Pia mater, spinal **W Cervical Spinal Cord** Dorsal root ganglion **X Thoracic Spinal Cord** Dorsal root ganglion **Y Lumbar Spinal Cord** Cauda equina Conus medullaris Dorsal root ganglion	**Ø Open** **3 Percutaneous** **4 Percutaneous Endoscopic**	**Z No Device**	**Z No Qualifier**

Ø Medical and Surgical
Ø Central Nervous System and Cranial Nerves
R Replacement Definition: Putting in or on biological or synthetic material that physically takes the place and/or function of all or a portion of a body part

Explanation: The body part may have been taken out or replaced, or may be taken out, physically eradicated, or rendered nonfunctional during the REPLACEMENT procedure. A REMOVAL procedure is coded for taking out the device used in a previous replacement procedure.

Body Part Character 4	Approach Character 5	Device Character 6	Qualifier Character 7
1 Cerebral Meninges Arachnoid mater, intracranial Leptomeninges, intracranial Pia mater, intracranial **2 Dura Mater** Diaphragma sellae Dura mater, intracranial Falx cerebri Tentorium cerebelli **6 Cerebral Ventricle** Aqueduct of Sylvius Cerebral aqueduct (Sylvius) Choroid plexus Ependyma Foramen of Monro (intraventricular) Fourth ventricle Interventricular foramen (Monro) Left lateral ventricle Right lateral ventricle Third ventricle **F Olfactory Nerve** First cranial nerve Olfactory bulb **G Optic Nerve** Optic chiasma Second cranial nerve **H Oculomotor Nerve** Third cranial nerve **J Trochlear Nerve** Fourth cranial nerve **K Trigeminal Nerve** Fifth cranial nerve Gasserian ganglion Mandibular nerve Maxillary nerve Ophthalmic nerve Trifacial nerve **L Abducens Nerve** Sixth cranial nerve **M Facial Nerve** Chorda tympani Geniculate ganglion Greater superficial petrosal nerve Nerve to the stapedius Parotid plexus Posterior auricular nerve Seventh cranial nerve Submandibular ganglion **N Acoustic Nerve** Cochlear nerve Eighth cranial nerve Scarpa's (vestibular) ganglion Spiral ganglion Vestibular (Scarpa's) ganglion Vestibular nerve Vestibulocochlear nerve **P Glossopharyngeal Nerve** Carotid sinus nerve Ninth cranial nerve Tympanic nerve **Q Vagus Nerve** Anterior vagal trunk Pharyngeal plexus Pneumogastric nerve Posterior vagal trunk Pulmonary plexus Recurrent laryngeal nerve Superior laryngeal nerve Tenth cranial nerve **R Accessory Nerve** Eleventh cranial nerve **S Hypoglossal Nerve** Twelfth cranial nerve **T Spinal Meninges** Arachnoid mater, spinal Denticulate (dentate) ligament Dura mater, spinal Filum terminale Leptomeninges, spinal Pia mater, spinal	**Ø Open** **4 Percutaneous Endoscopic**	**7 Autologous Tissue Substitute** **J Synthetic Substitute** **K Nonautologous Tissue Substitute**	**Z No Qualifier**

Ø Medical and Surgical
Ø Central Nervous System and Cranial Nerves
S Reposition Definition: Moving to its normal location, or other suitable location, all or a portion of a body part

Explanation: The body part is moved to a new location from an abnormal location, or from a normal location where it is not functioning correctly. The body part may or may not be cut out or off to be moved to the new location.

Body Part Character 4		Approach Character 5	Device Character 6	Qualifier Character 7
F Olfactory Nerve First cranial nerve Olfactory bulb **G Optic Nerve** Optic chiasma Second cranial nerve **H Oculomotor Nerve** Third cranial nerve **J Trochlear Nerve** Fourth cranial nerve **K Trigeminal Nerve** Fifth cranial nerve Gasserian ganglion Mandibular nerve Maxillary nerve Ophthalmic nerve Trifacial nerve **L Abducens Nerve** Sixth cranial nerve **M Facial Nerve** Chorda tympani Geniculate ganglion Greater superficial petrosal nerve Nerve to the stapedius Parotid plexus Posterior auricular nerve Seventh cranial nerve Submandibular ganglion	**N Acoustic Nerve** Cochlear nerve Eighth cranial nerve Scarpa's (vestibular) ganglion Spiral ganglion Vestibular (Scarpa's) ganglion Vestibular nerve Vestibulocochlear nerve **P Glossopharyngeal Nerve** Carotid sinus nerve Ninth cranial nerve Tympanic nerve **Q Vagus Nerve** Anterior vagal trunk Pharyngeal plexus Pneumogastric nerve Posterior vagal trunk Pulmonary plexus Recurrent laryngeal nerve Superior laryngeal nerve Tenth cranial nerve **R Accessory Nerve** Eleventh cranial nerve **S Hypoglossal Nerve** Twelfth cranial nerve **W Cervical Spinal Cord** Dorsal root ganglion **X Thoracic Spinal Cord** Dorsal root ganglion **Y Lumbar Spinal Cord** Cauda equina Conus medullaris Dorsal root ganglion	**Ø Open** **3 Percutaneous** **4 Percutaneous Endoscopic**	**Z No Device**	**Z No Qualifier**

Ø Medical and Surgical
Ø Central Nervous System and Cranial Nerves
T Resection Definition: Cutting out or off, without replacement, all of a body part

Explanation: None

Body Part Character 4	Approach Character 5	Device Character 6	Qualifier Character 7
7 Cerebral Hemisphere Frontal lobe Occipital lobe Parietal lobe Temporal lobe	**Ø Open** **3 Percutaneous** **4 Percutaneous Endoscopic**	**Z No Device**	**Z No Qualifier**

Ø Medical and Surgical
Ø Central Nervous System and Cranial Nerves
U Supplement Definition: Putting in or on biological or synthetic material that physically reinforces and/or augments the function of a portion of a body part

Explanation: The biological material is non-living, or is living and from the same individual. The body part may have been previously replaced, and the SUPPLEMENT procedure is performed to physically reinforce and/or augment the function of the replaced body part.

Body Part Character 4		Approach Character 5	Device Character 6	Qualifier Character 7
1 Cerebral Meninges Arachnoid mater, intracranial Leptomeninges, intracranial Pia mater, intracranial **2 Dura Mater** Diaphragma sellae Dura mater, intracranial Falx cerebri Tentorium cerebelli **6 Cerebral Ventricle** Aqueduct of Sylvius Cerebral aqueduct (Sylvius) Choroid plexus Ependyma Foramen of Monro (intraventricular) Fourth ventricle Interventricular foramen (Monro) Left lateral ventricle Right lateral ventricle Third ventricle **F Olfactory Nerve** First cranial nerve Olfactory bulb **G Optic Nerve** Optic chiasma Second cranial nerve **H Oculomotor Nerve** Third cranial nerve **J Trochlear Nerve** Fourth cranial nerve **K Trigeminal Nerve** Fifth cranial nerve Gasserian ganglion Mandibular nerve Maxillary nerve Ophthalmic nerve Trifacial nerve **L Abducens Nerve** Sixth cranial nerve	**M Facial Nerve** Chorda tympani Geniculate ganglion Greater superficial petrosal nerve Nerve to the stapedius Parotid plexus Posterior auricular nerve Seventh cranial nerve Submandibular ganglion **N Acoustic Nerve** Cochlear nerve Eighth cranial nerve Scarpa's (vestibular) ganglion Spiral ganglion Vestibular (Scarpa's) ganglion Vestibular nerve Vestibulocochlear nerve **P Glossopharyngeal Nerve** Carotid sinus nerve Ninth cranial nerve Tympanic nerve **Q Vagus Nerve** Anterior vagal trunk Pharyngeal plexus Pneumogastric nerve Posterior vagal trunk Pulmonary plexus Recurrent laryngeal nerve Superior laryngeal nerve Tenth cranial nerve **R Accessory Nerve** Eleventh cranial nerve **S Hypoglossal Nerve** Twelfth cranial nerve **T Spinal Meninges** Arachnoid mater, spinal Denticulate (dentate) ligament Dura mater, spinal Filum terminale Leptomeninges, spinal Pia mater, spinal	**Ø Open** **3 Percutaneous** **4 Percutaneous Endoscopic**	**7 Autologous Tissue Substitute** **J Synthetic Substitute** **K Nonautologous Tissue Substitute**	**Z No Qualifier**

Ø Medical and Surgical
Ø Central Nervous System and Cranial Nerves
W Revision

Definition: Correcting, to the extent possible, a portion of a malfunctioning device or the position of a displaced device

Explanation: Revision can include correcting a malfunctioning or displaced device by taking out or putting in components of the device such as a screw or pin

Body Part Character 4	Approach Character 5	Device Character 6	Qualifier Character 7
Ø Brain Cerebrum Corpus callosum Encephalon **V Spinal Cord** Dorsal root ganglion	**Ø** Open **3** Percutaneous **4** Percutaneous Endoscopic	**Ø** Drainage Device **2** Monitoring Device **3** Infusion Device **7** Autologous Tissue Substitute **J** Synthetic Substitute **K** Nonautologous Tissue Substitute **M** Neurostimulator Lead **Y** Other Device	**Z** No Qualifier
Ø Brain Cerebrum Corpus callosum Encephalon **V Spinal Cord** Dorsal root ganglion	**X** External	**Ø** Drainage Device **2** Monitoring Device **3** Infusion Device **7** Autologous Tissue Substitute **J** Synthetic Substitute **K** Nonautologous Tissue Substitute **M** Neurostimulator Lead	**Z** No Qualifier
6 Cerebral Ventricle Aqueduct of Sylvius Cerebral aqueduct (Sylvius) Choroid plexus Ependyma Foramen of Monro (intraventricular) Fourth ventricle Interventricular foramen (Monro) Left lateral ventricle Right lateral ventricle Third ventricle **U Spinal Canal** Epidural space, spinal Extradural space, spinal Subarachnoid space, spinal Subdural space, spinal Vertebral canal	**Ø** Open **3** Percutaneous **4** Percutaneous Endoscopic	**Ø** Drainage Device **2** Monitoring Device **3** Infusion Device **J** Synthetic Substitute **M** Neurostimulator Lead **Y** Other Device	**Z** No Qualifier
6 Cerebral Ventricle Aqueduct of Sylvius Cerebral aqueduct (Sylvius) Choroid plexus Ependyma Foramen of Monro (intraventricular) Fourth ventricle Interventricular foramen (Monro) Left lateral ventricle Right lateral ventricle Third ventricle **U Spinal Canal** Epidural space, spinal Extradural space, spinal Subarachnoid space, spinal Subdural space, spinal Vertebral canal	**X** External	**Ø** Drainage Device **2** Monitoring Device **3** Infusion Device **J** Synthetic Substitute **M** Neurostimulator Lead	**Z** No Qualifier
E Cranial Nerve	**Ø** Open **3** Percutaneous **4** Percutaneous Endoscopic	**Ø** Drainage Device **2** Monitoring Device **3** Infusion Device **7** Autologous Tissue Substitute **M** Neurostimulator Lead **Y** Other Device	**Z** No Qualifier
E Cranial Nerve	**X** External	**Ø** Drainage Device **2** Monitoring Device **3** Infusion Device **7** Autologous Tissue Substitute **M** Neurostimulator Lead	**Z** No Qualifier

Non-OR ØØW[Ø,V][3,4]YZ
Non-OR ØØW[Ø,V]X[Ø,2,3,7,J,K,M]Z
Non-OR ØØW[6,U][3,4]YZ
Non-OR ØØW[6,U]X[Ø,2,3,J,M]Z
Non-OR ØØWE[3,4]YZ
Non-OR ØØWEX[Ø,2,3,7,M]Z

Ø Medical and Surgical
Ø Central Nervous System and Cranial Nerves
X Transfer Definition: Moving, without taking out, all or a portion of a body part to another location to take over the function of all or a portion of a body part

Explanation: The body part transferred remains connected to its vascular and nervous supply

Body Part Character 4	Approach Character 5	Device Character 6	Qualifier Character 7
F Olfactory Nerve First cranial nerve Olfactory bulb **G Optic Nerve** Optic chiasma Second cranial nerve **H Oculomotor Nerve** Third cranial nerve **J Trochlear Nerve** Fourth cranial nerve **K Trigeminal Nerve** Fifth cranial nerve Gasserian ganglion Mandibular nerve Maxillary nerve Ophthalmic nerve Trifacial nerve **L Abducens Nerve** Sixth cranial nerve **M Facial Nerve** Chorda tympani Geniculate ganglion Greater superficial petrosal nerve Nerve to the stapedius Parotid plexus Posterior auricular nerve Seventh cranial nerve Submandibular ganglion **N Acoustic Nerve** Cochlear nerve Eighth cranial nerve Scarpa's (vestibular) ganglion Spiral ganglion Vestibular (Scarpa's) ganglion Vestibular nerve Vestibulocochlear nerve **P Glossopharyngeal Nerve** Carotid sinus nerve Ninth cranial nerve Tympanic nerve **Q Vagus Nerve** Anterior vagal trunk Pharyngeal plexus Pneumogastric nerve Posterior vagal trunk Pulmonary plexus Recurrent laryngeal nerve Superior laryngeal nerve Tenth cranial nerve **R Accessory Nerve** Eleventh cranial nerve **S Hypoglossal Nerve** Twelfth cranial nerve	**Ø Open** **4 Percutaneous Endoscopic**	**Z No Device**	**F Olfactory Nerve** **G Optic Nerve** **H Oculomotor Nerve** **J Trochlear Nerve** **K Trigeminal Nerve** **L Abducens Nerve** **M Facial Nerve** **N Acoustic Nerve** **P Glossopharyngeal Nerve** **Q Vagus Nerve** **R Accessory Nerve** **S Hypoglossal Nerve**

Peripheral Nervous System Ø12–Ø1X

Character Meanings

This Character Meaning table is provided as a guide to assist the user in the identification of character members that may be found in this section of code tables. It **SHOULD NOT** be used to build a PCS code.

Operation–Character 3	Body Part–Character 4	Approach–Character 5	Device–Character 6	Qualifier–Character 7
2 Change	Ø Cervical Plexus	Ø Open	Ø Drainage Device	1 Cervical Nerve
5 Destruction	1 Cervical Nerve	3 Percutaneous	1 Radioactive Element	2 Phrenic Nerve
8 Division	2 Phrenic Nerve	4 Percutaneous Endoscopic	2 Monitoring Device	4 Ulnar Nerve
9 Drainage	3 Brachial Plexus	X External	7 Autologous Tissue Substitute	5 Median Nerve
B Excision	4 Ulnar Nerve		J Synthetic Substitute	6 Radial Nerve
C Extirpation	5 Median Nerve		K Nonautologous Tissue Substitute	8 Thoracic Nerve
D Extraction	6 Radial Nerve		M Neurostimulator Lead	B Lumbar Nerve
H Insertion	8 Thoracic Nerve		Y Other Device	C Perineal Nerve
J Inspection	9 Lumbar Plexus		Z No Device	D Femoral Nerve
N Release	A Lumbosacral Plexus			F Sciatic Nerve
P Removal	B Lumbar Nerve			G Tibial Nerve
Q Repair	C Pudendal Nerve			H Peroneal Nerve
R Replacement	D Femoral Nerve			X Diagnostic
S Reposition	F Sciatic Nerve			Z No Qualifier
U Supplement	G Tibial Nerve			
W Revision	H Peroneal Nerve			
X Transfer	K Head and Neck Sympathetic Nerve			
	L Thoracic Sympathetic Nerve			
	M Abdominal Sympathetic Nerve			
	N Lumbar Sympathetic Nerve			
	P Sacral Sympathetic Nerve			
	Q Sacral Plexus			
	R Sacral Nerve			
	Y Peripheral Nerve			

AHA Coding Clinic for table Ø1B
2018, 2Q, 22 Excision of synovial cyst
2017, 2Q, 19 Thoracic outlet decompression with sympathectomy

AHA Coding Clinic for table Ø1H
2020, 4Q, 43-44 Insertion of radioactive element

AHA Coding Clinic for table Ø1N
2019, 1Q, 28 Decompressive laminectomy of both spinal cord and nerve roots
2018, 2Q, 22 Excision of synovial cyst
2017, 2Q, 19 Thoracic outlet decompression with sympathectomy
2016, 2Q, 16 Decompressive laminectomy/foraminotomy and lumbar discectomy
2016, 2Q, 17 Removal of longitudinal ligament to decompress cervical nerve root
2016, 2Q, 23 Thoracic outlet syndrome and release of brachial plexus
2015, 2Q, 34 Decompressive laminectomy
2014, 3Q, 33 Radial fracture treatment with open reduction internal fixation, and release of carpal ligament

AHA Coding Clinic for table Ø1Q
2019, 3Q, 32 Breast reconstruction with neurotization

AHA Coding Clinic for table Ø1S
2021, 3Q, 19 Elbow amputation and targeted muscle reinnervation

AHA Coding Clinic for table Ø1U
2019, 3Q, 32 Breast reconstruction with neurotization
2017, 4Q, 62 Added and revised device values - Nerve substitutes

Median and Ulnar Nerves

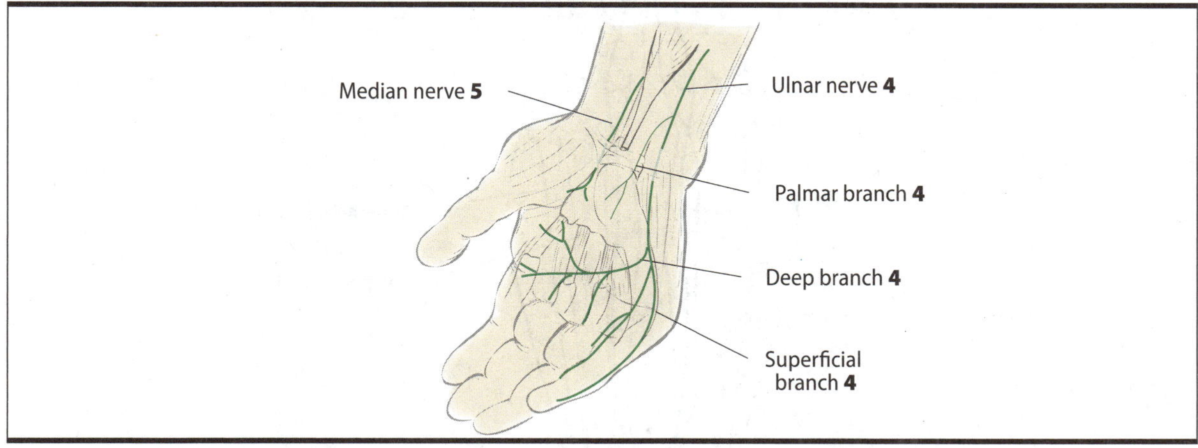

Peripheral Nervous System

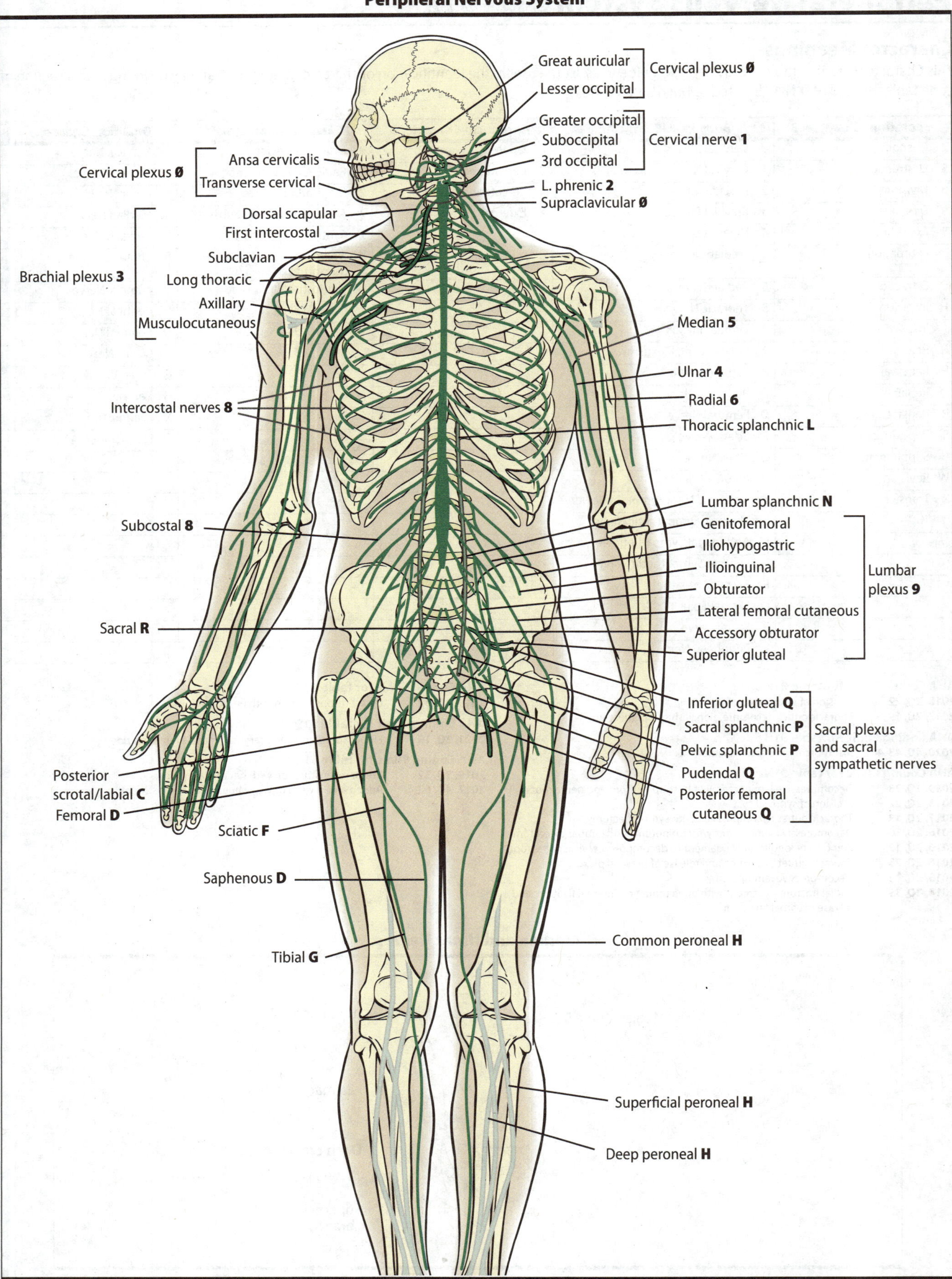

Ø Medical and Surgical
1 Peripheral Nervous System
2 Change Definition: Taking out or off a device from a body part and putting back an identical or similar device in or on the same body part without cutting or puncturing the skin or a mucous membrane

Explanation: All CHANGE procedures are coded using the approach EXTERNAL

Body Part Character 4	Approach Character 5	Device Character 6	Qualifier Character 7
Y Peripheral Nerve	X External	Ø Drainage Device Y Other Device	Z No Qualifier

Non-OR All body part, approach, device, and qualifier values

Ø Medical and Surgical
1 Peripheral Nervous System
5 Destruction Definition: Physical eradication of all or a portion of a body part by the direct use of energy, force, or a destructive agent

Explanation: None of the body part is physically taken out

Body Part Character 4	Approach Character 5	Device Character 6	Qualifier Character 7
Ø Cervical Plexus Ansa cervicalis Cutaneous (transverse) cervical nerve Great auricular nerve Lesser occipital nerve Supraclavicular nerve Transverse (cutaneous) cervical nerve 1 Cervical Nerve Greater occipital nerve Spinal nerve, cervical Suboccipital nerve Third occipital nerve 2 Phrenic Nerve Accessory phrenic nerve 3 Brachial Plexus Axillary nerve Dorsal scapular nerve First intercostal nerve Long thoracic nerve Musculocutaneous nerve Subclavius nerve Suprascapular nerve 4 Ulnar Nerve Cubital nerve 5 Median Nerve Anterior interosseous nerve Palmar cutaneous nerve 6 Radial Nerve Dorsal digital nerve Musculospiral nerve Palmar cutaneous nerve Posterior interosseous nerve 8 Thoracic Nerve Intercostal nerve Intercostobrachial nerve Spinal nerve, thoracic Subcostal nerve 9 Lumbar Plexus Accessory obturator nerve Genitofemoral nerve Iliohypogastric nerve Ilioinguinal nerve Lateral femoral cutaneous nerve Obturator nerve Superior gluteal nerve A Lumbosacral Plexus B Lumbar Nerve Lumbosacral trunk Spinal nerve, lumbar Superior clunic (cluneal) nerve C Pudendal Nerve Posterior labial nerve Posterior scrotal nerve D Femoral Nerve Anterior crural nerve Saphenous nerve F Sciatic Nerve Ischiatic nerve G Tibial Nerve Lateral plantar nerve Medial plantar nerve Medial popliteal nerve Medial sural cutaneous nerve H Peroneal Nerve Common fibular nerve Common peroneal nerve External popliteal nerve Lateral sural cutaneous nerve K Head and Neck Sympathetic Nerve Cavernous plexus Cervical ganglion Ciliary ganglion Internal carotid plexus Otic ganglion Pterygopalatine (sphenopalatine) ganglion Sphenopalatine (pterygopalatine) ganglion Stellate ganglion Submandibular ganglion Submaxillary ganglion L Thoracic Sympathetic Nerve Cardiac plexus Esophageal plexus Greater splanchnic nerve Inferior cardiac nerve Least splanchnic nerve Lesser splanchnic nerve Middle cardiac nerve Pulmonary plexus Superior cardiac nerve Thoracic aortic plexus Thoracic ganglion M Abdominal Sympathetic Nerve Abdominal aortic plexus Auerbach's (myenteric) plexus Celiac (solar) plexus Celiac ganglion Gastric plexus Hepatic plexus Inferior hypogastric plexus Inferior mesenteric ganglion Inferior mesenteric plexus Meissner's (submucous) plexus Myenteric (Auerbach's) plexus Pancreatic plexus Pelvic splanchnic nerve Renal nerve Renal plexus Solar (celiac) plexus Splenic plexus Submucous (Meissner's) plexus Superior hypogastric plexus Superior mesenteric ganglion Superior mesenteric plexus Suprarenal plexus N Lumbar Sympathetic Nerve Lumbar ganglion Lumbar splanchnic nerve P Sacral Sympathetic Nerve Ganglion impar (ganglion of Walther) Pelvic splanchnic nerve Sacral ganglion Sacral splanchnic nerve Q Sacral Plexus Inferior gluteal nerve Posterior femoral cutaneous nerve Pudendal nerve R Sacral Nerve Spinal nerve, sacral	Ø Open 3 Percutaneous 4 Percutaneous Endoscopic	Z No Device	Z No Qualifier

Non-OR Ø15[Ø,2,3,4,5,6,9,A,C,D,F,G,H,Q][Ø,3,4]ZZ

Non-OR Ø15[1,8,B,R]3ZZ

Ø Medical and Surgical
1 Peripheral Nervous System
8 Division

Definition: Cutting into a body part, without draining fluids and/or gases from the body part, in order to separate or transect a body part

Explanation: All or a portion of the body part is separated into two or more portions

Body Part Character 4	Approach Character 5	Device Character 6	Qualifier Character 7
Ø Cervical Plexus Ansa cervicalis Cutaneous (transverse) cervical nerve Great auricular nerve Lesser occipital nerve Supraclavicular nerve Transverse (cutaneous) cervical nervef **1 Cervical Nerve** Greater occipital nerve Spinal nerve, cervical Suboccipital nerve Third occipital nerve **2 Phrenic Nerve** Accessory phrenic nerve **3 Brachial Plexus** Axillary nerve Dorsal scapular nerve First intercostal nerve Long thoracic nerve Musculocutaneous nerve Subclavius nerve Suprascapular nerve **4 Ulnar Nerve** Cubital nerve **5 Median Nerve** Anterior interosseous nerve Palmar cutaneous nerve **6 Radial Nerve** Dorsal digital nerve Musculospiral nerve Palmar cutaneous nerve Posterior interosseous nerve **8 Thoracic Nerve** Intercostal nerve Intercostobrachial nerve Spinal nerve, thoracic Subcostal nerve **9 Lumbar Plexus** Accessory obturator nerve Genitofemoral nerve Iliohypogastric nerve Ilioinguinal nerve Lateral femoral cutaneous nerve Obturator nerve Superior gluteal nerve **A Lumbosacral Plexus** **B Lumbar Nerve** Lumbosacral trunk Spinal nerve, lumbar Superior clunic (cluneal) nerve **C Pudendal Nerve** Posterior labial nerve Posterior scrotal nerve **D Femoral Nerve** Anterior crural nerve Saphenous nerve **F Sciatic Nerve** Ischiatic nerve **G Tibial Nerve** Lateral plantar nerve Medial plantar nerve Medial popliteal nerve Medial sural cutaneous nerve **H Peroneal Nerve** Common fibular nerve Common peroneal nerve External popliteal nerve Lateral sural cutaneous nerve **K Head and Neck Sympathetic Nerve** Cavernous plexus Cervical ganglion Ciliary ganglion Internal carotid plexus Otic ganglion Pterygopalatine (sphenopalatine) ganglion Sphenopalatine (pterygopalatine) ganglion Stellate ganglion Submandibular ganglion Submaxillary ganglion **L Thoracic Sympathetic Nerve** Cardiac plexus Esophageal plexus Greater splanchnic nerve Inferior cardiac nerve Least splanchnic nerve Lesser splanchnic nerve Middle cardiac nerve Pulmonary plexus Superior cardiac nerve Thoracic aortic plexus Thoracic ganglion **M Abdominal Sympathetic Nerve** Abdominal aortic plexus Auerbach's (myenteric) plexus Celiac (solar) plexus Celiac ganglion Gastric plexus Hepatic plexus Inferior hypogastric plexus Inferior mesenteric ganglion Inferior mesenteric plexus Meissner's (submucous) plexus Myenteric (Auerbach's) plexus Pancreatic plexus Pelvic splanchnic nerve Renal nerve Renal plexus Solar (celiac) plexus Splenic plexus Submucous (Meissner's) plexus Superior hypogastric plexus Superior mesenteric ganglion Superior mesenteric plexus Suprarenal plexus **N Lumbar Sympathetic Nerve** Lumbar ganglion Lumbar splanchnic nerve **P Sacral Sympathetic Nerve** Ganglion impar (ganglion of Walther) Pelvic splanchnic nerve Sacral ganglion Sacral splanchnic nerve **Q Sacral Plexus** Inferior gluteal nerve Posterior femoral cutaneous nerve Pudendal nerve **R Sacral Nerve** Spinal nerve, sacral	**Ø Open** **3 Percutaneous** **4 Percutaneous Endoscopic**	**Z No Device**	**Z No Qualifier**

Ø Medical and Surgical
1 Peripheral Nervous System
9 Drainage Definition: Taking or letting out fluids and/or gases from a body part
Explanation: The qualifier DIAGNOSTIC is used to identify drainage procedures that are biopsies

Body Part Character 4	Approach Character 5	Device Character 6	Qualifier Character 7
Ø Cervical Plexus Ansa cervicalis Cutaneous (transverse) cervical nerve Great auricular nerve Lesser occipital nerve Supraclavicular nerve Transverse (cutaneous) cervical nerve 1 Cervical Nerve Greater occipital nerve Spinal nerve, cervical Suboccipital nerve Third occipital nerve 2 Phrenic Nerve Accessory phrenic nerve 3 Brachial Plexus Axillary nerve Dorsal scapular nerve First intercostal nerve Long thoracic nerve Musculocutaneous nerve Subclavius nerve Suprascapular nerve 4 Ulnar Nerve Cubital nerve 5 Median Nerve Anterior interosseous nerve Palmar cutaneous nerve 6 Radial Nerve Dorsal digital nerve Musculospiral nerve Palmar cutaneous nerve Posterior interosseous nerve 8 Thoracic Nerve Intercostal nerve Intercostobrachial nerve Spinal nerve, thoracic Subcostal nerve 9 Lumbar Plexus Accessory obturator nerve Genitofemoral nerve Iliohypogastric nerve Ilioinguinal nerve Lateral femoral cutaneous nerve Obturator nerve Superior gluteal nerve A Lumbosacral Plexus B Lumbar Nerve Lumbosacral trunk Spinal nerve, lumbar Superior clunic (cluneal) nerve C Pudendal Nerve Posterior labial nerve Posterior scrotal nerve D Femoral Nerve Anterior crural nerve Saphenous nerve F Sciatic Nerve Ischiatic nerve G Tibial Nerve Lateral plantar nerve Medial plantar nerve Medial popliteal nerve Medial sural cutaneous nerve H Peroneal Nerve Common fibular nerve Common peroneal nerve External popliteal nerve Lateral sural cutaneous nerve K Head and Neck Sympathetic Nerve Cavernous plexus Cervical ganglion Ciliary ganglion Internal carotid plexus Otic ganglion Pterygopalatine (sphenopalatine) ganglion Sphenopalatine (pterygopalatine) ganglion Stellate ganglion Submandibular ganglion Submaxillary ganglion L Thoracic Sympathetic Nerve Cardiac plexus Esophageal plexus Greater splanchnic nerve Inferior cardiac nerve Least splanchnic nerve Lesser splanchnic nerve Middle cardiac nerve Pulmonary plexus Superior cardiac nerve Thoracic aortic plexus Thoracic ganglion M Abdominal Sympathetic Nerve Abdominal aortic plexus Auerbach's (myenteric) plexus Celiac (solar) plexus Celiac ganglion Gastric plexus Hepatic plexus Inferior hypogastric plexus Inferior mesenteric ganglion Inferior mesenteric plexus Meissner's (submucous) plexus Myenteric (Auerbach's) plexus Pancreatic plexus Pelvic splanchnic nerve Renal nerve Renal plexus Solar (celiac) plexus Splenic plexus Submucous (Meissner's) plexus Superior hypogastric plexus Superior mesenteric ganglion Superior mesenteric plexus Suprarenal plexus N Lumbar Sympathetic Nerve Lumbar ganglion Lumbar splanchnic nerve P Sacral Sympathetic Nerve Ganglion impar (ganglion of Walther) Pelvic splanchnic nerve Sacral ganglion Sacral splanchnic nerve Q Sacral Plexus Inferior gluteal nerve Posterior femoral cutaneous nerve Pudendal nerve R Sacral Nerve Spinal nerve, sacral	Ø Open 3 Percutaneous 4 Percutaneous Endoscopic	Ø Drainage Device	Z No Qualifier

Non-OR Ø19[Ø,1,2,3,4,5,6,8,9,A,B,C,D,F,G,H,K,L,M,N,P,Q,R]3ØZ

Ø19 Continued on next page

Ø Medical and Surgical
1 Peripheral Nervous System
9 Drainage Definition: Taking or letting out fluids and/or gases from a body part
Explanation: The qualifier DIAGNOSTIC is used to identify drainage procedures that are biopsies

Ø19 Continued

Body Part Character 4		Approach Character 5	Device Character 6	Qualifier Character 7
Ø Cervical Plexus Ansa cervicalis Cutaneous (transverse) cervical nerve Great auricular nerve Lesser occipital nerve Supraclavicular nerve Transverse (cutaneous) cervical nerve **1 Cervical Nerve** Greater occipital nerve Spinal nerve, cervical Suboccipital nerve Third occipital nerve **2 Phrenic Nerve** Accessory phrenic nerve **3 Brachial Plexus** Axillary nerve Dorsal scapular nerve First intercostal nerve Long thoracic nerve Musculocutaneous nerve Subclavius nerve Suprascapular nerve **4 Ulnar Nerve** Cubital nerve **5 Median Nerve** Anterior interosseous nerve Palmar cutaneous nerve **6 Radial Nerve** Dorsal digital nerve Musculospiral nerve Palmar cutaneous nerve Posterior interosseous nerve **8 Thoracic Nerve** Intercostal nerve Intercostobrachial nerve Spinal nerve, thoracic Subcostal nerve **9 Lumbar Plexus** Accessory obturator nerve Genitofemoral nerve Iliohypogastric nerve Ilioinguinal nerve Lateral femoral cutaneous nerve Obturator nerve Superior gluteal nerve **A Lumbosacral Plexus** **B Lumbar Nerve** Lumbosacral trunk Spinal nerve, lumbar Superior clunic (cluneal) nerve **C Pudendal Nerve** Posterior labial nerve Posterior scrotal nerve **D Femoral Nerve** Anterior crural nerve Saphenous nerve **F Sciatic Nerve** Ischiatic nerve **G Tibial Nerve** Lateral plantar nerve Medial plantar nerve Medial popliteal nerve Medial sural cutaneous nerve	**H Peroneal Nerve** Common fibular nerve Common peroneal nerve External popliteal nerve Lateral sural cutaneous nerve **K Head and Neck Sympathetic Nerve** Cavernous plexus Cervical ganglion Ciliary ganglion Internal carotid plexus Otic ganglion Pterygopalatine (sphenopalatine) ganglion Sphenopalatine (pterygopalatine) ganglion Stellate ganglion Submandibular ganglion Submaxillary ganglion **L Thoracic Sympathetic Nerve** Cardiac plexus Esophageal plexus Greater splanchnic nerve Inferior cardiac nerve Least splanchnic nerve Lesser splanchnic nerve Middle cardiac nerve Pulmonary plexus Superior cardiac nerve Thoracic aortic plexus Thoracic ganglion **M Abdominal Sympathetic Nerve** Abdominal aortic plexus Auerbach's (myenteric) plexus Celiac (solar) plexus Celiac ganglion Gastric plexus Hepatic plexus Inferior hypogastric plexus Inferior mesenteric ganglion Inferior mesenteric plexus Meissner's (submucous) plexus Myenteric (Auerbach's) plexus Pancreatic plexus Pelvic splanchnic nerve Renal nerve Renal plexus Solar (celiac) plexus Splenic plexus Submucous (Meissner's) plexus Superior hypogastric plexus Superior mesenteric ganglion Superior mesenteric plexus Suprarenal plexus **N Lumbar Sympathetic Nerve** Lumbar ganglion Lumbar splanchnic nerve **P Sacral Sympathetic Nerve** Ganglion impar (ganglion of Walther) Pelvic splanchnic nerve Sacral ganglion Sacral splanchnic nerve **Q Sacral Plexus** Inferior gluteal nerve Posterior femoral cutaneous nerve Pudendal nerve **R Sacral Nerve** Spinal nerve, sacral	**Ø** Open **3** Percutaneous **4** Percutaneous Endoscopic	**Z** No Device	**X** Diagnostic **Z** No Qualifier

Non-OR Ø19[Ø,1,2,3,4,5,6,8,9,A,B,C,D,F,G,H,Q,R][3,4]ZX
Non-OR Ø19[Ø,1,2,3,4,5,6,8,9,A,B,C,D,F,G,H,K,L,M,N,P,Q,R]3ZZ

Ø Medical and Surgical
1 Peripheral Nervous System
B Excision

Definition: Cutting out or off, without replacement, a portion of a body part

Explanation: The qualifier DIAGNOSTIC is used to identify excision procedures that are biopsies

Body Part Character 4	Approach Character 5	Device Character 6	Qualifier Character 7
Ø Cervical Plexus Ansa cervicalis Cutaneous (transverse) cervical nerve Great auricular nerve Lesser occipital nerve Supraclavicular nerve Transverse (cutaneous) cervical nerve **1 Cervical Nerve** Greater occipital nerve Spinal nerve, cervical Suboccipital nerve Third occipital nerve **2 Phrenic Nerve** Accessory phrenic nerve **3 Brachial Plexus** Axillary nerve Dorsal scapular nerve First intercostal nerve Long thoracic nerve Musculocutaneous nerve Subclavius nerve Suprascapular nerve **4 Ulnar Nerve** Cubital nerve **5 Median Nerve** Anterior interosseous nerve Palmar cutaneous nerve **6 Radial Nerve** Dorsal digital nerve Musculospiral nerve Palmar cutaneous nerve Posterior interosseous nerve **8 Thoracic Nerve** Intercostal nerve Intercostobrachial nerve Spinal nerve, thoracic Subcostal nerve **9 Lumbar Plexus** Accessory obturator nerve Genitofemoral nerve Iliohypogastric nerve Ilioinguinal nerve Lateral femoral cutaneous nerve Obturator nerve Superior gluteal nerve **A Lumbosacral Plexus** **B Lumbar Nerve** Lumbosacral trunk Spinal nerve, lumbar Superior clunic (cluneal) nerve **C Pudendal Nerve** Posterior labial nerve Posterior scrotal nerve **D Femoral Nerve** Anterior crural nerve Saphenous nerve **F Sciatic Nerve** Ischiatic nerve **G Tibial Nerve** Lateral plantar nerve Medial plantar nerve Medial popliteal nerve Medial sural cutaneous nerve **H Peroneal Nerve** Common fibular nerve Common peroneal nerve External popliteal nerve Lateral sural cutaneous nerve **K Head and Neck Sympathetic Nerve** Cavernous plexus Cervical ganglion Ciliary ganglion Internal carotid plexus Otic ganglion Pterygopalatine (sphenopalatine) ganglion Sphenopalatine (pterygopalatine) ganglion Stellate ganglion Submandibular ganglion Submaxillary ganglion **L Thoracic Sympathetic Nerve** Cardiac plexus Esophageal plexus Greater splanchnic nerve Inferior cardiac nerve Least splanchnic nerve Lesser splanchnic nerve Middle cardiac nerve Pulmonary plexus Superior cardiac nerve Thoracic aortic plexus Thoracic ganglion **M Abdominal Sympathetic Nerve** Abdominal aortic plexus Auerbach's (myenteric) plexus Celiac (solar) plexus Celiac ganglion Gastric plexus Hepatic plexus Inferior hypogastric plexus Inferior mesenteric ganglion Inferior mesenteric plexus Meissner's (submucous) plexus Myenteric (Auerbach's) plexus Pancreatic plexus Pelvic splanchnic nerve Renal nerve Renal plexus Solar (celiac) plexus Splenic plexus Submucous (Meissner's) plexus Superior hypogastric plexus Superior mesenteric ganglion Superior mesenteric plexus Suprarenal plexus **N Lumbar Sympathetic Nerve** Lumbar ganglion Lumbar splanchnic nerve **P Sacral Sympathetic Nerve** Ganglion impar (ganglion of Walther) Pelvic splanchnic nerve Sacral ganglion Sacral splanchnic nerve **Q Sacral Plexus** Inferior gluteal nerve Posterior femoral cutaneous nerve Pudendal nerve **R Sacral Nerve** Spinal nerve, sacral	**Ø Open** **3 Percutaneous** **4 Percutaneous Endoscopic**	**Z No Device**	**X Diagnostic** **Z No Qualifier**

Non-OR Ø1B[Ø,1,2,3,4,5,6,8,9,A,B,C,D,F,G,H,Q,R][3,4]ZX

Ø Medical and Surgical
1 Peripheral Nervous System
C Extirpation Definition: Taking or cutting out solid matter from a body part

Explanation: The solid matter may be an abnormal byproduct of a biological function or a foreign body; it may be imbedded in a body part or in the lumen of a tubular body part. The solid matter may or may not have been previously broken into pieces.

Body Part Character 4	Approach Character 5	Device Character 6	Qualifier Character 7
Ø Cervical Plexus Ansa cervicalis; Cutaneous (transverse) cervical nerve; Great auricular nerve; Lesser occipital nerve; Supraclavicular nerve; Transverse (cutaneous) cervical nerve **1 Cervical Nerve** Greater occipital nerve; Spinal nerve, cervical; Suboccipital nerve; Third occipital nerve **2 Phrenic Nerve** Accessory phrenic nerve **3 Brachial Plexus** Axillary nerve; Dorsal scapular nerve; First intercostal nerve; Long thoracic nerve; Musculocutaneous nerve; Subclavius nerve; Suprascapular nerve **4 Ulnar Nerve** Cubital nerve **5 Median Nerve** Anterior interosseous nerve; Palmar cutaneous nerve **6 Radial Nerve** Dorsal digital nerve; Musculospiral nerve; Palmar cutaneous nerve; Posterior interosseous nerve **8 Thoracic Nerve** Intercostal nerve; Intercostobrachial nerve; Spinal nerve, thoracic; Subcostal nerve **9 Lumbar Plexus** Accessory obturator nerve; Genitofemoral nerve; Iliohypogastric nerve; Ilioinguinal nerve; Lateral femoral cutaneous nerve; Obturator nerve; Superior gluteal nerve **A Lumbosacral Plexus** **B Lumbar Nerve** Lumbosacral trunk; Spinal nerve, lumbar; Superior clunic (cluneal) nerve **C Pudendal Nerve** Posterior labial nerve; Posterior scrotal nerve **D Femoral Nerve** Anterior crural nerve; Saphenous nerve **F Sciatic Nerve** Ischiatic nerve **G Tibial Nerve** Lateral plantar nerve; Medial plantar nerve; Medial popliteal nerve; Medial sural cutaneous nerve **H Peroneal Nerve** Common fibular nerve; Common peroneal nerve; External popliteal nerve; Lateral sural cutaneous nerve **K Head and Neck Sympathetic Nerve** Cavernous plexus; Cervical ganglion; Ciliary ganglion; Internal carotid plexus; Otic ganglion; Pterygopalatine (sphenopalatine) ganglion; Sphenopalatine (pterygopalatine) ganglion; Stellate ganglion; Submandibular ganglion; Submaxillary ganglion **L Thoracic Sympathetic Nerve** Cardiac plexus; Esophageal plexus; Greater splanchnic nerve; Inferior cardiac nerve; Least splanchnic nerve; Lesser splanchnic nerve; Middle cardiac nerve; Pulmonary plexus; Superior cardiac nerve; Thoracic aortic plexus; Thoracic ganglion **M Abdominal Sympathetic Nerve** Abdominal aortic plexus; Auerbach's (myenteric) plexus; Celiac (solar) plexus; Celiac ganglion; Gastric plexus; Hepatic plexus; Inferior hypogastric plexus; Inferior mesenteric ganglion; Inferior mesenteric plexus; Meissner's (submucous) plexus; Myenteric (Auerbach's) plexus; Pancreatic plexus; Pelvic splanchnic nerve; Renal nerve; Renal plexus; Solar (celiac) plexus; Splenic plexus; Submucous (Meissner's) plexus; Superior hypogastric plexus; Superior mesenteric ganglion; Superior mesenteric plexus; Suprarenal plexus **N Lumbar Sympathetic Nerve** Lumbar ganglion; Lumbar splanchnic nerve **P Sacral Sympathetic Nerve** Ganglion impar (ganglion of Walther); Pelvic splanchnic nerve; Sacral ganglion; Sacral splanchnic nerve **Q Sacral Plexus** Inferior gluteal nerve; Posterior femoral cutaneous nerve; Pudendal nerve **R Sacral Nerve** Spinal nerve, sacral	**Ø Open** **3 Percutaneous** **4 Percutaneous Endoscopic**	**Z No Device**	**Z No Qualifier**

Ø Medical and Surgical
1 Peripheral Nervous System
D Extraction Definition: Pulling or stripping out or off all or a portion of a body part by the use of force
Explanation: The qualifier DIAGNOSTIC is used to identify extraction procedures that are biopsies

Body Part Character 4	Approach Character 5	Device Character 6	Qualifier Character 7
Ø Cervical Plexus Ansa cervicalis Cutaneous (transverse) cervical nerve Great auricular nerve Lesser occipital nerve Supraclavicular nerve Transverse (cutaneous) cervical nerve **1 Cervical Nerve** Greater occipital nerve Spinal nerve, cervical Suboccipital nerve Third occipital nerve **2 Phrenic Nerve** Accessory phrenic nerve **3 Brachial Plexus** Axillary nerve Dorsal scapular nerve First intercostal nerve Long thoracic nerve Musculocutaneous nerve Subclavius nerve Suprascapular nerve **4 Ulnar Nerve** Cubital nerve **5 Median Nerve** Anterior interosseous nerve Palmar cutaneous nerve **6 Radial Nerve** Dorsal digital nerve Musculospiral nerve Palmar cutaneous nerve Posterior interosseous nerve **8 Thoracic Nerve** Intercostal nerve Intercostobrachial nerve Spinal nerve, thoracic Subcostal nerve **9 Lumbar Plexus** Accessory obturator nerve Genitofemoral nerve Iliohypogastric nerve Ilioinguinal nerve Lateral femoral cutaneous nerve Obturator nerve Superior gluteal nerve **A Lumbosacral Plexus** **B Lumbar Nerve** Lumbosacral trunk Spinal nerve, lumbar Superior clunic (cluneal) nerve **C Pudendal Nerve]** Posterior labial nerve Posterior scrotal nerve **D Femoral Nerve** Anterior crural nerve Saphenous nerve **F Sciatic Nerve** Ischiatic nerve **G Tibial Nerve** Lateral plantar nerve Medial plantar nerve Medial popliteal nerve Medial sural cutaneous nerve **H Peroneal Nerve** Common fibular nerve Common peroneal nerve External popliteal nerve Lateral sural cutaneous nerve **K Head and Neck Sympathetic Nerve** Cavernous plexus Cervical ganglion Ciliary ganglion Internal carotid plexus Otic ganglion Pterygopalatine (sphenopalatine) ganglion Sphenopalatine (pterygopalatine) ganglion Stellate ganglion Submandibular ganglion Submaxillary ganglion **L Thoracic Sympathetic Nerve** Cardiac plexus Esophageal plexus Greater splanchnic nerve Inferior cardiac nerve Least splanchnic nerve Lesser splanchnic nerve Middle cardiac nerve Pulmonary plexus Superior cardiac nerve Thoracic aortic plexus Thoracic ganglion **M Abdominal Sympathetic Nerve** Abdominal aortic plexus Auerbach's (myenteric) plexus Celiac (solar) plexus Celiac ganglion Gastric plexus Hepatic plexus Inferior hypogastric plexus Inferior mesenteric ganglion Inferior mesenteric plexus Meissner's (submucous) plexus Myenteric (Auerbach's) plexus Pancreatic plexus Pelvic splanchnic nerve Renal nerve Renal plexus Solar (celiac) plexus Splenic plexus Submucous (Meissner's) plexus Superior hypogastric plexus Superior mesenteric ganglion Superior mesenteric plexus Suprarenal plexus **N Lumbar Sympathetic Nerve** Lumbar ganglion Lumbar splanchnic nerve **P Sacral Sympathetic Nerve** Ganglion impar (ganglion of Walther) Pelvic splanchnic nerve Sacral ganglion Sacral splanchnic nerve **Q Sacral Plexus** Inferior gluteal nerve Posterior femoral cutaneous nerve Pudendal nerve **R Sacral Nerve** Spinal nerve, sacral	**Ø Open** **3 Percutaneous** **4 Percutaneous Endoscopic**	**Z No Device**	**Z No Qualifier**

Ø Medical and Surgical
1 Peripheral Nervous System
H Insertion Definition: Putting in a nonbiological appliance that monitors, assists, performs, or prevents a physiological function but does not physically take the place of a body part

Explanation: None

Body Part Character 4	Approach Character 5	Device Character 6	Qualifier Character 7
Y Peripheral Nerve ⊞	Ø Open 3 Percutaneous 4 Percutaneous Endoscopic	1 Radioactive Element 2 Monitoring Device M Neurostimulator Lead Y Other Device	Z No Qualifier

Non-OR Ø1HY31Z
Non-OR Ø1HY[3,4]YZ

See Appendix L for Procedure Combinations
⊞ Ø1HY[Ø,3,4]MZ

Ø Medical and Surgical
1 Peripheral Nervous System
J Inspection Definition: Visually and/or manually exploring a body part

Explanation: Visual exploration may be performed with or without optical instrumentation. Manual exploration may be performed directly or through intervening body layers.

Body Part Character 4	Approach Character 5	Device Character 6	Qualifier Character 7
Y Peripheral Nerve	Ø Open 3 Percutaneous 4 Percutaneous Endoscopic	Z No Device	Z No Qualifier

Non-OR Ø1JY3ZZ

Ø Medical and Surgical
1 Peripheral Nervous System
N Release Definition: Freeing a body part from an abnormal physical constraint by cutting or by the use of force
Explanation: Some of the restraining tissue may be taken out but none of the body part is taken out

Body Part Character 4		Approach Character 5	Device Character 6	Qualifier Character 7
Ø Cervical Plexus Ansa cervicalis Cutaneous (transverse) cervical nerve Great auricular nerve Lesser occipital nerve Supraclavicular nerve Transverse (cutaneous) cervical nerve **1 Cervical Nerve** Greater occipital nerve Spinal nerve, cervical Suboccipital nerve Third occipital nerve **2 Phrenic Nerve** Accessory phrenic nerve **3 Brachial Plexus** Axillary nerve Dorsal scapular nerve First intercostal nerve Long thoracic nerve Musculocutaneous nerve Subclavius nerve Suprascapular nerve **4 Ulnar Nerve** Cubital nerve **5 Median Nerve** Anterior interosseous nerve Palmar cutaneous nerve **6 Radial Nerve** Dorsal digital nerve Musculospiral nerve Palmar cutaneous nerve Posterior interosseous nerve **8 Thoracic Nerve** Intercostal nerve Intercostobrachial nerve Spinal nerve, thoracic Subcostal nerve **9 Lumbar Plexus** Accessory obturator nerve Genitofemoral nerve Iliohypogastric nerve Ilioinguinal nerve Lateral femoral cutaneous nerve Obturator nerve Superior gluteal nerve **A Lumbosacral Plexus** **B Lumbar Nerve** Lumbosacral trunk Spinal nerve, lumbar Superior clunic (cluneal) nerve **C Pudendal Nerve** Posterior labial nerve Posterior scrotal nerve **D Femoral Nerve** Anterior crural nerve Saphenous nerve **F Sciatic Nerve** Ischiatic nerve **G Tibial Nerve** Lateral plantar nerve Medial plantar nerve Medial popliteal nerve Medial sural cutaneous nerve	**H Peroneal Nerve** Common fibular nerve Common peroneal nerve External popliteal nerve Lateral sural cutaneous nerve **K Head and Neck Sympathetic Nerve** Cavernous plexus Cervical ganglion Ciliary ganglion Internal carotid plexus Otic ganglion Pterygopalatine (sphenopalatine) ganglion Sphenopalatine (pterygopalatine) ganglion Stellate ganglion Submandibular ganglion Submaxillary ganglion **L Thoracic Sympathetic Nerve** Cardiac plexus Esophageal plexus Greater splanchnic nerve Inferior cardiac nerve Least splanchnic nerve Lesser splanchnic nerve Middle cardiac nerve Pulmonary plexus Superior cardiac nerve Thoracic aortic plexus Thoracic ganglion **M Abdominal Sympathetic Nerve** Abdominal aortic plexus Auerbach's (myenteric) plexus Celiac (solar) plexus Celiac ganglion Gastric plexus Hepatic plexus Inferior hypogastric plexus Inferior mesenteric ganglion Inferior mesenteric plexus Meissner's (submucous) plexus Myenteric (Auerbach's) plexus Pancreatic plexus Pelvic splanchnic nerve Renal nerve Renal plexus Solar (celiac) plexus Splenic plexus Submucous (Meissner's) plexus Superior hypogastric plexus Superior mesenteric ganglion Superior mesenteric plexus Suprarenal plexus **N Lumbar Sympathetic Nerve** Lumbar ganglion Lumbar splanchnic nerve **P Sacral Sympathetic Nerve** Ganglion impar (ganglion of Walther) Pelvic splanchnic nerve Sacral ganglion Sacral splanchnic nerve **Q Sacral Plexus** Inferior gluteal nerve Posterior femoral cutaneous nerve Pudendal nerve **R Sacral Nerve** Spinal nerve, sacral	**Ø Open** **3 Percutaneous** **4 Percutaneous Endoscopic**	**Z No Device**	**Z No Qualifier**

Ø Medical and Surgical
1 Peripheral Nervous System
P Removal Definition: Taking out or off a device from a body part

Explanation: If a device is taken out and a similar device put in without cutting or puncturing the skin or mucous membrane, the procedure is coded to the root operation CHANGE. Otherwise, the procedure for taking out a device is coded to the root operation REMOVAL.

Body Part Character 4	Approach Character 5	Device Character 6	Qualifier Character 7
Y Peripheral Nerve	Ø Open 3 Percutaneous 4 Percutaneous Endoscopic	Ø Drainage Device 2 Monitoring Device 7 Autologous Tissue Substitute M Neurostimulator Lead Y Other Device	Z No Qualifier
Y Peripheral Nerve	X External	Ø Drainage Device 2 Monitoring Device M Neurostimulator Lead	Z No Qualifier

Non-OR Ø1PY3[Ø,2]Z
Non-OR Ø1PY[3,4]YZ
Non-OR Ø1PYX[Ø,2,M]Z

Ø Medical and Surgical
1 Peripheral Nervous System
Q Repair Definition: Restoring, to the extent possible, a body part to its normal anatomic structure and function
Explanation: Used only when the method to accomplish the repair is not one of the other root operations

Body Part Character 4	Approach Character 5	Device Character 6	Qualifier Character 7
Ø Cervical Plexus Ansa cervicalis; Cutaneous (transverse) cervical nerve; Great auricular nerve; Lesser occipital nerve; Supraclavicular nerve; Transverse (cutaneous) cervical nerve **1 Cervical Nerve** Greater occipital nerve; Spinal nerve, cervical; Suboccipital nerve; Third occipital nerve **2 Phrenic Nerve** Accessory phrenic nerve **3 Brachial Plexus** Axillary nerve; Dorsal scapular nerve; First intercostal nerve; Long thoracic nerve; Musculocutaneous nerve; Subclavius nerve; Suprascapular nerve **4 Ulnar Nerve** Cubital nerve **5 Median Nerve** Anterior interosseous nerve; Palmar cutaneous nerve **6 Radial Nerve** Dorsal digital nerve; Musculospiral nerve; Palmar cutaneous nerve; Posterior interosseous nerve **8 Thoracic Nerve** Intercostal nerve; Intercostobrachial nerve; Spinal nerve, thoracic; Subcostal nerve **9 Lumbar Plexus** Accessory obturator nerve; Genitofemoral nerve; Iliohypogastric nerve; Ilioinguinal nerve; Lateral femoral cutaneous nerve; Obturator nerve; Superior gluteal nerve **A Lumbosacral Plexus** **B Lumbar Nerve** Lumbosacral trunk; Spinal nerve, lumbar; Superior clunic (cluneal) nerve **C Pudendal Nerve** Posterior labial nerve; Posterior scrotal nerve **D Femoral Nerve** Anterior crural nerve; Saphenous nerve **F Sciatic Nerve** Ischiatic nerve **G Tibial Nerve** Lateral plantar nerve; Medial plantar nerve; Medial popliteal nerve; Medial sural cutaneous nerve **H Peroneal Nerve** Common fibular nerve; Common peroneal nerve; External popliteal nerve; Lateral sural cutaneous nerve **K Head and Neck Sympathetic Nerve** Cavernous plexus; Cervical ganglion; Ciliary ganglion; Internal carotid plexus; Otic ganglion; Pterygopalatine (sphenopalatine) ganglion; Sphenopalatine (pterygopalatine) ganglion; Stellate ganglion; Submandibular ganglion; Submaxillary ganglion **L Thoracic Sympathetic Nerve** Cardiac plexus; Esophageal plexus; Greater splanchnic nerve; Inferior cardiac nerve; Least splanchnic nerve; Lesser splanchnic nerve; Middle cardiac nerve; Pulmonary plexus; Superior cardiac nerve; Thoracic aortic plexus; Thoracic ganglion **M Abdominal Sympathetic Nerve** Abdominal aortic plexus; Auerbach's (myenteric) plexus; Celiac (solar) plexus; Celiac ganglion; Gastric plexus; Hepatic plexus; Inferior hypogastric plexus; Inferior mesenteric ganglion; Inferior mesenteric plexus; Meissner's (submucous) plexus; Myenteric (Auerbach's) plexus; Pancreatic plexus; Pelvic splanchnic nerve; Renal nerve; Renal plexus; Solar (celiac) plexus; Splenic plexus; Submucous (Meissner's) plexus; Superior hypogastric plexus; Superior mesenteric ganglion; Superior mesenteric plexus; Suprarenal plexus **N Lumbar Sympathetic Nerve** Lumbar ganglion; Lumbar splanchnic nerve **P Sacral Sympathetic Nerve** Ganglion impar (ganglion of Walther); Pelvic splanchnic nerve; Sacral ganglion; Sacral splanchnic nerve **Q Sacral Plexus** Inferior gluteal nerve; Posterior femoral cutaneous nerve; Pudendal nerve **R Sacral Nerve** Spinal nerve, sacral	**Ø Open** **3 Percutaneous** **4 Percutaneous Endoscopic**	**Z No Device**	**Z No Qualifier**

Ø **Medical and Surgical**
1 **Peripheral Nervous System**
R **Replacement** Definition: Putting in or on biological or synthetic material that physically takes the place and/or function of all or a portion of a body part

Explanation: The body part may have been taken out or replaced, or may be taken out, physically eradicated, or rendered nonfunctional during the REPLACEMENT procedure. A REMOVAL procedure is coded for taking out the device used in a previous replacement procedure.

Body Part Character 4	Approach Character 5	Device Character 6	Qualifier Character 7
1 **Cervical Nerve** Greater occipital nerve Spinal nerve, cervical Suboccipital nerve Third occipital nerve 2 **Phrenic Nerve** Accessory phrenic nerve 4 **Ulnar Nerve** Cubital nerve 5 **Median Nerve** Anterior interosseous nerve Palmar cutaneous nerve 6 **Radial Nerve** Dorsal digital nerve Musculospiral nerve Palmar cutaneous nerve Posterior interosseous nerve 8 **Thoracic Nerve** Intercostal nerve Intercostobrachial nerve Spinal nerve, thoracic Subcostal nerve B **Lumbar Nerve** Lumbosacral trunk Spinal nerve, lumbar Superior clunic (cluneal) nerve C **Pudendal Nerve** Posterior labial nerve Posterior scrotal nerve D **Femoral Nerve** Anterior crural nerve Saphenous nerve F **Sciatic Nerve** Ischiatic nerve G **Tibial Nerve** Lateral plantar nerve Medial plantar nerve Medial popliteal nerve Medial sural cutaneous nerve H **Peroneal Nerve** Common fibular nerve Common peroneal nerve External popliteal nerve Lateral sural cutaneous nerve R **Sacral Nerve** Spinal nerve, sacral	Ø **Open** 4 **Percutaneous Endoscopic**	7 **Autologous Tissue Substitute** J **Synthetic Substitute** K **Nonautologous Tissue Substitute**	Z **No Qualifier**

Ø Medical and Surgical
1 Peripheral Nervous System
S Reposition Definition: Moving to its normal location, or other suitable location, all or a portion of a body part

Explanation: The body part is moved to a new location from an abnormal location, or from a normal location where it is not functioning correctly. The body part may or may not be cut out or off to be moved to the new location.

Body Part Character 4	Approach Character 5	Device Character 6	Qualifier Character 7
Ø Cervical Plexus Ansa cervicalis Cutaneous (transverse) cervical nerve Great auricular nerve Lesser occipital nerve Supraclavicular nerve Transverse (cutaneous) cervical nerve **1 Cervical Nerve** Greater occipital nerve Spinal nerve, cervical Suboccipital nerve Third occipital nerve **2 Phrenic Nerve** Accessory phrenic nerve **3 Brachial Plexus** Axillary nerve Dorsal scapular nerve First intercostal nerve Long thoracic nerve Musculocutaneous nerve Subclavius nerve Suprascapular nerve **4 Ulnar Nerve** Cubital nerve **5 Median Nerve** Anterior interosseous nerve Palmar cutaneous nerve **6 Radial Nerve** Dorsal digital nerve Musculospiral nerve Palmar cutaneous nerve Posterior interosseous nerve **8 Thoracic Nerve** Intercostal nerve Intercostobrachial nerve Spinal nerve, thoracic Subcostal nerve **9 Lumbar Plexus** Accessory obturator nerve Genitofemoral nerve Iliohypogastric nerve Ilioinguinal nerve Lateral femoral cutaneous nerve Obturator nerve Superior gluteal nerve **A Lumbosacral Plexus** **B Lumbar Nerve** Lumbosacral trunk Spinal nerve, lumbar Superior clunic (cluneal) nerve **C Pudendal Nerve** Posterior labial nerve Posterior scrotal nerve **D Femoral Nerve** Anterior crural nerve Saphenous nerve **F Sciatic Nerve** Ischiatic nerve **G Tibial Nerve** Lateral plantar nerve Medial plantar nerve Medial popliteal nerve Medial sural cutaneous nerve **H Peroneal Nerve** Common fibular nerve Common peroneal nerve External popliteal nerve Lateral sural cutaneous nerve **Q Sacral Plexus** Inferior gluteal nerve Posterior femoral cutaneous nerve Pudendal nerve **R Sacral Nerve** Spinal nerve, sacral	**Ø Open** **3 Percutaneous** **4 Percutaneous Endoscopic**	**Z No Device**	**Z No Qualifier**

Ø Medical and Surgical
1 Peripheral Nervous System
U Supplement Definition: Putting in or on biological or synthetic material that physically reinforces and/or augments the function of a portion of a body part

Explanation: The biological material is non-living, or is living and from the same individual. The body part may have been previously replaced, and the SUPPLEMENT procedure is performed to physically reinforce and/or augment the function of the replaced body part.

Body Part Character 4	Approach Character 5	Device Character 6	Qualifier Character 7
1 Cervical Nerve Greater occipital nerve Spinal nerve, cervical Suboccipital nerve Third occipital nerve **2 Phrenic Nerve** Accessory phrenic nerve **4 Ulnar Nerve** Cubital nerve **5 Median Nerve** Anterior interosseous nerve Palmar cutaneous nerve **6 Radial Nerve** Dorsal digital nerve Musculospiral nerve Palmar cutaneous nerve Posterior interosseous nerve **8 Thoracic Nerve** Intercostal nerve Intercostobrachial nerve Spinal nerve, thoracic Subcostal nerve **B Lumbar Nerve** Lumbosacral trunk Spinal nerve, lumbar Superior clunic (cluneal) nerve **C Pudendal Nerve** Posterior labial nerve Posterior scrotal nerve **D Femoral Nerve** Anterior crural nerve Saphenous nerve **F Sciatic Nerve** Ischiatic nerve **G Tibial Nerve** Lateral plantar nerve Medial plantar nerve Medial popliteal nerve Medial sural cutaneous nerve **H Peroneal Nerve** Common fibular nerve Common peroneal nerve External popliteal nerve Lateral sural cutaneous nerve **R Sacral Nerve** Spinal nerve, sacral	**Ø Open** **3 Percutaneous** **4 Percutaneous Endoscopic**	**7 Autologous Tissue Substitute** **J Synthetic Substitute** **K Nonautologous Tissue Substitute**	**Z No Qualifier**

Ø Medical and Surgical
1 Peripheral Nervous System
W Revision Definition: Correcting, to the extent possible, a portion of a malfunctioning device or the position of a displaced device

Explanation: Revision can include correcting a malfunctioning or displaced device by taking out or putting in components of the device such as a screw or pin

Body Part Character 4	Approach Character 5	Device Character 6	Qualifier Character 7
Y Peripheral Nerve	**Ø Open** **3 Percutaneous** **4 Percutaneous Endoscopic**	**Ø Drainage Device** **2 Monitoring Device** **7 Autologous Tissue Substitute** **M Neurostimulator Lead** **Y Other Device**	**Z No Qualifier**
Y Peripheral Nerve	**X External**	**Ø Drainage Device** **2 Monitoring Device** **7 Autologous Tissue Substitute** **M Neurostimulator Lead**	**Z No Qualifier**

Non-OR Ø1WY[3,4]YZ
Non-OR Ø1WYX[Ø,2,7,M]Z

Ø Medical and Surgical
1 Peripheral Nervous System
X Transfer Definition: Moving, without taking out, all or a portion of a body part to another location to take over the function of all or a portion of a body part
Explanation: The body part transferred remains connected to its vascular and nervous supply

Body Part Character 4	Approach Character 5	Device Character 6	Qualifier Character 7
1 Cervical Nerve Greater occipital nerve Spinal nerve, cervical Suboccipital nerve Third occipital nerve **2 Phrenic Nerve** Accessory phrenic nerve	**Ø Open** **4 Percutaneous Endoscopic**	**Z No Device**	**1 Cervical Nerve** **2 Phrenic Nerve**
4 Ulnar Nerve Cubital nerve **5 Median Nerve** Anterior interosseous nerve Palmar cutaneous nerve **6 Radial Nerve** Dorsal digital nerve Musculospiral nerve Palmar cutaneous nerve Posterior interosseous nerve	**Ø Open** **4 Percutaneous Endoscopic**	**Z No Device**	**4 Ulnar Nerve** **5 Median Nerve** **6 Radial Nerve**
8 Thoracic Nerve Intercostal nerve Intercostobrachial nerve Spinal nerve, thoracic Subcostal nerve	**Ø Open** **4 Percutaneous Endoscopic**	**Z No Device**	**8 Thoracic Nerve**
B Lumbar Nerve Lumbosacral trunk Spinal nerve, lumbar Superior clunic (cluneal) nerve **C Pudendal Nerve** Posterior labial nerve Posterior scrotal nerve	**Ø Open** **4 Percutaneous Endoscopic**	**Z No Device**	**B Lumbar Nerve** **C Perineal Nerve**
D Femoral Nerve Anterior crural nerve Saphenous nerve **F Sciatic Nerve** Ischiatic nerve **G Tibial Nerve** Lateral plantar nerve Medial plantar nerve Medial popliteal nerve Medial sural cutaneous nerve **H Peroneal Nerve** Common fibular nerve Common peroneal nerve External popliteal nerve Lateral sural cutaneous nerve	**Ø Open** **4 Percutaneous Endoscopic**	**Z No Device**	**D Femoral Nerve** **F Sciatic Nerve** **G Tibial Nerve** **H Peroneal Nerve**

Heart and Great Vessels Ø21–Ø2Y

Character Meanings

This Character Meaning table is provided as a guide to assist the user in the identification of character members that may be found in this section of code tables. It **SHOULD NOT** be used to build a PCS code.

Operation–Character 3	Body Part–Character 4	Approach–Character 5	Device–Character 6	Qualifier–Character 7
1 Bypass	Ø Coronary Artery, One Artery	Ø Open	Ø Monitoring Device, Pressure Sensor	Ø Allogeneic OR Ultrasonic
4 Creation	1 Coronary Artery, Two Arteries	3 Percutaneous	2 Monitoring Device	1 Syngeneic
5 Destruction	2 Coronary Artery, Three Arteries	4 Percutaneous Endoscopic	3 Infusion Device	2 Zooplastic OR Common Atrioventricular Valve
7 Dilation	3 Coronary Artery, Four or More Arteries	X External	4 Intraluminal Device, Drug-eluting	3 Coronary Artery
8 Division	4 Coronary Vein		5 Intraluminal Device, Drug-eluting, Two	4 Coronary Vein
B Excision	5 Atrial Septum		6 Intraluminal Device, Drug-eluting, Three	5 Coronary Circulation
C Extirpation	6 Atrium, Right		7 Intraluminal Device, Drug-eluting, Four or More OR Autologous Tissue Substitute	6 Bifurcation OR Atrium, Right
F Fragmentation	7 Atrium, Left		8 Zooplastic Tissue	7 Atrium, Left OR Orbital Atherectomy Technique
H Insertion	8 Conduction Mechanism		9 Autologous Venous Tissue	8 Internal Mammary, Right
J Inspection	9 Chordae Tendineae		A Autologous Arterial Tissue	9 Internal Mammary, Left
K Map	A Heart		C Extraluminal Device	A Innominate Artery
L Occlusion	B Heart, Right		D Intraluminal Device	B Subclavian
N Release	C Heart, Left		E Intraluminal Device, Two OR Intraluminal Device, Branched or Fenestrated, One or Two Arteries	C Thoracic Artery
P Removal	D Papillary Muscle		F Intraluminal Device, Three OR Intraluminal Device, Branched or Fenestrated, Three or More Arteries	D Carotid
Q Repair	F Aortic Valve		G Intraluminal Device, Four or More	E Atrioventricular Valve, Left
R Replacement	G Mitral Valve		J Synthetic Substitute OR Cardiac Lead, Pacemaker	F Abdominal Artery
S Reposition	H Pulmonary Valve		K Nonautologous Tissue Substitute OR Cardiac Lead, Defibrillator	G Atrioventricular Valve, Right OR Axillary Artery
T Resection	J Tricuspid Valve		L Biologic with Synthetic Substitute, Autoregulated Electrohydraulic	H Transapical OR Brachial Artery
U Supplement	K Ventricle, Right		M Cardiac Lead OR Synthetic Substitute, Pneumatic	J Truncal Valve OR Temporary OR Intraoperative
V Restriction	L Ventricle, Left		N Intracardiac Pacemaker	K Left Atrial Appendage
W Revision	M Ventricular Septum		Q Implantable Heart Assist System	L In Existing Conduit
Y Transplantation	N Pericardium		R Short-term External Heart Assist System	M Native Site
	P Pulmonary Trunk		T Intraluminal Device, Radioactive	N Rapid Deployment Technique
	Q Pulmonary Artery, Right		Y Other Device	P Pulmonary Trunk
	R Pulmonary Artery, Left		Z No Device	Q Pulmonary Artery, Right
	S Pulmonary Vein, Right			R Pulmonary Artery, Left
	T Pulmonary Vein, Left			S Pulmonary Vein, Right OR Biventricular
	V Superior Vena Cava			T Pulmonary Vein, Left OR Ductus Arteriosus
	W Thoracic Aorta, Descending			U Pulmonary Vein, Confluence
	X Thoracic Aorta, Ascending/Arch			V Lower Extremity Artery
	Y Great Vessel			W Aorta
				X Diagnostic
				Z No Qualifier

AHA Coding Clinic for Heart and Great Vessels

2022, 1Q, 10-13 Procedures performed on a continuous vessel, ICD-10-PCS Guideline B4.1c

AHA Coding Clinic for table Ø21

2023, 2Q, 22 Norwood procedure with excision of thymus
2022, 1Q, 54 Coronary artery bypass graft surgery
2021, 3Q, 22 Left internal mammary artery free graft between obtuse marginal saphenous vein graft and left anterior descending artery
2020, 4Q, 44-45 Atrium bypass qualifier
2020, 1Q, 24 Pulmonary artery unifocalization
2020, 1Q, 37 Bypass of ascending aorta to brachiocephalic artery
2019, 4Q, 23 Bypass thoracic aorta to innominate artery
2019, 3Q, 30 Aortic aneurysm repair with debranching of common carotid and brachiocephalic arteries
2018, 4Q, 45-46 Descending thoracic aorta bypass
2018, 3Q, 8 Coronary artery bypass graft surgery (revision versus total redo)
2018, 3Q, 26 Coronary artery bypass graft surgery with endarterectomy
2017, 4Q, 56 Added approach values - Percutaneous heart valve procedures
2017, 1Q, 19 Norwood Sano procedure
2016, 4Q, 80-81 Thoracic aorta, ascending/arch and descending
2016, 4Q, 82-83 Coronary artery, number of arteries
2016, 4Q, 102-109 Correction of congenital heart defects
2016, 4Q, 144 Repair of atrial septal defect and anomalous pulmonary venous return
2016, 4Q, 145 Modified Warden procedure for repair of septal defect and right partial anomalous pulmonary venous return
2016, 1Q, 27 Aortocoronary bypass graft utilizing Y-graft
2015, 4Q, 22, 24 Congenital heart corrective procedures
2015, 3Q, 16 Revision of previous truncus arteriosus surgery with ventricle to pulmonary artery conduit
2014, 3Q, 3 Blalock-Taussig shunt procedure
2014, 3Q, 8 Coronary artery bypass graft utilizing internal mammary as pedicle graft
2014, 3Q, 20 MAZE procedure performed with coronary artery bypass graft
2014, 3Q, 29 Fontan completion procedure stage II
2014, 3Q, 30 Creation of conduit from right ventricle to pulmonary artery
2014, 1Q, 10 Repair of thoracic aortic aneurysm & coronary artery bypass graft
2013, 2Q, 37 Coronary artery release performed during coronary artery bypass graft

AHA Coding Clinic for table Ø24

2016, 4Q, 101 Root operation Creation
2016, 4Q, 102-109 Correction of congenital heart defects

AHA Coding Clinic for table Ø25

2020, 1Q, 32 Ablation convergent procedure (catheter-based and thoracoscopic ablations)
2018, 3Q, 27 Alcohol septal ablation
2016, 4Q, 80-81 Thoracic aorta, ascending/arch and descending
2016, 3Q, 43-44 Peri-pulmonary catheter ablation
2016, 3Q, 44-45 Maze procedure
2016, 2Q, 17 Photodynamic therapy for treatment of malignant mesothelioma
2014, 4Q, 47 Catheter ablation of peripulmonary veins
2014, 3Q, 19 Ablation of ventricular tachycardia with Impella® support
2014, 3Q, 20 MAZE procedure performed with coronary artery bypass graft
2013, 2Q, 38 Catheter ablation to treat atrial fibrillation

AHA Coding Clinic for table Ø27

2018, 3Q, 7 Coronary brachytherapy with angioplasty
2018, 3Q, 10 Disruption of perma-catheter fibrin sheath via angioplasty of superior vena cava
2018, 2Q, 24 Coronary artery bifurcation
2017, 4Q, 32-33 Corrective surgery of left ventricular outflow tract obstruction
2016, 4Q, 80-81 Thoracic aorta, ascending/arch and descending
2016, 4Q, 82-83 Coronary artery, number of arteries
2016, 4Q, 84-85 Coronary artery, number of stents
2016, 4Q, 86-88 Coronary and peripheral artery bifurcation
2016, 1Q, 16 Pulmonary valvotomy and dilation of annulus
2015, 4Q, 13 New Section X codes—New Technology procedures
2015, 3Q, 9 Failed attempt to treat coronary artery occlusion
2015, 3Q, 10 Coronary angioplasty with unsuccessful stent insertion
2015, 3Q, 16 Revision of previous truncus arteriosus surgery with ventricle to pulmonary artery conduit
2015, 2Q, 3-5 Coronary artery intervention site
2014, 2Q, 4 Coronary angioplasty of bypassed vessel

AHA Coding Clinic for table Ø2B

2019, 3Q, 32 Endomyocardial biopsy and right heart catheterization
2019, 2Q, 20 Pericardiectomy for constrictive pericarditis
2017, 1Q, 38 Mitral valve repair and chordae tendineae transfer
2016, 4Q, 80-81 Thoracic aorta, ascending/arch and descending
2015, 2Q, 23 Annuloplasty ring

AHA Coding Clinic for table Ø2C

2021, 4Q, 41 Coronary orbital atherectomy
2019, 4Q, 25 Coronary artery to root operation Supplement
2018, 3Q, 26 Coronary artery bypass graft surgery with endarterectomy
2018, 2Q, 24 Coronary artery bifurcation
2017, 2Q, 23 Thrombectomy via Fogarty catheter
2016, 4Q, 80-81 Thoracic aorta, ascending/arch and descending
2016, 4Q, 82-83 Coronary artery, number of arteries
2016, 4Q, 86-87 Coronary and peripheral artery bifurcation
2016, 2Q, 24 Repair/decalcification of mitral valve
2016, 2Q, 25 Aortic valve surgery with excision of calcium deposits

AHA Coding Clinic for table Ø2F

2021, 4Q, 41-42 Coronary intravascular lithotripsy
2020, 4Q, 45-49 New fragmentation tables
2020, 4Q, 49-50 Intravascular ultrasound assisted thrombolysis
2020, 4Q, 50 Intravascular lithotripsy

AHA Coding Clinic for table Ø2H

2022, 3Q, 19 Placement of stent into aorta to secure debris
2022, 2Q, 25 Temporary-permanent pacemaker placement
2021, 2Q, 23 Clarification of lead placement in bundle of HIS
2019, 4Q, 23-24 Coronary artery Body Part to root operation Insertion
2019, 3Q, 19 Insertion of left ventricular catheter
2019, 3Q, 23 Placement of pacemaker lead in Bundle of HIS
2019, 1Q, 24 Replacement of left ventricular assist device with retention of outflow graft
2018, 4Q, 94 Insertion and removal of failed Watchman™ device
2018, 2Q, 3-5 Intra-aortic balloon pump
2018, 2Q, 19 Pacing lead attached to automatic implantable cardioverter defibrillator
2017, 4Q, 42-45 Insertion of external heart assist devices
2017, 4Q, 63-64 Added and revised device values - Vascular access reservoir
2017, 4Q, 104 Placement of Watchman™ left atrial appendage device
2017, 3Q, 11 Placement of peripherally inserted central catheter using 3CG ECG technology
2017, 2Q, 24 Tunneled catheter versus totally implantable catheter
2017, 2Q, 26 Exchange of tunneled catheter
2017, 1Q, 10-11 External heart assist device
2016, 4Q, 80-81 Thoracic aorta, ascending/arch and descending
2016, 4Q, 95 Intracardiac pacemaker
2016, 4Q, 137-138 Heart assist device systems
2016, 2Q, 15 Removal and replacement of tunneled internal jugular catheter
2015, 4Q, 14 New Section X codes—New Technology procedures
2015, 4Q, 26-31 Vascular access devices
2015, 3Q, 35 Swan Ganz catheterization
2015, 2Q, 31 Leadless pacemaker insertion
2015, 2Q, 33 Totally implantable central venous access device (Port-a-Cath)
2013, 3Q, 18 Placement of peripherally inserted central catheter (PICC)

AHA Coding Clinic for table Ø2J

2015, 3Q, 9 Failed attempt to treat coronary artery occlusion

AHA Coding Clinic for table Ø2K

2020, 1Q, 32 Ablation convergent procedure (catheter-based and thoracoscopic ablations)

AHA Coding Clinic for table Ø2L

2023, 1Q, 9 Temporary balloon occlusion of aorta
2018, 4Q, 94 Insertion and removal of failed Watchman™ device
2017, 4Q, 31 Resuscitative endovascular balloon occlusion of the aorta
2017, 4Q, 33-34 Occlusion/ligation of pulmonary trunk & right pulmonary artery
2016, 4Q, 102-109 Correction of congenital heart defects
2016, 2Q, 26 Embolization of pulmonary arteriovenous fistula
2015, 4Q, 23 Congenital heart corrective procedures
2014, 3Q, 20 MAZE procedure performed with coronary artery bypass graft

AHA Coding Clinic for table Ø2N

2021, 3Q, 26 Cavoatrial junction tear with repair and relief of cardiac tamponade
2019, 2Q, 13 Unroofing of anomalous coronary artery
2019, 2Q, 20 Pericardiectomy for constrictive pericarditis
2017, 4Q, 35 Release of myocardial bridge
2016, 4Q, 80-81 Thoracic aorta, ascending/arch and descending
2014, 3Q, 16 Repair of Tetralogy of Fallot

AHA Coding Clinic for table Ø2P

2022, 2Q, 25 Temporary-permanent pacemaker placement
2019, 1Q, 24 Replacement of left ventricular assist device with retention of outflow graft
2018, 4Q, 52-54 Percutaneous extracorporeal membrane oxygenation
2018, 4Q, 85 Externalization of lumboatrial shunt
2018, 4Q, 94 Insertion and removal of failed Watchman™ device
2018, 2Q, 3-5 Intra-aortic balloon pump
2017, 4Q, 42-45 Insertion of external heart assist devices
2017, 4Q, 104 Placement of Watchman™ left atrial appendage device
2017, 3Q, 18 Intra-aortic balloon pump removal
2017, 2Q, 24 Tunneled catheter versus totally implantable catheter
2017, 2Q, 26 Exchange of tunneled catheter
2017, 1Q, 11 External heart assist device
2017, 1Q, 13 SynCardia total artificial heart
2016, 4Q, 95-96 Intracardiac pacemaker
2016, 4Q, 137-139 Heart assist device systems
2016, 3Q, 19 Nonoperative removal of peripherally inserted central catheter

AHA Coding Clinic for table Ø2P (Continued)

2016, 2Q, 15	Removal and replacement of tunneled internal jugular catheter
2015, 4Q, 31	Vascular access devices
2015, 3Q, 33	Approach values for repositioning and removal of cardiac lead

AHA Coding Clinic for table Ø2Q

2022, 1Q, 40	Repair of common atrioventricular valve using Alfieri stitch
2022, 1Q, 41	Common atrioventricular valve repair with commissuroplasty sutures
2021, 3Q, 26	Cavoatrial junction tear with repair and relief of cardiac tamponade
2018, 1Q, 12	Percutaneous balloon valvuloplasty & cardiac catheterization with ventriculogram
2017, 1Q, 18	Sutureless repair of pulmonary vein stenosis
2016, 4Q, 80-81	Thoracic aorta, ascending/arch and descending
2016, 4Q, 82-83	Coronary artery, number of arteries
2016, 4Q, 101	Root operation Creation
2016, 4Q, 102-109	Correction of congenital heart defects
2015, 4Q, 23	Congenital heart corrective procedures
2015, 3Q, 16	Vascular ring surgery and double aortic arch
2015, 2Q, 23	Annuloplasty ring
2013, 3Q, 26	Transcatheter replacement of heart valve (TAVR) with measurements

AHA Coding Clinic for table Ø2R

2022, 4Q, 54-55	Rapid deployment technique for replacement of aortic valve using zooplastic tissue
2021, 4Q, 42-43	Total artificial heart systems
2021, 4Q, 43	Transcatheter replacement of pulmonary valve
2020, 1Q, 25	Elephant trunk repair of aortic dissection
2019, 4Q, 24	Coronary artery Body Part to root operation Insertion
2019, 4Q, 46	Cerebral embolic filtration
2019, 3Q, 23	Replacement of atrioventricular valve
2019, 3Q, 24	Valve sparing aortic root replacement with modified Gleason Vascutek® graft to ascending aorta
2019, 1Q, 31	Transcatheter aortic valve in valve replacement
2018, 3Q, 11	Transcatheter aortic valve replacement via transaortic approach
2018, 1Q, 12	Percutaneous balloon valvuloplasty & cardiac catheterization with ventriculogram
2017, 4Q, 55-56	Added approach values - Percutaneous heart valve procedures
2017, 1Q, 13	SynCardia total artificial heart
2016, 4Q, 80-81	Thoracic aorta, ascending/arch and descending
2016, 3Q, 32	Transcatheter tricuspid valve replacement
2014, 1Q, 10	Repair of thoracic aortic aneurysm & coronary artery bypass graft

AHA Coding Clinic for table Ø2S

2016, 4Q, 80-81	Thoracic aorta, ascending/arch and descending
2016, 4Q, 82-83	Coronary artery, number of arteries
2016, 4Q, 102-109	Correction of congenital heart defects
2015, 4Q, 23	Congenital heart corrective procedures

AHA Coding Clinic for table Ø2U

2023, 2Q, 21	Placement of Carillon Mitral Contour System®
2023, 2Q, 22	Norwood procedure with excision of thymus
2022, 1Q, 37	Insertion of amplatzer occluder device into atrium
2022, 1Q, 38	Reconstruction of aorto-mitral curtain using bovine pericardium
2021, 3Q, 28	Repair mitral valve with Pascal® system
2020, 4Q, 52	Transapical mitral valve repair with device
2020, 1Q, 24	Pulmonary artery unifocalization
2019, 4Q, 25	Coronary artery to root operation Supplement
2018, 1Q, 12	Percutaneous balloon valvuloplasty & cardiac catheterization with ventriculogram
2017, 4Q, 36	Alfieri stitch procedure
2017, 3Q, 7	Senning procedure (arterial switch)
2017, 1Q, 19	Norwood Sano procedure
2016, 4Q, 80-81	Thoracic aorta, ascending/arch and descending
2016, 4Q, 101	Root operation Creation
2016, 4Q, 102-109	Correction of congenital heart defects
2016, 2Q, 23	Repair of tetralogy of Fallot with autologous pericardial patch graft
2016, 2Q, 26	Aortic valve replacement with aortic root enlargement
2015, 4Q, 22-24	Congenital heart corrective procedures
2015, 3Q, 16	Revision of previous truncus arteriosus surgery with ventricle to pulmonary artery conduit
2015, 2Q, 23	Annuloplasty ring
2014, 3Q, 16	Repair of tetralogy of Fallot

AHA Coding Clinic for table Ø2V

2022, 1Q, 40	Repair of common atrioventricular valve using Alfieri stitch
2021, 4Q, 44	Restriction of left ventricle
2020, 1Q, 25	Elephant trunk repair of aortic dissection
2017, 4Q, 35-36	Alfieri stitch procedure
2016, 4Q, 80-81	Thoracic aorta, ascending/arch and descending
2016, 4Q, 89-92	Branched and fenestrated endograft repair of aneurysms

AHA Coding Clinic for table Ø2W

2019, 1Q, 24	Replacement of left ventricular assist device with retention of outflow graft
2018, 3Q, 8	Coronary artery bypass graft surgery (revision versus total redo)
2018, 3Q, 9	Fibrin sheath stripping of malfunctioning port-a-cath
2018, 1Q, 17	Repositioning of Impella short-term external heart assist device
2017, 4Q, 42-45	Insertion of external heart assist devices
2017, 4Q, 55-56	Added approach values - Percutaneous heart valve procedures
2016, 4Q, 85	Coronary artery, number of stents
2016, 4Q, 95-96	Intracardiac pacemaker
2015, 3Q, 32	Approach values for repositioning and removal of cardiac lead
2014, 3Q, 31	Closure of paravalvular leak using Amplatzer® vascular plug

AHA Coding Clinic for table Ø2Y

2023, 2Q, 32	Preparation of donor organ before transplantation
2013, 3Q, 18	Heart transplant surgery

Coronary Arteries

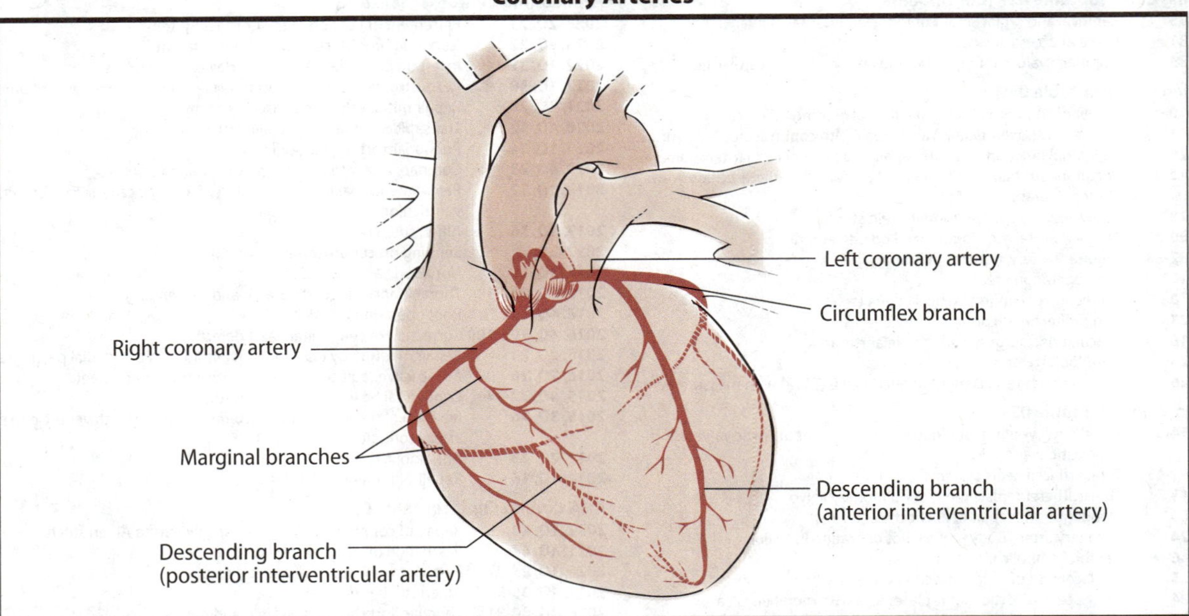

Heart Anatomy

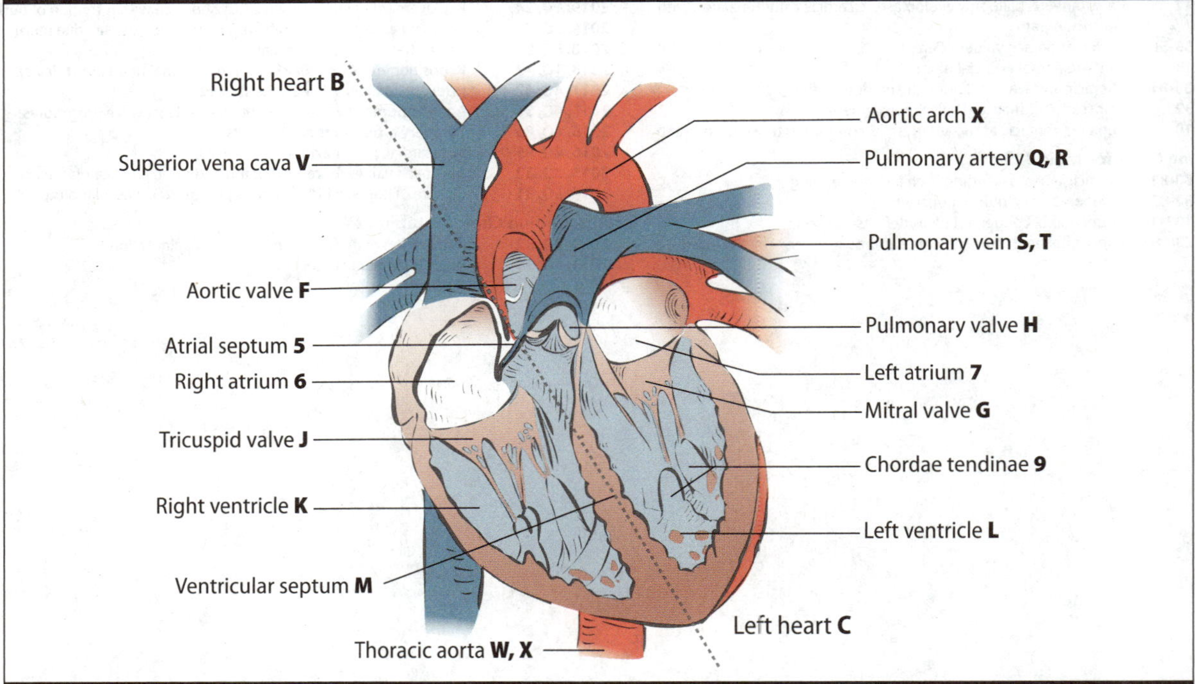

Ø Medical and Surgical
2 Heart and Great Vessels
1 Bypass Definition: Altering the route of passage of the contents of a tubular body part

Explanation: Rerouting contents of a body part to a downstream area of the normal route, to a similar route and body part, or to an abnormal route and dissimilar body part. Includes one or more anastomoses, with or without the use of a device.

Body Part Character 4	Approach Character 5	Device Character 6	Qualifier Character 7
Ø Coronary Artery, One Artery **1** Coronary Artery, Two Arteries **2** Coronary Artery, Three Arteries **3** Coronary Artery, Four or More Arteries	**Ø** Open	**8** Zooplastic Tissue **9** Autologous Venous Tissue **A** Autologous Arterial Tissue **J** Synthetic Substitute **K** Nonautologous Tissue Substitute	**3** Coronary Artery **8** Internal Mammary, Right **9** Internal Mammary, Left **C** Thoracic Artery **F** Abdominal Artery **W** Aorta
Ø Coronary Artery, One Artery **1** Coronary Artery, Two Arteries **2** Coronary Artery, Three Arteries **3** Coronary Artery, Four or More Arteries	**Ø** Open	**Z** No Device	**3** Coronary Artery **8** Internal Mammary, Right **9** Internal Mammary, Left **C** Thoracic Artery **F** Abdominal Artery
Ø Coronary Artery, One Artery **1** Coronary Artery, Two Arteries **2** Coronary Artery, Three Arteries **3** Coronary Artery, Four or More Arteries	**3** Percutaneous	**4** Intraluminal Device, Drug-eluting **D** Intraluminal Device	**4** Coronary Vein
Ø Coronary Artery, One Artery **1** Coronary Artery, Two Arteries **2** Coronary Artery, Three Arteries **3** Coronary Artery, Four or More Arteries	**4** Percutaneous Endoscopic	**4** Intraluminal Device, Drug-eluting **D** Intraluminal Device	**4** Coronary Vein
Ø Coronary Artery, One Artery **1** Coronary Artery, Two Arteries **2** Coronary Artery, Three Arteries **3** Coronary Artery, Four or More Arteries	**4** Percutaneous Endoscopic	**8** Zooplastic Tissue **9** Autologous Venous Tissue **A** Autologous Arterial Tissue **J** Synthetic Substitute **K** Nonautologous Tissue Substitute	**3** Coronary Artery **8** Internal Mammary, Right **9** Internal Mammary, Left **C** Thoracic Artery **F** Abdominal Artery **W** Aorta
Ø Coronary Artery, One Artery **1** Coronary Artery, Two Arteries **2** Coronary Artery, Three Arteries **3** Coronary Artery, Four or More Arteries	**4** Percutaneous Endoscopic	**Z** No Device	**3** Coronary Artery **8** Internal Mammary, Right **9** Internal Mammary, Left **C** Thoracic Artery **F** Abdominal Artery
6 Atrium, Right Atrium dextrum cordis Right auricular appendix Sinus venosus	**Ø** Open **4** Percutaneous Endoscopic	**8** Zooplastic Tissue **9** Autologous Venous Tissue **A** Autologous Arterial Tissue **J** Synthetic Substitute **K** Nonautologous Tissue Substitute	**P** Pulmonary Trunk **Q** Pulmonary Artery, Right **R** Pulmonary Artery, Left
6 Atrium, Right Atrium dextrum cordis Right auricular appendix Sinus venosus	**Ø** Open **4** Percutaneous Endoscopic	**Z** No Device	**7** Atrium, Left **P** Pulmonary Trunk **Q** Pulmonary Artery, Right **R** Pulmonary Artery, Left
6 Atrium, Right Atrium dextrum cordis Right auricular appendix Sinus venosus	**3** Percutaneous	**Z** No Device	**7** Atrium, Left
7 Atrium, Left Atrium pulmonale Left auricular appendix	**Ø** Open **4** Percutaneous Endoscopic	**8** Zooplastic Tissue **9** Autologous Venous Tissue **A** Autologous Arterial Tissue **J** Synthetic Substitute **K** Nonautologous Tissue Substitute **Z** No Device	**P** Pulmonary Trunk **Q** Pulmonary Artery, Right **R** Pulmonary Artery, Left **S** Pulmonary Vein, Right **T** Pulmonary Vein, Left **U** Pulmonary Vein, Confluence
7 Atrium, Left Atrium pulmonale Left auricular appendix	**3** Percutaneous	**J** Synthetic Substitute	**6** Atrium, Right
K Ventricle, Right Conus arteriosus **L** Ventricle, Left	**Ø** Open **4** Percutaneous Endoscopic	**8** Zooplastic Tissue **9** Autologous Venous Tissue **A** Autologous Arterial Tissue **J** Synthetic Substitute **K** Nonautologous Tissue Substitute	**P** Pulmonary Trunk **Q** Pulmonary Artery, Right **R** Pulmonary Artery, Left

HAC Ø21[Ø,1,2,3]Ø[8,9,A,J,K][3,8,9,C,F,W] when reported with SDx J98.51 or J98.59
HAC Ø21[Ø,1,2,3]ØZ[3,8,9,C,F] when reported with SDx J98.51 or J98.59
HAC Ø21[Ø,1,2,3]4[8,9,A,J,K][3,8,9,C,F,W] when reported with SDx J98.51 or J98.59
HAC Ø21[Ø,1,2,3]4Z[3,8,9,C,F] when reported with SDx J98.51 or J98.59

Ø21 Continued on next page

Ø21 Continued

Ø Medical and Surgical
2 Heart and Great Vessels
1 Bypass Definition: Altering the route of passage of the contents of a tubular body part

Explanation: Rerouting contents of a body part to a downstream area of the normal route, to a similar route and body part, or to an abnormal route and dissimilar body part. Includes one or more anastomoses, with or without the use of a device.

Body Part Character 4	Approach Character 5	Device Character 6	Qualifier Character 7
K Ventricle, Right Conus arteriosus **L** Ventricle, Left	**Ø** Open **4** Percutaneous Endoscopic	**Z** No Device	**5** Coronary Circulation **8** Internal Mammary, Right **9** Internal Mammary, Left **C** Thoracic Artery **F** Abdominal Artery **P** Pulmonary Trunk **Q** Pulmonary Artery, Right **R** Pulmonary Artery, Left **W** Aorta
P Pulmonary Trunk **Q** Pulmonary Artery, Right **R** Pulmonary Artery, Left Arterial canal (duct) Botallo's duct Pulmoaortic canal	**Ø** Open **4** Percutaneous Endoscopic	**8** Zooplastic Tissue **9** Autologous Venous Tissue **A** Autologous Arterial Tissue **J** Synthetic Substitute **K** Nonautologous Tissue Substitute **Z** No Device	**A** Innominate Artery **B** Subclavian **D** Carotid
V Superior Vena Cava Cavoatrial junction Precava	**Ø** Open **4** Percutaneous Endoscopic	**8** Zooplastic Tissue **9** Autologous Venous Tissue **A** Autologous Arterial Tissue **J** Synthetic Substitute **K** Nonautologous Tissue Substitute **Z** No Device	**P** Pulmonary Trunk **Q** Pulmonary Artery, Right **R** Pulmonary Artery, Left **S** Pulmonary Vein, Right **T** Pulmonary Vein, Left **U** Pulmonary Vein, Confluence
W Thoracic Aorta, Descending	**Ø** Open	**8** Zooplastic Tissue **9** Autologous Venous Tissue **A** Autologous Arterial Tissue **J** Synthetic Substitute **K** Nonautologous Tissue Substitute	**A** Innominate Artery **B** Subclavian **D** Carotid **F** Abdominal Artery **G** Axillary Artery **H** Brachial Artery **P** Pulmonary Trunk **Q** Pulmonary Artery, Right **R** Pulmonary Artery, Left **V** Lower Extremity Artery
W Thoracic Aorta, Descending	**Ø** Open	**Z** No Device	**A** Innominate Artery **B** Subclavian **D** Carotid **P** Pulmonary Trunk **Q** Pulmonary Artery, Right **R** Pulmonary Artery, Left
W Thoracic Aorta, Descending	**4** Percutaneous Endoscopic	**8** Zooplastic Tissue **9** Autologous Venous Tissue **A** Autologous Arterial Tissue **J** Synthetic Substitute **K** Nonautologous Tissue Substitute **Z** No Device	**A** Innominate Artery **B** Subclavian **D** Carotid **P** Pulmonary Trunk **Q** Pulmonary Artery, Right **R** Pulmonary Artery, Left
X Thoracic Aorta, Ascending/Arch Aortic arch Ascending aorta	**Ø** Open **4** Percutaneous Endoscopic	**8** Zooplastic Tissue **9** Autologous Venous Tissue **A** Autologous Arterial Tissue **J** Synthetic Substitute **K** Nonautologous Tissue Substitute **Z** No Device	**A** Innominate Artery **B** Subclavian **D** Carotid **P** Pulmonary Trunk **Q** Pulmonary Artery, Right **R** Pulmonary Artery, Left

Ø Medical and Surgical
2 Heart and Great Vessels
4 Creation Definition: Putting in or on biological or synthetic material to form a new body part that to the extent possible replicates the anatomic structure or function of an absent body part

Explanation: Used for gender reassignment surgery and corrective procedures in individuals with congenital anomalies

Body Part Character 4	Approach Character 5	Device Character 6	Qualifier Character 7
F Aortic Valve Aortic annulus	**Ø** Open	**7** Autologous Tissue **8** Zooplastic Tissue **J** Synthetic Substitute **K** Nonautologous Tissue Substitute	**J** Truncal Valve
G Mitral Valve Bicuspid valve Left atrioventricular valve Mitral annulus **J** Tricuspid Valve Right atrioventricular valve Tricuspid annulus	**Ø** Open	**7** Autologous Tissue **8** Zooplastic Tissue **J** Synthetic Substitute **K** Nonautologous Tissue Substitute	**2** Common Atrioventricular Valve

Ø Medical and Surgical
2 Heart and Great Vessels
5 Destruction Definition: Physical eradication of all or a portion of a body part by the direct use of energy, force, or a destructive agent
Explanation: None of the body part is physically taken out

Body Part Character 4	Approach Character 5	Device Character 6	Qualifier Character 7
4 Coronary Vein **5 Atrial Septum** Interatrial septum **6 Atrium, Right** Atrium dextrum cordis Right auricular appendix Sinus venosus **8 Conduction Mechanism** Atrioventricular node Bundle of His Bundle of Kent Sinoatrial node **9 Chordae Tendineae** **D Papillary Muscle** **F Aortic Valve** Aortic annulus **G Mitral Valve** Bicuspid valve Left atrioventricular valve Mitral annulus **H Pulmonary Valve** Pulmonary annulus Pulmonic valve **J Tricuspid Valve** Right atrioventricular valve Tricuspid annulus **K Ventricle, Right** Conus arteriosus **L Ventricle, Left** **M Ventricular Septum** Interventricular septum **N Pericardium** **P Pulmonary Trunk** **Q Pulmonary Artery, Right** **R Pulmonary Artery, Left** Arterial canal (duct) Botallo's duct Pulmoaortic canal **S Pulmonary Vein, Right** Right inferior pulmonary vein Right superior pulmonary vein **T Pulmonary Vein, Left** Left inferior pulmonary vein Left superior pulmonary vein **V Superior Vena Cava** Cavoatrial junction Precava **W Thoracic Aorta, Descending** **X Thoracic Aorta, Ascending/Arch** Aortic arch Ascending aorta	**Ø Open** **3 Percutaneous** **4 Percutaneous Endoscopic**	**Z No Device**	**Z No Qualifier**
7 Atrium, Left Atrium pulmonale Left auricular appendix	**Ø Open** **3 Percutaneous** **4 Percutaneous Endoscopic**	**Z No Device**	**K Left Atrial Appendage** **Z No Qualifier**

DRG Non-OR Ø257[Ø,3,4]ZK

Ø Medical and Surgical
2 Heart and Great Vessels
7 Dilation

Definition: Expanding an orifice or the lumen of a tubular body part

Explanation: The orifice can be a natural orifice or an artificially created orifice. Accomplished by stretching a tubular body part using intraluminal pressure or by cutting part of the orifice or wall of the tubular body part.

Body Part Character 4	Approach Character 5	Device Character 6	Qualifier Character 7
Ø Coronary Artery, One Artery 1 Coronary Artery, Two Arteries 2 Coronary Artery, Three Arteries 3 Coronary Artery, Four or More Arteries	Ø Open 3 Percutaneous 4 Percutaneous Endoscopic	4 Intraluminal Device, Drug-eluting 5 Intraluminal Device, Drug-eluting, Two 6 Intraluminal Device, Drug-eluting, Three 7 Intraluminal Device, Drug-eluting, Four or More D Intraluminal Device E Intraluminal Device, Two F Intraluminal Device, Three G Intraluminal Device, Four or More T Intraluminal Device, Radioactive Z No Device	6 Bifurcation Z No Qualifier
F Aortic Valve Aortic annulus G Mitral Valve Bicuspid valve Left atrioventricular valve Mitral annulus H Pulmonary Valve Pulmonary annulus Pulmonic valve J Tricuspid Valve Right atrioventricular valve Tricuspid annulus K Ventricle, Right Conus arteriosus L Ventricle, Left P Pulmonary Trunk Q Pulmonary Artery, Right S Pulmonary Vein, Right Right inferior pulmonary vein Right superior pulmonary vein T Pulmonary Vein, Left Left inferior pulmonary vein Left superior pulmonary vein V Superior Vena Cava Cavoatrial junction Precava W Thoracic Aorta, Descending X Thoracic Aorta, Ascending/Arch Aortic arch Ascending aorta	Ø Open 3 Percutaneous 4 Percutaneous Endoscopic	4 Intraluminal Device, Drug-eluting D Intraluminal Device Z No Device	Z No Qualifier
R Pulmonary Artery, Left Arterial canal (duct) Botallo's duct Pulmoaortic canal	Ø Open 3 Percutaneous 4 Percutaneous Endoscopic	4 Intraluminal Device, Drug-eluting D Intraluminal Device Z No Device	T Ductus Arteriosus Z No Qualifier

Ø Medical and Surgical
2 Heart and Great Vessels
8 Division

Definition: Cutting into a body part, without draining fluids and/or gases from the body part, in order to separate or transect a body part

Explanation: All or a portion of the body part is separated into two or more portions

Body Part Character 4	Approach Character 5	Device Character 6	Qualifier Character 7
8 Conduction Mechanism Atrioventricular node Bundle of His Bundle of Kent Sinoatrial node 9 Chordae Tendineae D Papillary Muscle	Ø Open 3 Percutaneous 4 Percutaneous Endoscopic	Z No Device	Z No Qualifier

Ø Medical and Surgical
2 Heart and Great Vessels
B Excision Definition: Cutting out or off, without replacement, a portion of a body part
Explanation: The qualifier DIAGNOSTIC is used to identify excision procedures that are biopsies

Body Part Character 4	Approach Character 5	Device Character 6	Qualifier Character 7
4 Coronary Vein **5 Atrial Septum** Interatrial septum **6 Atrium, Right** Atrium dextrum cordis Right auricular appendix Sinus venosus **8 Conduction Mechanism** Atrioventricular node Bundle of His Bundle of Kent Sinoatrial node **9 Chordae Tendineae** **D Papillary Muscle** **F Aortic Valve** Aortic annulus **G Mitral Valve** Bicuspid valve Left atrioventricular valve Mitral annulus **H Pulmonary Valve** Pulmonary annulus Pulmonic valve **J Tricuspid Valve** Right atrioventricular valve Tricuspid annulus **K Ventricle, Right** NC Conus arteriosus **L Ventricle, Left** NC **M Ventricular Septum** Interventricular septum **N Pericardium** **P Pulmonary Trunk** **Q Pulmonary Artery, Right** **R Pulmonary Artery, Left** Arterial canal (duct) Botallo's duct Pulmoaortic canal **S Pulmonary Vein, Right** Right inferior pulmonary vein Right superior pulmonary vein **T Pulmonary Vein, Left** Left inferior pulmonary vein Left superior pulmonary vein **V Superior Vena Cava** Cavoatrial junction Precava **W Thoracic Aorta, Descending** **X Thoracic Aorta, Ascending/Arch** Aortic arch Ascending aorta	**Ø Open** **3 Percutaneous** **4 Percutaneous Endoscopic**	**Z No Device**	**X Diagnostic** **Z No Qualifier**
7 Atrium, Left Atrium pulmonale Left auricular appendix	**Ø Open** **3 Percutaneous** **4 Percutaneous Endoscopic**	**Z No Device**	**K Left Atrial Appendage** **X Diagnostic** **Z No Qualifier**

DRG Non-OR Ø2B7[Ø,3,4]ZK
Non-OR Ø2B[4,5,6,8,9,D,F,G,H,J,K,L,M][Ø,3,4]ZX
NC Ø2B[K,L][Ø,3,4]ZZ

Ø Medical and Surgical
2 Heart and Great Vessels
C Extirpation Definition: Taking or cutting out solid matter from a body part

Explanation: The solid matter may be an abnormal byproduct of a biological function or a foreign body; it may be imbedded in a body part or in the lumen of a tubular body part. The solid matter may or may not have been previously broken into pieces.

Body Part Character 4	Approach Character 5	Device Character 6	Qualifier Character 7
Ø Coronary Artery, One Artery **1** Coronary Artery, Two Arteries **2** Coronary Artery, Three Arteries **3** Coronary Artery, Four or More Arteries	**Ø** Open **4** Percutaneous Endoscopic	**Z** No Device	**6** Bifurcation **Z** No Qualifier
Ø Coronary Artery, One Artery **1** Coronary Artery, Two Arteries **2** Coronary Artery, Three Arteries **3** Coronary Artery, Four or More Arteries	**3** Percutaneous	**Z** No Device	**6** Bifurcation **7** Orbital Atherectomy Technique **Z** No Qualifier
4 Coronary Vein **5** Atrial Septum Interatrial septum **6** Atrium, Right Atrium dextrum cordis Right auricular appendix Sinus venosus **7** Atrium, Left Atrium pulmonale Left auricular appendix **8** Conduction Mechanism Atrioventricular node Bundle of His Bundle of Kent Sinoatrial node **9** Chordae Tendineae **D** Papillary Muscle **F** Aortic Valve Aortic annulus **G** Mitral Valve Bicuspid valve Left atrioventricular valve Mitral annulus **H** Pulmonary Valve Pulmonary annulus Pulmonic valve **J** Tricuspid Valve Right atrioventricular valve Tricuspid annulus **K** Ventricle, Right Conus arteriosus **L** Ventricle, Left **M** Ventricular Septum Interventricular septum **N** Pericardium **P** Pulmonary Trunk **Q** Pulmonary Artery, Right **R** Pulmonary Artery, Left Arterial canal (duct) Botallo's duct Pulmoaortic canal **S** Pulmonary Vein, Right Right inferior pulmonary vein Right superior pulmonary vein **T** Pulmonary Vein, Left Left inferior pulmonary vein Left superior pulmonary vein **V** Superior Vena Cava Cavoatrial junction Precava **W** Thoracic Aorta, Descending **X** Thoracic Aorta, Ascending/Arch Aortic arch Ascending aorta	**Ø** Open **3** Percutaneous **4** Percutaneous Endoscopic	**Z** No Device	**Z** No Qualifier

Ø Medical and Surgical
2 Heart and Great Vessels
F Fragmentation Definition: Breaking solid matter in a body part into pieces

Explanation: Physical force (e.g., manual, ultrasonic) applied directly or indirectly is used to break the solid matter into pieces. The solid matter may be an abnormal byproduct of a biological function or a foreign body. The pieces of solid matter are not taken out.

Body Part Character 4	Approach Character 5	Device Character 6	Qualifier Character 7
Ø Coronary Artery, One Artery 1 Coronary Artery, Two Arteries 2 Coronary Artery, Three Arteries 3 Coronary Artery, Four or More Arteries	3 Percutaneous	Z No Device NT	Z No Qualifier
N Pericardium NC	Ø Open 3 Percutaneous 4 Percutaneous Endoscopic X External	Z No Device	Z No Qualifier
P Pulmonary Trunk Q Pulmonary Artery, Right R Pulmonary Artery, Left Arterial canal (duct) Botallo's duct Pulmoaortic canal S Pulmonary Vein, Right Right inferior pulmonary vein Right superior pulmonary vein T Pulmonary Vein, Left Left inferior pulmonary vein Left superior pulmonary vein	3 Percutaneous	Z No Device	Ø Ultrasonic Z No Qualifier

Non-OR Ø2FNXZZ
NC Ø2FNXZZ
NT Ø2F[Ø,1,2,3]3ZZ for Shockwave Coronary Intravascular Lithotripsy (IVL) System

Ø Medical and Surgical
2 Heart and Great Vessels
H Insertion Definition: Putting in a nonbiological appliance that monitors, assists, performs, or prevents a physiological function but does not physically take the place of a body part

Explanation: None

Body Part Character 4	Approach Character 5	Device Character 6	Qualifier Character 7
Ø Coronary Artery, One Artery 1 Coronary Artery, Two Arteries 2 Coronary Artery, Three Arteries 3 Coronary Artery, Four or More Arteries	Ø Open 3 Percutaneous 4 Percutaneous Endoscopic	D Intraluminal Device Y Other Device	Z No Qualifier
4 Coronary Vein 6 Atrium, Right Atrium dextrum cordis Right auricular appendix Sinus venosus 7 Atrium, Left Atrium pulmonale Left auricular appendix K Ventricle, Right Conus arteriosus L Ventricle, Left	Ø Open 3 Percutaneous 4 Percutaneous Endoscopic	Ø Monitoring Device, Pressure Sensor 2 Monitoring Device 3 Infusion Device D Intraluminal Device J Cardiac Lead, Pacemaker K Cardiac Lead, Defibrillator M Cardiac Lead N Intracardiac Pacemaker Y Other Device	Z No Qualifier
A Heart NC	Ø Open 3 Percutaneous 4 Percutaneous Endoscopic	Q Implantable Heart Assist System Y Other Device	Z No Qualifier
A Heart	Ø Open 3 Percutaneous 4 Percutaneous Endoscopic	R Short-term External Heart Assist System	J Intraoperative S Biventricular Z No Qualifier
N Pericardium	Ø Open 3 Percutaneous 4 Percutaneous Endoscopic	Ø Monitoring Device, Pressure Sensor 2 Monitoring Device J Cardiac Lead, Pacemaker K Cardiac Lead, Defibrillator M Cardiac Lead Y Other Device	Z No Qualifier
P Pulmonary Trunk Q Pulmonary Artery, Right R Pulmonary Artery, Left Arterial canal (duct) Botallo's duct Pulmoaortic canal S Pulmonary Vein, Right Right inferior pulmonary vein Right superior pulmonary vein T Pulmonary Vein, Left Left inferior pulmonary vein Left superior pulmonary vein V Superior Vena Cava Cavoatrial junction Precava	Ø Open 3 Percutaneous 4 Percutaneous Endoscopic	Ø Monitoring Device, Pressure Sensor 2 Monitoring Device 3 Infusion Device D Intraluminal Device Y Other Device	Z No Qualifier
W Thoracic Aorta, Descending	Ø Open 4 Percutaneous Endoscopic	Ø Monitoring Device, Pressure Sensor 2 Monitoring Device 3 Infusion Device D Intraluminal Device Y Other Device	Z No Qualifier
W Thoracic Aorta, Descending	3 Percutaneous	Ø Monitoring Device, Pressure Sensor 2 Monitoring Device 3 Infusion Device D Intraluminal Device R Short-term External Heart Assist System Y Other Device	Z No Qualifier

DRG Non-OR Ø2H[4,6,7,K,L][Ø,3,4][J,M]Z
DRG Non-OR Ø2HK32Z
DRG Non-OR Ø2HN[Ø,3,4][J,M]Z
Non-OR Ø2H[4,6,7,L]3[2,3]Z
Non-OR Ø2H[6,7]3MZ
Non-OR Ø2HK3[Ø,3]Z
Non-OR Ø2HN32Z
Non-OR Ø2HP[Ø,3,4][Ø,2,3]Z
Non-OR Ø2H[Q,R][Ø,3,4][2,3]Z
Non-OR Ø2H[S,T,V][Ø,3,4]3Z
Non-OR Ø2H[S,T,V]32Z
Non-OR Ø2HWØ[Ø,3]Z
Non-OR Ø2HW43Z
Non-OR Ø2HW3[Ø,2,3]Z
NC Ø2HA[3,4]QZ

HAC Ø2H43[J,K,M]Z when reported with SDx K68.11 or T81.4Ø-T81.49, T82.7 with 7th character A
HAC Ø2H[6,K]33Z when reported with SDx J95.811
HAC Ø2H[6,7]3[J,M]Z when reported with SDx K68.11 or T81.4Ø-T81.49, T82.7 with 7th character A
HAC Ø2H[K,L]3JZ when reported with SDx K68.11 or T81.4Ø-T81.49, T82.7 with 7th character A
HAC Ø2HN[Ø,3,4][J,M]Z when reported with SDx K68.11 or T81.4Ø-T81.49, T82.7 with 7th character A
HAC Ø2H[S,T,V][3,4]3Z when reported with SDx J95.811

See Appendix L for Procedure Combinations
Ø2H[4,6,7,K,L][Ø,3,4][J,K,M]Z
Ø2HA[Ø,4]R[S,Z]
Ø2HA3RS
Ø2HN[Ø,3,4][J,K,M]Z

Ø2H Continued on next page

Ø Medical and Surgical
2 Heart and Great Vessels
H Insertion Definition: Putting in a nonbiological appliance that monitors, assists, performs, or prevents a physiological function but does not physically take the place of a body part

Explanation: None

Ø2H Continued

Body Part Character 4	Approach Character 5	Device Character 6	Qualifier Character 7
X Thoracic Aorta, Ascending/Arch Aortic arch Ascending aorta	Ø Open 3 Percutaneous 4 Percutaneous Endoscopic	Ø Monitoring Device, Pressure Sensor 2 Monitoring Device 3 Infusion Device D Intraluminal Device	Z No Qualifier

Non-OR Ø2HX[Ø,3,4][Ø,3]Z

Ø Medical and Surgical
2 Heart and Great Vessels
J Inspection Definition: Visually and/or manually exploring a body part

Explanation: Visual exploration may be performed with or without optical instrumentation. Manual exploration may be performed directly or through intervening body layers.

Body Part Character 4	Approach Character 5	Device Character 6	Qualifier Character 7
A Heart Y Great Vessel	Ø Open 3 Percutaneous 4 Percutaneous Endoscopic	Z No Device	Z No Qualifier

Non-OR Ø2J[A,Y]3ZZ

Ø Medical and Surgical
2 Heart and Great Vessels
K Map Definition: Locating the route of passage of electrical impulses and/or locating functional areas in a body part

Explanation: Applicable only to the cardiac conduction mechanism and the central nervous system

Body Part Character 4	Approach Character 5	Device Character 6	Qualifier Character 7
8 Conduction Mechanism Atrioventricular node Bundle of His Bundle of Kent Sinoatrial node	Ø Open 3 Percutaneous 4 Percutaneous Endoscopic	Z No Device	Z No Qualifier

DRG Non-OR Ø2K8[Ø,3,4]ZZ

Ø Medical and Surgical
2 Heart and Great Vessels
L Occlusion Definition: Completely closing an orifice or the lumen of a tubular body part

Explanation: The orifice can be a natural orifice or an artificially created orifice

Body Part Character 4	Approach Character 5	Device Character 6	Qualifier Character 7
7 Atrium, Left Atrium pulmonale Left auricular appendix	Ø Open 3 Percutaneous 4 Percutaneous Endoscopic	C Extraluminal Device D Intraluminal Device Z No Device	K Left Atrial Appendage
H Pulmonary Valve Pulmonary annulus Pulmonic valve P Pulmonary Trunk Q Pulmonary Artery, Right S Pulmonary Vein, Right Right inferior pulmonary vein Right superior pulmonary vein T Pulmonary Vein, Left Left inferior pulmonary vein Left superior pulmonary vein V Superior Vena Cava Cavoatrial junction Precava	Ø Open 3 Percutaneous 4 Percutaneous Endoscopic	C Extraluminal Device D Intraluminal Device Z No Device	Z No Qualifier
R Pulmonary Artery, Left Arterial canal (duct) Botallo's duct Pulmoaortic canal	Ø Open 3 Percutaneous 4 Percutaneous Endoscopic	C Extraluminal Device D Intraluminal Device Z No Device	T Ductus Arteriosus Z No Qualifier
W Thoracic Aorta, Descending	Ø Open 3 Percutaneous	D Intraluminal Device	J Temporary

DRG Non-OR Ø2L7[Ø,3,4][C,D,Z]K

Ø Medical and Surgical
2 Heart and Great Vessels
N Release Definition: Freeing a body part from an abnormal physical constraint by cutting or by the use of force
Explanation: Some of the restraining tissue may be taken out but none of the body part is taken out

Body Part Character 4	Approach Character 5	Device Character 6	Qualifier Character 7
Ø Coronary Artery, One Artery **1** Coronary Artery, Two Arteries **2** Coronary Artery, Three Arteries **3** Coronary Artery, Four or More Arteries **4** Coronary Vein **5** Atrial Septum Interatrial septum **6** Atrium, Right Atrium dextrum cordis Right auricular appendix Sinus venosus **7** Atrium, Left Atrium pulmonale Left auricular appendix **8** Conduction Mechanism Atrioventricular node Bundle of His Bundle of Kent Sinoatrial node **9** Chordae Tendineae **D** Papillary Muscle **F** Aortic Valve Aortic annulus **G** Mitral Valve Bicuspid valve Left atrioventricular valve Mitral annulus **H** Pulmonary Valve Pulmonary annulus Pulmonic valve **J** Tricuspid Valve Right atrioventricular valve Tricuspid annulus **K** Ventricle, Right Conus arteriosus **L** Ventricle, Left **M** Ventricular Septum Interventricular septum **N** Pericardium **P** Pulmonary Trunk **Q** Pulmonary Artery, Right **R** Pulmonary Artery, Left Arterial canal (duct) Botallo's duct Pulmoaortic canal **S** Pulmonary Vein, Right Right inferior pulmonary vein Right superior pulmonary vein **T** Pulmonary Vein, Left Left inferior pulmonary vein Left superior pulmonary vein **V** Superior Vena Cava Cavoatrial junction Precava **W** Thoracic Aorta, Descending **X** Thoracic Aorta, Ascending/Arch Aortic arch Ascending aorta	**Ø** Open **3** Percutaneous **4** Percutaneous Endoscopic	**Z** No Device	**Z** No Qualifier

Ø Medical and Surgical
2 Heart and Great Vessels
P Removal Definition: Taking out or off a device from a body part

Explanation: If a device is taken out and a similar device put in without cutting or puncturing the skin or mucous membrane, the procedure is coded to the root operation CHANGE. Otherwise, the procedure for taking out a device is coded to the root operation REMOVAL.

Body Part Character 4	Approach Character 5	Device Character 6	Qualifier Character 7
A Heart	Ø Open 3 Percutaneous 4 Percutaneous Endoscopic	2 Monitoring Device 3 Infusion Device 7 Autologous Tissue Substitute 8 Zooplastic Tissue C Extraluminal Device D Intraluminal Device J Synthetic Substitute K Nonautologous Tissue Substitute M Cardiac Lead N Intracardiac Pacemaker Q Implantable Heart Assist System Y Other Device	Z No Qualifier
A Heart ⊞	Ø Open 3 Percutaneous 4 Percutaneous Endoscopic	R Short-term External Heart Assist System	S Biventricular Z No Qualifier
A Heart	X External	2 Monitoring Device 3 Infusion Device D Intraluminal Device M Cardiac Lead	Z No Qualifier
W Thoracic Aorta, Descending	3 Percutaneous	R Short-term External Heart Assist System	Z No Qualifier
Y Great Vessel	Ø Open 3 Percutaneous 4 Percutaneous Endoscopic	2 Monitoring Device 3 Infusion Device 7 Autologous Tissue Substitute 8 Zooplastic Tissue C Extraluminal Device D Intraluminal Device J Synthetic Substitute K Nonautologous Tissue Substitute Y Other Device	Z No Qualifier
Y Great Vessel	X External	2 Monitoring Device 3 Infusion Device D Intraluminal Device	Z No Qualifier

Non-OR Ø2PA3[2,3,D]Z
Non-OR Ø2PA[3,4]YZ
Non-OR Ø2PAX[2,3,D,M]Z
Non-OR Ø2PY3[2,3,D]Z
Non-OR Ø2PY[3,4]YZ
Non-OR Ø2PYX[2,3,D]Z
HAC Ø2PA[Ø,3,4]MZ when reported with SDx K68.11 or T81.4Ø-T81.49, T82.7 with 7th character A
HAC Ø2PAXMZ when reported with SDx K68.11 or T81.4Ø-T81.49, T82.7 with 7th character A

See Appendix L for Procedure Combinations
⊞ Ø2PA[Ø,3,4]RZ

Ø Medical and Surgical
2 Heart and Great Vessels
Q Repair Definition: Restoring, to the extent possible, a body part to its normal anatomic structure and function
Explanation: Used only when the method to accomplish the repair is not one of the other root operations

Body Part Character 4	Approach Character 5	Device Character 6	Qualifier Character 7
Ø Coronary Artery, One Artery **1 Coronary Artery, Two Arteries** **2 Coronary Artery, Three Arteries** **3 Coronary Artery, Four or More Arteries** **4 Coronary Vein** **5 Atrial Septum** Interatrial septum **6 Atrium, Right** Atrium dextrum cordis Right auricular appendix Sinus venosus **7 Atrium, Left** Atrium pulmonale Left auricular appendix **8 Conduction Mechanism** Atrioventricular node Bundle of His Bundle of Kent Sinoatrial node **9 Chordae Tendineae** **A Heart** **B Heart, Right** Right coronary sulcus **C Heart, Left** Left coronary sulcus Obtuse margin **D Papillary Muscle** **H Pulmonary Valve** Pulmonary annulus Pulmonic valve **K Ventricle, Right** Conus arteriosus **L Ventricle, Left** **M Ventricular Septum** Interventricular septum **N Pericardium** **P Pulmonary Trunk** **Q Pulmonary Artery, Right** **R Pulmonary Artery, Left** Arterial canal (duct) Botallo's duct Pulmoaortic canal **S Pulmonary Vein, Right** Right inferior pulmonary vein Right superior pulmonary vein **T Pulmonary Vein, Left** Left inferior pulmonary vein Left superior pulmonary vein **V Superior Vena Cava** Cavoatrial junction Precava **W Thoracic Aorta, Descending** **X Thoracic Aorta, Ascending/Arch** Aortic arch Ascending aorta	**Ø Open** **3 Percutaneous** **4 Percutaneous Endoscopic**	**Z No Device**	**Z No Qualifier**
F Aortic Valve Aortic annulus	**Ø Open** **3 Percutaneous** **4 Percutaneous Endoscopic**	**Z No Device**	**J Truncal Valve** **Z No Qualifier**
G Mitral Valve Bicuspid valve Left atrioventricular valve Mitral annulus	**Ø Open** **3 Percutaneous** **4 Percutaneous Endoscopic**	**Z No Device**	**E Atrioventricular Valve, Left** **Z No Qualifier**
J Tricuspid Valve Right atrioventricular valve Tricuspid annulus	**Ø Open** **3 Percutaneous** **4 Percutaneous Endoscopic**	**Z No Device**	**G Atrioventricular Valve, Right** **Z No Qualifier**

Ø Medical and Surgical
2 Heart and Great Vessels
R Replacement Definition: Putting in or on biological or synthetic material that physically takes the place and/or function of all or a portion of a body part

Explanation: The body part may have been taken out or replaced, or may be taken out, physically eradicated, or rendered nonfunctional during the REPLACEMENT procedure. A REMOVAL procedure is coded for taking out the device used in a previous replacement procedure.

Body Part Character 4	Approach Character 5	Device Character 6	Qualifier Character 7
5 Atrial Septum Interatrial septum **6 Atrium, Right** Atrium dextrum cordis Right auricular appendix Sinus venosus **7 Atrium, Left** Atrium pulmonale Left auricular appendix **9 Chordae Tendineae** **D Papillary Muscle** **K Ventricle, Right** ✚ Conus arteriosus **L Ventricle, Left** ✚ **M Ventricular Septum** Interventricular septum **N Pericardium** **P Pulmonary Trunk** **Q Pulmonary Artery, Right** **R Pulmonary Artery, Left** Arterial canal (duct) Botallo's duct Pulmoaortic canal **S Pulmonary Vein, Right** Right inferior pulmonary vein Right superior pulmonary vein **T Pulmonary Vein, Left** Left inferior pulmonary vein Left superior pulmonary vein **V Superior Vena Cava** Cavoatrial junction Precava **W Thoracic Aorta, Descending** **X Thoracic Aorta, Ascending/Arch** Aortic arch Ascending aorta	**Ø Open** **4 Percutaneous Endoscopic**	**7 Autologous Tissue Substitute** **8 Zooplastic Tissue** **J Synthetic Substitute** **K Nonautologous Tissue Substitute**	**Z No Qualifier**
A Heart	**Ø Open**	**L Biologic with Synthetic Substitute, Autoregulated Electrohydraulic** **M Synthetic Substitute, Pneumatic**	**Z No Qualifier**
F Aortic Valve Aortic annulus	**Ø Open** **4 Percutaneous Endoscopic**	**7 Autologous Tissue Substitute** **J Synthetic Substitute** **K Nonautologous Tissue Substitute**	**Z No Qualifier**
F Aortic Valve Aortic annulus	**Ø Open** **4 Percutaneous Endoscopic**	**8 Zooplastic Tissue**	**N Rapid Deployment Technique** **Z No Qualifier**
F Aortic Valve Aortic annulus	**3 Percutaneous**	**7 Autologous Tissue Substitute** **J Synthetic Substitute** **K Nonautologous Tissue Substitute**	**H Transapical** **Z No Qualifier**
F Aortic Valve Aortic annulus	**3 Percutaneous**	**8 Zooplastic Tissue**	**H Transapical** **N Rapid Deployment Technique** **Z No Qualifier**
G Mitral Valve Bicuspid valve Left atrioventricular valve Mitral annulus **J Tricuspid Valve** Right atrioventricular valve Tricuspid annulus	**Ø Open** **4 Percutaneous Endoscopic**	**7 Autologous Tissue Substitute** **8 Zooplastic Tissue** **J Synthetic Substitute** **K Nonautologous Tissue Substitute**	**Z No Qualifier**
G Mitral Valve Bicuspid valve Left atrioventricular valve Mitral annulus **J Tricuspid Valve** Right atrioventricular valve Tricuspid annulus	**3 Percutaneous**	**7 Autologous Tissue Substitute** **8 Zooplastic Tissue** **J Synthetic Substitute** **K Nonautologous Tissue Substitute**	**H Transapical** **Z No Qualifier**
H Pulmonary Valve Pulmonary annulus Pulmonic valve	**Ø Open** **4 Percutaneous Endoscopic**	**7 Autologous Tissue Substitute** **8 Zooplastic Tissue** **J Synthetic Substitute** **K Nonautologous Tissue Substitute**	**Z No Qualifier**
H Pulmonary Valve Pulmonary annulus Pulmonic valve	**3 Percutaneous**	**7 Autologous Tissue Substitute** **J Synthetic Substitute** **K Nonautologous Tissue Substitute**	**H Transapical** **Z No Qualifier**
H Pulmonary Valve Pulmonary annulus Pulmonic valve	**3 Percutaneous**	**8 Zooplastic Tissue** NT	**H Transapical** **L In Existing Conduit** **M Native Site** **Z No Qualifier**

NT Ø2RH38M for Harmony™ Transcatheter Pulmonary Valve (TPV) System

See Appendix L for Procedure Combinations

✚ Ø2R[K,L]ØJZ

NC Noncovered Procedure LC Limited Coverage QA Questionable OB Admit NT New Tech Add-on ✚ Combination Member ♂ Male ♀ Female

Ø Medical and Surgical
2 Heart and Great Vessels
S Reposition Definition: Moving to its normal location, or other suitable location, all or a portion of a body part

Explanation: The body part is moved to a new location from an abnormal location, or from a normal location where it is not functioning correctly. The body part may or may not be cut out or off to be moved to the new location.

Body Part Character 4	Approach Character 5	Device Character 6	Qualifier Character 7
Ø Coronary Artery, One Artery **1 Coronary Artery, Two Arteries** **P Pulmonary Trunk** **Q Pulmonary Artery, Right** **R Pulmonary Artery, Left** Arterial canal (duct) Botallo's duct Pulmoaortic canal **S Pulmonary Vein, Right** Right inferior pulmonary vein Right superior pulmonary vein **T Pulmonary Vein, Left** Left inferior pulmonary vein Left superior pulmonary vein **V Superior Vena Cava** Cavoatrial junction Precava **W Thoracic Aorta, Descending** **X Thoracic Aorta, Ascending/Arch** Aortic arch Ascending aorta	**Ø Open**	**Z No Device**	**Z No Qualifier**

Ø Medical and Surgical
2 Heart and Great Vessels
T Resection Definition: Cutting out or off, without replacement, all of a body part

Explanation: None

Body Part Character 4	Approach Character 5	Device Character 6	Qualifier Character 7
5 Atrial Septum Interatrial septum **8 Conduction Mechanism** Atrioventricular node Bundle of His Bundle of Kent Sinoatrial node **9 Chordae Tendineae** **D Papillary Muscle** **H Pulmonary Valve** Pulmonary annulus Pulmonic valve **M Ventricular Septum** Interventricular septum **N Pericardium**	**Ø Open** **3 Percutaneous** **4 Percutaneous Endoscopic**	**Z No Device**	**Z No Qualifier**

Ø Medical and Surgical
2 Heart and Great Vessels
U Supplement Definition: Putting in or on biological or synthetic material that physically reinforces and/or augments the function of a portion of a body part

Explanation: The biological material is non-living, or is living and from the same individual. The body part may have been previously replaced, and the SUPPLEMENT procedure is performed to physically reinforce and/or augment the function of the replaced body part.

Body Part Character 4	Approach Character 5	Device Character 6	Qualifier Character 7
Ø Coronary Artery, One Artery **1 Coronary Artery, Two Arteries** **2 Coronary Artery, Three Arteries** **3 Coronary Artery, Four or More Arteries** **5 Atrial Septum** Interatrial septum **6 Atrium, Right** Atrium dextrum cordis Right auricular appendix Sinus venosus **7 Atrium, Left** Atrium pulmonale Left auricular appendix **9 Chordae Tendineae** **A Heart** **D Papillary Muscle** **H Pulmonary Valve** Pulmonary annulus Pulmonic valve **K Ventricle, Right** Conus arteriosus **L Ventricle, Left** **M Ventricular Septum** Interventricular septum **N Pericardium** **P Pulmonary Trunk** **Q Pulmonary Artery, Right** **R Pulmonary Artery, Left** Arterial canal (duct) Botallo's duct Pulmoaortic canal **S Pulmonary Vein, Right** Right inferior pulmonary vein Right superior pulmonary vein **T Pulmonary Vein, Left** Left inferior pulmonary vein Left superior pulmonary vein **V Superior Vena Cava** Cavoatrial junction Precava **W Thoracic Aorta, Descending** **X Thoracic Aorta, Ascending/Arch** Aortic arch Ascending aorta	**Ø Open** **3 Percutaneous** **4 Percutaneous Endoscopic**	**7 Autologous Tissue Substitute** **8 Zooplastic Tissue** **J Synthetic Substitute** **K Nonautologous Tissue Substitute**	**Z No Qualifier**
F Aortic Valve Aortic annulus	**Ø Open** **3 Percutaneous** **4 Percutaneous Endoscopic**	**7 Autologous Tissue Substitute** **8 Zooplastic Tissue** **J Synthetic Substitute** **K Nonautologous Tissue Substitute**	**J Truncal Valve** **Z No Qualifier**
G Mitral Valve Bicuspid valve Left atrioventricular valve Mitral annulus	**Ø Open** **4 Percutaneous Endoscopic**	**7 Autologous Tissue Substitute** **8 Zooplastic Tissue** **J Synthetic Substitute** **K Nonautologous Tissue Substitute**	**E Atrioventricular Valve, Left** **Z No Qualifier**
G Mitral Valve Bicuspid valve Left atrioventricular valve Mitral annulus	**3 Percutaneous**	**7 Autologous Tissue Substitute** **8 Zooplastic Tissue** **K Nonautologous Tissue Substitute**	**E Atrioventricular Valve, Left** **Z No Qualifier**
G Mitral Valve Bicuspid valve Left atrioventricular valve Mitral annulus	**3 Percutaneous**	**J Synthetic Substitute**	**E Atrioventricular Valve, Left** **H Transapical** **Z No Qualifier**
J Tricuspid Valve Right atrioventricular valve Tricuspid annulus	**Ø Open** **3 Percutaneous** **4 Percutaneous Endoscopic**	**7 Autologous Tissue Substitute** **8 Zooplastic Tissue** **J Synthetic Substitute** **K Nonautologous Tissue Substitute**	**G Atrioventricular Valve, Right** **Z No Qualifier**

DRG Non-OR Ø2U7[3,4]JZ

Ø Medical and Surgical
2 Heart and Great Vessels
V Restriction Definition: Partially closing an orifice or the lumen of a tubular body part
Explanation: The orifice can be a natural orifice or an artificially created orifice

Body Part Character 4	Approach Character 5	Device Character 6	Qualifier Character 7
A Heart	**Ø Open** **3 Percutaneous** **4 Percutaneous Endoscopic**	**C Extraluminal Device** **Z No Device**	**Z No Qualifier**
G Mitral Valve Bicuspid valve Left atrioventricular valve Mitral annulus	**Ø Open** **3 Percutaneous** **4 Percutaneous Endoscopic**	**Z No Device**	**Z No Qualifier**
L Ventricle, Left **P Pulmonary Trunk** **Q Pulmonary Artery, Right** **S Pulmonary Vein, Right** Right inferior pulmonary vein Right superior pulmonary vein **T Pulmonary Vein, Left** Left inferior pulmonary vein Left superior pulmonary vein **V Superior Vena Cava** Cavoatrial junction Precava	**Ø Open** **3 Percutaneous** **4 Percutaneous Endoscopic**	**C Extraluminal Device** **D Intraluminal Device** **Z No Device**	**Z No Qualifier**
R Pulmonary Artery, Left Arterial canal (duct) Botallo's duct Pulmoaortic canal	**Ø Open** **3 Percutaneous** **4 Percutaneous Endoscopic**	**C Extraluminal Device** **D Intraluminal Device** **Z No Device**	**T Ductus Arteriosus** **Z No Qualifier**
W Thoracic Aorta, Descending **X Thoracic Aorta, Ascending/Arch** Aortic arch Ascending aorta	**Ø Open** **3 Percutaneous** **4 Percutaneous Endoscopic**	**C Extraluminal Device** **D Intraluminal Device** NT **E Intraluminal Device, Branched or Fenestrated, One or Two Arteries** NT **F Intraluminal Device, Branched or Fenestrated, Three or More Arteries** **Z No Device**	**Z No Qualifier**

NT Ø2VW3DZ with Ø2VX3EZ for GORE® TAG® Thoracic Branch Endoprosthesis

Ø Medical and Surgical
2 Heart and Great Vessels
W Revision Definition: Correcting, to the extent possible, a portion of a malfunctioning device or the position of a displaced device

Explanation: Revision can include correcting a malfunctioning or displaced device by taking out or putting in components of the device such as a screw or pin

Body Part Character 4	Approach Character 5	Device Character 6	Qualifier Character 7
5 Atrial Septum Interatrial septum M Ventricular Septum Interventricular septum	Ø Open 4 Percutaneous Endoscopic	J Synthetic Substitute	Z No Qualifier
A Heart LC ⊞	Ø Open 3 Percutaneous 4 Percutaneous Endoscopic	2 Monitoring Device 3 Infusion Device 7 Autologous Tissue Substitute 8 Zooplastic Tissue C Extraluminal Device D Intraluminal Device J Synthetic Substitute K Nonautologous Tissue Substitute M Cardiac Lead N Intracardiac Pacemaker Q Implantable Heart Assist System Y Other Device	Z No Qualifier
A Heart ⊞	Ø Open 3 Percutaneous 4 Percutaneous Endoscopic	R Short-term External Heart Assist System	S Biventricular Z No Qualifier
A Heart	X External	2 Monitoring Device 3 Infusion Device 7 Autologous Tissue Substitute 8 Zooplastic Tissue C Extraluminal Device D Intraluminal Device J Synthetic Substitute K Nonautologous Tissue Substitute M Cardiac Lead N Intracardiac Pacemaker Q Implantable Heart Assist System	Z No Qualifier
A Heart	X External	R Short-term External Heart Assist System	S Biventricular Z No Qualifier
F Aortic Valve Aortic annulus G Mitral Valve Bicuspid valve Left atrioventricular valve Mitral annulus H Pulmonary Valve Pulmonary annulus Pulmonic valve J Tricuspid Valve Right atrioventricular valve Tricuspid annulus	Ø Open 3 Percutaneous 4 Percutaneous Endoscopic	7 Autologous Tissue Substitute 8 Zooplastic Tissue J Synthetic Substitute K Nonautologous Tissue Substitute	Z No Qualifier
W Thoracic Aorta, Descending	3 Percutaneous	R Short-term External Heart Assist System	Z No Qualifier
Y Great Vessel	Ø Open 3 Percutaneous 4 Percutaneous Endoscopic	2 Monitoring Device 3 Infusion Device 7 Autologous Tissue Substitute 8 Zooplastic Tissue C Extraluminal Device D Intraluminal Device J Synthetic Substitute K Nonautologous Tissue Substitute Y Other Device	Z No Qualifier
Y Great Vessel	X External	2 Monitoring Device 3 Infusion Device 7 Autologous Tissue Substitute 8 Zooplastic Tissue C Extraluminal Device D Intraluminal Device J Synthetic Substitute K Nonautologous Tissue Substitute	Z No Qualifier

Non-OR Ø2WA3[2,3,D]Z
Non-OR Ø2WA[3,4]YZ
Non-OR Ø2WAX[2,3,7,8,C,D,J,K,M,N,Q]Z
Non-OR Ø2WAXRZ
Non-OR Ø2WY3[2,3]Z
Non-OR Ø2WY[3,4]YZ
Non-OR Ø2WYX[2,3,7,8,C,D,J,K]Z

HAC Ø2WA[Ø,3,4]MZ when reported with T81.4Ø–T81.49, T82.7 with 7th character A
LC Ø2WA[3,4]QZ

See Appendix L for Procedure Combinations
⊞ Ø2WA[Ø,3,4]QZ
⊞ Ø2WA[Ø,3,4]RZ

Ø Medical and Surgical
2 Heart and Great Vessels
Y Transplantation Definition: Putting in or on all or a portion of a living body part taken from another individual or animal to physically take the place and/or function of all or a portion of a similar body part
Explanation: The native body part may or may not be taken out, and the transplanted body part may take over all or a portion of its function

Body Part Character 4	Approach Character 5	Device Character 6	Qualifier Character 7
A Heart LC	Ø Open	Z No Device	Ø Allogeneic 1 Syngeneic 2 Zooplastic

LC Ø2YAØZ[Ø,1,2]

Upper Arteries Ø31–Ø3W

Character Meanings

This Character Meaning table is provided as a guide to assist the user in the identification of character members that may be found in this section of code tables. It **SHOULD NOT** be used to build a PCS code.

Operation–Character 3	Body Part–Character 4	Approach–Character 5	Device–Character 6	Qualifier–Character 7
1 Bypass	Ø Internal Mammary Artery, Right	Ø Open	Ø Drainage Device	Ø Upper Arm Artery, Right OR Ultrasonic
5 Destruction	1 Internal Mammary Artery, Left	3 Percutaneous	2 Monitoring Device	1 Upper Arm Artery, Left OR Drug-Coated Balloon
7 Dilation	2 Innominate Artery	4 Percutaneous Endoscopic	3 Infusion Device	2 Upper Arm Artery, Bilateral
9 Drainage	3 Subclavian Artery, Right	X External	4 Intraluminal Device, Drug-eluting	3 Lower Arm Artery, Right
B Excision	4 Subclavian Artery, Left		5 Intraluminal Device, Drug-eluting, Two	4 Lower Arm Artery, Left
C Extirpation	5 Axillary Artery, Right		6 Intraluminal Device, Drug-eluting, Three	5 Lower Arm Artery, Bilateral
F Fragmentation	6 Axillary Artery, Left		7 Intraluminal Device, Drug-eluting, Four or More OR Autologous Tissue Substitute	6 Upper Leg Artery, Right
H Insertion	7 Brachial Artery, Right		9 Autologous Venous Tissue	7 Upper Leg Artery, Left OR Stent Retriever
J Inspection	8 Brachial Artery, Left		A Autologous Arterial Tissue	8 Upper Leg Artery, Bilateral
L Occlusion	9 Ulnar Artery, Right		B Intraluminal Device, Bioactive	9 Lower Leg Artery, Right
N Release	A Ulnar Artery, Left		C Extraluminal Device	B Lower Leg Artery, Left
P Removal	B Radial Artery, Right		D Intraluminal Device	C Lower Leg Artery, Bilateral
Q Repair	C Radial Artery, Left		E Intraluminal Device, Two	D Upper Arm Vein
R Replacement	D Hand Artery, Right		F Intraluminal Device, Three	F Lower Arm Vein
S Reposition	F Hand Artery, Left		G Intraluminal Device, Four or More	G Intracranial Artery
U Supplement	G Intracranial Artery		H Intraluminal Device, Flow Diverter	J Extracranial Artery, Right
V Restriction	H Common Carotid Artery, Right		J Synthetic Substitute	K Extracranial Artery, Left
W Revision	J Common Carotid Artery, Left		K Nonautologous Tissue Substitute	M Pulmonary Artery, Right
	K Internal Carotid Artery, Right		M Stimulator Lead	N Pulmonary Artery, Left
	L Internal Carotid Artery, Left		Y Other Device	T Abdominal Artery
	M External Carotid Artery, Right		Z No Device	V Superior Vena Cava
	N External Carotid Artery, Left			W Lower Extremity Vein
	P Vertebral Artery, Right			X Diagnostic
	Q Vertebral Artery, Left			Y Upper Artery
	R Face Artery			Z No Qualifier
	S Temporal Artery, Right			
	T Temporal Artery, Left			
	U Thyroid Artery, Right			
	V Thyroid Artery, Left			
	Y Upper Artery			

AHA Coding Clinic for Upper Arteries

2022, 1Q, 10-13 Procedures performed on a continuous vessel, ICD-10-PCS Guideline B4.1c

AHA Coding Clinic for table Ø31

2021, 4Q, 45-46 Percutaneous bypass of brachial artery for arteriovenous fistula creation
2021, 3Q, 14 Arteriovenous fistula revision with graft to cephalic vein stump
2019, 4Q, 26 Upper artery bypass Qualifier
2019, 4Q, 26 Percutaneous approach upper artery bypass
2017, 4Q, 64-65 New qualifier values - Left to right carotid bypass
2017, 2Q, 22 Carotid artery to subclavian artery transposition
2017, 1Q, 31 Left to right common carotid artery bypass
2016, 3Q, 37 Insertion of arteriovenous graft using HeRO device
2016, 3Q, 39 Revision of arteriovenous graft
2013, 4Q, 125 Stage II cephalic vein transposition (superficialization) of arteriovenous fistula
2013, 1Q, 27 Creation of radial artery fistula

AHA Coding Clinic for table Ø37

2020, 4Q, 70-71 Cerebral embolic filtration extracorporeal flow reversal circuit
2019, 4Q, 27 Bifurcation Qualifier
2019, 3Q, 29 Transcarotid arterial catheterization
2018, 2Q, 24 Coronary artery bifurcation
2016, 4Q, 86 Peripheral artery, number of stents
2016, 4Q, 86-87 Coronary and peripheral artery bifurcation
2015, 1Q, 32 Deployment of stent for herniated/migrated coil in basilar artery

AHA Coding Clinic for table Ø3B

2016, 2Q, 12 Resection of malignant neoplasm of infratemporal fossa

AHA Coding Clinic for table Ø3C

2022, 1Q, 43 Cerebral thrombectomy with failed stent retriever deployment and aspiration of thrombus
2021, 2Q, 13 Thromboendarterectomy with deconstruction of internal carotid artery
2020, 3Q, 38 Thrombectomy of arteriovenous fistula with angioplasty and stent placement
2019, 4Q, 27 Bifurcation Qualifier
2018, 4Q, 47-48 Endovascular thrombectomy with stent retriever
2018, 2Q, 24 Coronary artery bifurcation
2017, 4Q, 64-65 New qualifier values - Left to right carotid bypass
2017, 2Q, 23 Thrombectomy via Fogarty catheter
2016, 4Q, 86-87 Coronary and peripheral artery bifurcation
2016, 2Q, 11 Carotid endarterectomy with patch angioplasty
2015, 1Q, 29 Discontinued carotid endarterectomy

AHA Coding Clinic for table Ø3F

2021, 4Q, 46 Fragmentation of intracranial artery
2020, 4Q, 45-49 New fragmentation tables
2020, 4Q, 49-50 Intravascular ultrasound assisted thrombolysis
2020, 4Q, 50 Intravascular lithotripsy

AHA Coding Clinic for table Ø3H

2020, 1Q, 25 Elephant trunk repair of aortic dissection
2016, 2Q, 32 Arterial catheter placement

AHA Coding Clinic for table Ø3J

2021, 1Q, 16 Placement of Sentinel™ embolic protection device with deployment of single filter
2015, 1Q, 29 Discontinued carotid endarterectomy

AHA Coding Clinic for table Ø3L

2021, 2Q, 13 Thromboendarterectomy with deconstruction of internal carotid artery
2016, 2Q, 30 Clipping (occlusion) of cerebral artery, decompressive craniectomy and storage of bone flap in abdominal wall
2014, 4Q, 20 Control of epistaxis
2014, 4Q, 37 Endovascular embolization of arteriovenous malformation using Onyx-18 liquid

AHA Coding Clinic for table Ø3Q

2017, 1Q, 31 Left to right common carotid artery bypass

AHA Coding Clinic for table Ø3S

2017, 2Q, 22 Carotid artery to subclavian artery transposition
2015, 3Q, 27 Moyamoya disease and hemispheric pial synangiosis with craniotomy

AHA Coding Clinic for table Ø3U

2023, 1Q, 35 Carotid artery endarterectomy with imbrication
2019, 1Q, 22 Cerebral artery fusiform aneurysm repair via wrapping
2016, 2Q, 11 Carotid endarterectomy with patch angioplasty

AHA Coding Clinic for table Ø3V

2023, 1Q, 34 Carotid artery pseudoaneurysm embolization using flow diverter stent and coils
2019, 4Q, 27-28 Aneurysm treatment using flow diverter stent
2019, 1Q, 22 Cerebral artery fusiform aneurysm repair via wrapping
2016, 1Q, 19 Embolization of superior hypophyseal aneurysm using stent-assisted coil

AHA Coding Clinic for table Ø3W

2016, 3Q, 39 Revision of arteriovenous graft
2015, 1Q, 32 Deployment of stent for herniated/migrated coil in basilar artery

Upper Arteries

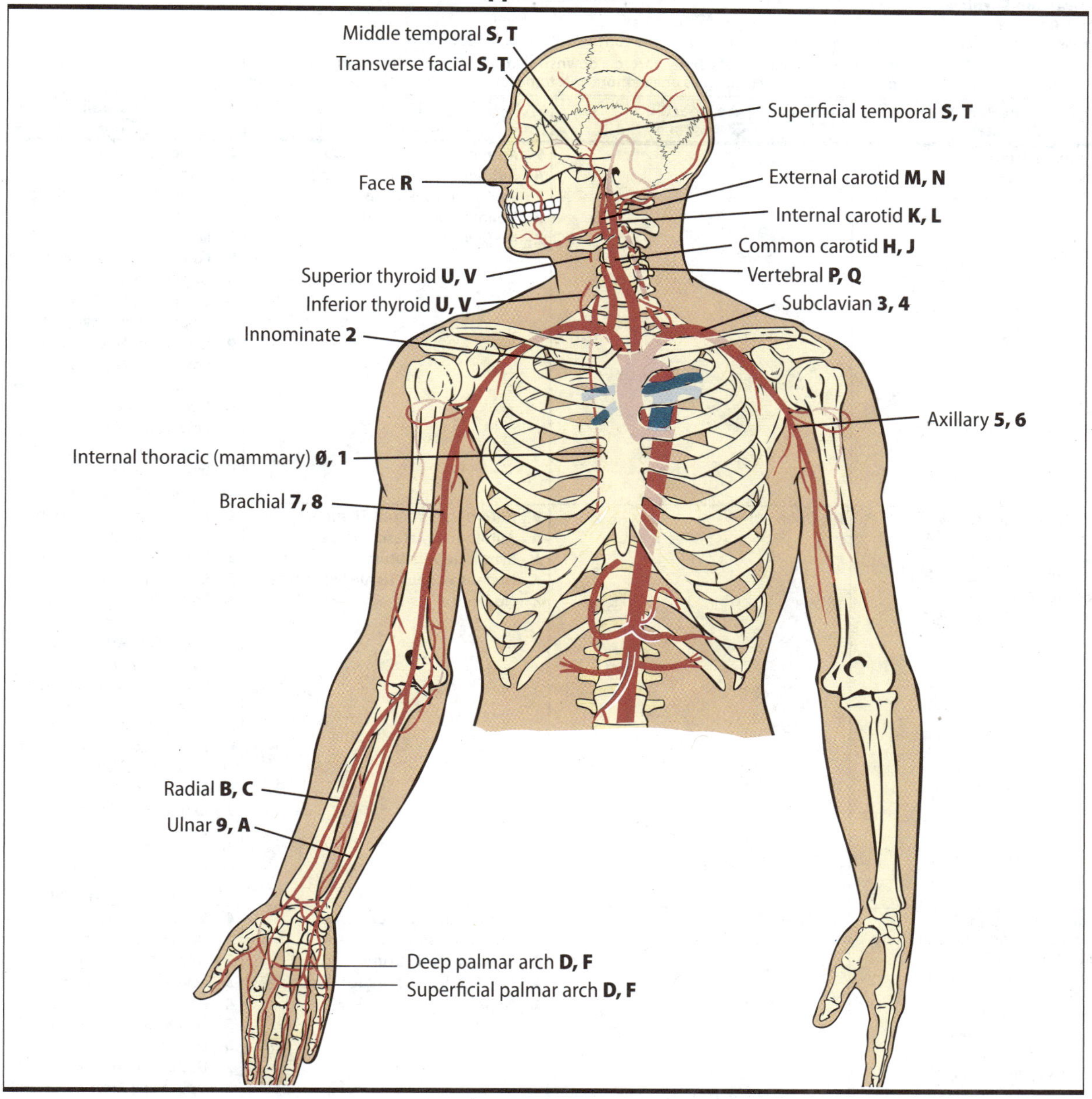

Middle temporal **S, T**
Transverse facial **S, T**
Superficial temporal **S, T**
Face **R**
External carotid **M, N**
Internal carotid **K, L**
Common carotid **H, J**
Superior thyroid **U, V**
Vertebral **P, Q**
Inferior thyroid **U, V**
Subclavian **3, 4**
Innominate **2**
Axillary **5, 6**
Internal thoracic (mammary) **Ø, 1**
Brachial **7, 8**
Radial **B, C**
Ulnar **9, A**
Deep palmar arch **D, F**
Superficial palmar arch **D, F**

Head and Neck Arteries

Middle cerebral **G**
Anterior cerebral **G**
Posterior communicating **G**
Anterior communicating **G**
Posterior cerebral **G**
Ophthalmic **G**
Basilar **G**
Internal carotid **K,L**
External carotid **M,N**
Vertebral **P,Q**
Common carotid **H,J**

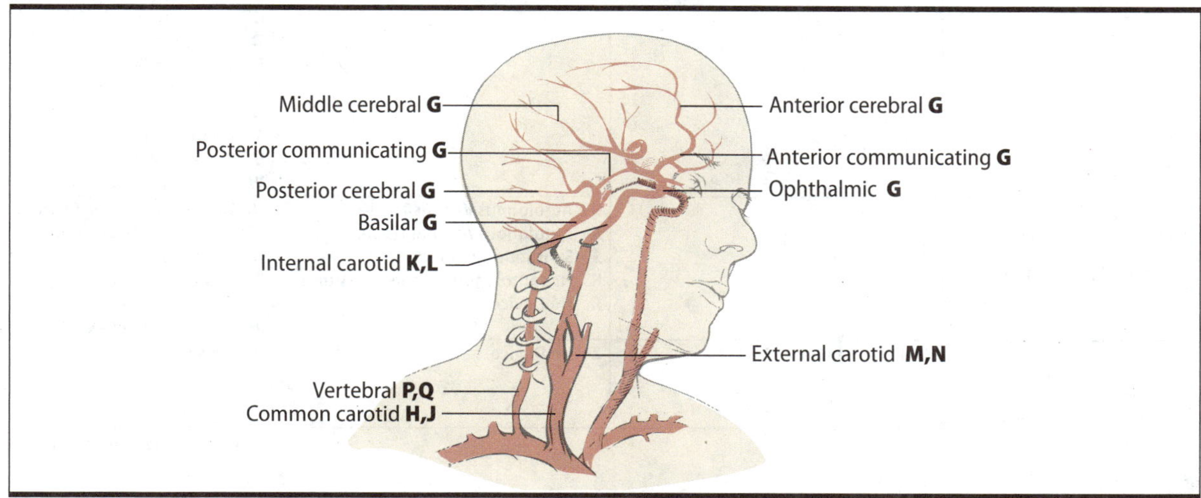

Ø Medical and Surgical
3 Upper Arteries
1 Bypass

Definition: Altering the route of passage of the contents of a tubular body part

Explanation: Rerouting contents of a body part to a downstream area of the normal route, to a similar route and body part, or to an abnormal route and dissimilar body part. Includes one or more anastomoses, with or without the use of a device.

Body Part Character 4	Approach Character 5	Device Character 6	Qualifier Character 7
2 Innominate Artery Brachiocephalic artery Brachiocephalic trunk	**Ø Open**	**9 Autologous Venous Tissue** **A Autologous Arterial Tissue** **J Synthetic Substitute** **K Nonautologous Tissue Substitute** **Z No Device**	**Ø Upper Arm Artery, Right** **1 Upper Arm Artery, Left** **2 Upper Arm Artery, Bilateral** **3 Lower Arm Artery, Right** **4 Lower Arm Artery, Left** **5 Lower Arm Artery, Bilateral** **6 Upper Leg Artery, Right** **7 Upper Leg Artery, Left** **8 Upper Leg Artery, Bilateral** **9 Lower Leg Artery, Right** **B Lower Leg Artery, Left** **C Lower Leg Artery, Bilateral** **D Upper Arm Vein** **F Lower Arm Vein** **J Extracranial Artery, Right** **K Extracranial Artery, Left** **W Lower Extremity Vein**
3 Subclavian Artery, Right Costocervical trunk Dorsal scapular artery Internal thoracic artery **4 Subclavian Artery, Left** *See 3 Subclavian Artery, Right*	**Ø Open**	**9 Autologous Venous Tissue** **A Autologous Arterial Tissue** **J Synthetic Substitute** **K Nonautologous Tissue Substitute** **Z No Device**	**Ø Upper Arm Artery, Right** **1 Upper Arm Artery, Left** **2 Upper Arm Artery, Bilateral** **3 Lower Arm Artery, Right** **4 Lower Arm Artery, Left** **5 Lower Arm Artery, Bilateral** **6 Upper Leg Artery, Right** **7 Upper Leg Artery, Left** **8 Upper Leg Artery, Bilateral** **9 Lower Leg Artery, Right** **B Lower Leg Artery, Left** **C Lower Leg Artery, Bilateral** **D Upper Arm Vein** **F Lower Arm Vein** **J Extracranial Artery, Right** **K Extracranial Artery, Left** **M Pulmonary Artery, Right** **N Pulmonary Artery, Left** **W Lower Extremity Vein**
5 Axillary Artery, Right Anterior circumflex humeral artery Lateral thoracic artery Posterior circumflex humeral artery Subscapular artery Superior thoracic artery Thoracoacromial artery **6 Axillary Artery, Left** *See 5 Axillary Artery, Right*	**Ø Open**	**9 Autologous Venous Tissue** **A Autologous Arterial Tissue** **J Synthetic Substitute** **K Nonautologous Tissue Substitute** **Z No Device**	**Ø Upper Arm Artery, Right** **1 Upper Arm Artery, Left** **2 Upper Arm Artery, Bilateral** **3 Lower Arm Artery, Right** **4 Lower Arm Artery, Left** **5 Lower Arm Artery, Bilateral** **6 Upper Leg Artery, Right** **7 Upper Leg Artery, Left** **8 Upper Leg Artery, Bilateral** **9 Lower Leg Artery, Right** **B Lower Leg Artery, Left** **C Lower Leg Artery, Bilateral** **D Upper Arm Vein** **F Lower Arm Vein** **J Extracranial Artery, Right** **K Extracranial Artery, Left** **T Abdominal Artery** **V Superior Vena Cava** **W Lower Extremity Vein**
7 Brachial Artery, Right Inferior ulnar collateral artery Profunda brachii Superior ulnar collateral artery	**Ø Open**	**9 Autologous Venous Tissue** **A Autologous Arterial Tissue** **J Synthetic Substitute** **K Nonautologous Tissue Substitute** **Z No Device**	**Ø Upper Arm Artery, Right** **3 Lower Arm Artery, Right** **D Upper Arm Vein** **F Lower Arm Vein** **V Superior Vena Cava** **W Lower Extremity Vein**
7 Brachial Artery, Right Inferior ulnar collateral artery Profunda brachii Superior ulnar collateral artery	**3 Percutaneous**	**Z No Device**	**F Lower Arm Vein**

Ø31 Continued on next page

Ø Medical and Surgical
3 Upper Arteries
1 Bypass Definition: Altering the route of passage of the contents of a tubular body part

Explanation: Rerouting contents of a body part to a downstream area of the normal route, to a similar route and body part, or to an abnormal route and dissimilar body part. Includes one or more anastomoses, with or without the use of a device.

Ø31 Continued

Body Part Character 4	Approach Character 5	Device Character 6	Qualifier Character 7
8 Brachial Artery, Left Inferior ulnar collateral artery Profunda brachii Superior ulnar collateral artery	**Ø Open**	**9 Autologous Venous Tissue** **A Autologous Arterial Tissue** **J Synthetic Substitute** **K Nonautologous Tissue Substitute** **Z No Device**	**1 Upper Arm Artery, Left** **4 Lower Arm Artery, Left** **D Upper Arm Vein** **F Lower Arm Vein** **V Superior Vena Cava** **W Lower Extremity Vein**
8 Brachial Artery, Left Inferior ulnar collateral artery Profunda brachii Superior ulnar collateral artery	**3 Percutaneous**	**Z No Device**	**F Lower Arm Vein**
9 Ulnar Artery, Right Anterior ulnar recurrent artery Common interosseous artery Posterior ulnar recurrent artery **B Radial Artery, Right** Radial recurrent artery	**Ø Open**	**9 Autologous Venous Tissue** **A Autologous Arterial Tissue** **J Synthetic Substitute** **K Nonautologous Tissue Substitute** **Z No Device**	**3 Lower Arm Artery, Right** **F Lower Arm Vein**
9 Ulnar Artery, Right Anterior ulnar recurrent artery Common interosseous artery Posterior ulnar recurrent artery **B Radial Artery, Right** Radial recurrent artery	**3 Percutaneous**	**Z No Device**	**F Lower Arm Vein**
A Ulnar Artery, Left Anterior ulnar recurrent artery Common interosseous artery Posterior ulnar recurrent artery **C Radial Artery, Left** Radial recurrent artery	**Ø Open**	**9 Autologous Venous Tissue** **A Autologous Arterial Tissue** **J Synthetic Substitute** **K Nonautologous Tissue Substitute** **Z No Device**	**4 Lower Arm Artery, Left** **F Lower Arm Vein**
A Ulnar Artery, Left Anterior ulnar recurrent artery Common interosseous artery Posterior ulnar recurrent artery **C Radial Artery, Left** Radial recurrent artery	**3 Percutaneous**	**Z No Device**	**F Lower Arm Vein**
G Intracranial Artery Anterior cerebral artery Anterior choroidal artery Anterior communicating artery Basilar artery Circle of Willis Internal carotid artery, intracranial portion Middle cerebral artery Middle meningeal artery, intracranial portion Ophthalmic artery Posterior cerebral artery Posterior communicating artery Posterior inferior cerebellar artery (PICA) Vertebral artery, intracranial portion **S Temporal Artery, Right** Middle temporal artery Superficial temporal artery Transverse facial artery **T Temporal Artery, Left** *See S Temporal Artery, Right*	**Ø Open**	**9 Autologous Venous Tissue** **A Autologous Arterial Tissue** **J Synthetic Substitute** **K Nonautologous Tissue Substitute** **Z No Device**	**G Intracranial Artery**
H Common Carotid Artery, Right **J Common Carotid Artery, Left**	**Ø Open**	**9 Autologous Venous Tissue** **A Autologous Arterial Tissue** **J Synthetic Substitute** **K Nonautologous Tissue Substitute** **Z No Device**	**G Intracranial Artery** **J Extracranial Artery, Right** **K Extracranial Artery, Left** **Y Upper Artery**

Ø31 Continued on next page

Ø31 Continued

Ø Medical and Surgical
3 Upper Arteries
1 Bypass

Definition: Altering the route of passage of the contents of a tubular body part

Explanation: Rerouting contents of a body part to a downstream area of the normal route, to a similar route and body part, or to an abnormal route and dissimilar body part. Includes one or more anastomoses, with or without the use of a device.

Body Part Character 4	Approach Character 5	Device Character 6	Qualifier Character 7
K Internal Carotid Artery, Right Caroticotympanic artery Carotid sinus **L Internal Carotid Artery, Left** Caroticotympanic artery Carotid sinus **M External Carotid Artery, Right** Ascending pharyngeal artery Internal maxillary artery Lingual artery Maxillary artery Occipital artery Posterior auricular artery Superior thyroid artery **N External Carotid Artery, Left** Ascending pharyngeal artery Internal maxillary artery Lingual artery Maxillary artery Occipital artery Posterior auricular artery Superior thyroid artery	**Ø Open**	**9 Autologous Venous Tissue** **A Autologous Arterial Tissue** **J Synthetic Substitute** **K Nonautologous Tissue Substitute** **Z No Device**	**J Extracranial Artery, Right** **K Extracranial Artery, Left**

Ø Medical and Surgical
3 Upper Arteries
5 Destruction

Definition: Physical eradication of all or a portion of a body part by the direct use of energy, force, or a destructive agent
Explanation: None of the body part is physically taken out

Body Part Character 4		Approach Character 5	Device Character 6	Qualifier Character 7
Ø Internal Mammary Artery, Right Anterior intercostal artery Internal thoracic artery Musculophrenic artery Pericardiophrenic artery Superior epigastric artery **1 Internal Mammary Artery, Left** *See Ø Internal Mammary Artery, Right* **2 Innominate Artery** Brachiocephalic artery Brachiocephalic trunk **3 Subclavian Artery, Right** Costocervical trunk Dorsal scapular artery Internal thoracic artery **4 Subclavian Artery, Left** *See 3 Subclavian Artery, Right* **5 Axillary Artery, Right** Anterior circumflex humeral artery Lateral thoracic artery Posterior circumflex humeral artery Subscapular artery Superior thoracic artery Thoracoacromial artery **6 Axillary Artery, Left** *See 5 Axillary Artery, Right* **7 Brachial Artery, Right** Inferior ulnar collateral artery Profunda brachii Superior ulnar collateral artery **8 Brachial Artery, Left** *See 7 Brachial Artery, Right* **9 Ulnar Artery, Right** Anterior ulnar recurrent artery Common interosseous artery Posterior ulnar recurrent artery **A Ulnar Artery, Left** *See 9 Ulnar Artery, Right* **B Radial Artery, Right** Radial recurrent artery **C Radial Artery, Left** *See B Radial Artery, Right* **D Hand Artery, Right** Deep palmar arch Princeps pollicis artery Radialis indicis Superficial palmar arch **F Hand Artery, Left** *See D Hand Artery, Right* **G Intracranial Artery** Anterior cerebral artery Anterior choroidal artery Anterior communicating artery Basilar artery Circle of Willis Internal carotid artery, intracranial portion Middle cerebral artery Middle meningeal artery, intracranial portion Ophthalmic artery Posterior cerebral artery Posterior communicating artery Posterior inferior cerebellar artery (PICA) Vertebral artery, intracranial portion	**H Common Carotid Artery, Right** **J Common Carotid Artery, Left** **K Internal Carotid Artery, Right** Caroticotympanic artery Carotid sinus **L Internal Carotid Artery, Left** *See K Internal Carotid Artery, Right* **M External Carotid Artery, Right** Ascending pharyngeal artery Internal maxillary artery Lingual artery Maxillary artery Occipital artery Posterior auricular artery Superior thyroid artery **N External Carotid Artery, Left** *See M External Carotid Artery, Right* **P Vertebral Artery, Right** Anterior spinal artery Posterior spinal artery **Q Vertebral Artery, Left** *See P Vertebral Artery, Right* **R Face Artery** Angular artery Ascending palatine artery External maxillary artery Facial artery Inferior labial artery Submental artery Superior labial artery **S Temporal Artery, Right** Middle temporal artery Superficial temporal artery Transverse facial artery **T Temporal Artery, Left** *See S Temporal Artery, Right* **U Thyroid Artery, Right** Cricothyroid artery Hyoid artery Sternocleidomastoid artery Superior laryngeal artery Superior thyroid artery Thyrocervical trunk **V Thyroid Artery, Left** *See U Thyroid Artery, Right* **Y Upper Artery** Aortic intercostal artery Bronchial artery Esophageal artery Subcostal artery	**Ø Open** **3 Percutaneous** **4 Percutaneous Endoscopic**	**Z No Device**	**Z No Qualifier**

Ø Medical and Surgical
3 Upper Arteries
7 Dilation

Definition: Expanding an orifice or the lumen of a tubular body part

Explanation: The orifice can be a natural orifice or an artificially created orifice. Accomplished by stretching a tubular body part using intraluminal pressure or by cutting part of the orifice or wall of the tubular body part.

Body Part Character 4	Approach Character 5	Device Character 6	Qualifier Character 7
Ø Internal Mammary Artery, Right Anterior intercostal artery Internal thoracic artery Musculophrenic artery Pericardiophrenic artery Superior epigastric artery **1 Internal Mammary Artery, Left** *See Ø Internal Mammary Artery, Right* **2 Innominate Artery** Brachiocephalic artery Brachiocephalic trunk **3 Subclavian Artery, Right** Costocervical trunk Dorsal scapular artery Internal thoracic artery **4 Subclavian Artery, Left** *See 3 Subclavian Artery, Right* **5 Axillary Artery, Right** Anterior circumflex humeral artery Lateral thoracic artery Posterior circumflex humeral artery Subscapular artery Superior thoracic artery Thoracoacromial artery **6 Axillary Artery, Left** *See 5 Axillary Artery, Right* **7 Brachial Artery, Right** Inferior ulnar collateral artery Profunda brachii Superior ulnar collateral artery **8 Brachial Artery, Left** *See 7 Brachial Artery, Right* **9 Ulnar Artery, Right** Anterior ulnar recurrent artery Common interosseous artery Posterior ulnar recurrent artery **A Ulnar Artery, Left** *See 9 Ulnar Artery, Right* **B Radial Artery, Right** Radial recurrent artery **C Radial Artery, Left** *See B Radial Artery, Right*	**Ø Open** **3 Percutaneous** **4 Percutaneous Endoscopic**	**4 Intraluminal Device, Drug-eluting** **5 Intraluminal Device, Drug-eluting, Two** **6 Intraluminal Device, Drug-eluting, Three** **7 Intraluminal Device, Drug-eluting, Four or More** **E Intraluminal Device, Two** **F Intraluminal Device, Three** **G Intraluminal Device, Four or More**	**Z No Qualifier**
Ø Internal Mammary Artery, Right Anterior intercostal artery Internal thoracic artery Musculophrenic artery Pericardiophrenic artery Superior epigastric artery **1 Internal Mammary Artery, Left** *See Ø Internal Mammary Artery, Right* **2 Innominate Artery** Brachiocephalic artery Brachiocephalic trunk **3 Subclavian Artery, Right** Costocervical trunk Dorsal scapular artery Internal thoracic artery **4 Subclavian Artery, Left** *See 3 Subclavian Artery, Right* **5 Axillary Artery, Right** Anterior circumflex humeral artery Lateral thoracic artery Posterior circumflex humeral artery Subscapular artery Superior thoracic artery Thoracoacromial artery **6 Axillary Artery, Left** *See 5 Axillary Artery, Right* **7 Brachial Artery, Right** Inferior ulnar collateral artery Profunda brachii Superior ulnar collateral artery **8 Brachial Artery, Left** *See 7 Brachial Artery, Right* **9 Ulnar Artery, Right** Anterior ulnar recurrent artery Common interosseous artery Posterior ulnar recurrent artery **A Ulnar Artery, Left** *See 9 Ulnar Artery, Right* **B Radial Artery, Right** Radial recurrent artery **C Radial Artery, Left** *See B Radial Artery, Right*	**Ø Open** **3 Percutaneous** **4 Percutaneous Endoscopic**	**D Intraluminal Device** **Z No Device**	**1 Drug-Coated Balloon** **Z No Qualifier**

Ø37 Continued on next page

Ø Medical and Surgical
3 Upper Arteries
7 Dilation

Ø37 Continued

Definition: Expanding an orifice or the lumen of a tubular body part

Explanation: The orifice can be a natural orifice or an artificially created orifice. Accomplished by stretching a tubular body part using intraluminal pressure or by cutting part of the orifice or wall of the tubular body part.

Body Part Character 4	Approach Character 5	Device Character 6	Qualifier Character 7
D Hand Artery, Right Deep palmar arch Princeps pollicis artery Radialis indicis Superficial palmar arch **F Hand Artery, Left** *See D Hand Artery, Right* **G Intracranial Artery** NC Anterior cerebral artery Anterior choroidal artery Anterior communicating artery Basilar artery Circle of Willis Internal carotid artery, intracranial portion Middle cerebral artery Middle meningeal artery, intracranial portion Ophthalmic artery Posterior cerebral artery Posterior communicating artery Posterior inferior cerebellar artery (PICA) Vertebral artery, intracranial portion **H Common Carotid Artery, Right** **J Common Carotid Artery, Left** **K Internal Carotid Artery, Right** Caroticotympanic artery Carotid sinus **L Internal Carotid Artery, Left** *See K Internal Carotid Artery, Right* **M External Carotid Artery, Right** Ascending pharyngeal artery Internal maxillary artery Lingual artery Maxillary artery Occipital artery Posterior auricular artery Superior thyroid artery **N External Carotid Artery, Left** *See M External Carotid Artery, Right* **P Vertebral Artery, Right** Anterior spinal artery Posterior spinal artery **Q Vertebral Artery, Left** *See P Vertebral Artery, Right* **R Face Artery** Angular artery Ascending palatine artery External maxillary artery Facial artery Inferior labial artery Submental artery Superior labial artery **S Temporal Artery, Right** Middle temporal artery Superficial temporal artery Transverse facial artery **T Temporal Artery, Left** *See S Temporal Artery, Right* **U Thyroid Artery, Right** Cricothyroid artery Hyoid artery Sternocleidomastoid artery Superior laryngeal artery Superior thyroid artery Thyrocervical trunk **V Thyroid Artery, Left** *See U Thyroid Artery, Right* **Y Upper Artery** Aortic intercostal artery Bronchial artery Esophageal artery Subcostal artery	**Ø Open** **3 Percutaneous** **4 Percutaneous Endoscopic**	**4 Intraluminal Device, Drug-eluting** **5 Intraluminal Device, Drug-eluting, Two** **6 Intraluminal Device, Drug-eluting, Three** **7 Intraluminal Device, Drug-eluting, Four or More** **D Intraluminal Device** **E Intraluminal Device, Two** **F Intraluminal Device, Three** **G Intraluminal Device, Four or More** **Z No Device**	**Z No Qualifier**

NC Ø37G[3,4]ZZ

Ø Medical and Surgical
3 Upper Arteries
9 Drainage

Definition: Taking or letting out fluids and/or gases from a body part

Explanation: The qualifier DIAGNOSTIC is used to identify drainage procedures that are biopsies

Body Part Character 4	Approach Character 5	Device Character 6	Qualifier Character 7
Ø Internal Mammary Artery, Right Anterior intercostal artery Internal thoracic artery Musculophrenic artery Pericardiophrenic artery Superior epigastric artery **1 Internal Mammary Artery, Left** *See Ø Internal Mammary Artery, Right above* **2 Innominate Artery** Brachiocephalic artery Brachiocephalic trunk **3 Subclavian Artery, Right** Costocervical trunk Dorsal scapular artery Internal thoracic artery **4 Subclavian Artery, Left** *See 3 Subclavian Artery, Right* **5 Axillary Artery, Right** Anterior circumflex humeral artery Lateral thoracic artery Posterior circumflex humeral artery Subscapular artery Superior thoracic artery Thoracoacromial artery **6 Axillary Artery, Left** *See 5 Axillary Artery, Right* **7 Brachial Artery, Right** Inferior ulnar collateral artery Profunda brachii Superior ulnar collateral artery **8 Brachial Artery, Left** *See 7 Brachial Artery, Right* **9 Ulnar Artery, Right** Anterior ulnar recurrent artery Common interosseous artery Posterior ulnar recurrent artery **A Ulnar Artery, Left** *See 9 Ulnar Artery, Right* **B Radial Artery, Right** Radial recurrent artery **C Radial Artery, Left** *See B Radial Artery, Right* **D Hand Artery, Right** Deep palmar arch Princeps pollicis artery Radialis indicis Superficial palmar arch **F Hand Artery, Left** *See D Hand Artery, Right* **G Intracranial Artery** Anterior cerebral artery Anterior choroidal artery Anterior communicating artery Basilar artery Circle of Willis Internal carotid artery, intracranial portion Middle cerebral artery Middle meningeal artery, intracranial portion Ophthalmic artery Posterior cerebral artery Posterior communicating artery Posterior inferior cerebellar artery (PICA) Vertebral artery, intracranial portion **H Common Carotid Artery, Right** **J Common Carotid Artery, Left** **K Internal Carotid Artery, Right** Caroticotympanic artery Carotid sinus **L Internal Carotid Artery, Left** *See K Internal Carotid Artery, Right* **M External Carotid Artery, Right** Ascending pharyngeal artery Internal maxillary artery Lingual artery Maxillary artery Occipital artery Posterior auricular artery Superior thyroid artery **N External Carotid Artery, Left** *See M External Carotid Artery, Right* **P Vertebral Artery, Right** Anterior spinal artery Posterior spinal artery **Q Vertebral Artery, Left** *See P Vertebral Artery, Right* **R Face Artery** Angular artery Ascending palatine artery External maxillary artery Facial artery Inferior labial artery Submental artery Superior labial artery **S Temporal Artery, Right** Middle temporal artery Superficial temporal artery Transverse facial artery **T Temporal Artery, Left** *See S Temporal Artery, Right* **U Thyroid Artery, Right** Cricothyroid artery Hyoid artery Sternocleidomastoid artery Superior laryngeal artery Superior thyroid artery Thyrocervical trunk **V Thyroid Artery, Left** *See U Thyroid Artery, Right* **Y Upper Artery** Aortic intercostal artery Bronchial artery Esophageal artery Subcostal artery	Ø Open 3 Percutaneous 4 Percutaneous Endoscopic	Ø Drainage Device	Z No Qualifier

Non-OR Ø39[Ø,1,2,3,4,5,6,7,8,9,A,B,C,D,F,G,H,J,K,L,M,N,P,Q,R,S,T,U,V,Y][Ø,3,4]ØZ

Ø39 Continued on next page

Ø Medical and Surgical
3 Upper Arteries
9 Drainage

Definition: Taking or letting out fluids and/or gases from a body part
Explanation: The qualifier DIAGNOSTIC is used to identify drainage procedures that are biopsies

Ø39 Continued

Body Part Character 4	Approach Character 5	Device Character 6	Qualifier Character 7
Ø Internal Mammary Artery, Right Anterior intercostal artery Internal thoracic artery Musculophrenic artery Pericardiophrenic artery Superior epigastric artery **1 Internal Mammary Artery, Left** *See Ø Internal Mammary Artery, Right* **2 Innominate Artery** Brachiocephalic artery Brachiocephalic trunk **3 Subclavian Artery, Right** Costocervical trunk Dorsal scapular artery Internal thoracic artery **4 Subclavian Artery, Left** *See 3 Subclavian Artery, Right* **5 Axillary Artery, Right** Anterior circumflex humeral artery Lateral thoracic artery Posterior circumflex humeral artery Subscapular artery Superior thoracic artery Thoracoacromial artery **6 Axillary Artery, Left** *See 5 Axillary Artery, Right* **7 Brachial Artery, Right** Inferior ulnar collateral artery Profunda brachii Superior ulnar collateral artery **8 Brachial Artery, Left** *See 7 Brachial Artery, Right* **9 Ulnar Artery, Right** Anterior ulnar recurrent artery Common interosseous artery Posterior ulnar recurrent artery **A Ulnar Artery, Left** *See 9 Ulnar Artery, Right* **B Radial Artery, Right** Radial recurrent artery **C Radial Artery, Left** *See B Radial Artery, Right* **D Hand Artery, Right** Deep palmar arch Princeps pollicis artery Radialis indicis Superficial palmar arch **F Hand Artery, Left** *See D Hand Artery, Right* **G Intracranial Artery** Anterior cerebral artery Anterior choroidal artery Anterior communicating artery Basilar artery Circle of Willis Internal carotid artery, intracranial portion Middle cerebral artery Middle meningeal artery, intracranial portion Ophthalmic artery Posterior cerebral artery Posterior communicating artery Posterior inferior cerebellar artery (PICA) Vertebral artery, intracranial portion **H Common Carotid Artery, Right** **J Common Carotid Artery, Left** **K Internal Carotid Artery, Right** Caroticotympanic artery Carotid sinus **L Internal Carotid Artery, Left** *See K Internal Carotid Artery, Right* **M External Carotid Artery, Right** Ascending pharyngeal artery Internal maxillary artery Lingual artery Maxillary artery Occipital artery Posterior auricular artery Superior thyroid artery **N External Carotid Artery, Left** *See M External Carotid Artery, Right* **P Vertebral Artery, Right** Anterior spinal artery Posterior spinal artery **Q Vertebral Artery, Left** *See P Vertebral Artery, Right* **R Face Artery** Angular artery Ascending palatine artery External maxillary artery Facial artery Inferior labial artery Submental artery Superior labial artery **S Temporal Artery, Right** Middle temporal artery Superficial temporal artery Transverse facial artery **T Temporal Artery, Left** *See S Temporal Artery, Right* **U Thyroid Artery, Right** Cricothyroid artery Hyoid artery Sternocleidomastoid artery Superior laryngeal artery Superior thyroid artery Thyrocervical trunk **V Thyroid Artery, Left** *See U Thyroid Artery, Right* **Y Upper Artery** Aortic intercostal artery Bronchial artery Esophageal artery Subcostal artery	Ø Open 3 Percutaneous 4 Percutaneous Endoscopic	Z No Device	X Diagnostic Z No Qualifier

Non-OR Ø39[Ø,1,2,3,4,5,6,7,8,9,A,B,C,D,F,G,H,J,K,L,M,N,P,Q,R,S,T,U,V,Y]3ZX
Non-OR Ø39[Ø,1,2,3,4,5,6,7,8,9,A,B,C,D,F,G,H,J,K,L,M,N,P,Q,R,S,T,U,V,Y][Ø,3,4]ZZ

Ø Medical and Surgical
3 Upper Arteries
B Excision

Definition: Cutting out or off, without replacement, a portion of a body part

Explanation: The qualifier DIAGNOSTIC is used to identify excision procedures that are biopsies

Body Part Character 4		Approach Character 5	Device Character 6	Qualifier Character 7
Ø Internal Mammary Artery, Right Anterior intercostal artery Internal thoracic artery Musculophrenic artery Pericardiophrenic artery Superior epigastric artery **1 Internal Mammary Artery, Left** ***See*** *Ø Internal Mammary Artery, Right* **2 Innominate Artery** Brachiocephalic artery Brachiocephalic trunk **3 Subclavian Artery, Right** Costocervical trunk Dorsal scapular artery Internal thoracic artery **4 Subclavian Artery, Left** ***See*** *3 Subclavian Artery, Right* **5 Axillary Artery, Right** Anterior circumflex humeral artery Lateral thoracic artery Posterior circumflex humeral artery Subscapular artery Superior thoracic artery Thoracoacromial artery **6 Axillary Artery, Left** ***See*** *5 Axillary Artery, Right* **7 Brachial Artery, Right** Inferior ulnar collateral artery Profunda brachii Superior ulnar collateral artery **8 Brachial Artery, Left** ***See*** *7 Brachial Artery, Right* **9 Ulnar Artery, Right** Anterior ulnar recurrent artery Common interosseous artery Posterior ulnar recurrent artery **A Ulnar Artery, Left** ***See*** *9 Ulnar Artery, Right* **B Radial Artery, Right** Radial recurrent artery **C Radial Artery, Left** ***See*** *B Radial Artery, Right* **D Hand Artery, Right** Deep palmar arch Princeps pollicis artery Radialis indicis Superficial palmar arch **F Hand Artery, Left** ***See*** *D Hand Artery, Right* **G Intracranial Artery** Anterior cerebral artery Anterior choroidal artery Anterior communicating artery Basilar artery Circle of Willis Internal carotid artery, intracranial portion Middle cerebral artery Middle meningeal artery, intracranial portion Ophthalmic artery Posterior cerebral artery Posterior communicating artery Posterior inferior cerebellar artery (PICA) Vertebral artery, intracranial portion	**H Common Carotid Artery, Right** **J Common Carotid Artery, Left** **K Internal Carotid Artery, Right** Caroticotympanic artery Carotid sinus **L Internal Carotid Artery, Left** ***See*** *K Internal Carotid Artery, Right* **M External Carotid Artery, Right** Ascending pharyngeal artery Internal maxillary artery Lingual artery Maxillary artery Occipital artery Posterior auricular artery Superior thyroid artery **N External Carotid Artery, Left** ***See*** *M External Carotid Artery, Right* **P Vertebral Artery, Right** Anterior spinal artery Posterior spinal artery **Q Vertebral Artery, Left** ***See*** *P Vertebral Artery, Right* **R Face Artery** Angular artery Ascending palatine artery External maxillary artery Facial artery Inferior labial artery Submental artery Superior labial artery **S Temporal Artery, Right** Middle temporal artery Superficial temporal artery Transverse facial artery **T Temporal Artery, Left** ***See*** *S Temporal Artery, Right* **U Thyroid Artery, Right** Cricothyroid artery Hyoid artery Sternocleidomastoid artery Superior laryngeal artery Superior thyroid artery Thyrocervical trunk **V Thyroid Artery, Left** ***See*** *U Thyroid Artery, Right* **Y Upper Artery** Aortic intercostal artery Bronchial artery Esophageal artery Subcostal artery	**Ø Open** **3 Percutaneous** **4 Percutaneous Endoscopic**	**Z No Device**	**X Diagnostic** **Z No Qualifier**

Ø Medical and Surgical
3 Upper Arteries
C Extirpation

Definition: Taking or cutting out solid matter from a body part

Explanation: The solid matter may be an abnormal byproduct of a biological function or a foreign body; it may be imbedded in a body part or in the lumen of a tubular body part. The solid matter may or may not have been previously broken into pieces.

Body Part Character 4		Approach Character 5	Device Character 6	Qualifier Character 7
Ø Internal Mammary Artery, Right Anterior intercostal artery Internal thoracic artery Musculophrenic artery Pericardiophrenic artery Superior epigastric artery **1 Internal Mammary Artery, Left** *See Ø Internal Mammary Artery, Right* **2 Innominate Artery** Brachiocephalic artery Brachiocephalic trunk **3 Subclavian Artery, Right** Costocervical trunk Dorsal scapular artery Internal thoracic artery **4 Subclavian Artery, Left** *See 3 Subclavian Artery, Right* **5 Axillary Artery, Right** Anterior circumflex humeral artery Lateral thoracic artery Posterior circumflex humeral artery Subscapular artery Superior thoracic artery Thoracoacromial artery **6 Axillary Artery, Left** *See 5 Axillary Artery, Right* **7 Brachial Artery, Right** Inferior ulnar collateral artery Profunda brachii Superior ulnar collateral artery **8 Brachial Artery, Left** *See 7 Brachial Artery, Right* **9 Ulnar Artery, Right** Anterior ulnar recurrent artery Common interosseous artery Posterior ulnar recurrent artery	**A Ulnar Artery, Left** *See 9 Ulnar Artery, Right* **B Radial Artery, Right** Radial recurrent artery **C Radial Artery, Left** *See B Radial Artery, Right* **D Hand Artery, Right** Deep palmar arch Princeps pollicis artery Radialis indicis Superficial palmar arch **F Hand Artery, Left** *See D Hand Artery, Right* **R Face Artery** Angular artery Ascending palatine artery External maxillary artery Facial artery Inferior labial artery Submental artery Superior labial artery **S Temporal Artery, Right** Middle temporal artery Superficial temporal artery Transverse facial artery **T Temporal Artery, Left** *See S Temporal Artery, Right* **U Thyroid Artery, Right** Cricothyroid artery Hyoid artery Sternocleidomastoid artery Superior laryngeal artery Superior thyroid artery Thyrocervical trunk **V Thyroid Artery, Left** *See U Thyroid Artery, Right* **Y Upper Artery** Aortic intercostal artery Bronchial artery Esophageal artery Subcostal artery	**Ø Open** **3 Percutaneous** **4 Percutaneous Endoscopic**	**Z No Device**	**Z No Qualifier**
G Intracranial Artery Anterior cerebral artery Anterior choroidal artery Anterior communicating artery Basilar artery Circle of Willis Internal carotid artery, intracranial portion Middle cerebral artery Middle meningeal artery, intracranial portion Ophthalmic artery Posterior cerebral artery Posterior communicating artery Posterior inferior cerebellar artery (PICA) Vertebral artery, intracranial portion **H Common Carotid Artery, Right** **J Common Carotid Artery, Left** **K Internal Carotid Artery, Right** Caroticotympanic artery Carotid sinus	**L Internal Carotid Artery, Left** *See K Internal Carotid Artery, Right* **M External Carotid Artery, Right** Ascending pharyngeal artery Internal maxillary artery Lingual artery Maxillary artery Occipital artery Posterior auricular artery Superior thyroid artery **N External Carotid Artery, Left** *See M External Carotid Artery, Right* **P Vertebral Artery, Right** Anterior spinal artery Posterior spinal artery **Q Vertebral Artery, Left** *See P Vertebral Artery, Right*	**Ø Open** **4 Percutaneous Endoscopic**	**Z No Device**	**Z No Qualifier**

Ø3C Continued on next page

Ø3C Continued

Ø Medical and Surgical
3 Upper Arteries
C Extirpation Definition: Taking or cutting out solid matter from a body part

Explanation: The solid matter may be an abnormal byproduct of a biological function or a foreign body; it may be imbedded in a body part or in the lumen of a tubular body part. The solid matter may or may not have been previously broken into pieces.

Body Part Character 4		Approach Character 5	Device Character 6	Qualifier Character 7
G Intracranial Artery Anterior cerebral artery Anterior choroidal artery Anterior communicating artery Basilar artery Circle of Willis Internal carotid artery, intracranial portion Middle cerebral artery Middle meningeal artery, intracranial portion Ophthalmic artery Posterior cerebral artery Posterior communicating artery Posterior inferior cerebellar artery (PICA) Vertebral artery, intracranial portion **H Common Carotid Artery, Right** **J Common Carotid Artery, Left** **K Internal Carotid Artery, Right** Caroticotympanic artery Carotid sinus	**L Internal Carotid Artery, Left** ***See** K Internal Carotid Artery, Right* **M External Carotid Artery, Right** Ascending pharyngeal artery Internal maxillary artery Lingual artery Maxillary artery Occipital artery Posterior auricular artery Superior thyroid artery **N External Carotid Artery, Left** ***See** M External Carotid Artery, Right* **P Vertebral Artery, Right** Anterior spinal artery Posterior spinal artery **Q Vertebral Artery, Left** ***See** P Vertebral Artery, Right*	**3** Percutaneous	**Z** No Device	**7** Stent Retriever **Z** No Qualifier

Ø Medical and Surgical
3 Upper Arteries
F Fragmentation Definition: Breaking solid matter in a body part into pieces

Explanation: Physical force (e.g., manual, ultrasonic) applied directly or indirectly is used to break the solid matter into pieces. The solid matter may be an abnormal byproduct of a biological function or a foreign body. The pieces of solid matter are not taken out.

Body Part Character 4		Approach Character 5	Device Character 6	Qualifier Character 7
2 Innominate Artery Brachiocephalic artery Brachiocephalic trunk **3 Subclavian Artery, Right** Costocervical trunk Dorsal scapular artery Internal thoracic artery **4 Subclavian Artery, Left** ***See** 3 Subclavian Artery, Right* **5 Axillary Artery, Right** Anterior circumflex humeral artery Lateral thoracic artery Posterior circumflex humeral artery Subscapular artery Superior thoracic artery Thoracoacromial artery **6 Axillary Artery, Left** ***See** 5 Axillary Artery, Right* **7 Brachial Artery, Right** Inferior ulnar collateral artery Profunda brachii Superior ulnar collateral artery **8 Brachial Artery, Left** ***See** 7 Brachial Artery, Right* **9 Ulnar Artery, Right** Anterior ulnar recurrent artery Common interosseous artery Posterior ulnar recurrent artery	**A Ulnar Artery, Left** ***See** 9 Ulnar Artery, Right* **B Radial Artery, Right** Radial recurrent artery **C Radial Artery, Left** ***See** B Radial Artery, Right* **G Intracranial Artery** Anterior cerebral artery Anterior choroidal artery Anterior communicating artery Basilar artery Circle of Willis Internal carotid artery, intracranial portion Middle cerebral artery Middle meningeal artery, intracranial portion Ophthalmic artery Posterior cerebral artery Posterior communicating artery Posterior inferior cerebellar artery (PICA) Vertebral artery, intracranial portion **Y Upper Artery** Aortic intercostal artery Bronchial artery Esophageal artery Subcostal artery	**3** Percutaneous	**Z** No Device	**Ø** Ultrasonic **Z** No Qualifier

Ø Medical and Surgical
3 Upper Arteries
H Insertion

Definition: Putting in a nonbiological appliance that monitors, assists, performs, or prevents a physiological function but does not physically take the place of a body part

Explanation: None

Body Part Character 4	Approach Character 5	Device Character 6	Qualifier Character 7
Ø Internal Mammary Artery, Right Anterior intercostal artery Internal thoracic artery Musculophrenic artery Pericardiophrenic artery Superior epigastric artery **1 Internal Mammary Artery, Left** *See Ø Internal Mammary Artery, Right* **2 Innominate Artery** Brachiocephalic artery Brachiocephalic trunk **3 Subclavian Artery, Right** Costocervical trunk Dorsal scapular artery Internal thoracic artery **4 Subclavian Artery, Left** *See 3 Subclavian Artery, Right* **5 Axillary Artery, Right** Anterior circumflex humeral artery Lateral thoracic artery Posterior circumflex humeral artery Subscapular artery Superior thoracic artery Thoracoacromial artery **6 Axillary Artery, Left** *See 5 Axillary Artery, Right* **7 Brachial Artery, Right** Inferior ulnar collateral artery Profunda brachii Superior ulnar collateral artery **8 Brachial Artery, Left** *See 7 Brachial Artery, Right* **9 Ulnar Artery, Right** Anterior ulnar recurrent artery Common interosseous artery Posterior ulnar recurrent artery **A Ulnar Artery, Left** *See 9 Ulnar Artery, Right* **B Radial Artery, Right** Radial recurrent artery **C Radial Artery, Left** *See B Radial Artery, Right* **D Hand Artery, Right** Deep palmar arch Princeps pollicis artery Radialis indicis Superficial palmar arch **F Hand Artery, Left** *See D Hand Artery, Right* **G Intracranial Artery** Anterior cerebral artery Anterior choroidal artery Anterior communicating artery Basilar artery Circle of Willis Internal carotid artery, intracranial portion Middle cerebral artery Middle meningeal artery, intracranial portion Ophthalmic artery Posterior cerebral artery Posterior communicating artery Posterior inferior cerebellar artery (PICA) Vertebral artery, intracranial portion **H Common Carotid Artery, Right** **J Common Carotid Artery, Left** **M External Carotid Artery, Right** Ascending pharyngeal artery Internal maxillary artery Lingual artery Maxillary artery Occipital artery Posterior auricular artery Superior thyroid artery **N External Carotid Artery, Left** *See M External Carotid Artery, Right* **P Vertebral Artery, Right** Anterior spinal artery Posterior spinal artery **Q Vertebral Artery, Left** *See P Vertebral Artery, Right* **R Face Artery** Angular artery Ascending palatine artery External maxillary artery Facial artery Inferior labial artery Submental artery Superior labial artery **S Temporal Artery, Right** Middle temporal artery Superficial temporal artery Transverse facial artery **T Temporal Artery, Left** *See S Temporal Artery, Right* **U Thyroid Artery, Right** Cricothyroid artery Hyoid artery Sternocleidomastoid artery Superior laryngeal artery Superior thyroid artery Thyrocervical trunk **V Thyroid Artery, Left** *See U Thyroid Artery, Right*	**Ø Open** **3 Percutaneous** **4 Percutaneous Endoscopic**	**3 Infusion Device** **D Intraluminal Device**	**Z No Qualifier**

Non-OR Ø3H[Ø,1,2,3,4,5,6,7,8,9,A,B,C,D,F,G,H,J,M,N,P,Q,R,S,T,U,V][Ø,3,4]3Z

Ø3H Continued on next page

Ø3H Continued

Ø Medical and Surgical
3 Upper Arteries
H Insertion

Definition: Putting in a nonbiological appliance that monitors, assists, performs, or prevents a physiological function but does not physically take the place of a body part

Explanation: None

Body Part Character 4	Approach Character 5	Device Character 6	Qualifier Character 7
K Internal Carotid Artery, Right Caroticotympanic artery Carotid sinus **L Internal Carotid Artery, Left** *See K Internal Carotid Artery, Right*	**Ø** Open **3** Percutaneous **4** Percutaneous Endoscope	**3** Infusion Device **D** Intraluminal Device **M** Stimulator Lead	**Z** No Qualifier
Y Upper Artery Aortic intercostal artery Bronchial artery Esophageal artery Subcostal artery	**Ø** Open **3** Percutaneous **4** Percutaneous Endoscopic	**2** Monitoring Device **3** Infusion Device **D** Intraluminal Device **Y** Other Device	**Z** No Qualifier

Non-OR Ø3H[K,L][Ø,3,4]3Z
Non-OR Ø3HY[Ø,3,4]3Z
Non-OR Ø3HY32Z
Non-OR Ø3HY[3,4]YZ

Ø Medical and Surgical
3 Upper Arteries
J Inspection

Definition: Visually and/or manually exploring a body part

Explanation: Visual exploration may be performed with or without optical instrumentation. Manual exploration may be performed directly or through intervening body layers.

Body Part Character 4	Approach Character 5	Device Character 6	Qualifier Character 7
Y Upper Artery Aortic intercostal artery Bronchial artery Esophageal artery Subcostal artery	**Ø** Open **3** Percutaneous **4** Percutaneous Endoscopic **X** External	**Z** No Device	**Z** No Qualifier

Non-OR Ø3JY[3,4,X]ZZ

Ø Medical and Surgical
3 Upper Arteries
L Occlusion

Definition: Completely closing an orifice or the lumen of a tubular body part
Explanation: The orifice can be a natural orifice or an artificially created orifice

Body Part Character 4	Approach Character 5	Device Character 6	Qualifier Character 7
Ø Internal Mammary Artery, Right Anterior intercostal artery Internal thoracic artery Musculophrenic artery Pericardiophrenic artery Superior epigastric artery **1 Internal Mammary Artery, Left** *See Ø Internal Mammary Artery, Left* **2 Innominate Artery** Brachiocephalic artery Brachiocephalic trunk **3 Subclavian Artery, Right** Costocervical trunk Dorsal scapular artery Internal thoracic artery **4 Subclavian Artery, Left** *See 3 Subclavian Artery, Right* **5 Axillary Artery, Right** Anterior circumflex humeral artery Lateral thoracic artery Posterior circumflex humeral artery Subscapular artery Superior thoracic artery Thoracoacromial artery **6 Axillary Artery, Left** *See 5 Axillary Artery, Right* **7 Brachial Artery, Right** Inferior ulnar collateral artery Profunda brachii Superior ulnar collateral artery **8 Brachial Artery, Left** *See 7 Brachial Artery, Right* **9 Ulnar Artery, Right** Anterior ulnar recurrent artery Common interosseous artery Posterior ulnar recurrent artery **A Ulnar Artery, Left** *See 9 Ulnar Artery, Right* **B Radial Artery, Right** Radial recurrent artery **C Radial Artery, Left** *See B Radial Artery, Right* **D Hand Artery, Right** Deep palmar arch Princeps pollicis artery Radialis indicis Superficial palmar arch **F Hand Artery, Left** *See D Hand Artery, Right* **R Face Artery** Angular artery Ascending palatine artery External maxillary artery Facial artery Inferior labial artery Submental artery Superior labial artery **S Temporal Artery, Right** Middle temporal artery Superficial temporal artery Transverse facial artery **T Temporal Artery, Left** *See S Temporal Artery, Right* **U Thyroid Artery, Right** Cricothyroid artery Hyoid artery Sternocleidomastoid artery Superior laryngeal artery Superior thyroid artery Thyrocervical trunk **V Thyroid Artery, Left** *See U Thyroid Artery, Right* **Y Upper Artery** Aortic intercostal artery Bronchial artery Esophageal artery Subcostal artery	**Ø** Open **3** Percutaneous **4** Percutaneous Endoscopic	**C** Extraluminal Device **D** Intraluminal Device **Z** No Device	**Z** No Qualifier
G Intracranial Artery Anterior cerebral artery Anterior choroidal artery Anterior communicating artery Basilar artery Circle of Willis Internal carotid artery, intracranial portion Middle cerebral artery Middle meningeal artery, intracranial portion Ophthalmic artery Posterior cerebral artery Posterior communicating artery Posterior inferior cerebellar artery (PICA) Vertebral artery, intracranial portion **H Common Carotid Artery, Right** **J Common Carotid Artery, Left** **K Internal Carotid Artery, Right** Caroticotympanic artery Carotid sinus **L Internal Carotid Artery, Left** *See K Internal Carotid Artery, Right* **M External Carotid Artery, Right** Ascending pharyngeal artery Internal maxillary artery Lingual artery Maxillary artery Occipital artery Posterior auricular artery Superior thyroid artery **N External Carotid Artery, Left** *See M External Carotid Artery, Right* **P Vertebral Artery, Right** Anterior spinal artery Posterior spinal artery **Q Vertebral Artery, Left** *See P Vertebral Artery, Right*	**Ø** Open **3** Percutaneous **4** Percutaneous Endoscopic	**B** Intraluminal Device, Bioactive **C** Extraluminal Device **D** Intraluminal Device **Z** No Device	**Z** No Qualifier

Ø Medical and Surgical
3 Upper Arteries
N Release

Definition: Freeing a body part from an abnormal physical constraint by cutting or by the use of force
Explanation: Some of the restraining tissue may be taken out but none of the body part is taken out

Body Part Character 4	Approach Character 5	Device Character 6	Qualifier Character 7
Ø Internal Mammary Artery, Right Anterior intercostal artery Internal thoracic artery Musculophrenic artery Pericardiophrenic artery Superior epigastric artery **1 Internal Mammary Artery, Left** *See Ø Internal Mammary Artery, Right* **2 Innominate Artery** Brachiocephalic artery Brachiocephalic trunk **3 Subclavian Artery, Right** Costocervical trunk Dorsal scapular artery Internal thoracic artery **4 Subclavian Artery, Left** *See 3 Subclavian Artery, Right* **5 Axillary Artery, Right** Anterior circumflex humeral artery Lateral thoracic artery Posterior circumflex humeral artery Subscapular artery Superior thoracic artery Thoracoacromial artery **6 Axillary Artery, Left** *See 5 Axillary Artery, Right* **7 Brachial Artery, Right** Inferior ulnar collateral artery Profunda brachii Superior ulnar collateral artery **8 Brachial Artery, Left** *See 7 Brachial Artery, Right* **9 Ulnar Artery, Right** Anterior ulnar recurrent artery Common interosseous artery Posterior ulnar recurrent artery **A Ulnar Artery, Left** *See 9 Ulnar Artery, Right* **B Radial Artery, Right** Radial recurrent artery **C Radial Artery, Left** *See B Radial Artery, Right* **D Hand Artery, Right** Deep palmar arch Princeps pollicis artery Radialis indicis Superficial palmar arch **F Hand Artery, Left** *See D Hand Artery, Right* **G Intracranial Artery** Anterior cerebral artery Anterior choroidal artery Anterior communicating artery Basilar artery Circle of Willis Internal carotid artery, intracranial portion Middle cerebral artery Middle meningeal artery, intracranial portion Ophthalmic artery Posterior cerebral artery Posterior communicating artery Posterior inferior cerebellar artery (PICA) Vertebral artery, intracranial portion **H Common Carotid Artery, Right** **J Common Carotid Artery, Left** **K Internal Carotid Artery, Right** Caroticotympanic artery Carotid sinus **L Internal Carotid Artery, Left** *See K Internal Carotid Artery, Right* **M External Carotid Artery, Right** Ascending pharyngeal artery Internal maxillary artery Lingual artery Maxillary artery Occipital artery Posterior auricular artery Superior thyroid artery **N External Carotid Artery, Left** *See M External Carotid Artery, Right* **P Vertebral Artery, Right** Anterior spinal artery Posterior spinal artery **Q Vertebral Artery, Left** *See P Vertebral Artery, Right* **R Face Artery** Angular artery Ascending palatine artery External maxillary artery Facial artery Inferior labial artery Submental artery Superior labial artery **S Temporal Artery, Right** Middle temporal artery Superficial temporal artery Transverse facial artery **T Temporal Artery, Left** *See S Temporal Artery, Right* **U Thyroid Artery, Right** Cricothyroid artery Hyoid artery Sternocleidomastoid artery Superior laryngeal artery Superior thyroid artery Thyrocervical trunk **V Thyroid Artery, Left** *See U Thyroid Artery, Right* **Y Upper Artery** Aortic intercostal artery Bronchial artery Esophageal artery Subcostal artery	**Ø Open** **3 Percutaneous** **4 Percutaneous Endoscopic**	**Z No Device**	**Z No Qualifier**

Ø Medical and Surgical
3 Upper Arteries
P Removal

Definition: Taking out or off a device from a body part

Explanation: If a device is taken out and a similar device put in without cutting or puncturing the skin or mucous membrane, the procedure is coded to the root operation CHANGE. Otherwise, the procedure for taking out a device is coded to the root operation REMOVAL.

Body Part Character 4	Approach Character 5	Device Character 6	Qualifier Character 7
Y Upper Artery Aortic intercostal artery Bronchial artery Esophageal artery Subcostal artery	**Ø Open** **3 Percutaneous** **4 Percutaneous Endoscopic**	**Ø Drainage Device** **2 Monitoring Device** **3 Infusion Device** **7 Autologous Tissue Substitute** **C Extraluminal Device** **D Intraluminal Device** **J Synthetic Substitute** **K Nonautologous Tissue Substitute** **M Stimulator Lead** **Y Other Device**	**Z No Qualifier**
Y Upper Artery Aortic intercostal artery Bronchial artery Esophageal artery Subcostal artery	**X External**	**Ø Drainage Device** **2 Monitoring Device** **3 Infusion Device** **D Intraluminal Device** **M Stimulator Lead**	**Z No Qualifier**

Non-OR Ø3PY3[Ø,2,3,D]Z
Non-OR Ø3PY[3,4]YZ
Non-OR Ø3PYX[Ø,2,3,D,M]Z

Ø Medical and Surgical
3 Upper Arteries
Q Repair

Definition: Restoring, to the extent possible, a body part to its normal anatomic structure and function
Explanation: Used only when the method to accomplish the repair is not one of the other root operations

Body Part Character 4	Approach Character 5	Device Character 6	Qualifier Character 7
Ø Internal Mammary Artery, Right Anterior intercostal artery Internal thoracic artery Musculophrenic artery Pericardiophrenic artery Superior epigastric artery **1 Internal Mammary Artery, Left** *See Ø Internal Mammary Artery, Right* **2 Innominate Artery** Brachiocephalic artery Brachiocephalic trunk **3 Subclavian Artery, Right** Costocervical trunk Dorsal scapular artery Internal thoracic artery **4 Subclavian Artery, Left** *See 3 Subclavian Artery, Right* **5 Axillary Artery, Right** Anterior circumflex humeral artery Lateral thoracic artery Posterior circumflex humeral artery Subscapular artery Superior thoracic artery Thoracoacromial artery **6 Axillary Artery, Left** *See 5 Axillary Artery, Right* **7 Brachial Artery, Right** Inferior ulnar collateral artery Profunda brachii Superior ulnar collateral artery **8 Brachial Artery, Left** *See 7 Brachial Artery, Right* **9 Ulnar Artery, Right** Anterior ulnar recurrent artery Common interosseous artery Posterior ulnar recurrent artery **A Ulnar Artery, Left** *See 9 Ulnar Artery, Right* **B Radial Artery, Right** Radial recurrent artery **C Radial Artery, Left** *See B Radial Artery, Right* **D Hand Artery, Right** Deep palmar arch Princeps pollicis artery Radialis indicis Superficial palmar arch **F Hand Artery, Left** *See D Hand Artery, Right* **G Intracranial Artery** Anterior cerebral artery Anterior choroidal artery Anterior communicating artery Basilar artery Circle of Willis Internal carotid artery, intracranial portion Middle cerebral artery Middle meningeal artery, intracranial portion Ophthalmic artery Posterior cerebral artery Posterior communicating artery Posterior inferior cerebellar artery (PICA) Vertebral artery, intracranial portion **H Common Carotid Artery, Right** **J Common Carotid Artery, Left** **K Internal Carotid Artery, Right** Caroticotympanic artery Carotid sinus **L Internal Carotid Artery, Left** *See K Internal Carotid Artery, Right* **M External Carotid Artery, Right** Ascending pharyngeal artery Internal maxillary artery Lingual artery Maxillary artery Occipital artery Posterior auricular artery Superior thyroid artery **N External Carotid Artery, Left** *See M External Carotid Artery, Right* **P Vertebral Artery, Right** Anterior spinal artery Posterior spinal artery **Q Vertebral Artery, Left** *See P Vertebral Artery, Right* **R Face Artery** Angular artery Ascending palatine artery External maxillary artery Facial artery Inferior labial artery Submental artery Superior labial artery **S Temporal Artery, Right** Middle temporal artery Superficial temporal artery Transverse facial artery **T Temporal Artery, Left** *See S Temporal Artery, Right* **U Thyroid Artery, Right** Cricothyroid artery Hyoid artery Sternocleidomastoid artery Superior laryngeal artery Superior thyroid artery Thyrocervical trunk **V Thyroid Artery, Left** *See U Thyroid Artery, Right* **Y Upper Artery** Aortic intercostal artery Bronchial artery Esophageal artery Subcostal artery	**Ø Open** **3 Percutaneous** **4 Percutaneous Endoscopic**	**Z No Device**	**Z No Qualifier**

Ø Medical and Surgical
3 Upper Arteries
R Replacement

Definition: Putting in or on biological or synthetic material that physically takes the place and/or function of all or a portion of a body part

Explanation: The body part may have been taken out or replaced, or may be taken out, physically eradicated, or rendered nonfunctional during the REPLACEMENT procedure. A REMOVAL procedure is coded for taking out the device used in a previous replacement procedure.

Body Part Character 4	Approach Character 5	Device Character 6	Qualifier Character 7
Ø Internal Mammary Artery, Right Anterior intercostal artery Internal thoracic artery Musculophrenic artery Pericardiophrenic artery Superior epigastric artery **1 Internal Mammary Artery, Left** **See** *Ø Internal Mammary Artery, Right* **2 Innominate Artery** Brachiocephalic artery Brachiocephalic trunk **3 Subclavian Artery, Right** Costocervical trunk Dorsal scapular artery Internal thoracic artery **4 Subclavian Artery, Left** **See** *3 Subclavian Artery, Right* **5 Axillary Artery, Right** Anterior circumflex humeral artery Lateral thoracic artery Posterior circumflex humeral artery Subscapular artery Superior thoracic artery Thoracoacromial artery **6 Axillary Artery, Left** **See** *5 Axillary Artery, Right* **7 Brachial Artery, Right** Inferior ulnar collateral artery Profunda brachii Superior ulnar collateral artery **8 Brachial Artery, Left** **See** *7 Brachial Artery, Right* **9 Ulnar Artery, Right** Anterior ulnar recurrent artery Common interosseous artery Posterior ulnar recurrent artery **A Ulnar Artery, Left** **See** *9 Ulnar Artery, Right* **B Radial Artery, Right** Radial recurrent artery **C Radial Artery, Left** **See** *B Radial Artery, Right* **D Hand Artery, Right** Deep palmar arch Princeps pollicis artery Radialis indicis Superficial palmar arch **F Hand Artery, Left** **See** *D Hand Artery, Right* **G Intracranial Artery** Anterior cerebral artery Anterior choroidal artery Anterior communicating artery Basilar artery Circle of Willis Internal carotid artery, intracranial portion Middle cerebral artery Middle meningeal artery, intracranial portion Ophthalmic artery Posterior cerebral artery Posterior communicating artery Posterior inferior cerebellar artery (PICA) Vertebral artery, intracranial portion **H Common Carotid Artery, Right** **J Common Carotid Artery, Left** **K Internal Carotid Artery, Right** Caroticotympanic artery Carotid sinus **L Internal Carotid Artery, Left** **See** *K Internal Carotid Artery, Right* **M External Carotid Artery, Right** Ascending pharyngeal artery Internal maxillary artery Lingual artery Maxillary artery Occipital artery Posterior auricular artery Superior thyroid artery **N External Carotid Artery, Left** **See** *M External Carotid Artery, Right* **P Vertebral Artery, Right** Anterior spinal artery Posterior spinal artery **Q Vertebral Artery, Left** **See** *P Vertebral Artery, Right* **R Face Artery** Angular artery Ascending palatine artery External maxillary artery Facial artery Inferior labial artery Submental artery Superior labial artery **S Temporal Artery, Right** Middle temporal artery Superficial temporal artery Transverse facial artery **T Temporal Artery, Left** **See** *S Temporal Artery, Right* **U Thyroid Artery, Right** Cricothyroid artery Hyoid artery Sternocleidomastoid artery Superior laryngeal artery Superior thyroid artery Thyrocervical trunk **V Thyroid Artery, Left** **See** *U Thyroid Artery, Right* **Y Upper Artery** Aortic intercostal artery Bronchial artery Esophageal artery Subcostal artery	**Ø Open** **4 Percutaneous Endoscopic**	**7 Autologous Tissue Substitute** **J Synthetic Substitute** **K Nonautologous Tissue Substitute**	**Z No Qualifier**

Ø Medical and Surgical
3 Upper Arteries
S Reposition Definition: Moving to its normal location, or other suitable location, all or a portion of a body part

Explanation: The body part is moved to a new location from an abnormal location, or from a normal location where it is not functioning correctly. The body part may or may not be cut out or off to be moved to the new location.

Body Part Character 4	Approach Character 5	Device Character 6	Qualifier Character 7
Ø Internal Mammary Artery, Right Anterior intercostal artery Internal thoracic artery Musculophrenic artery Pericardiophrenic artery Superior epigastric artery **1 Internal Mammary Artery, Left** *See Ø Internal Mammary Artery, Right* **2 Innominate Artery** Brachiocephalic artery Brachiocephalic trunk **3 Subclavian Artery, Right** Costocervical trunk Dorsal scapular artery Internal thoracic artery **4 Subclavian Artery, Left** *See 3 Subclavian Artery, Right* **5 Axillary Artery, Right** Anterior circumflex humeral artery Lateral thoracic artery Posterior circumflex humeral artery Subscapular artery Superior thoracic artery Thoracoacromial artery **6 Axillary Artery, Left** *See 5 Axillary Artery, Right* **7 Brachial Artery, Right** Inferior ulnar collateral artery Profunda brachii Superior ulnar collateral artery **8 Brachial Artery, Left** *See 7 Brachial Artery, Right* **9 Ulnar Artery, Right** Anterior ulnar recurrent artery Common interosseous artery Posterior ulnar recurrent artery **A Ulnar Artery, Left** *See 9 Ulnar Artery, Right* **B Radial Artery, Right** Radial recurrent artery **C Radial Artery, Left** *See B Radial Artery, Right* **D Hand Artery, Right** Deep palmar arch Princeps pollicis artery Radialis indicis Superficial palmar arch **F Hand Artery, Left** *See D Hand Artery, Right* **G Intracranial Artery** Anterior cerebral artery Anterior choroidal artery Anterior communicating artery Basilar artery Circle of Willis Internal carotid artery, intracranial portion Middle cerebral artery Middle meningeal artery, intracranial portion Ophthalmic artery Posterior cerebral artery Posterior communicating artery Posterior inferior cerebellar artery (PICA) Vertebral artery, intracranial portion **H Common Carotid Artery, Right** **J Common Carotid Artery, Left** **K Internal Carotid Artery, Right** Caroticotympanic artery Carotid sinus **L Internal Carotid Artery, Left** *See K Internal Carotid Artery, Right* **M External Carotid Artery, Right** Ascending pharyngeal artery Internal maxillary artery Lingual artery Maxillary artery Occipital artery Posterior auricular artery Superior thyroid artery **N External Carotid Artery, Left** *See M External Carotid Artery, Right* **P Vertebral Artery, Right** Anterior spinal artery Posterior spinal artery **Q Vertebral Artery, Left** *See P Vertebral Artery, Right* **R Face Artery** Angular artery Ascending palatine artery External maxillary artery Facial artery Inferior labial artery Submental artery Superior labial artery **S Temporal Artery, Right** Middle temporal artery Superficial temporal artery Transverse facial artery **T Temporal Artery, Left** *See S Temporal Artery, Right* **U Thyroid Artery, Right** Cricothyroid artery Hyoid artery Sternocleidomastoid artery Superior laryngeal artery Superior thyroid artery Thyrocervical trunk **V Thyroid Artery, Left** *See U Thyroid Artery, Right* **Y Upper Artery** Aortic intercostal artery Bronchial artery Esophageal artery Subcostal artery	**Ø Open** **3 Percutaneous** **4 Percutaneous Endoscopic**	**Z No Device**	**Z No Qualifier**

Ø Medical and Surgical
3 Upper Arteries
U Supplement

Definition: Putting in or on biological or synthetic material that physically reinforces and/or augments the function of a portion of a body part

Explanation: The biological material is non-living, or is living and from the same individual. The body part may have been previously replaced, and the SUPPLEMENT procedure is performed to physically reinforce and/or augment the function of the replaced body part.

Body Part Character 4	Approach Character 5	Device Character 6	Qualifier Character 7
Ø Internal Mammary Artery, Right Anterior intercostal artery Internal thoracic artery Musculophrenic artery Pericardiophrenic artery Superior epigastric artery **1 Internal Mammary Artery, Left** ***See*** *Ø Internal Mammary Artery, Right* **2 Innominate Artery** Brachiocephalic artery Brachiocephalic trunk **3 Subclavian Artery, Right** Costocervical trunk Dorsal scapular artery Internal thoracic artery **4 Subclavian Artery, Left** ***See*** *3 Subclavian Artery, Right* **5 Axillary Artery, Right** Anterior circumflex humeral artery Lateral thoracic artery Posterior circumflex humeral artery Subscapular artery Superior thoracic artery Thoracoacromial artery **6 Axillary Artery, Left** ***See*** *5 Axillary Artery, Right* **7 Brachial Artery, Right** Inferior ulnar collateral artery Profunda brachii Superior ulnar collateral artery **8 Brachial Artery, Left** ***See*** *7 Brachial Artery, Right* **9 Ulnar Artery, Right** Anterior ulnar recurrent artery Common interosseous artery Posterior ulnar recurrent artery **A Ulnar Artery, Left** ***See*** *9 Ulnar Artery, Right* **B Radial Artery, Right** Radial recurrent artery **C Radial Artery, Left** ***See*** *B Radial Artery, Right* **D Hand Artery, Right** Deep palmar arch Princeps pollicis artery Radialis indicis Superficial palmar arch **F Hand Artery, Left** ***See*** *D Hand Artery, Right* **G Intracranial Artery** Anterior cerebral artery Anterior choroidal artery Anterior communicating artery Basilar artery Circle of Willis Internal carotid artery, intracranial portion Middle cerebral artery Middle meningeal artery, intracranial portion Ophthalmic artery Posterior cerebral artery Posterior communicating artery Posterior inferior cerebellar artery (PICA) Vertebral artery, intracranial portion **H Common Carotid Artery, Right** **J Common Carotid Artery, Left** **K Internal Carotid Artery, Right** Caroticotympanic artery Carotid sinus **L Internal Carotid Artery, Left** ***See*** *K Internal Carotid Artery, Right* **M External Carotid Artery, Right** Ascending pharyngeal artery Internal maxillary artery Lingual artery Maxillary artery Occipital artery Posterior auricular artery Superior thyroid artery **N External Carotid Artery, Left** ***See*** *M External Carotid Artery, Right* **P Vertebral Artery, Right** Anterior spinal artery Posterior spinal artery **Q Vertebral Artery, Left** ***See*** *P Vertebral Artery, Right* **R Face Artery** Angular artery Ascending palatine artery External maxillary artery Facial artery Inferior labial artery Submental artery Superior labial artery **S Temporal Artery, Right** Middle temporal artery Superficial temporal artery Transverse facial artery **T Temporal Artery, Left** ***See*** *S Temporal Artery, Right* **U Thyroid Artery, Right** Cricothyroid artery Hyoid artery Sternocleidomastoid artery Superior laryngeal artery Superior thyroid artery Thyrocervical trunk **V Thyroid Artery, Left** ***See*** *U Thyroid Artery, Right* **Y Upper Artery** Aortic intercostal artery Bronchial artery Esophageal artery Subcostal artery	Ø Open 3 Percutaneous 4 Percutaneous Endoscopic	7 Autologous Tissue Substitute J Synthetic Substitute K Nonautologous Tissue Substitute	Z No Qualifier

Ø Medical and Surgical
3 Upper Arteries
V Restriction Definition: Partially closing an orifice or the lumen of a tubular body part
Explanation: The orifice can be a natural orifice or an artificially created orifice

Body Part Character 4		Approach Character 5	Device Character 6	Qualifier Character 7
Ø Internal Mammary Artery, Right Anterior intercostal artery Internal thoracic artery Musculophrenic artery Pericardiophrenic artery Superior epigastric artery **1 Internal Mammary Artery, Left** *See Ø Internal Mammary Artery, Right* **2 Innominate Artery** Brachiocephalic artery Brachiocephalic trunk **3 Subclavian Artery, Right** Costocervical trunk Dorsal scapular artery Internal thoracic artery **4 Subclavian Artery, Left** *See 3 Subclavian Artery, Right* **5 Axillary Artery, Right** Anterior circumflex humeral artery Lateral thoracic artery Posterior circumflex humeral artery Subscapular artery Superior thoracic artery Thoracoacromial artery **6 Axillary Artery, Left** *See 5 Axillary Artery, Right* **7 Brachial Artery, Right** Inferior ulnar collateral artery Profunda brachii Superior ulnar collateral artery **8 Brachial Artery, Left** *See 7 Brachial Artery, Right* **9 Ulnar Artery, Right** Anterior ulnar recurrent artery Common interosseous artery Posterior ulnar recurrent artery **A Ulnar Artery, Left** *See 9 Ulnar Artery, Right*	**B Radial Artery, Right** Radial recurrent artery **C Radial Artery, Left** *See B Radial Artery, Right* **D Hand Artery, Right** Deep palmar arch Princeps pollicis artery Radialis indicis Superficial palmar arch **F Hand Artery, Left** *See D Hand Artery, Right* **R Face Artery** Angular artery Ascending palatine artery External maxillary artery Facial artery Inferior labial artery Submental artery Superior labial artery **S Temporal Artery, Right** Middle temporal artery Superficial temporal artery Transverse facial artery **T Temporal Artery, Left** *See S Temporal Artery, Right* **U Thyroid Artery, Right** Cricothyroid artery Hyoid artery Sternocleidomastoid artery Superior laryngeal artery Superior thyroid artery Thyrocervical trunk **V Thyroid Artery, Left** *See U Thyroid Artery, Right* **Y Upper Artery** Aortic intercostal artery Bronchial artery Esophageal artery Subcostal artery	**Ø Open** **3 Percutaneous** **4 Percutaneous Endoscopic**	**C Extraluminal Device** **D Intraluminal Device** **Z No Device**	**Z No Qualifier**
G Intracranial Artery Anterior cerebral artery Anterior choroidal artery Anterior communicating artery Basilar artery Circle of Willis Internal carotid artery, intracranial portion Middle cerebral artery Middle meningeal artery, intracranial portion Ophthalmic artery Posterior cerebral artery Posterior communicating artery Posterior inferior cerebellar artery (PICA) Vertebral artery, intracranial portion **H Common Carotid Artery, Right** **J Common Carotid Artery, Left** **K Internal Carotid Artery, Right** Caroticotympanic artery Carotid sinus	**L Internal Carotid Artery, Left** *See K Internal Carotid Artery, Right* **M External Carotid Artery, Right** Ascending pharyngeal artery Internal maxillary artery Lingual artery Maxillary artery Occipital artery Posterior auricular artery Superior thyroid artery **N External Carotid Artery, Left** *See M External Carotid Artery, Right* **P Vertebral Artery, Right** Anterior spinal artery Posterior spinal artery **Q Vertebral Artery, Left** *See P Vertebral Artery, Right*	**Ø Open** **3 Percutaneous** **4 Percutaneous Endoscopic**	**B Intraluminal Device, Bioactive** **C Extraluminal Device** **D Intraluminal Device** **H Intraluminal Device, Flow Diverter** **Z No Device**	**Z No Qualifier**

Ø Medical and Surgical
3 Upper Arteries
W Revision

Definition: Correcting, to the extent possible, a portion of a malfunctioning device or the position of a displaced device

Explanation: Revision can include correcting a malfunctioning or displaced device by taking out or putting in components of the device such as a screw or pin

Body Part Character 4	Approach Character 5	Device Character 6	Qualifier Character 7
Y Upper Artery Aortic intercostal artery Bronchial artery Esophageal artery Subcostal artery	Ø Open 3 Percutaneous 4 Percutaneous Endoscopic	Ø Drainage Device 2 Monitoring Device 3 Infusion Device 7 Autologous Tissue Substitute C Extraluminal Device D Intraluminal Device J Synthetic Substitute K Nonautologous Tissue Substitute M Stimulator Lead Y Other Device	Z No Qualifier
Y Upper Artery Aortic intercostal artery Bronchial artery Esophageal artery Subcostal artery	X External	Ø Drainage Device 2 Monitoring Device 3 Infusion Device 7 Autologous Tissue Substitute C Extraluminal Device D Intraluminal Device J Synthetic Substitute K Nonautologous Tissue Substitute M Stimulator Lead	Z No Qualifier

Non-OR Ø3WY3[Ø,2,3]Z
Non-OR Ø3WY[3,4]YZ
Non-OR Ø3WYX[Ø,2,3,7,C,D,J,K,M]Z

Lower Arteries Ø41–Ø4W

Character Meanings

This Character Meaning table is provided as a guide to assist the user in the identification of character members that may be found in this section of code tables. It **SHOULD NOT** be used to build a PCS code.

Operation–Character 3	Body Part–Character 4	Approach–Character 5	Device–Character 6	Qualifier–Character 7
1 Bypass	Ø Abdominal Aorta	Ø Open	Ø Drainage Device	Ø Abdominal Aorta OR Ultrasonic
5 Destruction	1 Celiac Artery	3 Percutaneous	1 Radioactive Element	1 Celiac Artery OR Drug-Coated Balloon
7 Dilation	2 Gastric Artery	4 Percutaneous Endoscopic	2 Monitoring Device	2 Mesenteric Artery
9 Drainage	3 Hepatic Artery	X External	3 Infusion Device	3 Renal Artery, Right
B Excision	4 Splenic Artery		4 Intraluminal Device, Drug-eluting	4 Renal Artery, Left
C Extirpation	5 Superior Mesenteric Artery		5 Intraluminal Device, Drug-eluting, Two	5 Renal Artery, Bilateral
F Fragmentation	6 Colic Artery, Right		6 Intraluminal Device, Drug-eluting, Three	6 Common Iliac Artery, Right
H Insertion	7 Colic Artery, Left		7 Intraluminal Device, Drug-eluting, Four or More OR Autologous Tissue Substitute	7 Common Iliac Artery, Left
J Inspection	8 Colic Artery, Middle		9 Autologous Venous Tissue	8 Common Iliac Arteries, Bilateral
L Occlusion	9 Renal Artery, Right		A Autologous Arterial Tissue	9 Internal Iliac Artery, Right
N Release	A Renal Artery, Left		C Extraluminal Device	B Internal Iliac Artery, Left
P Removal	B Inferior Mesenteric Artery		D Intraluminal Device	C Internal Iliac Arteries, Bilateral
Q Repair	C Common Iliac Artery, Right		E Intraluminal Device, Two OR Intraluminal Device, Branched or Fenestrated, One or Two Arteries	D External Iliac Artery, Right
R Replacement	D Common Iliac Artery, Left		F Intraluminal Device, Three OR Intraluminal Device, Branched or Fenestrated, Three or More Arteries	F External Iliac Artery, Left
S Reposition	E Internal Iliac Artery, Right		G Intraluminal Device, Four or More	G External Iliac Arteries, Bilateral
U Supplement	F Internal Iliac Artery, Left		J Synthetic Substitute	H Femoral Artery, Right
V Restriction	H External Iliac Artery, Right		K Nonautologous Tissue Substitute	J Femoral Artery, Left OR Temporary
W Revision	J External Iliac Artery, Left		Y Other Device	K Femoral Arteries, Bilateral
	K Femoral Artery, Right		Z No Device	L Popliteal Artery
	L Femoral Artery, Left			M Peroneal Artery
	M Popliteal Artery, Right			N Posterior Tibial Artery
	N Popliteal Artery, Left			P Foot Artery
	P Anterior Tibial Artery, Right			Q Lower Extremity Artery
	Q Anterior Tibial Artery, Left			R Lower Artery
	R Posterior Tibial Artery, Right			S Lower Extremity Vein
	S Posterior Tibial Artery, Left			T Uterine Artery, Right
	T Peroneal Artery, Right			U Uterine Artery, Left
	U Peroneal Artery, Left			V Prostatic Artery, Right
	V Foot Artery, Right			W Prostatic Artery, Left
	W Foot Artery, Left			X Diagnostic
	Y Lower Artery			Z No Qualifier

AHA Coding Clinic for Lower Arteries

2022, 1Q, 10-13 Procedures performed on a continuous vessel, ICD-10-PCS Guideline B4.1c

AHA Coding Clinic for table Ø41

2022, 3Q, 5 Aortoiliac aneurysm repair
2019, 1Q, 23 Endovascular repair of shaggy aorta and deployment of chimney stent grafts
2018, 3Q, 25 Femoral artery to tibioperoneal trunk bypass
2017, 4Q, 46-47 New and revised body part values - Bypass hepatic artery to renal artery
2017, 3Q, 5 Femoral artery to posterior tibial artery bypass using autologous and synthetic grafts
2017, 3Q, 16 Abdominal aortic debranching with bypass of external iliac artery to bilateral renal arteries and superior mesenteric artery
2017, 1Q, 32 Peroneal artery to dorsalis pedis artery bypass using saphenous vein graft
2016, 2Q, 18 Femoral-tibial artery bypass and saphenous vein graft
2015, 3Q, 28 Bilateral renal artery bypass

AHA Coding Clinic for table Ø47

2020, 4Q, 50 Intravascular lithotripsy
2019, 4Q, 27 Bifurcation Qualifier
2019, 2Q, 14 Revision of occluded femoral-popliteal bypass graft
2018, 2Q, 24 Coronary artery bifurcation
2016, 4Q, 86 Peripheral artery, number of stents
2016, 4Q, 86-88 Coronary and peripheral artery bifurcation
2016, 3Q, 39 Infrarenal abdominal aortic aneurysm repair with iliac graft extension
2015, 4Q, 4-7, 15 Drug-coated balloon angioplasty in peripheral vessels
2015, 3Q, 9 Aborted endovascular stenting of superficial femoral artery

AHA Coding Clinic for table Ø4C

2021, 1Q, 15 Iliofemoral endarterectomy and furthest point of entry
2019, 4Q, 27 Bifurcation Qualifier
2019, 1Q, 23 Endovascular repair of shaggy aorta and deployment of chimney stent grafts
2018, 2Q, 24 Coronary artery bifurcation
2017, 2Q, 23 Thrombectomy via Fogarty catheter
2016, 4Q, 86-88 Coronary and peripheral artery bifurcation
2016, 1Q, 31 Iliofemoral endarterectomy with patch repair
2015, 1Q, 29 Discontinued carotid endarterectomy
2015, 1Q, 36 Percutaneous mechanical thrombectomy of femoropopliteal bypass graft

AHA Coding Clinic for table Ø4F

2020, 4Q, 45-49 New fragmentation tables
2020, 4Q, 49-50 Intravascular ultrasound assisted thrombolysis
2020, 4Q, 50-51 Intravascular lithotripsy

AHA Coding Clinic for table Ø4H

2022, 3Q, 19 Placement of stent into aorta to secure debris
2019, 3Q, 20 Removal and revision of ECMO component
2019, 1Q, 23 Endovascular repair of shaggy aorta and deployment of chimney stent grafts
2017, 1Q, 30 Insertion of umbilical artery catheter

AHA Coding Clinic for table Ø4J

2022, 4Q, 56 Embolization of prostatic artery

AHA Coding Clinic for table Ø4L

2023, 1Q, 9 Temporary balloon occlusion of aorta
2022, 4Q, 55-56 Embolization of prostatic artery
2020, 3Q, 43 Staged laparoscopic gastric conduit and placement of feeding tube
2018, 2Q, 18 Transverse rectus abdominis myocutaneous (TRAM) delay
2017, 4Q, 31 Resuscitative endovascular balloon occlusion of the aorta
2015, 2Q, 27 Uterine artery embolization using Gelfoam
2014, 3Q, 26 Coil embolization of gastroduodenal artery with chemoembolization of hepatic artery
2014, 1Q, 24 Endovascular embolization for gastrointestinal bleeding

AHA Coding Clinic for table Ø4N

2015, 2Q, 28 Release and replacement of celiac artery

AHA Coding Clinic for table Ø4P

2019, 3Q, 20 Removal and revision of ECMO component

AHA Coding Clinic for table Ø4Q

2014, 1Q, 21 Repair of femoral artery pseudoaneurysm

AHA Coding Clinic for table Ø4R

2022, 3Q, 5 Aortoiliac aneurysm repair
2019, 1Q, 22 Abdominal aortic aneurysm repair using tube graft
2015, 2Q, 28 Release and replacement of celiac artery

AHA Coding Clinic for table Ø4U

2019, 1Q, 22 Abdominal aortic aneurysm repair using tube graft
2016, 2Q, 18 Femoral-tibial artery bypass and saphenous vein graft
2016, 1Q, 31 Iliofemoral endarterectomy with patch repair
2014, 4Q, 37 Bovine patch arterioplasty
2014, 1Q, 22 Repair of pseudoaneurysm of femoral-popliteal bypass graft

AHA Coding Clinic for table Ø4V

2021, 3Q, 23 Transcatheter embolization of splenic artery
2019, 4Q, 27 Bifurcation Qualifier
2019, 1Q, 22 Abdominal aortic aneurysm repair using tube graft
2018, 2Q, 24 Coronary artery bifurcation
2016, 4Q, 86-87 Coronary and peripheral artery bifurcation
2016, 4Q, 89-93 Branched and fenestrated endograft repair of aneurysms
2016, 3Q, 39 Infrarenal abdominal aortic aneurysm repair with iliac graft extension
2014, 1Q, 9 Endovascular repair of abdominal aortic aneurysm

AHA Coding Clinic for table Ø4W

2020, 3Q, 5 Types of endoleaks following endovascular aneurysm repair
2019, 2Q, 14 Revision of occluded femoral-popliteal bypass graft
2015, 1Q, 36 Revision of femoropopliteal bypass graft
2014, 1Q, 9 Endovascular repair of endoleak
2014, 1Q, 22 Repair of pseudoaneurysm of femoral-popliteal bypass graft

Lower Arteries

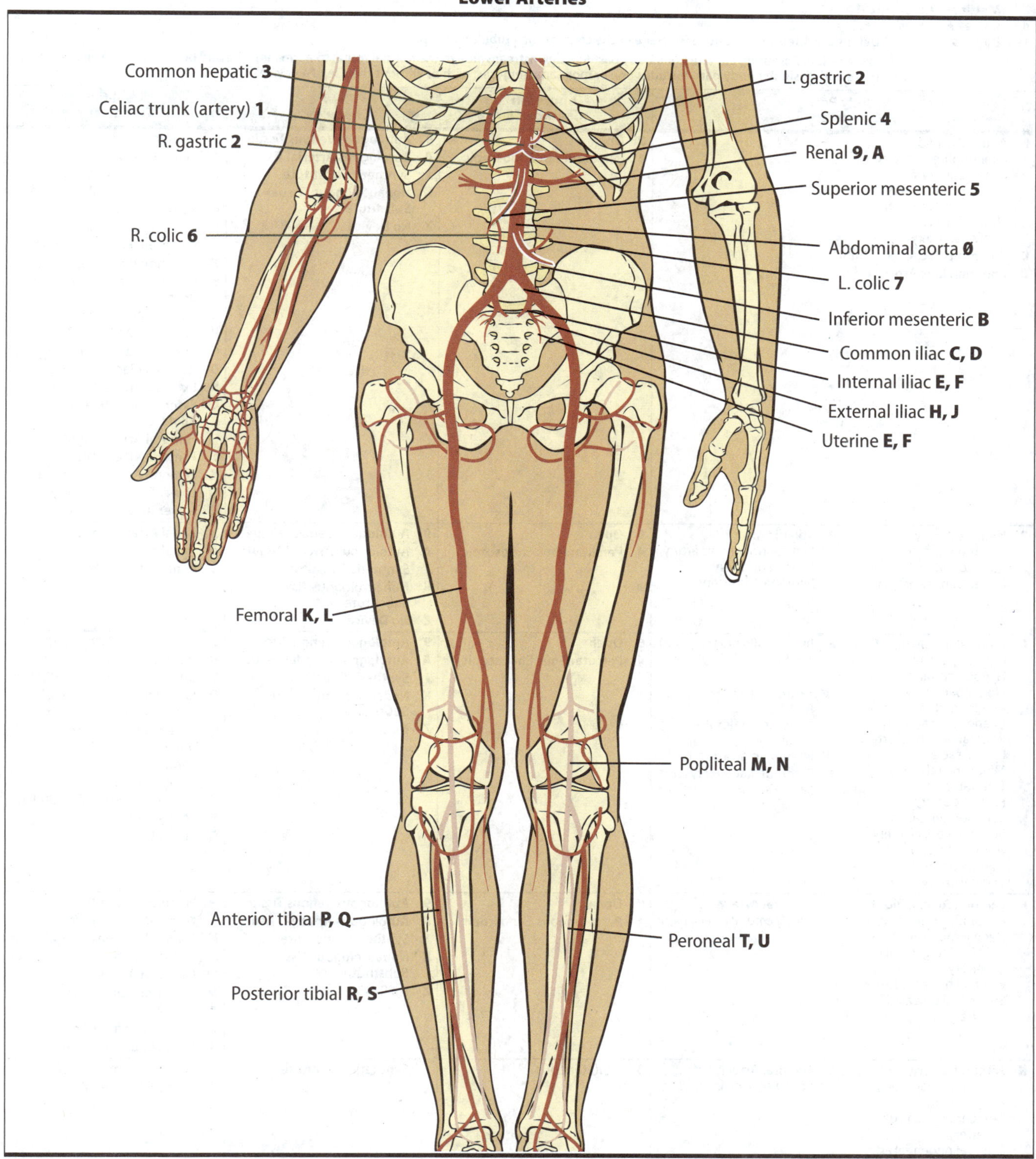

Ø Medical and Surgical
4 Lower Arteries
1 Bypass

Definition: Altering the route of passage of the contents of a tubular body part

Explanation: Rerouting contents of a body part to a downstream area of the normal route, to a similar route and body part, or to an abnormal route and dissimilar body part. Includes one or more anastomoses, with or without the use of a device.

Body Part Character 4	Approach Character 5	Device Character 6	Qualifier Character 7
Ø Abdominal Aorta Inferior phrenic artery Lumbar artery Median sacral artery Middle suprarenal artery Ovarian artery Testicular artery **C Common Iliac Artery, Right** **D Common Iliac Artery, Left**	**Ø** Open **4** Percutaneous Endoscopic	**9** Autologous Venous Tissue **A** Autologous Arterial Tissue **J** Synthetic Substitute **K** Nonautologous Tissue Substitute **Z** No Device	**Ø** Abdominal Aorta **1** Celiac Artery **2** Mesenteric Artery **3** Renal Artery, Right **4** Renal Artery, Left **5** Renal Artery, Bilateral **6** Common Iliac Artery, Right **7** Common Iliac Artery, Left **8** Common Iliac Arteries, Bilateral **9** Internal Iliac Artery, Right **B** Internal Iliac Artery, Left **C** Internal Iliac Arteries, Bilateral **D** External Iliac Artery, Right **F** External Iliac Artery, Left **G** External Iliac Arteries, Bilateral **H** Femoral Artery, Right **J** Femoral Artery, Left **K** Femoral Arteries, Bilateral **Q** Lower Extremity Artery **R** Lower Artery
3 Hepatic Artery Common hepatic artery Gastroduodenal artery Hepatic artery proper **4 Splenic Artery** Left gastroepiploic artery Pancreatic artery Short gastric artery	**Ø** Open **4** Percutaneous Endoscopic	**9** Autologous Venous Tissue **A** Autologous Arterial Tissue **J** Synthetic Substitute **K** Nonautologous Tissue Substitute **Z** No Device	**3** Renal Artery, Right **4** Renal Artery, Left **5** Renal Artery, Bilateral
E Internal Iliac Artery, Right Deferential artery Hypogastric artery Iliolumbar artery Inferior gluteal artery Inferior vesical artery Internal pudendal artery Lateral sacral artery Middle rectal artery Obturator artery Prostatic artery Superior gluteal artery Superior vesical artery Umbilical artery Uterine artery Vaginal artery **F Internal Iliac Artery, Left** *See* *E Internal Iliac Artery, Right* **H External Iliac Artery, Right** Deep circumflex iliac artery Inferior epigastric artery **J External Iliac Artery, Left** *See* *H External Iliac Artery, Right*	**Ø** Open **4** Percutaneous Endoscopic	**9** Autologous Venous Tissue **A** Autologous Arterial Tissue **J** Synthetic Substitute **K** Nonautologous Tissue Substitute **Z** No Device	**9** Internal Iliac Artery, Right **B** Internal Iliac Artery, Left **C** Internal Iliac Arteries, Bilateral **D** External Iliac Artery, Right **F** External Iliac Artery, Left **G** External Iliac Arteries, Bilateral **H** Femoral Artery, Right **J** Femoral Artery, Left **K** Femoral Arteries, Bilateral **P** Foot Artery **Q** Lower Extremity Artery
K Femoral Artery, Right Circumflex iliac artery Deep femoral artery Descending genicular artery External pudendal artery Superficial epigastric artery **L Femoral Artery, Left** *See* *K Femoral Artery, Right*	**Ø** Open **4** Percutaneous Endoscopic	**9** Autologous Venous Tissue **A** Autologous Arterial Tissue **J** Synthetic Substitute **K** Nonautologous Tissue Substitute **Z** No Device	**H** Femoral Artery, Right **J** Femoral Artery, Left **K** Femoral Arteries, Bilateral **L** Popliteal Artery **M** Peroneal Artery **N** Posterior Tibial Artery **P** Foot Artery **Q** Lower Extremity Artery **S** Lower Extremity Vein
K Femoral Artery, Right Circumflex iliac artery Deep femoral artery Descending genicular artery External pudendal artery Superficial epigastric artery **L Femoral Artery, Left** *See* *K Femoral Artery, Right*	**3** Percutaneous	**J** Synthetic Substitute	**Q** Lower Extremity Artery **S** Lower Extremity Vein
M Popliteal Artery, Right Inferior genicular artery Middle genicular artery Superior genicular artery Sural artery Tibioperoneal trunk **N Popliteal Artery, Left** *See* *M Popliteal Artery, Right*	**Ø** Open **4** Percutaneous Endoscopic	**9** Autologous Venous Tissue **A** Autologous Arterial Tissue **J** Synthetic Substitute **K** Nonautologous Tissue Substitute **Z** No Device	**L** Popliteal Artery **M** Peroneal Artery **P** Foot Artery **Q** Lower Extremity Artery **S** Lower Extremity Vein

Ø41 Continued on next page

Ø Medical and Surgical
4 Lower Arteries
1 Bypass

Ø41 Continued

Definition: Altering the route of passage of the contents of a tubular body part

Explanation: Rerouting contents of a body part to a downstream area of the normal route, to a similar route and body part, or to an abnormal route and dissimilar body part. Includes one or more anastomoses, with or without the use of a device.

Body Part Character 4		Approach Character 5	Device Character 6	Qualifier Character 7
M Popliteal Artery, Right Inferior genicular artery Middle genicular artery Superior genicular artery Sural artery Tibioperoneal trunk	**N Popliteal Artery, Left** *See M Popliteal Artery, Right*	3 Percutaneous	J Synthetic Substitute	Q Lower Extremity Artery S Lower Extremity Vein
P Anterior Tibial Artery, Right Anterior lateral malleolar artery Anterior medial malleolar artery Anterior tibial recurrent artery Dorsalis pedis artery Posterior tibial recurrent artery	**Q Anterior Tibial Artery, Left** *See P Anterior Tibial Artery, Right* **R Posterior Tibial Artery, Right** **S Posterior Tibial Artery, Left**	Ø Open 3 Percutaneous 4 Percutaneous Endoscopic	J Synthetic Substitute	Q Lower Extremity Artery S Lower Extremity Vein
T Peroneal Artery, Right Fibular artery **U Peroneal Artery, Left** *See T Peroneal Artery, Right*	**V Foot Artery, Right** Arcuate artery Dorsal metatarsal artery Lateral plantar artery Lateral tarsal artery Medial plantar artery **W Foot Artery, Left** *See V Foot Artery, Right*	Ø Open 4 Percutaneous Endoscopic	9 Autologous Venous Tissue A Autologous Arterial Tissue J Synthetic Substitute K Nonautologous Tissue Substitute Z No Device	P Foot Artery Q Lower Extremity Artery S Lower Extremity Vein
T Peroneal Artery, Right Fibular artery **U Peroneal Artery, Left** *See T Peroneal Artery, Right*	**V Foot Artery, Right** Arcuate artery Dorsal metatarsal artery Lateral plantar artery Lateral tarsal artery Medial plantar artery **W Foot Artery, Left** *See V Foot Artery, Right*	3 Percutaneous	J Synthetic Substitute	Q Lower Extremity Artery S Lower Extremity Vein

Ø Medical and Surgical
4 Lower Arteries
5 Destruction

Definition: Physical eradication of all or a portion of a body part by the direct use of energy, force, or a destructive agent

Explanation: None of the body part is physically taken out

Body Part Character 4	Approach Character 5	Device Character 6	Qualifier Character 7
Ø Abdominal Aorta Inferior phrenic artery Lumbar artery Median sacral artery Middle suprarenal artery Ovarian artery Testicular artery **1 Celiac Artery** Celiac trunk **2 Gastric Artery** Left gastric artery Right gastric artery **3 Hepatic Artery** Common hepatic artery Gastroduodenal artery Hepatic artery proper **4 Splenic Artery** Left gastroepiploic artery Pancreatic artery Short gastric artery **5 Superior Mesenteric Artery** Ileal artery Ileocolic artery Inferior pancreaticoduodenal artery Jejunal artery **6 Colic Artery, Right** **7 Colic Artery, Left** **8 Colic Artery, Middle** **9 Renal Artery, Right** Inferior suprarenal artery Renal segmental artery **A Renal Artery, Left** *See 9 Renal Artery, Right* **B Inferior Mesenteric Artery** Sigmoid artery Superior rectal artery **C Common Iliac Artery, Right** **D Common Iliac Artery, Left** **E Internal Iliac Artery, Right** Deferential artery Hypogastric artery Iliolumbar artery Inferior gluteal artery Inferior vesical artery Internal pudendal artery Lateral sacral artery Middle rectal artery Obturator artery Prostatic artery Superior gluteal artery Superior vesical artery Umbilical artery Uterine artery Vaginal artery **F Internal Iliac Artery, Left** *See E Internal Iliac Artery, Right* **H External Iliac Artery, Right** Deep circumflex iliac artery Inferior epigastric artery **J External Iliac Artery, Left** *See H External Iliac Artery, Right* **K Femoral Artery, Right** Circumflex iliac artery Deep femoral artery Descending genicular artery External pudendal artery Superficial epigastric artery **L Femoral Artery, Left** *See K Femoral Artery, Right* **M Popliteal Artery, Right** Inferior genicular artery Middle genicular artery Superior genicular artery Sural artery Tibioperoneal trunk **N Popliteal Artery, Left** *See M Popliteal Artery, Right* **P Anterior Tibial Artery, Right** Anterior lateral malleolar artery Anterior medial malleolar artery Anterior tibial recurrent artery Dorsalis pedis artery Posterior tibial recurrent artery **Q Anterior Tibial Artery, Left** *See P Anterior Tibial Artery, Right* **R Posterior Tibial Artery, Right** **S Posterior Tibial Artery, Left** **T Peroneal Artery, Right** Fibular artery **U Peroneal Artery, Left** *See T Peroneal Artery, Right* **V Foot Artery, Right** Arcuate artery Dorsal metatarsal artery Lateral plantar artery Lateral tarsal artery Medial plantar artery **W Foot Artery, Left** *See V Foot Artery, Right* **Y Lower Artery** Umbilical artery	**Ø Open** **3 Percutaneous** **4 Percutaneous Endoscopic**	**Z No Device**	**Z No Qualifier**

Ø Medical and Surgical
4 Lower Arteries
7 Dilation Definition: Expanding an orifice or the lumen of a tubular body part

Explanation: The orifice can be a natural orifice or an artificially created orifice. Accomplished by stretching a tubular body part using intraluminal pressure or by cutting part of the orifice or wall of the tubular body part.

Body Part Character 4	Approach Character 5	Device Character 6	Qualifier Character 7
Ø Abdominal Aorta Inferior phrenic artery Lumbar artery Median sacral artery Middle suprarenal artery Ovarian artery Testicular artery **1 Celiac Artery** Celiac trunk **2 Gastric Artery** Left gastric artery Right gastric artery **3 Hepatic Artery** Common hepatic artery Gastroduodenal artery Hepatic artery proper **4 Splenic Artery** Left gastroepiploic artery Pancreatic artery Short gastric artery **5 Superior Mesenteric Artery** Ileal artery Ileocolic artery Inferior pancreaticoduodenal artery Jejunal artery **6 Colic Artery, Right** **7 Colic Artery, Left** **8 Colic Artery, Middle** **9 Renal Artery, Right** Inferior suprarenal artery Renal segmental artery **A Renal Artery, Left** *See 9 Renal Artery, Right* **B Inferior Mesenteric Artery** Sigmoid artery Superior rectal artery **C Common Iliac Artery, Right** **D Common Iliac Artery, Left** **E Internal Iliac Artery, Right** Deferential artery Hypogastric artery Iliolumbar artery Inferior gluteal artery Inferior vesical artery Internal pudendal artery Lateral sacral artery Middle rectal artery Obturator artery Prostatic artery Superior gluteal artery Superior vesical artery Umbilical artery Uterine artery Vaginal artery **F Internal Iliac Artery, Left** *See E Internal Iliac Artery, Right* **H External Iliac Artery, Right** Deep circumflex iliac artery Inferior epigastric artery **J External Iliac Artery, Left** *See H External Iliac Artery, Right* **K Femoral Artery, Right** Circumflex iliac artery Deep femoral artery Descending genicular artery External pudendal artery Superficial epigastric artery **L Femoral Artery, Left** *See K Femoral Artery, Right* **M Popliteal Artery, Right** Inferior genicular artery Middle genicular artery Superior genicular artery Sural artery Tibioperoneal trunk **N Popliteal Artery, Left** *See M Popliteal Artery, Right* **P Anterior Tibial Artery, Right** Anterior lateral malleolar artery Anterior medial malleolar artery Anterior tibial recurrent artery Dorsalis pedis artery Posterior tibial recurrent artery **Q Anterior Tibial Artery, Left** *See P Anterior Tibial Artery, Right* **R Posterior Tibial Artery, Right** **S Posterior Tibial Artery, Left** **T Peroneal Artery, Right** Fibular artery **U Peroneal Artery, Left** *See T Peroneal Artery, Right* **V Foot Artery, Right** Arcuate artery Dorsal metatarsal artery Lateral plantar artery Lateral tarsal artery Medial plantar artery **W Foot Artery, Left** *See V Foot Artery, Right* **Y Lower Artery** Umbilical artery	**Ø Open** **3 Percutaneous** **4 Percutaneous Endoscopic**	**4 Intraluminal Device, Drug-eluting** **D Intraluminal Device** **Z No Device**	**1 Drug-Coated Balloon** **Z No Qualifier**

Ø47 Continued on next page

Ø47 Continued

Ø Medical and Surgical
4 Lower Arteries
7 Dilation

Definition: Expanding an orifice or the lumen of a tubular body part

Explanation: The orifice can be a natural orifice or an artificially created orifice. Accomplished by stretching a tubular body part using intraluminal pressure or by cutting part of the orifice or wall of the tubular body part.

Body Part Character 4	Approach Character 5	Device Character 6	Qualifier Character 7
Ø Abdominal Aorta Inferior phrenic artery Lumbar artery Median sacral artery Middle suprarenal artery Ovarian artery Testicular artery **1 Celiac Artery** Celiac trunk **2 Gastric Artery** Left gastric artery Right gastric artery **3 Hepatic Artery** Common hepatic artery Gastroduodenal artery Hepatic artery proper **4 Splenic Artery** Left gastroepiploic artery Pancreatic artery Short gastric artery **5 Superior Mesenteric Artery** Ileal artery Ileocolic artery Inferior pancreaticoduodenal artery Jejunal artery **6 Colic Artery, Right** **7 Colic Artery, Left** **8 Colic Artery, Middle** **9 Renal Artery, Right** Inferior suprarenal artery Renal segmental artery **A Renal Artery, Left** *See 9 Renal Artery, Right* **B Inferior Mesenteric Artery** Sigmoid artery Superior rectal artery **C Common Iliac Artery, Right** **D Common Iliac Artery, Left** **E Internal Iliac Artery, Right** Deferential artery Hypogastric artery Iliolumbar artery Inferior gluteal artery Inferior vesical artery Internal pudendal artery Lateral sacral artery Middle rectal artery Obturator artery Prostatic artery Superior gluteal artery Superior vesical artery Umbilical artery Uterine artery Vaginal artery **F Internal Iliac Artery, Left** *See E Internal Iliac Artery, Right* **H External Iliac Artery, Right** Deep circumflex iliac artery Inferior epigastric artery **J External Iliac Artery, Left** *See H External Iliac Artery, Right* **K Femoral Artery, Right** Circumflex iliac artery Deep femoral artery Descending genicular artery External pudendal artery Superficial epigastric artery **L Femoral Artery, Left** *See K Femoral Artery, Right* **M Popliteal Artery, Right** Inferior genicular artery Middle genicular artery Superior genicular artery Sural artery Tibioperoneal trunk **N Popliteal Artery, Left** *See M Popliteal Artery, Right* **P Anterior Tibial Artery, Right** Anterior lateral malleolar artery Anterior medial malleolar artery Anterior tibial recurrent artery Dorsalis pedis artery Posterior tibial recurrent artery **Q Anterior Tibial Artery, Left** *See P Anterior Tibial Artery, Right* **R Posterior Tibial Artery, Right** **S Posterior Tibial Artery, Left** **T Peroneal Artery, Right** Fibular artery **U Peroneal Artery, Left** *See T Peroneal Artery, Right* **V Foot Artery, Right** Arcuate artery Dorsal metatarsal artery Lateral plantar artery Lateral tarsal artery Medial plantar artery **W Foot Artery, Left** *See V Foot Artery, Right* **Y Lower Artery** Umbilical artery	**Ø Open** **3 Percutaneous** **4 Percutaneous Endoscopic**	**5 Intraluminal Device, Drug-eluting, Two** **6 Intraluminal Device, Drug-eluting, Three** **7 Intraluminal Device, Drug-eluting, Four or More** **E Intraluminal Device, Two** **F Intraluminal Device, Three** **G Intraluminal Device, Four or More**	**Z No Qualifier**

Ø Medical and Surgical
4 Lower Arteries
9 Drainage Definition: Taking or letting out fluids and/or gases from a body part
Explanation: The qualifier DIAGNOSTIC is used to identify drainage procedures that are biopsies

Body Part Character 4	Approach Character 5	Device Character 6	Qualifier Character 7
Ø Abdominal Aorta Inferior phrenic artery Lumbar artery Median sacral artery Middle suprarenal artery Ovarian artery Testicular artery **1 Celiac Artery** Celiac trunk **2 Gastric Artery** Left gastric artery Right gastric artery **3 Hepatic Artery** Common hepatic artery Gastroduodenal artery Hepatic artery proper **4 Splenic Artery** Left gastroepiploic artery Pancreatic artery Short gastric artery **5 Superior Mesenteric Artery** Ileal artery Ileocolic artery Inferior pancreaticoduodenal artery Jejunal artery **6 Colic Artery, Right** **7 Colic Artery, Left** **8 Colic Artery, Middle** **9 Renal Artery, Right** Inferior suprarenal artery Renal segmental artery **A Renal Artery, Left** ***See*** *9 Renal Artery, Right* **B Inferior Mesenteric Artery** Sigmoid artery Superior rectal artery **C Common Iliac Artery, Right** **D Common Iliac Artery, Left** **E Internal Iliac Artery, Right** Deferential artery Hypogastric artery Iliolumbar artery Inferior gluteal artery Inferior vesical artery Internal pudendal artery Lateral sacral artery Middle rectal artery Obturator artery Prostatic artery Superior gluteal artery Superior vesical artery Umbilical artery Uterine artery Vaginal artery **F Internal Iliac Artery, Left** ***See*** *E Internal Iliac Artery, Right* **H External Iliac Artery, Right** Deep circumflex iliac artery Inferior epigastric artery **J External Iliac Artery, Left** ***See*** *H External Iliac Artery, Right* **K Femoral Artery, Right** Circumflex iliac artery Deep femoral artery Descending genicular artery External pudendal artery Superficial epigastric artery **L Femoral Artery, Left** ***See*** *K Femoral Artery, Right* **M Popliteal Artery, Right** Inferior genicular artery Middle genicular artery Superior genicular artery Sural artery Tibioperoneal trunk **N Popliteal Artery, Left** ***See*** *M Popliteal Artery, Right* **P Anterior Tibial Artery, Right** Anterior lateral malleolar artery Anterior medial malleolar artery Anterior tibial recurrent artery Dorsalis pedis artery Posterior tibial recurrent artery **Q Anterior Tibial Artery, Left** ***See*** *P Anterior Tibial Artery, Right* **R Posterior Tibial Artery, Right** **S Posterior Tibial Artery, Left** **T Peroneal Artery, Right** Fibular artery **U Peroneal Artery, Left** ***See*** *T Peroneal Artery, Right* **V Foot Artery, Right** Arcuate artery Dorsal metatarsal artery Lateral plantar artery Lateral tarsal artery Medial plantar artery **W Foot Artery, Left** ***See*** *V Foot Artery, Right* **Y Lower Artery** Umbilical artery	Ø Open 3 Percutaneous 4 Percutaneous Endoscopic	Ø Drainage Device	Z No Qualifier

Non-OR Ø49[Ø,1,2,3,4,5,6,7,8,9,A,B,C,D,E,F,H,J,K,L,M,N,P,Q,R,S,T,U,V,W,Y][Ø,3,4]ØZ

Ø49 Continued on next page

Ø49 Continued

Ø Medical and Surgical
4 Lower Arteries
9 Drainage

Definition: Taking or letting out fluids and/or gases from a body part

Explanation: The qualifier DIAGNOSTIC is used to identify drainage procedures that are biopsies

Body Part Character 4		Approach Character 5	Device Character 6	Qualifier Character 7
Ø Abdominal Aorta Inferior phrenic artery Lumbar artery Median sacral artery Middle suprarenal artery Ovarian artery Testicular artery **1 Celiac Artery** Celiac trunk **2 Gastric Artery** Left gastric artery Right gastric artery **3 Hepatic Artery** Common hepatic artery Gastroduodenal artery Hepatic artery proper **4 Splenic Artery** Left gastroepiploic artery Pancreatic artery Short gastric artery **5 Superior Mesenteric Artery** Ileal artery Ileocolic artery Inferior pancreaticoduodenal artery Jejunal artery **6 Colic Artery, Right** **7 Colic Artery, Left** **8 Colic Artery, Middle** **9 Renal Artery, Right** Inferior suprarenal artery Renal segmental artery **A Renal Artery, Left** *See 9 Renal Artery, Right* **B Inferior Mesenteric Artery** Sigmoid artery Superior rectal artery **C Common Iliac Artery, Right** **D Common Iliac Artery, Left** **E Internal Iliac Artery, Right** Deferential artery Hypogastric artery Iliolumbar artery Inferior gluteal artery Inferior vesical artery Internal pudendal artery Lateral sacral artery Middle rectal artery Obturator artery Prostatic artery Superior gluteal artery Superior vesical artery Umbilical artery Uterine artery Vaginal artery	**F Internal Iliac Artery, Left** *See E Internal Iliac Artery, Right* **H External Iliac Artery, Right** Deep circumflex iliac artery Inferior epigastric artery **J External Iliac Artery, Left** *See H External Iliac Artery, Right* **K Femoral Artery, Right** Circumflex iliac artery Deep femoral artery Descending genicular artery External pudendal artery Superficial epigastric artery **L Femoral Artery, Left** *See K Femoral Artery, Right* **M Popliteal Artery, Right** Inferior genicular artery Middle genicular artery Superior genicular artery Sural artery Tibioperoneal trunk **N Popliteal Artery, Left** *See M Popliteal Artery, Right* **P Anterior Tibial Artery, Right** Anterior lateral malleolar artery Anterior medial malleolar artery Anterior tibial recurrent artery Dorsalis pedis artery Posterior tibial recurrent artery **Q Anterior Tibial Artery, Left** *See P Anterior Tibial Artery, Right* **R Posterior Tibial Artery, Right** **S Posterior Tibial Artery, Left** **T Peroneal Artery, Right** Fibular artery **U Peroneal Artery, Left** *See T Peroneal Artery, Right* **V Foot Artery, Right** Arcuate artery Dorsal metatarsal artery Lateral plantar artery Lateral tarsal artery Medial plantar artery **W Foot Artery, Left** *See V Foot Artery, Right* **Y Lower Artery** Umbilical artery	**Ø Open** **3 Percutaneous** **4 Percutaneous Endoscopic**	**Z No Device**	**X Diagnostic** **Z No Qualifier**

Non-OR Ø49[Ø,1,2,3,4,5,6,7,8,9,A,B,C,D,E,F,H,J,K,L,M,N,P,Q,R,S,T,U,V,W,Y]3ZX
Non-OR Ø49[Ø,1,2,3,4,5,6,7,8,9,A,B,C,D,E,F,H,J,K,L,M,N,P,Q,R,S,T,U,V,W,Y][Ø,3,4]ZZ

Ø Medical and Surgical
4 Lower Arteries
B Excision Definition: Cutting out or off, without replacement, a portion of a body part
Explanation: The qualifier DIAGNOSTIC is used to identify excision procedures that are biopsies

Body Part Character 4		Approach Character 5	Device Character 6	Qualifier Character 7
Ø Abdominal Aorta Inferior phrenic artery Lumbar artery Median sacral artery Middle suprarenal artery Ovarian artery Testicular artery **1 Celiac Artery** Celiac trunk **2 Gastric Artery** Left gastric artery Right gastric artery **3 Hepatic Artery** Common hepatic artery Gastroduodenal artery Hepatic artery proper **4 Splenic Artery** Left gastroepiploic artery Pancreatic artery Short gastric artery **5 Superior Mesenteric Artery** Ileal artery Ileocolic artery Inferior pancreaticoduodenal artery Jejunal artery **6 Colic Artery, Right** **7 Colic Artery, Left** **8 Colic Artery, Middle** **9 Renal Artery, Right** Inferior suprarenal artery Renal segmental artery **A Renal Artery, Left** ***See*** *9 Renal Artery, Right* **B Inferior Mesenteric Artery** Sigmoid artery Superior rectal artery **C Common Iliac Artery, Right** **D Common Iliac Artery, Left** **E Internal Iliac Artery, Right** Deferential artery Hypogastric artery Iliolumbar artery Inferior gluteal artery Inferior vesical artery Internal pudendal artery Lateral sacral artery Middle rectal artery Obturator artery Prostatic artery Superior gluteal artery Superior vesical artery Umbilical artery Uterine artery Vaginal artery	**F Internal Iliac Artery, Left** ***See*** *E Internal Iliac Artery, Right* **H External Iliac Artery, Right** Deep circumflex iliac artery Inferior epigastric artery **J External Iliac Artery, Left** ***See*** *H External Iliac Artery, Right* **K Femoral Artery, Right** Circumflex iliac artery Deep femoral artery Descending genicular artery External pudendal artery Superficial epigastric artery **L Femoral Artery, Left** ***See*** *K Femoral Artery, Right* **M Popliteal Artery, Right** Inferior genicular artery Middle genicular artery Superior genicular artery Sural artery Tibioperoneal trunk **N Popliteal Artery, Left** ***See*** *M Popliteal Artery, Right* **P Anterior Tibial Artery, Right** Anterior lateral malleolar artery Anterior medial malleolar artery Anterior tibial recurrent artery Dorsalis pedis artery Posterior tibial recurrent artery **Q Anterior Tibial Artery, Left** ***See*** *P Anterior Tibial Artery, Right* **R Posterior Tibial Artery, Right** **S Posterior Tibial Artery, Left** **T Peroneal Artery, Right** Fibular artery **U Peroneal Artery, Left** ***See*** *T Peroneal Artery, Right* **V Foot Artery, Right** Arcuate artery Dorsal metatarsal artery Lateral plantar artery Lateral tarsal artery Medial plantar artery **W Foot Artery, Left** ***See*** *V Foot Artery, Right* **Y Lower Artery** Umbilical artery	**Ø Open** **3 Percutaneous** **4 Percutaneous Endoscopic**	**Z No Device**	**X Diagnostic** **Z No Qualifier**

0 Medical and Surgical
4 Lower Arteries
C Extirpation

Definition: Taking or cutting out solid matter from a body part

Explanation: The solid matter may be an abnormal byproduct of a biological function or a foreign body; it may be imbedded in a body part or in the lumen of a tubular body part. The solid matter may or may not have been previously broken into pieces.

Body Part Character 4	Approach Character 5	Device Character 6	Qualifier Character 7
0 Abdominal Aorta Inferior phrenic artery Lumbar artery Median sacral artery Middle suprarenal artery Ovarian artery Testicular artery **1 Celiac Artery** Celiac trunk **2 Gastric Artery** Left gastric artery Right gastric artery **3 Hepatic Artery** Common hepatic artery Gastroduodenal artery Hepatic artery proper **4 Splenic Artery** Left gastroepiploic artery Pancreatic artery Short gastric artery **5 Superior Mesenteric Artery** Ileal artery Ileocolic artery Inferior pancreaticoduodenal artery Jejunal artery **6 Colic Artery, Right** **7 Colic Artery, Left** **8 Colic Artery, Middle** **9 Renal Artery, Right** Inferior suprarenal artery Renal segmental artery **A Renal Artery, Left** *See 9 Renal Artery, Right* **B Inferior Mesenteric Artery** Sigmoid artery Superior rectal artery **C Common Iliac Artery, Right** **D Common Iliac Artery, Left** **E Internal Iliac Artery, Right** Deferential artery Hypogastric artery Iliolumbar artery Inferior gluteal artery Inferior vesical artery Internal pudendal artery Lateral sacral artery Middle rectal artery Obturator artery Prostatic artery Superior gluteal artery Superior vesical artery Umbilical artery Uterine artery Vaginal artery **F Internal Iliac Artery, Left** *See E Internal Iliac Artery, Right* **H External Iliac Artery, Right** Deep circumflex iliac artery Inferior epigastric artery **J External Iliac Artery, Left** *See H External Iliac Artery, Right* **K Femoral Artery, Right** Circumflex iliac artery Deep femoral artery Descending genicular artery External pudendal artery Superficial epigastric artery **L Femoral Artery, Left** *See K Femoral Artery, Right* **M Popliteal Artery, Right** Inferior genicular artery Middle genicular artery Superior genicular artery Sural artery Tibioperoneal trunk **N Popliteal Artery, Left** *See M Popliteal Artery, Right* **P Anterior Tibial Artery, Right** Anterior lateral malleolar artery Anterior medial malleolar artery Anterior tibial recurrent artery Dorsalis pedis artery Posterior tibial recurrent artery **Q Anterior Tibial Artery, Left** *See P Anterior Tibial Artery, Right* **R Posterior Tibial Artery, Right** **S Posterior Tibial Artery, Left** **T Peroneal Artery, Right** Fibular artery **U Peroneal Artery, Left** *See T Peroneal Artery, Right* **V Foot Artery, Right** Arcuate artery Dorsal metatarsal artery Lateral plantar artery Lateral tarsal artery Medial plantar artery **W Foot Artery, Left** *See V Foot Artery, Right* **Y Lower Artery** Umbilical artery	**0 Open** **3 Percutaneous** **4 Percutaneous Endoscopic**	**Z No Device**	**Z No Qualifier**

Ø Medical and Surgical
4 Lower Arteries
F Fragmentation Definition: Breaking solid matter in a body part into pieces

Explanation: Physical force (e.g., manual, ultrasonic) applied directly or indirectly is used to break the solid matter into pieces. The solid matter may be an abnormal byproduct of a biological function or a foreign body. The pieces of solid matter are not taken out.

Body Part Character 4	Approach Character 5	Device Character 6	Qualifier Character 7
C Common Iliac Artery, Right **D Common Iliac Artery, Left** **E Internal Iliac Artery, Right** Deferential artery Hypogastric artery Iliolumbar artery Inferior gluteal artery Inferior vesical artery Internal pudendal artery Lateral sacral artery Middle rectal artery Obturator artery Prostatic artery Superior gluteal artery Superior vesical artery Umbilical artery Uterine artery Vaginal artery **F Internal Iliac Artery, Left** ***See*** *E Internal Iliac Artery, Right* **H External Iliac Artery, Right** Deep circumflex iliac artery Inferior epigastric artery **J External Iliac Artery, Left** ***See*** *H External Iliac Artery, Right* **K Femoral Artery, Right** Circumflex iliac artery Deep femoral artery Descending genicular artery External pudendal artery Superficial epigastric artery **L Femoral Artery, Left** ***See*** *K Femoral Artery, Right* **M Popliteal Artery, Right** Inferior genicular artery Middle genicular artery Superior genicular artery Sural artery Tibioperoneal trunk **N Popliteal Artery, Left** ***See*** *M Popliteal Artery, Right* **P Anterior Tibial Artery, Right** Anterior lateral malleolar artery Anterior medial malleolar artery Anterior tibial recurrent artery Dorsalis pedis artery Posterior tibial recurrent artery **Q Anterior Tibial Artery, Left** ***See*** *P Anterior Tibial Artery, Right* **R Posterior Tibial Artery, Right** **S Posterior Tibial Artery, Left** **T Peroneal Artery, Right** Fibular artery **U Peroneal Artery, Left** ***See*** *T Peroneal Artery, Right* **Y Lower Artery** Umbilical artery	**3 Percutaneous**	**Z No Device**	**Ø Ultrasonic** **Z No Qualifier**

Ø Medical and Surgical
4 Lower Arteries
H Insertion Definition: Putting in a nonbiological appliance that monitors, assists, performs, or prevents a physiological function but does not physically take the place of a body part

Explanation: None

Body Part Character 4		Approach Character 5	Device Character 6	Qualifier Character 7
Ø Abdominal Aorta Inferior phrenic artery Lumbar artery Median sacral artery Middle suprarenal artery Ovarian artery Testicular artery		Ø Open 3 Percutaneous 4 Percutaneous Endoscopic	2 Monitoring Device 3 Infusion Device D Intraluminal Device	Z No Qualifier
1 Celiac Artery Celiac trunk 2 Gastric Artery Left gastric artery Right gastric artery 3 Hepatic Artery Common hepatic artery Gastroduodenal artery Hepatic artery proper 4 Splenic Artery Left gastroepiploic artery Pancreatic artery Short gastric artery 5 Superior Mesenteric Artery Ileal artery Ileocolic artery Inferior pancreaticoduodenal artery Jejunal artery 6 Colic Artery, Right 7 Colic Artery, Left 8 Colic Artery, Middle 9 Renal Artery, Right Inferior suprarenal artery Renal segmental artery A Renal Artery, Left *See 9 Renal Artery, Right* B Inferior Mesenteric Artery Sigmoid artery Superior rectal artery C Common Iliac Artery, Right D Common Iliac Artery, Left E Internal Iliac Artery, Right Deferential artery Hypogastric artery Iliolumbar artery Inferior gluteal artery Inferior vesical artery Internal pudendal artery Lateral sacral artery Middle rectal artery Obturator artery Prostatic artery Superior gluteal artery Superior vesical artery Umbilical artery Uterine artery Vaginal artery	F Internal Iliac Artery, Left *See E Internal Iliac Artery, Right* H External Iliac Artery, Right Deep circumflex iliac artery Inferior epigastric artery J External Iliac Artery, Left *See H External Iliac Artery, Right* K Femoral Artery, Right Circumflex iliac artery Deep femoral artery Descending genicular artery External pudendal artery Superficial epigastric artery L Femoral Artery, Left *See K Femoral Artery, Right* M Popliteal Artery, Right Inferior genicular artery Middle genicular artery Superior genicular artery Sural artery Tibioperoneal trunk N Popliteal Artery, Left *See M Popliteal Artery, Right* P Anterior Tibial Artery, Right Anterior lateral malleolar artery Anterior medial malleolar artery Anterior tibial recurrent artery Dorsalis pedis artery Posterior tibial recurrent artery Q Anterior Tibial Artery, Left *See P Anterior Tibial Artery, Right* R Posterior Tibial Artery, Right S Posterior Tibial Artery, Left T Peroneal Artery, Right Fibular artery U Peroneal Artery, Left *See T Peroneal Artery, Right* V Foot Artery, Right Arcuate artery Dorsal metatarsal artery Lateral plantar artery Lateral tarsal artery Medial plantar artery W Foot Artery, Left *See V Foot Artery, Right*	Ø Open 3 Percutaneous 4 Percutaneous Endoscopic	3 Infusion Device D Intraluminal Device	Z No Qualifier
Y Lower Artery Umbilical artery		Ø Open 3 Percutaneous 4 Percutaneous Endoscopic	2 Monitoring Device 3 Infusion Device D Intraluminal Device Y Other Device	Z No Qualifier

Non-OR Ø4HØ[Ø,3,4][2,3]Z
Non-OR Ø4H[1,2,3,4,5,6,7,8,9,A,B,C,D,E,F,H,J,K,L,M,N,P,Q,R,S,T,U,V,W][Ø,3,4]3Z
Non-OR Ø4HY32Z
Non-OR Ø4HY[Ø,3,4]3Z
Non-OR Ø4HY[3,4]YZ

Ø Medical and Surgical
4 Lower Arteries
J Inspection

Definition: Visually and/or manually exploring a body part

Explanation: Visual exploration may be performed with or without optical instrumentation. Manual exploration may be performed directly or through intervening body layers.

Body Part Character 4	Approach Character 5	Device Character 6	Qualifier Character 7
Y Lower Artery Umbilical artery	**Ø** Open **3** Percutaneous **4** Percutaneous Endoscopic **X** External	**Z** No Device	**Z** No Qualifier

Non-OR Ø4JY[3,4,X]ZZ

Ø Medical and Surgical
4 Lower Arteries
L Occlusion

Definition: Completely closing an orifice or the lumen of a tubular body part

Explanation: The orifice can be a natural orifice or an artificially created orifice

Body Part Character 4	Approach Character 5	Device Character 6	Qualifier Character 7
Ø Abdominal Aorta Inferior phrenic artery Lumbar artery Median sacral artery Middle suprarenal artery Ovarian artery Testicular artery	**Ø** Open **3** Percutaneous	**C** Extraluminal Device **Z** No Device	**Z** No Qualifier
Ø Abdominal Aorta Inferior phrenic artery Lumbar artery Median sacral artery Middle suprarenal artery Ovarian artery Testicular artery	**Ø** Open **3** Percutaneous	**D** Intraluminal Device	**J** Temporary **Z** No Qualifier
Ø Abdominal Aorta Inferior phrenic artery Lumbar artery Median sacral artery Middle suprarenal artery Ovarian artery Testicular artery	**4** Percutaneous Endoscopic	**C** Extraluminal Device **D** Intraluminal Device **Z** No Device	**Z** No Qualifier

Ø4L Continued on next page

Ø4L Continued

Ø Medical and Surgical
4 Lower Arteries
L Occlusion Definition: Completely closing an orifice or the lumen of a tubular body part

Explanation: The orifice can be a natural orifice or an artificially created orifice

Body Part Character 4	Approach Character 5	Device Character 6	Qualifier Character 7
1 Celiac Artery Celiac trunk **2 Gastric Artery** Left gastric artery Right gastric artery **3 Hepatic Artery** Common hepatic artery Gastroduodenal artery Hepatic artery proper **4 Splenic Artery** Left gastroepiploic artery Pancreatic artery Short gastric artery **5 Superior Mesenteric Artery** Ileal artery Ileocolic artery Inferior pancreaticoduodenal artery Jejunal artery **6 Colic Artery, Right** **7 Colic Artery, Left** **8 Colic Artery, Middle** **9 Renal Artery, Right** Inferior suprarenal artery Renal segmental artery **A Renal Artery, Left** *See 9 Renal Artery, Right* **B Inferior Mesenteric Artery** Sigmoid artery Superior rectal artery **C Common Iliac Artery, Right** **D Common Iliac Artery, Left** **H External Iliac Artery, Right** Deep circumflex iliac artery Inferior epigastric artery **J External Iliac Artery, Left** *See H External Iliac Artery, Right* **K Femoral Artery, Right** Circumflex iliac artery Deep femoral artery Descending genicular artery External pudendal artery Superficial epigastric artery **L Femoral Artery, Left** *See K Femoral Artery, Right* **M Popliteal Artery, Right** Inferior genicular artery Middle genicular artery Superior genicular artery Sural artery Tibioperoneal trunk **N Popliteal Artery, Left** *See M Popliteal Artery, Right* **P Anterior Tibial Artery, Right** Anterior lateral malleolar artery Anterior medial malleolar artery Anterior tibial recurrent artery Dorsalis pedis artery Posterior tibial recurrent artery **Q Anterior Tibial Artery, Left** *See P Anterior Tibial Artery, Right* **R Posterior Tibial Artery, Right** **S Posterior Tibial Artery, Left** **T Peroneal Artery, Right** Fibular artery **U Peroneal Artery, Left** *See T Peroneal Artery, Right* **V Foot Artery, Right** Arcuate artery Dorsal metatarsal artery Lateral plantar artery Lateral tarsal artery Medial plantar artery **W Foot Artery, Left** *See V Foot Artery, Right* **Y Lower Artery** Umbilical artery	**Ø Open** **3 Percutaneous** **4 Percutaneous Endoscopic**	**C Extraluminal Device** **D Intraluminal Device** **Z No Device**	**Z No Qualifier**
E Internal Iliac Artery, Right Deferential artery Hypogastric artery Iliolumbar artery Inferior gluteal artery Inferior vesical artery Internal pudendal artery Lateral sacral artery Middle rectal artery Obturator artery Prostatic artery Superior gluteal artery Superior vesical artery Umbilical artery Uterine artery Vaginal artery	**Ø Open** **3 Percutaneous** **4 Percutaneous Endoscopic**	**C Extraluminal Device** **D Intraluminal Device** **Z No Device**	**T Uterine Artery, Right** ♀ **V Prostatic Artery, Right** ♂ **Z No Qualifier**
F Internal Iliac Artery, Left Deferential artery Hypogastric artery Iliolumbar artery Inferior gluteal artery Inferior vesical artery Internal pudendal artery Lateral sacral artery Middle rectal artery Obturator artery Prostatic artery Superior gluteal artery Superior vesical artery Umbilical artery Uterine artery Vaginal artery	**Ø Open** **3 Percutaneous** **4 Percutaneous Endoscopic**	**C Extraluminal Device** **D Intraluminal Device** **Z No Device**	**U Uterine Artery, Left** ♀ **W Prostatic Artery, Left** ♂ **Z No Qualifier**

♀ Ø4LE[Ø,3,4][C,D,Z]T
♀ Ø4LF[Ø,3,4][C,D,Z]U
♂ Ø4LE[Ø,3,4][C,D,Z]V
♂ Ø4LF[Ø,3,4][C,D,Z]W

Ø Medical and Surgical
4 Lower Arteries
N Release

Definition: Freeing a body part from an abnormal physical constraint by cutting or by the use of force
Explanation: Some of the restraining tissue may be taken out but none of the body part is taken out

Body Part Character 4	Approach Character 5	Device Character 6	Qualifier Character 7
Ø Abdominal Aorta Inferior phrenic artery Lumbar artery Median sacral artery Middle suprarenal artery Ovarian artery Testicular artery **1 Celiac Artery** Celiac trunk **2 Gastric Artery** Left gastric artery Right gastric artery **3 Hepatic Artery** Common hepatic artery Gastroduodenal artery Hepatic artery proper **4 Splenic Artery** Left gastroepiploic artery Pancreatic artery Short gastric artery **5 Superior Mesenteric Artery** Ileal artery Ileocolic artery Inferior pancreaticoduodenal artery Jejunal artery **6 Colic Artery, Right** **7 Colic Artery, Left** **8 Colic Artery, Middle** **9 Renal Artery, Right** Inferior suprarenal artery Renal segmental artery **A Renal Artery, Left** *See 9 Renal Artery, Right* **B Inferior Mesenteric Artery** Sigmoid artery Superior rectal artery **C Common Iliac Artery, Right** **D Common Iliac Artery, Left** **E Internal Iliac Artery, Right** Deferential artery Hypogastric artery Iliolumbar artery Inferior gluteal artery Inferior vesical artery Internal pudendal artery Lateral sacral artery Middle rectal artery Obturator artery Prostatic artery Superior gluteal artery Superior vesical artery Umbilical artery Uterine artery Vaginal artery **F Internal Iliac Artery, Left** *See E Internal Iliac Artery, Right* **H External Iliac Artery, Right** Deep circumflex iliac artery Inferior epigastric artery **J External Iliac Artery, Left** *See H External Iliac Artery, Right* **K Femoral Artery, Right** Circumflex iliac artery Deep femoral artery Descending genicular artery External pudendal artery Superficial epigastric artery **L Femoral Artery, Left** *See K Femoral Artery, Right* **M Popliteal Artery, Right** Inferior genicular artery Middle genicular artery Superior genicular artery Sural artery Tibioperoneal trunk **N Popliteal Artery, Left** *See M Popliteal Artery, Right* **P Anterior Tibial Artery, Right** Anterior lateral malleolar artery Anterior medial malleolar artery Anterior tibial recurrent artery Dorsalis pedis artery Posterior tibial recurrent artery **Q Anterior Tibial Artery, Left** *See P Anterior Tibial Artery, Right* **R Posterior Tibial Artery, Right** **S Posterior Tibial Artery, Left** **T Peroneal Artery, Right** Fibular artery **U Peroneal Artery, Left** *See T Peroneal Artery, Right* **V Foot Artery, Right** Arcuate artery Dorsal metatarsal artery Lateral plantar artery Lateral tarsal artery Medial plantar artery **W Foot Artery, Left** *See V Foot Artery, Right* **Y Lower Artery** Umbilical artery	**Ø Open** **3 Percutaneous** **4 Percutaneous Endoscopic**	**Z No Device**	**Z No Qualifier**

Ø Medical and Surgical
4 Lower Arteries
P Removal

Definition: Taking out or off a device from a body part

Explanation: If a device is taken out and a similar device put in without cutting or puncturing the skin or mucous membrane, the procedure is coded to the root operation CHANGE. Otherwise, the procedure for taking out a device is coded to the root operation REMOVAL.

Body Part Character 4	Approach Character 5	Device Character 6	Qualifier Character 7
Y Lower Artery Umbilical artery	**Ø Open** **3 Percutaneous** **4 Percutaneous Endoscopic**	**Ø Drainage Device** **2 Monitoring Device** **3 Infusion Device** **7 Autologous Tissue Substitute** **C Extraluminal Device** **D Intraluminal Device** **J Synthetic Substitute** **K Nonautologous Tissue Substitute** **Y Other Device**	**Z No Qualifier**
Y Lower Artery Umbilical artery	**X External**	**Ø Drainage Device** **1 Radioactive Element** **2 Monitoring Device** **3 Infusion Device** **D Intraluminal Device**	**Z No Qualifier**

Non-OR Ø4PY3[Ø,2,3,D]Z
Non-OR Ø4PY[3,4]YZ
Non-OR Ø4PYX[Ø,1,2,3,D]Z

Ø Medical and Surgical
4 Lower Arteries
Q Repair Definition: Restoring, to the extent possible, a body part to its normal anatomic structure and function
Explanation: Used only when the method to accomplish the repair is not one of the other root operations

Body Part Character 4	Approach Character 5	Device Character 6	Qualifier Character 7
Ø Abdominal Aorta Inferior phrenic artery Lumbar artery Median sacral artery Middle suprarenal artery Ovarian artery Testicular artery **1 Celiac Artery** Celiac trunk **2 Gastric Artery** Left gastric artery Right gastric artery **3 Hepatic Artery** Common hepatic artery Gastroduodenal artery Hepatic artery proper **4 Splenic Artery** Left gastroepiploic artery Pancreatic artery Short gastric artery **5 Superior Mesenteric Artery** Ileal artery Ileocolic artery Inferior pancreaticoduodenal artery Jejunal artery **6 Colic Artery, Right** **7 Colic Artery, Left** **8 Colic Artery, Middle** **9 Renal Artery, Right** Inferior suprarenal artery Renal segmental artery **A Renal Artery, Left** *See 9 Renal Artery, Right* **B Inferior Mesenteric Artery** Sigmoid artery Superior rectal artery **C Common Iliac Artery, Right** **D Common Iliac Artery, Left** **E Internal Iliac Artery, Right** Deferential artery Hypogastric artery Iliolumbar artery Inferior gluteal artery Inferior vesical artery Internal pudendal artery Lateral sacral artery Middle rectal artery Obturator artery Prostatic artery Superior gluteal artery Superior vesical artery Umbilical artery Uterine artery Vaginal artery **F Internal Iliac Artery, Left** *See E Internal Iliac Artery, Right* **H External Iliac Artery, Right** Deep circumflex iliac artery Inferior epigastric artery **J External Iliac Artery, Left** *See H External Iliac Artery, Right* **K Femoral Artery, Right** Circumflex iliac artery Deep femoral artery Descending genicular artery External pudendal artery Superficial epigastric artery **L Femoral Artery, Left** *See K Femoral Artery, Right* **M Popliteal Artery, Right** Inferior genicular artery Middle genicular artery Superior genicular artery Sural artery Tibioperoneal trunk **N Popliteal Artery, Left** *See M Popliteal Artery, Right* **P Anterior Tibial Artery, Right** Anterior lateral malleolar artery Anterior medial malleolar artery Anterior tibial recurrent artery Dorsalis pedis artery Posterior tibial recurrent artery **Q Anterior Tibial Artery, Left** *See P Anterior Tibial Artery, Right* **R Posterior Tibial Artery, Right** **S Posterior Tibial Artery, Left** **T Peroneal Artery, Right** Fibular artery **U Peroneal Artery, Left** *See T Peroneal Artery, Right* **V Foot Artery, Right** Arcuate artery Dorsal metatarsal artery Lateral plantar artery Lateral tarsal artery Medial plantar artery **W Foot Artery, Left** *See V Foot Artery, Right* **Y Lower Artery** Umbilical artery	**Ø Open** **3 Percutaneous** **4 Percutaneous Endoscopic**	**Z No Device**	**Z No Qualifier**

Ø Medical and Surgical
4 Lower Arteries
R Replacement

Definition: Putting in or on biological or synthetic material that physically takes the place and/or function of all or a portion of a body part

Explanation: The body part may have been taken out or replaced, or may be taken out, physically eradicated, or rendered nonfunctional during the REPLACEMENT procedure. A REMOVAL procedure is coded for taking out the device used in a previous replacement procedure.

Body Part Character 4	Approach Character 5	Device Character 6	Qualifier Character 7
Ø Abdominal Aorta Inferior phrenic artery Lumbar artery Median sacral artery Middle suprarenal artery Ovarian artery Testicular artery **1 Celiac Artery** Celiac trunk **2 Gastric Artery** Left gastric artery Right gastric artery **3 Hepatic Artery** Common hepatic artery Gastroduodenal artery Hepatic artery proper **4 Splenic Artery** Left gastroepiploic artery Pancreatic artery Short gastric artery **5 Superior Mesenteric Artery** Ileal artery Ileocolic artery Inferior pancreaticoduodenal artery Jejunal artery **6 Colic Artery, Right** **7 Colic Artery, Left** **8 Colic Artery, Middle** **9 Renal Artery, Right** Inferior suprarenal artery Renal segmental artery **A Renal Artery, Left** *See 9 Renal Artery, Right* **B Inferior Mesenteric Artery** Sigmoid artery Superior rectal artery **C Common Iliac Artery, Right** **D Common Iliac Artery, Left** **E Internal Iliac Artery, Right** Deferential artery Hypogastric artery Iliolumbar artery Inferior gluteal artery Inferior vesical artery Internal pudendal artery Lateral sacral artery Middle rectal artery Obturator artery Prostatic artery Superior gluteal artery Superior vesical artery Umbilical artery Uterine artery Vaginal artery **F Internal Iliac Artery, Left** *See E Internal Iliac Artery, Right* **H External Iliac Artery, Right** Deep circumflex iliac artery Inferior epigastric artery **J External Iliac Artery, Left** *See H External Iliac Artery, Right* **K Femoral Artery, Right** Circumflex iliac artery Deep femoral artery Descending genicular artery External pudendal artery Superficial epigastric artery **L Femoral Artery, Left** *See K Femoral Artery, Right* **M Popliteal Artery, Right** Inferior genicular artery Middle genicular artery Superior genicular artery Sural artery Tibioperoneal trunk **N Popliteal Artery, Left** *See M Popliteal Artery, Right* **P Anterior Tibial Artery, Right** Anterior lateral malleolar artery Anterior medial malleolar artery Anterior tibial recurrent artery Dorsalis pedis artery Posterior tibial recurrent artery **Q Anterior Tibial Artery, Left** *See P Anterior Tibial Artery, Right* **R Posterior Tibial Artery, Right** **S Posterior Tibial Artery, Left** **T Peroneal Artery, Right** Fibular artery **U Peroneal Artery, Left** *See T Peroneal Artery, Right* **V Foot Artery, Right** Arcuate artery Dorsal metatarsal artery Lateral plantar artery Lateral tarsal artery Medial plantar artery **W Foot Artery, Left** *See V Foot Artery, Right* **Y Lower Artery** Umbilical artery	**Ø Open** **4 Percutaneous Endoscopic**	**7 Autologous Tissue Substitute** **J Synthetic Substitute** **K Nonautologous Tissue Substitute**	**Z No Qualifier**

Ø Medical and Surgical
4 Lower Arteries
S Reposition

Definition: Moving to its normal location, or other suitable location, all or a portion of a body part

Explanation: The body part is moved to a new location from an abnormal location, or from a normal location where it is not functioning correctly. The body part may or may not be cut out or off to be moved to the new location.

Body Part Character 4	Approach Character 5	Device Character 6	Qualifier Character 7
Ø Abdominal Aorta Inferior phrenic artery Lumbar artery Median sacral artery Middle suprarenal artery Ovarian artery Testicular artery **1 Celiac Artery** Celiac trunk **2 Gastric Artery** Left gastric artery Right gastric artery **3 Hepatic Artery** Common hepatic artery Gastroduodenal artery Hepatic artery proper **4 Splenic Artery** Left gastroepiploic artery Pancreatic artery Short gastric artery **5 Superior Mesenteric Artery** Ileal artery Ileocolic artery Inferior pancreaticoduodenal artery Jejunal artery **6 Colic Artery, Right** **7 Colic Artery, Left** **8 Colic Artery, Middle** **9 Renal Artery, Right** Inferior suprarenal artery Renal segmental artery **A Renal Artery, Left** *See 9 Renal Artery, Right* **B Inferior Mesenteric Artery** Sigmoid artery Superior rectal artery **C Common Iliac Artery, Right** **D Common Iliac Artery, Left** **E Internal Iliac Artery, Right** Deferential artery Hypogastric artery Iliolumbar artery Inferior gluteal artery Inferior vesical artery Internal pudendal artery Lateral sacral artery Middle rectal artery Obturator artery Prostatic artery Superior gluteal artery Superior vesical artery Umbilical artery Uterine artery Vaginal artery **F Internal Iliac Artery, Left** *See E Internal Iliac Artery, Right* **H External Iliac Artery, Right** Deep circumflex iliac artery Inferior epigastric artery **J External Iliac Artery, Left** *See H External Iliac Artery, Right* **K Femoral Artery, Right** Circumflex iliac artery Deep femoral artery Descending genicular artery External pudendal artery Superficial epigastric artery **L Femoral Artery, Left** *See K Femoral Artery, Right* **M Popliteal Artery, Right** Inferior genicular artery Middle genicular artery Superior genicular artery Sural artery Tibioperoneal trunk **N Popliteal Artery, Left** *See M Popliteal Artery, Right* **P Anterior Tibial Artery, Right** Anterior lateral malleolar artery Anterior medial malleolar artery Anterior tibial recurrent artery Dorsalis pedis artery Posterior tibial recurrent artery **Q Anterior Tibial Artery, Left** *See P Anterior Tibial Artery, Right* **R Posterior Tibial Artery, Right** **S Posterior Tibial Artery, Left** **T Peroneal Artery, Right** Fibular artery **U Peroneal Artery, Left** *See T Peroneal Artery, Right* **V Foot Artery, Right** Arcuate artery Dorsal metatarsal artery Lateral plantar artery Lateral tarsal artery Medial plantar artery **W Foot Artery, Left** *See V Foot Artery, Right* **Y Lower Artery** Umbilical artery	**Ø Open** **3 Percutaneous** **4 Percutaneous Endoscopic**	**Z No Device**	**Z No Qualifier**

Ø Medical and Surgical
4 Lower Arteries
U Supplement

Definition: Putting in or on biological or synthetic material that physically reinforces and/or augments the function of a portion of a body part

Explanation: The biological material is non-living, or is living and from the same individual. The body part may have been previously replaced, and the SUPPLEMENT procedure is performed to physically reinforce and/or augment the function of the replaced body part.

Body Part Character 4	Approach Character 5	Device Character 6	Qualifier Character 7
Ø Abdominal Aorta Inferior phrenic artery Lumbar artery Median sacral artery Middle suprarenal artery Ovarian artery Testicular artery **1 Celiac Artery** Celiac trunk **2 Gastric Artery** Left gastric artery Right gastric artery **3 Hepatic Artery** Common hepatic artery Gastroduodenal artery Hepatic artery proper **4 Splenic Artery** Left gastroepiploic artery Pancreatic artery Short gastric artery **5 Superior Mesenteric Artery** Ileal artery Ileocolic artery Inferior pancreaticoduodenal artery Jejunal artery **6 Colic Artery, Right** **7 Colic Artery, Left** **8 Colic Artery, Middle** **9 Renal Artery, Right** Inferior suprarenal artery Renal segmental artery **A Renal Artery, Left** *See 9 Renal Artery, Right* **B Inferior Mesenteric Artery** Sigmoid artery Superior rectal artery **C Common Iliac Artery, Right** **D Common Iliac Artery, Left** **E Internal Iliac Artery, Right** Deferential artery Hypogastric artery Iliolumbar artery Inferior gluteal artery Inferior vesical artery Internal pudendal artery Lateral sacral artery Middle rectal artery Obturator artery Prostatic artery Superior gluteal artery Superior vesical artery Umbilical artery Uterine artery Vaginal artery **F Internal Iliac Artery, Left** *See E Internal Iliac Artery, Right* **H External Iliac Artery, Right** Deep circumflex iliac artery Inferior epigastric artery **J External Iliac Artery, Left** *See H External Iliac Artery, Right* **K Femoral Artery, Right** Circumflex iliac artery Deep femoral artery Descending genicular artery External pudendal artery Superficial epigastric artery **L Femoral Artery, Left** *See K Femoral Artery, Right* **M Popliteal Artery, Right** Inferior genicular artery Middle genicular artery Superior genicular artery Sural artery Tibioperoneal trunk **N Popliteal Artery, Left** *See M Popliteal Artery, Right* **P Anterior Tibial Artery, Right** Anterior lateral malleolar artery Anterior medial malleolar artery Anterior tibial recurrent artery Dorsalis pedis artery Posterior tibial recurrent artery **Q Anterior Tibial Artery, Left** *See P Anterior Tibial Artery, Right* **R Posterior Tibial Artery, Right** **S Posterior Tibial Artery, Left** **T Peroneal Artery, Right** Fibular artery **U Peroneal Artery, Left** *See T Peroneal Artery, Right* **V Foot Artery, Right** Arcuate artery Dorsal metatarsal artery Lateral plantar artery Lateral tarsal artery Medial plantar artery **W Foot Artery, Left** *See V Foot Artery, Right* **Y Lower Artery** Umbilical artery	**Ø Open** **3 Percutaneous** **4 Percutaneous Endoscopic**	**7 Autologous Tissue Substitute** **J Synthetic Substitute** **K Nonautologous Tissue Substitute**	**Z No Qualifier**

Ø Medical and Surgical
4 Lower Arteries
V Restriction

Definition: Partially closing an orifice or the lumen of a tubular body part
Explanation: The orifice can be a natural orifice or an artificially created orifice

Body Part Character 4	Approach Character 5	Device Character 6	Qualifier Character 7
Ø Abdominal Aorta Inferior phrenic artery Lumbar artery Median sacral artery Middle suprarenal artery Ovarian artery Testicular artery	**Ø Open** **3 Percutaneous** **4 Percutaneous Endoscopic**	**C Extraluminal Device** **E Intraluminal Device, Branched or Fenestrated, One or Two Arteries** **F Intraluminal Device, Branched or Fenestrated, Three or More Arteries** **Z No Device**	**Z No Qualifier**
Ø Abdominal Aorta Inferior phrenic artery Lumbar artery Median sacral artery Middle suprarenal artery Ovarian artery Testicular artery	**Ø Open** **3 Percutaneous** **4 Percutaneous Endoscopic**	**D Intraluminal Device**	**J Temporary** **Z No Qualifier**
1 Celiac Artery Celiac trunk **2 Gastric Artery** Left gastric artery Right gastric artery **3 Hepatic Artery** Common hepatic artery Gastroduodenal artery Hepatic artery proper **4 Splenic Artery** Left gastroepiploic artery Pancreatic artery Short gastric artery **5 Superior Mesenteric Artery** Ileal artery Ileocolic artery Inferior pancreaticoduodenal artery Jejunal artery **6 Colic Artery, Right** **7 Colic Artery, Left** **8 Colic Artery, Middle** **9 Renal Artery, Right** Inferior suprarenal artery Renal segmental artery **A Renal Artery, Left** *See 9 Renal Artery, Right* **B Inferior Mesenteric Artery** Sigmoid artery Superior rectal artery **E Internal Iliac Artery, Right** Deferential artery Hypogastric artery Iliolumbar artery Inferior gluteal artery Inferior vesical artery Internal pudendal artery Lateral sacral artery Middle rectal artery Obturator artery Prostatic artery Superior gluteal artery Superior vesical artery Umbilical artery Uterine artery Vaginal artery **F Internal Iliac Artery, Left** *See E Internal Iliac Artery, Right* **H External Iliac Artery, Right** Deep circumflex iliac artery Inferior epigastric artery **J External Iliac Artery, Left** *See H External Iliac Artery, Right* **K Femoral Artery, Right** Circumflex iliac artery Deep femoral artery Descending genicular artery External pudendal artery Superficial epigastric artery **L Femoral Artery, Left** *See K Femoral Artery, Right* **M Popliteal Artery, Right** Inferior genicular artery Middle genicular artery Superior genicular artery Sural artery Tibioperoneal trunk **N Popliteal Artery, Left** *See M Popliteal Artery, Right* **P Anterior Tibial Artery, Right** Anterior lateral malleolar artery Anterior medial malleolar artery Anterior tibial recurrent artery Dorsalis pedis artery Posterior tibial recurrent artery **Q Anterior Tibial Artery, Left** *See P Anterior Tibial Artery, Right* **R Posterior Tibial Artery, Right** **S Posterior Tibial Artery, Left** **T Peroneal Artery, Right** Fibular artery **U Peroneal Artery, Left** *See T Peroneal Artery, Right* **V Foot Artery, Right** Arcuate artery Dorsal metatarsal artery Lateral plantar artery Lateral tarsal artery Medial plantar artery **W Foot Artery, Left** *See V Foot Artery, Right* **Y Lower Artery** Umbilical artery	**Ø Open** **3 Percutaneous** **4 Percutaneous Endoscopic**	**C Extraluminal Device** **D Intraluminal Device** **Z No Device**	**Z No Qualifier**
C Common Iliac Artery, Right **D Common Iliac Artery, Left**	**Ø Open** **3 Percutaneous** **4 Percutaneous Endoscopic**	**C Extraluminal Device** **D Intraluminal Device** **E Intraluminal Device, Branched or Fenestrated, One or Two Arteries** **Z No Device**	**Z No Qualifier**

Ø Medical and Surgical
4 Lower Arteries
W Revision

Definition: Correcting, to the extent possible, a portion of a malfunctioning device or the position of a displaced device

Explanation: Revision can include correcting a malfunctioning or displaced device by taking out or putting in components of the device such as a screw or pin

Body Part Character 4	Approach Character 5	Device Character 6	Qualifier Character 7
Y Lower Artery Umbilical artery	Ø Open 3 Percutaneous 4 Percutaneous Endoscopic	Ø Drainage Device 2 Monitoring Device 3 Infusion Device 7 Autologous Tissue Substitute C Extraluminal Device D Intraluminal Device J Synthetic Substitute K Nonautologous Tissue Substitute Y Other Device	Z No Qualifier
Y Lower Artery Umbilical artery	X External	Ø Drainage Device 2 Monitoring Device 3 Infusion Device 7 Autologous Tissue Substitute C Extraluminal Device D Intraluminal Device J Synthetic Substitute K Nonautologous Tissue Substitute	Z No Qualifier

Non-OR Ø4WY3[Ø,2,3]Z
Non-OR Ø4WY[3,4]YZ
Non-OR Ø4WYX[Ø,2,3,7,C,D,J,K]Z

Upper Veins Ø51–Ø5W

Character Meanings

This Character Meaning table is provided as a guide to assist the user in the identification of character members that may be found in this section of code tables. It **SHOULD NOT** be used to build a PCS code.

Operation–Character 3		Body Part–Character 4		Approach–Character 5		Device–Character 6		Qualifier–Character 7	
1	Bypass	Ø	Azygos Vein	Ø	Open	Ø	Drainage Device	Ø	Ultrasonic
5	Destruction	1	Hemiazygos Vein	3	Percutaneous	2	Monitoring Device	1	Drug-Coated Balloon
7	Dilation	3	Innominate Vein, Right	4	Percutaneous Endoscopic	3	Infusion Device	X	Diagnostic
9	Drainage	4	Innominate Vein, Left	X	External	7	Autologous Tissue Substitute	Y	Upper Vein
B	Excision	5	Subclavian Vein, Right			9	Autologous Venous Tissue	Z	No Qualifier
C	Extirpation	6	Subclavian Vein, Left			A	Autologous Arterial Tissue		
D	Extraction	7	Axillary Vein, Right			C	Extraluminal Device		
F	Fragmentation	8	Axillary Vein, Left			D	Intraluminal Device		
H	Insertion	9	Brachial Vein, Right			J	Synthetic Substitute		
J	Inspection	A	Brachial Vein, Left			K	Nonautologous Tissue Substitute		
L	Occlusion	B	Basilic Vein, Right			M	Neurostimulator Lead		
N	Release	C	Basilic Vein, Left			Y	Other Device		
P	Removal	D	Cephalic Vein, Right			Z	No Device		
Q	Repair	F	Cephalic Vein, Left						
R	Replacement	G	Hand Vein, Right						
S	Reposition	H	Hand Vein, Left						
U	Supplement	L	Intracranial Vein						
V	Restriction	M	Internal Jugular Vein, Right						
W	Revision	N	Internal Jugular Vein, Left						
		P	External Jugular Vein, Right						
		Q	External Jugular Vein, Left						
		R	Vertebral Vein, Right						
		S	Vertebral Vein, Left						
		T	Face Vein, Right						
		V	Face Vein, Left						
		Y	Upper Vein						

AHA Coding Clinic for Upper Veins
2022, 1Q, 10-13 Procedures performed on a continuous vessel, ICD-10-PCS Guideline B4.1c

AHA Coding Clinic for table Ø51
2020, 1Q, 28 Free flap microvascular breast reconstruction
2017, 3Q, 15 Bypass of innominate vein to atrial appendage

AHA Coding Clinic for table Ø57
2020, 3Q, 38 Thrombectomy of arteriovenous fistula with angioplasty and stent placement

AHA Coding Clinic for table Ø59
2018, 3Q, 7 Catheter placement for treatment of congestive heart failure

AHA Coding Clinic for table Ø5B
2021, 2Q, 15 Excision of pituitary macroadenoma within cavernous sinus
2020, 3Q, 40 Excision of ulceration of arteriovenous fistula
2020, 1Q, 24 Resection of vascular malformation, likely cavernoma
2016, 2Q, 12 Resection of malignant neoplasm of infratemporal fossa

AHA Coding Clinic for table Ø5C
2020, 3Q, 37 Repair of aneurysm of arteriovenous fistula with endovenectomy
2020, 3Q, 38 Thrombectomy of arteriovenous fistula with angioplasty and stent placement

AHA Coding Clinic for table Ø5F
2020, 4Q, 45-49 New fragmentation tables
2020, 4Q, 49-50 Intravascular ultrasound assisted thrombolysis
2020, 4Q, 50 Intravascular lithotripsy

AHA Coding Clinic for table Ø5H
2016, 4Q, 97-98 Phrenic neurostimulator

AHA Coding Clinic for table Ø5P
2016, 4Q, 97-98 Phrenic neurostimulator

AHA Coding Clinic for table Ø5Q
2017, 3Q, 15 Bypass of innominate vein to atrial appendage

AHA Coding Clinic for table Ø5S
2013, 4Q, 125 Stage II cephalic vein transposition (superficialization) of arteriovenous fistula

AHA Coding Clinic for table Ø5V
2020, 3Q, 37 Repair of aneurysm of arteriovenous fistula with endovenectomy

AHA Coding Clinic for table Ø5W
2016, 4Q, 97-98 Phrenic neurostimulator

Head and Neck Veins

Superficial temporal **L**
Superior sagittal sinus **L**
Inferior sagittal sinus **L**
Superior ophthalmic **L**
Straight sinus **L**
Transverse sinus **L**
Retromandibular **T, V**
Occipital sinus **L**
Facial **T, V**
Posterior auricular **P, Q**
Lingual **T, V**
Deep cervical **R, S**
Thyroid **P, Q**
Anterior jugular **P, Q**
External jugular **P, Q**
External jugular **P, Q**
Vertebral **R, S**
Brachiocephalic **3, 4**
Subclavian **5, 6**

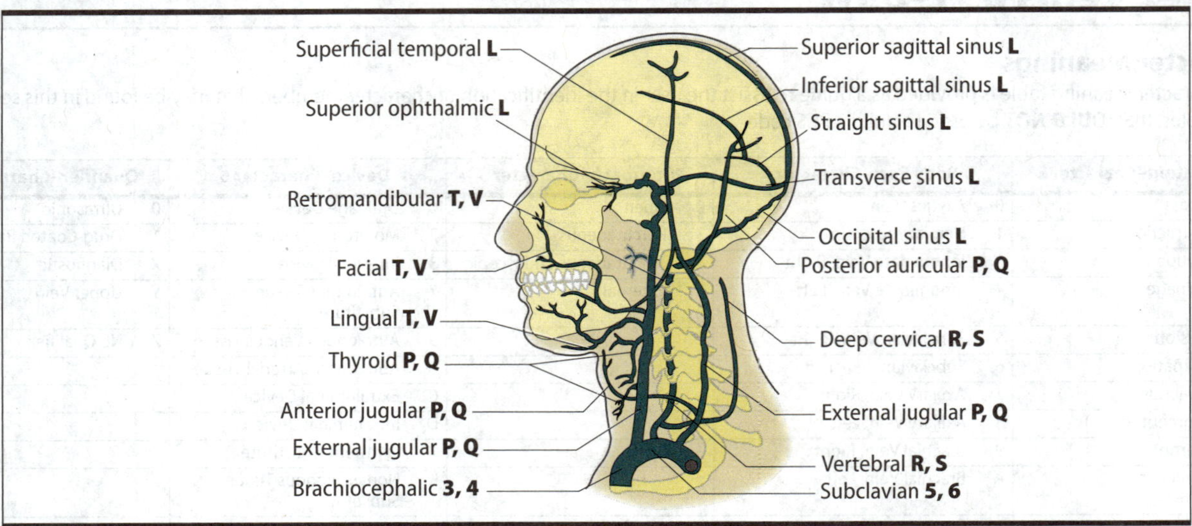

Upper Veins

Superficial temporal **L**
Vertebral **R, S**
Internal jugular **M, N**
External jugular **P, Q**
Subclavian **5, 6**
Innominate **3, 4**
Azygos **Ø**
Axillary **7,8**
Hemiazygos **1**
Brachial **9, A**
Cephalic **D, F**
Basilic **B, C**
Radial **9, A**
Ulnar **9, A**
Digital **G, H**

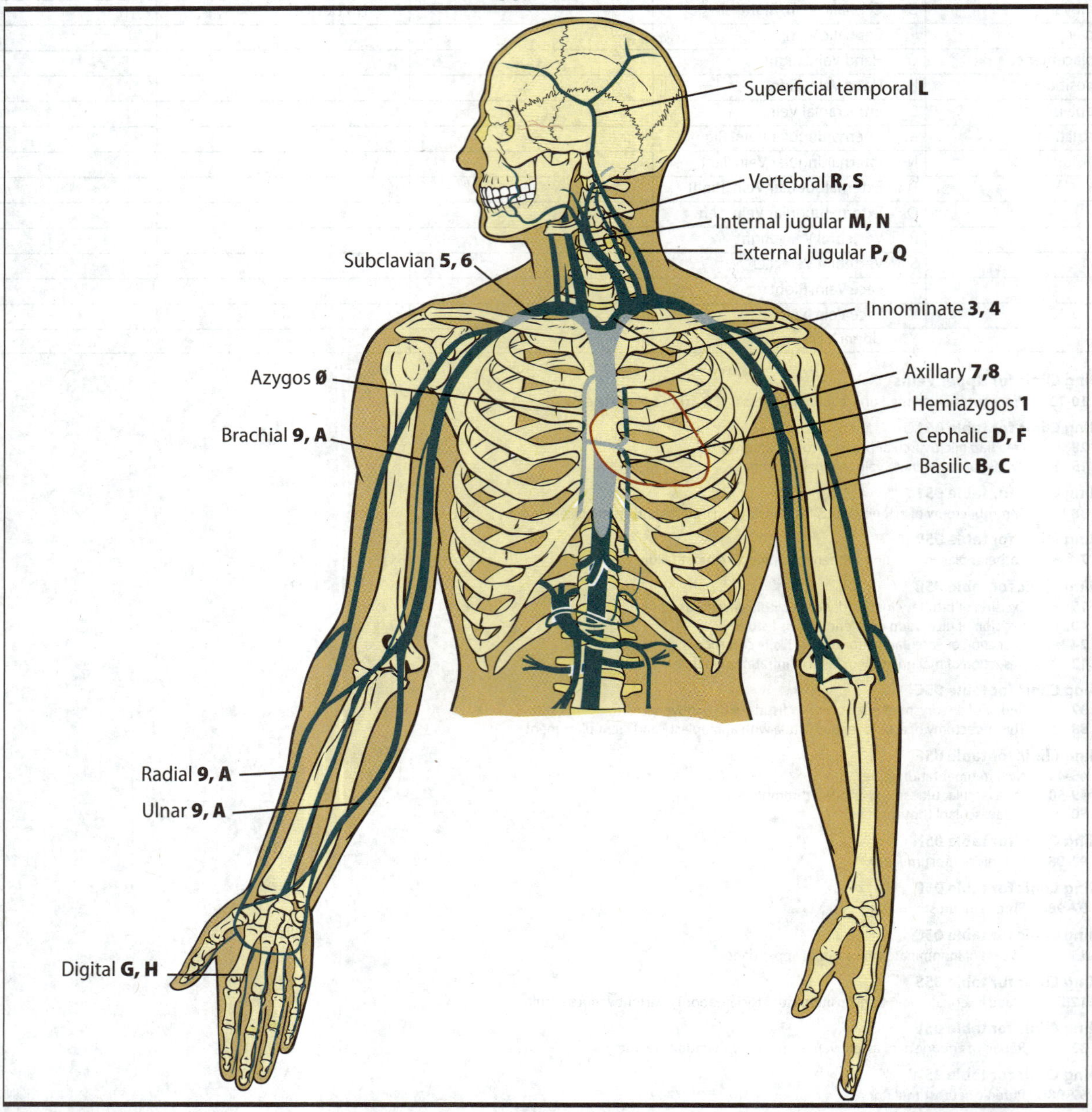

Ø Medical and Surgical
5 Upper Veins
1 Bypass

Definition: Altering the route of passage of the contents of a tubular body part

Explanation: Rerouting contents of a body part to a downstream area of the normal route, to a similar route and body part, or to an abnormal route and dissimilar body part. Includes one or more anastomoses, with or without the use of a device.

Body Part Character 4	Approach Character 5	Device Character 6	Qualifier Character 7
Ø Azygos Vein Right ascending lumbar vein Right subcostal vein **1 Hemiazygos Vein** Left ascending lumbar vein Left subcostal vein **3 Innominate Vein, Right** Brachiocephalic vein Inferior thyroid vein **4 Innominate Vein, Left** *See 3 Innominate Vein, Right* **5 Subclavian Vein, Right** **6 Subclavian Vein, Left** **7 Axillary Vein, Right** **8 Axillary Vein, Left** **9 Brachial Vein, Right** Radial vein Ulnar vein **A Brachial Vein, Left** *See 9 Brachial Vein, Right* **B Basilic Vein, Right** Median antebrachial vein Median cubital vein **C Basilic Vein, Left** *See B Basilic Vein, Right* **D Cephalic Vein, Right** Accessory cephalic vein **F Cephalic Vein, Left** *See D Cephalic Vein, Right* **G Hand Vein, Right** Dorsal metacarpal vein Palmar (volar) digital vein Palmar (volar) metacarpal vein Superficial palmar venous arch Volar (palmar) digital vein Volar (palmar) metacarpal vein **H Hand Vein, Left** *See G Hand Vein, Right* **L Intracranial Vein** Anterior cerebral vein Basal (internal) cerebral vein Dural venous sinus Great cerebral vein Inferior cerebellar vein Inferior cerebral vein Internal (basal) cerebral vein Middle cerebral vein Ophthalmic vein Superior cerebellar vein Superior cerebral vein **M Internal Jugular Vein, Right** **N Internal Jugular Vein, Left** **P External Jugular Vein, Right** Posterior auricular vein **Q External Jugular Vein, Left** *See P External Jugular Vein, Right* **R Vertebral Vein, Right** Deep cervical vein Suboccipital venous plexus **S Vertebral Vein, Left** *See R Vertebral Vein, Right* **T Face Vein, Right** Angular vein Anterior facial vein Common facial vein Deep facial vein Frontal vein Posterior facial (retromandibular) vein Supraorbital vein **V Face Vein, Left** *See T Face Vein, Right*	**Ø Open** **4 Percutaneous Endoscopic**	**7 Autologous Tissue Substitute** **9 Autologous Venous Tissue** **A Autologous Arterial Tissue** **J Synthetic Substitute** **K Nonautologous Tissue Substitute** **Z No Device**	**Y Upper Vein**

Ø Medical and Surgical
5 Upper Veins
5 Destruction Definition: Physical eradication of all or a portion of a body part by the direct use of energy, force, or a destructive agent

Explanation: None of the body part is physically taken out

Body Part Character 4	Approach Character 5	Device Character 6	Qualifier Character 7
Ø Azygos Vein Right ascending lumbar vein Right subcostal vein **1 Hemiazygos Vein** Left ascending lumbar vein Left subcostal vein **3 Innominate Vein, Right** Brachiocephalic vein Inferior thyroid vein **4 Innominate Vein, Left** *See 3 Innominate Vein, Right* **5 Subclavian Vein, Right** **6 Subclavian Vein, Left** **7 Axillary Vein, Right** **8 Axillary Vein, Left** **9 Brachial Vein, Right** Radial vein Ulnar vein **A Brachial Vein, Left** *See 9 Brachial Vein, Right* **B Basilic Vein, Right** Median antebrachial vein Median cubital vein **C Basilic Vein, Left** *See B Basilic Vein, Right* **D Cephalic Vein, Right** Accessory cephalic vein **F Cephalic Vein, Left** *See D Cephalic Vein, Right* **G Hand Vein, Right** Dorsal metacarpal vein Palmar (volar) digital vein Palmar (volar) metacarpal vein Superficial palmar venous arch Volar (palmar) digital vein Volar (palmar) metacarpal vein **H Hand Vein, Left** *See G Hand Vein, Right* **L Intracranial Vein** Anterior cerebral vein Basal (internal) cerebral vein Dural venous sinus Great cerebral vein Inferior cerebellar vein Inferior cerebral vein Internal (basal) cerebral vein Middle cerebral vein Ophthalmic vein Superior cerebellar vein Superior cerebral vein **M Internal Jugular Vein, Right** **N Internal Jugular Vein, Left** **P External Jugular Vein, Right** Posterior auricular vein **Q External Jugular Vein, Left** *See P External Jugular Vein, Right* **R Vertebral Vein, Right** Deep cervical vein Suboccipital venous plexus **S Vertebral Vein, Left** *See R Vertebral Vein, Right* **T Face Vein, Right** Angular vein Anterior facial vein Common facial vein Deep facial vein Frontal vein Posterior facial (retromandibular) vein Supraorbital vein **V Face Vein, Left** *See T Face Vein, Right* **Y Upper Vein**	**Ø Open** **3 Percutaneous** **4 Percutaneous Endoscopic**	**Z No Device**	**Z No Qualifier**

Ø Medical and Surgical
5 Upper Veins
7 Dilation

Definition: Expanding an orifice or the lumen of a tubular body part

Explanation: The orifice can be a natural orifice or an artificially created orifice. Accomplished by stretching a tubular body part using intraluminal pressure or by cutting part of the orifice or wall of the tubular body part.

Body Part Character 4	Approach Character 5	Device Character 6	Qualifier Character 7
Ø Azygos Vein Right ascending lumbar vein Right subcostal vein **1 Hemiazygos Vein** Left ascending lumbar vein Left subcostal vein **G Hand Vein, Right** Dorsal metacarpal vein Palmar (volar) digital vein Palmar (volar) metacarpal vein Superficial palmar venous arch Volar (palmar) digital vein Volar (palmar) metacarpal vein **H Hand Vein, Left** *See G Hand Vein, Right* **L Intracranial Vein** NC Anterior cerebral vein Basal (internal) cerebral vein Dural venous sinus Great cerebral vein Inferior cerebellar vein Inferior cerebral vein Internal (basal) cerebral vein Middle cerebral vein Ophthalmic vein Superior cerebellar vein Superior cerebral vein **M Internal Jugular Vein, Right** **N Internal Jugular Vein, Left** **P External Jugular Vein, Right** Posterior auricular vein **Q External Jugular Vein, Left** *See P External Jugular Vein, Right* **R Vertebral Vein, Right** Deep cervical vein Suboccipital venous plexus **S Vertebral Vein, Left** *See R Vertebral Vein, Right* **T Face Vein, Right** Angular vein Anterior facial vein Common facial vein Deep facial vein Frontal vein Posterior facial (retromandibular) vein Supraorbital vein **V Face Vein, Left** *See T Face Vein, Right* **Y Upper Vein**	**Ø Open** **3 Percutaneous** **4 Percutaneous Endoscopic**	**D Intraluminal Device** **Z No Device**	**Z No Qualifier**
3 Innominate Vein, Right Brachiocephalic vein Inferior thyroid vein **4 Innominate Vein, Left** *See 3 Innominate Vein, Right* **5 Subclavian Vein, Right** **6 Subclavian Vein, Left** **7 Axillary Vein, Right** **8 Axillary Vein, Left** **9 Brachial Vein, Right** Radial vein Ulnar vein **A Brachial Vein, Left** *See 9 Brachial Vein, Right* **B Basilic Vein, Right** Median antebrachial vein Median cubital vein **C Basilic Vein, Left** *See B Basilic Vein, Right* **D Cephalic Vein, Right** Accessory cephalic vein **F Cephalic Vein, Left** *See D Cephalic Vein, Right*	**Ø Open** **3 Percutaneous** **4 Percutaneous Endoscopic**	**D Intraluminal Device** **Z No Device**	**1 Drug-Coated Balloon** **Z No Qualifier**

NC Ø57L[3,4]ZZ

Ø Medical and Surgical
5 Upper Veins
9 Drainage

Definition: Taking or letting out fluids and/or gases from a body part

Explanation: The qualifier DIAGNOSTIC is used to identify drainage procedures that are biopsies

Body Part Character 4	Approach Character 5	Device Character 6	Qualifier Character 7
Ø Azygos Vein Right ascending lumbar vein Right subcostal vein **1 Hemiazygos Vein** Left ascending lumbar vein Left subcostal vein **3 Innominate Vein, Right** Brachiocephalic vein Inferior thyroid vein **4 Innominate Vein, Left** *See 3 Innominate Vein, Right* **5 Subclavian Vein, Right** **6 Subclavian Vein, Left** **7 Axillary Vein, Right** **8 Axillary Vein, Left** **9 Brachial Vein, Right** Radial vein Ulnar vein **A Brachial Vein, Left** *See 9 Brachial Vein, Right* **B Basilic Vein, Right** Median antebrachial vein Median cubital vein **C Basilic Vein, Left** *See B Basilic Vein, Right* **D Cephalic Vein, Right** Accessory cephalic vein **F Cephalic Vein, Left** *See D Cephalic Vein, Right* **G Hand Vein, Right** Dorsal metacarpal vein Palmar (volar) digital vein Palmar (volar) metacarpal vein Superficial palmar venous arch Volar (palmar) digital vein Volar (palmar) metacarpal vein **H Hand Vein, Left** *See G Hand Vein, Right* **L Intracranial Vein** Anterior cerebral vein Basal (internal) cerebral vein Dural venous sinus Great cerebral vein Inferior cerebellar vein Inferior cerebral vein Internal (basal) cerebral vein Middle cerebral vein Ophthalmic vein Superior cerebellar vein Superior cerebral vein **M Internal Jugular Vein, Right** **N Internal Jugular Vein, Left** **P External Jugular Vein, Right** Posterior auricular vein **Q External Jugular Vein, Left** *See P External Jugular Vein, Right* **R Vertebral Vein, Right** Deep cervical vein Suboccipital venous plexus **S Vertebral Vein, Left** *See R Vertebral Vein, Right* **T Face Vein, Right** Angular vein Anterior facial vein Common facial vein Deep facial vein Frontal vein Posterior facial (retromandibular) vein Supraorbital vein **V Face Vein, Left** *See T Face Vein, Right* **Y Upper Vein**	**Ø** Open **3** Percutaneous **4** Percutaneous Endoscopic	**Ø** Drainage Device	**Z** No Qualifier
Ø Azygos Vein Right ascending lumbar vein Right subcostal vein **1 Hemiazygos Vein** Left ascending lumbar vein Left subcostal vein **3 Innominate Vein, Right** Brachiocephalic vein Inferior thyroid vein **4 Innominate Vein, Left** *See 3 Innominate Vein, Right* **5 Subclavian Vein, Right** **6 Subclavian Vein, Left** **7 Axillary Vein, Right** **8 Axillary Vein, Left** **9 Brachial Vein, Right** Radial vein Ulnar vein **A Brachial Vein, Left** *See 9 Brachial Vein, Right* **B Basilic Vein, Right** Median antebrachial vein Median cubital vein **C Basilic Vein, Left** *See B Basilic Vein, Right* **D Cephalic Vein, Right** Accessory cephalic vein **F Cephalic Vein, Left** *See D Cephalic Vein, Right* **G Hand Vein, Right** Dorsal metacarpal vein Palmar (volar) digital vein Palmar (volar) metacarpal vein Superficial palmar venous arch Volar (palmar) digital vein Volar (palmar) metacarpal vein **H Hand Vein, Left** *See G Hand Vein, Right* **L Intracranial Vein** Anterior cerebral vein Basal (internal) cerebral vein Dural venous sinus Great cerebral vein Inferior cerebellar vein Inferior cerebral vein Internal (basal) cerebral vein Middle cerebral vein Ophthalmic vein Superior cerebellar vein Superior cerebral vein **M Internal Jugular Vein, Right** **N Internal Jugular Vein, Left** **P External Jugular Vein, Right** Posterior auricular vein **Q External Jugular Vein, Left** *See P External Jugular Vein, Right* **R Vertebral Vein, Right** Deep cervical vein Suboccipital venous plexus **S Vertebral Vein, Left** *See R Vertebral Vein, Right* **T Face Vein, Right** Angular vein Anterior facial vein Common facial vein Deep facial vein Frontal vein Posterior facial (retromandibular) vein Supraorbital vein **V Face Vein, Left** *See T Face Vein, Right* **Y Upper Vein**	**Ø** Open **3** Percutaneous **4** Percutaneous Endoscopic	**Z** No Device	**X** Diagnostic **Z** No Qualifier

Non-OR Ø59[Ø,1,3,4,5,6,7,8,9,A,B,C,D,F,G,H,L,M,N,P,Q,R,S,T,V,Y][Ø,3,4]ØZ
Non-OR Ø59[Ø,1,3,4,5,6,7,8,9,A,B,C,D,F,G,H,L,M,N,P,Q,R,S,T,V,Y]3ZX
Non-OR Ø59[Ø,1,3,4,5,6,7,8,9,A,B,C,D,F,G,H,L,M,N,P,Q,R,S,T,V,Y][Ø,3,4]ZZ

Ø Medical and Surgical
5 Upper Veins
B Excision

Definition: Cutting out or off, without replacement, a portion of a body part

Explanation: The qualifier DIAGNOSTIC is used to identify excision procedures that are biopsies

Body Part Character 4	Approach Character 5	Device Character 6	Qualifier Character 7
Ø Azygos Vein Right ascending lumbar vein Right subcostal vein **1 Hemiazygos Vein** Left ascending lumbar vein Left subcostal vein **3 Innominate Vein, Right** Brachiocephalic vein Inferior thyroid vein **4 Innominate Vein, Left** *See 3 Innominate Vein, Right* **5 Subclavian Vein, Right** **6 Subclavian Vein, Left** **7 Axillary Vein, Right** **8 Axillary Vein, Left** **9 Brachial Vein, Right** Radial vein Ulnar vein **A Brachial Vein, Left** *See 9 Brachial Vein, Right* **B Basilic Vein, Right** Median antebrachial vein Median cubital vein **C Basilic Vein, Left** *See B Basilic Vein, Right* **D Cephalic Vein, Right** Accessory cephalic vein **F Cephalic Vein, Left** *See D Cephalic Vein, Right* **G Hand Vein, Right** Dorsal metacarpal vein Palmar (volar) digital vein Palmar (volar) metacarpal vein Superficial palmar venous arch Volar (palmar) digital vein Volar (palmar) metacarpal vein **H Hand Vein, Left** *See G Hand Vein, Right* **L Intracranial Vein** Anterior cerebral vein Basal (internal) cerebral vein Dural venous sinus Great cerebral vein Inferior cerebellar vein Inferior cerebral vein Internal (basal) cerebral vein Middle cerebral vein Ophthalmic vein Superior cerebellar vein Superior cerebral vein **M Internal Jugular Vein, Right** **N Internal Jugular Vein, Left** **P External Jugular Vein, Right** Posterior auricular vein **Q External Jugular Vein, Left** *See P External Jugular Vein, Right* **R Vertebral Vein, Right** Deep cervical vein Suboccipital venous plexus **S Vertebral Vein, Left** *See R Vertebral Vein, Right* **T Face Vein, Right** Angular vein Anterior facial vein Common facial vein Deep facial vein Frontal vein Posterior facial (retromandibular) vein Supraorbital vein **V Face Vein, Left** *See T Face Vein, Right* **Y Upper Vein**	**Ø Open** **3 Percutaneous** **4 Percutaneous Endoscopic**	**Z No Device**	**X Diagnostic** **Z No Qualifier**

Ø Medical and Surgical
5 Upper Veins
C Extirpation Definition: Taking or cutting out solid matter from a body part

Explanation: The solid matter may be an abnormal byproduct of a biological function or a foreign body; it may be imbedded in a body part or in the lumen of a tubular body part. The solid matter may or may not have been previously broken into pieces.

Body Part Character 4	Approach Character 5	Device Character 6	Qualifier Character 7
Ø Azygos Vein Right ascending lumbar vein Right subcostal vein **1 Hemiazygos Vein** Left ascending lumbar vein Left subcostal vein **3 Innominate Vein, Right** Brachiocephalic vein Inferior thyroid vein **4 Innominate Vein, Left** *See 3 Innominate Vein, Right* **5 Subclavian Vein, Right** **6 Subclavian Vein, Left** **7 Axillary Vein, Right** **8 Axillary Vein, Left** **9 Brachial Vein, Right** Radial vein Ulnar vein **A Brachial Vein, Left** *See 9 Brachial Vein, Right* **B Basilic Vein, Right** Median antebrachial vein Median cubital vein **C Basilic Vein, Left** *See B Basilic Vein, Right* **D Cephalic Vein, Right** Accessory cephalic vein **F Cephalic Vein, Left** *See D Cephalic Vein, Right* **G Hand Vein, Right** Dorsal metacarpal vein Palmar (volar) digital vein Palmar (volar) metacarpal vein Superficial palmar venous arch Volar (palmar) digital vein Volar (palmar) metacarpal vein **H Hand Vein, Left** *See G Hand Vein, Right* **L Intracranial Vein** Anterior cerebral vein Basal (internal) cerebral vein Dural venous sinus Great cerebral vein Inferior cerebellar vein Inferior cerebral vein Internal (basal) cerebral vein Middle cerebral vein Ophthalmic vein Superior cerebellar vein Superior cerebral vein **M Internal Jugular Vein, Right** **N Internal Jugular Vein, Left** **P External Jugular Vein, Right** Posterior auricular vein **Q External Jugular Vein, Left** *See P External Jugular Vein, Right* **R Vertebral Vein, Right** Deep cervical vein Suboccipital venous plexus **S Vertebral Vein, Left** *See R Vertebral Vein, Right* **T Face Vein, Right** Angular vein Anterior facial vein Common facial vein Deep facial vein Frontal vein Posterior facial (retromandibular) vein Supraorbital vein **V Face Vein, Left** *See T Face Vein, Right* **Y Upper Vein**	**Ø Open** **3 Percutaneous** **4 Percutaneous Endoscopic**	**Z No Device**	**Z No Qualifier**

Ø Medical and Surgical
5 Upper Veins
D Extraction Definition: Pulling or stripping out or off all or a portion of a body part by the use of force

Explanation: The qualifier DIAGNOSTIC is used to identify extraction procedures that are biopsies

Body Part Character 4	Approach Character 5	Device Character 6	Qualifier Character 7
9 Brachial Vein, Right Radial vein Ulnar vein **A Brachial Vein, Left** *See 9 Brachial Vein, Right* **B Basilic Vein, Right** Median antebrachial vein Median cubital vein **C Basilic Vein, Left** *See B Basilic Vein, Right* **D Cephalic Vein, Right** Accessory cephalic vein **F Cephalic Vein, Left** *See D Cephalic Vein, Right* **G Hand Vein, Right** Dorsal metacarpal vein Palmar (volar) digital vein Palmar (volar) metacarpal vein Superficial palmar venous arch Volar (palmar) digital vein Volar (palmar) metacarpal vein **H Hand Vein, Left** *See G Hand Vein, Right* **Y Upper Vein**	**Ø Open** **3 Percutaneous**	**Z No Device**	**Z No Qualifier**

Ø Medical and Surgical
5 Upper Veins
F Fragmentation Definition: Breaking solid matter in a body part into pieces

Explanation: Physical force (e.g., manual, ultrasonic) applied directly or indirectly is used to break the solid matter into pieces. The solid matter may be an abnormal byproduct of a biological function or a foreign body. The pieces of solid matter are not taken out.

Body Part Character 4	Approach Character 5	Device Character 6	Qualifier Character 7
3 Innominate Vein, Right Brachiocephalic vein Inferior thyroid vein **4 Innominate Vein, Left** *See 3 Innominate Vein, Right* **5 Subclavian Vein, Right** **6 Subclavian Vein, Left** **7 Axillary Vein, Right** **8 Axillary Vein, Left** **9 Brachial Vein, Right** Radial vein Ulnar vein **A Brachial Vein, Left** *See 9 Brachial Vein, Right* **B Basilic Vein, Right** Median antebrachial vein Median cubital vein **C Basilic Vein, Left** *See B Basilic Vein, Right* **D Cephalic Vein, Right** Accessory cephalic vein **F Cephalic Vein, Left** *See D Cephalic Vein, Right* **Y Upper Vein**	**3 Percutaneous**	**Z No Device**	**Ø Ultrasonic** **Z No Qualifier**

Ø Medical and Surgical
5 Upper Veins
H Insertion

Definition: Putting in a nonbiological appliance that monitors, assists, performs, or prevents a physiological function but does not physically take the place of a body part

Explanation: None

Body Part Character 4	Approach Character 5	Device Character 6	Qualifier Character 7
Ø Azygos Vein ⊞ Right ascending lumbar vein Right subcostal vein	**Ø** Open **3** Percutaneous **4** Percutaneous Endoscopic	**2** Monitoring Device **3** Infusion Device **D** Intraluminal Device **M** Neurostimulator Lead	**Z** No Qualifier
1 Hemiazygos Vein Left ascending lumbar vein Left subcostal vein **5 Subclavian Vein, Right** **6 Subclavian Vein, Left** **7 Axillary Vein, Right** **8 Axillary Vein, Left** **9 Brachial Vein, Right** Radial vein Ulnar vein **A Brachial Vein, Left** *See 9 Brachial Vein, Right* **B Basilic Vein, Right** Median antebrachial vein Median cubital vein **C Basilic Vein, Left** *See B Basilic Vein, Right* **D Cephalic Vein, Right** Accessory cephalic vein **F Cephalic Vein, Left** *See D Cephalic Vein, Right* **G Hand Vein, Right** Dorsal metacarpal vein Palmar (volar) digital vein Palmar (volar) metacarpal vein Superficial palmar venous arch Volar (palmar) digital vein Volar (palmar) metacarpal vein **H Hand Vein, Left** *See G Hand Vein, Right* **L Intracranial Vein** Anterior cerebral vein Basal (internal) cerebral vein Dural venous sinus Great cerebral vein Inferior cerebellar vein Inferior cerebral vein Internal (basal) cerebral vein Middle cerebral vein Ophthalmic vein Superior cerebellar vein Superior cerebral vein **M Internal Jugular Vein, Right** **N Internal Jugular Vein, Left** **P External Jugular Vein, Right** Posterior auricular vein **Q External Jugular Vein, Left** *See P External Jugular Vein, Right* **R Vertebral Vein, Right** Deep cervical vein Suboccipital venous plexus **S Vertebral Vein, Left** *See R Vertebral Vein, Right* **T Face Vein, Right** Angular vein Anterior facial vein Common facial vein Deep facial vein Frontal vein Posterior facial (retromandibular) vein Supraorbital vein **V Face Vein, Left** *See T Face Vein, Right*	**Ø** Open **3** Percutaneous **4** Percutaneous Endoscopic	**3** Infusion Device **D** Intraluminal Device	**Z** No Qualifier
3 Innominate Vein, Right ⊞ Brachiocephalic vein Inferior thyroid vein **4 Innominate Vein, Left** ⊞ *See 3 Innominate Vein, Right*	**Ø** Open **3** Percutaneous **4** Percutaneous Endoscopic	**3** Infusion Device **D** Intraluminal Device **M** Neurostimulator Lead	**Z** No Qualifier
Y Upper Vein	**Ø** Open **3** Percutaneous **4** Percutaneous Endoscopic	**2** Monitoring Device **3** Infusion Device **D** Intraluminal Device **Y** Other Device	**Z** No Qualifier

Non-OR Ø5HØ[Ø,3,4]3Z
Non-OR Ø5H[1,5,6,7,8,9,A,B,C,D,F,G,H,L,M,N,P,Q,R,S,T,V][Ø,3,4]3Z
Non-OR Ø5H[3,4][Ø,3,4]3Z
Non-OR Ø5HY[Ø,3,4]3Z
Non-OR Ø5HY32Z
Non-OR Ø5HY[3,4]YZ
HAC Ø5HØ[3,4]3Z when reported with SDx J95.811
HAC Ø5H[1,5,6][3,4]3Z when reported with SDx J95.811
HAC Ø5H[M,N,P,Q]33Z when reported with SDx J95.811
HAC Ø5H[3,4][3,4]3Z when reported with SDx J95.811

See Appendix L for Procedure Combinations
⊞ Ø5HØ[Ø,3,4]MZ
⊞ Ø5H[3,4][Ø,3,4]MZ

Ø Medical and Surgical
5 Upper Veins
J Inspection

Definition: Visually and/or manually exploring a body part

Explanation: Visual exploration may be performed with or without optical instrumentation. Manual exploration may be performed directly or through intervening body layers.

Body Part Character 4	Approach Character 5	Device Character 6	Qualifier Character 7
Y Upper Vein	**Ø** Open **3** Percutaneous **4** Percutaneous Endoscopic **X** External	**Z** No Device	**Z** No Qualifier

Non-OR Ø5JY[3,X]ZZ

Ø Medical and Surgical
5 Upper Veins
L Occlusion

Definition: Completely closing an orifice or the lumen of a tubular body part
Explanation: The orifice can be a natural orifice or an artificially created orifice

Body Part Character 4	Approach Character 5	Device Character 6	Qualifier Character 7
Ø Azygos Vein Right ascending lumbar vein Right subcostal vein **1 Hemiazygos Vein** Left ascending lumbar vein Left subcostal vein **3 Innominate Vein, Right** Brachiocephalic vein Inferior thyroid vein **4 Innominate Vein, Left** *See 3 Innominate Vein, Right* **5 Subclavian Vein, Right** **6 Subclavian Vein, Left** **7 Axillary Vein, Right** **8 Axillary Vein, Left** **9 Brachial Vein, Right** Radial vein Ulnar vein **A Brachial Vein, Left** *See 9 Brachial Vein, Right* **B Basilic Vein, Right** Median antebrachial vein Median cubital vein **C Basilic Vein, Left** *See B Basilic Vein, Right* **D Cephalic Vein, Right** Accessory cephalic vein **F Cephalic Vein, Left** *See D Cephalic Vein, Right* **G Hand Vein, Right** Dorsal metacarpal vein Palmar (volar) digital vein Palmar (volar) metacarpal vein Superficial palmar venous arch Volar (palmar) digital vein Volar (palmar) metacarpal vein **H Hand Vein, Left** *See G Hand Vein, Right* **L Intracranial Vein** Anterior cerebral vein Basal (internal) cerebral vein Dural venous sinus Great cerebral vein Inferior cerebellar vein Inferior cerebral vein Internal (basal) cerebral vein Middle cerebral vein Ophthalmic vein Superior cerebellar vein Superior cerebral vein **M Internal Jugular Vein, Right** **N Internal Jugular Vein, Left** **P External Jugular Vein, Right** Posterior auricular vein **Q External Jugular Vein, Left** *See P External Jugular Vein, Right* **R Vertebral Vein, Right** Deep cervical vein Suboccipital venous plexus **S Vertebral Vein, Left** *See R Vertebral Vein, Right* **T Face Vein, Right** Angular vein Anterior facial vein Common facial vein Deep facial vein Frontal vein Posterior facial (retromandibular) vein Supraorbital vein **V Face Vein, Left** *See T Face Vein, Right* **Y Upper Vein**	**Ø Open** **3 Percutaneous** **4 Percutaneous Endoscopic**	**C Extraluminal Device** **D Intraluminal Device** **Z No Device**	**Z No Qualifier**

Ø Medical and Surgical
5 Upper Veins
N Release

Definition: Freeing a body part from an abnormal physical constraint by cutting or by the use of force
Explanation: Some of the restraining tissue may be taken out but none of the body part is taken out

Body Part Character 4	Approach Character 5	Device Character 6	Qualifier Character 7
Ø Azygos Vein Right ascending lumbar vein Right subcostal vein **1 Hemiazygos Vein** Left ascending lumbar vein Left subcostal vein **3 Innominate Vein, Right** Brachiocephalic vein Inferior thyroid vein **4 Innominate Vein, Left** *See 3 Innominate Vein, Right* **5 Subclavian Vein, Right** **6 Subclavian Vein, Left** **7 Axillary Vein, Right** **8 Axillary Vein, Left** **9 Brachial Vein, Right** Radial vein Ulnar vein **A Brachial Vein, Left** *See 9 Brachial Vein, Right* **B Basilic Vein, Right** Median antebrachial vein Median cubital vein **C Basilic Vein, Left** *See B Basilic Vein, Right* **D Cephalic Vein, Right** Accessory cephalic vein **F Cephalic Vein, Left** *See D Cephalic Vein, Right* **G Hand Vein, Right** Dorsal metacarpal vein Palmar (volar) digital vein Palmar (volar) metacarpal vein Superficial palmar venous arch Volar (palmar) digital vein Volar (palmar) metacarpal vein **H Hand Vein, Left** *See G Hand Vein, Right* **L Intracranial Vein** Anterior cerebral vein Basal (internal) cerebral vein Dural venous sinus Great cerebral vein Inferior cerebellar vein Inferior cerebral vein Internal (basal) cerebral vein Middle cerebral vein Ophthalmic vein Superior cerebellar vein Superior cerebral vein **M Internal Jugular Vein, Right** **N Internal Jugular Vein, Left** **P External Jugular Vein, Right** Posterior auricular vein **Q External Jugular Vein, Left** *See P External Jugular Vein, Right* **R Vertebral Vein, Right** Deep cervical vein Suboccipital venous plexus **S Vertebral Vein, Left** *See R Vertebral Vein, Right* **T Face Vein, Right** Angular vein Anterior facial vein Common facial vein Deep facial vein Frontal vein Posterior facial (retromandibular) vein Supraorbital vein **V Face Vein, Left** *See T Face Vein, Right* **Y Upper Vein**	**Ø Open** **3 Percutaneous** **4 Percutaneous Endoscopic**	**Z No Device**	**Z No Qualifier**

Ø Medical and Surgical
5 Upper Veins
P Removal

Definition: Taking out or off a device from a body part

Explanation: If a device is taken out and a similar device put in without cutting or puncturing the skin or mucous membrane, the procedure is coded to the root operation CHANGE. Otherwise, the procedure for taking out a device is coded to the root operation REMOVAL.

Body Part Character 4	Approach Character 5	Device Character 6	Qualifier Character 7
Ø Azygos Vein Right ascending lumbar vein Right subcostal vein	**Ø Open** **3 Percutaneous** **4 Percutaneous Endoscopic** **X External**	**2 Monitoring Device** **M Neurostimulator Lead**	**Z No Qualifier**
3 Innominate Vein, Right Brachiocephalic vein Inferior thyroid vein **4 Innominate Vein, Left** *See 3 Innominate Vein, Right*	**Ø Open** **3 Percutaneous** **4 Percutaneous Endoscopic** **X External**	**M Neurostimulator Lead**	**Z No Qualifier**
Y Upper Vein	**Ø Open** **3 Percutaneous** **4 Percutaneous Endoscopic**	**Ø Drainage Device** **2 Monitoring Device** **3 Infusion Device** **7 Autologous Tissue Substitute** **C Extraluminal Device** **D Intraluminal Device** **J Synthetic Substitute** **K Nonautologous Tissue Substitute** **Y Other Device**	**Z No Qualifier**
Y Upper Vein	**X External**	**Ø Drainage Device** **2 Monitoring Device** **3 Infusion Device** **D Intraluminal Device**	**Z No Qualifier**

Non-OR Ø5PØ[Ø,3,4,X]2Z
Non-OR Ø5PY3[Ø,2,3]Z
Non-OR Ø5PY[3,4]YZ
Non-OR Ø5PYX[Ø,2,3,D]Z

Ø Medical and Surgical
5 Upper Veins
Q Repair Definition: Restoring, to the extent possible, a body part to its normal anatomic structure and function
Explanation: Used only when the method to accomplish the repair is not one of the other root operations

Body Part Character 4	Approach Character 5	Device Character 6	Qualifier Character 7
Ø Azygos Vein Right ascending lumbar vein Right subcostal vein **1 Hemiazygos Vein** Left ascending lumbar vein Left subcostal vein **3 Innominate Vein, Right** Brachiocephalic vein Inferior thyroid vein **4 Innominate Vein, Left** *See 3 Innominate Vein, Right* **5 Subclavian Vein, Right** **6 Subclavian Vein, Left** **7 Axillary Vein, Right** **8 Axillary Vein, Left** **9 Brachial Vein, Right** Radial vein Ulnar vein **A Brachial Vein, Left** *See 9 Brachial Vein, Right* **B Basilic Vein, Right** Median antebrachial vein Median cubital vein **C Basilic Vein, Left** *See B Basilic Vein, Right* **D Cephalic Vein, Right** Accessory cephalic vein **F Cephalic Vein, Left** *See D Cephalic Vein, Right* **G Hand Vein, Right** Dorsal metacarpal vein Palmar (volar) digital vein Palmar (volar) metacarpal vein Superficial palmar venous arch Volar (palmar) digital vein Volar (palmar) metacarpal vein **H Hand Vein, Left** *See G Hand Vein, Right* **L Intracranial Vein** Anterior cerebral vein Basal (internal) cerebral vein Dural venous sinus Great cerebral vein Inferior cerebellar vein Inferior cerebral vein Internal (basal) cerebral vein Middle cerebral vein Ophthalmic vein Superior cerebellar vein Superior cerebral vein **M Internal Jugular Vein, Right** **N Internal Jugular Vein, Left** **P External Jugular Vein, Right** Posterior auricular vein **Q External Jugular Vein, Left** *See P External Jugular Vein, Right* **R Vertebral Vein, Right** Deep cervical vein Suboccipital venous plexus **S Vertebral Vein, Left** *See R Vertebral Vein, Right* **T Face Vein, Right** Angular vein Anterior facial vein Common facial vein Deep facial vein Frontal vein Posterior facial (retromandibular) vein Supraorbital vein **V Face Vein, Left** *See T Face Vein, Right* **Y Upper Vein**	**Ø Open** **3 Percutaneous** **4 Percutaneous Endoscopic**	**Z No Device**	**Z No Qualifier**

Ø Medical and Surgical
5 Upper Veins
R Replacement Definition: Putting in or on biological or synthetic material that physically takes the place and/or function of all or a portion of a body part

Explanation: The body part may have been taken out or replaced, or may be taken out, physically eradicated, or rendered nonfunctional during the REPLACEMENT procedure. A REMOVAL procedure is coded for taking out the device used in a previous replacement procedure.

Body Part Character 4	Approach Character 5	Device Character 6	Qualifier Character 7
Ø Azygos Vein Right ascending lumbar vein Right subcostal vein **1 Hemiazygos Vein** Left ascending lumbar vein Left subcostal vein **3 Innominate Vein, Right** Brachiocephalic vein Inferior thyroid vein **4 Innominate Vein, Left** *See 3 Innominate Vein, Right* **5 Subclavian Vein, Right** **6 Subclavian Vein, Left** **7 Axillary Vein, Right** **8 Axillary Vein, Left** **9 Brachial Vein, Right** Radial vein Ulnar vein **A Brachial Vein, Left** *See 9 Brachial Vein, Right* **B Basilic Vein, Right** Median antebrachial vein Median cubital vein **C Basilic Vein, Left** *See B Basilic Vein, Right* **D Cephalic Vein, Right** Accessory cephalic vein **F Cephalic Vein, Left** *See D Cephalic Vein, Right* **G Hand Vein, Right** Dorsal metacarpal vein Palmar (volar) digital vein Palmar (volar) metacarpal vein Superficial palmar venous arch Volar (palmar) digital vein Volar (palmar) metacarpal vein **H Hand Vein, Left** *See G Hand Vein, Right* **L Intracranial Vein** Anterior cerebral vein Basal (internal) cerebral vein Dural venous sinus Great cerebral vein Inferior cerebellar vein Inferior cerebral vein Internal (basal) cerebral vein Middle cerebral vein Ophthalmic vein Superior cerebellar vein Superior cerebral vein **M Internal Jugular Vein, Right** **N Internal Jugular Vein, Left** **P External Jugular Vein, Right** Posterior auricular vein **Q External Jugular Vein, Left** *See P External Jugular Vein, Right* **R Vertebral Vein, Right** Deep cervical vein Suboccipital venous plexus **S Vertebral Vein, Left** *See R Vertebral Vein, Right* **T Face Vein, Right** Angular vein Anterior facial vein Common facial vein Deep facial vein Frontal vein Posterior facial (retromandibular) vein Supraorbital vein **V Face Vein, Left** *See T Face Vein, Right* **Y Upper Vein**	**Ø Open** **4 Percutaneous Endoscopic**	**7 Autologous Tissue Substitute** **J Synthetic Substitute** **K Nonautologous Tissue Substitute**	**Z No Qualifier**

Ø Medical and Surgical
5 Upper Veins
S Reposition

Definition: Moving to its normal location, or other suitable location, all or a portion of a body part

Explanation: The body part is moved to a new location from an abnormal location, or from a normal location where it is not functioning correctly. The body part may or may not be cut out or off to be moved to the new location.

Body Part Character 4	Approach Character 5	Device Character 6	Qualifier Character 7
Ø Azygos Vein Right ascending lumbar vein Right subcostal vein **1 Hemiazygos Vein** Left ascending lumbar vein Left subcostal vein **3 Innominate Vein, Right** Brachiocephalic vein Inferior thyroid vein **4 Innominate Vein, Left** *See 3 Innominate Vein, Right* **5 Subclavian Vein, Right** **6 Subclavian Vein, Left** **7 Axillary Vein, Right** **8 Axillary Vein, Left** **9 Brachial Vein, Right** Radial vein Ulnar vein **A Brachial Vein, Left** *See 9 Brachial Vein, Right* **B Basilic Vein, Right** Median antebrachial vein Median cubital vein **C Basilic Vein, Left** *See B Basilic Vein, Right* **D Cephalic Vein, Right** Accessory cephalic vein **F Cephalic Vein, Left** *See D Cephalic Vein, Right* **G Hand Vein, Right** Dorsal metacarpal vein Palmar (volar) digital vein Palmar (volar) metacarpal vein Superficial palmar venous arch Volar (palmar) digital vein Volar (palmar) metacarpal vein **H Hand Vein, Left** *See G Hand Vein, Right* **L Intracranial Vein** Anterior cerebral vein Basal (internal) cerebral vein Dural venous sinus Great cerebral vein Inferior cerebellar vein Inferior cerebral vein Internal (basal) cerebral vein Middle cerebral vein Ophthalmic vein Superior cerebellar vein Superior cerebral vein **M Internal Jugular Vein, Right** **N Internal Jugular Vein, Left** **P External Jugular Vein, Right** Posterior auricular vein **Q External Jugular Vein, Left** *See P External Jugular Vein, Right* **R Vertebral Vein, Right** Deep cervical vein Suboccipital venous plexus **S Vertebral Vein, Left** *See R Vertebral Vein, Right* **T Face Vein, Right** Angular vein Anterior facial vein Common facial vein Deep facial vein Frontal vein Posterior facial (retromandibular) vein Supraorbital vein **V Face Vein, Left** *See T Face Vein, Right* **Y Upper Vein**	**Ø Open** **3 Percutaneous** **4 Percutaneous Endoscopic**	**Z No Device**	**Z No Qualifier**

Ø Medical and Surgical
5 Upper Veins
U Supplement Definition: Putting in or on biological or synthetic material that physically reinforces and/or augments the function of a portion of a body part

Explanation: The biological material is non-living, or is living and from the same individual. The body part may have been previously replaced, and the SUPPLEMENT procedure is performed to physically reinforce and/or augment the function of the replaced body part.

Body Part Character 4	Approach Character 5	Device Character 6	Qualifier Character 7
Ø Azygos Vein Right ascending lumbar vein Right subcostal vein **1 Hemiazygos Vein** Left ascending lumbar vein Left subcostal vein **3 Innominate Vein, Right** Brachiocephalic vein Inferior thyroid vein **4 Innominate Vein, Left** *See 3 Innominate Vein, Right* **5 Subclavian Vein, Right** **6 Subclavian Vein, Left** **7 Axillary Vein, Right** **8 Axillary Vein, Left** **9 Brachial Vein, Right** Radial vein Ulnar vein **A Brachial Vein, Left** *See 9 Brachial Vein, Right* **B Basilic Vein, Right** Median antebrachial vein Median cubital vein **C Basilic Vein, Left** *See B Basilic Vein, Right* **D Cephalic Vein, Right** Accessory cephalic vein **F Cephalic Vein, Left** *See D Cephalic Vein, Right* **G Hand Vein, Right** Dorsal metacarpal vein Palmar (volar) digital vein Palmar (volar) metacarpal vein Superficial palmar venous arch Volar (palmar) digital vein Volar (palmar) metacarpal vein **H Hand Vein, Left** *See G Hand Vein, Right* **L Intracranial Vein** Anterior cerebral vein Basal (internal) cerebral vein Dural venous sinus Great cerebral vein Inferior cerebellar vein Inferior cerebral vein Internal (basal) cerebral vein Middle cerebral vein Ophthalmic vein Superior cerebellar vein Superior cerebral vein **M Internal Jugular Vein, Right** **N Internal Jugular Vein, Left** **P External Jugular Vein, Right** Posterior auricular vein **Q External Jugular Vein, Left** *See P External Jugular Vein, Right* **R Vertebral Vein, Right** Deep cervical vein Suboccipital venous plexus **S Vertebral Vein, Left** *See R Vertebral Vein, Right* **T Face Vein, Right** Angular vein Anterior facial vein Common facial vein Deep facial vein Frontal vein Posterior facial (retromandibular) vein Supraorbital vein **V Face Vein, Left** *See T Face Vein, Right* **Y Upper Vein**	**Ø Open** **3 Percutaneous** **4 Percutaneous Endoscopic**	**7 Autologous Tissue Substitute** **J Synthetic Substitute** **K Nonautologous Tissue Substitute**	**Z No Qualifier**

Ø Medical and Surgical
5 Upper Veins
V Restriction Definition: Partially closing an orifice or the lumen of a tubular body part

Explanation: The orifice can be a natural orifice or an artificially created orifice

Body Part Character 4	Approach Character 5	Device Character 6	Qualifier Character 7
Ø Azygos Vein Right ascending lumbar vein Right subcostal vein **1 Hemiazygos Vein** Left ascending lumbar vein Left subcostal vein **3 Innominate Vein, Right** Brachiocephalic vein Inferior thyroid vein **4 Innominate Vein, Left** *See 3 Innominate Vein, Right* **5 Subclavian Vein, Right** **6 Subclavian Vein, Left** **7 Axillary Vein, Right** **8 Axillary Vein, Left** **9 Brachial Vein, Right** Radial vein Ulnar vein **A Brachial Vein, Left** *See 9 Brachial Vein, Right* **B Basilic Vein, Right** Median antebrachial vein Median cubital vein **C Basilic Vein, Left** *See B Basilic Vein, Right* **D Cephalic Vein, Right** Accessory cephalic vein **F Cephalic Vein, Left** *See D Cephalic Vein, Right* **G Hand Vein, Right** Dorsal metacarpal vein Palmar (volar) digital vein Palmar (volar) metacarpal vein Superficial palmar venous arch Volar (palmar) digital vein Volar (palmar) metacarpal vein **H Hand Vein, Left** *See G Hand Vein, Right* **L Intracranial Vein** Anterior cerebral vein Basal (internal) cerebral vein Dural venous sinus Great cerebral vein Inferior cerebellar vein Inferior cerebral vein Internal (basal) cerebral vein Middle cerebral vein Ophthalmic vein Superior cerebellar vein Superior cerebral vein **M Internal Jugular Vein, Right** **N Internal Jugular Vein, Left** **P External Jugular Vein, Right** Posterior auricular vein **Q External Jugular Vein, Left** *See P External Jugular Vein, Right* **R Vertebral Vein, Right** Deep cervical vein Suboccipital venous plexus **S Vertebral Vein, Left** *See R Vertebral Vein, Right* **T Face Vein, Right** Angular vein Anterior facial vein Common facial vein Deep facial vein Frontal vein Posterior facial (retromandibular) vein Supraorbital vein **V Face Vein, Left** *See T Face Vein, Right* **Y Upper Vein**	**Ø Open** **3 Percutaneous** **4 Percutaneous Endoscopic**	**C Extraluminal Device** **D Intraluminal Device** **Z No Device**	**Z No Qualifier**

Ø Medical and Surgical
5 Upper Veins
W Revision

Definition: Correcting, to the extent possible, a portion of a malfunctioning device or the position of a displaced device

Explanation: Revision can include correcting a malfunctioning or displaced device by taking out or putting in components of the device such as a screw or pin

Body Part Character 4	Approach Character 5	Device Character 6	Qualifier Character 7
Ø Azygos Vein Right ascending lumbar vein Right subcostal vein	**Ø Open** **3 Percutaneous** **4 Percutaneous Endoscopic** **X External**	**2 Monitoring Device** **M Neurostimulator Lead**	**Z No Qualifier**
3 Innominate Vein, Right Brachiocephalic vein Inferior thyroid vein **4 Innominate Vein, Left** *See* *3 Innominate Vein, Right*	**Ø Open** **3 Percutaneous** **4 Percutaneous Endoscopic** **X External**	**M Neurostimulator Lead**	**Z No Qualifier**
Y Upper Vein	**Ø Open** **3 Percutaneous** **4 Percutaneous Endoscopic**	**Ø Drainage Device** **2 Monitoring Device** **3 Infusion Device** **7 Autologous Tissue Substitute** **C Extraluminal Device** **D Intraluminal Device** **J Synthetic Substitute** **K Nonautologous Tissue Substitute** **Y Other Device**	**Z No Qualifier**
Y Upper Vein	**X External**	**Ø Drainage Device** **2 Monitoring Device** **3 Infusion Device** **7 Autologous Tissue Substitute** **C Extraluminal Device** **D Intraluminal Device** **J Synthetic Substitute** **K Nonautologous Tissue Substitute**	**Z No Qualifier**

Non-OR Ø5WØXMZ
Non-OR Ø5W[3,4]XMZ
Non-OR Ø5WY3[Ø,2,3]Z
Non-OR Ø5WY[3,4]YZ
Non-OR Ø5WYX[Ø,2,3,7,C,D,J,K]Z

Lower Veins Ø61–Ø6W

Character Meanings

This Character Meaning table is provided as a guide to assist the user in the identification of character members that may be found in this section of code tables. It **SHOULD NOT** be used to build a PCS code.

Operation–Character 3	Body Part–Character 4	Approach–Character 5	Device–Character 6	Qualifier–Character 7
1 Bypass	Ø Inferior Vena Cava	Ø Open	Ø Drainage Device	Ø Ultrasonic
5 Destruction	1 Splenic Vein	3 Percutaneous	2 Monitoring Device	4 Hepatic Vein
7 Dilation	2 Gastric Vein	4 Percutaneous Endoscopic	3 Infusion Device	5 Superior Mesenteric Vein
9 Drainage	3 Esophageal Vein	7 Via Natural or Artificial Opening	7 Autologous Tissue Substitute	6 Inferior Mesenteric Vein
B Excision	4 Hepatic Vein	8 Via Natural or Artificial Opening Endoscopic	9 Autologous Venous Tissue	9 Renal Vein, Right
C Extirpation	5 Superior Mesenteric Vein	X External	A Autologous Arterial Tissue	B Renal Vein, Left
D Extraction	6 Inferior Mesenteric Vein		C Extraluminal Device	C Hemorrhoidal Plexus
F Fragmentation	7 Colic Vein		D Intraluminal Device	P Pulmonary Trunk
H Insertion	8 Portal Vein		J Synthetic Substitute	Q Pulmonary Artery, Right
J Inspection	9 Renal Vein, Right		K Nonautologous Tissue Substitute	R Pulmonary Artery, Left
L Occlusion	B Renal Vein, Left		Y Other Device	T Via Umbilical Vein
N Release	C Common Iliac Vein, Right		Z No Device	X Diagnostic
P Removal	D Common Iliac Vein, Left			Y Lower Vein
Q Repair	F External Iliac Vein, Right			Z No Qualifier
R Replacement	G External Iliac Vein, Left			
S Reposition	H Hypogastric Vein, Right			
U Supplement	J Hypogastric Vein, Left			
V Restriction	M Femoral Vein, Right			
W Revision	N Femoral Vein, Left			
	P Saphenous Vein, Right			
	Q Saphenous Vein, Left			
	T Foot Vein, Right			
	V Foot Vein, Left			
	Y Lower Vein			

AHA Coding Clinic for Lower Veins

2022, 1Q, 10-13 Procedures performed on a continuous vessel, ICD-10-PCS Guideline B4.1c

AHA Coding Clinic for table Ø61

2017, 4Q, 36-38 Fontan completion procedure
2017, 4Q, 66-67 New qualifier values - Portal to hepatic shunt

AHA Coding Clinic for table Ø6B

2020, 1Q, 28 Free flap microvascular breast reconstruction
2017, 3Q, 5 Femoral artery to posterior tibial artery bypass using autologous and synthetic grafts
2017, 1Q, 31 Left to right common carotid artery bypass
2017, 1Q, 32 Peroneal artery to dorsalis pedis artery bypass using saphenous vein graft
2016, 3Q, 31 Femoral to peroneal artery bypass with in-situ saphenous vein graft and lysis of valves
2016, 2Q, 18 Femoral-tibial artery bypass and saphenous vein graft
2016, 1Q, 27 Aortocoronary bypass graft utilizing Y-graft
2014, 3Q, 8 Excision of saphenous vein for coronary artery bypass graft
2014, 3Q, 20 MAZE procedure performed with coronary artery bypass graft
2014, 1Q, 10 Repair of thoracic aortic aneurysm & coronary artery bypass graft

AHA Coding Clinic for table Ø6F

2020, 4Q, 45-49 New fragmentation tables
2020, 4Q, 49-50 Intravascular ultrasound assisted thrombolysis
2020, 4Q, 50 Intravascular lithotripsy

AHA Coding Clinic for table Ø6H

2021, 3Q, 18 Placement and removal of cannulas for extracorporeal membrane oxygenation
2017, 3Q, 11 Placement of peripherally inserted central catheter using 3CG ECG technology
2017, 1Q, 31 Umbilical vein catheterization
2017, 1Q, 31 Central catheter placement in femoral vein
2013, 3Q, 18 Heart transplant surgery

AHA Coding Clinic for table Ø6L

2021, 4Q, 47 Endoscopic banding of hemorrhoidal plexus
2021, 4Q, 49 Division of liver for staged hepatectomy
2020, 3Q, 44 Cardiophrenic vein embolization
2019, 4Q, 28 Transorifice occlusion of gastric varices
2018, 2Q, 18 Transverse rectus abdominis myocutaneous (TRAM) delay
2017, 4Q, 57-58 Added approach values - Transorifice esophageal vein banding
2013, 4Q, 112 Endoscopic banding of esophageal varices

AHA Coding Clinic for table Ø6P

2021, 3Q, 18 Placement and removal of cannulas for extracorporeal membrane oxygenation

AHA Coding Clinic for table Ø6V

2018, 3Q, 11 Transvenous transcatheter placement of valve in inferior vena cava
2018, 1Q, 10 Revision of transjugular intrahepatic portosystemic shunt

AHA Coding Clinic for table Ø6W

2019, 2Q, 39 Transjugular intrahepatic portosystemic shunt revision
2018, 1Q, 10 Revision of transjugular intrahepatic portosystemic shunt
2014, 3Q, 25 Revision of transjugular intrahepatic portosystemic shunt (TIPS)

Lower Veins

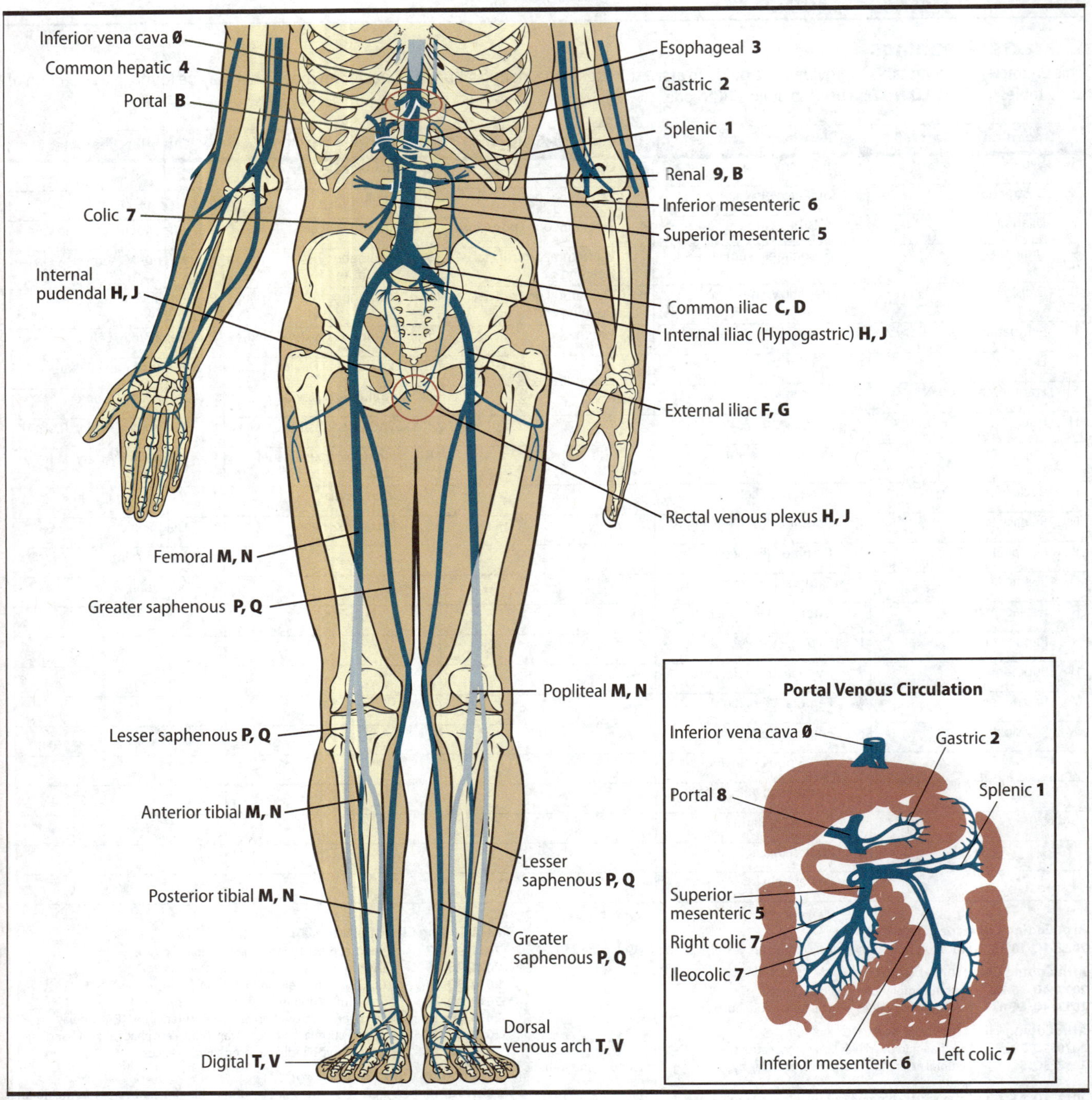

Inferior vena cava Ø
Common hepatic 4
Portal B
Colic 7
Internal pudendal H, J
Esophageal 3
Gastric 2
Splenic 1
Renal 9, B
Inferior mesenteric 6
Superior mesenteric 5
Common iliac C, D
Internal iliac (Hypogastric) H, J
External iliac F, G
Rectal venous plexus H, J
Femoral M, N
Greater saphenous P, Q
Popliteal M, N
Lesser saphenous P, Q
Anterior tibial M, N
Lesser saphenous P, Q
Posterior tibial M, N
Greater saphenous P, Q
Dorsal venous arch T, V
Digital T, V

Portal Venous Circulation

Inferior vena cava Ø
Gastric 2
Splenic 1
Portal 8
Superior mesenteric 5
Right colic 7
Ileocolic 7
Inferior mesenteric 6
Left colic 7

Ø Medical and Surgical
6 Lower Veins
1 Bypass

Definition: Altering the route of passage of the contents of a tubular body part

Explanation: Rerouting contents of a body part to a downstream area of the normal route, to a similar route and body part, or to an abnormal route and dissimilar body part. Includes one or more anastomoses, with or without the use of a device.

Body Part Character 4	Approach Character 5	Device Character 6	Qualifier Character 7
Ø Inferior Vena Cava Postcava Right inferior phrenic vein Right ovarian vein Right second lumbar vein Right suprarenal vein Right testicular vein	**Ø Open** **4 Percutaneous Endoscopic**	**7 Autologous Tissue Substitute** **9 Autologous Venous Tissue** **A Autologous Arterial Tissue** **J Synthetic Substitute** **K Nonautologous Tissue Substitute** **Z No Device**	**5 Superior Mesenteric Vein** **6 Inferior Mesenteric Vein** **P Pulmonary Trunk** **Q Pulmonary Artery, Right** **R Pulmonary Artery, Left** **Y Lower Vein**
1 Splenic Vein Left gastroepiploic vein Pancreatic vein	**Ø Open** **4 Percutaneous Endoscopic**	**7 Autologous Tissue Substitute** **9 Autologous Venous Tissue** **A Autologous Arterial Tissue** **J Synthetic Substitute** **K Nonautologous Tissue Substitute** **Z No Device**	**9 Renal Vein, Right** **B Renal Vein, Left** **Y Lower Vein**
2 Gastric Vein **3 Esophageal Vein** **4 Hepatic Vein** **5 Superior Mesenteric Vein** Right gastroepiploic vein **6 Inferior Mesenteric Vein** Sigmoid vein Superior rectal vein **7 Colic Vein** Ileocolic vein Left colic vein Middle colic vein Right colic vein **9 Renal Vein, Right** **B Renal Vein, Left** Left inferior phrenic vein Left ovarian vein Left second lumbar vein Left suprarenal vein Left testicular vein **C Common Iliac Vein, Right** **D Common Iliac Vein, Left** **F External Iliac Vein, Right** **G External Iliac Vein, Left** **H Hypogastric Vein, Right** Gluteal vein Internal iliac vein Internal pudendal vein Lateral sacral vein Middle hemorrhoidal vein Obturator vein Uterine vein Vaginal vein Vesical vein **J Hypogastric Vein, Left** *See H Hypogastric Vein, Right* **M Femoral Vein, Right** Deep femoral (profunda femoris) vein Popliteal vein Profunda femoris (deep femoral) vein **N Femoral Vein, Left** *See M Femoral Vein, Right* **P Saphenous Vein, Right** External pudendal vein Great(er) saphenous vein Lesser saphenous vein Small saphenous vein Superficial circumflex iliac vein Superficial epigastric vein **Q Saphenous Vein, Left** *See P Saphenous Vein, Right* **T Foot Vein, Right** Common digital vein Dorsal metatarsal vein Dorsal venous arch Plantar digital vein Plantar metatarsal vein Plantar venous arch **V Foot Vein, Left** *See T Foot Vein, Right*	**Ø Open** **4 Percutaneous Endoscopic**	**7 Autologous Tissue Substitute** **9 Autologous Venous Tissue** **A Autologous Arterial Tissue** **J Synthetic Substitute** **K Nonautologous Tissue Substitute** **Z No Device**	**Y Lower Vein**
8 Portal Vein Hepatic portal vein	**Ø Open**	**7 Autologous Tissue Substitute** **9 Autologous Venous Tissue** **A Autologous Arterial Tissue** **J Synthetic Substitute** **K Nonautologous Tissue Substitute** **Z No Device**	**9 Renal Vein, Right** **B Renal Vein, Left** **Y Lower Vein**
8 Portal Vein Hepatic portal vein	**3 Percutaneous**	**J Synthetic Substitute**	**4 Hepatic Vein** **Y Lower Vein**
8 Portal Vein Hepatic portal vein	**4 Percutaneous Endoscopic**	**7 Autologous Tissue Substitute** **9 Autologous Venous Tissue** **A Autologous Arterial Tissue** **K Nonautologous Tissue Substitute** **Z No Device**	**9 Renal Vein, Right** **B Renal Vein, Left** **Y Lower Vein**
8 Portal Vein Hepatic portal vein	**4 Percutaneous Endoscopic**	**J Synthetic Substitute**	**4 Hepatic Vein** **9 Renal Vein, Right** **B Renal Vein, Left** **Y Lower Vein**

Ø Medical and Surgical
6 Lower Veins
5 Destruction

Definition: Physical eradication of all or a portion of a body part by the direct use of energy, force, or a destructive agent
Explanation: None of the body part is physically taken out

Body Part Character 4	Approach Character 5	Device Character 6	Qualifier Character 7
Ø Inferior Vena Cava Postcava Right inferior phrenic vein Right ovarian vein Right second lumbar vein Right suprarenal vein Right testicular vein **1 Splenic Vein** Left gastroepiploic vein Pancreatic vein **2 Gastric Vein** **3 Esophageal Vein** **4 Hepatic Vein** **5 Superior Mesenteric Vein** Right gastroepiploic vein **6 Inferior Mesenteric Vein** Sigmoid vein Superior rectal vein **7 Colic Vein** Ileocolic vein Left colic vein Middle colic vein Right colic vein **8 Portal Vein** Hepatic portal vein **9 Renal Vein, Right** **B Renal Vein, Left** Left inferior phrenic vein Left ovarian vein Left second lumbar vein Left suprarenal vein Left testicular vein **C Common Iliac Vein, Right** **D Common Iliac Vein, Left** **F External Iliac Vein, Right** **G External Iliac Vein, Left** **H Hypogastric Vein, Right** Gluteal vein Internal iliac vein Internal pudendal vein Lateral sacral vein Middle hemorrhoidal vein Obturator vein Uterine vein Vaginal vein Vesical vein **J Hypogastric Vein, Left** *See H Hypogastric Vein, Right* **M Femoral Vein, Right** Deep femoral (profunda femoris) vein Popliteal vein Profunda femoris (deep femoral) vein **N Femoral Vein, Left** *See M Femoral Vein, Right* **P Saphenous Vein, Right** External pudendal vein Great(er) saphenous vein Lesser saphenous vein Small saphenous vein Superficial circumflex iliac vein Superficial epigastric vein **Q Saphenous Vein, Left** *See P Saphenous Vein, Right* **T Foot Vein, Right** Common digital vein Dorsal metatarsal vein Dorsal venous arch Plantar digital vein Plantar metatarsal vein Plantar venous arch **V Foot Vein, Left** *See T Foot Vein, Right*	**Ø Open** **3 Percutaneous** **4 Percutaneous Endoscopic**	**Z No Device**	**Z No Qualifier**
Y Lower Vein	**Ø Open** **3 Percutaneous** **4 Percutaneous Endoscopic**	**Z No Device**	**C Hemorrhoidal Plexus** **Z No Qualifier**

Ø Medical and Surgical
6 Lower Veins
7 Dilation

Definition: Expanding an orifice or the lumen of a tubular body part

Explanation: The orifice can be a natural orifice or an artificially created orifice. Accomplished by stretching a tubular body part using intraluminal pressure or by cutting part of the orifice or wall of the tubular body part.

Body Part Character 4	Approach Character 5	Device Character 6	Qualifier Character 7
Ø Inferior Vena Cava Postcava Right inferior phrenic vein Right ovarian vein Right second lumbar vein Right suprarenal vein Right testicular vein **1 Splenic Vein** Left gastroepiploic vein Pancreatic vein **2 Gastric Vein** **3 Esophageal Vein** **4 Hepatic Vein** **5 Superior Mesenteric Vein** Right gastroepiploic vein **6 Inferior Mesenteric Vein** Sigmoid vein Superior rectal vein **7 Colic Vein** Ileocolic vein Left colic vein Middle colic vein Right colic vein **8 Portal Vein** Hepatic portal vein **9 Renal Vein, Right** **B Renal Vein, Left** Left inferior phrenic vein Left ovarian vein Left second lumbar vein Left suprarenal vein Left testicular vein **C Common Iliac Vein, Right** **D Common Iliac Vein, Left** **F External Iliac Vein, Right** **G External Iliac Vein, Left** **H Hypogastric Vein, Right** Gluteal vein Internal iliac vein Internal pudendal vein Lateral sacral vein Middle hemorrhoidal vein Obturator vein Uterine vein Vaginal vein Vesical vein **J Hypogastric Vein, Left** *See H Hypogastric Vein, Right* **M Femoral Vein, Right** Deep femoral (profunda femoris) vein Popliteal vein Profunda femoris (deep femoral) vein **N Femoral Vein, Left** *See M Femoral Vein, Right* **P Saphenous Vein, Right** External pudendal vein Great(er) saphenous vein Lesser saphenous vein Small saphenous vein Superficial circumflex iliac vein Superficial epigastric vein **Q Saphenous Vein, Left** *See P Saphenous Vein, Right* **T Foot Vein, Right** Common digital vein Dorsal metatarsal vein Dorsal venous arch Plantar digital vein Plantar metatarsal vein Plantar venous arch **V Foot Vein, Left** *See T Foot Vein, Right* **Y Lower Vein**	**Ø Open** **3 Percutaneous** **4 Percutaneous Endoscopic**	**D Intraluminal Device** **Z No Device**	**Z No Qualifier**

Ø Medical and Surgical
6 Lower Veins
9 Drainage

Definition: Taking or letting out fluids and/or gases from a body part
Explanation: The qualifier DIAGNOSTIC is used to identify drainage procedures that are biopsies

Body Part Character 4	Approach Character 5	Device Character 6	Qualifier Character 7
Ø Inferior Vena Cava Postcava Right inferior phrenic vein Right ovarian vein Right second lumbar vein Right suprarenal vein Right testicular vein **1 Splenic Vein** Left gastroepiploic vein Pancreatic vein **2 Gastric Vein** **3 Esophageal Vein** **4 Hepatic Vein** **5 Superior Mesenteric Vein** Right gastroepiploic vein **6 Inferior Mesenteric Vein** Sigmoid vein Superior rectal vein **7 Colic Vein** Ileocolic vein Left colic vein Middle colic vein Right colic vein **8 Portal Vein** Hepatic portal vein **9 Renal Vein, Right** **B Renal Vein, Left** Left inferior phrenic vein Left ovarian vein Left second lumbar vein Left suprarenal vein Left testicular vein **C Common Iliac Vein, Right** **D Common Iliac Vein, Left** **F External Iliac Vein, Right** **G External Iliac Vein, Left** **H Hypogastric Vein, Right** Gluteal vein Internal iliac vein Internal pudendal vein Lateral sacral vein Middle hemorrhoidal vein Obturator vein Uterine vein Vaginal vein Vesical vein **J Hypogastric Vein, Left** *See H Hypogastric Vein, Right* **M Femoral Vein, Right** Deep femoral (profunda femoris) vein Popliteal vein Profunda femoris (deep femoral) vein **N Femoral Vein, Left** *See M Femoral Vein, Right* **P Saphenous Vein, Right** External pudendal vein Great(er) saphenous vein Lesser saphenous vein Small saphenous vein Superficial circumflex iliac vein Superficial epigastric vein **Q Saphenous Vein, Left** *See P Saphenous Vein, Right* **T Foot Vein, Right** Common digital vein Dorsal metatarsal vein Dorsal venous arch Plantar digital vein Plantar metatarsal vein Plantar venous arch **V Foot Vein, Left** *See T Foot Vein, Right* **Y Lower Vein**	**Ø Open** **3 Percutaneous** **4 Percutaneous Endoscopic**	**Ø Drainage Device**	**Z No Qualifier**

Non-OR Ø69[Ø,1,2,4,5,6,7,8,9,B,C,D,F,G,H,J,M,N,P,Q,T,V,Y][Ø,3,4]ØZ
Non-OR Ø6933ØZ

Ø69 Continued on next page

Ø Medical and Surgical
6 Lower Veins
9 Drainage

Ø69 Continued

Definition: Taking or letting out fluids and/or gases from a body part

Explanation: The qualifier DIAGNOSTIC is used to identify drainage procedures that are biopsies

Body Part Character 4	Approach Character 5	Device Character 6	Qualifier Character 7
Ø Inferior Vena Cava Postcava Right inferior phrenic vein Right ovarian vein Right second lumbar vein Right suprarenal vein Right testicular vein 1 Splenic Vein Left gastroepiploic vein Pancreatic vein 2 Gastric Vein 3 Esophageal Vein 4 Hepatic Vein 5 Superior Mesenteric Vein Right gastroepiploic vein 6 Inferior Mesenteric Vein Sigmoid vein Superior rectal vein 7 Colic Vein Ileocolic vein Left colic vein Middle colic vein Right colic vein 8 Portal Vein Hepatic portal vein 9 Renal Vein, Right B Renal Vein, Left Left inferior phrenic vein Left ovarian vein Left second lumbar vein Left suprarenal vein Left testicular vein C Common Iliac Vein, Right D Common Iliac Vein, Left F External Iliac Vein, Right G External Iliac Vein, Left H Hypogastric Vein, Right Gluteal vein Internal iliac vein Internal pudendal vein Lateral sacral vein Middle hemorrhoidal vein Obturator vein Uterine vein Vaginal vein Vesical vein J Hypogastric Vein, Left *See H Hypogastric Vein, Right* M Femoral Vein, Right Deep femoral (profunda femoris) vein Popliteal vein Profunda femoris (deep femoral) vein N Femoral Vein, Left *See M Femoral Vein, Right* P Saphenous Vein, Right External pudendal vein Great(er) saphenous vein Lesser saphenous vein Small saphenous vein Superficial circumflex iliac vein Superficial epigastric vein Q Saphenous Vein, Left *See P Saphenous Vein, Right* T Foot Vein, Right Common digital vein Dorsal metatarsal vein Dorsal venous arch Plantar digital vein Plantar metatarsal vein Plantar venous arch V Foot Vein, Left *See T Foot Vein, Right* Y Lower Vein	Ø Open 3 Percutaneous 4 Percutaneous Endoscopic	Z No Device	X Diagnostic Z No Qualifier

Non-OR Ø69 Ø,1,2,3,4,5,6,7,8,9,B,C,D,F,G,H,J,M,N,P,Q,T,V,Y]3ZX
Non-OR Ø69 Ø,1,2,4,5,6,7,8,9,B,C,D,F,G,H,J,M,N,P,Q,T,V,Y][Ø,3,4]ZZ
Non-OR Ø6933ZZ

Ø Medical and Surgical
6 Lower Veins
B Excision

Definition: Cutting out or off, without replacement, a portion of a body part
Explanation: The qualifier DIAGNOSTIC is used to identify excision procedures that are biopsies

Body Part Character 4	Approach Character 5	Device Character 6	Qualifier Character 7
Ø Inferior Vena Cava Postcava Right inferior phrenic vein Right ovarian vein Right second lumbar vein Right suprarenal vein Right testicular vein **1 Splenic Vein** Left gastroepiploic vein Pancreatic vein **2 Gastric Vein** **3 Esophageal Vein** **4 Hepatic Vein** **5 Superior Mesenteric Vein** Right gastroepiploic vein **6 Inferior Mesenteric Vein** Sigmoid vein Superior rectal vein **7 Colic Vein** Ileocolic vein Left colic vein Middle colic vein Right colic vein **8 Portal Vein** Hepatic portal vein **9 Renal Vein, Right** **B Renal Vein, Left** Left inferior phrenic vein Left ovarian vein Left second lumbar vein Left suprarenal vein Left testicular vein **C Common Iliac Vein, Right** **D Common Iliac Vein, Left** **F External Iliac Vein, Right** **G External Iliac Vein, Left** **H Hypogastric Vein, Right** Gluteal vein Internal iliac vein Internal pudendal vein Lateral sacral vein Middle hemorrhoidal vein Obturator vein Uterine vein Vaginal vein Vesical vein **J Hypogastric Vein, Left** *See H Hypogastric Vein, Right* **M Femoral Vein, Right** Deep femoral (profunda femoris) vein Popliteal vein Profunda femoris (deep femoral) vein **N Femoral Vein, Left** *See M Femoral Vein, Right* **P Saphenous Vein, Right** External pudendal vein Great(er) saphenous vein Lesser saphenous vein Small saphenous vein Superficial circumflex iliac vein Superficial epigastric vein **Q Saphenous Vein, Left** *See P Saphenous Vein, Right* **T Foot Vein, Right** Common digital vein Dorsal metatarsal vein Dorsal venous arch Plantar digital vein Plantar metatarsal vein Plantar venous arch **V Foot Vein, Left** *See T Foot Vein, Right*	**Ø Open** **3 Percutaneous** **4 Percutaneous Endoscopic**	**Z No Device**	**X Diagnostic** **Z No Qualifier**
Y Lower Vein	**Ø Open** **3 Percutaneous** **4 Percutaneous Endoscopic**	**Z No Device**	**C Hemorrhoidal Plexus** **X Diagnostic** **Z No Qualifier**

Ø Medical and Surgical
6 Lower Veins
C Extirpation

Definition: Taking or cutting out solid matter from a body part

Explanation: The solid matter may be an abnormal byproduct of a biological function or a foreign body; it may be imbedded in a body part or in the lumen of a tubular body part. The solid matter may or may not have been previously broken into pieces.

Body Part Character 4	Approach Character 5	Device Character 6	Qualifier Character 7
Ø Inferior Vena Cava Postcava Right inferior phrenic vein Right ovarian vein Right second lumbar vein Right suprarenal vein Right testicular vein **1 Splenic Vein** Left gastroepiploic vein Pancreatic vein **2 Gastric Vein** **3 Esophageal Vein** **4 Hepatic Vein** **5 Superior Mesenteric Vein** Right gastroepiploic vein **6 Inferior Mesenteric Vein** Sigmoid vein Superior rectal vein **7 Colic Vein** Ileocolic vein Left colic vein Middle colic vein Right colic vein **8 Portal Vein** Hepatic portal vein **9 Renal Vein, Right** **B Renal Vein, Left** Left inferior phrenic vein Left ovarian vein Left second lumbar vein Left suprarenal vein Left testicular vein **C Common Iliac Vein, Right** **D Common Iliac Vein, Left** **F External Iliac Vein, Right** **G External Iliac Vein, Left** **H Hypogastric Vein, Right** Gluteal vein Internal iliac vein Internal pudendal vein Lateral sacral vein Middle hemorrhoidal vein Obturator vein Uterine vein Vaginal vein Vesical vein **J Hypogastric Vein, Left** *See H Hypogastric Vein, Right* **M Femoral Vein, Right** Deep femoral (profunda femoris) vein Popliteal vein Profunda femoris (deep femoral) vein **N Femoral Vein, Left** *See M Femoral Vein, Right* **P Saphenous Vein, Right** External pudendal vein Great(er) saphenous vein Lesser saphenous vein Small saphenous vein Superficial circumflex iliac vein Superficial epigastric vein **Q Saphenous Vein, Left** *See P Saphenous Vein, Right* **T Foot Vein, Right** Common digital vein Dorsal metatarsal vein Dorsal venous arch Plantar digital vein Plantar metatarsal vein Plantar venous arch **V Foot Vein, Left** *See T Foot Vein, Right* **Y Lower Vein**	Ø Open 3 Percutaneous 4 Percutaneous Endoscopic	Z No Device	Z No Qualifier

Ø Medical and Surgical
6 Lower Veins
D Extraction

Definition: Pulling or stripping out or off all or a portion of a body part by the use of force
Explanation: The qualifier DIAGNOSTIC is used to identify extraction procedures that are biopsies

Body Part Character 4	Approach Character 5	Device Character 6	Qualifier Character 7
M Femoral Vein, Right Deep femoral (profunda femoris) vein Popliteal vein Profunda femoris (deep femoral) vein **N Femoral Vein, Left** *See M Femoral Vein, Right* **P Saphenous Vein, Right** External pudendal vein Great(er) saphenous vein Lesser saphenous vein Small saphenous vein Superficial circumflex iliac vein Superficial epigastric vein **Q Saphenous Vein, Left** *See P Saphenous Vein, Right* **T Foot Vein, Right** Common digital vein Dorsal metatarsal vein Dorsal venous arch Plantar digital vein Plantar metatarsal vein Plantar venous arch **V Foot Vein, Left** *See T Foot Vein, Right* **Y Lower Vein**	**Ø Open** **3 Percutaneous** **4 Percutaneous Endoscopic**	**Z No Device**	**Z No Qualifier**

Ø Medical and Surgical
6 Lower Veins
F Fragmentation

Definition: Breaking solid matter in a body part into pieces
Explanation: Physical force (e.g., manual, ultrasonic) applied directly or indirectly is used to break the solid matter into pieces. The solid matter may be an abnormal byproduct of a biological function or a foreign body. The pieces of solid matter are not taken out.

Body Part Character 4	Approach Character 5	Device Character 6	Qualifier Character 7
C Common Iliac Vein, Right **D Common Iliac Vein, Left** **F External Iliac Vein, Right** **G External Iliac Vein, Left** **H Hypogastric Vein, Right** Gluteal vein Internal iliac vein Internal pudendal vein Lateral sacral vein Middle hemorrhoidal vein Obturator vein Uterine vein Vaginal vein Vesical vein **J Hypogastric Vein, Left** *See H Hypogastric Vein, Right* **M Femoral Vein, Right** Deep femoral (profunda femoris) vein Popliteal vein Profunda femoris (deep femoral) vein **N Femoral Vein, Left** *See M Femoral Vein, Right* **P Saphenous Vein, Right** External pudendal vein Great(er) saphenous vein Lesser saphenous vein Small saphenous vein Superficial circumflex iliac vein Superficial epigastric vein **Q Saphenous Vein, Left** *See P Saphenous Vein, Right* **Y Lower Vein**	**3 Percutaneous**	**Z No Device**	**Ø Ultrasonic** **Z No Qualifier**

Ø Medical and Surgical
6 Lower Veins
H Insertion Definition: Putting in a nonbiological appliance that monitors, assists, performs, or prevents a physiological function but does not physically take the place of a body part

Explanation: None

Body Part Character 4	Approach Character 5	Device Character 6	Qualifier Character 7
Ø Inferior Vena Cava Postcava Right inferior phrenic vein Right ovarian vein Right second lumbar vein Right suprarenal vein Right testicular vein	Ø Open 3 Percutaneous	3 Infusion Device	T Via Umbilical Vein Z No Qualifier
Ø Inferior Vena Cava Postcava Right inferior phrenic vein Right ovarian vein Right second lumbar vein Right suprarenal vein Right testicular vein	Ø Open 3 Percutaneous	D Intraluminal Device	Z No Qualifier
Ø Inferior Vena Cava Postcava Right inferior phrenic vein Right ovarian vein Right second lumbar vein Right suprarenal vein Right testicular vein	4 Percutaneous Endoscopic	3 Infusion Device D Intraluminal Device	Z No Qualifier
1 Splenic Vein Left gastroepiploic vein Pancreatic vein **2 Gastric Vein** **3 Esophageal Vein** **4 Hepatic Vein** **5 Superior Mesenteric Vein** Right gastroepiploic vein **6 Inferior Mesenteric Vein** Sigmoid vein Superior rectal vein **7 Colic Vein** Ileocolic vein Left colic vein Middle colic vein Right colic vein **8 Portal Vein** Hepatic portal vein **9 Renal Vein, Right** **B Renal Vein, Left** Left inferior phrenic vein Left ovarian vein Left second lumbar vein Left suprarenal vein Left testicular vein **C Common Iliac Vein, Right** **D Common Iliac Vein, Left** **F External Iliac Vein, Right** **G External Iliac Vein, Left** **H Hypogastric Vein, Right** Gluteal vein Internal iliac vein Internal pudendal vein Lateral sacral vein Middle hemorrhoidal vein Obturator vein Uterine vein Vaginal vein Vesical vein **J Hypogastric Vein, Left** *See H Hypogastric Vein, Right* **M Femoral Vein, Right** Deep femoral (profunda femoris) vein Popliteal vein Profunda femoris (deep femoral) vein **N Femoral Vein, Left** *See M Femoral Vein, Right* **P Saphenous Vein, Right** External pudendal vein Great(er) saphenous vein Lesser saphenous vein Small saphenous vein Superficial circumflex iliac vein Superficial epigastric vein **Q Saphenous Vein, Left** *See P Saphenous Vein, Right* **T Foot Vein, Right** Common digital vein Dorsal metatarsal vein Dorsal venous arch Plantar digital vein Plantar metatarsal vein Plantar venous arch **V Foot Vein, Left** *See T Foot Vein, Right*	Ø Open 3 Percutaneous 4 Percutaneous Endoscopic	3 Infusion Device D Intraluminal Device	Z No Qualifier
Y Lower Vein	Ø Open 3 Percutaneous 4 Percutaneous Endoscopic	2 Monitoring Device 3 Infusion Device D Intraluminal Device Y Other Device	Z No Qualifier

Non-OR	Ø6HØ[Ø,3]3[T,Z]
Non-OR	Ø6HØ3DZ
Non-OR	Ø6HØ43Z
Non-OR	Ø6H[1,2,3,4,5,6,7,8,9,B,C,D,F,G,H,J,M,N,P,Q,T,V][Ø,3,4]3Z
Non-OR	Ø6HY[Ø,3,4]3Z
Non-OR	Ø6HY32Z
Non-OR	Ø6HY[3,4]YZ

Ø Medical and Surgical
6 Lower Veins
J Inspection

Definition: Visually and/or manually exploring a body part

Explanation: Visual exploration may be performed with or without optical instrumentation. Manual exploration may be performed directly or through intervening body layers.

Body Part Character 4	Approach Character 5	Device Character 6	Qualifier Character 7
Y Lower Vein	Ø Open 3 Percutaneous 4 Percutaneous Endoscopic X External	Z No Device	Z No Qualifier

Non-OR Ø6JY[3,X]ZZ

Ø Medical and Surgical
6 Lower Veins
L Occlusion

Definition: Completely closing an orifice or the lumen of a tubular body part

Explanation: The orifice can be a natural orifice or an artificially created orifice

Body Part Character 4	Approach Character 5	Device Character 6	Qualifier Character 7
Ø Inferior Vena Cava Postcava Right inferior phrenic vein Right ovarian vein Right second lumbar vein Right suprarenal vein Right testicular vein **1 Splenic Vein** Left gastroepiploic vein Pancreatic vein **4 Hepatic Vein** **5 Superior Mesenteric Vein** Right gastroepiploic vein **6 Inferior Mesenteric Vein** Sigmoid vein Superior rectal vein **7 Colic Vein** Ileocolic vein Left colic vein Middle colic vein Right colic vein **8 Portal Vein** Hepatic portal vein **9 Renal Vein, Right** **B Renal Vein, Left** Left inferior phrenic vein Left ovarian vein Left second lumbar vein Left suprarenal vein Left testicular vein **C Common Iliac Vein, Right** **D Common Iliac Vein, Left** **F External Iliac Vein, Right** **G External Iliac Vein, Left** **H Hypogastric Vein, Right** Gluteal vein Internal iliac vein Internal pudendal vein Lateral sacral vein Middle hemorrhoidal vein Obturator vein Uterine vein Vaginal vein Vesical vein **J Hypogastric Vein, Left** ***See** H Hypogastric Vein, Right* **M Femoral Vein, Right** Deep femoral (profunda femoris) vein Popliteal vein Profunda femoris (deep femoral) vein **N Femoral Vein, Left** ***See** M Femoral Vein, Right* **P Saphenous Vein, Right** External pudendal vein Great(er) saphenous vein Lesser saphenous vein Small saphenous vein Superficial circumflex iliac vein Superficial epigastric vein **Q Saphenous Vein, Left** ***See** P Saphenous Vein, Right* **T Foot Vein, Right** Common digital vein Dorsal metatarsal vein Dorsal venous arch Plantar digital vein Plantar metatarsal vein Plantar venous arch **V Foot Vein, Left** ***See** T Foot Vein, Right*	Ø Open 3 Percutaneous 4 Percutaneous Endoscopic	C Extraluminal Device D Intraluminal Device Z No Device	Z No Qualifier
2 Gastric Vein 3 Esophageal Vein	Ø Open 3 Percutaneous 4 Percutaneous Endoscopic 7 Via Natural or Artificial Opening 8 Via Natural or Artificial Opening Endoscopic	C Extraluminal Device D Intraluminal Device Z No Device	Z No Qualifier
Y Lower Vein	Ø Open 3 Percutaneous 4 Percutaneous Endoscopic 7 Via Natural or Artificial Opening 8 Via Natural or Artificial Opening Endoscopic	C Extraluminal Device D Intraluminal Device Z No Device	C Hemorrhoidal Plexus Z No Qualifier

Non-OR Ø6L2[7,8][C,D,Z]Z
Non-OR Ø6L3[3,4,7,8][C,D,Z]Z

Ø Medical and Surgical
6 Lower Veins
N Release

Definition: Freeing a body part from an abnormal physical constraint by cutting or by the use of force
Explanation: Some of the restraining tissue may be taken out but none of the body part is taken out

Body Part Character 4	Approach Character 5	Device Character 6	Qualifier Character 7
Ø Inferior Vena Cava Postcava Right inferior phrenic vein Right ovarian vein Right second lumbar vein Right suprarenal vein Right testicular vein **1 Splenic Vein** Left gastroepiploic vein Pancreatic vein **2 Gastric Vein** **3 Esophageal Vein** **4 Hepatic Vein** **5 Superior Mesenteric Vein** Right gastroepiploic vein **6 Inferior Mesenteric Vein** Sigmoid vein Superior rectal vein **7 Colic Vein** Ileocolic vein Left colic vein Middle colic vein Right colic vein **8 Portal Vein** Hepatic portal vein **9 Renal Vein, Right** **B Renal Vein, Left** Left inferior phrenic vein Left ovarian vein Left second lumbar vein Left suprarenal vein Left testicular vein **C Common Iliac Vein, Right** **D Common Iliac Vein, Left** **F External Iliac Vein, Right** **G External Iliac Vein, Left** **H Hypogastric Vein, Right** Gluteal vein Internal iliac vein Internal pudendal vein Lateral sacral vein Middle hemorrhoidal vein Obturator vein Uterine vein Vaginal vein Vesical vein **J Hypogastric Vein, Left** *See H Hypogastric Vein, Right* **M Femoral Vein, Right** Deep femoral (profunda femoris) vein Popliteal vein Profunda femoris (deep femoral) vein **N Femoral Vein, Left** *See M Femoral Vein, Right* **P Saphenous Vein, Right** External pudendal vein Great(er) saphenous vein Lesser saphenous vein Small saphenous vein Superficial circumflex iliac vein Superficial epigastric vein **Q Saphenous Vein, Left** *See P Saphenous Vein, Right* **T Foot Vein, Right** Common digital vein Dorsal metatarsal vein Dorsal venous arch Plantar digital vein Plantar metatarsal vein Plantar venous arch **V Foot Vein, Left** *See T Foot Vein, Right* **Y Lower Vein**	**Ø** Open **3** Percutaneous **4** Percutaneous Endoscopic	**Z** No Device	**Z** No Qualifier

Ø Medical and Surgical
6 Lower Veins
P Removal

Definition: Taking out or off a device from a body part
Explanation: If a device is taken out and a similar device put in without cutting or puncturing the skin or mucous membrane, the procedure is coded to the root operation CHANGE. Otherwise, the procedure for taking out a device is coded to the root operation REMOVAL.

Body Part Character 4	Approach Character 5	Device Character 6	Qualifier Character 7
Y Lower Vein	**Ø** Open **3** Percutaneous **4** Percutaneous Endoscopic	**Ø** Drainage Device **2** Monitoring Device **3** Infusion Device **7** Autologous Tissue Substitute **C** Extraluminal Device **D** Intraluminal Device **J** Synthetic Substitute **K** Nonautologous Tissue Substitute **Y** Other Device	**Z** No Qualifier
Y Lower Vein	**X** External	**Ø** Drainage Device **2** Monitoring Device **3** Infusion Device **D** Intraluminal Device	**Z** No Qualifier

Non-OR Ø6PY3[Ø,2,3]Z
Non-OR Ø6PY[3,4]YZ
Non-OR Ø6PYX[Ø,2,3,D]Z

Ø Medical and Surgical
6 Lower Veins
Q Repair

Definition: Restoring, to the extent possible, a body part to its normal anatomic structure and function

Explanation: Used only when the method to accomplish the repair is not one of the other root operations

Body Part Character 4	Approach Character 5	Device Character 6	Qualifier Character 7
Ø Inferior Vena Cava Postcava Right inferior phrenic vein Right ovarian vein Right second lumbar vein Right suprarenal vein Right testicular vein **1 Splenic Vein** Left gastroepiploic vein Pancreatic vein **2 Gastric Vein** **3 Esophageal Vein** **4 Hepatic Vein** **5 Superior Mesenteric Vein** Right gastroepiploic vein **6 Inferior Mesenteric Vein** Sigmoid vein Superior rectal vein **7 Colic Vein** Ileocolic vein Left colic vein Middle colic vein Right colic vein **8 Portal Vein** Hepatic portal vein **9 Renal Vein, Right** **B Renal Vein, Left** Left inferior phrenic vein Left ovarian vein Left second lumbar vein Left suprarenal vein Left testicular vein **C Common Iliac Vein, Right** **D Common Iliac Vein, Left** **F External Iliac Vein, Right** **G External Iliac Vein, Left** **H Hypogastric Vein, Right** Gluteal vein Internal iliac vein Internal pudendal vein Lateral sacral vein Middle hemorrhoidal vein Obturator vein Uterine vein Vaginal vein Vesical vein **J Hypogastric Vein, Left** *See H Hypogastric Vein, Right* **M Femoral Vein, Right** Deep femoral (profunda femoris) vein Popliteal vein Profunda femoris (deep femoral) vein **N Femoral Vein, Left** *See M Femoral Vein, Right* **P Saphenous Vein, Right** External pudendal vein Great(er) saphenous vein Lesser saphenous vein Small saphenous vein Superficial circumflex iliac vein Superficial epigastric vein **Q Saphenous Vein, Left** *See P Saphenous Vein, Right* **T Foot Vein, Right** Common digital vein Dorsal metatarsal vein Dorsal venous arch Plantar digital vein Plantar metatarsal vein Plantar venous arch **V Foot Vein, Left** *See T Foot Vein, Right* **Y Lower Vein**	**Ø Open** **3 Percutaneous** **4 Percutaneous Endoscopic**	**Z No Device**	**Z No Qualifier**

Ø Medical and Surgical
6 Lower Veins
R Replacement Definition: Putting in or on biological or synthetic material that physically takes the place and/or function of all or a portion of a body part

Explanation: The body part may have been taken out or replaced, or may be taken out, physically eradicated, or rendered nonfunctional during the REPLACEMENT procedure. A REMOVAL procedure is coded for taking out the device used in a previous replacement procedure.

Body Part Character 4	Approach Character 5	Device Character 6	Qualifier Character 7
Ø Inferior Vena Cava Postcava Right inferior phrenic vein Right ovarian vein Right second lumbar vein Right suprarenal vein Right testicular vein **1 Splenic Vein** Left gastroepiploic vein Pancreatic vein **2 Gastric Vein** **3 Esophageal Vein** **4 Hepatic Vein** **5 Superior Mesenteric Vein** Right gastroepiploic vein **6 Inferior Mesenteric Vein** Sigmoid vein Superior rectal vein **7 Colic Vein** Ileocolic vein Left colic vein Middle colic vein Right colic vein **8 Portal Vein** Hepatic portal vein **9 Renal Vein, Right** **B Renal Vein, Left** Left inferior phrenic vein Left ovarian vein Left second lumbar vein Left suprarenal vein Left testicular vein **C Common Iliac Vein, Right** **D Common Iliac Vein, Left** **F External Iliac Vein, Right** **G External Iliac Vein, Left** **H Hypogastric Vein, Right** Gluteal vein Internal iliac vein Internal pudendal vein Lateral sacral vein Middle hemorrhoidal vein Obturator vein Uterine vein Vaginal vein Vesical vein **J Hypogastric Vein, Left** *See H Hypogastric Vein, Right* **M Femoral Vein, Right** Deep femoral (profunda femoris) vein Popliteal vein Profunda femoris (deep femoral) vein **N Femoral Vein, Left** *See M Femoral Vein, Right* **P Saphenous Vein, Right** External pudendal vein Great(er) saphenous vein Lesser saphenous vein Small saphenous vein Superficial circumflex iliac vein Superficial epigastric vein **Q Saphenous Vein, Left** *See P Saphenous Vein, Right* **T Foot Vein, Right** Common digital vein Dorsal metatarsal vein Dorsal venous arch Plantar digital vein Plantar metatarsal vein Plantar venous arch **V Foot Vein, Left** *See T Foot Vein, Right* **Y Lower Vein**	**Ø Open** **4 Percutaneous Endoscopic**	**7 Autologous Tissue Substitute** **J Synthetic Substitute** **K Nonautologous Tissue Substitute**	**Z No Qualifier**

Ø Medical and Surgical
6 Lower Veins
S Reposition

Definition: Moving to its normal location, or other suitable location, all or a portion of a body part

Explanation: The body part is moved to a new location from an abnormal location, or from a normal location where it is not functioning correctly. The body part may or may not be cut out or off to be moved to the new location.

Body Part Character 4	Approach Character 5	Device Character 6	Qualifier Character 7
Ø Inferior Vena Cava Postcava Right inferior phrenic vein Right ovarian vein Right second lumbar vein Right suprarenal vein Right testicular vein **1 Splenic Vein** Left gastroepiploic vein Pancreatic vein **2 Gastric Vein** **3 Esophageal Vein** **4 Hepatic Vein** **5 Superior Mesenteric Vein** Right gastroepiploic vein **6 Inferior Mesenteric Vein** Sigmoid vein Superior rectal vein **7 Colic Vein** Ileocolic vein Left colic vein Middle colic vein Right colic vein **8 Portal Vein** Hepatic portal vein **9 Renal Vein, Right** **B Renal Vein, Left** Left inferior phrenic vein Left ovarian vein Left second lumbar vein Left suprarenal vein Left testicular vein **C Common Iliac Vein, Right** **D Common Iliac Vein, Left** **F External Iliac Vein, Right** **G External Iliac Vein, Left** **H Hypogastric Vein, Right** Gluteal vein Internal iliac vein Internal pudendal vein Lateral sacral vein Middle hemorrhoidal vein Obturator vein Uterine vein Vaginal vein Vesical vein **J Hypogastric Vein, Left** *See H Hypogastric Vein, Right* **M Femoral Vein, Right** Deep femoral (profunda femoris) vein Popliteal vein Profunda femoris (deep femoral) vein **N Femoral Vein, Left** *See M Femoral Vein, Right* **P Saphenous Vein, Right** External pudendal vein Great(er) saphenous vein Lesser saphenous vein Small saphenous vein Superficial circumflex iliac vein Superficial epigastric vein **Q Saphenous Vein, Left** *See P Saphenous Vein, Right* **T Foot Vein, Right** Common digital vein Dorsal metatarsal vein Dorsal venous arch Plantar digital vein Plantar metatarsal vein Plantar venous arch **V Foot Vein, Left** *See T Foot Vein, Right* **Y Lower Vein**	**Ø Open** **3 Percutaneous** **4 Percutaneous Endoscopic**	**Z No Device**	**Z No Qualifier**

Ø Medical and Surgical
6 Lower Veins
U Supplement Definition: Putting in or on biological or synthetic material that physically reinforces and/or augments the function of a portion of a body part

Explanation: The biological material is non-living, or is living and from the same individual. The body part may have been previously replaced, and the SUPPLEMENT procedure is performed to physically reinforce and/or augment the function of the replaced body part.

Body Part Character 4	Approach Character 5	Device Character 6	Qualifier Character 7
Ø Inferior Vena Cava Postcava Right inferior phrenic vein Right ovarian vein Right second lumbar vein Right suprarenal vein Right testicular vein **1 Splenic Vein** Left gastroepiploic vein Pancreatic vein **2 Gastric Vein** **3 Esophageal Vein** **4 Hepatic Vein** **5 Superior Mesenteric Vein** Right gastroepiploic vein **6 Inferior Mesenteric Vein** Sigmoid vein Superior rectal vein **7 Colic Vein** Ileocolic vein Left colic vein Middle colic vein Right colic vein **8 Portal Vein** Hepatic portal vein **9 Renal Vein, Right** **B Renal Vein, Left** Left inferior phrenic vein Left ovarian vein Left second lumbar vein Left suprarenal vein Left testicular vein **C Common Iliac Vein, Right** **D Common Iliac Vein, Left** **F External Iliac Vein, Right** **G External Iliac Vein, Left** **H Hypogastric Vein, Right** Gluteal vein Internal iliac vein Internal pudendal vein Lateral sacral vein Middle hemorrhoidal vein Obturator vein Uterine vein Vaginal vein Vesical vein **J Hypogastric Vein, Left** ***See*** *H Hypogastric Vein, Right* **M Femoral Vein, Right** Deep femoral (profunda femoris) vein Popliteal vein Profunda femoris (deep femoral) vein **N Femoral Vein, Left** ***See*** *M Femoral Vein, Right* **P Saphenous Vein, Right** External pudendal vein Great(er) saphenous vein Lesser saphenous vein Small saphenous vein Superficial circumflex iliac vein Superficial epigastric vein **Q Saphenous Vein, Left** ***See*** *P Saphenous Vein, Right* **T Foot Vein, Right** Common digital vein Dorsal metatarsal vein Dorsal venous arch Plantar digital vein Plantar metatarsal vein Plantar venous arch **V Foot Vein, Left** ***See*** *T Foot Vein, Right* **Y Lower Vein**	**Ø Open** **3 Percutaneous** **4 Percutaneous Endoscopic**	**7 Autologous Tissue Substitute** **J Synthetic Substitute** **K Nonautologous Tissue Substitute**	**Z No Qualifier**

Ø Medical and Surgical
6 Lower Veins
V Restriction Definition: Partially closing an orifice or the lumen of a tubular body part
Explanation: The orifice can be a natural orifice or an artificially created orifice

Body Part Character 4	Approach Character 5	Device Character 6	Qualifier Character 7
Ø Inferior Vena Cava Postcava Right inferior phrenic vein Right ovarian vein Right second lumbar vein Right suprarenal vein Right testicular vein **1 Splenic Vein** Left gastroepiploic vein Pancreatic vein **2 Gastric Vein** **3 Esophageal Vein** **4 Hepatic Vein** **5 Superior Mesenteric Vein** Right gastroepiploic vein **6 Inferior Mesenteric Vein** Sigmoid vein Superior rectal vein **7 Colic Vein** Ileocolic vein Left colic vein Middle colic vein Right colic vein **8 Portal Vein** Hepatic portal vein **9 Renal Vein, Right** **B Renal Vein, Left** Left inferior phrenic vein Left ovarian vein Left second lumbar vein Left suprarenal vein Left testicular vein **C Common Iliac Vein, Right** **D Common Iliac Vein, Left** **F External Iliac Vein, Right** **G External Iliac Vein, Left** **H Hypogastric Vein, Right** Gluteal vein Internal iliac vein Internal pudendal vein Lateral sacral vein Middle hemorrhoidal vein Obturator vein Uterine vein Vaginal vein Vesical vein **J Hypogastric Vein, Left** *See H Hypogastric Vein, Right* **M Femoral Vein, Right** Deep femoral (profunda femoris) vein Popliteal vein Profunda femoris (deep femoral) vein **N Femoral Vein, Left** *See M Femoral Vein, Right* **P Saphenous Vein, Right** External pudendal vein Great(er) saphenous vein Lesser saphenous vein Small saphenous vein Superficial circumflex iliac vein Superficial epigastric vein **Q Saphenous Vein, Left** *See P Saphenous Vein, Right* **T Foot Vein, Right** Common digital vein Dorsal metatarsal vein Dorsal venous arch Plantar digital vein Plantar metatarsal vein Plantar venous arch **V Foot Vein, Left** *See T Foot Vein, Right* **Y Lower Vein**	**Ø Open** **3 Percutaneous** **4 Percutaneous Endoscopic**	**C Extraluminal Device** **D Intraluminal Device** **Z No Device**	**Z No Qualifier**

Ø Medical and Surgical
6 Lower Veins
W Revision

Definition: Correcting, to the extent possible, a portion of a malfunctioning device or the position of a displaced device

Explanation: Revision can include correcting a malfunctioning or displaced device by taking out or putting in components of the device such as a screw or pin

Body Part Character 4	Approach Character 5	Device Character 6	Qualifier Character 7
Y Lower Vein	Ø Open 3 Percutaneous 4 Percutaneous Endoscopic	Ø Drainage Device 2 Monitoring Device 3 Infusion Device 7 Autologous Tissue Substitute C Extraluminal Device D Intraluminal Device J Synthetic Substitute K Nonautologous Tissue Substitute Y Other Device	Z No Qualifier
Y Lower Vein	X External	Ø Drainage Device 2 Monitoring Device 3 Infusion Device 7 Autologous Tissue Substitute C Extraluminal Device D Intraluminal Device J Synthetic Substitute K Nonautologous Tissue Substitute	Z No Qualifier

Non-OR Ø6WY3[Ø,2,3]Z
Non-OR Ø6WY[3,4]YZ
Non-OR Ø6WYX[Ø,2,3,7,C,D,J,K]Z

Lymphatic and Hemic Systems Ø72–Ø7Y

Character Meanings*

This Character Meaning table is provided as a guide to assist the user in the identification of character members that may be found in this section of code tables. It **SHOULD NOT** be used to build a PCS code.

Operation–Character 3		Body Part–Character 4		Approach–Character 5		Device–Character 6		Qualifier–Character 7	
2	Change	Ø	Lymphatic, Head	Ø	Open	Ø	Drainage Device	Ø	Allogeneic
5	Destruction	1	Lymphatic, Right Neck	3	Percutaneous	1	Radioactive Element	1	Syngeneic
9	Drainage	2	Lymphatic, Left Neck	4	Percutaneous Endoscopic	3	Infusion Device	2	Zooplastic
B	Excision	3	Lymphatic, Right Upper Extremity	8	Via Natural or Artificial Opening Endoscopic	7	Autologous Tissue Substitute	X	Diagnostic
C	Extirpation	4	Lymphatic, Left Upper Extremity	X	External	C	Extraluminal Device	Z	No Qualifier
D	Extraction	5	Lymphatic, Right Axillary			D	Intraluminal Device		
H	Insertion	6	Lymphatic, Left Axillary			J	Synthetic Substitute		
J	Inspection	7	Lymphatic, Thorax			K	Nonautologous Tissue Substitute		
L	Occlusion	8	Lymphatic, Internal Mammary, Right			Y	Other Device		
N	Release	9	Lymphatic, Internal Mammary, Left			Z	No Device		
P	Removal	B	Lymphatic, Mesenteric						
Q	Repair	C	Lymphatic, Pelvis						
S	Reposition	D	Lymphatic, Aortic						
T	Resection	F	Lymphatic, Right Lower Extremity						
U	Supplement	G	Lymphatic, Left Lower Extremity						
V	Restriction	H	Lymphatic, Right Inguinal						
W	Revision	J	Lymphatic, Left Inguinal						
Y	Transplantation	K	Thoracic Duct						
		L	Cisterna Chyli						
		M	Thymus						
		N	Lymphatic						
		P	Spleen						
		Q	Bone Marrow, Sternum						
		R	Bone Marrow, Iliac						
		S	Bone Marrow, Vertebral						
		T	Bone Marrow						

* Includes lymph vessels and lymph nodes.

AHA Coding Clinic for table Ø79

2021, 4Q, 47 Extraction of bone marrow from other sites
2018, 4Q, 84 Fine needle aspiration biopsy of lymphatic tissue
2017, 1Q, 34 Lymphovenous bypass following mastectomy
2014, 1Q, 26 Transbronchial needle aspiration lymph node biopsy
2013, 4Q, 111 Transbronchial needle aspiration lymph node biopsy

AHA Coding Clinic for table Ø7B

2022, 1Q, 14 Reduction mammoplasty for breast symmetry
2019, 1Q, 3-8 Whipple procedure
2018, 4Q, 84 Fine needle aspiration biopsy of lymphatic tissue
2018, 1Q, 22 Resection of lymph node chains
2016, 1Q, 30 Axillary lymph node resection with modified radical mastectomy
2014, 3Q, 10 Selective excision of paratracheal lymph nodes
2014, 1Q, 20 Fiducial marker placement
2014, 1Q, 26 Transbronchial endoscopic lymph node aspiration biopsy

AHA Coding Clinic for table Ø7D

2022, 1Q, 54 Extraction of bone marrow from other sites
2021, 4Q, 47 Extraction of bone marrow from other sites
2018, 4Q, 84 Fine needle aspiration biopsy of lymphatic tissue
2013, 4Q, 111 Root operation for bone marrow biopsy

AHA Coding Clinic for table Ø7H

2020, 4Q, 43-44 Insertion of radioactive element
2020, 4Q, 53 Bone marrow body part

AHA Coding Clinic for table Ø7Q

2017, 1Q, 34 Lymphovenous bypass following mastectomy

AHA Coding Clinic for table Ø7S

2019, 3Q, 29 Thymus transplant for T-Cell production

AHA Coding Clinic for table Ø7T

2023, 2Q, 22 Norwood procedure with excision of thymus
2018, 1Q, 22 Resection of lymph node chains
2016, 2Q, 12 Resection of malignant neoplasm of infratemporal fossa
2016, 1Q, 30 Axillary lymph node resection with modified radical mastectomy
2015, 4Q, 13 New Section X codes—New Technology procedures
2014, 3Q, 9 Radical resection of level I lymph nodes
2014, 3Q, 16 Repair of Tetralogy of Fallot

AHA Coding Clinic for table Ø7Y

2023, 2Q, 32 Preparation of donor organ before transplantation
2019, 3Q, 29 Thymus transplant for T-Cell production

Lymphatic System

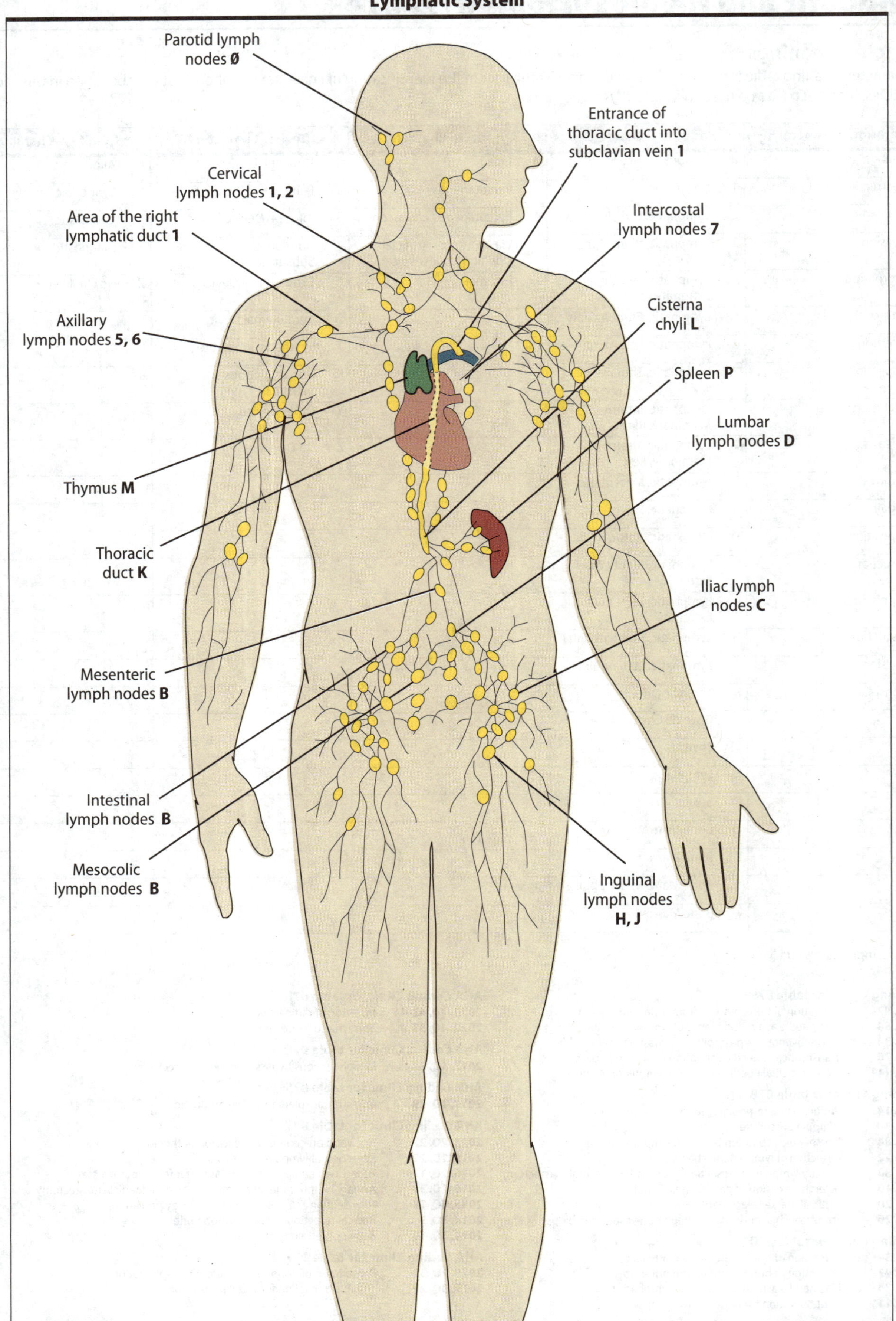

Ø Medical and Surgical
7 Lymphatic and Hemic Systems
2 Change Definition: Taking out or off a device from a body part and putting back an identical or similar device in or on the same body part without cutting or puncturing the skin or a mucous membrane

Explanation: All CHANGE procedures are coded using the approach EXTERNAL

Body Part Character 4		Approach Character 5	Device Character 6	Qualifier Character 7
K Thoracic Duct Left jugular trunk Left subclavian trunk L Cisterna Chyli Intestinal lymphatic trunk Lumbar lymphatic trunk	M Thymus Thymus gland N Lymphatic P Spleen Accessory spleen T Bone Marrow	X External	Ø Drainage Device Y Other Device	Z No Qualifier

Non-OR All body part, approach, device, and qualifier values

Ø Medical and Surgical
7 Lymphatic and Hemic Systems
5 Destruction Definition: Physical eradication of all or a portion of a body part by the direct use of energy, force, or a destructive agent

Explanation: None of the body part is physically taken out

Body Part Character 4		Approach Character 5	Device Character 6	Qualifier Character 7
Ø Lymphatic, Head Buccinator lymph node Infraauricular lymph node Infraparotid lymph node Parotid lymph node Preauricular lymph node Submandibular lymph node Submaxillary lymph node Submental lymph node Subparotid lymph node Suprahyoid lymph node **1 Lymphatic, Right Neck** Cervical lymph node Jugular lymph node Mastoid (postauricular) lymph node Occipital lymph node Postauricular (mastoid) lymph node Retropharyngeal lymph node Right jugular trunk Right lymphatic duct Right subclavian trunk Supraclavicular (Virchow's) lymph node Virchow's (supraclavicular) lymph node **2 Lymphatic, Left Neck** Cervical lymph node Jugular lymph node Mastoid (postauricular) lymph node Occipital lymph node Postauricular (mastoid) lymph node Retropharyngeal lymph node Supraclavicular (Virchow's) lymph node Virchow's (supraclavicular) lymph node **3 Lymphatic, Right Upper Extremity** Cubital lymph node Deltopectoral (infraclavicular) lymph node Epitrochlear lymph node Infraclavicular (deltopectoral) lymph node Supratrochlear lymph node **4 Lymphatic, Left Upper Extremity** *See 3 Lymphatic, Right Upper Extremity* **5 Lymphatic, Right Axillary** Anterior (pectoral) lymph node Apical (subclavicular) lymph node Brachial (lateral) lymph node Central axillary lymph node Lateral (brachial) lymph node Pectoral (anterior) lymph node Posterior (subscapular) lymph node Subclavicular (apical) lymph node Subscapular (posterior) lymph node	**6 Lymphatic, Left Axillary** *See 5 Lymphatic, Right Axillary* **7 Lymphatic, Thorax** Intercostal lymph node Mediastinal lymph node Parasternal lymph node Paratracheal lymph node Tracheobronchial lymph node **8 Lymphatic, Internal Mammary, Right** **9 Lymphatic, Internal Mammary, Left** **B Lymphatic, Mesenteric** Inferior mesenteric lymph node Pararectal lymph node Superior mesenteric lymph node **C Lymphatic, Pelvis** Common iliac (subaortic) lymph node Gluteal lymph node Iliac lymph node Inferior epigastric lymph node Obturator lymph node Sacral lymph node Subaortic (common iliac) lymph node Suprainguinal lymph node **D Lymphatic, Aortic** Celiac lymph node Gastric lymph node Hepatic lymph node Lumbar lymph node Pancreaticosplenic lymph node Paraaortic lymph node Retroperitoneal lymph node **F Lymphatic, Right Lower Extremity** Femoral lymph node Popliteal lymph node **G Lymphatic, Left Lower Extremity** *See F Lymphatic, Right Lower Extremity* **H Lymphatic, Right Inguinal** **J Lymphatic, Left Inguinal** **K Thoracic Duct** Left jugular trunk Left subclavian trunk **L Cisterna Chyli** Intestinal lymphatic trunk Lumbar lymphatic trunk **M Thymus** Thymus gland **P Spleen** Accessory spleen	Ø Open 3 Percutaneous 4 Percutaneous Endoscopic	Z No Device	Z No Qualifier

Ø Medical and Surgical
7 Lymphatic and Hemic Systems
9 Drainage Definition: Taking or letting out fluids and/or gases from a body part
Explanation: The qualifier DIAGNOSTIC is used to identify drainage procedures that are biopsies

Body Part Character 4		Approach Character 5	Device Character 6	Qualifier Character 7
Ø Lymphatic, Head Buccinator lymph node Infraauricular lymph node Infraparotid lymph node Parotid lymph node Preauricular lymph node Submandibular lymph node Submaxillary lymph node Submental lymph node Subparotid lymph node Suprahyoid lymph node **1 Lymphatic, Right Neck** Cervical lymph node Jugular lymph node Mastoid (postauricular) lymph node Occipital lymph node Postauricular (mastoid) lymph node Retropharyngeal lymph node Right jugular trunk Right lymphatic duct Right subclavian trunk Supraclavicular (Virchow's) lymph node Virchow's (supraclavicular) lymph node **2 Lymphatic, Left Neck** Cervical lymph node Jugular lymph node Mastoid (postauricular) lymph node Occipital lymph node Postauricular (mastoid) lymph node Retropharyngeal lymph node Supraclavicular (Virchow's) lymph node Virchow's (supraclavicular) lymph node **3 Lymphatic, Right Upper Extremity** Cubital lymph node Deltopectoral (infraclavicular) lymph node Epitrochlear lymph node Infraclavicular (deltopectoral) lymph node Supratrochlear lymph node **4 Lymphatic, Left Upper Extremity** ***See*** *3 Lymphatic, Right Upper Extremity* **5 Lymphatic, Right Axillary** Anterior (pectoral) lymph node Apical (subclavicular) lymph node Brachial (lateral) lymph node Central axillary lymph node Lateral (brachial) lymph node Pectoral (anterior) lymph node Posterior (subscapular) lymph node Subclavicular (apical) lymph node Subscapular (posterior) lymph node	**6 Lymphatic, Left Axillary** ***See*** *5 Lymphatic, Right Axillary* **7 Lymphatic, Thorax** Intercostal lymph node Mediastinal lymph node Parasternal lymph node Paratracheal lymph node Tracheobronchial lymph node **8 Lymphatic, Internal Mammary, Right** **9 Lymphatic, Internal Mammary, Left** **B Lymphatic, Mesenteric** Inferior mesenteric lymph node Pararectal lymph node Superior mesenteric lymph node **C Lymphatic, Pelvis** Common iliac (subaortic) lymph node Gluteal lymph node Iliac lymph node Inferior epigastric lymph node Obturator lymph node Sacral lymph node Subaortic (common iliac) lymph node Suprainguinal lymph node **D Lymphatic, Aortic** Celiac lymph node Gastric lymph node Hepatic lymph node Lumbar lymph node Pancreaticosplenic lymph node Paraaortic lymph node Retroperitoneal lymph node **F Lymphatic, Right Lower Extremity** Femoral lymph node Popliteal lymph node **G Lymphatic, Left Lower Extremity** ***See*** *F Lymphatic, Right Lower Extremity* **H Lymphatic, Right Inguinal** **J Lymphatic, Left Inguinal** **K Thoracic Duct** Left jugular trunk Left subclavian trunk **L Cisterna Chyli** Intestinal lymphatic trunk Lumbar lymphatic trunk	**Ø Open** **3 Percutaneous** **4 Percutaneous Endoscopic** **8 Via Natural or Artificial Opening Endoscopic**	**Ø Drainage Device**	**Z No Qualifier**

Non-OR Ø79[Ø,1,2,3,4,5,6,7,8,9,B,C,D,F,G,H,J,K,L][3,8]ØZ

Ø79 Continued on next page

Ø Medical and Surgical
7 Lymphatic and Hemic Systems
9 Drainage Definition: Taking or letting out fluids and/or gases from a body part
Explanation: The qualifier DIAGNOSTIC is used to identify drainage procedures that are biopsies

Ø79 Continued

Body Part Character 4	Approach Character 5	Device Character 6	Qualifier Character 7
Ø Lymphatic, Head Buccinator lymph node Infraauricular lymph node Infraparotid lymph node Parotid lymph node Preauricular lymph node Submandibular lymph node Submaxillary lymph node Submental lymph node Subparotid lymph node Suprahyoid lymph node **1 Lymphatic, Right Neck** Cervical lymph node Jugular lymph node Mastoid (postauricular) lymph node Occipital lymph node Postauricular (mastoid) lymph node Retropharyngeal lymph node Right jugular trunk Right lymphatic duct Right subclavian trunk Supraclavicular (Virchow's) lymph node Virchow's (supraclavicular) lymph node **2 Lymphatic, Left Neck** Cervical lymph node Jugular lymph node Mastoid (postauricular) lymph node Occipital lymph node Postauricular (mastoid) lymph node Retropharyngeal lymph node Supraclavicular (Virchow's) lymph node Virchow's (supraclavicular) lymph node **3 Lymphatic, Right Upper Extremity** Cubital lymph node Deltopectoral (infraclavicular) lymph node Epitrochlear lymph node Infraclavicular (deltopectoral) lymph node Supratrochlear lymph node **4 Lymphatic, Left Upper Extremity** *See 3 Lymphatic, Right Upper Extremity* **5 Lymphatic, Right Axillary** Anterior (pectoral) lymph node Apical (subclavicular) lymph node Brachial (lateral) lymph node Central axillary lymph node Lateral (brachial) lymph node Pectoral (anterior) lymph node Posterior (subscapular) lymph node Subclavicular (apical) lymph node Subscapular (posterior) lymph node **6 Lymphatic, Left Axillary** *See 5 Lymphatic, Right Axillary* **7 Lymphatic, Thorax** Intercostal lymph node Mediastinal lymph node Parasternal lymph node Paratracheal lymph node Tracheobronchial lymph node **8 Lymphatic, Internal Mammary, Right** **9 Lymphatic, Internal Mammary, Left** **B Lymphatic, Mesenteric** Inferior mesenteric lymph node Pararectal lymph node Superior mesenteric lymph node **C Lymphatic, Pelvis** Common iliac (subaortic) lymph node Gluteal lymph node Iliac lymph node Inferior epigastric lymph node Obturator lymph node Sacral lymph node Subaortic (common iliac) lymph node Suprainguinal lymph node **D Lymphatic, Aortic** Celiac lymph node Gastric lymph node Hepatic lymph node Lumbar lymph node Pancreaticosplenic lymph node Paraaortic lymph node Retroperitoneal lymph node **F Lymphatic, Right Lower Extremity** Femoral lymph node Popliteal lymph node **G Lymphatic, Left Lower Extremity** *See F Lymphatic, Right Lower Extremity* **H Lymphatic, Right Inguinal** **J Lymphatic, Left Inguinal** **K Thoracic Duct** Left jugular trunk Left subclavian trunk **L Cisterna Chyli** Intestinal lymphatic trunk Lumbar lymphatic trunk	Ø Open 3 Percutaneous 4 Percutaneous Endoscopic 8 Via Natural or Artificial Opening Endoscopic	Z No Device	X Diagnostic Z No Qualifier
M Thymus Thymus gland **P Spleen** Accessory spleen **T Bone Marrow**	Ø Open 3 Percutaneous 4 Percutaneous Endoscopic	Ø Drainage Device	Z No Qualifier
M Thymus Thymus gland **P Spleen** Accessory spleen **T Bone Marrow**	Ø Open 3 Percutaneous 4 Percutaneous Endoscopic	Z No Device	X Diagnostic Z No Qualifier

Non-OR Ø79[Ø,1,2,3,4,5,6,7,8,9,B,C,D,F,G,H,J,K,L]8ZX
Non-OR Ø79[Ø,1,2,3,4,5,6,7,8,9,B,C,D,F,G,H,J,K,L][3,8]ZZ
Non-OR Ø79M3ØZ
Non-OR Ø79P[3,4]ØZ
Non-OR Ø79T[Ø,3,4]ØZ
Non-OR Ø79M3ZZ
Non-OR Ø79P[3,4]Z[X,Z]
Non-OR Ø79T[Ø,3,4]Z[X,Z]

Ø Medical and Surgical
7 Lymphatic and Hemic Systems
B Excision Definition: Cutting out or off, without replacement, a portion of a body part
Explanation: The qualifier DIAGNOSTIC is used to identify excision procedures that are biopsies

Body Part Character 4	Approach Character 5	Device Character 6	Qualifier Character 7
Ø Lymphatic, Head Buccinator lymph node Infraauricular lymph node Infraparotid lymph node Parotid lymph node Preauricular lymph node Submandibular lymph node Submaxillary lymph node Submental lymph node Subparotid lymph node Suprahyoid lymph node **1 Lymphatic, Right Neck** Cervical lymph node Jugular lymph node Mastoid (postauricular) lymph node Occipital lymph node Postauricular (mastoid) lymph node Retropharyngeal lymph node Right jugular trunk Right lymphatic duct Right subclavian trunk Supraclavicular (Virchow's) lymph node Virchow's (supraclavicular) lymph node **2 Lymphatic, Left Neck** Cervical lymph node Jugular lymph node Mastoid (postauricular) lymph node Occipital lymph node Postauricular (mastoid) lymph node Retropharyngeal lymph node Supraclavicular (Virchow's) lymph node Virchow's (supraclavicular) lymph node **3 Lymphatic, Right Upper Extremity** Cubital lymph node Deltopectoral (infraclavicular) lymph node Epitrochlear lymph node Infraclavicular (deltopectoral) lymph node Supratrochlear lymph node **4 Lymphatic, Left Upper Extremity** *See 3 Lymphatic, Right Upper Extremity* **5 Lymphatic, Right Axillary** Anterior (pectoral) lymph node Apical (subclavicular) lymph node Brachial (lateral) lymph node Central axillary lymph node Lateral (brachial) lymph node Pectoral (anterior) lymph node Posterior (subscapular) lymph node Subclavicular (apical) lymph node Subscapular (posterior) lymph node **6 Lymphatic, Left Axillary** *See 5 Lymphatic, Right Axillary* **7 Lymphatic, Thorax** Intercostal lymph node Mediastinal lymph node Parasternal lymph node Paratracheal lymph node Tracheobronchial lymph node **8 Lymphatic, Internal Mammary, Right** **9 Lymphatic, Internal Mammary, Left** **B Lymphatic, Mesenteric** Inferior mesenteric lymph node Pararectal lymph node Superior mesenteric lymph node **C Lymphatic, Pelvis** Common iliac (subaortic) lymph node Gluteal lymph node Iliac lymph node Inferior epigastric lymph node Obturator lymph node Sacral lymph node Subaortic (common iliac) lymph node Suprainguinal lymph node **D Lymphatic, Aortic** Celiac lymph node Gastric lymph node Hepatic lymph node Lumbar lymph node Pancreaticosplenic lymph node Paraaortic lymph node Retroperitoneal lymph node **F Lymphatic, Right Lower Extremity** Femoral lymph node Popliteal lymph node **G Lymphatic, Left Lower Extremity** *See F Lymphatic, Right Lower Extremity* **H Lymphatic, Right Inguinal** ⊞ **J Lymphatic, Left Inguinal** ⊞ **K Thoracic Duct** Left jugular trunk Left subclavian trunk **L Cisterna Chyli** Intestinal lymphatic trunk Lumbar lymphatic trunk **M Thymus** Thymus gland **P Spleen** Accessory spleen	**Ø Open** **3 Percutaneous** **4 Percutaneous Endoscopic**	**Z No Device**	**X Diagnostic** **Z No Qualifier**

Non-OR Ø7BP[3,4]ZX

See Appendix L for Procedure Combinations
⊞ Ø7B[H,J][Ø,4]ZZ

Ø Medical and Surgical
7 Lymphatic and Hemic Systems
C Extirpation Definition: Taking or cutting out solid matter from a body part

Explanation: The solid matter may be an abnormal byproduct of a biological function or a foreign body; it may be imbedded in a body part or in the lumen of a tubular body part. The solid matter may or may not have been previously broken into pieces.

Body Part Character 4	Approach Character 5	Device Character 6	Qualifier Character 7
Ø Lymphatic, Head Buccinator lymph node Infraauricular lymph node Infraparotid lymph node Parotid lymph node Preauricular lymph node Submandibular lymph node Submaxillary lymph node Submental lymph node Subparotid lymph node Suprahyoid lymph node **1 Lymphatic, Right Neck** Cervical lymph node Jugular lymph node Mastoid (postauricular) lymph node Occipital lymph node Postauricular (mastoid) lymph node Retropharyngeal lymph node Right jugular trunk Right lymphatic duct Right subclavian trunk Supraclavicular (Virchow's) lymph node Virchow's (supraclavicular) lymph node **2 Lymphatic, Left Neck** Cervical lymph node Jugular lymph node Mastoid (postauricular) lymph node Occipital lymph node Postauricular (mastoid) lymph node Retropharyngeal lymph node Supraclavicular (Virchow's) lymph node Virchow's (supraclavicular) lymph node **3 Lymphatic, Right Upper Extremity** Cubital lymph node Deltopectoral (infraclavicular) lymph node Epitrochlear lymph node Infraclavicular (deltopectoral) lymph node Supratrochlear lymph node **4 Lymphatic, Left Upper Extremity** *See 3 Lymphatic, Right Upper Extremity* **5 Lymphatic, Right Axillary** Anterior (pectoral) lymph node Apical (subclavicular) lymph node Brachial (lateral) lymph node Central axillary lymph node Lateral (brachial) lymph node Pectoral (anterior) lymph node Posterior (subscapular) lymph node Subclavicular (apical) lymph node Subscapular (posterior) lymph node **6 Lymphatic, Left Axillary** *See 5 Lymphatic, Right Axillary* **7 Lymphatic, Thorax** Intercostal lymph node Mediastinal lymph node Parasternal lymph node Paratracheal lymph node Tracheobronchial lymph node **8 Lymphatic, Internal Mammary, Right** **9 Lymphatic, Internal Mammary, Left** **B Lymphatic, Mesenteric** Inferior mesenteric lymph node Pararectal lymph node Superior mesenteric lymph node **C Lymphatic, Pelvis** Common iliac (subaortic) lymph node Gluteal lymph node Iliac lymph node Inferior epigastric lymph node Obturator lymph node Sacral lymph node Subaortic (common iliac) lymph node Suprainguinal lymph node **D Lymphatic, Aortic** Celiac lymph node Gastric lymph node Hepatic lymph node Lumbar lymph node Pancreaticosplenic lymph node Paraaortic lymph node Retroperitoneal lymph node **F Lymphatic, Right Lower Extremity** Femoral lymph node Popliteal lymph node **G Lymphatic, Left Lower Extremity** *See F Lymphatic, Right Lower Extremity* **H Lymphatic, Right Inguinal** **J Lymphatic, Left Inguinal** **K Thoracic Duct** Left jugular trunk Left subclavian trunk **L Cisterna Chyli** Intestinal lymphatic trunk Lumbar lymphatic trunk **M Thymus** Thymus gland **P Spleen** Accessory spleen	**Ø Open** **3 Percutaneous** **4 Percutaneous Endoscopic**	**Z No Device**	**Z No Qualifier**

Non-OR Ø7CP[3,4]ZZ

Ø Medical and Surgical
7 Lymphatic and Hemic Systems
D Extraction Definition: Pulling or stripping out or off all or a portion of a body part by the use of force
Explanation: The qualifier DIAGNOSTIC is used to identify extraction procedures that are biopsies

Body Part Character 4	Approach Character 5	Device Character 6	Qualifier Character 7
Ø Lymphatic, Head Buccinator lymph node Infraauricular lymph node Infraparotid lymph node Parotid lymph node Preauricular lymph node Submandibular lymph node Submaxillary lymph node Submental lymph node Subparotid lymph node Suprahyoid lymph node **1 Lymphatic, Right Neck** Cervical lymph node Jugular lymph node Mastoid (postauricular) lymph node Occipital lymph node Postauricular (mastoid) lymph node Retropharyngeal lymph node Right jugular trunk Right lymphatic duct Right subclavian trunk Supraclavicular (Virchow's) lymph node Virchow's (supraclavicular) lymph node **2 Lymphatic, Left Neck** Cervical lymph node Jugular lymph node Mastoid (postauricular) lymph node Occipital lymph node Postauricular (mastoid) lymph node Retropharyngeal lymph node Supraclavicular (Virchow's) lymph node Virchow's (supraclavicular) lymph node **3 Lymphatic, Right Upper Extremity** Cubital lymph node Deltopectoral (infraclavicular) lymph node Epitrochlear lymph node Infraclavicular (deltopectoral) lymph node Supratrochlear lymph node **4 Lymphatic, Left Upper Extremity** *See 3 Lymphatic, Right Upper Extremity* **5 Lymphatic, Right Axillary** Anterior (pectoral) lymph node Apical (subclavicular) lymph node Brachial (lateral) lymph node Central axillary lymph node Lateral (brachial) lymph node Pectoral (anterior) lymph node Posterior (subscapular) lymph node Subclavicular (apical) lymph node Subscapular (posterior) lymph node **6 Lymphatic, Left Axillary** *See 5 Lymphatic, Right Axillary* **7 Lymphatic, Thorax** Intercostal lymph node Mediastinal lymph node Parasternal lymph node Paratracheal lymph node Tracheobronchial lymph node **8 Lymphatic, Internal Mammary, Right** **9 Lymphatic, Internal Mammary, Left** **B Lymphatic, Mesenteric** Inferior mesenteric lymph node Pararectal lymph node Superior mesenteric lymph node **C Lymphatic, Pelvis** Common iliac (subaortic) lymph node Gluteal lymph node Iliac lymph node Inferior epigastric lymph node Obturator lymph node Sacral lymph node Subaortic (common iliac) lymph node Suprainguinal lymph node **D Lymphatic, Aortic** Celiac lymph node Gastric lymph node Hepatic lymph node Lumbar lymph node Pancreaticosplenic lymph node Paraaortic lymph node Retroperitoneal lymph node **F Lymphatic, Right Lower Extremity** Femoral lymph node Popliteal lymph node **G Lymphatic, Left Lower Extremity** *See F Lymphatic, Right Lower Extremity* **H Lymphatic, Right Inguinal** **J Lymphatic, Left Inguinal** **K Thoracic Duct** Left jugular trunk Left subclavian trunk **L Cisterna Chyli** Intestinal lymphatic trunk Lumbar lymphatic trunk	**3 Percutaneous** **4 Percutaneous Endoscopic** **8 Via Natural or Artificial Opening Endoscopic**	**Z No Device**	**X Diagnostic**
M Thymus Thymus gland **P Spleen** Accessory spleen	**3 Percutaneous** **4 Percutaneous Endoscopic**	**Z No Device**	**X Diagnostic**
Q Bone Marrow, Sternum **R Bone Marrow, Iliac** **S Bone Marrow, Vertebral** **T Bone Marrow**	**Ø Open** **3 Percutaneous**	**Z No Device**	**X Diagnostic** **Z No Qualifier**

Non-OR All body part, approach, device, and qualifier values

Ø Medical and Surgical
7 Lymphatic and Hemic Systems
H Insertion Definition: Putting in a nonbiological appliance that monitors, assists, performs, or prevents a physiological function but does not physically take the place of a body part

Explanation: None

Body Part Character 4	Approach Character 5	Device Character 6	Qualifier Character 7
K Thoracic Duct Left jugular trunk Left subclavian trunk L Cisterna Chyli Intestinal lymphatic trunk Lumbar lymphatic trunk M Thymus Thymus gland N Lymphatic P Spleen Accessory spleen T Bone Marrow	Ø Open 3 Percutaneous 4 Percutaneous Endoscopic	1 Radioactive Element 3 Infusion Device Y Other Device	Z No Qualifier

Non-OR Ø7H[K,L,M,N,P][Ø,4]3Z
Non-OR Ø7H[K,L,M,N,P,T]3[1,3,Y]Z
Non-OR Ø7H[N,P]4YZ
Non-OR Ø7HT[Ø,4][1,3,Y]Z

Ø Medical and Surgical
7 Lymphatic and Hemic Systems
J Inspection Definition: Visually and/or manually exploring a body part

Explanation: Visual exploration may be performed with or without optical instrumentation. Manual exploration may be performed directly or through intervening body layers.

Body Part Character 4	Approach Character 5	Device Character 6	Qualifier Character 7
K Thoracic Duct Left jugular trunk Left subclavian trunk L Cisterna Chyli Intestinal lymphatic trunk Lumbar lymphatic trunk M Thymus Thymus gland T Bone Marrow	Ø Open 3 Percutaneous 4 Percutaneous Endoscopic	Z No Device	Z No Qualifier
N Lymphatic	Ø Open 3 Percutaneous 4 Percutaneous Endoscopic 8 Via Natural or Artificial Opening Endoscopic X External	Z No Device	Z No Qualifier
P Spleen Accessory spleen	Ø Open 3 Percutaneous 4 Percutaneous Endoscopic X External	Z No Device	Z No Qualifier

Non-OR Ø7J[K,L,M]3ZZ
Non-OR Ø7JT[Ø,3,4]ZZ
Non-OR Ø7JN[3,8,X]ZZ
Non-OR Ø7JP[3,4,X]ZZ

Ø Medical and Surgical
7 Lymphatic and Hemic Systems
L Occlusion Definition: Completely closing an orifice or the lumen of a tubular body part
Explanation: The orifice can be a natural orifice or an artificially created orifice

Body Part Character 4		Approach Character 5	Device Character 6	Qualifier Character 7
Ø Lymphatic, Head Buccinator lymph node Infraauricular lymph node Infraparotid lymph node Parotid lymph node Preauricular lymph node Submandibular lymph node Submaxillary lymph node Submental lymph node Subparotid lymph node Suprahyoid lymph node **1 Lymphatic, Right Neck** Cervical lymph node Jugular lymph node Mastoid (postauricular) lymph node Occipital lymph node Postauricular (mastoid) lymph node Retropharyngeal lymph node Right jugular trunk Right lymphatic duct Right subclavian trunk Supraclavicular (Virchow's) lymph node Virchow's (supraclavicular) lymph node **2 Lymphatic, Left Neck** Cervical lymph node Jugular lymph node Mastoid (postauricular) lymph node Occipital lymph node Postauricular (mastoid) lymph node Retropharyngeal lymph node Supraclavicular (Virchow's) lymph node Virchow's (supraclavicular) lymph node **3 Lymphatic, Right Upper Extremity** Cubital lymph node Deltopectoral (infraclavicular) lymph node Epitrochlear lymph node Infraclavicular (deltopectoral) lymph node Supratrochlear lymph node **4 Lymphatic, Left Upper Extremity** *See 3 Lymphatic, Right Upper Extremity* **5 Lymphatic, Right Axillary** Anterior (pectoral) lymph node Apical (subclavicular) lymph node Brachial (lateral) lymph node Central axillary lymph node Lateral (brachial) lymph node Pectoral (anterior) lymph node Posterior (subscapular) lymph node Subclavicular (apical) lymph node Subscapular (posterior) lymph node	**6 Lymphatic, Left Axillary** *See 5 Lymphatic, Right Axillary* **7 Lymphatic, Thorax** Intercostal lymph node Mediastinal lymph node Parasternal lymph node Paratracheal lymph node Tracheobronchial lymph node **8 Lymphatic, Internal Mammary, Right** **9 Lymphatic, Internal Mammary, Left** **B Lymphatic, Mesenteric** Inferior mesenteric lymph node Pararectal lymph node Superior mesenteric lymph node **C Lymphatic, Pelvis** Common iliac (subaortic) lymph node Gluteal lymph node Iliac lymph node Inferior epigastric lymph node Obturator lymph node Sacral lymph node Subaortic (common iliac) lymph node Suprainguinal lymph node **D Lymphatic, Aortic** Celiac lymph node Gastric lymph node Hepatic lymph node Lumbar lymph node Pancreaticosplenic lymph node Paraaortic lymph node Retroperitoneal lymph node **F Lymphatic, Right Lower Extremity** Femoral lymph node Popliteal lymph node **G Lymphatic, Left Lower Extremity** *See F Lymphatic, Right Lower Extremity* **H Lymphatic, Right Inguinal** **J Lymphatic, Left Inguinal** **K Thoracic Duct** Left jugular trunk Left subclavian trunk **L Cisterna Chyli** Intestinal lymphatic trunk Lumbar lymphatic trunk	**Ø Open** **3 Percutaneous** **4 Percutaneous Endoscopic**	**C Extraluminal Device** **D Intraluminal Device** **Z No Device**	**Z No Qualifier**

Ø Medical and Surgical
7 Lymphatic and Hemic Systems
N Release Definition: Freeing a body part from an abnormal physical constraint by cutting or by the use of force
Explanation: Some of the restraining tissue may be taken out but none of the body part is taken out

Body Part Character 4	Approach Character 5	Device Character 6	Qualifier Character 7
Ø Lymphatic, Head Buccinator lymph node Infraauricular lymph node Infraparotid lymph node Parotid lymph node Preauricular lymph node Submandibular lymph node Submaxillary lymph node Submental lymph node Subparotid lymph node Suprahyoid lymph node **1 Lymphatic, Right Neck** Cervical lymph node Jugular lymph node Mastoid (postauricular) lymph node Occipital lymph node Postauricular (mastoid) lymph node Retropharyngeal lymph node Right jugular trunk Right lymphatic duct Right subclavian trunk Supraclavicular (Virchow's) lymph node Virchow's (supraclavicular) lymph node **2 Lymphatic, Left Neck** Cervical lymph node Jugular lymph node Mastoid (postauricular) lymph node Occipital lymph node Postauricular (mastoid) lymph node Retropharyngeal lymph node Supraclavicular (Virchow's) lymph node Virchow's (supraclavicular) lymph node **3 Lymphatic, Right Upper Extremity** Cubital lymph node Deltopectoral (infraclavicular) lymph node Epitrochlear lymph node Infraclavicular (deltopectoral) lymph node Supratrochlear lymph node **4 Lymphatic, Left Upper Extremity** *See 3 Lymphatic, Right Upper Extremity* **5 Lymphatic, Right Axillary** Anterior (pectoral) lymph node Apical (subclavicular) lymph node Brachial (lateral) lymph node Central axillary lymph node Lateral (brachial) lymph node Pectoral (anterior) lymph node Posterior (subscapular) lymph node Subclavicular (apical) lymph node Subscapular (posterior) lymph node **6 Lymphatic, Left Axillary** *See 5 Lymphatic, Right Axillary* **7 Lymphatic, Thorax** Intercostal lymph node Mediastinal lymph node Parasternal lymph node Paratracheal lymph node Tracheobronchial lymph node **8 Lymphatic, Internal Mammary, Right** **9 Lymphatic, Internal Mammary, Left** **B Lymphatic, Mesenteric** Inferior mesenteric lymph node Pararectal lymph node Superior mesenteric lymph node **C Lymphatic, Pelvis** Common iliac (subaortic) lymph node Gluteal lymph node Iliac lymph node Inferior epigastric lymph node Obturator lymph node Sacral lymph node Subaortic (common iliac) lymph node Suprainguinal lymph node **D Lymphatic, Aortic** Celiac lymph node Gastric lymph node Hepatic lymph node Lumbar lymph node Pancreaticosplenic lymph node Paraaortic lymph node Retroperitoneal lymph node **F Lymphatic, Right Lower Extremity** Femoral lymph node Popliteal lymph node **G Lymphatic, Left Lower Extremity** *See F Lymphatic, Right Lower Extremity* **H Lymphatic, Right Inguinal** **J Lymphatic, Left Inguinal** **K Thoracic Duct** Left jugular trunk Left subclavian trunk **L Cisterna Chyli** Intestinal lymphatic trunk Lumbar lymphatic trunk **M Thymus** Thymus gland **P Spleen** Accessory spleen	**Ø Open** **3 Percutaneous** **4 Percutaneous Endoscopic**	**Z No Device**	**Z No Qualifier**

Ø Medical and Surgical
7 Lymphatic and Hemic Systems
P Removal Definition: Taking out or off a device from a body part

Explanation: If a device is taken out and a similar device put in without cutting or puncturing the skin or mucous membrane, the procedure is coded to the root operation CHANGE. Otherwise, the procedure for taking out a device is coded to the root operation REMOVAL.

Body Part Character 4	Approach Character 5	Device Character 6	Qualifier Character 7
K Thoracic Duct Left jugular trunk Left subclavian trunk **L Cisterna Chyli** Intestinal lymphatic trunk Lumbar lymphatic trunk **N Lymphatic**	**Ø** Open **3** Percutaneous **4** Percutaneous Endoscopic	**Ø** Drainage Device **3** Infusion Device **7** Autologous Tissue Substitute **C** Extraluminal Device **D** Intraluminal Device **J** Synthetic Substitute **K** Nonautologous Tissue Substitute **Y** Other Device	**Z** No Qualifier
K Thoracic Duct Left jugular trunk Left subclavian trunk **L Cisterna Chyli** Intestinal lymphatic trunk Lumbar lymphatic trunk **N Lymphatic**	**X** External	**Ø** Drainage Device **3** Infusion Device **D** Intraluminal Device	**Z** No Qualifier
M Thymus Thymus gland **P Spleen** Accessory spleen	**Ø** Open **3** Percutaneous **4** Percutaneous Endoscopic	**Ø** Drainage Device **3** Infusion Device **Y** Other Device	**Z** No Qualifier
M Thymus Thymus gland **P Spleen** Accessory spleen	**X** External	**Ø** Drainage Device **3** Infusion Device	**Z** No Qualifier
T Bone Marrow	**Ø** Open **3** Percutaneous **4** Percutaneous Endoscopic **X** External	**Ø** Drainage Device	**Z** No Qualifier

Non-OR Ø7P[K,L,N][3,4]YZ
Non-OR Ø7P[K,L,N]X[Ø,3,D]Z
Non-OR Ø7P[M,P][3,4]YZ
Non-OR Ø7P[M,P]X[Ø,3]Z
Non-OR Ø7PT[Ø,3,4,X]ØZ

Ø Medical and Surgical
7 Lymphatic and Hemic Systems
Q Repair Definition: Restoring, to the extent possible, a body part to its normal anatomic structure and function
Explanation: Used only when the method to accomplish the repair is not one of the other root operations

Body Part Character 4	Approach Character 5	Device Character 6	Qualifier Character 7
Ø Lymphatic, Head Buccinator lymph node Infraauricular lymph node Infraparotid lymph node Parotid lymph node Preauricular lymph node Submandibular lymph node Submaxillary lymph node Submental lymph node Subparotid lymph node Suprahyoid lymph node **1 Lymphatic, Right Neck** Cervical lymph node Jugular lymph node Mastoid (postauricular) lymph node Occipital lymph node Postauricular (mastoid) lymph node Retropharyngeal lymph node Right jugular trunk Right lymphatic duct Right subclavian trunk Supraclavicular (Virchow's) lymph node Virchow's (supraclavicular) lymph node **2 Lymphatic, Left Neck** Cervical lymph node Jugular lymph node Mastoid (postauricular) lymph node Occipital lymph node Postauricular (mastoid) lymph node Retropharyngeal lymph node Supraclavicular (Virchow's) lymph node Virchow's (supraclavicular) lymph node **3 Lymphatic, Right Upper Extremity** Cubital lymph node Deltopectoral (infraclavicular) lymph node Epitrochlear lymph node Infraclavicular (deltopectoral) lymph node Supratrochlear lymph node **4 Lymphatic, Left Upper Extremity** *See 3 Lymphatic, Right Upper Extremity* **5 Lymphatic, Right Axillary** Anterior (pectoral) lymph node Apical (subclavicular) lymph node Brachial (lateral) lymph node Central axillary lymph node Lateral (brachial) lymph node Pectoral (anterior) lymph node Posterior (subscapular) lymph node Subclavicular (apical) lymph node Subscapular (posterior) lymph node **6 Lymphatic, Left Axillary** *See 5 Lymphatic, Right Axillary* **7 Lymphatic, Thorax** Intercostal lymph node Mediastinal lymph node Parasternal lymph node Paratracheal lymph node Tracheobronchial lymph node **8 Lymphatic, Internal Mammary, Right** **9 Lymphatic, Internal Mammary, Left** **B Lymphatic, Mesenteric** Inferior mesenteric lymph node Pararectal lymph node Superior mesenteric lymph node **C Lymphatic, Pelvis** Common iliac (subaortic) lymph node Gluteal lymph node Iliac lymph node Inferior epigastric lymph node Obturator lymph node Sacral lymph node Subaortic (common iliac) lymph node Suprainguinal lymph node **D Lymphatic, Aortic** Celiac lymph node Gastric lymph node Hepatic lymph node Lumbar lymph node Pancreaticosplenic lymph node Paraaortic lymph node Retroperitoneal lymph node **F Lymphatic, Right Lower Extremity** Femoral lymph node Popliteal lymph node **G Lymphatic, Left Lower Extremity** *See F Lymphatic, Right Lower Extremity* **H Lymphatic, Right Inguinal** **J Lymphatic, Left Inguinal** **K Thoracic Duct** Left jugular trunk Left subclavian trunk **L Cisterna Chyli** Intestinal lymphatic trunk Lumbar lymphatic trunk	**Ø Open** **3 Percutaneous** **4 Percutaneous Endoscopic** **8 Via Natural or Artificial Opening Endoscopic**	**Z No Device**	**Z No Qualifier**
M Thymus Thymus gland **P Spleen** Accessory spleen	**Ø Open** **3 Percutaneous** **4 Percutaneous Endoscopic**	**Z No Device**	**Z No Qualifier**

Ø Medical and Surgical
7 Lymphatic and Hemic Systems
S Reposition Definition: Moving to its normal location, or other suitable location, all or a portion of a body part

Explanation: The body part is moved to a new location from an abnormal location, or from a normal location where it is not functioning correctly. The body part may or may not be cut out or off to be moved to the new location.

Body Part Character 4	Approach Character 5	Device Character 6	Qualifier Character 7
M Thymus Thymus gland **P Spleen** Accessory spleen	**Ø Open**	**Z No Device**	**Z No Qualifier**

Ø Medical and Surgical
7 Lymphatic and Hemic Systems
T Resection Definition: Cutting out or off, without replacement, all of a body part

Explanation: None

Body Part Character 4	Approach Character 5	Device Character 6	Qualifier Character 7
Ø Lymphatic, Head Buccinator lymph node Infraauricular lymph node Infraparotid lymph node Parotid lymph node Preauricular lymph node Submandibular lymph node Submaxillary lymph node Submental lymph node Subparotid lymph node Suprahyoid lymph node **1 Lymphatic, Right Neck** Cervical lymph node Jugular lymph node Mastoid (postauricular) lymph node Occipital lymph node Postauricular (mastoid) lymph node Retropharyngeal lymph node Right jugular trunk Right lymphatic duct Right subclavian trunk Supraclavicular (Virchow's) lymph node Virchow's (supraclavicular) lymph node **2 Lymphatic, Left Neck** Cervical lymph node Jugular lymph node Mastoid (postauricular) lymph node Occipital lymph node Postauricular (mastoid) lymph node Retropharyngeal lymph node Supraclavicular (Virchow's) lymph node Virchow's (supraclavicular) lymph node **3 Lymphatic, Right Upper Extremity** Cubital lymph node Deltopectoral (infraclavicular) lymph node Epitrochlear lymph node Infraclavicular (deltopectoral) lymph node Supratrochlear lymph node **4 Lymphatic, Left Upper Extremity** *See 3 Lymphatic, Right Upper Extremity* **5 Lymphatic, Right Axillary** ⊞ Anterior (pectoral) lymph node Apical (subclavicular) lymph node Brachial (lateral) lymph node Central axillary lymph node Lateral (brachial) lymph node Pectoral (anterior) lymph node Posterior (subscapular) lymph node Subclavicular (apical) lymph node Subscapular (posterior) lymph node **6 Lymphatic, Left Axillary** ⊞ *See 5 Lymphatic, Right Axillary* **7 Lymphatic, Thorax** ⊞ Intercostal lymph node Mediastinal lymph node Parasternal lymph node Paratracheal lymph node Tracheobronchial lymph node **8 Lymphatic, Internal Mammary, Right** ⊞ **9 Lymphatic, Internal Mammary, Left** ⊞ **B Lymphatic, Mesenteric** Inferior mesenteric lymph node Pararectal lymph node Superior mesenteric lymph node **C Lymphatic, Pelvis** Common iliac (subaortic) lymph node Gluteal lymph node Iliac lymph node Inferior epigastric lymph node Obturator lymph node Sacral lymph node Subaortic (common iliac) lymph node Suprainguinal lymph node **D Lymphatic, Aortic** Celiac lymph node Gastric lymph node Hepatic lymph node Lumbar lymph node Pancreaticosplenic lymph node Paraaortic lymph node Retroperitoneal lymph node **F Lymphatic, Right Lower Extremity** Femoral lymph node Popliteal lymph node **G Lymphatic, Left Lower Extremity** *See F Lymphatic, Right Lower Extremity* **H Lymphatic, Right Inguinal** **J Lymphatic, Left Inguinal** **K Thoracic Duct** Left jugular trunk Left subclavian trunk **L Cisterna Chyli** Intestinal lymphatic trunk Lumbar lymphatic trunk **M Thymus** Thymus gland **P Spleen** Accessory spleen	**Ø Open** **4 Percutaneous Endoscopic**	**Z No Device**	**Z No Qualifier**

See Appendix L for Procedure Combinations
⊞ Ø7T[5,6,7,8,9]ØZZ

Ø Medical and Surgical
7 Lymphatic and Hemic Systems
U Supplement Definition: Putting in or on biological or synthetic material that physically reinforces and/or augments the function of a portion of a body part

Explanation: The biological material is non-living, or is living and from the same individual. The body part may have been previously replaced, and the SUPPLEMENT procedure is performed to physically reinforce and/or augment the function of the replaced body part.

Body Part Character 4	Approach Character 5	Device Character 6	Qualifier Character 7
Ø Lymphatic, Head Buccinator lymph node Infraauricular lymph node Infraparotid lymph node Parotid lymph node Preauricular lymph node Submandibular lymph node Submaxillary lymph node Submental lymph node Subparotid lymph node Suprahyoid lymph node **1 Lymphatic, Right Neck** Cervical lymph node Jugular lymph node Mastoid (postauricular) lymph node Occipital lymph node Postauricular (mastoid) lymph node Retropharyngeal lymph node Right jugular trunk Right lymphatic duct Right subclavian trunk Supraclavicular (Virchow's) lymph node Virchow's (supraclavicular) lymph node **2 Lymphatic, Left Neck** Cervical lymph node Jugular lymph node Mastoid (postauricular) lymph node Occipital lymph node Postauricular (mastoid) lymph node Retropharyngeal lymph node Supraclavicular (Virchow's) lymph node Virchow's (supraclavicular) lymph node **3 Lymphatic, Right Upper Extremity** Cubital lymph node Deltopectoral (infraclavicular) lymph node Epitrochlear lymph node Infraclavicular (deltopectoral) lymph node Supratrochlear lymph node **4 Lymphatic, Left Upper Extremity** ***See** 3 Lymphatic, Right Upper Extremity* **5 Lymphatic, Right Axillary** Anterior (pectoral) lymph node Apical (subclavicular) lymph node Brachial (lateral) lymph node Central axillary lymph node Lateral (brachial) lymph node Pectoral (anterior) lymph node Posterior (subscapular) lymph node Subclavicular (apical) lymph node Subscapular (posterior) lymph node **6 Lymphatic, Left Axillary** ***See** 5 Lymphatic, Right Axillary* **7 Lymphatic, Thorax** Intercostal lymph node Mediastinal lymph node Parasternal lymph node Paratracheal lymph node Tracheobronchial lymph node **8 Lymphatic, Internal Mammary, Right** **9 Lymphatic, Internal Mammary, Left** **B Lymphatic, Mesenteric** Inferior mesenteric lymph node Pararectal lymph node Superior mesenteric lymph node **C Lymphatic, Pelvis** Common iliac (subaortic) lymph node Gluteal lymph node Iliac lymph node Inferior epigastric lymph node Obturator lymph node Sacral lymph node Subaortic (common iliac) lymph node Suprainguinal lymph node **D Lymphatic, Aortic** Celiac lymph node Gastric lymph node Hepatic lymph node Lumbar lymph node Pancreaticosplenic lymph node Paraaortic lymph node Retroperitoneal lymph node **F Lymphatic, Right Lower Extremity** Femoral lymph node Popliteal lymph node **G Lymphatic, Left Lower Extremity** ***See** F Lymphatic, Right Lower Extremity* **H Lymphatic, Right Inguinal** **J Lymphatic, Left Inguinal** **K Thoracic Duct** Left jugular trunk Left subclavian trunk **L Cisterna Chyli** Intestinal lymphatic trunk Lumbar lymphatic trunk	**Ø Open** **4 Percutaneous Endoscopic**	**7 Autologous Tissue Substitute** **J Synthetic Substitute** **K Nonautologous Tissue Substitute**	**Z No Qualifier**

Ø Medical and Surgical
7 Lymphatic and Hemic Systems
V Restriction Definition: Partially closing an orifice or the lumen of a tubular body part
Explanation: The orifice can be a natural orifice or an artificially created orifice

Body Part Character 4		Approach Character 5	Device Character 6	Qualifier Character 7
Ø Lymphatic, Head Buccinator lymph node Infraauricular lymph node Infraparotid lymph node Parotid lymph node Preauricular lymph node Submandibular lymph node Submaxillary lymph node Submental lymph node Subparotid lymph node Suprahyoid lymph node **1 Lymphatic, Right Neck** Cervical lymph node Jugular lymph node Mastoid (postauricular) lymph node Occipital lymph node Postauricular (mastoid) lymph node Retropharyngeal lymph node Right jugular trunk Right lymphatic duct Right subclavian trunk Supraclavicular (Virchow's) lymph node Virchow's (supraclavicular) lymph node **2 Lymphatic, Left Neck** Cervical lymph node Jugular lymph node Mastoid (postauricular) lymph node Occipital lymph node Postauricular (mastoid) lymph node Retropharyngeal lymph node Supraclavicular (Virchow's) lymph node Virchow's (supraclavicular) lymph node **3 Lymphatic, Right Upper Extremity** Cubital lymph node Deltopectoral (infraclavicular) lymph node Epitrochlear lymph node Infraclavicular (deltopectoral) lymph node Supratrochlear lymph node **4 Lymphatic, Left Upper Extremity** *See 3 Lymphatic, Right Upper Extremity* **5 Lymphatic, Right Axillary** Anterior (pectoral) lymph node Apical (subclavicular) lymph node Brachial (lateral) lymph node Central axillary lymph node Lateral (brachial) lymph node Pectoral (anterior) lymph node Posterior (subscapular) lymph node Subclavicular (apical) lymph node Subscapular (posterior) lymph node	**6 Lymphatic, Left Axillary** *See 5 Lymphatic, Right Axillary* **7 Lymphatic, Thorax** Intercostal lymph node Mediastinal lymph node Parasternal lymph node Paratracheal lymph node Tracheobronchial lymph node **8 Lymphatic, Internal Mammary, Right** **9 Lymphatic, Internal Mammary, Left** **B Lymphatic, Mesenteric** Inferior mesenteric lymph node Pararectal lymph node Superior mesenteric lymph node **C Lymphatic, Pelvis** Common iliac (subaortic) lymph node Gluteal lymph node Iliac lymph node Inferior epigastric lymph node Obturator lymph node Sacral lymph node Subaortic (common iliac) lymph node Suprainguinal lymph node **D Lymphatic, Aortic** Celiac lymph node Gastric lymph node Hepatic lymph node Lumbar lymph node Pancreaticosplenic lymph node Paraaortic lymph node Retroperitoneal lymph node **F Lymphatic, Right Lower Extremity** Femoral lymph node Popliteal lymph node **G Lymphatic, Left Lower Extremity** *See F Lymphatic, Right Lower Extremity* **H Lymphatic, Right Inguinal** **J Lymphatic, Left Inguinal** **K Thoracic Duct** Left jugular trunk Left subclavian trunk **L Cisterna Chyli** Intestinal lymphatic trunk Lumbar lymphatic trunk	**Ø Open** **3 Percutaneous** **4 Percutaneous Endoscopic**	**C Extraluminal Device** **D Intraluminal Device** **Z No Device**	**Z No Qualifier**

Ø Medical and Surgical
7 Lymphatic and Hemic Systems
W Revision Definition: Correcting, to the extent possible, a portion of a malfunctioning device or the position of a displaced device

Explanation: Revision can include correcting a malfunctioning or displaced device by taking out or putting in components of the device such as a screw or pin

Body Part Character 4	Approach Character 5	Device Character 6	Qualifier Character 7
K Thoracic Duct Left jugular trunk Left subclavian trunk **L** Cisterna Chyli Intestinal lymphatic trunk Lumbar lymphatic trunk **N** Lymphatic	**Ø** Open **3** Percutaneous **4** Percutaneous Endoscopic	**Ø** Drainage Device **3** Infusion Device **7** Autologous Tissue Substitute **C** Extraluminal Device **D** Intraluminal Device **J** Synthetic Substitute **K** Nonautologous Tissue Substitute **Y** Other Device	**Z** No Qualifier
K Thoracic Duct Left jugular trunk Left subclavian trunk **L** Cisterna Chyli Intestinal lymphatic trunk Lumbar lymphatic trunk **N** Lymphatic	**X** External	**Ø** Drainage Device **3** Infusion Device **7** Autologous Tissue Substitute **C** Extraluminal Device **D** Intraluminal Device **J** Synthetic Substitute **K** Nonautologous Tissue Substitute	**Z** No Qualifier
M Thymus Thymus gland **P** Spleen Accessory spleen	**Ø** Open **3** Percutaneous **4** Percutaneous Endoscopic	**Ø** Drainage Device **3** Infusion Device **Y** Other Device	**Z** No Qualifier
M Thymus Thymus gland **P** Spleen Accessory spleen	**X** External	**Ø** Drainage Device **3** Infusion Device	**Z** No Qualifier
T Bone Marrow	**Ø** Open **3** Percutaneous **4** Percutaneous Endoscopic **X** External	**Ø** Drainage Device	**Z** No Qualifier

Non-OR Ø7W[K,L,N][3,4]YZ
Non-OR Ø7W[K,L,N]X[Ø,3,7,C,D,J,K]Z
Non-OR Ø7W[M,P][3,4]YZ
Non-OR Ø7W[M,P]X[Ø,3]Z
Non-OR Ø7WT[Ø,3,4,X]ØZ

Ø Medical and Surgical
7 Lymphatic and Hemic Systems
Y Transplantation Definition: Putting in or on all or a portion of a living body part taken from another individual or animal to physically take the place and/or function of all or a portion of a similar body part

Explanation: The native body part may or may not be taken out, and the transplanted body part may take over all or a portion of its function

Body Part Character 4	Approach Character 5	Device Character 6	Qualifier Character 7
M Thymus Thymus gland **P** Spleen Accessory spleen	**Ø** Open	**Z** No Device	**Ø** Allogeneic **1** Syngeneic **2** Zooplastic

Eye Ø8Ø–Ø8X

Character Meanings

This Character Meaning table is provided as a guide to assist the user in the identification of character members that may be found in this section of code tables. It **SHOULD NOT** be used to build a PCS code.

Operation–Character 3	Body Part–Character 4	Approach–Character 5	Device–Character 6	Qualifier–Character 7
Ø Alteration	Ø Eye, Right	Ø Open	Ø Drainage Device OR Synthetic Substitute, Intraocular Telescope	3 Nasal Cavity
1 Bypass	1 Eye, Left	3 Percutaneous	1 Radioactive Element	4 Sclera
2 Change	2 Anterior Chamber, Right	7 Via Natural or Artificial Opening	3 Infusion Device	X Diagnostic
5 Destruction	3 Anterior Chamber, Left	8 Via Natural or Artificial Opening Endoscopic	5 Epiretinal Visual Prosthesis	Z No Qualifier
7 Dilation	4 Vitreous, Right	X External	7 Autologous Tissue Substitute	
9 Drainage	5 Vitreous, Left		C Extraluminal Device	
B Excision	6 Sclera, Right		D Intraluminal Device	
C Extirpation	7 Sclera, Left		J Synthetic Substitute	
D Extraction	8 Cornea, Right		K Nonautologous Tissue Substitute	
F Fragmentation	9 Cornea, Left		Y Other Device	
H Insertion	A Choroid, Right		Z No Device	
J Inspection	B Choroid, Left			
L Occlusion	C Iris, Right			
M Reattachment	D Iris, Left			
N Release	E Retina, Right			
P Removal	F Retina, Left			
Q Repair	G Retinal Vessel, Right			
R Replacement	H Retinal Vessel, Left			
S Reposition	J Lens, Right			
T Resection	K Lens, Left			
U Supplement	L Extraocular Muscle, Right			
V Restriction	M Extraocular Muscle, Left			
W Revision	N Upper Eyelid, Right			
X Transfer	P Upper Eyelid, Left			
	Q Lower Eyelid, Right			
	R Lower Eyelid, Left			
	S Conjunctiva, Right			
	T Conjunctiva, Left			
	V Lacrimal Gland, Right			
	W Lacrimal Gland, Left			
	X Lacrimal Duct, Right			
	Y Lacrimal Duct, Left			

AHA Coding Clinic for table Ø81
2019, 1Q, 27 Glaucoma tube shunt

AHA Coding Clinic for table Ø89
2016, 2Q, 21 Laser trabeculoplasty

AHA Coding Clinic for table Ø8B
2014, 4Q, 35 Vitrectomy with air/fluid exchange
2014, 4Q, 36 Pars plans vitrectomy without mention of instillation of oil, air or fluid

AHA Coding Clinic for table Ø8J
2015, 1Q, 35 Attempted removal of foreign body from cornea

AHA Coding Clinic for table Ø8N
2015, 2Q, 24 Penetrating keratoplasty and anterior segment reconstruction

AHA Coding Clinic for table Ø8Q
2018, 3Q, 13 Repair of ruptured globe

AHA Coding Clinic for table Ø8R
2015, 2Q, 24 Penetrating keratoplasty and anterior segment reconstruction
2015, 2Q, 25 Penetrating keratoplasty and placement of viscoelastic eye with paracentesis

AHA Coding Clinic for table Ø8T
2015, 2Q, 12 Orbital exenteration

AHA Coding Clinic for table Ø8U
2014, 3Q, 31 Corneal amniotic membrane transplantation

Eye

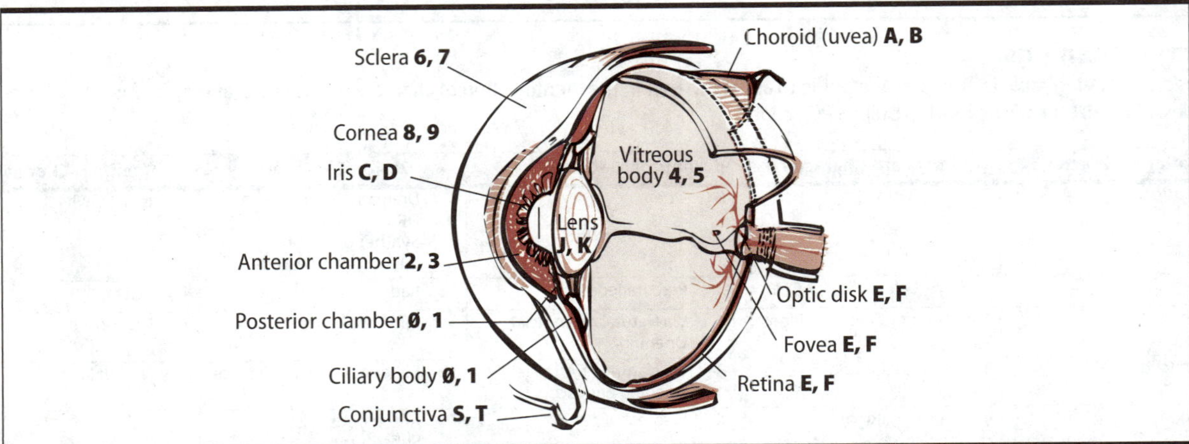

Eye Musculature

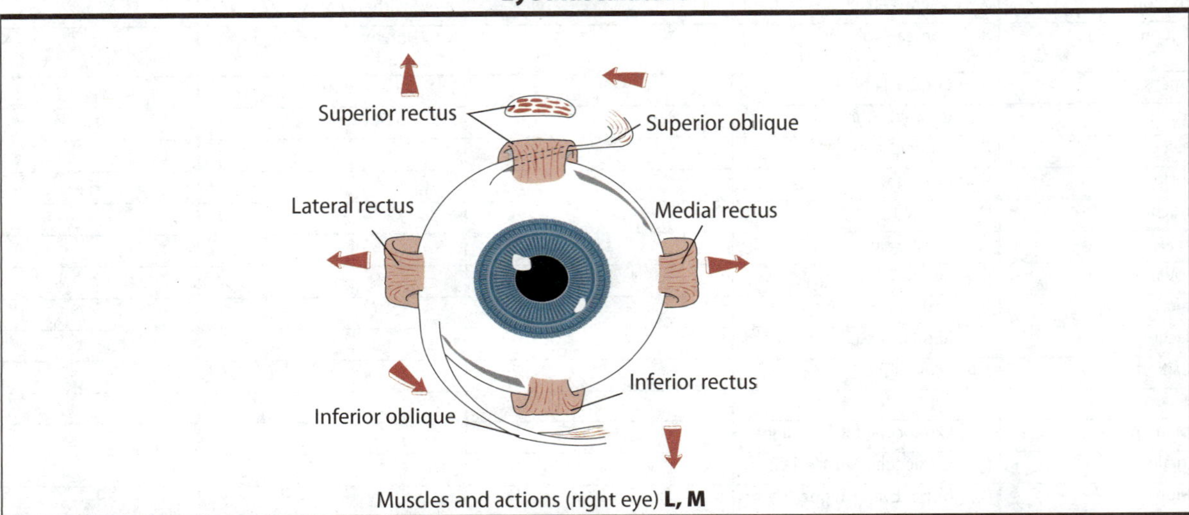

Muscles and actions (right eye) **L, M**

Lacrimal System

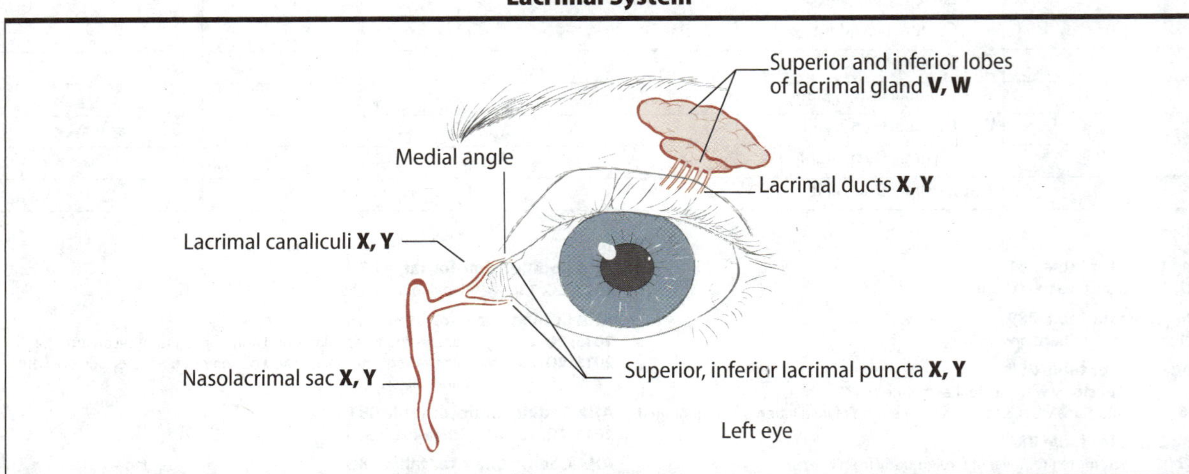

Left eye

Ø Medical and Surgical
8 Eye
Ø Alteration

Definition: Modifying the anatomic structure of a body part without affecting the function of the body part

Explanation: Principal purpose is to improve appearance

Body Part Character 4	Approach Character 5	Device Character 6	Qualifier Character 7
N Upper Eyelid, Right Lateral canthus Levator palpebrae superioris muscle Orbicularis oculi muscle Superior tarsal plate P Upper Eyelid, Left *See N Upper Eyelid, Right* Q Lower Eyelid, Right Inferior tarsal plate Medial canthus R Lower Eyelid, Left *See Q Lower Eyelid, Right*	Ø Open 3 Percutaneous X External	7 Autologous Tissue Substitute J Synthetic Substitute K Nonautologous Tissue Substitute Z No Device	Z No Qualifier

Non-OR All body part, approach, device, and qualifier values

Ø Medical and Surgical
8 Eye
1 Bypass

Definition: Altering the route of passage of the contents of a tubular body part

Explanation: Rerouting contents of a body part to a downstream area of the normal route, to a similar route and body part, or to an abnormal route and dissimilar body part. Includes one or more anastomoses, with or without the use of a device.

Body Part Character 4	Approach Character 5	Device Character 6	Qualifier Character 7
2 Anterior Chamber, Right Aqueous humour 3 Anterior Chamber, Left *See 2 Anterior Chamber, Right*	3 Percutaneous	J Synthetic Substitute K Nonautologous Tissue Substitute Z No Device	4 Sclera
X Lacrimal Duct, Right Lacrimal canaliculus Lacrimal punctum Lacrimal sac Nasolacrimal duct Y Lacrimal Duct, Left *See X Lacrimal Duct, Right*	Ø Open 3 Percutaneous	J Synthetic Substitute K Nonautologous Tissue Substitute Z No Device	3 Nasal Cavity

Ø Medical and Surgical
8 Eye
2 Change

Definition: Taking out or off a device from a body part and putting back an identical or similar device in or on the same body part without cutting or puncturing the skin or a mucous membrane

Explanation: All CHANGE procedures are coded using the approach EXTERNAL

Body Part Character 4	Approach Character 5	Device Character 6	Qualifier Character 7
Ø Eye, Right Ciliary body Posterior chamber 1 Eye, Left *See Ø Eye, Right*	X External	Ø Drainage Device Y Other Device	Z No Qualifier

Non-OR All body part, approach, device, and qualifier values

Ø Medical and Surgical
8 Eye
5 Destruction

Definition: Physical eradication of all or a portion of a body part by the direct use of energy, force, or a destructive agent

Explanation: None of the body part is physically taken out

Body Part Character 4		Approach Character 5	Device Character 6	Qualifier Character 7
Ø Eye, Right Ciliary body Posterior chamber **1 Eye, Left** *See Ø Eye, Right* **6 Sclera, Right** **7 Sclera, Left**	**8 Cornea, Right** **9 Cornea, Left** **S Conjunctiva, Right** Plica semilunaris **T Conjunctiva, Left** *See S Conjunctiva, Right*	**X External**	**Z No Device**	**Z No Qualifier**
2 Anterior Chamber, Right Aqueous humour **3 Anterior Chamber, Left** *See 2 Anterior Chamber, Right* **4 Vitreous, Right** Vitreous body **5 Vitreous, Left** *See 4 Vitreous, Right* **C Iris, Right** **D Iris, Left**	**E Retina, Right** Fovea Macula Optic disc **F Retina, Left** *See E Retina, Right* **G Retinal Vessel, Right** **H Retinal Vessel, Left** **J Lens, Right** Zonule of Zinn **K Lens, Left** *See J Lens, Right*	**3 Percutaneous**	**Z No Device**	**Z No Qualifier**
A Choroid, Right **B Choroid, Left** **L Extraocular Muscle, Right** Inferior oblique muscle Inferior rectus muscle Lateral rectus muscle Medial rectus muscle Superior oblique muscle Superior rectus muscle	**M Extraocular Muscle, Left** *See L Extraocular Muscle, Right* **V Lacrimal Gland, Right** **W Lacrimal Gland, Left**	**Ø Open** **3 Percutaneous**	**Z No Device**	**Z No Qualifier**
N Upper Eyelid, Right Lateral canthus Levator palpebrae superioris muscle Orbicularis oculi muscle Superior tarsal plate **P Upper Eyelid, Left** *See N Upper Eyelid, Right*	**Q Lower Eyelid, Right** Inferior tarsal plate Medial canthus **R Lower Eyelid, Left** *See Q Lower Eyelid, Right*	**Ø Open** **3 Percutaneous** **X External**	**Z No Device**	**Z No Qualifier**
X Lacrimal Duct, Right Lacrimal canaliculus Lacrimal punctum Lacrimal sac Nasolacrimal duct	**Y Lacrimal Duct, Left** *See X Lacrimal Duct, Right*	**Ø Open** **3 Percutaneous** **7 Via Natural or Artificial Opening** **8 Via Natural or Artificial Opening Endoscopic**	**Z No Device**	**Z No Qualifier**

Non-OR Ø85[E,F]3ZZ

Ø Medical and Surgical
8 Eye
7 Dilation

Definition: Expanding an orifice or the lumen of a tubular body part

Explanation: The orifice can be a natural orifice or an artificially created orifice. Accomplished by stretching a tubular body part using intraluminal pressure or by cutting part of the orifice or wall of the tubular body part.

Body Part Character 4	Approach Character 5	Device Character 6	Qualifier Character 7
X Lacrimal Duct, Right Lacrimal canaliculus Lacrimal punctum Lacrimal sac Nasolacrimal duct **Y Lacrimal Duct, Left** *See X Lacrimal Duct, Right*	**Ø Open** **3 Percutaneous** **7 Via Natural or Artificial Opening** **8 Via Natural or Artificial Opening Endoscopic**	**D Intraluminal Device** **Z No Device**	**Z No Qualifier**

Ø Medical and Surgical
8 Eye
9 Drainage

Definition: Taking or letting out fluids and/or gases from a body part
Explanation: The qualifier DIAGNOSTIC is used to identify drainage procedures that are biopsies

Body Part Character 4		Approach Character 5	Device Character 6	Qualifier Character 7
Ø Eye, Right Ciliary body Posterior chamber **1 Eye, Left** *See Ø Eye, Right* **6 Sclera, Right** **7 Sclera, Left**	**8 Cornea, Right** **9 Cornea, Left** **S Conjunctiva, Right** Plica semilunaris **T Conjunctiva, Left** *See S Conjunctiva, Right*	X External	Ø Drainage Device	Z No Qualifier
Ø Eye, Right Ciliary body Posterior chamber **1 Eye, Left** *See Ø Eye, Right* **6 Sclera, Right** **7 Sclera, Left**	**8 Cornea, Right** **9 Cornea, Left** **S Conjunctiva, Right** Plica semilunaris **T Conjunctiva, Left** *See S Conjunctiva, Right*	X External	Z No Device	X Diagnostic Z No Qualifier
2 Anterior Chamber, Right Aqueous humour **3 Anterior Chamber, Left** *See 2 Anterior Chamber, Right* **4 Vitreous, Right** Vitreous body **5 Vitreous, Left** *See 4 Vitreous, Right* **C Iris, Right** **D Iris, Left**	**E Retina, Right** Fovea Macula Optic disc **F Retina, Left** *See E Retina, Right* **G Retinal Vessel, Right** **H Retinal Vessel, Left** **J Lens, Right** Zonule of Zinn **K Lens, Left** *See J Lens, Right*	3 Percutaneous	Ø Drainage Device	Z No Qualifier
2 Anterior Chamber, Right Aqueous humour **3 Anterior Chamber, Left** *See 2 Anterior Chamber, Right* **4 Vitreous, Right** Vitreous body **5 Vitreous, Left** *See 4 Vitreous, Right* **C Iris, Right** **D Iris, Left**	**E Retina, Right** Fovea Macula Optic disc **F Retina, Left** *See E Retina, Right* **G Retinal Vessel, Right** **H Retinal Vessel, Left** **J Lens, Right** Zonule of Zinn **K Lens, Left** *See J Lens, Right*	3 Percutaneous	Z No Device	X Diagnostic Z No Qualifier
A Choroid, Right **B Choroid, Left** **L Extraocular Muscle, Right** Inferior oblique muscle Inferior rectus muscle Lateral rectus muscle Medial rectus muscle Superior oblique muscle Superior rectus muscle	**M Extraocular Muscle, Left** *See L Extraocular Muscle, Right* **V Lacrimal Gland, Right** **W Lacrimal Gland, Left**	Ø Open 3 Percutaneous	Ø Drainage Device	Z No Qualifier
A Choroid, Right **B Choroid, Left** **L Extraocular Muscle, Right** Inferior oblique muscle Inferior rectus muscle Lateral rectus muscle Medial rectus muscle Superior oblique muscle Superior rectus muscle	**M Extraocular Muscle, Left** *See L Extraocular Muscle, Right* **V Lacrimal Gland, Right** **W Lacrimal Gland, Left**	Ø Open 3 Percutaneous	Z No Device	X Diagnostic Z No Qualifier
N Upper Eyelid, Right Lateral canthus Levator palpebrae superioris muscle Orbicularis oculi muscle Superior tarsal plate **P Upper Eyelid, Left** *See N Upper Eyelid, Right*	**Q Lower Eyelid, Right** Inferior tarsal plate Medial canthus **R Lower Eyelid, Left** *See Q Lower Eyelid, Right*	Ø Open 3 Percutaneous X External	Ø Drainage Device	Z No Qualifier

Non-OR Ø89[Ø,1,6,7,8,9,S,T]XZ[X,Z]
Non-OR Ø89[N,P,Q,R][Ø,3,X]ØZ

Ø89 Continued on next page

Ø89 Continued

Ø Medical and Surgical
8 Eye
9 Drainage

Definition: Taking or letting out fluids and/or gases from a body part
Explanation: The qualifier DIAGNOSTIC is used to identify drainage procedures that are biopsies

Body Part Character 4		Approach Character 5	Device Character 6	Qualifier Character 7
N Upper Eyelid, Right Lateral canthus Levator palpebrae superioris muscle Orbicularis oculi muscle Superior tarsal plate **P Upper Eyelid, Left** *See N Upper Eyelid, Right*	**Q Lower Eyelid, Right** Inferior tarsal plate Medial canthus **R Lower Eyelid, Left** *See Q Lower Eyelid, Right*	**Ø Open** **3 Percutaneous** **X External**	**Z No Device**	**X Diagnostic** **Z No Qualifier**
X Lacrimal Duct, Right Lacrimal canaliculus Lacrimal punctum Lacrimal sac Nasolacrimal duct	**Y Lacrimal Duct, Left** *See X Lacrimal Duct, Right*	**Ø Open** **3 Percutaneous** **7 Via Natural or Artificial Opening** **8 Via Natural or Artificial Opening Endoscopic**	**Ø Drainage Device**	**Z No Qualifier**
X Lacrimal Duct, Right Lacrimal canaliculus Lacrimal punctum Lacrimal sac Nasolacrimal duct	**Y Lacrimal Duct, Left** *See X Lacrimal Duct, Right*	**Ø Open** **3 Percutaneous** **7 Via Natural or Artificial Opening** **8 Via Natural or Artificial Opening Endoscopic**	**Z No Device**	**X Diagnostic** **Z No Qualifier**

Non-OR Ø89[N,P,Q,R]ØZZ
Non-OR Ø89[N,P,Q,R][3,X]Z[X,Z]

Ø Medical and Surgical
8 Eye
B Excision

Definition: Cutting out or off, without replacement, a portion of a body part
Explanation: The qualifier DIAGNOSTIC is used to identify excision procedures that are biopsies

Body Part Character 4		Approach Character 5	Device Character 6	Qualifier Character 7
Ø Eye, Right Ciliary body Posterior chamber **1 Eye, Left** *See Ø Eye, Right* **N Upper Eyelid, Right** Lateral canthus Levator palpebrae superioris muscle Orbicularis oculi muscle Superior tarsal plate	**P Upper Eyelid, Left** *See N Upper Eyelid, Right* **Q Lower Eyelid, Right** Inferior tarsal plate Medial canthus **R Lower Eyelid, Left** *See Q Lower Eyelid, Right*	**Ø Open** **3 Percutaneous** **X External**	**Z No Device**	**X Diagnostic** **Z No Qualifier**
4 Vitreous, Right Vitreous body **5 Vitreous, Left** *See 4 Vitreous, Right* **C Iris, Right** **D Iris, Left** **E Retina, Right** Fovea Macula Optic disc	**F Retina, Left** *See E Retina, Right* **J Lens, Right** Zonule of Zinn **K Lens, Left** *See J Lens, Right*	**3 Percutaneous**	**Z No Device**	**X Diagnostic** **Z No Qualifier**
6 Sclera, Right **7 Sclera, Left** **8 Cornea, Right** **9 Cornea, Left**	**S Conjunctiva, Right** Plica semilunaris **T Conjunctiva, Left** *See S Conjunctiva, Right*	**X External**	**Z No Device**	**X Diagnostic** **Z No Qualifier**
A Choroid, Right **B Choroid, Left** **L Extraocular Muscle, Right** Inferior oblique muscle Inferior rectus muscle Lateral rectus muscle Medial rectus muscle Superior oblique muscle Superior rectus muscle	**M Extraocular Muscle, Left** *See L Extraocular Muscle, Right* **V Lacrimal Gland, Right** **W Lacrimal Gland, Left**	**Ø Open** **3 Percutaneous**	**Z No Device**	**X Diagnostic** **Z No Qualifier**
X Lacrimal Duct, Right Lacrimal canaliculus Lacrimal punctum Lacrimal sac Nasolacrimal duct	**Y Lacrimal Duct, Left** *See X Lacrimal Duct, Right*	**Ø Open** **3 Percutaneous** **7 Via Natural or Artificial Opening** **8 Via Natural or Artificial Opening Endoscopic**	**Z No Device**	**X Diagnostic** **Z No Qualifier**

Ø Medical and Surgical
8 Eye
C Extirpation

Definition: Taking or cutting out solid matter from a body part

Explanation: The solid matter may be an abnormal byproduct of a biological function or a foreign body; it may be imbedded in a body part or in the lumen of a tubular body part. The solid matter may or may not have been previously broken into pieces.

Body Part Character 4	Approach Character 5	Device Character 6	Qualifier Character 7
Ø Eye, Right Ciliary body Posterior chamber **1 Eye, Left** *See Ø Eye, Right* **6 Sclera, Right** **7 Sclera, Left** **8 Cornea, Right** **9 Cornea, Left** **S Conjunctiva, Right** Plica semilunaris **T Conjunctiva, Left** *See S Conjunctiva, Right*	**X External**	**Z No Device**	**Z No Qualifier**
2 Anterior Chamber, Right Aqueous humour **3 Anterior Chamber, Left** *See 2 Anterior Chamber, Right* **4 Vitreous, Right** Vitreous body **5 Vitreous, Left** *See 4 Vitreous, Right* **C Iris, Right** **D Iris, Left** **E Retina, Right** Fovea Macula Optic disc **F Retina, Left** *See* E Retina, Right **G Retinal Vessel, Right** **H Retinal Vessel, Left** **J Lens, Right** Zonule of Zinn **K Lens, Left** *See J Lens, Right*	**3 Percutaneous** **X External**	**Z No Device**	**Z No Qualifier**
A Choroid, Right **B Choroid, Left** **L Extraocular Muscle, Right** Inferior oblique muscle Inferior rectus muscle Lateral rectus muscle Medial rectus muscle Superior oblique muscle Superior rectus muscle **M Extraocular Muscle, Left** *See L Extraocular Muscle, Right* **N Upper Eyelid, Right** Lateral canthus Levator palpebrae superioris muscle Orbicularis oculi muscle Superior tarsal plate **P Upper Eyelid, Left** *See N Upper Eyelid, Right* **Q Lower Eyelid, Right** Inferior tarsal plate Medial canthus **R Lower Eyelid, Left** *See Q Lower Eyelid, Right* **V Lacrimal Gland, Right** **W Lacrimal Gland, Left**	**Ø Open** **3 Percutaneous** **X External**	**Z No Device**	**Z No Qualifier**
X Lacrimal Duct, Right Lacrimal canaliculus Lacrimal punctum Lacrimal sac Nasolacrimal duct **Y Lacrimal Duct, Left** *See X Lacrimal Duct, Right*	**Ø Open** **3 Percutaneous** **7 Via Natural or Artificial Opening** **8 Via Natural or Artificial Opening Endoscopic**	**Z No Device**	**Z No Qualifier**

Non-OR Ø8C[Ø,1,6,7,S,T]XZZ
Non-OR Ø8C[2,3]XZZ
Non-OR Ø8C[N,P,Q,R][Ø,3,X]ZZ

Ø Medical and Surgical
8 Eye
D Extraction

Definition: Pulling or stripping out or off all or a portion of a body part by the use of force

Explanation: The qualifier DIAGNOSTIC is used to identify extraction procedures that are biopsies

Body Part Character 4	Approach Character 5	Device Character 6	Qualifier Character 7
8 Cornea, Right **9** Cornea, Left	**X** External	**Z** No Device	**X** Diagnostic **Z** No Qualifier
J Lens, Right Zonule of Zinn **K** Lens, Left *See J Lens, Right*	**3** Percutaneous	**Z** No Device	**Z** No Qualifier

Ø Medical and Surgical
8 Eye
F Fragmentation

Definition: Breaking solid matter in a body part into pieces

Explanation: Physical force (e.g., manual, ultrasonic) applied directly or indirectly is used to break the solid matter into pieces. The solid matter may be an abnormal byproduct of a biological function or a foreign body. The pieces of solid matter are not taken out.

Body Part Character 4	Approach Character 5	Device Character 6	Qualifier Character 7
4 Vitreous, Right NC Vitreous body **5** Vitreous, Left NC *See 4 Vitreous, Right*	**3** Percutaneous **X** External	**Z** No Device	**Z** No Qualifier

Non-OR Ø8F[4,5]XZZ
NC Ø8F[4,5]XZZ

Ø Medical and Surgical
8 Eye
H Insertion

Definition: Putting in a nonbiological appliance that monitors, assists, performs, or prevents a physiological function but does not physically take the place of a body part

Explanation: None

Body Part Character 4	Approach Character 5	Device Character 6	Qualifier Character 7
Ø Eye, Right Ciliary body Posterior chamber **1** Eye, Left *See Ø Eye, Right*	**Ø** Open	**5** Epiretinal Visual Prosthesis **Y** Other Device	**Z** No Qualifier
Ø Eye, Right Ciliary body Posterior chamber **1** Eye, Left *See Ø Eye, Right*	**3** Percutaneous	**1** Radioactive Element **3** Infusion Device **Y** Other Device	**Z** No Qualifier
Ø Eye, Right Ciliary body Posterior chamber **1** Eye, Left *See Ø Eye, Right*	**7** Via Natural or Artificial Opening **8** Via Natural or Artificial Opening Endoscopic	**Y** Other Device	**Z** No Qualifier
Ø Eye, Right Ciliary body Posterior chamber **1** Eye, Left *See Ø Eye, Right*	**X** External	**1** Radioactive Element **3** Infusion Device	**Z** No Qualifier

Non-OR Ø8H[Ø,1]3YZ
Non-OR Ø8H[Ø,1][7,8]YZ

Ø Medical and Surgical
8 Eye
J Inspection

Definition: Visually and/or manually exploring a body part

Explanation: Visual exploration may be performed with or without optical instrumentation. Manual exploration may be performed directly or through intervening body layers.

Body Part Character 4	Approach Character 5	Device Character 6	Qualifier Character 7
Ø Eye, Right Ciliary body Posterior chamber **1 Eye, Left** *See Ø Eye, Right* **J Lens, Right** Zonule of Zinn **K Lens, Left** *See J Lens, Right*	**X** External	**Z** No Device	**Z** No Qualifier
L Extraocular Muscle, Right Inferior oblique muscle Inferior rectus muscle Lateral rectus muscle Medial rectus muscle Superior oblique muscle Superior rectus muscle **M Extraocular Muscle, Left** *See L Extraocular Muscle, Right*	**Ø** Open **X** External	**Z** No Device	**Z** No Qualifier

Non-OR Ø8J[Ø,1,J,K]XZZ
Non-OR Ø8J[L,M]XZZ

Ø Medical and Surgical
8 Eye
L Occlusion

Definition: Completely closing an orifice or the lumen of a tubular body part

Explanation: The orifice can be a natural orifice or an artificially created orifice

Body Part Character 4	Approach Character 5	Device Character 6	Qualifier Character 7
X Lacrimal Duct, Right Lacrimal canaliculus Lacrimal punctum Lacrimal sac Nasolacrimal duct **Y Lacrimal Duct, Left** *See X Lacrimal Duct, Right*	**Ø** Open **3** Percutaneous	**C** Extraluminal Device **D** Intraluminal Device **Z** No Device	**Z** No Qualifier
X Lacrimal Duct, Right Lacrimal canaliculus Lacrimal punctum Lacrimal sac Nasolacrimal duct **Y Lacrimal Duct, Left** *See X Lacrimal Duct, Right*	**7** Via Natural or Artificial Opening **8** Via Natural or Artificial Opening Endoscopic	**D** Intraluminal Device **Z** No Device	**Z** No Qualifier

Ø Medical and Surgical
8 Eye
M Reattachment

Definition: Putting back in or on all or a portion of a separated body part to its normal location or other suitable location

Explanation: Vascular circulation and nervous pathways may or may not be reestablished

Body Part Character 4	Approach Character 5	Device Character 6	Qualifier Character 7
N Upper Eyelid, Right Lateral canthus Levator palpebrae superioris muscle Orbicularis oculi muscle Superior tarsal plate **P Upper Eyelid, Left** *See N Upper Eyelid, Right* **Q Lower Eyelid, Right** Inferior tarsal plate Medial canthus **R Lower Eyelid, Left** *See Q Lower Eyelid, Right*	**X** External	**Z** No Device	**Z** No Qualifier

Ø Medical and Surgical
8 Eye
N Release Definition: Freeing a body part from an abnormal physical constraint by cutting or by the use of force
Explanation: Some of the restraining tissue may be taken out but none of the body part is taken out

Body Part Character 4	Approach Character 5	Device Character 6	Qualifier Character 7
Ø Eye, Right Ciliary body Posterior chamber **1 Eye, Left** *See Ø Eye, Right* **6 Sclera, Right** **7 Sclera, Left** **8 Cornea, Right** **9 Cornea, Left** **S Conjunctiva, Right** Plica semilunaris **T Conjunctiva, Left** *See S Conjunctiva, Right*	**X External**	**Z No Device**	**Z No Qualifier**
2 Anterior Chamber, Right Aqueous humour **3 Anterior Chamber, Left** *See 2 Anterior Chamber, Right* **4 Vitreous, Right** Vitreous body **5 Vitreous, Left** *See 4 Vitreous, Right* **C Iris, Right** **D Iris, Left** **E Retina, Right** Fovea Macula Optic disc **F Retina, Left** *See E Retina, Right* **G Retinal Vessel, Right** **H Retinal Vessel, Left** **J Lens, Right** Zonule of Zinn **K Lens, Left** *See J Lens, Right*	**3 Percutaneous**	**Z No Device**	**Z No Qualifier**
A Choroid, Right **B Choroid, Left** **L Extraocular Muscle, Right** Inferior oblique muscle Inferior rectus muscle Lateral rectus muscle Medial rectus muscle Superior oblique muscle Superior rectus muscle **M Extraocular Muscle, Left** *See L Extraocular Muscle, Right* **V Lacrimal Gland, Right** **W Lacrimal Gland, Left**	**Ø Open** **3 Percutaneous**	**Z No Device**	**Z No Qualifier**
N Upper Eyelid, Right Lateral canthus Levator palpebrae superioris muscle Orbicularis oculi muscle Superior tarsal plate **P Upper Eyelid, Left** *See N Upper Eyelid, Right* **Q Lower Eyelid, Right** Inferior tarsal plate Medial canthus **R Lower Eyelid, Left** *See Q Lower Eyelid, Right*	**Ø Open** **3 Percutaneous** **X External**	**Z No Device**	**Z No Qualifier**
X Lacrimal Duct, Right Lacrimal canaliculus Lacrimal punctum Lacrimal sac Nasolacrimal duct **Y Lacrimal Duct, Left** *See X Lacrimal Duct, Right*	**Ø Open** **3 Percutaneous** **7 Via Natural or Artificial Opening** **8 Via Natural or Artificial Opening Endoscopic**	**Z No Device**	**Z No Qualifier**

Ø Medical and Surgical
8 Eye
P Removal

Definition: Taking out or off a device from a body part

Explanation: If a device is taken out and a similar device put in without cutting or puncturing the skin or mucous membrane, the procedure is coded to the root operation CHANGE. Otherwise, the procedure for taking out a device is coded to the root operation REMOVAL.

Body Part Character 4	Approach Character 5	Device Character 6	Qualifier Character 7
Ø Eye, Right Ciliary body Posterior chamber **1 Eye, Left** *See Ø Eye, Right*	**Ø Open** **3 Percutaneous** **7 Via Natural or Artificial Opening** **8 Via Natural or Artificial Opening Endoscopic**	**Ø Drainage Device** **1 Radioactive Element** **3 Infusion Device** **7 Autologous Tissue Substitute** **C Extraluminal Device** **D Intraluminal Device** **J Synthetic Substitute** **K Nonautologous Tissue Substitute** **Y Other Device**	**Z No Qualifier**
Ø Eye, Right Ciliary body Posterior chamber **1 Eye, Left** *See Ø Eye, Right*	**X External**	**Ø Drainage Device** **1 Radioactive Element** **3 Infusion Device** **7 Autologous Tissue Substitute** **C Extraluminal Device** **D Intraluminal Device** **J Synthetic Substitute** **K Nonautologous Tissue Substitute**	**Z No Qualifier**
J Lens, Right Zonule of Zinn **K Lens, Left** *See J Lens, Right*	**3 Percutaneous**	**J Synthetic Substitute** **Y Other Device**	**Z No Qualifier**
L Extraocular Muscle, Right Inferior oblique muscle Inferior rectus muscle Lateral rectus muscle Medial rectus muscle Superior oblique muscle Superior rectus muscle **M Extraocular Muscle, Left** *See L Extraocular Muscle, Right*	**Ø Open** **3 Percutaneous**	**Ø Drainage Device** **7 Autologous Tissue Substitute** **J Synthetic Substitute** **K Nonautologous Tissue Substitute** **Y Other Device**	**Z No Qualifier**

Non-OR Ø8P[Ø,1]3YZ
Non-OR Ø8P[Ø,1][7,8][Ø,3,D,Y]Z
Non-OR Ø8P[Ø,1]X[Ø,1,3,C,D,J]Z
Non-OR Ø8P[J,K]3YZ
Non-OR Ø8P[L,M]3YZ

Ø Medical and Surgical
8 Eye
Q Repair

Definition: Restoring, to the extent possible, a body part to its normal anatomic structure and function
Explanation: Used only when the method to accomplish the repair is not one of the other root operations

Body Part Character 4	Approach Character 5	Device Character 6	Qualifier Character 7
Ø Eye, Right Ciliary body Posterior chamber **1 Eye, Left** *See Ø Eye, Right* **6 Sclera, Right** **7 Sclera, Left** **8 Cornea, Right** NC **9 Cornea, Left** NC **S Conjunctiva, Right** Plica semilunaris **T Conjunctiva, Left** *See S Conjunctiva, Right*	**X External**	**Z No Device**	**Z No Qualifier**
2 Anterior Chamber, Right Aqueous humour **3 Anterior Chamber, Left** *See 2 Anterior Chamber, Right* **4 Vitreous, Right** Vitreous body **5 Vitreous, Left** *See 4 Vitreous, Right* **C Iris, Right** **D Iris, Left** **E Retina, Right** Fovea Macula Optic disc **F Retina, Left** *See E Retina, Right* **G Retinal Vessel, Right** **H Retinal Vessel, Left** **J Lens, Right** Zonule of Zinn **K Lens, Left** *See J Lens, Right*	**3 Percutaneous**	**Z No Device**	**Z No Qualifier**
A Choroid, Right **B Choroid, Left** **L Extraocular Muscle, Right** Inferior oblique muscle Inferior rectus muscle Lateral rectus muscle Medial rectus muscle Superior oblique muscle Superior rectus muscle **M Extraocular Muscle, Left** *See L Extraocular Muscle, Right* **V Lacrimal Gland, Right** **W Lacrimal Gland, Left**	**Ø Open** **3 Percutaneous**	**Z No Device**	**Z No Qualifier**
N Upper Eyelid, Right Lateral canthus Levator palpebrae superioris muscle Orbicularis oculi muscle Superior tarsal plate **P Upper Eyelid, Left** *See N Upper Eyelid, Right* **Q Lower Eyelid, Right** Inferior tarsal plate Medial canthus **R Lower Eyelid, Left** *See Q Lower Eyelid, Right*	**Ø Open** **3 Percutaneous** **X External**	**Z No Device**	**Z No Qualifier**
X Lacrimal Duct, Right Lacrimal canaliculus Lacrimal punctum Lacrimal sac Nasolacrimal duct **Y Lacrimal Duct, Left** *See X Lacrimal Duct, Right*	**Ø Open** **3 Percutaneous** **7 Via Natural or Artificial Opening** **8 Via Natural or Artificial Opening Endoscopic**	**Z No Device**	**Z No Qualifier**

Non-OR Ø8Q[N,P,Q,R][Ø,3,X]ZZ
NC Ø8Q[8,9]XZZ

Ø Medical and Surgical
8 Eye
R Replacement

Definition: Putting in or on biological or synthetic material that physically takes the place and/or function of all or a portion of a body part

Explanation: The body part may have been taken out or replaced, or may be taken out, physically eradicated, or rendered nonfunctional during the REPLACEMENT procedure. A REMOVAL procedure is coded for taking out the device used in a previous replacement procedure.

Body Part Character 4	Approach Character 5	Device Character 6	Qualifier Character 7
Ø Eye, Right Ciliary body Posterior chamber **1 Eye, Left** *See Ø Eye, Right* **A Choroid, Right** **B Choroid, Left**	**Ø Open** **3 Percutaneous**	**7 Autologous Tissue Substitute** **J Synthetic Substitute** **K Nonautologous Tissue Substitute**	**Z No Qualifier**
4 Vitreous, Right Vitreous body **5 Vitreous, Left** *See 4 Vitreous, Right* **C Iris, Right** **D Iris, Left** **G Retinal Vessel, Right** **H Retinal Vessel, Left**	**3 Percutaneous**	**7 Autologous Tissue Substitute** **J Synthetic Substitute** **K Nonautologous Tissue Substitute**	**Z No Qualifier**
6 Sclera, Right **7 Sclera, Left** **S Conjunctiva, Right** Plica semilunaris **T Conjunctiva, Left** *See S Conjunctiva, Right*	**X External**	**7 Autologous Tissue Substitute** **J Synthetic Substitute** **K Nonautologous Tissue Substitute**	**Z No Qualifier**
8 Cornea, Right **9 Cornea, Left**	**3 Percutaneous** **X External**	**7 Autologous Tissue Substitute** **J Synthetic Substitute** **K Nonautologous Tissue Substitute**	**Z No Qualifier**
J Lens, Right Zonule of Zinn **K Lens, Left** *See J Lens, Right*	**3 Percutaneous**	**Ø Synthetic Substitute, Intraocular Telescope** **7 Autologous Tissue Substitute** **J Synthetic Substitute** **K Nonautologous Tissue Substitute**	**Z No Qualifier**
N Upper Eyelid, Right Lateral canthus Levator palpebrae superioris muscle Orbicularis oculi muscle Superior tarsal plate **P Upper Eyelid, Left** *See N Upper Eyelid, Right* **Q Lower Eyelid, Right** Inferior tarsal plate Medial canthus **R Lower Eyelid, Left** *See Q Lower Eyelid, Right*	**Ø Open** **3 Percutaneous** **X External**	**7 Autologous Tissue Substitute** **J Synthetic Substitute** **K Nonautologous Tissue Substitute**	**Z No Qualifier**
X Lacrimal Duct, Right Lacrimal canaliculus Lacrimal punctum Lacrimal sac Nasolacrimal duct **Y Lacrimal Duct, Left** *See X Lacrimal Duct, Right*	**Ø Open** **3 Percutaneous** **7 Via Natural or Artificial Opening** **8 Via Natural or Artificial Opening Endoscopic**	**7 Autologous Tissue Substitute** **J Synthetic Substitute** **K Nonautologous Tissue Substitute**	**Z No Qualifier**

Ø Medical and Surgical
8 Eye
S Reposition

Definition: Moving to its normal location, or other suitable location, all or a portion of a body part

Explanation: The body part is moved to a new location from an abnormal location, or from a normal location where it is not functioning correctly. The body part may or may not be cut out or off to be moved to the new location.

Body Part Character 4	Approach Character 5	Device Character 6	Qualifier Character 7
C Iris, Right **D Iris, Left** **G Retinal Vessel, Right** **H Retinal Vessel, Left** **J Lens, Right** Zonule of Zinn **K Lens, Left** *See J Lens, Right*	**3 Percutaneous**	**Z No Device**	**Z No Qualifier**
L Extraocular Muscle, Right Inferior oblique muscle Inferior rectus muscle Lateral rectus muscle Medial rectus muscle Superior oblique muscle Superior rectus muscle **M Extraocular Muscle, Left** *See L Extraocular Muscle, Right* **V Lacrimal Gland, Right** **W Lacrimal Gland, Left**	**Ø Open** **3 Percutaneous**	**Z No Device**	**Z No Qualifier**
N Upper Eyelid, Right Lateral canthus Levator palpebrae superioris muscle Orbicularis oculi muscle Superior tarsal plate **P Upper Eyelid, Left** *See N Upper Eyelid, Right* **Q Lower Eyelid, Right** Inferior tarsal plate Medial canthus **R Lower Eyelid, Left** *See Q Lower Eyelid, Right*	**Ø Open** **3 Percutaneous** **X External**	**Z No Device**	**Z No Qualifier**
X Lacrimal Duct, Right Lacrimal canaliculus Lacrimal punctum Lacrimal sac Nasolacrimal duct **Y Lacrimal Duct, Left** *See X Lacrimal Duct, Right*	**Ø Open** **3 Percutaneous** **7 Via Natural or Artificial Opening** **8 Via Natural or Artificial Opening Endoscopic**	**Z No Device**	**Z No Qualifier**

Ø Medical and Surgical
8 Eye
T Resection

Definition: Cutting out or off, without replacement, all of a body part

Explanation: None

Body Part Character 4	Approach Character 5	Device Character 6	Qualifier Character 7
Ø Eye, Right Ciliary body Posterior chamber **1 Eye, Left** *See Ø Eye, Right* **8 Cornea, Right** **9 Cornea, Left**	**X External**	**Z No Device**	**Z No Qualifier**
4 Vitreous, Right Vitreous body **5 Vitreous, Left** *See 4 Vitreous, Right* **C Iris, Right** **D Iris, Left** **J Lens, Right** Zonule of Zinn **K Lens, Left** *See J Lens, Right*	**3 Percutaneous**	**Z No Device**	**Z No Qualifier**
L Extraocular Muscle, Right Inferior oblique muscle Inferior rectus muscle Lateral rectus muscle Medial rectus muscle Superior oblique muscle Superior rectus muscle **M Extraocular Muscle, Left** *See L Extraocular Muscle, Right* **V Lacrimal Gland, Right** **W Lacrimal Gland, Left**	**Ø Open** **3 Percutaneous**	**Z No Device**	**Z No Qualifier**
N Upper Eyelid, Right Lateral canthus Levator palpebrae superioris muscle Orbicularis oculi muscle Superior tarsal plate **P Upper Eyelid, Left** *See N Upper Eyelid, Right* **Q Lower Eyelid, Right** Inferior tarsal plate Medial canthus **R Lower Eyelid, Left** *See Q Lower Eyelid, Right*	**Ø Open** **X External**	**Z No Device**	**Z No Qualifier**
X Lacrimal Duct, Right Lacrimal canaliculus Lacrimal punctum Lacrimal sac Nasolacrimal duct **Y Lacrimal Duct, Left** *See X Lacrimal Duct, Right*	**Ø Open** **3 Percutaneous** **7 Via Natural or Artificial Opening** **8 Via Natural or Artificial Opening Endoscopic**	**Z No Device**	**Z No Qualifier**

Ø Medical and Surgical
8 Eye
U Supplement

Definition: Putting in or on biological or synthetic material that physically reinforces and/or augments the function of a portion of a body part

Explanation: The biological material is non-living, or is living and from the same individual. The body part may have been previously replaced, and the SUPPLEMENT procedure is performed to physically reinforce and/or augment the function of the replaced body part.

Body Part Character 4	Approach Character 5	Device Character 6	Qualifier Character 7
Ø Eye, Right Ciliary body Posterior chamber **1 Eye, Left** *See Ø Eye, Right* **C Iris, Right** **D Iris, Left** **E Retina, Right** Fovea Macula Optic disc **F Retina, Left** *See E Retina, Right* **G Retinal Vessel, Right** **H Retinal Vessel, Left** **L Extraocular Muscle, Right** Inferior oblique muscle Inferior rectus muscle Lateral rectus muscle Medial rectus muscle Superior oblique muscle Superior rectus muscle **M Extraocular Muscle, Left** *See L Extraocular Muscle, Right*	**Ø Open** **3 Percutaneous**	**7 Autologous Tissue Substitute** **J Synthetic Substitute** **K Nonautologous Tissue Substitute**	**Z No Qualifier**
8 Cornea, Right NC **9 Cornea, Left** NC **N Upper Eyelid, Right** Lateral canthus Levator palpebrae superioris muscle Orbicularis oculi muscle Superior tarsal plate **P Upper Eyelid, Left** *See N Upper Eyelid, Right* **Q Lower Eyelid, Right** Inferior tarsal plate Medial canthus **R Lower Eyelid, Left** *See Q Lower Eyelid, Right*	**Ø Open** **3 Percutaneous** **X External**	**7 Autologous Tissue Substitute** **J Synthetic Substitute** **K Nonautologous Tissue Substitute**	**Z No Qualifier**
X Lacrimal Duct, Right Lacrimal canaliculus Lacrimal punctum Lacrimal sac Nasolacrimal duct **Y Lacrimal Duct, Left** *See X Lacrimal Duct, Right*	**Ø Open** **3 Percutaneous** **7 Via Natural or Artificial Opening** **8 Via Natural or Artificial Opening Endoscopic**	**7 Autologous Tissue Substitute** **J Synthetic Substitute** **K Nonautologous Tissue Substitute**	**Z No Qualifier**

NC Ø8U[8,9][Ø,3,X]KZ

Ø Medical and Surgical
8 Eye
V Restriction

Definition: Partially closing an orifice or the lumen of a tubular body part

Explanation: The orifice can be a natural orifice or an artificially created orifice

Body Part Character 4	Approach Character 5	Device Character 6	Qualifier Character 7
X Lacrimal Duct, Right Lacrimal canaliculus Lacrimal punctum Lacrimal sac Nasolacrimal duct **Y Lacrimal Duct, Left** *See X Lacrimal Duct, Right*	**Ø Open** **3 Percutaneous**	**C Extraluminal Device** **D Intraluminal Device** **Z No Device**	**Z No Qualifier**
X Lacrimal Duct, Right Lacrimal canaliculus Lacrimal punctum Lacrimal sac Nasolacrimal duct **Y Lacrimal Duct, Left** *See X Lacrimal Duct, Right*	**7 Via Natural or Artificial Opening** **8 Via Natural or Artificial Opening Endoscopic**	**D Intraluminal Device** **Z No Device**	**Z No Qualifier**

Ø Medical and Surgical
8 Eye
W Revision

Definition: Correcting, to the extent possible, a portion of a malfunctioning device or the position of a displaced device

Explanation: Revision can include correcting a malfunctioning or displaced device by taking out or putting in components of the device such as a screw or pin

Body Part Character 4	Approach Character 5	Device Character 6	Qualifier Character 7
Ø Eye, Right Ciliary body Posterior chamber **1 Eye, Left** *See Ø Eye, Right*	**Ø Open** **3 Percutaneous** **7 Via Natural or Artificial Opening** **8 Via Natural or Artificial Opening Endoscopic**	**Ø Drainage Device** **3 Infusion Device** **7 Autologous Tissue Substitute** **C Extraluminal Device** **D Intraluminal Device** **J Synthetic Substitute** **K Nonautologous Tissue Substitute** **Y Other Device**	**Z No Qualifier**
Ø Eye, Right Ciliary body Posterior chamber **1 Eye, Left** *See Ø Eye, Right*	**X External**	**Ø Drainage Device** **3 Infusion Device** **7 Autologous Tissue Substitute** **C Extraluminal Device** **D Intraluminal Device** **J Synthetic Substitute** **K Nonautologous Tissue Substitute**	**Z No Qualifier**
J Lens, Right Zonule of Zinn **K Lens, Left** *See J Lens, Right*	**3 Percutaneous**	**J Synthetic Substitute** **Y Other Device**	**Z No Qualifier**
J Lens, Right Zonule of Zinn **K Lens, Left** *See J Lens, Right*	**X External**	**J Synthetic Substitute**	**Z No Qualifier**
L Extraocular Muscle, Right Inferior oblique muscle Inferior rectus muscle Lateral rectus muscle Medial rectus muscle Superior oblique muscle Superior rectus muscle **M Extraocular Muscle, Left** *See L Extraocular Muscle, Right*	**Ø Open** **3 Percutaneous**	**Ø Drainage Device** **7 Autologous Tissue Substitute** **J Synthetic Substitute** **K Nonautologous Tissue Substitute** **Y Other Device**	**Z No Qualifier**

Non-OR Ø8W[Ø,1][3,7,8]YZ
Non-OR Ø8W[Ø,1]X[Ø,3,7,C,D,J,K]Z
Non-OR Ø8W[J,K]3YZ
Non-OR Ø8W[J,K]XJZ
Non-OR Ø8W[L,M]3YZ

Ø Medical and Surgical
8 Eye
X Transfer

Definition: Moving, without taking out, all or a portion of a body part to another location to take over the function of all or a portion of a body part

Explanation: The body part transferred remains connected to its vascular and nervous supply

Body Part Character 4	Approach Character 5	Device Character 6	Qualifier Character 7
L Extraocular Muscle, Right Inferior oblique muscle Inferior rectus muscle Lateral rectus muscle Medial rectus muscle Superior oblique muscle Superior rectus muscle **M Extraocular Muscle, Left** *See L Extraocular Muscle, Right*	**Ø Open** **3 Percutaneous**	**Z No Device**	**Z No Qualifier**

Ear, Nose, Sinus Ø9Ø–Ø9W

Character Meanings*

This Character Meaning table is provided as a guide to assist the user in the identification of character members that may be found in this section of code tables. It **SHOULD NOT** be used to build a PCS code.

Operation–Character 3		Body Part–Character 4		Approach–Character 5		Device–Character 6		Qualifier–Character 7	
Ø	Alteration	Ø	External Ear, Right	Ø	Open	Ø	Drainage Device	Ø	Endolymphatic
1	Bypass	1	External Ear, Left	3	Percutaneous	1	Radioactive Element	X	Diagnostic
2	Change	2	External Ear, Bilateral	4	Percutaneous Endoscopic	4	Hearing Device, Bone Conduction	Z	No Qualifier
3	Control	3	External Auditory Canal, Right	7	Via Natural or Artificial Opening	5	Hearing Device, Single Channel Cochlear Prosthesis		
5	Destruction	4	External Auditory Canal, Left	8	Via Natural or Artificial Opening Endoscopic	6	Hearing Device, Multiple Channel Cochlear Prosthesis		
7	Dilation	5	Middle Ear, Right	X	External	7	Autologous Tissue Substitute		
8	Division	6	Middle Ear, Left			B	Intraluminal Device, Airway		
9	Drainage	7	Tympanic Membrane, Right			D	Intraluminal Device		
B	Excision	8	Tympanic Membrane, Left			J	Synthetic Substitute		
C	Extirpation	9	Auditory Ossicle, Right			K	Nonautologous Tissue Substitute		
D	Extraction	A	Auditory Ossicle, Left			S	Hearing Device		
H	Insertion	B	Mastoid Sinus, Right			Y	Other Device		
J	Inspection	C	Mastoid Sinus, Left			Z	No Device		
M	Reattachment	D	Inner Ear, Right						
N	Release	E	Inner Ear, Left						
P	Removal	F	Eustachian Tube, Right						
Q	Repair	G	Eustachian Tube, Left						
R	Replacement	H	Ear, Right						
S	Reposition	J	Ear, Left						
T	Resection	K	Nasal Mucosa and Soft Tissue						
U	Supplement	L	Nasal Turbinate						
W	Revision	M	Nasal Septum						
		N	Nasopharynx						
		P	Accessory Sinus						
		Q	Maxillary Sinus, Right						
		R	Maxillary Sinus, Left						
		S	Frontal Sinus, Right						
		T	Frontal Sinus, Left						
		U	Ethmoid Sinus, Right						
		V	Ethmoid Sinus, Left						
		W	Sphenoid Sinus, Right						
		X	Sphenoid Sinus, Left						
		Y	Sinus						

* Includes sinus ducts.

AHA Coding Clinic for table Ø93
2018, 4Q, 38 Control of epistaxis

AHA Coding Clinic for table Ø95
2018, 1Q, 19 Control of epistaxis via silver nitrate cauterization

AHA Coding Clinic for table Ø9B
2023, 2Q, 19 Sigmoid sinus dehiscence with mastoidectomy with resurfacing

AHA Coding Clinic for table Ø9H
2022, 2Q, 17 Congenital nasal pyriform aperture stenosis and repair
2020, 4Q, 43-44 Insertion of radioactive element

AHA Coding Clinic for table Ø9Q
2018, 1Q, 19 Control of epistaxis via silver nitrate cauterization
2017, 4Q, 106 Control of bleeding of external naris using suture
2014, 4Q, 20 Control of epistaxis
2014, 3Q, 22 Transsphenoidal removal of pituitary tumor and fat graft placement
2013, 4Q, 114 Balloon sinuplasty

AHA Coding Clinic for table Ø9U
2022, 1Q, 48 Repair of facial fractures of frontal sinus and orbital roof
2019, 4Q, 28-29 Sinus supplement

Ear, Nose, Sinus

Ear Anatomy

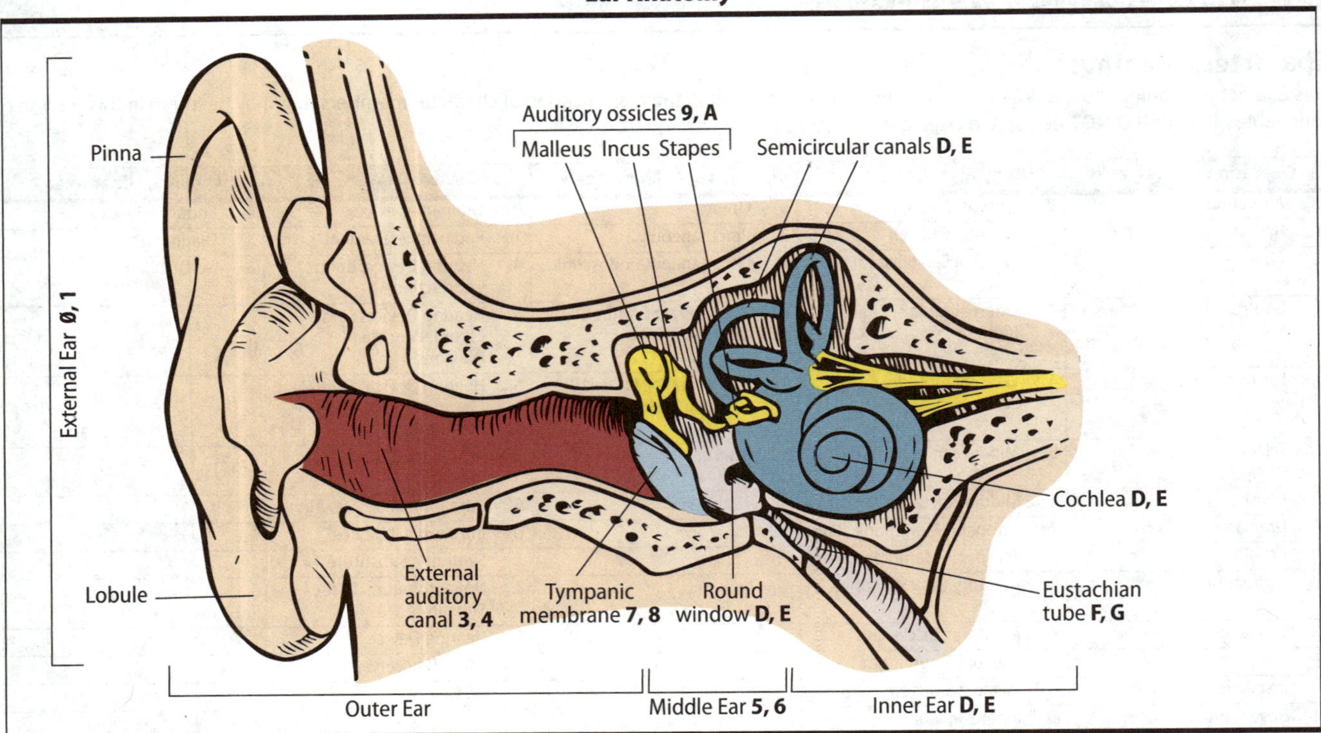

Nasal Turbinates

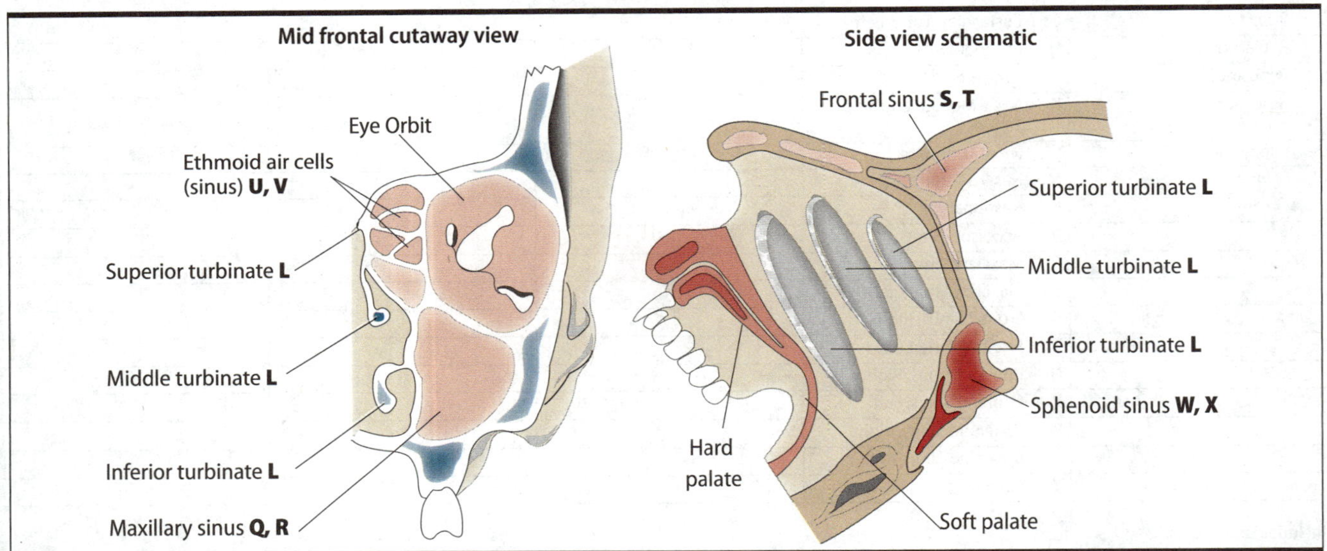

Paranasal Sinuses

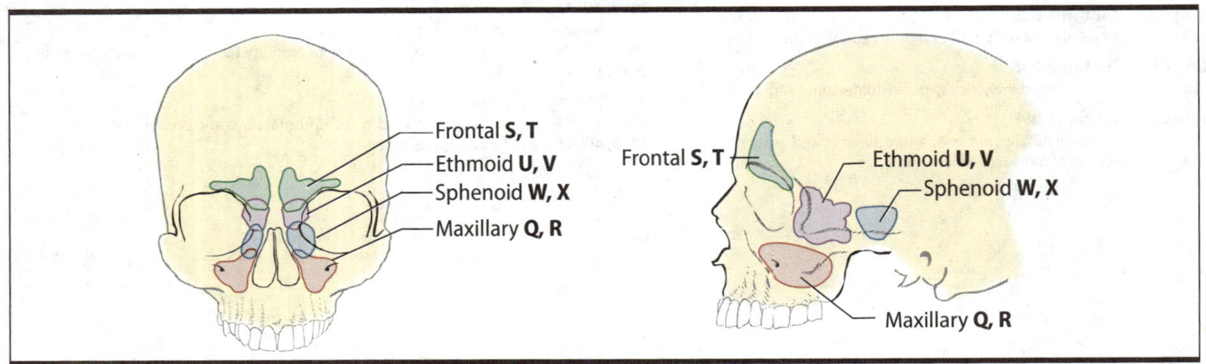

Ø Medical and Surgical
9 Ear, Nose, Sinus
Ø Alteration

Definition: Modifying the anatomic structure of a body part without affecting the function of the body part

Explanation: Principal purpose is to improve appearance

Body Part Character 4		Approach Character 5	Device Character 6	Qualifier Character 7
Ø External Ear, Right Antihelix Antitragus Auricle Earlobe Helix Pinna Tragus **1 External Ear, Left** *See Ø External Ear, Right*	**2 External Ear, Bilateral** *See Ø External Ear, Right* **K Nasal Mucosa and Soft Tissue** Columella External naris Greater alar cartilage Internal naris Lateral nasal cartilage Lesser alar cartilage Nasal cavity Nostril	**Ø Open** **3 Percutaneous** **4 Percutaneous Endoscopic** **X External**	**7 Autologous Tissue Substitute** **J Synthetic Substitute** **K Nonautologous Tissue Substitute** **Z No Device**	**Z No Qualifier**

Ø Medical and Surgical
9 Ear, Nose, Sinus
1 Bypass

Definition: Altering the route of passage of the contents of a tubular body part

Explanation: Rerouting contents of a body part to a downstream area of the normal route, to a similar route and body part, or to an abnormal route and dissimilar body part. Includes one or more anastomoses, with or without the use of a device.

Body Part Character 4	Approach Character 5	Device Character 6	Qualifier Character 7
D Inner Ear, Right Bony labyrinth Bony vestibule Cochlea Round window Semicircular canal **E Inner Ear, Left** *See D Inner Ear, Right*	**Ø Open**	**7 Autologous Tissue Substitute** **J Synthetic Substitute** **K Nonautologous Tissue Substitute** **Z No Device**	**Ø Endolymphatic**

Ø Medical and Surgical
9 Ear, Nose, Sinus
2 Change

Definition: Taking out or off a device from a body part and putting back an identical or similar device in or on the same body part without cutting or puncturing the skin or a mucous membrane

Explanation: All CHANGE procedures are coded using the approach EXTERNAL

Body Part Character 4	Approach Character 5	Device Character 6	Qualifier Character 7
H Ear, Right **J Ear, Left** **K Nasal Mucosa and Soft Tissue** Columella External naris Greater alar cartilage Internal naris Lateral nasal cartilage Lesser alar cartilage Nasal cavity Nostril **Y Sinus**	**X External**	**Ø Drainage Device** **Y Other Device**	**Z No Qualifier**

Non-OR All body part, approach, device, and qualifier values

Ø Medical and Surgical
9 Ear, Nose, Sinus
3 Control

Definition: Stopping, or attempting to stop, postprocedural or other acute bleeding

Explanation: None

Body Part Character 4	Approach Character 5	Device Character 6	Qualifier Character 7
K Nasal Mucosa and Soft Tissue Columella External naris Greater alar cartilage Internal naris Lateral nasal cartilage Lesser alar cartilage Nasal cavity Nostril	**7 Via Natural or Artificial Opening** **8 Via Natural or Artificial Opening Endoscopic**	**Z No Device**	**Z No Qualifier**

Non-OR Ø93K[7,8]ZZ

Ø Medical and Surgical
9 Ear, Nose, Sinus
5 Destruction Definition: Physical eradication of all or a portion of a body part by the direct use of energy, force, or a destructive agent

Explanation: None of the body part is physically taken out

Body Part Character 4		Approach Character 5	Device Character 6	Qualifier Character 7
Ø External Ear, Right Antihelix Antitragus Auricle Earlobe Helix Pinna Tragus	**1 External Ear, Left** *See Ø External Ear, Right*	**Ø Open** **3 Percutaneous** **4 Percutaneous Endoscopic** **X External**	**Z No Device**	**Z No Qualifier**
3 External Auditory Canal, Right External auditory meatus	**4 External Auditory Canal, Left** *See 3 External Auditory Canal, Right*	**Ø Open** **3 Percutaneous** **4 Percutaneous Endoscopic** **7 Via Natural or Artificial Opening** **8 Via Natural or Artificial Opening Endoscopic** **X External**	**Z No Device**	**Z No Qualifier**
5 Middle Ear, Right Oval window Tympanic cavity **6 Middle Ear, Left** *See 5 Middle Ear, Right* **9 Auditory Ossicle, Right** Incus Malleus Stapes **A Auditory Ossicle, Left** *See 9 Auditory Ossicle, Right*	**D Inner Ear, Right** Bony labyrinth Bony vestibule Cochlea Round window Semicircular canal **E Inner Ear, Left** *See D Inner Ear, Right*	**Ø Open** **8 Via Natural or Artificial Opening Endoscopic**	**Z No Device**	**Z No Qualifier**
7 Tympanic Membrane, Right Pars flaccida **8 Tympanic Membrane, Left** *See 7 Tympanic Membrane, Right* **F Eustachian Tube, Right** Auditory tube Pharyngotympanic tube **G Eustachian Tube, Left** *See F Eustachian Tube, Right*	**L Nasal Turbinate** Inferior turbinate Middle turbinate Nasal concha Superior turbinate **N Nasopharynx** Choana Fossa of Rosenmuller Pharyngeal recess Rhinopharynx	**Ø Open** **3 Percutaneous** **4 Percutaneous Endoscopic** **7 Via Natural or Artificial Opening** **8 Via Natural or Artificial Opening Endoscopic**	**Z No Device**	**Z No Qualifier**
B Mastoid Sinus, Right Mastoid air cells **C Mastoid Sinus, Left** *See B Mastoid Sinus, Right* **M Nasal Septum** Quadrangular cartilage Septal cartilage Vomer bone **P Accessory Sinus** **Q Maxillary Sinus, Right** Antrum of Highmore	**R Maxillary Sinus, Left** *See Q Maxillary Sinus, Right* **S Frontal Sinus, Right** **T Frontal Sinus, Left** **U Ethmoid Sinus, Right** Ethmoidal air cell **V Ethmoid Sinus, Left** *See U Ethmoid Sinus, Right* **W Sphenoid Sinus, Right** **X Sphenoid Sinus, Left**	**Ø Open** **3 Percutaneous** **4 Percutaneous Endoscopic** **8 Via Natural or Artificial Opening Endoscopic**	**Z No Device**	**Z No Qualifier**
K Nasal Mucosa and Soft Tissue Columella External naris Greater alar cartilage Internal naris Lateral nasal cartilage Lesser alar cartilage Nasal cavity Nostril		**Ø Open** **3 Percutaneous** **4 Percutaneous Endoscopic** **8 Via Natural or Artificial Opening Endoscopic** **X External**	**Z No Device**	**Z No Qualifier**

Non-OR Ø95[Ø,1][Ø,3,4,X]ZZ
Non-OR Ø95[3,4][Ø,3,4,7,8,X]ZZ
Non-OR Ø95[F,G][Ø,3,4,7,8]ZZ
Non-OR Ø95M[Ø,3,4,8]ZZ
Non-OR Ø95K[Ø,3,4,8,X]ZZ

0 Medical and Surgical
9 Ear, Nose, Sinus
7 Dilation

Definition: Expanding an orifice or the lumen of a tubular body part

Explanation: The orifice can be a natural orifice or an artificially created orifice. Accomplished by stretching a tubular body part using intraluminal pressure or by cutting part of the orifice or wall of the tubular body part.

Body Part Character 4	Approach Character 5	Device Character 6	Qualifier Character 7
F Eustachian Tube, Right Auditory tube Pharyngotympanic tube G Eustachian Tube, Left *See F Eustachian Tube, Right*	0 Open 7 Via Natural or Artificial Opening 8 Via Natural or Artificial Opening Endoscopic	D Intraluminal Device Z No Device	Z No Qualifier
F Eustachian Tube, Right Auditory tube Pharyngotympanic tube G Eustachian Tube, Left *See F Eustachian Tube, Right*	3 Percutaneous 4 Percutaneous Endoscopic	Z No Device	Z No Qualifier

Non-OR All body part, approach, device, and qualifier values

0 Medical and Surgical
9 Ear, Nose, Sinus
8 Division

Definition: Cutting into a body part, without draining fluids and/or gases from the body part, in order to separate or transect a body part

Explanation: All or a portion of the body part is separated into two or more portions

Body Part Character 4	Approach Character 5	Device Character 6	Qualifier Character 7
L Nasal Turbinate Inferior turbinate Middle turbinate Nasal concha Superior turbinate	0 Open 3 Percutaneous 4 Percutaneous Endoscopic 7 Via Natural or Artificial Opening 8 Via Natural or Artificial Opening Endoscopic	Z No Device	Z No Qualifier

Ø Medical and Surgical
9 Ear, Nose, Sinus
9 Drainage Definition: Taking or letting out fluids and/or gases from a body part
Explanation: The qualifier DIAGNOSTIC is used to identify drainage procedures that are biopsies

Body Part Character 4		Approach Character 5	Device Character 6	Qualifier Character 7
Ø External Ear, Right Antihelix Antitragus Auricle Earlobe Helix Pinna Tragus	**1 External Ear, Left** *See Ø External Ear, Right*	**Ø Open** **3 Percutaneous** **4 Percutaneous Endoscopic** **X External**	**Ø Drainage Device**	**Z No Qualifier**
Ø External Ear, Right Antihelix Antitragus Auricle Earlobe Helix Pinna Tragus	**1 External Ear, Left** *See Ø External Ear, Right*	**Ø Open** **3 Percutaneous** **4 Percutaneous Endoscopic** **X External**	**Z No Device**	**X Diagnostic** **Z No Qualifier**
3 External Auditory Canal, Right External auditory meatus **4 External Auditory Canal, Left** *See 3 External Auditory Canal, Right*	**K Nasal Mucosa and Soft Tissue** Columella External naris Greater alar cartilage Internal naris Lateral nasal cartilage Lesser alar cartilage Nasal cavity Nostril	**Ø Open** **3 Percutaneous** **4 Percutaneous Endoscopic** **7 Via Natural or Artificial Opening** **8 Via Natural or Artificial Opening Endoscopic** **X External**	**Ø Drainage Device**	**Z No Qualifier**
3 External Auditory Canal, Right External auditory meatus **4 External Auditory Canal, Left** *See 3 External Auditory Canal, Right*	**K Nasal Mucosa and Soft Tissue** Columella External naris Greater alar cartilage Internal naris Lateral nasal cartilage Lesser alar cartilage Nasal cavity Nostril	**Ø Open** **3 Percutaneous** **4 Percutaneous Endoscopic** **7 Via Natural or Artificial Opening** **8 Via Natural or Artificial Opening Endoscopic** **X External**	**Z No Device**	**X Diagnostic** **Z No Qualifier**
5 Middle Ear, Right Oval window Tympanic cavity **6 Middle Ear, Left** *See 5 Middle Ear, Right* **9 Auditory Ossicle, Right** Incus Malleus Stapes	**A Auditory Ossicle, Left** *See 9 Auditory Ossicle, Right* **D Inner Ear, Right** Bony labyrinth Bony vestibule Cochlea Round window Semicircular canal **E Inner Ear, Left** *See D Inner Ear, Right*	**Ø Open** **7 Via Natural or Artificial Opening** **8 Via Natural or Artificial Opening Endoscopic**	**Ø Drainage Device**	**Z No Qualifier**
5 Middle Ear, Right Oval window Tympanic cavity **6 Middle Ear, Left** *See 5 Middle Ear, Right* **9 Auditory Ossicle, Right** Incus Malleus Stapes	**A Auditory Ossicle, Left** *See 9 Auditory Ossicle, Right* **D Inner Ear, Right** Bony labyrinth Bony vestibule Cochlea Round window Semicircular canal **E Inner Ear, Left** *See D Inner Ear, Right*	**Ø Open** **7 Via Natural or Artificial Opening** **8 Via Natural or Artificial Opening Endoscopic**	**Z No Device**	**X Diagnostic** **Z No Qualifier**

Non-OR Ø99[Ø,1][Ø,3,4,X]ØZ
Non-OR Ø99[Ø,1][Ø,3,4,X]Z[X,Z]
Non-OR Ø99[3,4,K][Ø,3,4,7,8,X]ØZ
Non-OR Ø99[3,4,K][Ø,3,4,7,8,X]Z[X,Z]
Non-OR Ø99[5,6]8ØZ
Non-OR Ø99[9,A,D,E][7,8]ØZ
Non-OR Ø99[5,6]ØZZ
Non-OR Ø99[5,6,9,A,D,E][7,8]Z[X,Z]

Ø99 Continued on next page

Ø Medical and Surgical
9 Ear, Nose, Sinus
9 Drainage Definition: Taking or letting out fluids and/or gases from a body part
Explanation: The qualifier DIAGNOSTIC is used to identify drainage procedures that are biopsies

Ø99 Continued

Body Part Character 4	Approach Character 5	Device Character 6	Qualifier Character 7
7 Tympanic Membrane, Right Pars flaccida **8 Tympanic Membrane, Left** *See 7 Tympanic Membrane, Right* **B Mastoid Sinus, Right** Mastoid air cells **C Mastoid Sinus, Left** *See B Mastoid Sinus, Right* **F Eustachian Tube, Right** Auditory tube Pharyngotympanic tube **G Eustachian Tube, Left** *See F Eustachian Tube, Right* **L Nasal Turbinate** Inferior turbinate Middle turbinate Nasal concha Superior turbinate **M Nasal Septum** Quadrangular cartilage Septal cartilage Vomer bone **N Nasopharynx** Choana Fossa of Rosenmuller Pharyngeal recess Rhinopharynx **P Accessory Sinus** **Q Maxillary Sinus, Right** Antrum of Highmore **R Maxillary Sinus, Left** *See Q Maxillary Sinus, Right* **S Frontal Sinus, Right** **T Frontal Sinus, Left** **U Ethmoid Sinus, Right** Ethmoidal air cell **V Ethmoid Sinus, Left** *See U Ethmoid Sinus, Right* **W Sphenoid Sinus, Right** **X Sphenoid Sinus, Left**	**Ø Open** **3 Percutaneous** **4 Percutaneous Endoscopic** **7 Via Natural or Artificial Opening** **8 Via Natural or Artificial Opening Endoscopic**	**Ø Drainage Device**	**Z No Qualifier**
7 Tympanic Membrane, Right Pars flaccida **8 Tympanic Membrane, Left** *See 7 Tympanic Membrane, Right* **B Mastoid Sinus, Right** Mastoid air cells **C Mastoid Sinus, Left** *See B Mastoid Sinus, Right* **F Eustachian Tube, Right** Auditory tube Pharyngotympanic tube **G Eustachian Tube, Left** *See F Eustachian Tube, Right* **L Nasal Turbinate** Inferior turbinate Middle turbinate Nasal concha Superior turbinate **M Nasal Septum** Quadrangular cartilage Septal cartilage Vomer bone **N Nasopharynx** Choana Fossa of Rosenmuller Pharyngeal recess Rhinopharynx **P Accessory Sinus** **Q Maxillary Sinus, Right** Antrum of Highmore **R Maxillary Sinus, Left** *See Q Maxillary Sinus, Right* **S Frontal Sinus, Right** **T Frontal Sinus, Left** **U Ethmoid Sinus, Right** Ethmoidal air cell **V Ethmoid Sinus, Left** *See U Ethmoid Sinus, Right* **W Sphenoid Sinus, Right** **X Sphenoid Sinus, Left**	**Ø Open** **3 Percutaneous** **4 Percutaneous Endoscopic** **7 Via Natural or Artificial Opening** **8 Via Natural or Artificial Opening Endoscopic**	**Z No Device**	**X Diagnostic** **Z No Qualifier**

Non-OR Ø99[B,C][3,7,8]ØZ
Non-OR Ø99[F,G,L,M][Ø,3,4,7,8]ØZ
Non-OR Ø99N3ØZ
Non-OR Ø99[P,Q,R,S,T,U,V,W,X][3,4,7,8]ØZ
Non-OR Ø99[7,8][Ø,3,4,7,8]ZZ
Non-OR Ø99[7,8][7,8]ZX
Non-OR Ø99[B,C]3ZZ
Non-OR Ø99[B,C][7,8]Z[X,Z]
Non-OR Ø99[F,G][Ø,3,4,7,8]ZZ
Non-OR Ø99[F,G][7,8]ZX
Non-OR Ø99[L,M][Ø,3,4,7,8]Z[X,Z]
Non-OR Ø99N[Ø,3,4,7,8]ZX
Non-OR Ø99N3ZZ
Non-OR Ø99[P,Q,R,S,T,U,V,W,X][3,4,7,8]Z[X,Z]

Ø Medical and Surgical
9 Ear, Nose, Sinus
B Excision

Definition: Cutting out or off, without replacement, a portion of a body part
Explanation: The qualifier DIAGNOSTIC is used to identify excision procedures that are biopsies

Body Part Character 4	Approach Character 5	Device Character 6	Qualifier Character 7
Ø External Ear, Right Antihelix Antitragus Auricle Earlobe Helix Pinna Tragus **1 External Ear, Left** *See Ø External Ear, Right*	**Ø Open** **3 Percutaneous** **4 Percutaneous Endoscopic** **X External**	**Z No Device**	**X Diagnostic** **Z No Qualifier**
3 External Auditory Canal, Right External auditory meatus **4 External Auditory Canal, Left** *See 3 External Auditory Canal, Right*	**Ø Open** **3 Percutaneous** **4 Percutaneous Endoscopic** **7 Via Natural or Artificial Opening** **8 Via Natural or Artificial Opening Endoscopic** **X External**	**Z No Device**	**X Diagnostic** **Z No Qualifier**
5 Middle Ear, Right Oval window Tympanic cavity **6 Middle Ear, Left** *See 5 Middle Ear, Right* **9 Auditory Ossicle, Right** Incus Malleus Stapes **A Auditory Ossicle, Left** *See 9 Auditory Ossicle, Right* **D Inner Ear, Right** Bony labyrinth Bony vestibule Cochlea Round window Semicircular canal **E Inner Ear, Left** *See D Inner Ear, Right*	**Ø Open** **8 Via Natural or Artificial Opening Endoscopic**	**Z No Device**	**X Diagnostic** **Z No Qualifier**
7 Tympanic Membrane, Right Pars flaccida **8 Tympanic Membrane, Left** *See 7 Tympanic Membrane, Right* **F Eustachian Tube, Right** Auditory tube Pharyngotympanic tube **G Eustachian Tube, Left** *See F Eustachian Tube, Right* **L Nasal Turbinate** Inferior turbinate Middle turbinate Nasal concha Superior turbinate **N Nasopharynx** Choana Fossa of Rosenmuller Pharyngeal recess Rhinopharynx	**Ø Open** **3 Percutaneous** **4 Percutaneous Endoscopic** **7 Via Natural or Artificial Opening** **8 Via Natural or Artificial Opening Endoscopic**	**Z No Device**	**X Diagnostic** **Z No Qualifier**
B Mastoid Sinus, Right Mastoid air cells **C Mastoid Sinus, Left** *See B Mastoid Sinus, Right* **M Nasal Septum** Quadrangular cartilage Septal cartilage Vomer bone **P Accessory Sinus** **Q Maxillary Sinus, Right** Antrum of Highmore **R Maxillary Sinus, Left** *See Q Maxillary Sinus, Right* **S Frontal Sinus, Right** **T Frontal Sinus, Left** **U Ethmoid Sinus, Right** Ethmoidal air cell **V Ethmoid Sinus, Left** *See U Ethmoid Sinus, Right* **W Sphenoid Sinus, Right** **X Sphenoid Sinus, Left**	**Ø Open** **3 Percutaneous** **4 Percutaneous Endoscopic** **8 Via Natural or Artificial Opening Endoscopic**	**Z No Device**	**X Diagnostic** **Z No Qualifier**
K Nasal Mucosa and Soft Tissue Columella External naris Greater alar cartilage Internal naris Lateral nasal cartilage Lesser alar cartilage Nasal cavity Nostril	**Ø Open** **3 Percutaneous** **4 Percutaneous Endoscopic** **8 Via Natural or Artificial Opening Endoscopic** **X External**	**Z No Device**	**X Diagnostic** **Z No Qualifier**

Non-OR Ø9B[Ø,1][Ø,3,4,X]Z[X,Z]
Non-OR Ø9B[3,4][Ø,3,4,7,8,X]Z[X,Z]
Non-OR Ø9B[F,G,L,N][Ø,3,4,7,8]Z[X,Z]
Non-OR Ø9BM[Ø,3,4,8]ZX
Non-OR Ø9B[P,Q,R,S,T,U,V,W,X][3,4,8]ZX
Non-OR Ø9BK8Z[X,Z]

Ø Medical and Surgical
9 Ear, Nose, Sinus
C Extirpation

Definition: Taking or cutting out solid matter from a body part

Explanation: The solid matter may be an abnormal byproduct of a biological function or a foreign body; it may be imbedded in a body part or in the lumen of a tubular body part. The solid matter may or may not have been previously broken into pieces.

Body Part Character 4		Approach Character 5	Device Character 6	Qualifier Character 7
Ø External Ear, Right Antihelix Antitragus Auricle Earlobe Helix Pinna Tragus	**1 External Ear, Left** *See Ø External Ear, Right*	**Ø Open** **3 Percutaneous** **4 Percutaneous Endoscopic** **X External**	**Z No Device**	**Z No Qualifier**
3 External Auditory Canal, Right External auditory meatus	**4 External Auditory Canal, Left** *See 3 External Auditory Canal, Right*	**Ø Open** **3 Percutaneous** **4 Percutaneous Endoscopic** **7 Via Natural or Artificial Opening** **8 Via Natural or Artificial Opening Endoscopic** **X External**	**Z No Device**	**Z No Qualifier**
5 Middle Ear, Right Oval window Tympanic cavity **6 Middle Ear, Left** *See 5 Middle Ear, Right* **9 Auditory Ossicle, Right** Incus Malleus Stapes	**A Auditory Ossicle, Left** *See 9 Auditory Ossicle, Right* **D Inner Ear, Right** Bony labyrinth Bony vestibule Cochlea Round window Semicircular canal **E Inner Ear, Left** *See D Inner Ear, Right*	**Ø Open** **8 Via Natural or Artificial Opening Endoscopic**	**Z No Device**	**Z No Qualifier**
7 Tympanic Membrane, Right Pars flaccida **8 Tympanic Membrane, Left** *See 7 Tympanic Membrane, Right* **F Eustachian Tube, Right** Auditory tube Pharyngotympanic tube **G Eustachian Tube, Left** *See F Eustachian Tube, Right*	**L Nasal Turbinate** Inferior turbinate Middle turbinate Nasal concha Superior turbinate **N Nasopharynx** Choana Fossa of Rosenmuller Pharyngeal recess Rhinopharynx	**Ø Open** **3 Percutaneous** **4 Percutaneous Endoscopic** **7 Via Natural or Artificial Opening** **8 Via Natural or Artificial Opening Endoscopic**	**Z No Device**	**Z No Qualifier**
B Mastoid Sinus, Right Mastoid air cells **C Mastoid Sinus, Left** *See B Mastoid Sinus, Right* **M Nasal Septum** Quadrangular cartilage Septal cartilage Vomer bone **P Accessory Sinus** **Q Maxillary Sinus, Right** Antrum of Highmore	**R Maxillary Sinus, Left** *See Q Maxillary Sinus, Right* **S Frontal Sinus, Right** **T Frontal Sinus, Left** **U Ethmoid Sinus, Right** Ethmoidal air cell **V Ethmoid Sinus, Left** *See U Ethmoid Sinus, Right* **W Sphenoid Sinus, Right** **X Sphenoid Sinus, Left**	**Ø Open** **3 Percutaneous** **4 Percutaneous Endoscopic** **8 Via Natural or Artificial Opening Endoscopic**	**Z No Device**	**Z No Qualifier**
K Nasal Mucosa and Soft Tissue Columella External naris Greater alar cartilage Internal naris Lateral nasal cartilage Lesser alar cartilage Nasal cavity Nostril		**Ø Open** **3 Percutaneous** **4 Percutaneous Endoscopic** **8 Via Natural or Artificial Opening Endoscopic** **X External**	**Z No Device**	**Z No Qualifier**

Non-OR Ø9C[Ø,1][Ø,3,4,X]ZZ
Non-OR Ø9C[3,4][Ø,3,4,7,8,X]ZZ
Non-OR Ø9C[7,8,F,G,L][Ø,3,4,7,8]ZZ
Non-OR Ø9CM[Ø,3,4,8]ZZ
Non-OR Ø9CK8ZZ

Ø Medical and Surgical
9 Ear, Nose, Sinus
D Extraction

Definition: Pulling or stripping out or off all or a portion of a body part by the use of force
Explanation: The qualifier DIAGNOSTIC is used to identify extraction procedures that are biopsies

Body Part Character 4	Approach Character 5	Device Character 6	Qualifier Character 7
7 Tympanic Membrane, Right Pars flaccida **8 Tympanic Membrane, Left** *See 7 Tympanic Membrane, Right* **L Nasal Turbinate** Inferior turbinate Middle turbinate Nasal concha Superior turbinate	**Ø Open** **3 Percutaneous** **4 Percutaneous Endoscopic** **7 Via Natural or Artificial Opening** **8 Via Natural or Artificial Opening Endoscopic**	**Z No Device**	**Z No Qualifier**
9 Auditory Ossicle, Right Incus Malleus Stapes **A Auditory Ossicle, Left** *See 9 Auditory Ossicle, Right*	**Ø Open**	**Z No Device**	**Z No Qualifier**
B Mastoid Sinus, Right Mastoid air cells **C Mastoid Sinus, Left** *See B Mastoid Sinus, Right* **M Nasal Septum** Quadrangular cartilage Septal cartilage Vomer bone **P Accessory Sinus** **Q Maxillary Sinus, Right** Antrum of Highmore **R Maxillary Sinus, Left** *See Q Maxillary Sinus, Right* **S Frontal Sinus, Right** **T Frontal Sinus, Left** **U Ethmoid Sinus, Right** Ethmoidal air cell **V Ethmoid Sinus, Left** *See U Ethmoid Sinus, Right* **W Sphenoid Sinus, Right** **X Sphenoid Sinus, Left**	**Ø Open** **3 Percutaneous** **4 Percutaneous Endoscopic**	**Z No Device**	**Z No Qualifier**

Ø Medical and Surgical
9 Ear, Nose, Sinus
H Insertion

Definition: Putting in a nonbiological appliance that monitors, assists, performs, or prevents a physiological function but does not physically take the place of a body part
Explanation: None

Body Part Character 4	Approach Character 5	Device Character 6	Qualifier Character 7
D Inner Ear, Right Bony labyrinth Bony vestibule Cochlea Round window Semicircular canal **E Inner Ear, Left** *See D Inner Ear, Right*	**Ø Open** **3 Percutaneous** **4 Percutaneous Endoscopic**	**1 Radioactive Element** **4 Hearing Device, Bone Conduction** **5 Hearing Device, Single Channel Cochlear Prosthesis** **6 Hearing Device, Multiple Channel Cochlear Prosthesis** **S Hearing Device**	**Z No Qualifier**
H Ear, Right **J Ear, Left** **K Nasal Mucosa and Soft Tissue** Columella External naris Greater alar cartilage Internal naris Lateral nasal cartilage Lesser alar cartilage Nasal cavity Nostril **Y Sinus**	**Ø Open** **3 Percutaneous** **4 Percutaneous Endoscopic** **7 Via Natural or Artificial Opening** **8 Via Natural or Artificial Opening Endoscopic**	**1 Radioactive Element** **Y Other Device**	**Z No Qualifier**
N Nasopharynx Choana Fossa of Rosenmuller Pharyngeal recess Rhinopharynx	**7 Via Natural or Artificial Opening** **8 Via Natural or Artificial Opening Endoscopic**	**1 Radioactive Element** **B Intraluminal Device, Airway**	**Z No Qualifier**

Non-OR Ø9H[H,J,K]Ø1Z
Non-OR Ø9HKØYZ
Non-OR Ø9H[H,J,K,Y][3,4,7,8][1,Y]Z
Non-OR Ø9HN[7,8][1,B]Z

Ø Medical and Surgical
9 Ear, Nose, Sinus
J Inspection Definition: Visually and/or manually exploring a body part

Explanation: Visual exploration may be performed with or without optical instrumentation. Manual exploration may be performed directly or through intervening body layers.

Body Part Character 4	Approach Character 5	Device Character 6	Qualifier Character 7
7 Tympanic Membrane, Right Pars flaccida **8 Tympanic Membrane, Left** *See 7 Tympanic Membrane, Right* **H Ear, Right** **J Ear, Left**	**Ø Open** **3 Percutaneous** **4 Percutaneous Endoscopic** **7 Via Natural or Artificial Opening** **8 Via Natural or Artificial Opening Endoscopic** **X External**	**Z No Device**	**Z No Qualifier**
D Inner Ear, Right Bony labyrinth Bony vestibule Cochlea Round window Semicircular canal **E Inner Ear, Left** *See D Inner Ear, Right* **K Nasal Mucosa and Soft Tissue** Columella External naris Greater alar cartilage Internal naris Lateral nasal cartilage Lesser alar cartilage Nasal cavity Nostril **Y Sinus**	**Ø Open** **3 Percutaneous** **4 Percutaneous Endoscopic** **8 Via Natural or Artificial Opening Endoscopic** **X External**	**Z No Device**	**Z No Qualifier**

Non-OR Ø9J[7,8][3,7,8,X]ZZ
Non-OR Ø9J[H,J][Ø,3,4,7,8,X]ZZ
Non-OR Ø9J[D,E][3,8,X]ZZ
Non-OR Ø9J[K,Y][Ø,3,4,8,X]ZZ

Ø Medical and Surgical
9 Ear, Nose, Sinus
M Reattachment Definition: Putting back in or on all or a portion of a separated body part to its normal location or other suitable location

Explanation: Vascular circulation and nervous pathways may or may not be reestablished

Body Part Character 4	Approach Character 5	Device Character 6	Qualifier Character 7
Ø External Ear, Right Antihelix Antitragus Auricle Earlobe Helix Pinna Tragus **1 External Ear, Left** *See Ø External Ear, Right* **K Nasal Mucosa and Soft Tissue** Columella External naris Greater alar cartilage Internal naris Lateral nasal cartilage Lesser alar cartilage Nasal cavity Nostril	**X External**	**Z No Device**	**Z No Qualifier**

Ø Medical and Surgical
9 Ear, Nose, Sinus
N Release

Definition: Freeing a body part from an abnormal physical constraint by cutting or by the use of force
Explanation: Some of the restraining tissue may be taken out but none of the body part is taken out

Body Part Character 4		Approach Character 5	Device Character 6	Qualifier Character 7
Ø External Ear, Right Antihelix Antitragus Auricle Earlobe Helix Pinna Tragus	**1 External Ear, Left** *See Ø External Ear, Right*	**Ø Open** **3 Percutaneous** **4 Percutaneous Endoscopic** **X External**	**Z No Device**	**Z No Qualifier**
3 External Auditory Canal, Right External auditory meatus	**4 External Auditory Canal, Left** *See 3 External Auditory Canal, Right*	**Ø Open** **3 Percutaneous** **4 Percutaneous Endoscopic** **7 Via Natural or Artificial Opening** **8 Via Natural or Artificial Opening Endoscopic** **X External**	**Z No Device**	**Z No Qualifier**
5 Middle Ear, Right Oval window Tympanic cavity **6 Middle Ear, Left** *See 5 Middle Ear, Right* **9 Auditory Ossicle, Right** Incus Malleus Stapes	**A Auditory Ossicle, Left** *See 9 Auditory Ossicle, Right* **D Inner Ear, Right** Bony labyrinth Bony vestibule Cochlea Round window Semicircular canal **E Inner Ear, Left** *See D Inner Ear, Right*	**Ø Open** **8 Via Natural or Artificial Opening Endoscopic**	**Z No Device**	**Z No Qualifier**
7 Tympanic Membrane, Right Pars flaccida **8 Tympanic Membrane, Left** *See 7 Tympanic Membrane, Right* **F Eustachian Tube, Right** Auditory tube Pharyngotympanic tube **G Eustachian Tube, Left** *See F Eustachian Tube, Right*	**L Nasal Turbinate** Inferior turbinate Middle turbinate Nasal concha Superior turbinate **N Nasopharynx** Choana Fossa of Rosenmuller Pharyngeal recess Rhinopharynx	**Ø Open** **3 Percutaneous** **4 Percutaneous Endoscopic** **7 Via Natural or Artificial Opening** **8 Via Natural or Artificial Opening Endoscopic**	**Z No Device**	**Z No Qualifier**
B Mastoid Sinus, Right Mastoid air cells **C Mastoid Sinus, Left** *See B Mastoid Sinus, Right* **M Nasal Septum** Quadrangular cartilage Septal cartilage Vomer bone **P Accessory Sinus** **Q Maxillary Sinus, Right** Antrum of Highmore	**R Maxillary Sinus, Left** *See Q Maxillary Sinus, Right* **S Frontal Sinus, Right** **T Frontal Sinus, Left** **U Ethmoid Sinus, Right** Ethmoidal air cell **V Ethmoid Sinus, Left** *See U Ethmoid Sinus, Right* **W Sphenoid Sinus, Right** **X Sphenoid Sinus, Left**	**Ø Open** **3 Percutaneous** **4 Percutaneous Endoscopic** **8 Via Natural or Artificial Opening Endoscopic**	**Z No Device**	**Z No Qualifier**
K Nasal Mucosa and Soft Tissue Columella External naris Greater alar cartilage Internal naris Lateral nasal cartilage Lesser alar cartilage Nasal cavity Nostril		**Ø Open** **3 Percutaneous** **4 Percutaneous Endoscopic** **8 Via Natural or Artificial Opening Endoscopic** **X External**	**Z No Device**	**Z No Qualifier**

Non-OR Ø9N[Ø,1]XZZ
Non-OR Ø9N[3,4]XZZ
Non-OR Ø9N[F,G,L][Ø,3,4,7,8]ZZ
Non-OR Ø9NM[Ø,3,4,8]ZZ
Non-OR Ø9NK[Ø,3,4,8,X]ZZ

Ø Medical and Surgical
9 Ear, Nose, Sinus
P Removal Definition: Taking out or off a device from a body part

Explanation: If a device is taken out and a similar device put in without cutting or puncturing the skin or mucous membrane, the procedure is coded to the root operation CHANGE. Otherwise, the procedure for taking out a device is coded to the root operation REMOVAL.

Body Part Character 4	Approach Character 5	Device Character 6	Qualifier Character 7
7 Tympanic Membrane, Right Pars flaccida **8 Tympanic Membrane, Left** *See 7 Tympanic Membrane, Right*	**Ø Open** **7 Via Natural or Artificial Opening** **8 Via Natural or Artificial Opening Endoscopic** **X External**	**Ø Drainage Device**	**Z No Qualifier**
D Inner Ear, Right Bony labyrinth Bony vestibule Cochlea Round window Semicircular canal **E Inner Ear, Left** *See D Inner Ear, Right*	**Ø Open** **7 Via Natural or Artificial Opening** **8 Via Natural or Artificial Opening Endoscopic**	**S Hearing Device**	**Z No Qualifier**
H Ear, Right **J Ear, Left** **K Nasal Mucosa and Soft Tissue** Columella External naris Greater alar cartilage Internal naris Lateral nasal cartilage Lesser alar cartilage Nasal cavity Nostril	**Ø Open** **3 Percutaneous** **4 Percutaneous Endoscopic** **7 Via Natural or Artificial Opening** **8 Via Natural or Artificial Opening Endoscopic**	**Ø Drainage Device** **7 Autologous Tissue Substitute** **D Intraluminal Device** **J Synthetic Substitute** **K Nonautologous Tissue Substitute** **Y Other Device**	**Z No Qualifier**
H Ear, Right **J Ear, Left** **K Nasal Mucosa and Soft Tissue** Columella External naris Greater alar cartilage Internal naris Lateral nasal cartilage Lesser alar cartilage Nasal cavity Nostril	**X External**	**Ø Drainage Device** **7 Autologous Tissue Substitute** **D Intraluminal Device** **J Synthetic Substitute** **K Nonautologous Tissue Substitute**	**Z No Qualifier**
Y Sinus	**Ø Open** **3 Percutaneous** **4 Percutaneous Endoscopic**	**Ø Drainage Device** **Y Other Device**	**Z No Qualifier**
Y Sinus	**7 Via Natural or Artificial Opening** **8 Via Natural or Artificial Opening Endoscopic**	**Y Other Device**	**Z No Qualifier**
Y Sinus	**X External**	**Ø Drainage Device**	**Z No Qualifier**

Non-OR Ø9P[7,8][Ø,7,8,X]ØZ
Non-OR Ø9P[H,J][3,4][Ø,J,K,Y]Z
Non-OR Ø9P[H,J][7,8][Ø,D,Y]Z
Non-OR Ø9PK[Ø,3,4,7,8][Ø,7,D,J,K,Y]Z
Non-OR Ø9P[H,J]X[Ø,7,D,J,K]Z
Non-OR Ø9PKX[Ø,7,D,J,K]Z
Non-OR Ø9PY[3,4]YZ
Non-OR Ø9PY[7,8]YZ
Non-OR Ø9PYXØZ

Ø Medical and Surgical
9 Ear, Nose, Sinus
Q Repair

Definition: Restoring, to the extent possible, a body part to its normal anatomic structure and function
Explanation: Used only when the method to accomplish the repair is not one of the other root operations

Body Part Character 4		Approach Character 5	Device Character 6	Qualifier Character 7
Ø External Ear, Right Antihelix Antitragus Auricle Earlobe Helix Pinna Tragus	**1 External Ear, Left** *See Ø External Ear, Right* **2 External Ear, Bilateral** *See Ø External Ear, Right*	**Ø Open** **3 Percutaneous** **4 Percutaneous Endoscopic** **X External**	**Z No Device**	**Z No Qualifier**
3 External Auditory Canal, Right External auditory meatus **4 External Auditory Canal, Left** *See 3 External Auditory Canal, Right*	**F Eustachian Tube, Right** Auditory tube Pharyngotympanic tube **G Eustachian Tube, Left** *See F Eustachian Tube, Right*	**Ø Open** **3 Percutaneous** **4 Percutaneous Endoscopic** **7 Via Natural or Artificial Opening** **8 Via Natural or Artificial Opening Endoscopic** **X External**	**Z No Device**	**Z No Qualifier**
5 Middle Ear, Right Oval window Tympanic cavity **6 Middle Ear, Left** *See 5 Middle Ear, Right* **9 Auditory Ossicle, Right** Incus Malleus Stapes	**A Auditory Ossicle, Left** *See 9 Auditory Ossicle, Right* **D Inner Ear, Right** Bony labyrinth Bony vestibule Cochlea Round window Semicircular canal **E Inner Ear, Left** *See D Inner Ear, Right*	**Ø Open** **8 Via Natural or Artificial Opening Endoscopic**	**Z No Device**	**Z No Qualifier**
7 Tympanic Membrane, Right Pars flaccida **8 Tympanic Membrane, Left** *See 7 Tympanic Membrane, Right* **L Nasal Turbinate** Inferior turbinate Middle turbinate Nasal concha Superior turbinate	**N Nasopharynx** Choana Fossa of Rosenmuller Pharyngeal recess Rhinopharynx	**Ø Open** **3 Percutaneous** **4 Percutaneous Endoscopic** **7 Via Natural or Artificial Opening** **8 Via Natural or Artificial Opening Endoscopic**	**Z No Device**	**Z No Qualifier**
B Mastoid Sinus, Right Mastoid air cells **C Mastoid Sinus, Left** *See B Mastoid Sinus, Right* **M Nasal Septum** Quadrangular cartilage Septal cartilage Vomer bone **P Accessory Sinus** **Q Maxillary Sinus, Right** Antrum of Highmore	**R Maxillary Sinus, Left** *See Q Maxillary Sinus, Right* **S Frontal Sinus, Right** **T Frontal Sinus, Left** **U Ethmoid Sinus, Right** Ethmoidal air cell **V Ethmoid Sinus, Left** *See U Ethmoid Sinus, Right* **W Sphenoid Sinus, Right** **X Sphenoid Sinus, Left**	**Ø Open** **3 Percutaneous** **4 Percutaneous Endoscopic** **8 Via Natural or Artificial Opening Endoscopic**	**Z No Device**	**Z No Qualifier**
K Nasal Mucosa and Soft Tissue Columella External naris Greater alar cartilage Internal naris Lateral nasal cartilage Lesser alar cartilage Nasal cavity Nostril		**Ø Open** **3 Percutaneous** **4 Percutaneous Endoscopic** **8 Via Natural or Artificial Opening Endoscopic** **X External**	**Z No Device**	**Z No Qualifier**

Non-OR Ø9Q[Ø,1,2]XZZ
Non-OR Ø9Q[3,4]XZZ
Non-OR Ø9Q[F,G][Ø,3,4,7,8,X]ZZ
Non-OR Ø9QKXZZ

Ø Medical and Surgical
9 Ear, Nose, Sinus
R Replacement

Definition: Putting in or on biological or synthetic material that physically takes the place and/or function of all or a portion of a body part

Explanation: The body part may have been taken out or replaced, or may be taken out, physically eradicated, or rendered nonfunctional during the REPLACEMENT procedure. A REMOVAL procedure is coded for taking out the device used in a previous replacement procedure.

Body Part Character 4	Approach Character 5	Device Character 6	Qualifier Character 7
Ø External Ear, Right Antihelix Antitragus Auricle Earlobe Helix Pinna Tragus **1 External Ear, Left** *See Ø External Ear, Right* **2 External Ear, Bilateral** *See Ø External Ear, Right* **K Nasal Mucosa and Soft Tissue** Columella External naris Greater alar cartilage Internal naris Lateral nasal cartilage Lesser alar cartilage Nasal cavity Nostril	**Ø Open** **X External**	**7 Autologous Tissue Substitute** **J Synthetic Substitute** **K Nonautologous Tissue Substitute**	**Z No Qualifier**
5 Middle Ear, Right Oval window Tympanic cavity **6 Middle Ear, Left** *See 5 Middle Ear, Right* **9 Auditory Ossicle, Right** Incus Malleus Stapes **A Auditory Ossicle, Left** *See 9 Auditory Ossicle, Right* **D Inner Ear, Right** Bony labyrinth Bony vestibule Cochlea Round window Semicircular canal **E Inner Ear, Left** *See D Inner Ear, Right*	**Ø Open**	**7 Autologous Tissue Substitute** **J Synthetic Substitute** **K Nonautologous Tissue Substitute**	**Z No Qualifier**
7 Tympanic Membrane, Right Pars flaccida **8 Tympanic Membrane, Left** *See 7 Tympanic Membrane, Right* **N Nasopharynx** Choana Fossa of Rosenmuller Pharyngeal recess Rhinopharynx	**Ø Open** **7 Via Natural or Artificial Opening** **8 Via Natural or Artificial Opening Endoscopic**	**7 Autologous Tissue Substitute** **J Synthetic Substitute** **K Nonautologous Tissue Substitute**	**Z No Qualifier**
L Nasal Turbinate Inferior turbinate Middle turbinate Nasal concha Superior turbinate	**Ø Open** **3 Percutaneous** **4 Percutaneous Endoscopic** **7 Via Natural or Artificial Opening** **8 Via Natural or Artificial Opening Endoscopic**	**7 Autologous Tissue Substitute** **J Synthetic Substitute** **K Nonautologous Tissue Substitute**	**Z No Qualifier**
M Nasal Septum Quadrangular cartilage Septal cartilage Vomer bone	**Ø Open** **3 Percutaneous** **4 Percutaneous Endoscopic**	**7 Autologous Tissue Substitute** **J Synthetic Substitute** **K Nonautologous Tissue Substitute**	**Z No Qualifier**

Ø Medical and Surgical
9 Ear, Nose, Sinus
S Reposition

Definition: Moving to its normal location, or other suitable location, all or a portion of a body part

Explanation: The body part is moved to a new location from an abnormal location, or from a normal location where it is not functioning correctly. The body part may or may not be cut out or off to be moved to the new location.

Body Part Character 4	Approach Character 5	Device Character 6	Qualifier Character 7
Ø External Ear, Right Antihelix Antitragus Auricle Earlobe Helix Pinna Tragus **1 External Ear, Left** *See Ø External Ear, Right* **2 External Ear, Bilateral** *See Ø External Ear, Right* **K Nasal Mucosa and Soft Tissue** Columella External naris Greater alar cartilage Internal naris Lateral nasal cartilage Lesser alar cartilage Nasal cavity Nostril	**Ø Open** **4 Percutaneous Endoscopic** **X External**	**Z No Device**	**Z No Qualifier**
7 Tympanic Membrane, Right Pars flaccida **8 Tympanic Membrane, Left** *See 7 Tympanic Membrane, Right* **F Eustachian Tube, Right** Auditory tube Pharyngotympanic tube **G Eustachian Tube, Left** *See F Eustachian Tube, Right* **L Nasal Turbinate** Inferior turbinate Middle turbinate Nasal concha Superior turbinate	**Ø Open** **4 Percutaneous Endoscopic** **7 Via Natural or Artificial Opening** **8 Via Natural or Artificial Opening Endoscopic**	**Z No Device**	**Z No Qualifier**
9 Auditory Ossicle, Right Incus Malleus Stapes **A Auditory Ossicle, Left** *See 9 Auditory Ossicle, Right* **M Nasal Septum** Quadrangular cartilage Septal cartilage Vomer bone	**Ø Open** **4 Percutaneous Endoscopic**	**Z No Device**	**Z No Qualifier**

Non-OR Ø9S[F,G][Ø,4,7,8]ZZ

Ø Medical and Surgical
9 Ear, Nose, Sinus
T Resection Definition: Cutting out or off, without replacement, all of a body part
Explanation: None

Body Part Character 4		Approach Character 5	Device Character 6	Qualifier Character 7
Ø External Ear, Right Antihelix Antitragus Auricle Earlobe Helix Pinna Tragus	**1 External Ear, Left** *See Ø External Ear, Right*	**Ø Open** **4 Percutaneous Endoscopic** **X External**	**Z No Device**	**Z No Qualifier**
5 Middle Ear, Right Oval window Tympanic cavity **6 Middle Ear, Left** *See 5 Middle Ear, Right* **9 Auditory Ossicle, Right** Incus Malleus Stapes	**A Auditory Ossicle, Left** *See 9 Auditory Ossicle, Right* **D Inner Ear, Right** Bony labyrinth Bony vestibule Cochlea Round window Semicircular canal **E Inner Ear, Left** *See D Inner Ear, Right*	**Ø Open** **8 Via Natural or Artificial Opening Endoscopic**	**Z No Device**	**Z No Qualifier**
7 Tympanic Membrane, Right Pars flaccida **8 Tympanic Membrane, Left** *See 7 Tympanic Membrane, Right* **F Eustachian Tube, Right** Auditory tube Pharyngotympanic tube **G Eustachian Tube, Left** *See F Eustachian Tube, Right*	**L Nasal Turbinate** Inferior turbinate Middle turbinate Nasal concha Superior turbinate **N Nasopharynx** Choana Fossa of Rosenmuller Pharyngeal recess Rhinopharynx	**Ø Open** **4 Percutaneous Endoscopic** **7 Via Natural or Artificial Opening** **8 Via Natural or Artificial Opening Endoscopic**	**Z No Device**	**Z No Qualifier**
B Mastoid Sinus, Right Mastoid air cells **C Mastoid Sinus, Left** *See B Mastoid Sinus, Right* **M Nasal Septum** Quadrangular cartilage Septal cartilage Vomer bone **P Accessory Sinus** **Q Maxillary Sinus, Right** Antrum of Highmore	**R Maxillary Sinus, Left** *See Q Maxillary Sinus, Right* **S Frontal Sinus, Right** **T Frontal Sinus, Left** **U Ethmoid Sinus, Right** Ethmoidal air cell **V Ethmoid Sinus, Left** *See U Ethmoid Sinus, Right* **W Sphenoid Sinus, Right** **X Sphenoid Sinus, Left**	**Ø Open** **4 Percutaneous Endoscopic** **8 Via Natural or Artificial Opening Endoscopic**	**Z No Device**	**Z No Qualifier**
K Nasal Mucosa and Soft Tissue Columella External naris Greater alar cartilage Internal naris Lateral nasal cartilage Lesser alar cartilage Nasal cavity Nostril		**Ø Open** **4 Percutaneous Endoscopic** **8 Via Natural or Artificial Opening Endoscopic** **X External**	**Z No Device**	**Z No Qualifier**

Non-OR Ø9T[F,G][Ø,4,7,8]ZZ

Ø Medical and Surgical
9 Ear, Nose, Sinus
U Supplement

Definition: Putting in or on biological or synthetic material that physically reinforces and/or augments the function of a portion of a body part

Explanation: The biological material is non-living, or is living and from the same individual. The body part may have been previously replaced, and the SUPPLEMENT procedure is performed to physically reinforce and/or augment the function of the replaced body part.

Body Part Character 4	Approach Character 5	Device Character 6	Qualifier Character 7
Ø External Ear, Right Antihelix, Antitragus, Auricle, Earlobe, Helix, Pinna, Tragus **1 External Ear, Left** *See Ø External Ear, Right* **2 External Ear, Bilateral** *See Ø External Ear, Right*	**Ø Open** **X External**	**7 Autologous Tissue Substitute** **J Synthetic Substitute** **K Nonautologous Tissue Substitute**	**Z No Qualifier**
5 Middle Ear, Right Oval window, Tympanic cavity **6 Middle Ear, Left** *See 5 Middle Ear, Right* **9 Auditory Ossicle, Right** Incus, Malleus, Stapes **A Auditory Ossicle, Left** *See 9 Auditory Ossicle, Right* **D Inner Ear, Right** Bony labyrinth, Bony vestibule, Cochlea, Round window, Semicircular canal **E Inner Ear, Left** *See D Inner Ear, Right*	**Ø Open** **8 Via Natural or Artificial Opening Endoscopic**	**7 Autologous Tissue Substitute** **J Synthetic Substitute** **K Nonautologous Tissue Substitute**	**Z No Qualifier**
7 Tympanic Membrane, Right Pars flaccida **8 Tympanic Membrane, Left** *See 7 Tympanic Membrane, Right* **N Nasopharynx** Choana, Fossa of Rosenmuller, Pharyngeal recess, Rhinopharynx	**Ø Open** **7 Via Natural or Artificial Opening** **8 Via Natural or Artificial Opening Endoscopic**	**7 Autologous Tissue Substitute** **J Synthetic Substitute** **K Nonautologous Tissue Substitute**	**Z No Qualifier**
B Mastoid Sinus, Right Mastoid air cells **C Mastoid Sinus, Left** *See B Mastoid Sinus, Right* **L Nasal Turbinate** Inferior turbinate, Middle turbinate, Nasal concha, Superior turbinate **P Accessory Sinus** **Q Maxillary Sinus, Right** Antrum of Highmore **R Maxillary Sinus, Left** *See Q Maxillary Sinus, Right* **S Frontal Sinus, Right** **T Frontal Sinus, Left** **U Ethmoid Sinus, Right** Ethmoidal air cell **V Ethmoid Sinus, Left** *See U Ethmoid Sinus, Right* **W Sphenoid Sinus, Right** **X Sphenoid Sinus, Left**	**Ø Open** **3 Percutaneous** **4 Percutaneous Endoscopic** **7 Via Natural or Artificial Opening** **8 Via Natural or Artificial Opening Endoscopic**	**7 Autologous Tissue Substitute** **J Synthetic Substitute** **K Nonautologous Tissue Substitute**	**Z No Qualifier**
K Nasal Mucosa and Soft Tissue Columella, External naris, Greater alar cartilage, Internal naris, Lateral nasal cartilage, Lesser alar cartilage, Nasal cavity, Nostril	**Ø Open** **8 Via Natural or Artificial Opening Endoscopic** **X External**	**7 Autologous Tissue Substitute** **J Synthetic Substitute** **K Nonautologous Tissue Substitute**	**Z No Qualifier**
M Nasal Septum Quadrangular cartilage, Septal cartilage, Vomer bone	**Ø Open** **3 Percutaneous** **4 Percutaneous Endoscopic** **8 Via Natural or Artificial Opening Endoscopic**	**7 Autologous Tissue Substitute** **J Synthetic Substitute** **K Nonautologous Tissue Substitute**	**Z No Qualifier**

Ø Medical and Surgical
9 Ear, Nose, Sinus
W Revision

Definition: Correcting, to the extent possible, a portion of a malfunctioning device or the position of a displaced device

Explanation: Revision can include correcting a malfunctioning or displaced device by taking out or putting in components of the device such as a screw or pin

Body Part Character 4	Approach Character 5	Device Character 6	Qualifier Character 7
7 Tympanic Membrane, Right Pars flaccida **8 Tympanic Membrane, Left** *See 7 Tympanic Membrane, Right* **9 Auditory Ossicle, Right** Incus Malleus Stapes **A Auditory Ossicle, Left** *See 9 Auditory Ossicle, Right*	**Ø Open** **7 Via Natural or Artificial Opening** **8 Via Natural or Artificial Opening Endoscopic**	**7 Autologous Tissue Substitute** **J Synthetic Substitute** **K Nonautologous Tissue Substitute**	**Z No Qualifier**
D Inner Ear, Right Bony labyrinth Bony vestibule Cochlea Round window Semicircular canal **E Inner Ear, Left** *See D Inner Ear, Right*	**Ø Open** **7 Via Natural or Artificial Opening** **8 Via Natural or Artificial Opening Endoscopic**	**S Hearing Device**	**Z No Qualifier**
H Ear, Right **J Ear, Left** **K Nasal Mucosa and Soft Tissue** Columella External naris Greater alar cartilage Internal naris Lateral nasal cartilage Lesser alar cartilage Nasal cavity Nostril	**Ø Open** **3 Percutaneous** **4 Percutaneous Endoscopic** **7 Via Natural or Artificial Opening** **8 Via Natural or Artificial Opening Endoscopic**	**Ø Drainage Device** **7 Autologous Tissue Substitute** **D Intraluminal Device** **J Synthetic Substitute** **K Nonautologous Tissue Substitute** **Y Other Device**	**Z No Qualifier**
H Ear, Right **J Ear, Left** **K Nasal Mucosa and Soft Tissue** Columella External naris Greater alar cartilage Internal naris Lateral nasal cartilage Lesser alar cartilage Nasal cavity Nostril	**X External**	**Ø Drainage Device** **7 Autologous Tissue Substitute** **D Intraluminal Device** **J Synthetic Substitute** **K Nonautologous Tissue Substitute**	**Z No Qualifier**
Y Sinus	**Ø Open** **3 Percutaneous** **4 Percutaneous Endoscopic**	**Ø Drainage Device** **Y Other Device**	**Z No Qualifier**
Y Sinus	**7 Via Natural or Artificial Opening** **8 Via Natural or Artificial Opening Endoscopic**	**Y Other Device**	**Z No Qualifier**
Y Sinus	**X External**	**Ø Drainage Device**	**Z No Qualifier**

Non-OR Ø9W[H,J][3,4][J,K,Y]Z
Non-OR Ø9W[H,J][7,8][D,Y]Z
Non-OR Ø9WK[Ø,3,4,7,8][Ø,7,D,J,K,Y]Z
Non-OR Ø9W[H,J,K]X[Ø,7,D,J,K]Z
Non-OR Ø9WY[3,4]YZ
Non-OR Ø9WY[7,8]YZ
Non-OR Ø9WYXØZ

Respiratory System ØB1–ØBY

Character Meanings

This Character Meaning table is provided as a guide to assist the user in the identification of character members that may be found in this section of code tables. It **SHOULD NOT** be used to build a PCS code.

Operation–Character 3	Body Part–Character 4	Approach–Character 5	Device–Character 6	Qualifier–Character 7
1 Bypass	Ø Tracheobronchial Tree	Ø Open	Ø Drainage Device	Ø Allogeneic
2 Change	1 Trachea	3 Percutaneous	1 Radioactive Element	1 Syngeneic
5 Destruction	2 Carina	4 Percutaneous Endoscopic	2 Monitoring Device	2 Zooplastic
7 Dilation	3 Main Bronchus, Right	7 Via Natural or Artificial Opening	3 Infusion Device	3 Laser Interstitial Thermal Therapy
9 Drainage	4 Upper Lobe Bronchus, Right	8 Via Natural or Artificial Opening Endoscopic	7 Autologous Tissue Substitute	4 Cutaneous
B Excision	5 Middle Lobe Bronchus, Right	X External	C Extraluminal Device	6 Esophagus
C Extirpation	6 Lower Lobe Bronchus, Right		D Intraluminal Device	X Diagnostic
D Extraction	7 Main Bronchus, Left		E Intraluminal Device, Endotracheal Airway	Z No Qualifier
F Fragmentation	8 Upper Lobe Bronchus, Left		F Tracheostomy Device	
H Insertion	9 Lingula Bronchus		G Intraluminal Device, Endobronchial Valve	
J Inspection	B Lower Lobe Bronchus, Left		J Synthetic Substitute	
L Occlusion	C Upper Lung Lobe, Right		K Nonautologous Tissue Substitute	
M Reattachment	D Middle Lung Lobe, Right		M Diaphragmatic Pacemaker Lead	
N Release	F Lower Lung Lobe, Right		Y Other Device	
P Removal	G Upper Lung Lobe, Left		Z No Device	
Q Repair	H Lung Lingula			
R Replacement	J Lower Lung Lobe, Left			
S Reposition	K Lung, Right			
T Resection	L Lung, Left			
U Supplement	M Lungs, Bilateral			
V Restriction	N Pleura, Right			
W Revision	P Pleura, Left			
Y Transplantation	Q Pleura			
	T Diaphragm			

AHA Coding Clinic for table ØB5
2022, 4Q, 53-54 Laser interstitial thermal therapy
2016, 2Q, 17 Photodynamic therapy for treatment of malignant mesothelioma
2015, 2Q, 31 Thoracoscopic talc pleurodesis

AHA Coding Clinic for table ØB7
2020, 3Q, 43 Tracheobronchomalacia with placement of tracheobronchial stent

AHA Coding Clinic for table ØB9
2017, 3Q, 15 Bronchoscopy with suctioning for removal of retained secretions
2017, 1Q, 51 Bronchoalveolar lavage
2016, 1Q, 26 Bronchoalveolar lavage, endobronchial biopsy and transbronchial biopsy
2016, 1Q, 27 Fiberoptic bronchoscopy with brushings and bronchoalveolar lavage

AHA Coding Clinic for table ØBB
2022, 2Q, 19 Transbronchial lung biopsy using alligator forceps
2016, 1Q, 26 Bronchoalveolar lavage, endobronchial biopsy and transbronchial biopsy
2016, 1Q, 27 Fiberoptic bronchoscopy with brushings and bronchoalveolar lavage
2014, 1Q, 20 Fiducial marker placement

AHA Coding Clinic for table ØBC
2017, 3Q, 14 Bronchoscopy with suctioning and washings for removal of mucus plug

AHA Coding Clinic for table ØBD
2020, 3Q, 40 Transbronchial cryobiopsy of upper, middle and lower lobes of lung
2018, 3Q, 28 Lung decortication for empyema

AHA Coding Clinic for table ØBH
2022, 3Q, 22 Approach value for placement of endotracheal tube
2019, 3Q, 33 Insertion of endobronchial valve
2014, 4Q, 3-10 Mechanical ventilation

AHA Coding Clinic for table ØBJ
2015, 2Q, 31 Thoracoscopic talc pleurodesis
2014, 1Q, 20 Fiducial marker placement

AHA Coding Clinic for table ØBL
2019, 3Q, 33 Insertion of endobronchial valve

AHA Coding Clinic for table ØBN
2019, 2Q, 20 Pericardiectomy for constrictive pericarditis
2018, 3Q, 28 Lung decortication
2018, 3Q, 28 Lung decortication for empyema
2015, 3Q, 15 Vascular ring surgery with release of esophagus and trachea

AHA Coding Clinic for table ØBQ
2020, 3Q, 41 Plication of diaphragm
2016, 2Q, 22 Esophageal lengthening Collis gastroplasty with Nissen fundoplication and hiatal hernia
2014, 3Q, 28 Laparoscopic Nissen fundoplication and diaphragmatic hernia repair

AHA Coding Clinic for table ØBU
2020, 3Q, 43 Tracheobronchomalacia with placement of tracheobronchial stent
2015, 1Q, 28 Repair of bronchopleural fistula using omental pedicle graft

AHA Coding Clinic for table ØBV
2020, 3Q, 41 Plication of diaphragm

AHA Coding Clinic for table ØBY
2023, 2Q, 32 Preparation of donor organ before transplantation

Respiratory System

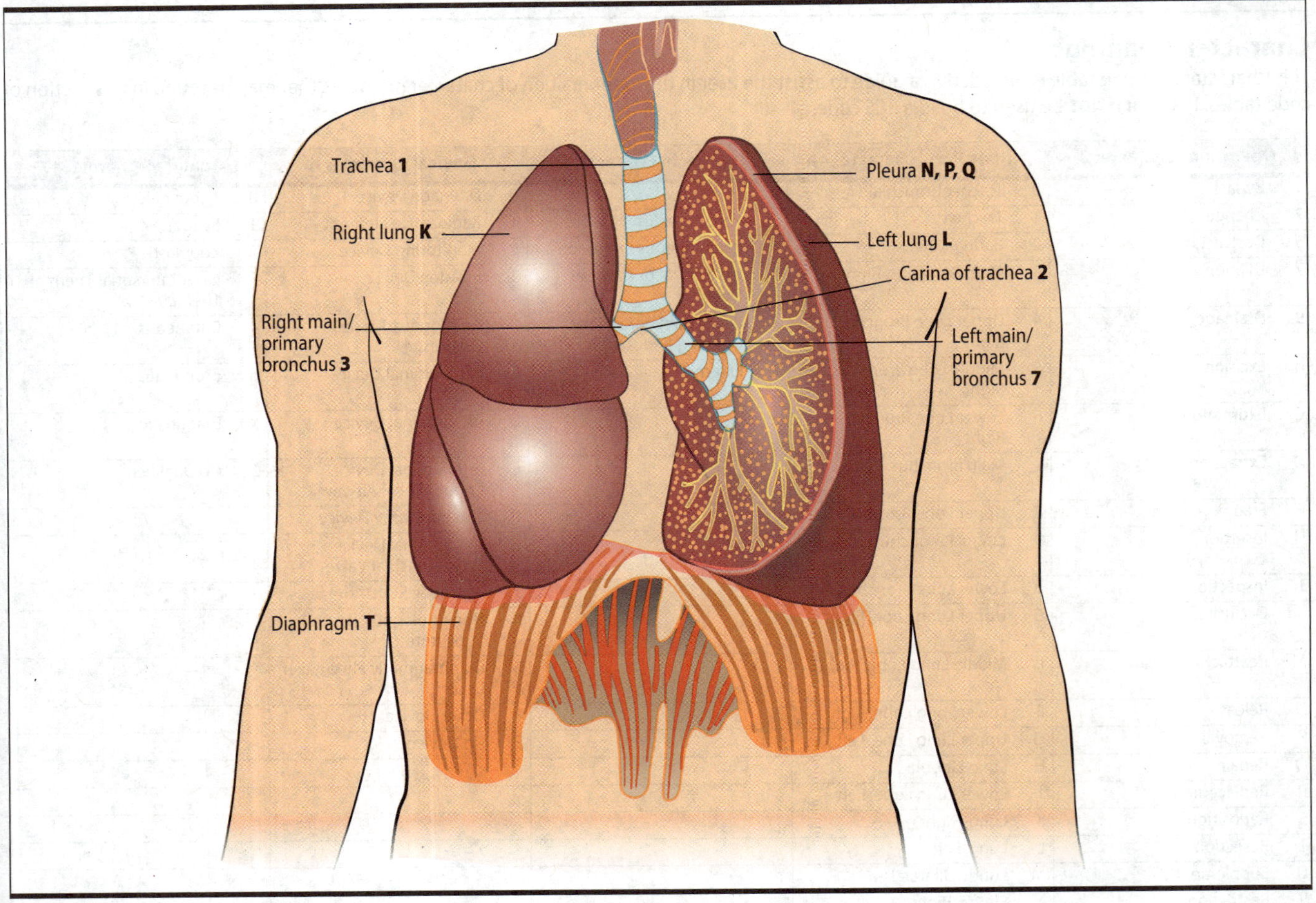

Trachea 1
Pleura N, P, Q
Right lung K
Left lung L
Carina of trachea 2
Right main/
primary
bronchus 3
Left main/
primary
bronchus 7
Diaphragm T

Right Lung Bronchi

Right lung K
R. main
bronchus 3
Trachea 1
R. upper lobe
bronchus 4
Tracheobronchial tree Ø
R. middle lobe
bronchus 5
Carini 2
R. lower lobe
bronchus 6

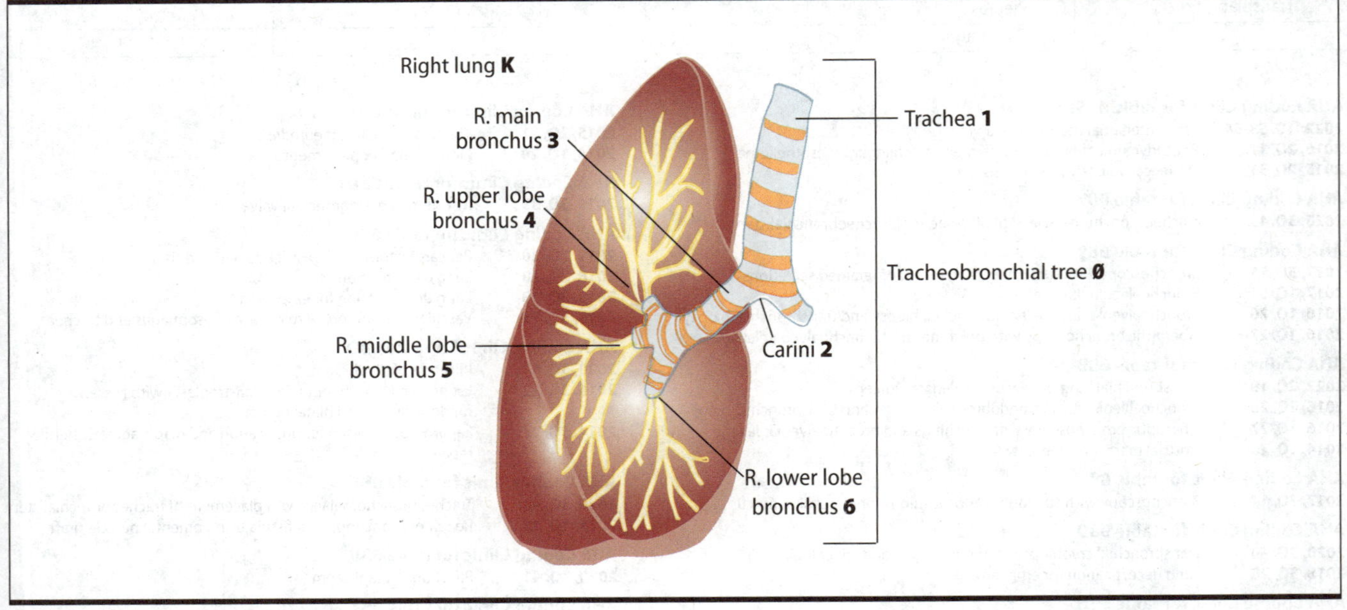

Ø Medical and Surgical
B Respiratory System
1 Bypass

Definition: Altering the route of passage of the contents of a tubular body part

Explanation: Rerouting contents of a body part to a downstream area of the normal route, to a similar route and body part, or to an abnormal route and dissimilar body part. Includes one or more anastomoses, with or without the use of a device.

Body Part Character 4	Approach Character 5	Device Character 6	Qualifier Character 7
1 Trachea Cricoid cartilage	Ø Open	D Intraluminal Device	6 Esophagus
1 Trachea Cricoid cartilage	Ø Open	F Tracheostomy Device Z No Device	4 Cutaneous
1 Trachea Cricoid cartilage	3 Percutaneous 4 Percutaneous Endoscopic	F Tracheostomy Device Z No Device	4 Cutaneous

DRG Non-OR ØB113[F,Z]4
Non-OR ØB11ØD6

Ø Medical and Surgical
B Respiratory System
2 Change

Definition: Taking out or off a device from a body part and putting back an identical or similar device in or on the same body part without cutting or puncturing the skin or a mucous membrane

Explanation: All CHANGE procedures are coded using the approach EXTERNAL

Body Part Character 4	Approach Character 5	Device Character 6	Qualifier Character 7
Ø Tracheobronchial Tree K Lung, Right L Lung, Left Q Pleura T Diaphragm	X External	Ø Drainage Device Y Other Device	Z No Qualifier
1 Trachea Cricoid cartilage	X External	Ø Drainage Device E Intraluminal Device, Endotracheal Airway F Tracheostomy Device Y Other Device	Z No Qualifier

Non-OR All body part, approach, device, and qualifier values

Ø Medical and Surgical
B Respiratory System
5 Destruction Definition: Physical eradication of all or a portion of a body part by the direct use of energy, force, or a destructive agent

Explanation: None of the body part is physically taken out

Body Part Character 4	Approach Character 5	Device Character 6	Qualifier Character 7
1 Trachea Cricoid cartilage **2** Carina **3** Main Bronchus, Right Bronchus intermedius Intermediate bronchus **4** Upper Lobe Bronchus, Right **5** Middle Lobe Bronchus, Right **6** Lower Lobe Bronchus, Right **7** Main Bronchus, Left **8** Upper Lobe Bronchus, Left **9** Lingula Bronchus **B** Lower Lobe Bronchus, Left	**Ø** Open **3** Percutaneous **4** Percutaneous Endoscopic **7** Via Natural or Artificial Opening **8** Via Natural or Artificial Opening Endoscopic	**Z** No Device	**Z** No Qualifier
C Upper Lung Lobe, Right **D** Middle Lung Lobe, Right **F** Lower Lung Lobe, Right **G** Upper Lung Lobe, Left **H** Lung Lingula **J** Lower Lung Lobe, Left **K** Lung, Right **L** Lung, Left **M** Lungs, Bilateral	**Ø** Open **3** Percutaneous **4** Percutaneous Endoscopic	**Z** No Device	**3** Laser Interstitial Thermal Therapy **Z** No Qualifier
C Upper Lung Lobe, Right **D** Middle Lung Lobe, Right **F** Lower Lung Lobe, Right **G** Upper Lung Lobe, Left **H** Lung Lingula **J** Lower Lung Lobe, Left **K** Lung, Right **L** Lung, Left **M** Lungs, Bilateral	**7** Via Natural or Artificial Opening **8** Via Natural or Artificial Opening Endoscopic	**Z** No Device	**Z** No Qualifier
N Pleura, Right **P** Pleura, Left **T** Diaphragm	**Ø** Open **3** Percutaneous **4** Percutaneous Endoscopic	**Z** No Device	**Z** No Qualifier

Non-OR ØB5[3,4,5,6,7,8,9,B]4ZZ
Non-OR ØB5[C,D,F,G,H,J,K,L,M]8ZZ

Ø Medical and Surgical
B Respiratory System
7 Dilation Definition: Expanding an orifice or the lumen of a tubular body part

Explanation: The orifice can be a natural orifice or an artificially created orifice. Accomplished by stretching a tubular body part using intraluminal pressure or by cutting part of the orifice or wall of the tubular body part.

Body Part Character 4	Approach Character 5	Device Character 6	Qualifier Character 7
1 Trachea Cricoid cartilage **2** Carina **3** Main Bronchus, Right Bronchus intermedius Intermediate bronchus **4** Upper Lobe Bronchus, Right **5** Middle Lobe Bronchus, Right **6** Lower Lobe Bronchus, Right **7** Main Bronchus, Left **8** Upper Lobe Bronchus, Left **9** Lingula Bronchus **B** Lower Lobe Bronchus, Left	**Ø** Open **3** Percutaneous **4** Percutaneous Endoscopic **7** Via Natural or Artificial Opening **8** Via Natural or Artificial Opening Endoscopic	**D** Intraluminal Device **Z** No Device	**Z** No Qualifier

Non-OR ØB7[3,4,5,6,7,8,9,B][Ø,3,4,7,8][D,Z]Z

Ø Medical and Surgical
B Respiratory System
9 Drainage Definition: Taking or letting out fluids and/or gases from a body part
Explanation: The qualifier DIAGNOSTIC is used to identify drainage procedures that are biopsies

Body Part Character 4	Approach Character 5	Device Character 6	Qualifier Character 7
1 Trachea Cricoid cartilage 2 Carina 3 Main Bronchus, Right Bronchus intermedius Intermediate bronchus 4 Upper Lobe Bronchus, Right 5 Middle Lobe Bronchus, Right 6 Lower Lobe Bronchus, Right 7 Main Bronchus, Left 8 Upper Lobe Bronchus, Left 9 Lingula Bronchus B Lower Lobe Bronchus, Left C Upper Lung Lobe, Right D Middle Lung Lobe, Right F Lower Lung Lobe, Right G Upper Lung Lobe, Left H Lung Lingula J Lower Lung Lobe, Left K Lung, Right L Lung, Left M Lungs, Bilateral	Ø Open 3 Percutaneous 4 Percutaneous Endoscopic 7 Via Natural or Artificial Opening 8 Via Natural or Artificial Opening Endoscopic	Ø Drainage Device	Z No Qualifier
1 Trachea Cricoid cartilage 2 Carina 3 Main Bronchus, Right Bronchus intermedius Intermediate bronchus 4 Upper Lobe Bronchus, Right 5 Middle Lobe Bronchus, Right 6 Lower Lobe Bronchus, Right 7 Main Bronchus, Left 8 Upper Lobe Bronchus, Left 9 Lingula Bronchus B Lower Lobe Bronchus, Left C Upper Lung Lobe, Right D Middle Lung Lobe, Right F Lower Lung Lobe, Right G Upper Lung Lobe, Left H Lung Lingula J Lower Lung Lobe, Left K Lung, Right L Lung, Left M Lungs, Bilateral	Ø Open 3 Percutaneous 4 Percutaneous Endoscopic 7 Via Natural or Artificial Opening 8 Via Natural or Artificial Opening Endoscopic	Z No Device	X Diagnostic Z No Qualifier
N Pleura, Right P Pleura, Left	Ø Open 3 Percutaneous 4 Percutaneous Endoscopic 8 Via Natural or Artificial Opening Endoscopic	Ø Drainage Device	Z No Qualifier
N Pleura, Right P Pleura, Left	Ø Open 3 Percutaneous 4 Percutaneous Endoscopic 8 Via Natural or Artificial Opening Endoscopic	Z No Device	X Diagnostic Z No Qualifier
T Diaphragm	Ø Open 3 Percutaneous 4 Percutaneous Endoscopic	Ø Drainage Device	Z No Qualifier
T Diaphragm	Ø Open 3 Percutaneous 4 Percutaneous Endoscopic	Z No Device	X Diagnostic Z No Qualifier

Non-OR ØB9[1,2,3,4,5,6,7,8,9,B][7,8]ØZ
Non-OR ØB9[1,2,3,4,5,6,7,8,9,B][3,4]ZX
Non-OR ØB9[1,2,3,4,5,6,7,8,9,B][7,8]Z[X,Z]
Non-OR ØB9[C,D,F,G,H,J,K,L,M][3,4,7]ZX
Non-OR ØB9[C,D,F,G,H,J,K,L,M]8Z[X,Z]
Non-OR ØB9[N,P][Ø,3,8]ØZ
Non-OR ØB9[N,P][Ø,3,8]Z[X,Z]
Non-OR ØB9[N,P]4ZX
Non-OR ØB9T[3,4]ØZ
Non-OR ØB9T[3,4]Z[X,Z]

Ø Medical and Surgical
B Respiratory System
B Excision

Definition: Cutting out or off, without replacement, a portion of a body part

Explanation: The qualifier DIAGNOSTIC is used to identify excision procedures that are biopsies

Body Part Character 4	Approach Character 5	Device Character 6	Qualifier Character 7
1 Trachea Cricoid cartilage **2** Carina **3** Main Bronchus, Right Bronchus intermedius Intermediate bronchus **4** Upper Lobe Bronchus, Right **5** Middle Lobe Bronchus, Right **6** Lower Lobe Bronchus, Right **7** Main Bronchus, Left **8** Upper Lobe Bronchus, Left **9** Lingula Bronchus **B** Lower Lobe Bronchus, Left **C** Upper Lung Lobe, Right **D** Middle Lung Lobe, Right **F** Lower Lung Lobe, Right **G** Upper Lung Lobe, Left **H** Lung Lingula **J** Lower Lung Lobe, Left **K** Lung, Right **L** Lung, Left **M** Lungs, Bilateral	**Ø** Open **3** Percutaneous **4** Percutaneous Endoscopic **7** Via Natural or Artificial Opening **8** Via Natural or Artificial Opening Endoscopic	**Z** No Device	**X** Diagnostic **Z** No Qualifier
N Pleura, Right **P** Pleura, Left	**Ø** Open **3** Percutaneous **4** Percutaneous Endoscopic **8** Via Natural or Artificial Opening Endoscopic	**Z** No Device	**X** Diagnostic **Z** No Qualifier
T Diaphragm	**Ø** Open **3** Percutaneous **4** Percutaneous Endoscopic	**Z** No Device	**X** Diagnostic **Z** No Qualifier

Non-OR ØBB[1,2,3,4,5,6,7,8,9,B][3,4,7,8]ZX
Non-OR ØBB[3,4,5,6,7,8,9,B,M][4,8]ZZ
Non-OR ØBB[C,D,F,G,H,J,K,L,M]3ZX
Non-OR ØBB[C,D,F,G,H,J,K,L]8ZZ
Non-OR ØBB[N,P]3ZX

Ø Medical and Surgical
B Respiratory System
C Extirpation

Definition: Taking or cutting out solid matter from a body part

Explanation: The solid matter may be an abnormal byproduct of a biological function or a foreign body; it may be imbedded in a body part or in the lumen of a tubular body part. The solid matter may or may not have been previously broken into pieces.

Body Part Character 4	Approach Character 5	Device Character 6	Qualifier Character 7
1 Trachea Cricoid cartilage **2** Carina **3** Main Bronchus, Right Bronchus intermedius Intermediate bronchus **4** Upper Lobe Bronchus, Right **5** Middle Lobe Bronchus, Right **6** Lower Lobe Bronchus, Right **7** Main Bronchus, Left **8** Upper Lobe Bronchus, Left **9** Lingula Bronchus **B** Lower Lobe Bronchus, Left **C** Upper Lung Lobe, Right **D** Middle Lung Lobe, Right **F** Lower Lung Lobe, Right **G** Upper Lung Lobe, Left **H** Lung Lingula **J** Lower Lung Lobe, Left **K** Lung, Right **L** Lung, Left **M** Lungs, Bilateral	**Ø** Open **3** Percutaneous **4** Percutaneous Endoscopic **7** Via Natural or Artificial Opening **8** Via Natural or Artificial Opening Endoscopic	**Z** No Device	**Z** No Qualifier
N Pleura, Right **P** Pleura, Left **T** Diaphragm	**Ø** Open **3** Percutaneous **4** Percutaneous Endoscopic	**Z** No Device	**Z** No Qualifier

Non-OR ØBC[1,2,3,4,5,6,7,8,9,B][7,8]ZZ
Non-OR ØBC[N,P]3ZZ

Ø Medical and Surgical
B Respiratory System
D Extraction Definition: Pulling or stripping out or off all or a portion of a body part by the use of force
Explanation: The qualifier DIAGNOSTIC is used to identify extraction procedures that are biopsies

Body Part Character 4	Approach Character 5	Device Character 6	Qualifier Character 7
1 Trachea Cricoid cartilage 2 Carina 3 Main Bronchus, Right Bronchus intermedius Intermediate bronchus 4 Upper Lobe Bronchus, Right 5 Middle Lobe Bronchus, Right 6 Lower Lobe Bronchus, Right 7 Main Bronchus, Left 8 Upper Lobe Bronchus, Left 9 Lingula Bronchus B Lower Lobe Bronchus, Left C Upper Lung Lobe, Right D Middle Lung Lobe, Right F Lower Lung Lobe, Right G Upper Lung Lobe, Left H Lung Lingula J Lower Lung Lobe, Left K Lung, Right L Lung, Left M Lungs, Bilateral	4 Percutaneous Endoscopic 8 Via Natural or Artificial Opening Endoscopic	Z No Device	X Diagnostic
N Pleura, Right P Pleura, Left	Ø Open 3 Percutaneous 4 Percutaneous Endoscopic	Z No Device	X Diagnostic Z No Qualifier

Non-OR ØBD[1,2,3,4,5,6,7,8,9,B,C,D,F,G,H,J,K,L,M][4,8]ZX

Ø Medical and Surgical
B Respiratory System
F Fragmentation Definition: Breaking solid matter in a body part into pieces
Explanation: Physical force (e.g., manual, ultrasonic) applied directly or indirectly is used to break the solid matter into pieces. The solid matter may be an abnormal byproduct of a biological function or a foreign body. The pieces of solid matter are not taken out.

Body Part Character 4	Approach Character 5	Device Character 6	Qualifier Character 7
1 Trachea NC Cricoid cartilage 2 Carina NC 3 Main Bronchus, Right NC Bronchus intermedius Intermediate bronchus 4 Upper Lobe Bronchus, Right NC 5 Middle Lobe Bronchus, Right NC 6 Lower Lobe Bronchus, Right NC 7 Main Bronchus, Left NC 8 Upper Lobe Bronchus, Left NC 9 Lingula Bronchus NC B Lower Lobe Bronchus, Left NC	Ø Open 3 Percutaneous 4 Percutaneous Endoscopic 7 Via Natural or Artificial Opening 8 Via Natural or Artificial Opening Endoscopic X External	Z No Device	Z No Qualifier

Non-OR ØBF[1,2,3,4,5,6,7,8,9,B]XZZ
Non-OR ØBF[3,4,5,6,7,8,9,B][7,8]ZZ
NC ØBF[1,2,3,4,5,6,7,8,9,B]XZZ

Ø Medical and Surgical
B Respiratory System
H Insertion

Definition: Putting in a nonbiological appliance that monitors, assists, performs, or prevents a physiological function but does not physically take the place of a body part

Explanation: None

Body Part Character 4	Approach Character 5	Device Character 6	Qualifier Character 7
Ø Tracheobronchial Tree	Ø Open 3 Percutaneous 4 Percutaneous Endoscopic 7 Via Natural or Artificial Opening 8 Via Natural or Artificial Opening Endoscopic	1 Radioactive Element 2 Monitoring Device 3 Infusion Device D Intraluminal Device Y Other Device	Z No Qualifier
1 Trachea Cricoid cartilage	Ø Open	2 Monitoring Device D Intraluminal Device Y Other Device	Z No Qualifier
1 Trachea Cricoid cartilage	3 Percutaneous	D Intraluminal Device E Intraluminal Device, Endotracheal Airway Y Other Device	Z No Qualifier
1 Trachea Cricoid cartilage	4 Percutaneous Endoscopic	D Intraluminal Device Y Other Device	Z No Qualifier
1 Trachea Cricoid cartilage	7 Via Natural or Artificial Opening 8 Via Natural or Artificial Opening Endoscopic	2 Monitoring Device D Intraluminal Device E Intraluminal Device, Endotracheal Airway Y Other Device	Z No Qualifier
3 Main Bronchus, Right Bronchus intermedius Intermediate bronchus 4 Upper Lobe Bronchus, Right 5 Middle Lobe Bronchus, Right 6 Lower Lobe Bronchus, Right 7 Main Bronchus, Left 8 Upper Lobe Bronchus, Left 9 Lingula Bronchus B Lower Lobe Bronchus, Left	Ø Open 3 Percutaneous 4 Percutaneous Endoscopic 7 Via Natural or Artificial Opening 8 Via Natural or Artificial Opening Endoscopic	G Intraluminal Device, Endobronchial Valve	Z No Qualifier
K Lung, Right L Lung, Left	Ø Open 3 Percutaneous 4 Percutaneous Endoscopic 7 Via Natural or Artificial Opening 8 Via Natural or Artificial Opening Endoscopic	1 Radioactive Element 2 Monitoring Device 3 Infusion Device Y Other Device	Z No Qualifier
Q Pleura	Ø Open 3 Percutaneous 4 Percutaneous Endoscopic 7 Via Natural or Artificial Opening 8 Via Natural or Artificial Opening Endoscopic	Y Other Device	Z No Qualifier
T Diaphragm	Ø Open 3 Percutaneous 4 Percutaneous Endoscopic	2 Monitoring Device M Diaphragmatic Pacemaker Lead Y Other Device	Z No Qualifier
T Diaphragm	7 Via Natural or Artificial Opening 8 Via Natural or Artificial Opening Endoscopic	Y Other Device	Z No Qualifier

DRG Non-OR ØBH[3,4,5,6,7,8,9,B]8GZ
Non-OR ØBHØ3YZ
Non-OR ØBHØ[7,8][2,3,D,Y]Z
Non-OR ØBH13[E,Y]Z
Non-OR ØBH1[7,8][2,D,E,Y]Z
Non-OR ØBH[K,L]3YZ
Non-OR ØBH[K,L]7[2,3,Y]Z
Non-OR ØBH[K,L]8[2,3]Z
Non-OR ØBHQ[3,7]YZ
Non-OR ØBHT3YZ
Non-OR ØBHT[7,8]YZ

Ø Medical and Surgical
B Respiratory System
J Inspection Definition: Visually and/or manually exploring a body part

Explanation: Visual exploration may be performed with or without optical instrumentation. Manual exploration may be performed directly or through intervening body layers.

Body Part Character 4	Approach Character 5	Device Character 6	Qualifier Character 7
Ø Tracheobronchial Tree 1 Trachea Cricoid cartilage K Lung, Right L Lung, Left Q Pleura T Diaphragm	Ø Open 3 Percutaneous 4 Percutaneous Endoscopic 7 Via Natural or Artificial Opening 8 Via Natural or Artificial Opening Endoscopic X External	Z No Device	Z No Qualifier

Non-OR ØBJ[Ø,K,L,Q,T][3,7,8,X]ZZ
Non-OR ØBJ1[3,4,7,8,X]ZZ

Ø Medical and Surgical
B Respiratory System
L Occlusion Definition: Completely closing an orifice or the lumen of a tubular body part

Explanation: The orifice can be a natural orifice or an artificially created orifice

Body Part Character 4	Approach Character 5	Device Character 6	Qualifier Character 7
1 Trachea Cricoid cartilage 2 Carina 3 Main Bronchus, Right Bronchus intermedius Intermediate bronchus 4 Upper Lobe Bronchus, Right 5 Middle Lobe Bronchus, Right 6 Lower Lobe Bronchus, Right 7 Main Bronchus, Left 8 Upper Lobe Bronchus, Left 9 Lingula Bronchus B Lower Lobe Bronchus, Left	Ø Open 3 Percutaneous 4 Percutaneous Endoscopic	C Extraluminal Device D Intraluminal Device Z No Device	Z No Qualifier
1 Trachea Cricoid cartilage 2 Carina 3 Main Bronchus, Right Bronchus intermedius Intermediate bronchus 4 Upper Lobe Bronchus, Right 5 Middle Lobe Bronchus, Right 6 Lower Lobe Bronchus, Right 7 Main Bronchus, Left 8 Upper Lobe Bronchus, Left 9 Lingula Bronchus B Lower Lobe Bronchus, Left	7 Via Natural or Artificial Opening 8 Via Natural or Artificial Opening Endoscopic	D Intraluminal Device Z No Device	Z No Qualifier

Ø Medical and Surgical
B Respiratory System
M Reattachment Definition: Putting back in or on all or a portion of a separated body part to its normal location or other suitable location
Explanation: Vascular circulation and nervous pathways may or may not be reestablished

Body Part Character 4	Approach Character 5	Device Character 6	Qualifier Character 7
1 Trachea Cricoid cartilage **2 Carina** **3 Main Bronchus, Right** Bronchus intermedius Intermediate bronchus **4 Upper Lobe Bronchus, Right** **5 Middle Lobe Bronchus, Right** **6 Lower Lobe Bronchus, Right** **7 Main Bronchus, Left** **8 Upper Lobe Bronchus, Left** **9 Lingula Bronchus** **B Lower Lobe Bronchus, Left** **C Upper Lung Lobe, Right** **D Middle Lung Lobe, Right** **F Lower Lung Lobe, Right** **G Upper Lung Lobe, Left** **H Lung Lingula** **J Lower Lung Lobe, Left** **K Lung, Right** **L Lung, Left** **T Diaphragm**	**Ø Open**	**Z No Device**	**Z No Qualifier**

Ø Medical and Surgical
B Respiratory System
N Release Definition: Freeing a body part from an abnormal physical constraint by cutting or by the use of force
Explanation: Some of the restraining tissue may be taken out but none of the body part is taken out

Body Part Character 4	Approach Character 5	Device Character 6	Qualifier Character 7
1 Trachea Cricoid cartilage **2 Carina** **3 Main Bronchus, Right** Bronchus intermedius Intermediate bronchus **4 Upper Lobe Bronchus, Right** **5 Middle Lobe Bronchus, Right** **6 Lower Lobe Bronchus, Right** **7 Main Bronchus, Left** **8 Upper Lobe Bronchus, Left** **9 Lingula Bronchus** **B Lower Lobe Bronchus, Left** **C Upper Lung Lobe, Right** **D Middle Lung Lobe, Right** **F Lower Lung Lobe, Right** **G Upper Lung Lobe, Left** **H Lung Lingula** **J Lower Lung Lobe, Left** **K Lung, Right** **L Lung, Left** **M Lungs, Bilateral**	**Ø Open** **3 Percutaneous** **4 Percutaneous Endoscopic** **7 Via Natural or Artificial Opening** **8 Via Natural or Artificial Opening Endoscopic**	**Z No Device**	**Z No Qualifier**
N Pleura, Right **P Pleura, Left** **T Diaphragm**	**Ø Open** **3 Percutaneous** **4 Percutaneous Endoscopic**	**Z No Device**	**Z No Qualifier**

Ø Medical and Surgical
B Respiratory System
P Removal Definition: Taking out or off a device from a body part

Explanation: If a device is taken out and a similar device put in without cutting or puncturing the skin or mucous membrane, the procedure is coded to the root operation CHANGE. Otherwise, the procedure for taking out a device is coded to the root operation REMOVAL.

Body Part Character 4	Approach Character 5	Device Character 6	Qualifier Character 7
Ø Tracheobronchial Tree	Ø Open 3 Percutaneous 4 Percutaneous Endoscopic 7 Via Natural or Artificial Opening 8 Via Natural or Artificial Opening Endoscopic	Ø Drainage Device 1 Radioactive Element 2 Monitoring Device 3 Infusion Device 7 Autologous Tissue Substitute C Extraluminal Device D Intraluminal Device J Synthetic Substitute K Nonautologous Tissue Substitute Y Other Device	Z No Qualifier
Ø Tracheobronchial Tree	X External	Ø Drainage Device 1 Radioactive Element 2 Monitoring Device 3 Infusion Device D Intraluminal Device	Z No Qualifier
1 Trachea Cricoid cartilage	Ø Open 3 Percutaneous 4 Percutaneous Endoscopic 7 Via Natural or Artificial Opening 8 Via Natural or Artificial Opening Endoscopic	Ø Drainage Device 2 Monitoring Device 7 Autologous Tissue Substitute C Extraluminal Device D Intraluminal Device F Tracheostomy Device J Synthetic Substitute K Nonautologous Tissue Substitute	Z No Qualifier
1 Trachea Cricoid cartilage	X External	Ø Drainage Device 2 Monitoring Device D Intraluminal Device F Tracheostomy Device	Z No Qualifier
K Lung, Right L Lung, Left	Ø Open 3 Percutaneous 4 Percutaneous Endoscopic 7 Via Natural or Artificial Opening 8 Via Natural or Artificial Opening Endoscopic	Ø Drainage Device 1 Radioactive Element 2 Monitoring Device 3 Infusion Device Y Other Device	Z No Qualifier
K Lung, Right L Lung, Left	X External	Ø Drainage Device 1 Radioactive Element 2 Monitoring Device 3 Infusion Device	Z No Qualifier
Q Pleura	Ø Open 3 Percutaneous 4 Percutaneous Endoscopic 7 Via Natural or Artificial Opening 8 Via Natural or Artificial Opening Endoscopic	Ø Drainage Device 1 Radioactive Element 2 Monitoring Device Y Other Device	Z No Qualifier
Q Pleura	X External	Ø Drainage Device 1 Radioactive Element 2 Monitoring Device	Z No Qualifier
T Diaphragm	Ø Open 3 Percutaneous 4 Percutaneous Endoscopic 7 Via Natural or Artificial Opening 8 Via Natural or Artificial Opening Endoscopic	Ø Drainage Device 2 Monitoring Device 7 Autologous Tissue Substitute J Synthetic Substitute K Nonautologous Tissue Substitute M Diaphragmatic Pacemaker Lead Y Other Device	Z No Qualifier
T Diaphragm	X External	Ø Drainage Device 2 Monitoring Device M Diaphragmatic Pacemaker Lead	Z No Qualifier

Non-OR ØBPØ[3,4]YZ
Non-OR ØBPØ[7,8][Ø,2,3,D,Y]Z
Non-OR ØBPØX[Ø,1,2,3,D]Z
Non-OR ØBP1[Ø,3,4]FZ
Non-OR ØBP1[7,8][Ø,2,D,F]Z
Non-OR ØBP1X[Ø,2,D,F]Z
Non-OR ØBP[K,L]3YZ
Non-OR ØBPK7[Ø,1,2,3,Y]Z
Non-OR ØBPK8[Ø,1,2,3]Z
Non-OR ØBPL7[Ø,2,3,Y]Z
Non-OR ØBPL8[Ø,2,3]Z
Non-OR ØBP[K,L]X[Ø,1,2,3]Z
Non-OR ØBPQ[Ø,3,4,7,8][Ø,1,2,]Z
Non-OR ØBPQ[3,7]YZ
Non-OR ØBPQX[Ø,1,2]Z
Non-OR ØBPT3YZ
Non-OR ØBPT[7,8][Ø,2,Y]Z
Non-OR ØBPTX[Ø,2,M]Z

Ø Medical and Surgical
B Respiratory System
Q Repair Definition: Restoring, to the extent possible, a body part to its normal anatomic structure and function
Explanation: Used only when the method to accomplish the repair is not one of the other root operations

Body Part Character 4	Approach Character 5	Device Character 6	Qualifier Character 7
1 Trachea Cricoid cartilage **2** Carina **3** Main Bronchus, Right Bronchus intermedius Intermediate bronchus **4** Upper Lobe Bronchus, Right **5** Middle Lobe Bronchus, Right **6** Lower Lobe Bronchus, Right **7** Main Bronchus, Left **8** Upper Lobe Bronchus, Left **9** Lingula Bronchus **B** Lower Lobe Bronchus, Left **C** Upper Lung Lobe, Right **D** Middle Lung Lobe, Right **F** Lower Lung Lobe, Right **G** Upper Lung Lobe, Left **H** Lung Lingula **J** Lower Lung Lobe, Left **K** Lung, Right **L** Lung, Left **M** Lungs, Bilateral	**Ø** Open **3** Percutaneous **4** Percutaneous Endoscopic **7** Via Natural or Artificial Opening **8** Via Natural or Artificial Opening Endoscopic	**Z** No Device	**Z** No Qualifier
N Pleura, Right **P** Pleura, Left **T** Diaphragm	**Ø** Open **3** Percutaneous **4** Percutaneous Endoscopic	**Z** No Device	**Z** No Qualifier

Ø Medical and Surgical
B Respiratory System
R Replacement Definition: Putting in or on biological or synthetic material that physically takes the place and/or function of all or a portion of a body part
Explanation: The body part may have been taken out or replaced, or may be taken out, physically eradicated, or rendered nonfunctional during the REPLACEMENT procedure. A REMOVAL procedure is coded for taking out the device used in a previous replacement procedure.

Body Part Character 4	Approach Character 5	Device Character 6	Qualifier Character 7
1 Trachea Cricoid cartilage **2** Carina **3** Main Bronchus, Right Bronchus intermedius Intermediate bronchus **4** Upper Lobe Bronchus, Right **5** Middle Lobe Bronchus, Right **6** Lower Lobe Bronchus, Right **7** Main Bronchus, Left **8** Upper Lobe Bronchus, Left **9** Lingula Bronchus **B** Lower Lobe Bronchus, Left **T** Diaphragm	**Ø** Open **4** Percutaneous Endoscopic	**7** Autologous Tissue Substitute **J** Synthetic Substitute **K** Nonautologous Tissue Substitute	**Z** No Qualifier

Ø Medical and Surgical
B Respiratory System
S Reposition

Definition: Moving to its normal location, or other suitable location, all or a portion of a body part

Explanation: The body part is moved to a new location from an abnormal location, or from a normal location where it is not functioning correctly. The body part may or may not be cut out or off to be moved to the new location.

Body Part Character 4	Approach Character 5	Device Character 6	Qualifier Character 7
1 Trachea Cricoid cartilage **2 Carina** **3 Main Bronchus, Right** Bronchus intermedius Intermediate bronchus **4 Upper Lobe Bronchus, Right** **5 Middle Lobe Bronchus, Right** **6 Lower Lobe Bronchus, Right** **7 Main Bronchus, Left** **8 Upper Lobe Bronchus, Left** **9 Lingula Bronchus** **B Lower Lobe Bronchus, Left** **C Upper Lung Lobe, Right** **D Middle Lung Lobe, Right** **F Lower Lung Lobe, Right** **G Upper Lung Lobe, Left** **H Lung Lingula** **J Lower Lung Lobe, Left** **K Lung, Right** **L Lung, Left** **T Diaphragm**	**Ø Open**	**Z No Device**	**Z No Qualifier**

Ø Medical and Surgical
B Respiratory System
T Resection

Definition: Cutting out or off, without replacement, all of a body part

Explanation: None

Body Part Character 4	Approach Character 5	Device Character 6	Qualifier Character 7
1 Trachea Cricoid cartilage **2 Carina** **3 Main Bronchus, Right** Bronchus intermedius Intermediate bronchus **4 Upper Lobe Bronchus, Right** **5 Middle Lobe Bronchus, Right** **6 Lower Lobe Bronchus, Right** **7 Main Bronchus, Left** **8 Upper Lobe Bronchus, Left** **9 Lingula Bronchus** **B Lower Lobe Bronchus, Left** **C Upper Lung Lobe, Right** **D Middle Lung Lobe, Right** **F Lower Lung Lobe, Right** **G Upper Lung Lobe, Left** **H Lung Lingula** **J Lower Lung Lobe, Left** **K Lung, Right** **L Lung, Left** **M Lungs, Bilateral** **T Diaphragm**	**Ø Open** **4 Percutaneous Endoscopic**	**Z No Device**	**Z No Qualifier**

Ø Medical and Surgical
B Respiratory System
U Supplement

Definition: Putting in or on biological or synthetic material that physically reinforces and/or augments the function of a portion of a body part

Explanation: The biological material is non-living, or is living and from the same individual. The body part may have been previously replaced, and the SUPPLEMENT procedure is performed to physically reinforce and/or augment the function of the replaced body part.

Body Part Character 4	Approach Character 5	Device Character 6	Qualifier Character 7
1 Trachea Cricoid cartilage **2 Carina** **3 Main Bronchus, Right** Bronchus intermedius Intermediate bronchus **4 Upper Lobe Bronchus, Right** **5 Middle Lobe Bronchus, Right** **6 Lower Lobe Bronchus, Right** **7 Main Bronchus, Left** **8 Upper Lobe Bronchus, Left** **9 Lingula Bronchus** **B Lower Lobe Bronchus, Left**	**Ø Open** **4 Percutaneous Endoscopic** **8 Via Natural or Artificial Opening Endoscopic**	**7 Autologous Tissue Substitute** **J Synthetic Substitute** **K Nonautologous Tissue Substitute**	**Z No Qualifier**
T Diaphragm	**Ø Open** **4 Percutaneous Endoscopic**	**7 Autologous Tissue Substitute** **J Synthetic Substitute** **K Nonautologous Tissue Substitute**	**Z No Qualifier**

Ø Medical and Surgical
B Respiratory System
V Restriction

Definition: Partially closing an orifice or the lumen of a tubular body part

Explanation: The orifice can be a natural orifice or an artificially created orifice

Body Part Character 4	Approach Character 5	Device Character 6	Qualifier Character 7
1 Trachea Cricoid cartilage **2 Carina** **3 Main Bronchus, Right** Bronchus intermedius Intermediate bronchus **4 Upper Lobe Bronchus, Right** **5 Middle Lobe Bronchus, Right** **6 Lower Lobe Bronchus, Right** **7 Main Bronchus, Left** **8 Upper Lobe Bronchus, Left** **9 Lingula Bronchus** **B Lower Lobe Bronchus, Left**	**Ø Open** **3 Percutaneous** **4 Percutaneous Endoscopic**	**C Extraluminal Device** **D Intraluminal Device** **Z No Device**	**Z No Qualifier**
1 Trachea Cricoid cartilage **2 Carina** **3 Main Bronchus, Right** Bronchus intermedius Intermediate bronchus **4 Upper Lobe Bronchus, Right** **5 Middle Lobe Bronchus, Right** **6 Lower Lobe Bronchus, Right** **7 Main Bronchus, Left** **8 Upper Lobe Bronchus, Left** **9 Lingula Bronchus** **B Lower Lobe Bronchus, Left**	**7 Via Natural or Artificial Opening** **8 Via Natural or Artificial Opening Endoscopic**	**D Intraluminal Device** **Z No Device**	**Z No Qualifier**

Ø Medical and Surgical
B Respiratory System
W Revision

Definition: Correcting, to the extent possible, a portion of a malfunctioning device or the position of a displaced device

Explanation: Revision can include correcting a malfunctioning or displaced device by taking out or putting in components of the device such as a screw or pin

Body Part Character 4	Approach Character 5	Device Character 6	Qualifier Character 7
Ø Tracheobronchial Tree	Ø Open 3 Percutaneous 4 Percutaneous Endoscopic 7 Via Natural or Artificial Opening 8 Via Natural or Artificial Opening Endoscopic	Ø Drainage Device 2 Monitoring Device 3 Infusion Device 7 Autologous Tissue Substitute C Extraluminal Device D Intraluminal Device J Synthetic Substitute K Nonautologous Tissue Substitute Y Other Device	Z No Qualifier
Ø Tracheobronchial Tree	X External	Ø Drainage Device 2 Monitoring Device 3 Infusion Device 7 Autologous Tissue Substitute C Extraluminal Device D Intraluminal Device J Synthetic Substitute K Nonautologous Tissue Substitute	Z No Qualifier
1 Trachea Cricoid cartilage	Ø Open 3 Percutaneous 4 Percutaneous Endoscopic 7 Via Natural or Artificial Opening 8 Via Natural or Artificial Opening Endoscopic X External	Ø Drainage Device 2 Monitoring Device 7 Autologous Tissue Substitute C Extraluminal Device D Intraluminal Device F Tracheostomy Device J Synthetic Substitute K Nonautologous Tissue Substitute	Z No Qualifier
K Lung, Right L Lung, Left	Ø Open 3 Percutaneous 4 Percutaneous Endoscopic 7 Via Natural or Artificial Opening 8 Via Natural or Artificial Opening Endoscopic	Ø Drainage Device 2 Monitoring Device 3 Infusion Device Y Other Device	Z No Qualifier
K Lung, Right L Lung, Left	X External	Ø Drainage Device 2 Monitoring Device 3 Infusion Device	Z No Qualifier
Q Pleura	Ø Open 3 Percutaneous 4 Percutaneous Endoscopic 7 Via Natural or Artificial Opening 8 Via Natural or Artificial Opening Endoscopic	Ø Drainage Device 2 Monitoring Device Y Other Device	Z No Qualifier
Q Pleura	X External	Ø Drainage Device 2 Monitoring Device	Z No Qualifier
T Diaphragm	Ø Open 3 Percutaneous 4 Percutaneous Endoscopic 7 Via Natural or Artificial Opening 8 Via Natural or Artificial Opening Endoscopic	Ø Drainage Device 2 Monitoring Device 7 Autologous Tissue Substitute J Synthetic Substitute K Nonautologous Tissue Substitute M Diaphragmatic Pacemaker Lead Y Other Device	Z No Qualifier
T Diaphragm	X External	Ø Drainage Device 2 Monitoring Device 7 Autologous Tissue Substitute J Synthetic Substitute K Nonautologous Tissue Substitute M Diaphragmatic Pacemaker Lead	Z No Qualifier

Non-OR ØBWØ[3,4]YZ
Non-OR ØBWØ[7,8][2,3,D,Y]Z
Non-OR ØBWØX[Ø,2,3,7,C,D,J,K]Z
Non-OR ØBW1X[Ø,2,7,C,D,F,J,K]Z
Non-OR ØBW[K,L]3YZ
Non-OR ØBW[K,L]7[Ø,2,3,Y]Z
Non-OR ØBW[K,L]8[Ø,2,3]Z
Non-OR ØBW[K,L]X[Ø,2,3]Z
Non-OR ØBWQ[Ø,3,4,7,8][Ø,2]Z
Non-OR ØBWQ[Ø,3,7]YZ
Non-OR ØBWQX[Ø,2]Z
Non-OR ØBWT[3,7,8]YZ
Non-OR ØBWTX[Ø,2,7,J,K,M]Z

Ø Medical and Surgical
B Respiratory System
Y Transplantation Definition: Putting in or on all or a portion of a living body part taken from another individual or animal to physically take the place and/or function of all or a portion of a similar body part

Explanation: The native body part may or may not be taken out, and the transplanted body part may take over all or a portion of its function

Body Part Character 4	Approach Character 5	Device Character 6	Qualifier Character 7
C Upper Lung Lobe, Right LC D Middle Lung Lobe, Right LC F Lower Lung Lobe, Right LC G Upper Lung Lobe, Left LC H Lung Lingula LC J Lower Lung Lobe, Left LC K Lung, Right LC L Lung, Left LC M Lungs, Bilateral LC	Ø Open	Z No Device	Ø Allogeneic 1 Syngeneic 2 Zooplastic

LC ØBY[C,D,F,G,H,J,K,L,M]ØZ[Ø,1,2]

Mouth and Throat ØCØ–ØCX

Character Meanings

This Character Meaning table is provided as a guide to assist the user in the identification of character members that may be found in this section of code tables. It **SHOULD NOT** be used to build a PCS code.

Operation–Character 3		Body Part–Character 4		Approach–Character 5		Device–Character 6		Qualifier–Character 7	
Ø	Alteration	Ø	Upper Lip	Ø	Open	Ø	Drainage Device	Ø	Single
2	Change	1	Lower Lip	3	Percutaneous	1	Radioactive Element	1	Multiple
5	Destruction	2	Hard Palate	4	Percutaneous Endoscopic	5	External Fixation Device	2	All
7	Dilation	3	Soft Palate	7	Via Natural or Artificial Opening	7	Autologous Tissue Substitute	X	Diagnostic
9	Drainage	4	Buccal Mucosa	8	Via Natural or Artificial Opening Endoscopic	B	Intraluminal Device, Airway	Z	No Qualifier
B	Excision	5	Upper Gingiva	X	External	C	Extraluminal Device		
C	Extirpation	6	Lower Gingiva			D	Intraluminal Device		
D	Extraction	7	Tongue			J	Synthetic Substitute		
F	Fragmentation	8	Parotid Gland, Right			K	Nonautologous Tissue Substitute		
H	Insertion	9	Parotid Gland, Left			Y	Other Device		
J	Inspection	A	Salivary Gland			Z	No Device		
L	Occlusion	B	Parotid Duct, Right						
M	Reattachment	C	Parotid Duct, Left						
N	Release	D	Sublingual Gland, Right						
P	Removal	F	Sublingual Gland, Left						
Q	Repair	G	Submaxillary Gland, Right						
R	Replacement	H	Submaxillary Gland, Left						
S	Reposition	J	Minor Salivary Gland						
T	Resection	M	Pharynx						
U	Supplement	N	Uvula						
V	Restriction	P	Tonsils						
W	Revision	Q	Adenoids						
X	Transfer	R	Epiglottis						
		S	Larynx						
		T	Vocal Cord, Right						
		V	Vocal Cord, Left						
		W	Upper Tooth						
		X	Lower Tooth						
		Y	Mouth and Throat						

AHA Coding Clinic for table ØC9
2017, 2Q, 16 Incision and drainage of floor of mouth

AHA Coding Clinic for table ØCB
2017, 2Q, 16 Excision of floor of mouth
2016, 3Q, 28 Lingual tonsillectomy, tongue base excision and epiglottopexy
2016, 2Q, 19 Biopsy of the base of tongue
2014, 3Q, 21 Superficial parotidectomy

AHA Coding Clinic for table ØCC
2016, 2Q, 20 Sialendoscopy with stone removal

AHA Coding Clinic for table ØCH
2020, 4Q, 43-44 Insertion of radioactive element

AHA Coding Clinic for table ØCQ
2017, 1Q, 20 Preparatory nasal adhesion repair before definitive cleft palate repair

AHA Coding Clinic for table ØCR
2014, 3Q, 25 Excision of soft palate with placement of surgical obturator
2014, 2Q, 5 Oasis acellular matrix graft
2014, 2Q, 6 Composite grafting (synthetic versus nonautologous tissue substitute)

AHA Coding Clinic for table ØCS
2022, 2Q, 24 Palatoplasty with intravelar veloplasty
2016, 3Q, 28 Lingual tonsillectomy, tongue base excision and epiglottopexy

AHA Coding Clinic for table ØCT
2016, 2Q, 12 Resection of malignant neoplasm of infratemporal fossa
2014, 3Q, 21 Superficial parotidectomy
2014, 3Q, 23 Le Fort I osteotomy

Salivary Glands

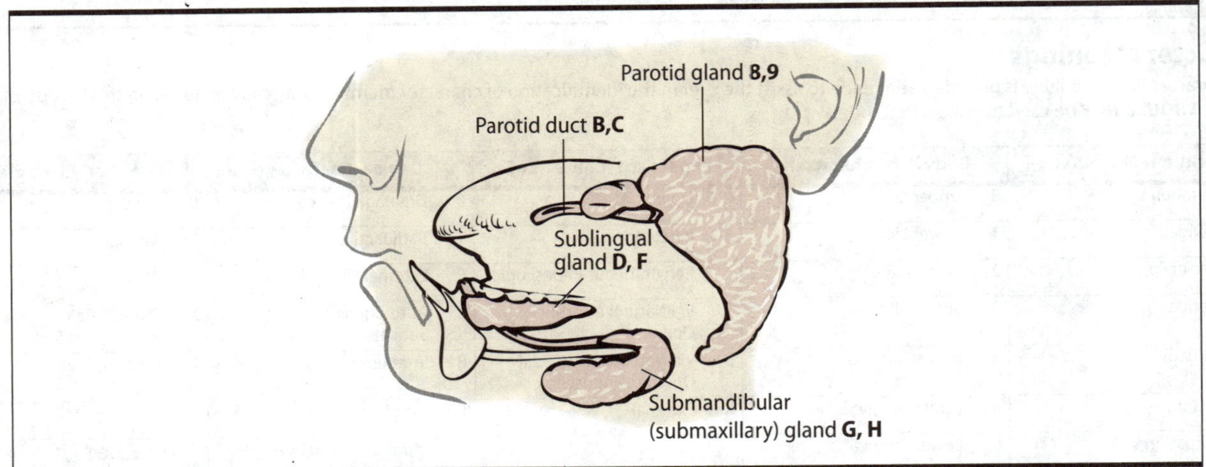

Oral Anatomy

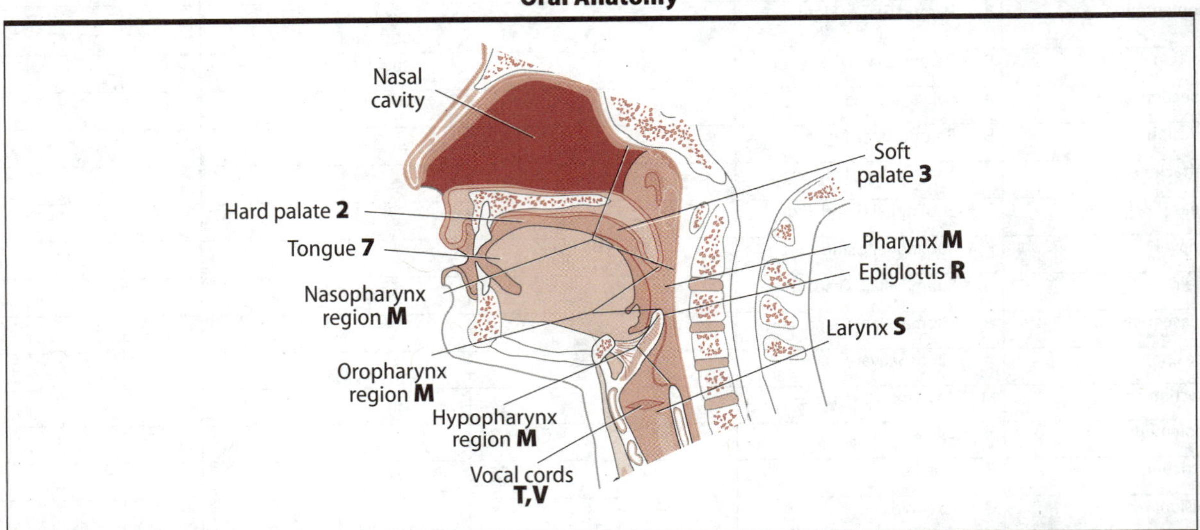

Mouth Frontal View (Upper)

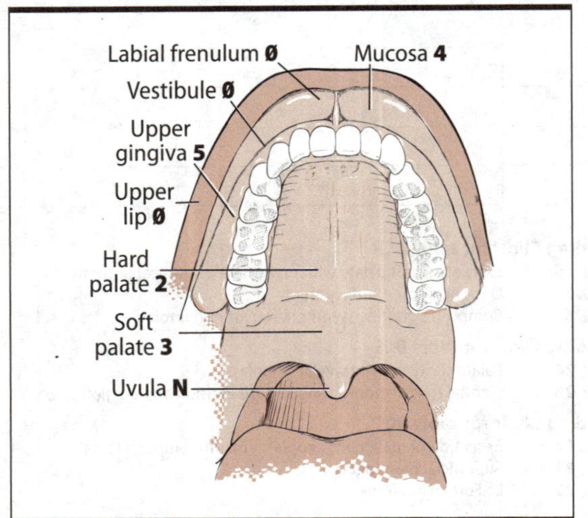

Mouth Frontal View (Lower)

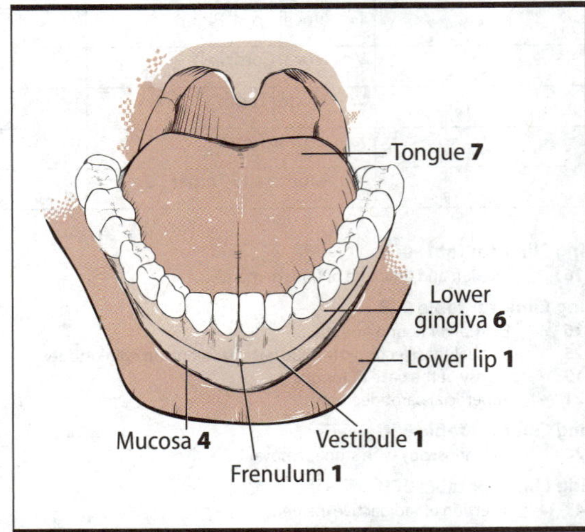

Ø Medical and Surgical
C Mouth and Throat
Ø Alteration Definition: Modifying the anatomic structure of a body part without affecting the function of the body part

Explanation: Principal purpose is to improve appearance

Body Part Character 4	Approach Character 5	Device Character 6	Qualifier Character 7
Ø Upper Lip Frenulum labii superioris Labial gland Vermilion border 1 Lower Lip Frenulum labii inferioris Labial gland Vermilion border	X External	7 Autologous Tissue Substitute J Synthetic Substitute K Nonautologous Tissue Substitute Z No Device	Z No Qualifier

Ø Medical and Surgical
C Mouth and Throat
2 Change Definition: Taking out or off a device from a body part and putting back an identical or similar device in or on the same body part without cutting or puncturing the skin or a mucous membrane

Explanation: All CHANGE procedures are coded using the approach EXTERNAL

Body Part Character 4	Approach Character 5	Device Character 6	Qualifier Character 7
A Salivary Gland S Larynx Aryepiglottic fold Arytenoid cartilage Corniculate cartilage Cuneiform cartilage False vocal cord Glottis Rima glottidis Thyroid cartilage Ventricular fold Y Mouth and Throat	X External	Ø Drainage Device Y Other Device	Z No Qualifier

Non-OR All body part, approach, device, and qualifier values

Ø Medical and Surgical
C Mouth and Throat
5 Destruction Definition: Physical eradication of all or a portion of a body part by the direct use of energy, force, or a destructive agent

Explanation: None of the body part is physically taken out

Body Part Character 4		Approach Character 5	Device Character 6	Qualifier Character 7
Ø Upper Lip Frenulum labii superioris Labial gland Vermilion border **1 Lower Lip** Frenulum labii inferioris Labial gland Vermilion border **2 Hard Palate** **3 Soft Palate** **4 Buccal Mucosa** Buccal gland Molar gland Palatine gland	**5 Upper Gingiva** **6 Lower Gingiva** **7 Tongue** Frenulum linguae **N Uvula** Palatine uvula **P Tonsils** Palatine tonsil **Q Adenoids** Pharyngeal tonsil	**Ø Open** **3 Percutaneous** **X External**	**Z No Device**	**Z No Qualifier**
8 Parotid Gland, Right **9 Parotid Gland, Left** **B Parotid Duct, Right** Stensen's duct **C Parotid Duct, Left** *See B Parotid Duct, Right* **D Sublingual Gland, Right**	**F Sublingual Gland, Left** **G Submaxillary Gland, Right** Submandibular gland **H Submaxillary Gland, Left** *See G Submaxillary Gland, Right* **J Minor Salivary Gland** Anterior lingual gland	**Ø Open** **3 Percutaneous**	**Z No Device**	**Z No Qualifier**
M Pharynx Base of tongue Hypopharynx Laryngopharynx Lingual tonsil Oropharynx Piriform recess (sinus) Tongue, base of **R Epiglottis** Glossoepiglottic fold	**S Larynx** Aryepiglottic fold Arytenoid cartilage Corniculate cartilage Cuneiform cartilage False vocal cord Glottis Rima glottidis Thyroid cartilage Ventricular fold **T Vocal Cord, Right** Vocal fold **V Vocal Cord, Left** *See T Vocal Cord, Right*	**Ø Open** **3 Percutaneous** **4 Percutaneous Endoscopic** **7 Via Natural or Artificial Opening** **8 Via Natural or Artificial Opening Endoscopic**	**Z No Device**	**Z No Qualifier**
W Upper Tooth **X Lower Tooth**		**Ø Open** **X External**	**Z No Device**	**Ø Single** **1 Multiple** **2 All**

Non-OR ØC5[5,6][Ø,3,X]ZZ
Non-OR ØC5[W,X][Ø,X]Z[Ø,1,2]

Ø Medical and Surgical
C Mouth and Throat
7 Dilation Definition: Expanding an orifice or the lumen of a tubular body part

Explanation: The orifice can be a natural orifice or an artificially created orifice. Accomplished by stretching a tubular body part using intraluminal pressure or by cutting part of the orifice or wall of the tubular body part.

Body Part Character 4	Approach Character 5	Device Character 6	Qualifier Character 7
B Parotid Duct, Right Stensen's duct **C Parotid Duct, Left** *See B Parotid Duct, Right*	**Ø Open** **3 Percutaneous** **7 Via Natural or Artificial Opening**	**D Intraluminal Device** **Z No Device**	**Z No Qualifier**
M Pharynx Base of tongue Hypopharynx Laryngopharynx Lingual tonsil Oropharynx Piriform recess (sinus) Tongue, base of	**7 Via Natural or Artificial Opening** **8 Via Natural or Artificial Opening Endoscopic**	**D Intraluminal Device** **Z No Device**	**Z No Qualifier**
S Larynx Aryepiglottic fold Arytenoid cartilage Corniculate cartilage Cuneiform cartilage False vocal cord Glottis Rima glottidis Thyroid cartilage Ventricular fold	**Ø Open** **3 Percutaneous** **4 Percutaneous Endoscopic** **7 Via Natural or Artificial Opening** **8 Via Natural or Artificial Opening Endoscopic**	**D Intraluminal Device** **Z No Device**	**Z No Qualifier**

Non-OR ØC7[B,C][Ø,3,7][D,Z]Z
Non-OR ØC7M[7,8][D,Z]Z

Ø Medical and Surgical
C Mouth and Throat
9 Drainage

Definition: Taking or letting out fluids and/or gases from a body part

Explanation: The qualifier DIAGNOSTIC is used to identify drainage procedures that are biopsies

Body Part Character 4	Approach Character 5	Device Character 6	Qualifier Character 7
Ø Upper Lip Frenulum labii superioris Labial gland Vermilion border **1 Lower Lip** Frenulum labii inferioris Labial gland Vermilion border **2 Hard Palate** **3 Soft Palate** **4 Buccal Mucosa** Buccal gland Molar gland Palatine gland **5 Upper Gingiva** **6 Lower Gingiva** **7 Tongue** Frenulum linguae **N Uvula** Palatine uvula **P Tonsils** Palatine tonsil **Q Adenoids** Pharyngeal tonsil	**Ø Open** **3 Percutaneous** **X External**	**Ø Drainage Device**	**Z No Qualifier**
Ø Upper Lip Frenulum labii superioris Labial gland Vermilion border **1 Lower Lip** Frenulum labii inferioris Labial gland Vermilion border **2 Hard Palate** **3 Soft Palate** **4 Buccal Mucosa** Buccal gland Molar gland Palatine gland **5 Upper Gingiva** **6 Lower Gingiva** **7 Tongue** Frenulum linguae **N Uvula** Palatine uvula **P Tonsils** Palatine tonsil **Q Adenoids** Pharyngeal tonsil	**Ø Open** **3 Percutaneous** **X External**	**Z No Device**	**X Diagnostic** **Z No Qualifier**
8 Parotid Gland, Right **9 Parotid Gland, Left** **B Parotid Duct, Right** Stensen's duct **C Parotid Duct, Left** *See B Parotid Duct, Right* **D Sublingual Gland, Right** **F Sublingual Gland, Left** **G Submaxillary Gland, Right** Submandibular gland **H Submaxillary Gland, Left** *See G Submaxillary Gland, Right* **J Minor Salivary Gland** Anterior lingual gland	**Ø Open** **3 Percutaneous**	**Ø Drainage Device**	**Z No Qualifier**
8 Parotid Gland, Right **9 Parotid Gland, Left** **B Parotid Duct, Right** Stensen's duct **C Parotid Duct, Left** *See B Parotid Duct, Right* **D Sublingual Gland, Right** **F Sublingual Gland, Left** **G Submaxillary Gland, Right** Submandibular gland **H Submaxillary Gland, Left** *See G Submaxillary Gland, Right* **J Minor Salivary Gland** Anterior lingual gland	**Ø Open** **3 Percutaneous**	**Z No Device**	**X Diagnostic** **Z No Qualifier**
M Pharynx Base of tongue Hypopharynx Laryngopharynx Lingual tonsil Oropharynx Piriform recess (sinus) Tongue, base of **R Epiglottis** Glossoepiglottic fold **S Larynx** Aryepiglottic fold Arytenoid cartilage Corniculate cartilage Cuneiform cartilage False vocal cord Glottis Rima glottidis Thyroid cartilage Ventricular fold **T Vocal Cord, Right** Vocal fold **V Vocal Cord, Left** *See T Vocal Cord, Right*	**Ø Open** **3 Percutaneous** **4 Percutaneous Endoscopic** **7 Via Natural or Artificial Opening** **8 Via Natural or Artificial Opening Endoscopic**	**Ø Drainage Device**	**Z No Qualifier**

Non-OR ØC9[Ø,1,2,3,4,7,N,P,Q]3ØZ
Non-OR ØC9[5,6][Ø,3,X]ØZ
Non-OR ØC9[Ø,1,4][Ø,3,X]ZX
Non-OR ØC9[Ø,1,2,3,4,7,N,P,Q]3ZZ
Non-OR ØC9[5,6][Ø,3,X]Z[X,Z]
Non-OR ØC97[3,X]ZX
Non-OR ØC9[8,9,B,C,D,F,G,H,J][Ø,3]ØZ
Non-OR ØC9[8,9,B,C,D,F,G,H,J]3ZX
Non-OR ØC9[8,9,G,H]3ZZ
Non-OR ØC9[B,C,D, F,J][Ø,3]ZZ
Non-OR ØC9[M,R,S,T,V]3ØZ

ØC9 Continued on next page

Mouth and Throat

ØC9 Continued

Ø Medical and Surgical
C Mouth and Throat
9 Drainage

Definition: Taking or letting out fluids and/or gases from a body part
Explanation: The qualifier DIAGNOSTIC is used to identify drainage procedures that are biopsies

Body Part Character 4	Approach Character 5	Device Character 6	Qualifier Character 7
M Pharynx Base of tongue, Hypopharynx, Laryngopharynx, Lingual tonsil, Oropharynx, Piriform recess (sinus), Tongue, base of **R Epiglottis** Glossoepiglottic fold **S Larynx** Aryepiglottic fold, Arytenoid cartilage, Corniculate cartilage, Cuneiform cartilage, False vocal cord, Glottis, Rima glottidis, Thyroid cartilage, Ventricular fold **T Vocal Cord, Right** Vocal fold **V Vocal Cord, Left** *See T Vocal Cord, Right*	**Ø Open** **3 Percutaneous** **4 Percutaneous Endoscopic** **7 Via Natural or Artificial Opening** **8 Via Natural or Artificial Opening Endoscopic**	**Z No Device**	**X Diagnostic** **Z No Qualifier**
W Upper Tooth **X Lower Tooth**	**Ø Open** **X External**	**Ø Drainage Device** **Z No Device**	**Ø Single** **1 Multiple** **2 All**

Non-OR ØC9M[Ø,3,4,7,8]ZX
Non-OR ØC9[M,R,S,T,V]3ZZ
Non-OR ØC9[R,S,T,V][3,4,7,8]ZX
Non-OR ØC9[W,X][Ø,X][Ø,Z][Ø,1,2]

Ø Medical and Surgical
C Mouth and Throat
B Excision

Definition: Cutting out or off, without replacement, a portion of a body part
Explanation: The qualifier DIAGNOSTIC is used to identify excision procedures that are biopsies

Body Part Character 4	Approach Character 5	Device Character 6	Qualifier Character 7
Ø Upper Lip Frenulum labii superioris, Labial gland, Vermilion border **1 Lower Lip** Frenulum labii inferioris, Labial gland, Vermilion border **2 Hard Palate** **3 Soft Palate** **4 Buccal Mucosa** Buccal gland, Molar gland, Palatine gland **5 Upper Gingiva** **6 Lower Gingiva** **7 Tongue** Frenulum linguae **N Uvula** Palatine uvula **P Tonsils** Palatine tonsil **Q Adenoids** Pharyngeal tonsil	**Ø Open** **3 Percutaneous** **X External**	**Z No Device**	**X Diagnostic** **Z No Qualifier**
8 Parotid Gland, Right **9 Parotid Gland, Left** **B Parotid Duct, Right** Stensen's duct **C Parotid Duct, Left** *See B Parotid Duct, Right* **D Sublingual Gland, Right** **F Sublingual Gland, Left** **G Submaxillary Gland, Right** Submandibular gland **H Submaxillary Gland, Left** *See G Submaxillary Gland, Right* **J Minor Salivary Gland** Anterior lingual gland	**Ø Open** **3 Percutaneous**	**Z No Device**	**X Diagnostic** **Z No Qualifier**
M Pharynx Base of tongue, Hypopharynx, Laryngopharynx, Lingual tonsil, Oropharynx, Piriform recess (sinus), Tongue, base of **R Epiglottis** Glossoepiglottic fold **S Larynx** Aryepiglottic fold, Arytenoid cartilage, Corniculate cartilage, Cuneiform cartilage, False vocal cord, Glottis, Rima glottidis, Thyroid cartilage, Ventricular fold **T Vocal Cord, Right** Vocal fold **V Vocal Cord, Left** *See T Vocal Cord, Right*	**Ø Open** **3 Percutaneous** **4 Percutaneous Endoscopic** **7 Via Natural or Artificial Opening** **8 Via Natural or Artificial Opening Endoscopic**	**Z No Device**	**X Diagnostic** **Z No Qualifier**
W Upper Tooth **X Lower Tooth**	**Ø Open** **X External**	**Z No Device**	**Ø Single** **1 Multiple** **2 All**

Non-OR ØCB[Ø,1,4][Ø,3,X]ZX
Non-OR ØCB[5,6][Ø,3,X]Z[X,Z]
Non-OR ØCB7[3,X]ZX
Non-OR ØCB[8,9,B,C,D,F,G,H,J]3ZX
Non-OR ØCBM[Ø,3,4,7,8]ZX
Non-OR ØCB[R,S,T,V][3,4,7,8]ZX
Non-OR ØCB[W,X][Ø,X]Z[Ø,1,2]

Ø Medical and Surgical
C Mouth and Throat
C Extirpation Definition: Taking or cutting out solid matter from a body part

Explanation: The solid matter may be an abnormal byproduct of a biological function or a foreign body; it may be imbedded in a body part or in the lumen of a tubular body part. The solid matter may or may not have been previously broken into pieces.

Body Part Character 4	Approach Character 5	Device Character 6	Qualifier Character 7
Ø Upper Lip Frenulum labii superioris, Labial gland, Vermilion border **1 Lower Lip** Frenulum labii inferioris, Labial gland, Vermilion border **2 Hard Palate** **3 Soft Palate** **4 Buccal Mucosa** Buccal gland, Molar gland, Palatine gland **5 Upper Gingiva** **6 Lower Gingiva** **7 Tongue** Frenulum linguae **N Uvula** Palatine uvula **P Tonsils** Palatine tonsil **Q Adenoids** Pharyngeal tonsil	**Ø** Open **3** Percutaneous **X** External	**Z** No Device	**Z** No Qualifier
8 Parotid Gland, Right **9 Parotid Gland, Left** **B Parotid Duct, Right** Stensen's duct **C Parotid Duct, Left** *See B Parotid Duct, Right* **D Sublingual Gland, Right** **F Sublingual Gland, Left** **G Submaxillary Gland, Right** Submandibular gland **H Submaxillary Gland, Left** *See G Submaxillary Gland, Right* **J Minor Salivary Gland** Anterior lingual gland	**Ø** Open **3** Percutaneous	**Z** No Device	**Z** No Qualifier
M Pharynx Base of tongue, Hypopharynx, Laryngopharynx, Lingual tonsil, Oropharynx, Piriform recess (sinus), Tongue, base of **R Epiglottis** Glossoepiglottic fold **S Larynx** Aryepiglottic fold, Arytenoid cartilage, Corniculate cartilage, Cuneiform cartilage, False vocal cord, Glottis, Rima glottidis, Thyroid cartilage, Ventricular fold **T Vocal Cord, Right** Vocal fold **V Vocal Cord, Left** *See T Vocal Cord, Right*	**Ø** Open **3** Percutaneous **4** Percutaneous Endoscopic **7** Via Natural or Artificial Opening **8** Via Natural or Artificial Opening Endoscopic	**Z** No Device	**Z** No Qualifier
W Upper Tooth **X Lower Tooth**	**Ø** Open **X** External	**Z** No Device	**Ø** Single **1** Multiple **2** All

Non-OR ØCC[Ø,1,2,3,4,7,N,P,Q]XZZ
Non-OR ØCC[5,6][Ø,3,X]ZZ
Non-OR ØCC[8,9,G,H]3ZZ
Non-OR ØCC[B,C,D, F,J][Ø,3]ZZ
Non-OR ØCC[M,S][7,8]ZZ
Non-OR ØCC[W,X][Ø,X]Z[Ø,1,2]

Ø Medical and Surgical
C Mouth and Throat
D Extraction Definition: Pulling or stripping out or off all or a portion of a body part by the use of force

Explanation: The qualifier DIAGNOSTIC is used to identify extraction procedures that are biopsies

Body Part Character 4	Approach Character 5	Device Character 6	Qualifier Character 7
T Vocal Cord, Right Vocal fold **V** Vocal Cord, Left *See T Vocal Cord, Right*	**Ø** Open **3** Percutaneous **4** Percutaneous Endoscopic **7** Via Natural or Artificial Opening **8** Via Natural or Artificial Opening Endoscopic	**Z** No Device	**Z** No Qualifier
W Upper Tooth **X Lower Tooth**	**X** External	**Z** No Device	**Ø** Single **1** Multiple **2** All

Non-OR ØCD[W,X]XZ[Ø,1,2]

Ø Medical and Surgical
C Mouth and Throat
F Fragmentation Definition: Breaking solid matter in a body part into pieces

Explanation: Physical force (e.g., manual, ultrasonic) applied directly or indirectly is used to break the solid matter into pieces. The solid matter may be an abnormal byproduct of a biological function or a foreign body. The pieces of solid matter are not taken out.

Body Part Character 4	Approach Character 5	Device Character 6	Qualifier Character 7
B Parotid Duct, Right NC Stensen's duct **C** Parotid Duct, Left NC *See B Parotid Duct, Right*	**Ø** Open **3** Percutaneous **7** Via Natural or Artificial Opening **X** External	**Z** No Device	**Z** No Qualifier

Non-OR All body part, approach, device, and qualifier values
NC ØCF[B,C]XZZ

Ø Medical and Surgical
C Mouth and Throat
H Insertion Definition: Putting in a nonbiological appliance that monitors, assists, performs, or prevents a physiological function but does not physically take the place of a body part

Explanation: None

Body Part Character 4	Approach Character 5	Device Character 6	Qualifier Character 7
7 Tongue Frenulum linguae	**Ø** Open **3** Percutaneous **X** External	**1** Radioactive Element	**Z** No Qualifier
A Salivary Gland **S** Larynx Aryepiglottic fold Arytenoid cartilage Corniculate cartilage Cuneiform cartilage False vocal cord Glottis Rima glottidis Thyroid cartilage Ventricular fold	**Ø** Open **3** Percutaneous **7** Via Natural or Artificial Opening **8** Via Natural or Artificial Opening Endoscopic	**1** Radioactive Element **Y** Other Device	**Z** No Qualifier
Y Mouth and Throat	**Ø** Open **3** Percutaneous	**1** Radioactive Element **Y** Other Device	**Z** No Qualifier
Y Mouth and Throat	**7** Via Natural or Artificial Opening **8** Via Natural or Artificial Opening Endoscopic	**1** Radioactive Element **B** Intraluminal Device, Airway **Y** Other Device	**Z** No Qualifier

Non-OR ØCH[A,S]Ø1Z
Non-OR ØCHSØYZ
Non-OR ØCH[A,S][3,7,8][1,Y]Z
Non-OR ØCHY[Ø,3][1,Y]Z
Non-OR ØCHY[7,8][1,B,Y]Z

Ø Medical and Surgical
C Mouth and Throat
J Inspection Definition: Visually and/or manually exploring a body part

Explanation: Visual exploration may be performed with or without optical instrumentation. Manual exploration may be performed directly or through intervening body layers.

Body Part Character 4	Approach Character 5	Device Character 6	Qualifier Character 7
A Salivary Gland	**Ø** Open **3** Percutaneous **X** External	**Z** No Device	**Z** No Qualifier
S Larynx Aryepiglottic fold Arytenoid cartilage Corniculate cartilage Cuneiform cartilage False vocal cord Glottis Rima glottidis Thyroid cartilage Ventricular fold **Y** Mouth and Throat	**Ø** Open **3** Percutaneous **4** Percutaneous Endoscopic **7** Via Natural or Artificial Opening **8** Via Natural or Artificial Opening Endoscopic **X** External	**Z** No Device	**Z** No Qualifier

Non-OR All body part, approach, device, and qualifier values

Ø Medical and Surgical
C Mouth and Throat
L Occlusion

Definition: Completely closing an orifice or the lumen of a tubular body part
Explanation: The orifice can be a natural orifice or an artificially created orifice

Body Part Character 4	Approach Character 5	Device Character 6	Qualifier Character 7
B Parotid Duct, Right Stensen's duct **C** Parotid Duct, Left *See B Parotid Duct, Right*	**Ø** Open **3** Percutaneous **4** Percutaneous Endoscopic	**C** Extraluminal Device **D** Intraluminal Device **Z** No Device	**Z** No Qualifier
B Parotid Duct, Right Stensen's duct **C** Parotid Duct, Left *See B Parotid Duct, Right*	**7** Via Natural or Artificial Opening **8** Via Natural or Artificial Opening Endoscopic	**D** Intraluminal Device **Z** No Device	**Z** No Qualifier

Ø Medical and Surgical
C Mouth and Throat
M Reattachment

Definition: Putting back in or on all or a portion of a separated body part to its normal location or other suitable location
Explanation: Vascular circulation and nervous pathways may or may not be reestablished

Body Part Character 4	Approach Character 5	Device Character 6	Qualifier Character 7
Ø Upper Lip Frenulum labii superioris Labial gland Vermilion border **1** Lower Lip Frenulum labii inferioris Labial gland Vermilion border **3** Soft Palate **7** Tongue Frenulum linguae **N** Uvula Palatine uvula	**Ø** Open	**Z** No Device	**Z** No Qualifier
W Upper Tooth **X** Lower Tooth	**Ø** Open **X** External	**Z** No Device	**Ø** Single **1** Multiple **2** All

Non-OR ØCM[W,X][Ø,X]Z[Ø,1,2]

Ø Medical and Surgical
C Mouth and Throat
N Release Definition: Freeing a body part from an abnormal physical constraint by cutting or by the use of force
Explanation: Some of the restraining tissue may be taken out but none of the body part is taken out

Body Part Character 4	Approach Character 5	Device Character 6	Qualifier Character 7
Ø Upper Lip Frenulum labii superioris, Labial gland, Vermilion border **1 Lower Lip** Frenulum labii inferioris, Labial gland, Vermilion border **2 Hard Palate** **3 Soft Palate** **4 Buccal Mucosa** Buccal gland, Molar gland, Palatine gland **5 Upper Gingiva** **6 Lower Gingiva** **7 Tongue** Frenulum linguae **N Uvula** Palatine uvula **P Tonsils** Palatine tonsil **Q Adenoids** Pharyngeal tonsil	**Ø Open** **3 Percutaneous** **X External**	**Z No Device**	**Z No Qualifier**
8 Parotid Gland, Right **9 Parotid Gland, Left** **B Parotid Duct, Right** Stensen's duct **C Parotid Duct, Left** *See B Parotid Duct, Right* **D Sublingual Gland, Right** **F Sublingual Gland, Left** **G Submaxillary Gland, Right** Submandibular gland **H Submaxillary Gland, Left** *See G Submaxillary Gland, Right* **J Minor Salivary Gland** Anterior lingual gland	**Ø Open** **3 Percutaneous**	**Z No Device**	**Z No Qualifier**
M Pharynx Base of tongue, Hypopharynx, Laryngopharynx, Lingual tonsil, Oropharynx, Piriform recess (sinus), Tongue, base of **R Epiglottis** Glossoepiglottic fold **S Larynx** Aryepiglottic fold, Arytenoid cartilage, Corniculate cartilage, Cuneiform cartilage, False vocal cord, Glottis, Rima glottidis, Thyroid cartilage, Ventricular fold **T Vocal Cord, Right** Vocal fold **V Vocal Cord, Left** *See T Vocal Cord, Right*	**Ø Open** **3 Percutaneous** **4 Percutaneous Endoscopic** **7 Via Natural or Artificial Opening** **8 Via Natural or Artificial Opening Endoscopic**	**Z No Device**	**Z No Qualifier**
W Upper Tooth **X Lower Tooth**	**Ø Open** **X External**	**Z No Device**	**Ø Single** **1 Multiple** **2 All**

Non-OR ØCN[Ø,1,5,6,7][Ø,3,X]ZZ
Non-OR ØCN[W,X][Ø,X]Z[Ø,1,2]

Ø Medical and Surgical
C Mouth and Throat
P Removal Definition: Taking out or off a device from a body part

Explanation: If a device is taken out and a similar device put in without cutting or puncturing the skin or mucous membrane, the procedure is coded to the root operation CHANGE. Otherwise, the procedure for taking out a device is coded to the root operation REMOVAL.

Body Part Character 4	Approach Character 5	Device Character 6	Qualifier Character 7
A Salivary Gland	**Ø** Open **3** Percutaneous	**Ø** Drainage Device **C** Extraluminal Device **Y** Other Device	**Z** No Qualifier
A Salivary Gland	**7** Via Natural or Artificial Opening **8** Via Natural or Artificial Opening Endoscopic	**Y** Other Device	**Z** No Qualifier
S Larynx Aryepiglottic fold Arytenoid cartilage Corniculate cartilage Cuneiform cartilage False vocal cord Glottis Rima glottidis Thyroid cartilage Ventricular fold	**Ø** Open **3** Percutaneous **7** Via Natural or Artificial Opening **8** Via Natural or Artificial Opening Endoscopic	**Ø** Drainage Device **7** Autologous Tissue Substitute **D** Intraluminal Device **J** Synthetic Substitute **K** Nonautologous Tissue Substitute **Y** Other Device	**Z** No Qualifier
S Larynx Aryepiglottic fold Arytenoid cartilage Corniculate cartilage Cuneiform cartilage False vocal cord Glottis Rima glottidis Thyroid cartilage Ventricular fold	**X** External	**Ø** Drainage Device **7** Autologous Tissue Substitute **D** Intraluminal Device **J** Synthetic Substitute **K** Nonautologous Tissue Substitute	**Z** No Qualifier
Y Mouth and Throat	**Ø** Open **3** Percutaneous **7** Via Natural or Artificial Opening **8** Via Natural or Artificial Opening Endoscopic	**Ø** Drainage Device **1** Radioactive Element **7** Autologous Tissue Substitute **D** Intraluminal Device **J** Synthetic Substitute **K** Nonautologous Tissue Substitute **Y** Other Device	**Z** No Qualifier
Y Mouth and Throat	**X** External	**Ø** Drainage Device **1** Radioactive Element **7** Autologous Tissue Substitute **D** Intraluminal Device **J** Synthetic Substitute **K** Nonautologous Tissue Substitute	**Z** No Qualifier

Non-OR ØCPA[Ø,3][Ø,C,Y]Z
Non-OR ØCPA[7,8]YZ
Non-OR ØCPS3YZ
Non-OR ØCPS[7,8][Ø,D,Y]Z
Non-OR ØCPSX[Ø,7,D,J,K]Z
Non-OR ØCPY3YZ
Non-OR ØCPY[7,8][Ø,D,Y]Z
Non-OR ØCPYX[Ø,1,7,D,J,K]Z

Ø Medical and Surgical
C Mouth and Throat
Q Repair Definition: Restoring, to the extent possible, a body part to its normal anatomic structure and function
Explanation: Used only when the method to accomplish the repair is not one of the other root operations

Body Part Character 4	Approach Character 5	Device Character 6	Qualifier Character 7
Ø Upper Lip Frenulum labii superioris Labial gland Vermilion border **1 Lower Lip** Frenulum labii inferioris Labial gland Vermilion border **2 Hard Palate** **3 Soft Palate** **4 Buccal Mucosa** Buccal gland Molar gland Palatine gland **5 Upper Gingiva** **6 Lower Gingiva** **7 Tongue** Frenulum linguae **N Uvula** Palatine uvula **P Tonsils** Palatine tonsil **Q Adenoids** Pharyngeal tonsil	**Ø Open** **3 Percutaneous** **X External**	**Z No Device**	**Z No Qualifier**
8 Parotid Gland, Right **9 Parotid Gland, Left** **B Parotid Duct, Right** Stensen's duct **C Parotid Duct, Left** *See B Parotid Duct, Right* **D Sublingual Gland, Right** **F Sublingual Gland, Left** **G Submaxillary Gland, Right** Submandibular gland **H Submaxillary Gland, Left** *See G Submaxillary Gland, Right* **J Minor Salivary Gland** Anterior lingual gland	**Ø Open** **3 Percutaneous**	**Z No Device**	**Z No Qualifier**
M Pharynx Base of tongue Hypopharynx Laryngopharynx Lingual tonsil Oropharynx Piriform recess (sinus) Tongue, base of **R Epiglottis** Glossoepiglottic fold **S Larynx** Aryepiglottic fold Arytenoid cartilage Corniculate cartilage Cuneiform cartilage False vocal cord Glottis Rima glottidis Thyroid cartilage Ventricular fold **T Vocal Cord, Right** Vocal fold **V Vocal Cord, Left** *See T Vocal Cord, Right*	**Ø Open** **3 Percutaneous** **4 Percutaneous Endoscopic** **7 Via Natural or Artificial Opening** **8 Via Natural or Artificial Opening Endoscopic**	**Z No Device**	**Z No Qualifier**
W Upper Tooth **X Lower Tooth**	**Ø Open** **X External**	**Z No Device**	**Ø Single** **1 Multiple** **2 All**

Non-OR ØCQ[Ø,1,4,7]XZZ
Non-OR ØCQ[5,6][Ø,3,X]ZZ
Non-OR ØCQ[W,X][Ø,X]Z[Ø,1,2]

Ø Medical and Surgical
C Mouth and Throat
R Replacement

Definition: Putting in or on biological or synthetic material that physically takes the place and/or function of all or a portion of a body part

Explanation: The body part may have been taken out or replaced, or may be taken out, physically eradicated, or rendered nonfunctional during the REPLACEMENT procedure. A REMOVAL procedure is coded for taking out the device used in a previous replacement procedure.

Body Part Character 4	Approach Character 5	Device Character 6	Qualifier Character 7
Ø Upper Lip Frenulum labii superioris Labial gland Vermilion border **1 Lower Lip** Frenulum labii inferioris Labial gland Vermilion border **2 Hard Palate** **3 Soft Palate** **4 Buccal Mucosa** Buccal gland Molar gland Palatine gland **5 Upper Gingiva** **6 Lower Gingiva** **7 Tongue** Frenulum linguae **N Uvula** Palatine uvula	**Ø Open** **3 Percutaneous** **X External**	**7 Autologous Tissue Substitute** **J Synthetic Substitute** **K Nonautologous Tissue Substitute**	**Z No Qualifier**
B Parotid Duct, Right Stensen's duct **C Parotid Duct, Left** *See B Parotid Duct, Right*	**Ø Open** **3 Percutaneous**	**7 Autologous Tissue Substitute** **J Synthetic Substitute** **K Nonautologous Tissue Substitute**	**Z No Qualifier**
M Pharynx Base of tongue Hypopharynx Laryngopharynx Lingual tonsil Oropharynx Piriform recess (sinus) Tongue, base of **R Epiglottis** Glossoepiglottic fold **S Larynx** Aryepiglottic fold Arytenoid cartilage Corniculate cartilage Cuneiform cartilage False vocal cord Glottis Rima glottidis Thyroid cartilage Ventricular fold **T Vocal Cord, Right** Vocal fold **V Vocal Cord, Left** *See T Vocal Cord, Right*	**Ø Open** **7 Via Natural or Artificial Opening** **8 Via Natural or Artificial Opening Endoscopic**	**7 Autologous Tissue Substitute** **J Synthetic Substitute** **K Nonautologous Tissue Substitute**	**Z No Qualifier**
W Upper Tooth **X Lower Tooth**	**Ø Open** **X External**	**7 Autologous Tissue Substitute** **J Synthetic Substitute** **K Nonautologous Tissue Substitute**	**Ø Single** **1 Multiple** **2 All**

Non-OR ØCR[W,X][Ø,X][7,J,K][Ø,1,2]

Ø Medical and Surgical
C Mouth and Throat
S Reposition Definition: Moving to its normal location, or other suitable location, all or a portion of a body part

Explanation: The body part is moved to a new location from an abnormal location, or from a normal location where it is not functioning correctly. The body part may or may not be cut out or off to be moved to the new location.

Body Part Character 4	Approach Character 5	Device Character 6	Qualifier Character 7
Ø Upper Lip Frenulum labii superioris Labial gland Vermilion border **1 Lower Lip** Frenulum labii inferioris Labial gland Vermilion border **2 Hard Palate** **3 Soft Palate** **7 Tongue** Frenulum linguae **N Uvula** Palatine uvula	**Ø Open** **X External**	**Z No Device**	**Z No Qualifier**
B Parotid Duct, Right Stensen's duct **C Parotid Duct, Left** *See B Parotid Duct, Right*	**Ø Open** **3 Percutaneous**	**Z No Device**	**Z No Qualifier**
R Epiglottis Glossoepiglottic fold **S Larynx** **T Vocal Cord, Right** Vocal fold **V Vocal Cord, Left** *See T Vocal Cord, Right*	**Ø Open** **7 Via Natural or Artificial Opening** **8 Via Natural or Artificial Opening Endoscopic**	**Z No Device**	**Z No Qualifier**
W Upper Tooth **X Lower Tooth**	**Ø Open** **X External**	**5 External Fixation Device** **Z No Device**	**Ø Single** **1 Multiple** **2 All**

Non-OR ØCS[W,X][Ø,X][5,Z][Ø,1,2]

Ø Medical and Surgical
C Mouth and Throat
T Resection Definition: Cutting out or off, without replacement, all of a body part

Explanation: None

Body Part Character 4	Approach Character 5	Device Character 6	Qualifier Character 7
Ø Upper Lip Frenulum labii superioris Labial gland Vermilion border **1 Lower Lip** Frenulum labii inferioris Labial gland Vermilion border **2 Hard Palate** **3 Soft Palate** **7 Tongue** Frenulum linguae **N Uvula** Palatine uvula **P Tonsils** Palatine tonsil **Q Adenoids** Pharyngeal tonsil	**Ø Open** **X External**	**Z No Device**	**Z No Qualifier**
8 Parotid Gland, Right **9 Parotid Gland, Left** **B Parotid Duct, Right** Stensen's duct **C Parotid Duct, Left** ***See*** *B Parotid Duct, Right* **D Sublingual Gland, Right** **F Sublingual Gland, Left** **G Submaxillary Gland, Right** Submandibular gland **H Submaxillary Gland, Left** ***See*** *G Submaxillary Gland, Right* **J Minor Salivary Gland** Anterior lingual gland	**Ø Open**	**Z No Device**	**Z No Qualifier**
M Pharynx Base of tongue Hypopharynx Laryngopharynx Lingual tonsil Oropharynx Piriform recess (sinus) Tongue, base of **R Epiglottis** Glossoepiglottic fold **S Larynx** Aryepiglottic fold Arytenoid cartilage Corniculate cartilage Cuneiform cartilage False vocal cord Glottis Rima glottidis Thyroid cartilage Ventricular fold **T Vocal Cord, Right** Vocal fold **V Vocal Cord, Left** ***See*** *T Vocal Cord, Right*	**Ø Open** **4 Percutaneous Endoscopic** **7 Via Natural or Artificial Opening** **8 Via Natural or Artificial Opening Endoscopic**	**Z No Device**	**Z No Qualifier**
W Upper Tooth **X Lower Tooth**	**Ø Open**	**Z No Device**	**Ø Single** **1 Multiple** **2 All**

Non-OR ØCT[W,X]ØZ[Ø,1,2]

Ø Medical and Surgical
C Mouth and Throat
U Supplement Definition: Putting in or on biological or synthetic material that physically reinforces and/or augments the function of a portion of a body part

Explanation: The biological material is non-living, or is living and from the same individual. The body part may have been previously replaced, and the SUPPLEMENT procedure is performed to physically reinforce and/or augment the function of the replaced body part.

Body Part Character 4	Approach Character 5	Device Character 6	Qualifier Character 7
Ø Upper Lip Frenulum labii superioris Labial gland Vermilion border **1 Lower Lip** Frenulum labii inferioris Labial gland Vermilion border **2 Hard Palate** **3 Soft Palate** **4 Buccal Mucosa** Buccal gland Molar gland Palatine gland **5 Upper Gingiva** **6 Lower Gingiva** **7 Tongue** Frenulum linguae **N Uvula** Palatine uvula	**Ø Open** **3 Percutaneous** **X External**	**7 Autologous Tissue Substitute** **J Synthetic Substitute** **K Nonautologous Tissue Substitute**	**Z No Qualifier**
M Pharynx Base of tongue Hypopharynx Laryngopharynx Lingual tonsil Oropharynx Piriform recess (sinus) Tongue, base of **R Epiglottis** Glossoepiglottic fold **S Larynx** Aryepiglottic fold Arytenoid cartilage Corniculate cartilage Cuneiform cartilage False vocal cord Glottis Rima glottidis Thyroid cartilage Ventricular fold **T Vocal Cord, Right** Vocal fold **V Vocal Cord, Left** *See T Vocal Cord, Right*	**Ø Open** **7 Via Natural or Artificial Opening** **8 Via Natural or Artificial Opening Endoscopic**	**7 Autologous Tissue Substitute** **J Synthetic Substitute** **K Nonautologous Tissue Substitute**	**Z No Qualifier**

Non-OR ØCU2[Ø,3]JZ

Ø Medical and Surgical
C Mouth and Throat
V Restriction Definition: Partially closing an orifice or the lumen of a tubular body part

Explanation: The orifice can be a natural orifice or an artificially created orifice

Body Part Character 4	Approach Character 5	Device Character 6	Qualifier Character 7
B Parotid Duct, Right Stensen's duct **C Parotid Duct, Left** *See B Parotid Duct, Right*	**Ø Open** **3 Percutaneous**	**C Extraluminal Device** **D Intraluminal Device** **Z No Device**	**Z No Qualifier**
B Parotid Duct, Right Stensen's duct **C Parotid Duct, Left** *See B Parotid Duct, Right*	**7 Via Natural or Artificial Opening** **8 Via Natural or Artificial Opening Endoscopic**	**D Intraluminal Device** **Z No Device**	**Z No Qualifier**

Ø Medical and Surgical
C Mouth and Throat
W Revision

Definition: Correcting, to the extent possible, a portion of a malfunctioning device or the position of a displaced device

Explanation: Revision can include correcting a malfunctioning or displaced device by taking out or putting in components of the device such as a screw or pin

Body Part Character 4	Approach Character 5	Device Character 6	Qualifier Character 7
A Salivary Gland	**Ø** Open **3** Percutaneous	**Ø** Drainage Device **C** Extraluminal Device **Y** Other Device	**Z** No Qualifier
A Salivary Gland	**7** Via Natural or Artificial Opening **8** Via Natural or Artificial Opening Endoscopic	**Y** Other Device	**Z** No Qualifier
A Salivary Gland	**X** External	**Ø** Drainage Device **C** Extraluminal Device	**Z** No Qualifier
S Larynx Aryepiglottic fold Arytenoid cartilage Corniculate cartilage Cuneiform cartilage False vocal cord Glottis Rima glottidis Thyroid cartilage Ventricular fold	**Ø** Open **3** Percutaneous **7** Via Natural or Artificial Opening **8** Via Natural or Artificial Opening Endoscopic	**Ø** Drainage Device **7** Autologous Tissue Substitute **D** Intraluminal Device **J** Synthetic Substitute **K** Nonautologous Tissue Substitute **Y** Other Device	**Z** No Qualifier
S Larynx Aryepiglottic fold Arytenoid cartilage Corniculate cartilage Cuneiform cartilage False vocal cord Glottis Rima glottidis Thyroid cartilage Ventricular fold	**X** External	**Ø** Drainage Device **7** Autologous Tissue Substitute **D** Intraluminal Device **J** Synthetic Substitute **K** Nonautologous Tissue Substitute	**Z** No Qualifier
Y Mouth and Throat	**Ø** Open **3** Percutaneous **7** Via Natural or Artificial Opening **8** Via Natural or Artificial Opening Endoscopic	**Ø** Drainage Device **1** Radioactive Element **7** Autologous Tissue Substitute **D** Intraluminal Device **J** Synthetic Substitute **K** Nonautologous Tissue Substitute **Y** Other Device	**Z** No Qualifier
Y Mouth and Throat	**X** External	**Ø** Drainage Device **1** Radioactive Element **7** Autologous Tissue Substitute **D** Intraluminal Device **J** Synthetic Substitute **K** Nonautologous Tissue Substitute	**Z** No Qualifier

Non-OR ØCWA[Ø,3][Ø,C,Y]Z
Non-OR ØCWA[7,8]YZ
Non-OR ØCWAX[Ø,C]Z
Non-OR ØCWS[3,7,8]YZ
Non-OR ØCWSX[Ø,7,D,J,K]Z
Non-OR ØCWYØ7Z
Non-OR ØCWY[3,7,8]YZ
Non-OR ØCWYX[Ø,1,7,D,J,K]Z

Ø Medical and Surgical
C Mouth and Throat
X Transfer Definition: Moving, without taking out, all or a portion of a body part to another location to take over the function of all or a portion of a body part
Explanation: The body part transferred remains connected to its vascular and nervous supply

Body Part Character 4	Approach Character 5	Device Character 6	Qualifier Character 7
Ø Upper Lip Frenulum labii superioris Labial gland Vermilion border **1 Lower Lip** Frenulum labii inferioris Labial gland Vermilion border **3 Soft Palate** **4 Buccal Mucosa** Buccal gland Molar gland Palatine gland **5 Upper Gingiva** **6 Lower Gingiva** **7 Tongue** Frenulum linguae	**Ø Open** **X External**	**Z No Device**	**Z No Qualifier**

Gastrointestinal System ØD1–ØDY

Character Meanings

This Character Meaning table is provided as a guide to assist the user in the identification of character members that may be found in this section of code tables. It **SHOULD NOT** be used to build a PCS code.

Operation–Character 3		Body Part–Character 4		Approach–Character 5		Device–Character 6		Qualifier–Character 7	
1	Bypass	Ø	Upper Intestinal Tract	Ø	Open	Ø	Drainage Device	Ø	Allogeneic
2	Change	1	Esophagus, Upper	3	Percutaneous	1	Radioactive Element	1	Syngeneic
5	Destruction	2	Esophagus, Middle	4	Percutaneous Endoscopic	2	Monitoring Device	2	Zooplastic
7	Dilation	3	Esophagus, Lower	7	Via Natural or Artificial Opening	3	Infusion Device	3	Vertical OR Laser Interstitial Thermal Therapy
8	Division	4	Esophagogastric Junction	8	Via Natural or Artificial Opening Endoscopic	7	Autologous Tissue Substitute	4	Cutaneous
9	Drainage	5	Esophagus	F	Via Natural or Artificial Opening with Percutaneous Endoscopic Assistance	B	Intraluminal Device, Airway	5	Esophagus
B	Excision	6	Stomach	X	External	C	Extraluminal Device	6	Stomach
C	Extirpation	7	Stomach, Pylorus			D	Intraluminal Device	7	Vagina
D	Extraction	8	Small Intestine			J	Synthetic Substitute OR Magnetic Lengthening Device	8	Small Intestine
F	Fragmentation	9	Duodenum			K	Nonautologous Tissue Substitute	9	Duodenum
H	Insertion	A	Jejunum			L	Artificial Sphincter	A	Jejunum
J	Inspection	B	Ileum			M	Stimulator Lead	B	Ileum OR Bladder
L	Occlusion	C	Ileocecal Valve			U	Feeding Device	C	Ureter, Right
M	Reattachment	D	Lower Intestinal Tract			Y	Other Device	D	Ureter, Left
N	Release	E	Large Intestine			Z	No Device	E	Large Intestine
P	Removal	F	Large Intestine, Right					F	Ureters, Bilateral
Q	Repair	G	Large Intestine, Left					H	Cecum
R	Replacement	H	Cecum					K	Ascending Colon
S	Reposition	J	Appendix					L	Transverse Colon
T	Resection	K	Ascending Colon					M	Descending Colon
U	Supplement	L	Transverse Colon					N	Sigmoid Colon
V	Restriction	M	Descending Colon					P	Rectum
W	Revision	N	Sigmoid Colon					Q	Anus
X	Transfer	P	Rectum					X	Diagnostic
Y	Transplantation	Q	Anus					Z	No Qualifier
		R	Anal Sphincter						
		U	Omentum						
		V	Mesentery						
		W	Peritoneum						

AHA Coding Clinic for Gastrointestinal System

2022, 1Q, 11 Procedures performed on a continuous vessel, ICD-10-PCS Guideline B4.1c

AHA Coding Clinic for table ØD1

2021, 1Q, 19 Kock pouch revision surgery
2019, 4Q, 29 Intestinal bypass
2017, 2Q, 17 Billroth II (distal gastrectomy and gastrojejunostomy)
2016, 2Q, 31 Laparoscopic biliopancreatic diversion with duodenal switch
2014, 4Q, 41 Abdominoperineal resection (APR) with flap closure of perineum and colostomy

AHA Coding Clinic for table ØD2

2022, 1Q, 45 Insertion, removal and replacement of endoluminal vacuum application
2019, 1Q, 26 Exchange of clogged gastrojejunostomy tube

AHA Coding Clinic for table ØD5

2022, 4Q, 53-54 Laser interstitial thermal therapy
2017, 1Q, 34 Debulking of tumor and peritoneum ablation

AHA Coding Clinic for table ØD7

2020, 3Q, 45 Dilation versus drainage of perirectal cyst
2017, 3Q, 23 Laparoscopic pyloromyotomy
2014, 4Q, 40 Dilation of gastrojejunostomy anastomosis stricture

AHA Coding Clinic for table ØD8

2019, 2Q, 15 Reversal of Roux-en-Y bypass
2017, 3Q, 22 Laparoscopic esophagomyotomy (Heller type) and Toupet fundoplication
2017, 3Q, 23 Laparoscopic pyloromyotomy

AHA Coding Clinic for table ØD9

2020, 3Q, 45 Dilation versus drainage of perirectal cyst
2015, 2Q, 29 Insertion of nasogastric tube for drainage and feeding

AHA Coding Clinic for table ØDB

2023, 2Q, 23 V-Y anoplasty and excision of mucosal ectropion
2023, 1Q, 32 Zenker's diverticulectomy
2021, 3Q, 28 Retrieval of capsule via small bowel excision
2021, 2Q, 11 Serosal injury with excision of small intestine
2021, 1Q, 20 Rectal suction biopsy
2021, 1Q, 22 Total proctocolectomy with creation of J-pouch
2019, 2Q, 15 Reversal of Roux-en-Y bypass
2019, 1Q, 3-8 Whipple procedure
2019, 1Q, 27 Excision of pelvic sidewall mass
2017, 2Q, 17 Billroth II (distal gastrectomy and gastrojejunostomy)
2017, 1Q, 16 Hepatic flexure versus transverse colon
2016, 3Q, 3-7 Stoma creation & takedown procedures
2016, 2Q, 31 Laparoscopic biliopancreatic diversion with duodenal switch
2016, 1Q, 22 Perineal proctectomy
2016, 1Q, 24 Endoscopic brush biopsy of esophagus
2014, 4Q, 40 Abdominoperineal resection (APR) with flap closure of perineum and colostomy
2014, 3Q, 28 Ileostomy takedown and parastomal hernia repair
2014, 3Q, 32 Pyloric-sparing Whipple procedure

AHA Coding Clinic for table ØDD

2021, 1Q, 20 Rectal suction biopsy
2017, 4Q, 41-42 Extraction procedures

AHA Coding Clinic for table ØDH

2022, 1Q, 44 Insertion, removal and replacement of endoluminal vacuum application
2020, 4Q, 43-44 Insertion of radioactive element
2020, 3Q, 43 Staged laparoscopic gastric conduit and placement of feeding tube
2019, 2Q, 18 Endoscopic wound VAC placement
2016, 3Q, 26 Insertion of gastrostomy tube
2013, 4Q,117 Percutaneous endoscopic placement of gastrostomy tube

AHA Coding Clinic for table ØDJ

2019, 1Q, 25 Laparoscopic appendectomy converted to open procedure
2019, 1Q, 25 Milking of inspissated material from ileum to colon
2017, 2Q, 15 Low anterior resection with sigmoidoscopy
2016, 2Q, 20 Capsule endoscopy of small intestine
2015, 3Q, 24 Esophagogastroduodenoscopy with epinephrine injection for control of bleeding

AHA Coding Clinic for table ØDL

2013, 4Q, 112 Endoscopic banding of esophageal varices

AHA Coding Clinic for table ØDN

2017, 4Q, 49-50 New and revised body part values - Repositioning of the intestine
2017, 1Q, 35 Lysis of omental and peritoneal adhesions
2015, 3Q, 15 Vascular ring surgery with release of esophagus and trachea
2015, 3Q, 16 Vascular ring surgery and double aortic arch

AHA Coding Clinic for table ØDP

2019, 2Q, 18 Removal of wound VAC

AHA Coding Clinic for table ØDQ

2023, 2Q, 23 V-Y anoplasty and excision of mucosal ectropion
2019, 2Q, 15 Reversal of Roux-en-Y bypass
2018, 2Q, 25 Third and fourth degree obstetric lacerations
2018, 1Q, 11 Repair of internal hernia at Petersen space
2017, 3Q, 17 Posterior sagittal anorectoplasty
2016, 3Q, 3-7 Stoma creation & takedown procedures
2016, 3Q, 26 Insertion of gastrostomy tube
2016, 1Q, 7 Obstetrical perineal laceration repair
2016, 1Q, 8 Obstetrical perineal laceration repair
2014, 4Q, 20 Control of bleeding duodenal ulcer

AHA Coding Clinic for table ØDS

2019, 1Q, 30 Laparoscopic-assisted rectopexy with manual reduction of prolapse
2017, 4Q, 49-50 New and revised body part values - Repositioning of the intestine
2017, 3Q, 9 Ileocolic intussusception reduction via air enema
2017, 3Q, 17 Posterior sagittal anorectoplasty
2016, 3Q, 3-5 Stoma creation & takedown procedures

AHA Coding Clinic for table ØDT

2022, 1Q, 49 Robotic-assisted low anterior resection of colon
2021, 1Q, 22 Total proctocolectomy with creation of J-pouch
2020, 4Q, 100 Robotic-assisted sigmoid colectomy with extension of incision for specimen removal
2019, 1Q, 3-8 Whipple procedure
2019, 1Q, 14 Esophagectomy with colon interposition
2017, 4Q, 49-50 New and revised body part values - Repositioning of the intestine
2014, 4Q, 40 Abdominoperineal resection (APR) with flap closure of perineum and colostomy
2014, 4Q, 42 Right colectomy with side-to-side functional end-to-end anastomosis
2014, 3Q, 6 Ileocecectomy including cecum, terminal ileum and appendix
2014, 3Q, 6 Right colectomy

AHA Coding Clinic for table ØDU

2023, 2Q, 23 V-Y anoplasty and excision of mucosal ectropion
2021, 2Q, 20 Malone antegrade continence enema procedure
2021, 1Q, 22 Total proctocolectomy with creation of J-pouch
2019, 1Q, 30 Laparoscopic-assisted rectopexy with manual reduction of prolapse

AHA Coding Clinic for table ØDV

2017, 3Q, 22 Laparoscopic esophagomyotomy (Heller type) and Toupet fundoplication
2016, 2Q, 22 Esophageal lengthening Collis gastroplasty with Nissen fundoplication and hiatal hernia
2014, 3Q, 28 Laparoscopic Nissen fundoplication and diaphragmatic hernia repair

AHA Coding Clinic for table ØDW

2021, 1Q, 19 Kock pouch revision surgery
2018, 1Q, 20 Adjustment of gastric band

AHA Coding Clinic for table ØDX

2022, 4Q, 56-57 Bladder augmentation
2022, 4Q, 58 Ileal ureter
2019, 4Q, 29-30 Transfer large intestine to vagina
2019, 1Q, 14 Esophagectomy with colon interposition
2017, 2Q, 18 Esophagectomy and esophagogastrectomy with cervical esophagogastrostomy
2016, 2Q, 22 Esophageal lengthening Collis gastroplasty with Nissen fundoplication and hiatal hernia
2015, 1Q, 28 Repair of bronchopleural fistula using omental pedicle graft

AHA Coding Clinic for table ØDY

2023, 2Q, 32 Preparation of donor organ before transplantation

Upper Intestinal Tract (Ø) and Lower Intestinal Tract (D)

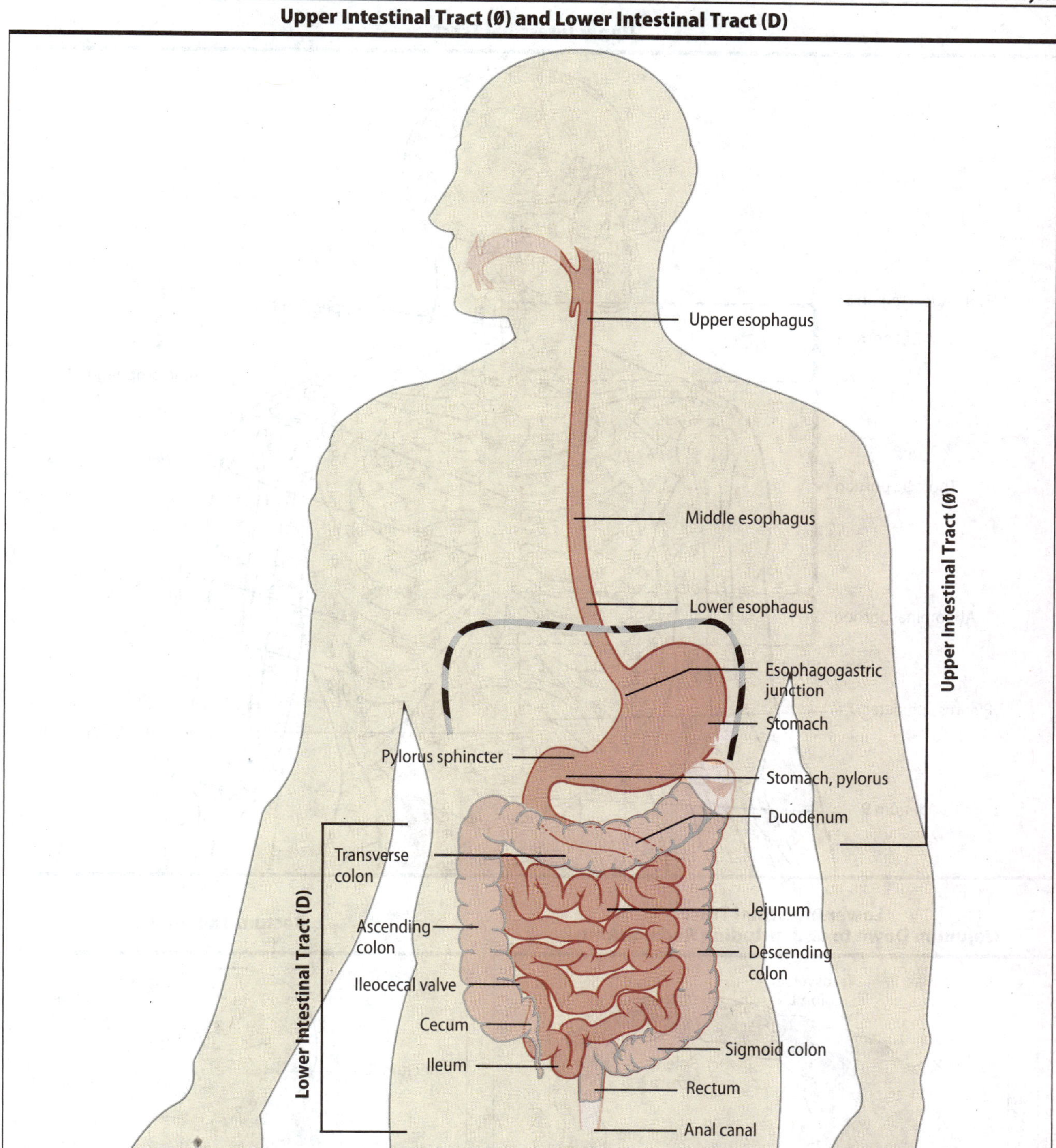

Upper Intestinal Tract

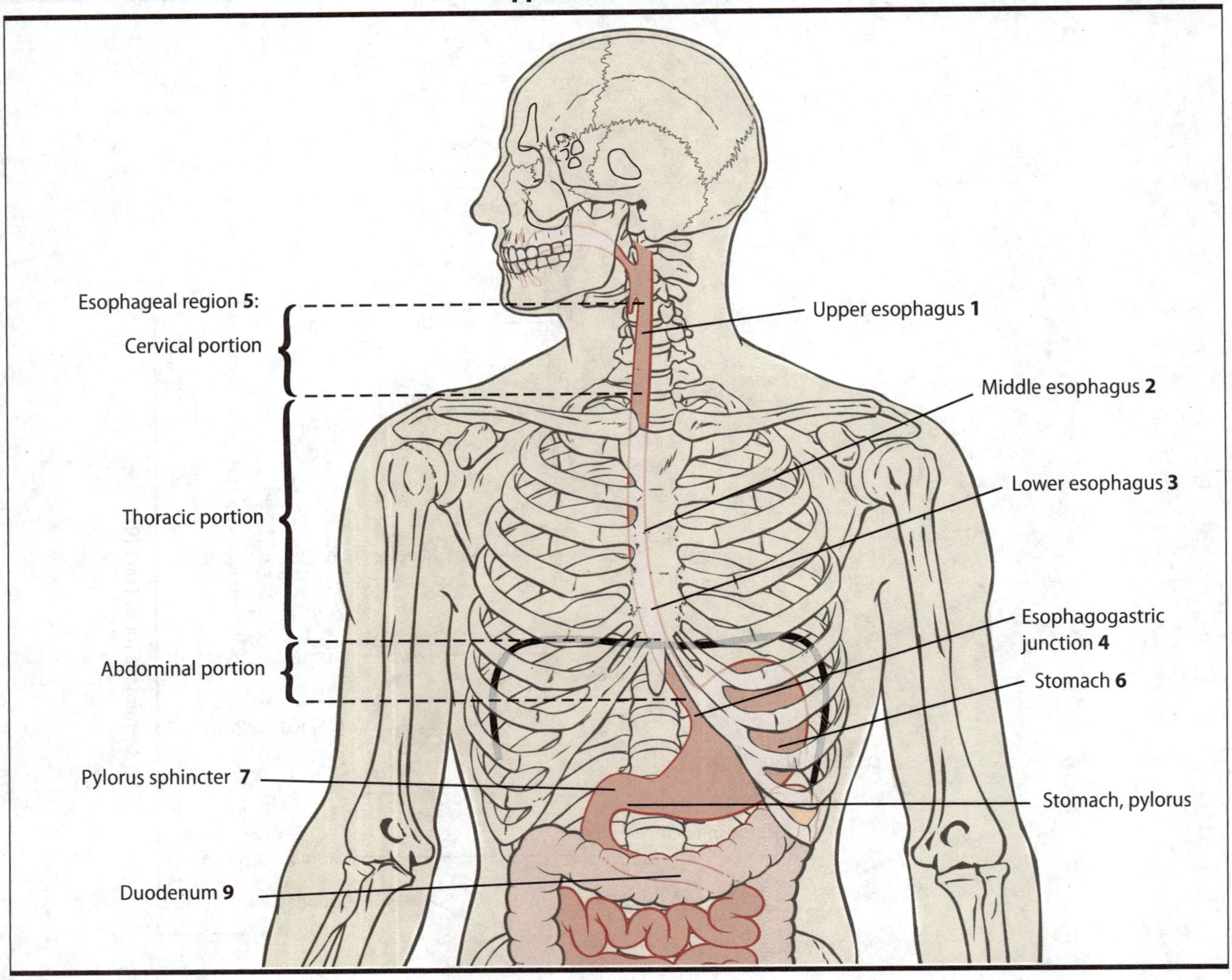

Esophageal region **5**:
Cervical portion
Thoracic portion
Abdominal portion
Upper esophagus **1**
Middle esophagus **2**
Lower esophagus **3**
Esophagogastric junction **4**
Stomach **6**
Pylorus sphincter **7**
Stomach, pylorus
Duodenum **9**

Lower Intestinal Tract (Jejunum Down to and Including Rectum/Anus)

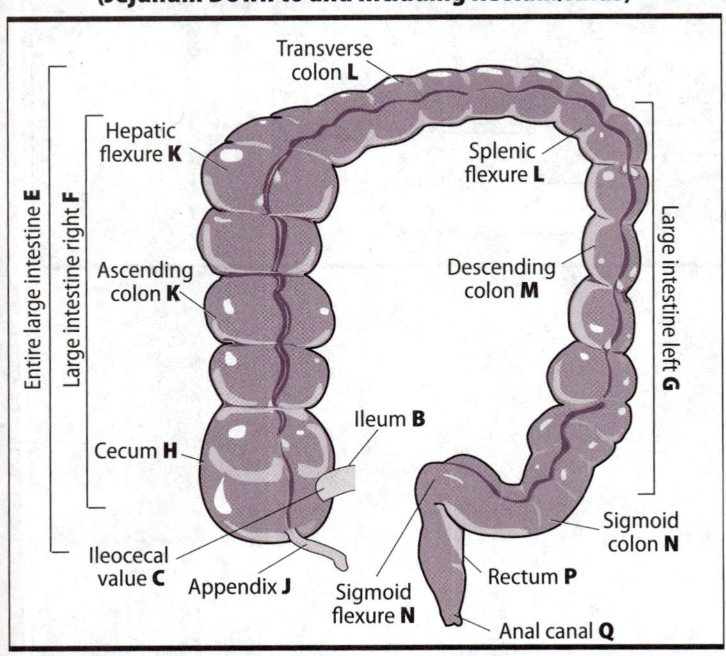

Rectum and Anus

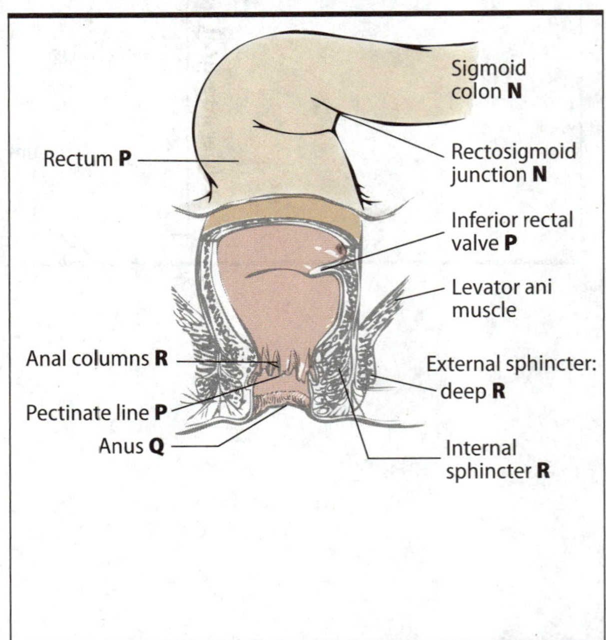

Ø Medical and Surgical
D Gastrointestinal System
1 Bypass Definition: Altering the route of passage of the contents of a tubular body part

Explanation: Rerouting contents of a body part to a downstream area of the normal route, to a similar route and body part, or to an abnormal route and dissimilar body part. Includes one or more anastomoses, with or without the use of a device.

Body Part Character 4	Approach Character 5	Device Character 6	Qualifier Character 7
1 Esophagus, Upper Cervical esophagus 2 Esophagus, Middle Thoracic esophagus 3 Esophagus, Lower Abdominal esophagus 5 Esophagus	Ø Open 4 Percutaneous Endoscopic 8 Via Natural or Artificial Opening Endoscopic	7 Autologous Tissue Substitute J Synthetic Substitute K Nonautologous Tissue Substitute Z No Device	4 Cutaneous 6 Stomach 9 Duodenum A Jejunum B Ileum
1 Esophagus, Upper Cervical esophagus 2 Esophagus, Middle Thoracic esophagus 3 Esophagus, Lower Abdominal esophagus 5 Esophagus	3 Percutaneous	J Synthetic Substitute	4 Cutaneous
6 Stomach 9 Duodenum	Ø Open 4 Percutaneous Endoscopic 8 Via Natural or Artificial Opening Endoscopic	7 Autologous Tissue Substitute J Synthetic Substitute K Nonautologous Tissue Substitute Z No Device	4 Cutaneous 9 Duodenum A Jejunum B Ileum L Transverse Colon
6 Stomach 9 Duodenum	3 Percutaneous	J Synthetic Substitute	4 Cutaneous
8 Small Intestine	Ø Open 4 Percutaneous Endoscopic 8 Via Natural or Artificial Opening Endoscopic	7 Autologous Tissue Substitute J Synthetic Substitute K Nonautologous Tissue Substitute Z No Device	4 Cutaneous 8 Small Intestine H Cecum K Ascending Colon L Transverse Colon M Descending Colon N Sigmoid Colon P Rectum Q Anus
A Jejunum Duodenojejunal flexure	Ø Open 4 Percutaneous Endoscopic 8 Via Natural or Artificial Opening Endoscopic	7 Autologous Tissue Substitute J Synthetic Substitute K Nonautologous Tissue Substitute Z No Device	4 Cutaneous A Jejunum B Ileum H Cecum K Ascending Colon L Transverse Colon M Descending Colon N Sigmoid Colon P Rectum Q Anus
A Jejunum Duodenojejunal flexure	3 Percutaneous	J Synthetic Substitute	4 Cutaneous
B Ileum	Ø Open 4 Percutaneous Endoscopic 8 Via Natural or Artificial Opening Endoscopic	7 Autologous Tissue Substitute J Synthetic Substitute K Nonautologous Tissue Substitute Z No Device	4 Cutaneous B Ileum H Cecum K Ascending Colon L Transverse Colon M Descending Colon N Sigmoid Colon P Rectum Q Anus
B Ileum	3 Percutaneous	J Synthetic Substitute	4 Cutaneous
E Large Intestine	Ø Open 4 Percutaneous Endoscopic 8 Via Natural or Artificial Opening Endoscopic	7 Autologous Tissue Substitute J Synthetic Substitute K Nonautologous Tissue Substitute Z No Device	4 Cutaneous E Large Intestine P Rectum
H Cecum	Ø Open 4 Percutaneous Endoscopic 8 Via Natural or Artificial Opening Endoscopic	7 Autologous Tissue Substitute J Synthetic Substitute K Nonautologous Tissue Substitute Z No Device	4 Cutaneous H Cecum K Ascending Colon L Transverse Colon M Descending Colon N Sigmoid Colon P Rectum
H Cecum	3 Percutaneous	J Synthetic Substitute	4 Cutaneous

Non-OR ØD16[Ø,4,8][7,J,K,Z]4
Non-OR ØD163J4
HAC ØD16[Ø,4,8][7,J,K,Z][9,A,B,L] when reported with PDx E66.Ø1 and SDx K68.11, K95.Ø1, K95.81 or T81.4Ø–T81.49 with 7th character A

ØD1 Continued on next page

ØD1 Continued

Ø Medical and Surgical
D Gastrointestinal System
1 Bypass Definition: Altering the route of passage of the contents of a tubular body part

Explanation: Rerouting contents of a body part to a downstream area of the normal route, to a similar route and body part, or to an abnormal route and dissimilar body part. Includes one or more anastomoses, with or without the use of a device.

Body Part Character 4	Approach Character 5	Device Character 6	Qualifier Character 7
K Ascending Colon	Ø Open 4 Percutaneous Endoscopic 8 Via Natural or Artificial Opening Endoscopic	7 Autologous Tissue Substitute J Synthetic Substitute K Nonautologous Tissue Substitute Z No Device	4 Cutaneous K Ascending Colon L Transverse Colon M Descending Colon N Sigmoid Colon P Rectum
K Ascending Colon	3 Percutaneous	J Synthetic Substitute	4 Cutaneous
L Transverse Colon Hepatic flexure Splenic flexure	Ø Open 4 Percutaneous Endoscopic 8 Via Natural or Artificial Opening Endoscopic	7 Autologous Tissue Substitute J Synthetic Substitute K Nonautologous Tissue Substitute Z No Device	4 Cutaneous L Transverse Colon M Descending Colon N Sigmoid Colon P Rectum
L Transverse Colon Hepatic flexure Splenic flexure	3 Percutaneous	J Synthetic Substitute	4 Cutaneous
M Descending Colon	Ø Open 4 Percutaneous Endoscopic 8 Via Natural or Artificial Opening Endoscopic	7 Autologous Tissue Substitute J Synthetic Substitute K Nonautologous Tissue Substitute Z No Device	4 Cutaneous M Descending Colon N Sigmoid Colon P Rectum
M Descending Colon	3 Percutaneous	J Synthetic Substitute	4 Cutaneous
N Sigmoid Colon Rectosigmoid junction Sigmoid flexure	Ø Open 4 Percutaneous Endoscopic 8 Via Natural or Artificial Opening Endoscopic	7 Autologous Tissue Substitute J Synthetic Substitute K Nonautologous Tissue Substitute Z No Device	4 Cutaneous N Sigmoid Colon P Rectum
N Sigmoid Colon Rectosigmoid junction Sigmoid flexure	3 Percutaneous	J Synthetic Substitute	4 Cutaneous

Ø Medical and Surgical
D Gastrointestinal System
2 Change Definition: Taking out or off a device from a body part and putting back an identical or similar device in or on the same body part without cutting or puncturing the skin or a mucous membrane

Explanation: All CHANGE procedures are coded using the approach EXTERNAL

Body Part Character 4	Approach Character 5	Device Character 6	Qualifier Character 7
Ø Upper Intestinal Tract D Lower Intestinal Tract	X External	Ø Drainage Device U Feeding Device Y Other Device	Z No Qualifier
U Omentum Gastrocolic ligament Gastrocolic omentum Gastrohepatic omentum Gastrophrenic ligament Gastrosplenic ligament Greater Omentum Hepatogastric ligament Lesser Omentum V Mesentery Mesoappendix Mesocolon W Peritoneum Epiploic foramen	X External	Ø Drainage Device Y Other Device	Z No Qualifier

Non-OR All body part, approach, device, and qualifier values

Ø Medical and Surgical
D Gastrointestinal System
5 Destruction Definition: Physical eradication of all or a portion of a body part by the direct use of energy, force, or a destructive agent
Explanation: None of the body part is physically taken out

Body Part Character 4	Approach Character 5	Device Character 6	Qualifier Character 7
1 Esophagus, Upper Cervical esophagus **2 Esophagus, Middle** Thoracic esophagus **3 Esophagus, Lower** Abdominal esophagus **4 Esophagogastric Junction** Cardia Cardioesophageal junction Gastroesophageal (GE) junction **5 Esophagus** **6 Stomach** **7 Stomach, Pylorus** Pyloric antrum Pyloric canal Pyloric sphincter **8 Small Intestine** **9 Duodenum** **A Jejunum** Duodenojejunal flexure **B Ileum** **C Ileocecal Valve** **E Large Intestine** **F Large Intestine, Right** **G Large Intestine, Left** **H Cecum** **J Appendix** Appendiceal orifice Vermiform appendix **K Ascending Colon** **L Transverse Colon** Hepatic flexure Splenic flexure **M Descending Colon** **N Sigmoid Colon** Rectosigmoid junction Sigmoid flexure **P Rectum** Anorectal junction	**Ø Open** **3 Percutaneous** **4 Percutaneous Endoscopic**	**Z No Device**	**3 Laser Interstitial Thermal Therapy** **Z No Qualifier**
1 Esophagus, Upper Cervical esophagus **2 Esophagus, Middle** Thoracic esophagus **3 Esophagus, Lower** Abdominal esophagus **4 Esophagogastric Junction** Cardia Cardioesophageal junction Gastroesophageal (GE) junction **5 Esophagus** **6 Stomach** **7 Stomach, Pylorus** Pyloric antrum Pyloric canal Pyloric sphincter **8 Small Intestine** **9 Duodenum** **A Jejunum** Duodenojejunal flexure **B Ileum** **C Ileocecal Valve** **E Large Intestine** **F Large Intestine, Right** **G Large Intestine, Left** **H Cecum** **J Appendix** Appendiceal orifice Vermiform appendix **K Ascending Colon** **L Transverse Colon** Hepatic flexure Splenic flexure **M Descending Colon** **N Sigmoid Colon** Rectosigmoid junction Sigmoid flexure **P Rectum** Anorectal junction	**7 Via Natural or Artificial Opening** **8 Via Natural or Artificial Opening Endoscopic**	**Z No Device**	**Z No Qualifier**
Q Anus Anal orifice	**Ø Open** **3 Percutaneous** **4 Percutaneous Endoscopic**	**Z No Device**	**3 Laser Interstitial Thermal Therapy** **Z No Qualifier**
Q Anus Anal orifice	**7 Via Natural or Artificial Opening** **8 Via Natural or Artificial Opening Endoscopic** **X External**	**Z No Device**	**Z No Qualifier**
R Anal Sphincter External anal sphincter Internal anal sphincter **U Omentum** Gastrocolic ligament Gastrocolic omentum Gastrohepatic omentum Gastrophrenic ligament Gastrosplenic ligament Greater Omentum Hepatogastric ligament Lesser Omentum **V Mesentery** Mesoappendix Mesocolon **W Peritoneum** Epiploic foramen	**Ø Open** **3 Percutaneous** **4 Percutaneous Endoscopic**	**Z No Device**	**Z No Qualifier**

DRG Non-OR ØD5[1,2,3,4,5,6,7,9,E,F,G,H,K,L,M,N]4Z3
DRG Non-OR ØD5P[Ø,3,4]Z3
DRG Non-OR ØD5Q4Z3

Non-OR ØD5[1,2,3,4,5,6,7,9,E,F,G,H,K,L,M,N]4ZZ
Non-OR ØD5P[Ø,3,4]ZZ
Non-OR ØD5[1,2,3,4,5,6,7,8,9,A,B,C,E,F,G,H,K,L,M,N]8ZZ
Non-OR ØD5P[7,8]ZZ
Non-OR ØD5Q4ZZ
Non-OR ØD5Q8ZZ
Non-OR ØD5R4ZZ

NC Noncovered Procedure LC Limited Coverage QA Questionable OB Admit NT New Tech Add-on ⊞ Combination Member ♂ Male ♀ Female

Ø Medical and Surgical
D Gastrointestinal System
7 Dilation Definition: Expanding an orifice or the lumen of a tubular body part

Explanation: The orifice can be a natural orifice or an artificially created orifice. Accomplished by stretching a tubular body part using intraluminal pressure or by cutting part of the orifice or wall of the tubular body part.

Body Part Character 4	Approach Character 5	Device Character 6	Qualifier Character 7
1 Esophagus, Upper Cervical esophagus **2 Esophagus, Middle** Thoracic esophagus **3 Esophagus, Lower** Abdominal esophagus **4 Esophagogastric Junction** Cardia Cardioesophageal junction Gastroesophageal (GE) junction **5 Esophagus** **6 Stomach** **7 Stomach, Pylorus** Pyloric antrum Pyloric canal Pyloric sphincter **8 Small Intestine** **9 Duodenum** **A Jejunum** Duodenojejunal flexure **B Ileum** **C Ileocecal Valve** **E Large Intestine** **F Large Intestine, Right** **G Large Intestine, Left** **H Cecum** **K Ascending Colon** **L Transverse Colon** Hepatic flexure Splenic flexure **M Descending Colon** **N Sigmoid Colon** Rectosigmoid junction Sigmoid flexure **P Rectum** Anorectal junction **Q Anus** Anal orifice	**Ø Open** **3 Percutaneous** **4 Percutaneous Endoscopic** **7 Via Natural or Artificial Opening** **8 Via Natural or Artificial Opening Endoscopic**	**D Intraluminal Device** **Z No Device**	**Z No Qualifier**

Non-OR ØD7[1,2,3,4,5,6,8,9,A,B,C,E,F,G,H,K,L,M,N,P,Q][7,8][D,Z]Z
Non-OR ØD77[4,8]DZ
Non-OR ØD777[D,Z]Z
Non-OR ØD7[8,9,A,B,C,E,F,G,H,K,L,M,N][Ø,3,4]DZ

Ø Medical and Surgical
D Gastrointestinal System
8 Division Definition: Cutting into a body part, without draining fluids and/or gases from the body part, in order to separate or transect a body part

Explanation: All or a portion of the body part is separated into two or more portions

Body Part Character 4	Approach Character 5	Device Character 6	Qualifier Character 7
4 Esophagogastric Junction Cardia Cardioesophageal junction Gastroesophageal (GE) junction **7 Stomach, Pylorus** Pyloric antrum Pyloric canal Pyloric sphincter	**Ø Open** **3 Percutaneous** **4 Percutaneous Endoscopic** **7 Via Natural or Artificial Opening** **8 Via Natural or Artificial Opening Endoscopic**	**Z No Device**	**Z No Qualifier**
R Anal Sphincter External anal sphincter Internal anal sphincter	**Ø Open** **3 Percutaneous**	**Z No Device**	**Z No Qualifier**

Ø Medical and Surgical
D Gastrointestinal System
9 Drainage Definition: Taking or letting out fluids and/or gases from a body part
Explanation: The qualifier DIAGNOSTIC is used to identify drainage procedures that are biopsies

Body Part Character 4	Approach Character 5	Device Character 6	Qualifier Character 7
1 Esophagus, Upper Cervical esophagus **2 Esophagus, Middle** Thoracic esophagus **3 Esophagus, Lower** Abdominal esophagus **4 Esophagogastric Junction** Cardia Cardioesophageal junction Gastroesophageal (GE) junction **5 Esophagus** **6 Stomach** **7 Stomach, Pylorus** Pyloric antrum Pyloric canal Pyloric sphincter **8 Small Intestine** **9 Duodenum** **A Jejunum** Duodenojejunal flexure **B Ileum** **C Ileocecal Valve** **E Large Intestine** **F Large Intestine, Right** **G Large Intestine, Left** **H Cecum** **J Appendix** Appendiceal orifice Vermiform appendix **K Ascending Colon** **L Transverse Colon** Hepatic flexure Splenic flexure **M Descending Colon** **N Sigmoid Colon** Rectosigmoid junction Sigmoid flexure **P Rectum** Anorectal junction	**Ø Open** **3 Percutaneous** **4 Percutaneous Endoscopic** **7 Via Natural or Artificial Opening** **8 Via Natural or Artificial Opening Endoscopic**	**Ø Drainage Device**	**Z No Qualifier**
1 Esophagus, Upper Cervical esophagus **2 Esophagus, Middle** Thoracic esophagus **3 Esophagus, Lower** Abdominal esophagus **4 Esophagogastric Junction** Cardia Cardioesophageal junction Gastroesophageal (GE) junction **5 Esophagus** **6 Stomach** **7 Stomach, Pylorus** Pyloric antrum Pyloric canal Pyloric sphincter **8 Small Intestine** **9 Duodenum** **A Jejunum** Duodenojejunal flexure **B Ileum** **C Ileocecal Valve** **E Large Intestine** **F Large Intestine, Right** **G Large Intestine, Left** **H Cecum** **J Appendix** Appendiceal orifice Vermiform appendix **K Ascending Colon** **L Transverse Colon** Hepatic flexure Splenic flexure **M Descending Colon** **N Sigmoid Colon** Rectosigmoid junction Sigmoid flexure **P Rectum** Anorectal junction	**Ø Open** **3 Percutaneous** **4 Percutaneous Endoscopic** **7 Via Natural or Artificial Opening** **8 Via Natural or Artificial Opening Endoscopic**	**Z No Device**	**X Diagnostic** **Z No Qualifier**
Q Anus Anal orifice	**Ø Open** **3 Percutaneous** **4 Percutaneous Endoscopic** **7 Via Natural or Artificial Opening** **8 Via Natural or Artificial Opening Endoscopic** **X External**	**Ø Drainage Device**	**Z No Qualifier**
Q Anus Anal orifice	**Ø Open** **3 Percutaneous** **4 Percutaneous Endoscopic** **7 Via Natural or Artificial Opening** **8 Via Natural or Artificial Opening Endoscopic** **X External**	**Z No Device**	**X Diagnostic** **Z No Qualifier**

Non-OR ØD9[1,2,3,4,5,C,J]3ØZ
Non-OR ØD9[6,7,8,9,A,B,E,F,G,H,K,L,M,N,P][3,7,8]ØZ
Non-OR ØD9[1,2,3,4,5,6,7,8,9,A,B,C,E,F,G,H,K,L,M,N,P][3,4,7,8]ZX
Non-OR ØD9[1,2,3,4,5,6,7,8,9,A,B,C,E,F,G,H,J,K,L,M,N,P]3ZZ
Non-OR ØD9Q3ØZ
Non-OR ØD9Q[Ø,3,4,7,8,X]ZX
Non-OR ØD9Q3ZZ

ØD9 Continued on next page

Gastrointestinal System

ØD9 Continued

Ø Medical and Surgical
D Gastrointestinal System
9 Drainage Definition: Taking or letting out fluids and/or gases from a body part

Explanation: The qualifier DIAGNOSTIC is used to identify drainage procedures that are biopsies

Body Part Character 4	Approach Character 5	Device Character 6	Qualifier Character 7
R Anal Sphincter External anal sphincter Internal anal sphincter **U Omentum** Gastrocolic ligament Gastrocolic omentum Gastrohepatic omentum Gastrophrenic ligament Gastrosplenic ligament Greater Omentum Hepatogastric ligament Lesser Omentum **V Mesentery** Mesoappendix Mesocolon **W Peritoneum** Epiploic foramen	**Ø** Open **3** Percutaneous **4** Percutaneous Endoscopic	**Ø** Drainage Device	**Z** No Qualifier
R Anal Sphincter External anal sphincter Internal anal sphincter **U Omentum** Gastrocolic ligament Gastrocolic omentum Gastrohepatic omentum Gastrophrenic ligament Gastrosplenic ligament Greater Omentum Hepatogastric ligament Lesser Omentum **V Mesentery** Mesoappendix Mesocolon **W Peritoneum** Epiploic foramen	**Ø** Open **3** Percutaneous **4** Percutaneous Endoscopic	**Z** No Device	**X** Diagnostic **Z** No Qualifier

Non-OR ØD9[R,W]3ØZ
Non-OR ØD9[U,V][3,4]ØZ
Non-OR ØD9[R,U,V,W]3Z[X,Z]
Non-OR ØD9R[Ø,4]ZX
Non-OR ØD9[U,V]4ZZ

Ø Medical and Surgical
D Gastrointestinal System
B Excision

Definition: Cutting out or off, without replacement, a portion of a body part

Explanation: The qualifier DIAGNOSTIC is used to identify excision procedures that are biopsies

Body Part Character 4	Approach Character 5	Device Character 6	Qualifier Character 7
1 Esophagus, Upper Cervical esophagus 2 Esophagus, Middle Thoracic esophagus 3 Esophagus, Lower Abdominal esophagus 4 Esophagogastric Junction Cardia Cardioesophageal junction Gastroesophageal (GE) junction 5 Esophagus 7 Stomach, Pylorus Pyloric antrum Pyloric canal Pyloric sphincter 8 Small Intestine 9 Duodenum A Jejunum Duodenojejunal flexure B Ileum C Ileocecal Valve E Large Intestine F Large Intestine, Right H Cecum J Appendix Appendiceal orifice Vermiform appendix K Ascending Colon P Rectum Anorectal junction	Ø Open 3 Percutaneous 4 Percutaneous Endoscopic 7 Via Natural or Artificial Opening 8 Via Natural or Artificial Opening Endoscopic	Z No Device	X Diagnostic Z No Qualifier
6 Stomach	Ø Open 3 Percutaneous 4 Percutaneous Endoscopic 7 Via Natural or Artificial Opening 8 Via Natural or Artificial Opening Endoscopic	Z No Device	3 Vertical X Diagnostic Z No Qualifier
G Large Intestine, Left L Transverse Colon Hepatic flexure Splenic flexure M Descending Colon N Sigmoid Colon Rectosigmoid junction Sigmoid flexure	Ø Open 3 Percutaneous 4 Percutaneous Endoscopic 7 Via Natural or Artificial Opening 8 Via Natural or Artificial Opening Endoscopic	Z No Device	X Diagnostic Z No Qualifier
G Large Intestine, Left L Transverse Colon Hepatic flexure Splenic flexure M Descending Colon N Sigmoid Colon Rectosigmoid junction Sigmoid flexure	F Via Natural or Artificial Opening with Percutaneous Endoscopic Assistance	Z No Device	Z No Qualifier
Q Anus Anal orifice	Ø Open 3 Percutaneous 4 Percutaneous Endoscopic 7 Via Natural or Artificial Opening 8 Via Natural or Artificial Opening Endoscopic X External	Z No Device	X Diagnostic Z No Qualifier
R Anal Sphincter External anal sphincter Internal anal sphincter U Omentum Gastrocolic ligament Gastrocolic omentum Gastrohepatic omentum Gastrophrenic ligament Gastrosplenic ligament Greater Omentum Hepatogastric ligament Lesser Omentum V Mesentery Mesoappendix Mesocolon W Peritoneum Epiploic foramen	Ø Open 3 Percutaneous 4 Percutaneous Endoscopic	Z No Device	X Diagnostic Z No Qualifier

Non-OR ØDB[1,2,3,4,5,7,8,9,A,B,C,E,F,H,K,P][3,4,7,8]ZX
Non-OR ØDB[1,2,3,5,7,9][4,8]ZZ
Non-OR ØDB[4,E,F,H,K,P]8ZZ
Non-OR ØDB6[3,7]ZX
Non-OR ØDB68Z[X,Z]
Non-OR ØDB[G,L,M,N][3,4,7,8]ZX
Non-OR ØDB[G,L,M,N]8ZZ
Non-OR ØDBQ[Ø,3,4,7,8,X]ZX
Non-OR ØDBQ8ZZ
Non-OR ØDBR[Ø,3,4]ZX
Non-OR ØDB[U,V,W][3,4]ZX

Ø Medical and Surgical
D Gastrointestinal System
C Extirpation Definition: Taking or cutting out solid matter from a body part

Explanation: The solid matter may be an abnormal byproduct of a biological function or a foreign body; it may be imbedded in a body part or in the lumen of a tubular body part. The solid matter may or may not have been previously broken into pieces.

Body Part Character 4	Approach Character 5	Device Character 6	Qualifier Character 7
1 Esophagus, Upper Cervical esophagus **2 Esophagus, Middle** Thoracic esophagus **3 Esophagus, Lower** Abdominal esophagus **4 Esophagogastric Junction** Cardia Cardioesophageal junction Gastroesophageal (GE) junction **5 Esophagus** **6 Stomach** **7 Stomach, Pylorus** Pyloric antrum Pyloric canal Pyloric sphincter **8 Small Intestine** **9 Duodenum** **A Jejunum** Duodenojejunal flexure **B Ileum** **C Ileocecal Valve** **E Large Intestine** **F Large Intestine, Right** **G Large Intestine, Left** **H Cecum** **J Appendix** Appendiceal orifice Vermiform appendix **K Ascending Colon** **L Transverse Colon** Hepatic flexure Splenic flexure **M Descending Colon** **N Sigmoid Colon** Rectosigmoid junction Sigmoid flexure **P Rectum** Anorectal junction	**Ø Open** **3 Percutaneous** **4 Percutaneous Endoscopic** **7 Via Natural or Artificial Opening** **8 Via Natural or Artificial Opening Endoscopic**	**Z No Device**	**Z No Qualifier**
Q Anus Anal orifice	**Ø Open** **3 Percutaneous** **4 Percutaneous Endoscopic** **7 Via Natural or Artificial Opening** **8 Via Natural or Artificial Opening Endoscopic** **X External**	**Z No Device**	**Z No Qualifier**
R Anal Sphincter External anal sphincter Internal anal sphincter **U Omentum** Gastrocolic ligament Gastrocolic omentum Gastrohepatic omentum Gastrophrenic ligament Gastrosplenic ligament Greater Omentum Hepatogastric ligament Lesser Omentum **V Mesentery** Mesoappendix Mesocolon **W Peritoneum** Epiploic foramen	**Ø Open** **3 Percutaneous** **4 Percutaneous Endoscopic**	**Z No Device**	**Z No Qualifier**

Non-OR ØDC[1,2,3,4,5,6,7,8,9,A,B,C,E,F,G,H,K,L,M,N,P][7,8]ZZ
Non-OR ØDCQ[7,8,X]ZZ

Ø Medical and Surgical
D Gastrointestinal System
D Extraction Definition: Pulling or stripping out or off all or a portion of a body part by the use of force
Explanation: The qualifier DIAGNOSTIC is used to identify extraction procedures that are biopsies

Body Part Character 4	Approach Character 5	Device Character 6	Qualifier Character 7
1 Esophagus, Upper Cervical esophagus 2 Esophagus, Middle Thoracic esophagus 3 Esophagus, Lower Abdominal esophagus 4 Esophagogastric Junction Cardia Cardioesophageal junction Gastroesophageal (GE) junction 5 Esophagus 6 Stomach 7 Stomach, Pylorus Pyloric antrum Pyloric canal Pyloric sphincter 8 Small Intestine 9 Duodenum A Jejunum Duodenojejunal flexure B Ileum C Ileocecal Valve E Large Intestine F Large Intestine, Right G Large Intestine, Left H Cecum J Appendix Appendiceal orifice Vermiform appendix K Ascending Colon L Transverse Colon Hepatic flexure Splenic flexure M Descending Colon N Sigmoid Colon Rectosigmoid junction Sigmoid flexure P Rectum Anorectal junction	3 Percutaneous 4 Percutaneous Endoscopic 8 Via Natural or Artificial Opening Endoscopic	Z No Device	X Diagnostic
Q Anus Anal orifice	3 Percutaneous 4 Percutaneous Endoscopic 8 Via Natural or Artificial Opening Endoscopic X External	Z No Device	X Diagnostic

Non-OR ØDD[1,2,3,4,5,6,7,8,9,A,B,C,E,F,G,H,K,L,M,N,P][3,4,8]ZX
Non-OR ØDDQ[3,4,8,X]ZX

Ø Medical and Surgical
D Gastrointestinal System
F Fragmentation Definition: Breaking solid matter in a body part into pieces

Explanation: Physical force (e.g., manual, ultrasonic) applied directly or indirectly is used to break the solid matter into pieces. The solid matter may be an abnormal byproduct of a biological function or a foreign body. The pieces of solid matter are not taken out.

Body Part Character 4	Approach Character 5	Device Character 6	Qualifier Character 7
5 Esophagus NC 6 Stomach NC 8 Small Intestine NC 9 Duodenum NC A Jejunum NC Duodenojejunal flexure B Ileum NC E Large Intestine NC F Large Intestine, Right NC G Large Intestine, Left NC H Cecum NC J Appendix NC Appendiceal orifice Vermiform appendix K Ascending Colon NC L Transverse Colon NC Hepatic flexure Splenic flexure M Descending Colon NC N Sigmoid Colon NC Rectosigmoid junction Sigmoid flexure P Rectum NC Anorectal junction Q Anus NC Anal orifice	Ø Open 3 Percutaneous 4 Percutaneous Endoscopic 7 Via Natural or Artificial Opening 8 Via Natural or Artificial Opening Endoscopic X External	Z No Device	Z No Qualifier

Non-OR ØDF[5,6,8,9,A,B,E,F,G,H,J,K,L,M,N,P,Q]XZZ
NC ØDF[5,6,8,9,A,B,E,F,G,H,J,K,L,M,N,P,Q]XZZ

Ø Medical and Surgical
D Gastrointestinal System
H Insertion Definition: Putting in a nonbiological appliance that monitors, assists, performs, or prevents a physiological function but does not physically take the place of a body part

Explanation: None

Body Part Character 4	Approach Character 5	Device Character 6	Qualifier Character 7
Ø Upper Intestinal Tract D Lower Intestinal Tract	Ø Open 3 Percutaneous 4 Percutaneous Endoscopic 7 Via Natural or Artificial Opening 8 Via Natural or Artificial Opening Endoscopic	Y Other Device	Z No Qualifier
1 Esophagus, Upper 2 Esophagus, Middle 3 Esophagus, Lower	7 Via Natural or Artificial Opening	J Magnetic Lengthening Device	Z No Qualifier
5 Esophagus	Ø Open 3 Percutaneous 4 Percutaneous Endoscopic	1 Radioactive Element 2 Monitoring Device 3 Infusion Device D Intraluminal Device U Feeding Device Y Other Device	Z No Qualifier
5 Esophagus	7 Via Natural or Artificial Opening 8 Via Natural or Artificial Opening Endoscopic	1 Radioactive Element 2 Monitoring Device 3 Infusion Device B Intraluminal Device, Airway D Intraluminal Device U Feeding Device Y Other Device	Z No Qualifier
6 Stomach ⊞	Ø Open 3 Percutaneous 4 Percutaneous Endoscopic	1 Radioactive Element 2 Monitoring Device 3 Infusion Device D Intraluminal Device M Stimulator Lead U Feeding Device Y Other Device	Z No Qualifier
6 Stomach	7 Via Natural or Artificial Opening 8 Via Natural or Artificial Opening Endoscopic	1 Radioactive Element 2 Monitoring Device 3 Infusion Device D Intraluminal Device U Feeding Device Y Other Device	Z No Qualifier
8 Small Intestine 9 Duodenum A Jejunum Duodenojejunal flexure B Ileum	Ø Open 3 Percutaneous 4 Percutaneous Endoscopic 7 Via Natural or Artificial Opening 8 Via Natural or Artificial Opening Endoscopic	1 Radioactive Element 2 Monitoring Device 3 Infusion Device D Intraluminal Device U Feeding Device	Z No Qualifier
E Large Intestine P Rectum Anorectal junction	Ø Open 3 Percutaneous 4 Percutaneous Endoscopic 7 Via Natural or Artificial Opening 8 Via Natural or Artificial Opening Endoscopic	1 Radioactive Element D Intraluminal Device	Z No Qualifier
Q Anus Anal orifice	Ø Open 3 Percutaneous 4 Percutaneous Endoscopic	D Intraluminal Device L Artificial Sphincter	Z No Qualifier
Q Anus Anal orifice	7 Via Natural or Artificial Opening 8 Via Natural or Artificial Opening Endoscopic	D Intraluminal Device	Z No Qualifier
R Anal Sphincter External anal sphincter Internal anal sphincter	Ø Open 3 Percutaneous 4 Percutaneous Endoscopic	M Stimulator Lead	Z No Qualifier

Non-OR ØDH[Ø,D][Ø,3,4,7,8]YZ
Non-OR ØDH5[Ø,3,4][D,U]Z
Non-OR ØDH5[3,4]YZ
Non-OR ØDH5[7,8][2,3,B,D,U,Y]Z
Non-OR ØDH631Z
Non-OR ØDH6[Ø,3,4]UZ
Non-OR ØDH6[3,4]YZ
Non-OR ØDH6[7,8][1,2,3,D,U,Y]Z
Non-OR ØDH[8,9,A,B][Ø,3,4,7,8][1,D,U]Z
Non-OR ØDH[8,9,A,B][7,8][2,3]Z
Non-OR ØDHE[Ø,3,4,7,8][1,D]Z
Non-OR ØDHP[Ø,3,4,7,8]DZ

See Appendix L for Procedure Combinations
⊞ ØDH6[Ø,3,4]MZ

Ø Medical and Surgical
D Gastrointestinal System
J Inspection

Definition: Visually and/or manually exploring a body part

Explanation: Visual exploration may be performed with or without optical instrumentation. Manual exploration may be performed directly or through intervening body layers.

Body Part Character 4	Approach Character 5	Device Character 6	Qualifier Character 7
Ø Upper Intestinal Tract 6 Stomach D Lower Intestinal Tract	Ø Open 3 Percutaneous 4 Percutaneous Endoscopic 7 Via Natural or Artificial Opening 8 Via Natural or Artificial Opening Endoscopic X External	Z No Device	Z No Qualifier
U Omentum Gastrocolic ligament Gastrocolic omentum Gastrohepatic omentum Gastrophrenic ligament Gastrosplenic ligament Greater Omentum Hepatogastric ligament Lesser Omentum V Mesentery Mesoappendix Mesocolon W Peritoneum Epiploic foramen	Ø Open 3 Percutaneous 4 Percutaneous Endoscopic X External	Z No Device	Z No Qualifier

Non-OR ØDJ[Ø,6,D][3,7,8,X]ZZ
Non-OR ØDJ[U,V,W][3,X]ZZ

Ø Medical and Surgical
D Gastrointestinal System
L Occlusion Definition: Completely closing an orifice or the lumen of a tubular body part
Explanation: The orifice can be a natural orifice or an artificially created orifice

Body Part Character 4	Approach Character 5	Device Character 6	Qualifier Character 7
1 Esophagus, Upper Cervical esophagus **2 Esophagus, Middle** Thoracic esophagus **3 Esophagus, Lower** Abdominal esophagus **4 Esophagogastric Junction** Cardia, Cardioesophageal junction, Gastroesophageal (GE) junction **5 Esophagus** **6 Stomach** **7 Stomach, Pylorus** Pyloric antrum, Pyloric canal, Pyloric sphincter **8 Small Intestine** **9 Duodenum** **A Jejunum** Duodenojejunal flexure **B Ileum** **C Ileocecal Valve** **E Large Intestine** **F Large Intestine, Right** **G Large Intestine, Left** **H Cecum** **K Ascending Colon** **L Transverse Colon** Hepatic flexure, Splenic flexure **M Descending Colon** **N Sigmoid Colon** Rectosigmoid junction, Sigmoid flexure **P Rectum** Anorectal junction	**Ø Open** **3 Percutaneous** **4 Percutaneous Endoscopic**	**C Extraluminal Device** **D Intraluminal Device** **Z No Device**	**Z No Qualifier**
1 Esophagus, Upper Cervical esophagus **2 Esophagus, Middle** Thoracic esophagus **3 Esophagus, Lower** Abdominal esophagus **4 Esophagogastric Junction** Cardia, Cardioesophageal junction, Gastroesophageal (GE) junction **5 Esophagus** **6 Stomach** **7 Stomach, Pylorus** Pyloric antrum, Pyloric canal, Pyloric sphincter **8 Small Intestine** **9 Duodenum** **A Jejunum** Duodenojejunal flexure **B Ileum** **C Ileocecal Valve** **E Large Intestine** **F Large Intestine, Right** **G Large Intestine, Left** **H Cecum** **K Ascending Colon** **L Transverse Colon** Hepatic flexure, Splenic flexure **M Descending Colon** **N Sigmoid Colon** Rectosigmoid junction, Sigmoid flexure **P Rectum** Anorectal junction	**7 Via Natural or Artificial Opening** **8 Via Natural or Artificial Opening Endoscopic**	**D Intraluminal Device** **Z No Device**	**Z No Qualifier**
Q Anus Anal orifice	**Ø Open** **3 Percutaneous** **4 Percutaneous Endoscopic** **X External**	**C Extraluminal Device** **D Intraluminal Device** **Z No Device**	**Z No Qualifier**
Q Anus Anal orifice	**7 Via Natural or Artificial Opening** **8 Via Natural or Artificial Opening Endoscopic**	**D Intraluminal Device** **Z No Device**	**Z No Qualifier**

Non-OR ØDL[1,2,3,4,5][Ø,3,4][C,D,Z]Z
Non-OR ØDL[1,2,3,4,5][7,8][D,Z]Z

Gastrointestinal System

ØDL–ØDL

Ø Medical and Surgical
D Gastrointestinal System
M Reattachment Definition: Putting back in or on all or a portion of a separated body part to its normal location or other suitable location
Explanation: Vascular circulation and nervous pathways may or may not be reestablished

Body Part Character 4	Approach Character 5	Device Character 6	Qualifier Character 7
5 Esophagus **6 Stomach** **8 Small Intestine** **9 Duodenum** **A Jejunum** Duodenojejunal flexure **B Ileum** **E Large Intestine** **F Large Intestine, Right** **G Large Intestine, Left** **H Cecum** **K Ascending Colon** **L Transverse Colon** Hepatic flexure Splenic flexure **M Descending Colon** **N Sigmoid Colon** Rectosigmoid junction Sigmoid flexure **P Rectum** Anorectal junction	**Ø Open** **4 Percutaneous Endoscopic**	**Z No Device**	**Z No Qualifier**

Ø Medical and Surgical
D Gastrointestinal System
N Release Definition: Freeing a body part from an abnormal physical constraint by cutting or by the use of force
Explanation: Some of the restraining tissue may be taken out but none of the body part is taken out

Body Part Character 4	Approach Character 5	Device Character 6	Qualifier Character 7
1 Esophagus, Upper Cervical esophagus **2 Esophagus, Middle** Thoracic esophagus **3 Esophagus, Lower** Abdominal esophagus **4 Esophagogastric Junction** Cardia Cardioesophageal junction Gastroesophageal (GE) junction **5 Esophagus** **6 Stomach** **7 Stomach, Pylorus** Pyloric antrum Pyloric canal Pyloric sphincter **8 Small Intestine** **9 Duodenum** **A Jejunum** Duodenojejunal flexure **B Ileum** **C Ileocecal Valve** **E Large Intestine** **F Large Intestine, Right** **G Large Intestine, Left** **H Cecum** **J Appendix** Appendiceal orifice Vermiform appendix **K Ascending Colon** **L Transverse Colon** Hepatic flexure Splenic flexure **M Descending Colon** **N Sigmoid Colon** Rectosigmoid junction Sigmoid flexure **P Rectum** Anorectal junction	**Ø Open** **3 Percutaneous** **4 Percutaneous Endoscopic** **7 Via Natural or Artificial Opening** **8 Via Natural or Artificial Opening Endoscopic**	**Z No Device**	**Z No Qualifier**
Q Anus Anal orifice	**Ø Open** **3 Percutaneous** **4 Percutaneous Endoscopic** **7 Via Natural or Artificial Opening** **8 Via Natural or Artificial Opening Endoscopic** **X External**	**Z No Device**	**Z No Qualifier**
R Anal Sphincter External anal sphincter Internal anal sphincter **U Omentum** Gastrocolic ligament Gastrocolic omentum Gastrohepatic omentum Gastrophrenic ligament Gastrosplenic ligament Greater Omentum Hepatogastric ligament Lesser Omentum **V Mesentery** Mesoappendix Mesocolon **W Peritoneum** Epiploic foramen	**Ø Open** **3 Percutaneous** **4 Percutaneous Endoscopic**	**Z No Device**	**Z No Qualifier**

Non-OR ØDN[8,9,A,B,E,F,G,H,K,L,M,N][7,8]ZZ

Ø Medical and Surgical
D Gastrointestinal System
P Removal Definition: Taking out or off a device from a body part

Explanation: If a device is taken out and a similar device put in without cutting or puncturing the skin or mucous membrane, the procedure is coded to the root operation CHANGE. Otherwise, the procedure for taking out a device is coded to the root operation REMOVAL.

Body Part Character 4	Approach Character 5	Device Character 6	Qualifier Character 7
Ø Upper Intestinal Tract D Lower Intestinal Tract	Ø Open 3 Percutaneous 4 Percutaneous Endoscopic 7 Via Natural or Artificial Opening 8 Via Natural or Artificial Opening Endoscopic	Ø Drainage Device 2 Monitoring Device 3 Infusion Device 7 Autologous Tissue Substitute C Extraluminal Device D Intraluminal Device J Synthetic Substitute K Nonautologous Tissue Substitute U Feeding Device Y Other Device	Z No Qualifier
Ø Upper Intestinal Tract D Lower Intestinal Tract	X External	Ø Drainage Device 2 Monitoring Device 3 Infusion Device D Intraluminal Device U Feeding Device	Z No Qualifier
5 Esophagus	Ø Open 3 Percutaneous 4 Percutaneous Endoscopic	1 Radioactive Element 2 Monitoring Device 3 Infusion Device U Feeding Device Y Other Device	Z No Qualifier
5 Esophagus	7 Via Natural or Artificial Opening 8 Via Natural or Artificial Opening Endoscopic	1 Radioactive Element D Intraluminal Device Y Other Device	Z No Qualifier
5 Esophagus	X External	1 Radioactive Element 2 Monitoring Device 3 Infusion Device D Intraluminal Device U Feeding Device	Z No Qualifier
6 Stomach	Ø Open 3 Percutaneous 4 Percutaneous Endoscopic	Ø Drainage Device 2 Monitoring Device 3 Infusion Device 7 Autologous Tissue Substitute C Extraluminal Device D Intraluminal Device J Synthetic Substitute K Nonautologous Tissue Substitute M Stimulator Lead U Feeding Device Y Other Device	Z No Qualifier
6 Stomach	7 Via Natural or Artificial Opening 8 Via Natural or Artificial Opening Endoscopic	Ø Drainage Device 2 Monitoring Device 3 Infusion Device 7 Autologous Tissue Substitute C Extraluminal Device D Intraluminal Device J Synthetic Substitute K Nonautologous Tissue Substitute U Feeding Device Y Other Device	Z No Qualifier
6 Stomach	X External	Ø Drainage Device 2 Monitoring Device 3 Infusion Device D Intraluminal Device U Feeding Device	Z No Qualifier

Non-OR ØDP[Ø,D][3,4]YZ
Non-OR ØDP[Ø,D][7,8][Ø,2,3,D,U,Y]Z
Non-OR ØDP[Ø,D]X[Ø,2,3,D,U]Z
Non-OR ØDP5[3,4]YZ
Non-OR ØDP5[7,8][1,D,Y]Z
Non-OR ØDP5X[1,2,3,D,U]Z
Non-OR ØDP6[3,4]YZ
Non-OR ØDP6[7,8][Ø,2,3,D,U,Y]Z
Non-OR ØDP6X[Ø,2,3,D,U]Z

ØDP Continued on next page

ØDP Continued

Ø Medical and Surgical
D Gastrointestinal System
P Removal

Definition: Taking out or off a device from a body part

Explanation: If a device is taken out and a similar device put in without cutting or puncturing the skin or mucous membrane, the procedure is coded to the root operation CHANGE. Otherwise, the procedure for taking out a device is coded to the root operation REMOVAL.

Body Part Character 4	Approach Character 5	Device Character 6	Qualifier Character 7
P Rectum Anorectal junction	**Ø Open** **3 Percutaneous** **4 Percutaneous Endoscopic** **7 Via Natural or Artificial Opening** **8 Via Natural or Artificial Opening Endoscopic** **X External**	**1 Radioactive Element**	**Z No Qualifier**
Q Anus Anal orifice	**Ø Open** **3 Percutaneous** **4 Percutaneous Endoscopic** **7 Via Natural or Artificial Opening** **8 Via Natural or Artificial Opening Endoscopic**	**L Artificial Sphincter**	**Z No Qualifier**
R Anal Sphincter External anal sphincter Internal anal sphincter	**Ø Open** **3 Percutaneous** **4 Percutaneous Endoscopic**	**M Stimulator Lead**	**Z No Qualifier**
U Omentum Gastrocolic ligament Gastrocolic omentum Gastrohepatic omentum Gastrophrenic ligament Gastrosplenic ligament Greater Omentum Hepatogastric ligament Lesser Omentum **V Mesentery** Mesoappendix Mesocolon **W Peritoneum** Epiploic foramen	**Ø Open** **3 Percutaneous** **4 Percutaneous Endoscopic**	**Ø Drainage Device** **1 Radioactive Element** **7 Autologous Tissue Substitute** **J Synthetic Substitute** **K Nonautologous Tissue Substitute**	**Z No Qualifier**

Non-OR ØDPP[7,8,X]1Z

Ø Medical and Surgical
D Gastrointestinal System
Q Repair

Definition: Restoring, to the extent possible, a body part to its normal anatomic structure and function

Explanation: Used only when the method to accomplish the repair is not one of the other root operations

Body Part Character 4	Approach Character 5	Device Character 6	Qualifier Character 7
1 Esophagus, Upper Cervical esophagus **2 Esophagus, Middle** Thoracic esophagus **3 Esophagus, Lower** Abdominal esophagus **4 Esophagogastric Junction** Cardia Cardioesophageal junction Gastroesophageal (GE) junction **5 Esophagus** **6 Stomach** **7 Stomach, Pylorus** Pyloric antrum Pyloric canal Pyloric sphincter **8 Small Intestine** ⊞ **9 Duodenum** ⊞ **A Jejunum** ⊞ Duodenojejunal flexure **B Ileum** ⊞ **C Ileocecal Valve** **E Large Intestine** ⊞ **F Large Intestine, Right** ⊞ **G Large Intestine, Left** ⊞ **H Cecum** ⊞ **J Appendix** Appendiceal orifice Vermiform appendix **K Ascending Colon** ⊞ **L Transverse Colon** ⊞ Hepatic flexure Splenic flexure **M Descending Colon** ⊞ **N Sigmoid Colon** ⊞ Rectosigmoid junction Sigmoid flexure **P Rectum** Anorectal junction	**Ø Open** **3 Percutaneous** **4 Percutaneous Endoscopic** **7 Via Natural or Artificial Opening** **8 Via Natural or Artificial Opening Endoscopic**	**Z No Device**	**Z No Qualifier**
Q Anus Anal orifice	**Ø Open** **3 Percutaneous** **4 Percutaneous Endoscopic** **7 Via Natural or Artificial Opening** **8 Via Natural or Artificial Opening Endoscopic** **X External**	**Z No Device**	**Z No Qualifier**
R Anal Sphincter External anal sphincter Internal anal sphincter **U Omentum** Gastrocolic ligament Gastrocolic omentum Gastrohepatic omentum Gastrophrenic ligament Gastrosplenic ligament Greater Omentum Hepatogastric ligament Lesser Omentum **V Mesentery** Mesoappendix Mesocolon **W Peritoneum** Epiploic foramen	**Ø Open** **3 Percutaneous** **4 Percutaneous Endoscopic**	**Z No Device**	**Z No Qualifier**

See Appendix L for Procedure Combinations

⊞ ØDQ[8,9,A,B,E,F,G,H,K,L,M,N]ØZZ

Ø Medical and Surgical
D Gastrointestinal System
R Replacement Definition: Putting in or on biological or synthetic material that physically takes the place and/or function of all or a portion of a body part

Explanation: The body part may have been taken out or replaced, or may be taken out, physically eradicated, or rendered nonfunctional during the REPLACEMENT procedure. A REMOVAL procedure is coded for taking out the device used in a previous replacement procedure.

Body Part Character 4	Approach Character 5	Device Character 6	Qualifier Character 7
5 Esophagus	**Ø Open** **4 Percutaneous Endoscopic** **7 Via Natural or Artificial Opening** **8 Via Natural or Artificial Opening Endoscopic**	**7 Autologous Tissue Substitute** **J Synthetic Substitute** **K Nonautologous Tissue Substitute**	**Z No Qualifier**
R Anal Sphincter External anal sphincter Internal anal sphincter **U Omentum** Gastrocolic ligament Gastrocolic omentum Gastrohepatic omentum Gastrophrenic ligament Gastrosplenic ligament Greater Omentum Hepatogastric ligament Lesser Omentum **V Mesentery** Mesoappendix Mesocolon **W Peritoneum** Epiploic foramen	**Ø Open** **4 Percutaneous Endoscopic**	**7 Autologous Tissue Substitute** **J Synthetic Substitute** **K Nonautologous Tissue Substitute**	**Z No Qualifier**

Ø Medical and Surgical
D Gastrointestinal System
S Reposition Definition: Moving to its normal location, or other suitable location, all or a portion of a body part

Explanation: The body part is moved to a new location from an abnormal location, or from a normal location where it is not functioning correctly. The body part may or may not be cut out or off to be moved to the new location.

Body Part Character 4	Approach Character 5	Device Character 6	Qualifier Character 7
5 Esophagus **6 Stomach** **9 Duodenum** **A Jejunum** Duodenojejunal flexure **B Ileum** **H Cecum** **K Ascending Colon** **L Transverse Colon** Hepatic flexure Splenic flexure **M Descending Colon** **N Sigmoid Colon** Rectosigmoid junction Sigmoid flexure **P Rectum** Anorectal junction **Q Anus** Anal orifice	**Ø Open** **4 Percutaneous Endoscopic** **7 Via Natural or Artificial Opening** **8 Via Natural or Artificial Opening Endoscopic** **X External**	**Z No Device**	**Z No Qualifier**
8 Small Intestine **E Large Intestine**	**Ø Open** **4 Percutaneous Endoscopic** **7 Via Natural or Artificial Opening** **8 Via Natural or Artificial Opening Endoscopic**	**Z No Device**	**Z No Qualifier**

Non-OR ØDS[5,6,9,A,B,H,K,L,M,N,P,Q]XZZ

Ø Medical and Surgical
D Gastrointestinal System
T Resection Definition: Cutting out or off, without replacement, all of a body part
Explanation: None

Body Part Character 4	Approach Character 5	Device Character 6	Qualifier Character 7
1 Esophagus, Upper Cervical esophagus **2 Esophagus, Middle** Thoracic esophagus **3 Esophagus, Lower** Abdominal esophagus **4 Esophagogastric Junction** Cardia Cardioesophageal junction Gastroesophageal (GE) junction **5 Esophagus** **6 Stomach** **7 Stomach, Pylorus** Pyloric antrum Pyloric canal Pyloric sphincter **8 Small Intestine** **9 Duodenum** ⊞ **A Jejunum** Duodenojejunal flexure **B Ileum** **C Ileocecal Valve** **E Large Intestine** **F Large Intestine, Right** **H Cecum** **J Appendix** Appendiceal orifice Vermiform appendix **K Ascending Colon** **P Rectum** Anorectal junction **Q Anus** Anal orifice	**Ø Open** **4 Percutaneous Endoscopic** **7 Via Natural or Artificial Opening** **8 Via Natural or Artificial Opening Endoscopic**	**Z No Device**	**Z No Qualifier**
G Large Intestine, Left **L Transverse Colon** Hepatic flexure Splenic flexure **M Descending Colon** **N Sigmoid Colon** Rectosigmoid junction Sigmoid flexure	**Ø Open** **4 Percutaneous Endoscopic** **7 Via Natural or Artificial Opening** **8 Via Natural or Artificial Opening Endoscopic** **F Via Natural or Artificial Opening with Percutaneous Endoscopic Assistance**	**Z No Device**	**Z No Qualifier**
R Anal Sphincter External anal sphincter Internal anal sphincter **U Omentum** Gastrocolic ligament Gastrocolic omentum Gastrohepatic omentum Gastrophrenic ligament Gastrosplenic ligament Greater Omentum Hepatogastric ligament Lesser Omentum	**Ø Open** **4 Percutaneous Endoscopic**	**Z No Device**	**Z No Qualifier**

See Appendix L for Procedure Combinations
⊞ ØDT9ØZZ

Ø Medical and Surgical
D Gastrointestinal System
U Supplement

Definition: Putting in or on biological or synthetic material that physically reinforces and/or augments the function of a portion of a body part

Explanation: The biological material is non-living, or is living and from the same individual. The body part may have been previously replaced, and the SUPPLEMENT procedure is performed to physically reinforce and/or augment the function of the replaced body part.

Body Part Character 4	Approach Character 5	Device Character 6	Qualifier Character 7
1 Esophagus, Upper Cervical esophagus **2 Esophagus, Middle** Thoracic esophagus **3 Esophagus, Lower** Abdominal esophagus **4 Esophagogastric Junction** Cardia Cardioesophageal junction Gastroesophageal (GE) junction **5 Esophagus** **6 Stomach** **7 Stomach, Pylorus** Pyloric antrum Pyloric canal Pyloric sphincter **8 Small Intestine** **9 Duodenum** **A Jejunum** Duodenojejunal flexure **B Ileum** **C Ileocecal Valve** **E Large Intestine** **F Large Intestine, Right** **G Large Intestine, Left** **H Cecum** **K Ascending Colon** **L Transverse Colon** Hepatic flexure Splenic flexure **M Descending Colon** **N Sigmoid Colon** Rectosigmoid junction Sigmoid flexure **P Rectum** Anorectal junction	**Ø Open** **4 Percutaneous Endoscopic** **7 Via Natural or Artificial Opening** **8 Via Natural or Artificial Opening Endoscopic**	**7 Autologous Tissue Substitute** **J Synthetic Substitute** **K Nonautologous Tissue Substitute**	**Z No Qualifier**
Q Anus Anal orifice	**Ø Open** **4 Percutaneous Endoscopic** **7 Via Natural or Artificial Opening** **8 Via Natural or Artificial Opening Endoscopic** **X External**	**7 Autologous Tissue Substitute** **J Synthetic Substitute** **K Nonautologous Tissue Substitute**	**Z No Qualifier**
R Anal Sphincter External anal sphincter Internal anal sphincter **U Omentum** Gastrocolic ligament Gastrocolic omentum Gastrohepatic omentum Gastrophrenic ligament Gastrosplenic ligament Greater Omentum Hepatogastric ligament Lesser Omentum **V Mesentery** Mesoappendix Mesocolon **W Peritoneum** Epiploic foramen	**Ø Open** **4 Percutaneous Endoscopic**	**7 Autologous Tissue Substitute** **J Synthetic Substitute** **K Nonautologous Tissue Substitute**	**Z No Qualifier**

Ø Medical and Surgical
D Gastrointestinal System
V Restriction Definition: Partially closing an orifice or the lumen of a tubular body part

Explanation: The orifice can be a natural orifice or an artificially created orifice

Body Part Character 4		Approach Character 5	Device Character 6	Qualifier Character 7
1 Esophagus, Upper Cervical esophagus **2 Esophagus, Middle** Thoracic esophagus **3 Esophagus, Lower** Abdominal esophagus **4 Esophagogastric Junction** Cardia, Cardioesophageal junction, Gastroesophageal (GE) junction **5 Esophagus** **6 Stomach** **7 Stomach, Pylorus** Pyloric antrum, Pyloric canal, Pyloric sphincter **8 Small Intestine**	**9 Duodenum** **A Jejunum** Duodenojejunal flexure **B Ileum** **C Ileocecal Valve** **E Large Intestine** **F Large Intestine, Right** **G Large Intestine, Left** **H Cecum** **K Ascending Colon** **L Transverse Colon** Hepatic flexure, Splenic flexure **M Descending Colon** **N Sigmoid Colon** Rectosigmoid junction, Sigmoid flexure **P Rectum** Anorectal junction	**Ø Open** **3 Percutaneous** **4 Percutaneous Endoscopic**	**C Extraluminal Device** **D Intraluminal Device** **Z No Device**	**Z No Qualifier**
1 Esophagus, Upper Cervical esophagus **2 Esophagus, Middle** Thoracic esophagus **3 Esophagus, Lower** Abdominal esophagus **4 Esophagogastric Junction** Cardia, Cardioesophageal junction, Gastroesophageal (GE) junction **5 Esophagus** **6 Stomach** NC **7 Stomach, Pylorus** Pyloric antrum, Pyloric canal, Pyloric sphincter **8 Small Intestine**	**9 Duodenum** **A Jejunum** Duodenojejunal flexure **B Ileum** **C Ileocecal Valve** **E Large Intestine** **F Large Intestine, Right** **G Large Intestine, Left** **H Cecum** **K Ascending Colon** **L Transverse Colon** Hepatic flexure, Splenic flexure **M Descending Colon** **N Sigmoid Colon** Rectosigmoid junction, Sigmoid flexure **P Rectum** Anorectal junction	**7 Via Natural or Artificial Opening** **8 Via Natural or Artificial Opening Endoscopic**	**D Intraluminal Device** **Z No Device**	**Z No Qualifier**
Q Anus Anal orifice		**Ø Open** **3 Percutaneous** **4 Percutaneous Endoscopic** **X External**	**C Extraluminal Device** **D Intraluminal Device** **Z No Device**	**Z No Qualifier**
Q Anus Anal orifice		**7 Via Natural or Artificial Opening** **8 Via Natural or Artificial Opening Endoscopic**	**D Intraluminal Device** **Z No Device**	**Z No Qualifier**

Non-OR ØDV6[7,8]DZ
HAC ØDV64CZ when reported with PDx E66.Ø1 and SDx K68.11, K95.Ø1, K95.81, or T81.4Ø–T81.49 with 7th character A
NC ØDV6[7,8]DZ

Ø Medical and Surgical
D Gastrointestinal System
W Revision

Definition: Correcting, to the extent possible, a portion of a malfunctioning device or the position of a displaced device

Explanation: Revision can include correcting a malfunctioning or displaced device by taking out or putting in components of the device such as a screw or pin

Body Part Character 4	Approach Character 5	Device Character 6	Qualifier Character 7
Ø Upper Intestinal Tract D Lower Intestinal Tract	Ø Open 3 Percutaneous 4 Percutaneous Endoscopic 7 Via Natural or Artificial Opening 8 Via Natural or Artificial Opening Endoscopic	Ø Drainage Device 2 Monitoring Device 3 Infusion Device 7 Autologous Tissue Substitute C Extraluminal Device D Intraluminal Device J Synthetic Substitute K Nonautologous Tissue Substitute U Feeding Device Y Other Device	Z No Qualifier
Ø Upper Intestinal Tract D Lower Intestinal Tract	X External	Ø Drainage Device 2 Monitoring Device 3 Infusion Device 7 Autologous Tissue Substitute C Extraluminal Device D Intraluminal Device J Synthetic Substitute K Nonautologous Tissue Substitute U Feeding Device	Z No Qualifier
5 Esophagus	Ø Open 3 Percutaneous 4 Percutaneous Endoscopic	Y Other Device	Z No Qualifier
5 Esophagus	7 Via Natural or Artificial Opening 8 Via Natural or Artificial Opening Endoscopic	D Intraluminal Device Y Other Device	Z No Qualifier
5 Esophagus	X External	D Intraluminal Device	Z No Qualifier
6 Stomach	Ø Open 3 Percutaneous 4 Percutaneous Endoscopic	Ø Drainage Device 2 Monitoring Device 3 Infusion Device 7 Autologous Tissue Substitute C Extraluminal Device D Intraluminal Device J Synthetic Substitute K Nonautologous Tissue Substitute M Stimulator Lead U Feeding Device Y Other Device	Z No Qualifier
6 Stomach	7 Via Natural or Artificial Opening 8 Via Natural or Artificial Opening Endoscopic	Ø Drainage Device 2 Monitoring Device 3 Infusion Device 7 Autologous Tissue Substitute C Extraluminal Device D Intraluminal Device J Synthetic Substitute K Nonautologous Tissue Substitute U Feeding Device Y Other Device	Z No Qualifier
6 Stomach	X External	Ø Drainage Device 2 Monitoring Device 3 Infusion Device 7 Autologous Tissue Substitute C Extraluminal Device D Intraluminal Device J Synthetic Substitute K Nonautologous Tissue Substitute U Feeding Device	Z No Qualifier

Non-OR ØDW[Ø,D][3,4,7,8]YZ
Non-OR ØDW[Ø,D]8UZ
Non-OR ØDW[Ø,D]X[Ø,2,3,7,C,D,J,K,U]Z
Non-OR ØDW5[Ø,3,4]YZ
Non-OR ØDW5[7,8]YZ
Non-OR ØDW5XDZ
Non-OR ØDW6[3,4]YZ
Non-OR ØDW68UZ
Non-OR ØDW6[7,8]YZ
Non-OR ØDW6X[Ø,2,3,7,C,D,J,K,U]Z

ØDW Continued on next page

Ø Medical and Surgical
D Gastrointestinal System
W Revision

ØDW Continued

Definition: Correcting, to the extent possible, a portion of a malfunctioning device or the position of a displaced device

Explanation: Revision can include correcting a malfunctioning or displaced device by taking out or putting in components of the device such as a screw or pin

Body Part Character 4	Approach Character 5	Device Character 6	Qualifier Character 7
8 Small Intestine E Large Intestine	Ø Open 4 Percutaneous Endoscopic 7 Via Natural or Artificial Opening 8 Via Natural or Artificial Opening Endoscopic	7 Autologous Tissue Substitute J Synthetic Substitute K Nonautologous Tissue Substitute	Z No Qualifier
Q Anus Anal orifice	Ø Open 3 Percutaneous 4 Percutaneous Endoscopic 7 Via Natural or Artificial Opening 8 Via Natural or Artificial Opening Endoscopic	L Artificial Sphincter	Z No Qualifier
R Anal Sphincter External anal sphincter Internal anal sphincter	Ø Open 3 Percutaneous 4 Percutaneous Endoscopic	M Stimulator Lead	Z No Qualifier
U Omentum Gastrocolic ligament Gastrocolic omentum Gastrohepatic omentum Gastrophrenic ligament Gastrosplenic ligament Greater Omentum Hepatogastric ligament Lesser Omentum V Mesentery Mesoappendix Mesocolon W Peritoneum Epiploic foramen	Ø Open 3 Percutaneous 4 Percutaneous Endoscopic	Ø Drainage Device 7 Autologous Tissue Substitute J Synthetic Substitute K Nonautologous Tissue Substitute	Z No Qualifier

Non-OR ØDW[U,V,W][Ø,3,4]ØZ

Ø Medical and Surgical
D Gastrointestinal System
X Transfer

Definition: Moving, without taking out, all or a portion of a body part to another location to take over the function of all or a portion of a body part

Explanation: The body part transferred remains connected to its vascular and nervous supply

Body Part Character 4	Approach Character 5	Device Character 6	Qualifier Character 7
6 Stomach	Ø Open 4 Percutaneous Endoscopic	Z No Device	5 Esophagus
8 Small Intestine	Ø Open 4 Percutaneous Endoscopic	Z No Device	5 Esophagus B Bladder C Ureter, Right D Ureter, Left F Ureters, Bilateral
E Large Intestine	Ø Open 4 Percutaneous Endoscopic	Z No Device	5 Esophagus 7 Vagina ♀ B Bladder

♀ ØDXE[Ø,4]Z7

Ø Medical and Surgical
D Gastrointestinal System
Y Transplantation

Definition: Putting in or on all or a portion of a living body part taken from another individual or animal to physically take the place and/or function of all or a portion of a similar body part

Explanation: The native body part may or may not be taken out, and the transplanted body part may take over all or a portion of its function

Body Part Character 4	Approach Character 5	Device Character 6	Qualifier Character 7
5 Esophagus 6 Stomach 8 Small Intestine LC E Large Intestine LC	Ø Open	Z No Device	Ø Allogeneic 1 Syngeneic 2 Zooplastic

Non-OR ØDY5ØZ[Ø,1,2]
LC ØDY[8,E]ØZ[Ø,1,2]

Hepatobiliary System and Pancreas ØF1–ØFY

Character Meanings

This Character Meaning table is provided as a guide to assist the user in the identification of character members that may be found in this section of code tables. It **SHOULD NOT** be used to build a PCS code.

Operation–Character 3	Body Part–Character 4	Approach–Character 5	Device–Character 6	Qualifier–Character 7
1 Bypass	Ø Liver	Ø Open	Ø Drainage Device	Ø Allogeneic
2 Change	1 Liver, Right Lobe	3 Percutaneous	1 Radioactive Element	1 Syngeneic
5 Destruction	2 Liver, Left Lobe	4 Percutaneous Endoscopic	2 Monitoring Device	2 Zooplastic
7 Dilation	4 Gallbladder	7 Via Natural or Artificial Opening	3 Infusion Device	3 Duodenum OR Laser Interstitial Thermal Therapy
8 Division	5 Hepatic Duct, Right	8 Via Natural or Artificial Opening Endoscopic	7 Autologous Tissue Substitute	4 Stomach
9 Drainage	6 Hepatic Duct, Left	X External	C Extraluminal Device	5 Hepatic Duct, Right
B Excision	7 Hepatic Duct, Common		D Intraluminal Device	6 Hepatic Duct, Left
C Extirpation	8 Cystic Duct		J Synthetic Substitute	7 Hepatic Duct, Caudate
D Extraction	9 Common Bile Duct		K Nonautologous Tissue Substitute	8 Cystic Duct
F Fragmentation	B Hepatobiliary Duct		Y Other Device	9 Common Bile Duct
H Insertion	C Ampulla of Vater		Z No Device	B Small Intestine
J Inspection	D Pancreatic Duct			C Large Intestine
L Occlusion	F Pancreatic Duct, Accessory			F Irreversible Electroporation
M Reattachment	G Pancreas			X Diagnostic
N Release				Z No Qualifier
P Removal				
Q Repair				
R Replacement				
S Reposition				
T Resection				
U Supplement				
V Restriction				
W Revision				
Y Transplantation				

AHA Coding Clinic for table ØF1
2020, 4Q, 53 Bypass pancreatic duct to stomach

AHA Coding Clinic for table ØF5
2022, 4Q, 53-54 Laser interstitial thermal therapy
2018, 4Q, 39 Irreversible electroporation

AHA Coding Clinic for table ØF7
2016, 3Q, 27 Endoscopic retrograde cholangiopancreatography with sphincterotomy and insertion of pancreatic stent
2016, 1Q, 25 Endoscopic retrograde cholangiopancreatography with brush biopsy of pancreatic and common bile ducts
2015, 1Q, 32 Percutaneous transhepatic biliary drainage catheter placement
2014, 3Q, 15 Drainage of pancreatic pseudocyst

AHA Coding Clinic for table ØF8
2021, 4Q, 48-49 Division of liver for staged hepatectomy

AHA Coding Clinic for table ØF9
2023, 2Q, 22 Direct endoscopic necrosectomy
2020, 3Q, 34 Cystogastrostomy with stent insertion
2015, 1Q, 32 Percutaneous transhepatic biliary drainage catheter placement
2014, 3Q, 15 Drainage of pancreatic pseudocyst

AHA Coding Clinic for table ØFB
2023, 2Q, 22 Direct endoscopic necrosectomy
2023, 1Q, 38 Ex-vivo liver tumor resection and autotransplantation
2019, 1Q, 3-8 Whipple procedure
2016, 3Q, 41 Open cholecystectomy with needle biopsy of liver
2016, 1Q, 23 Endoscopic ultrasound with aspiration biopsy of common hepatic duct
2016, 1Q, 25 Endoscopic retrograde cholangiopancreatography with brush biopsy of pancreatic and common bile ducts
2014, 3Q, 32 Pyloric-sparing Whipple procedure

AHA Coding Clinic for table ØFC
2023, 2Q, 22 Direct endoscopic necrosectomy
2016, 3Q, 27 Endoscopic retrograde cholangiopancreatography with sphincterotomy and insertion of pancreatic stent

AHA Coding Clinic for table ØFD
2023, 2Q, 22 Direct endoscopic necrosectomy

AHA Coding Clinic for table ØFH
2022, 2Q, 26 Radioembolization of right hepatic lobe
2020, 4Q, 43-44 Insertion of radioactive element

AHA Coding Clinic for table ØFQ
2016, 3Q, 27 Revision of common bile duct anastomosis
2013, 4Q, 109 Separating conjoined twins

AHA Coding Clinic for table ØFT
2021, 4Q, 49 Division of liver for staged hepatectomy
2019, 1Q, 3-8 Whipple procedure
2012, 4Q, 99 Domino liver transplant

AHA Coding Clinic for table ØFY
2023, 2Q, 32 Preparation of donor organ before transplantation
2023, 1Q, 38 Ex-vivo liver tumor resection and autotransplantation
2014, 3Q, 13 Orthotopic liver transplant with end to side cavoplasty
2012, 4Q, 99 Domino liver transplant

Liver

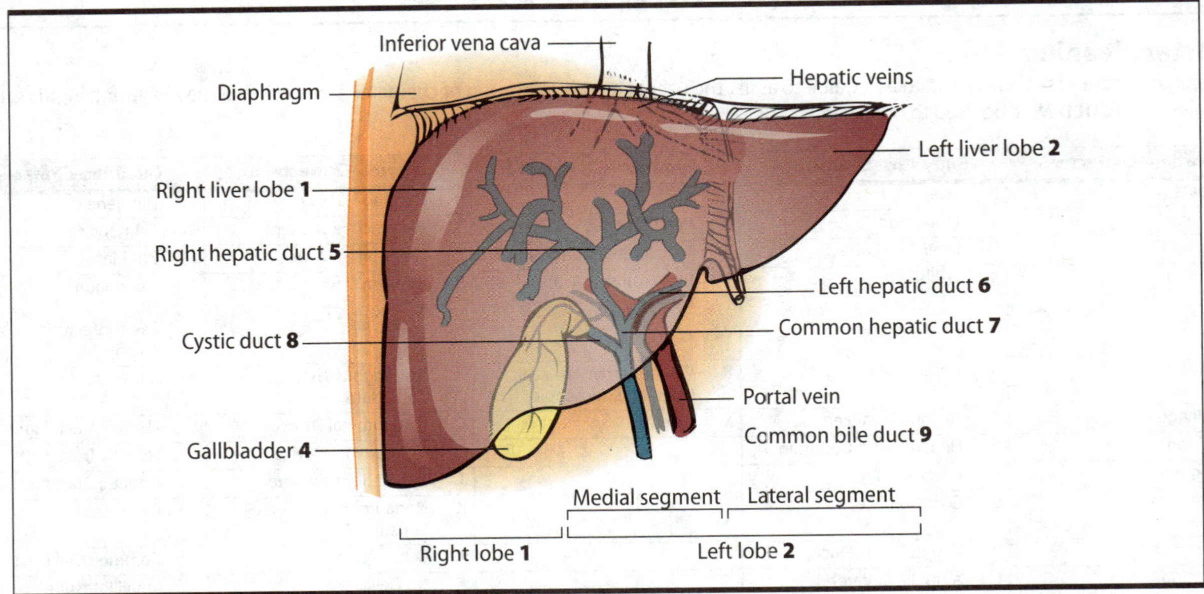

Pancreas

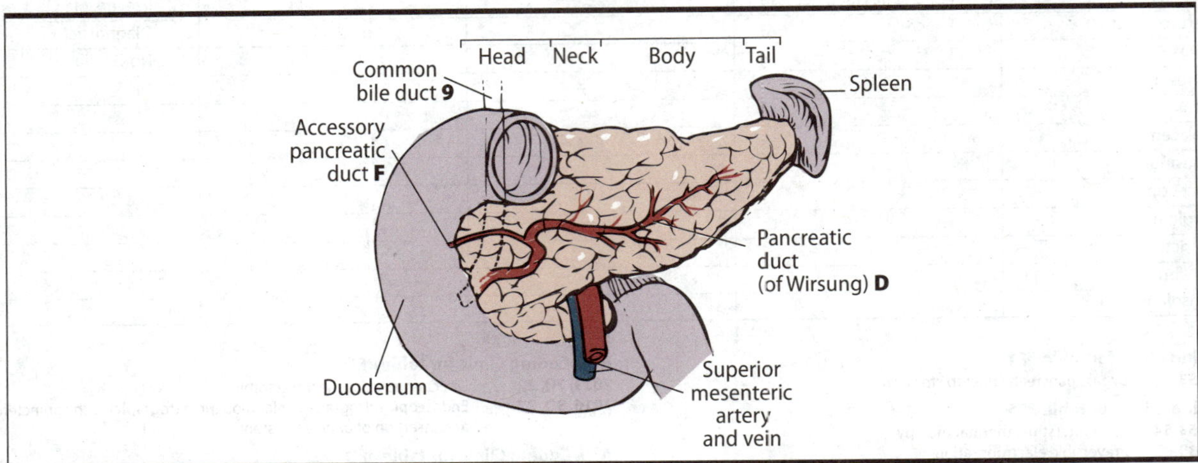

Gallbladder and Ducts

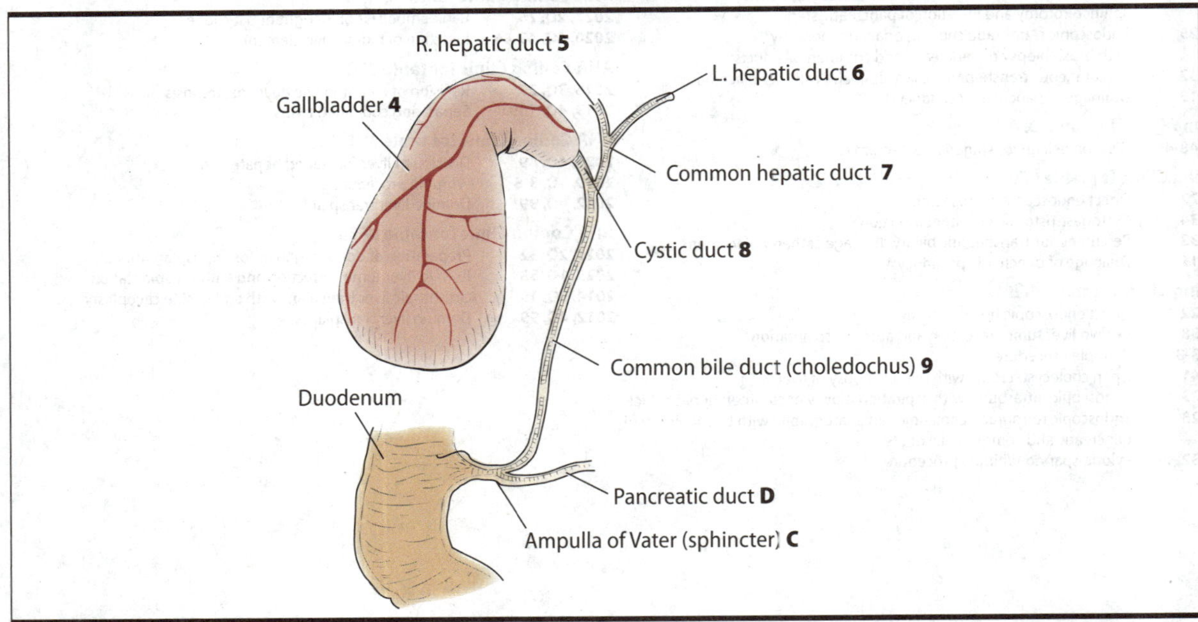

Ø Medical and Surgical
F Hepatobiliary System and Pancreas
1 Bypass Definition: Altering the route of passage of the contents of a tubular body part

Explanation: Rerouting contents of a body part to a downstream area of the normal route, to a similar route and body part, or to an abnormal route and dissimilar body part. Includes one or more anastomoses, with or without the use of a device.

Body Part Character 4	Approach Character 5	Device Character 6	Qualifier Character 7
4 Gallbladder 5 Hepatic Duct, Right 6 Hepatic Duct, Left 7 Hepatic Duct, Common 8 Cystic Duct 9 Common Bile Duct	Ø Open 4 Percutaneous Endoscopic	D Intraluminal Device Z No Device	3 Duodenum 4 Stomach 5 Hepatic Duct, Right 6 Hepatic Duct, Left 7 Hepatic Duct, Caudate 8 Cystic Duct 9 Common Bile Duct B Small Intestine
D Pancreatic Duct Duct of Wirsung	Ø Open 4 Percutaneous Endoscopic	D Intraluminal Device Z No Device	3 Duodenum 4 Stomach B Small Intestine C Large Intestine
F Pancreatic Duct, Accessory Duct of Santorini G Pancreas	Ø Open 4 Percutaneous Endoscopic	D Intraluminal Device Z No Device	3 Duodenum B Small Intestine C Large Intestine

Ø Medical and Surgical
F Hepatobiliary System and Pancreas
2 Change Definition: Taking out or off a device from a body part and putting back an identical or similar device in or on the same body part without cutting or puncturing the skin or a mucous membrane

Explanation: All CHANGE procedures are coded using the approach EXTERNAL

Body Part Character 4	Approach Character 5	Device Character 6	Qualifier Character 7
Ø Liver Quadrate lobe 4 Gallbladder B Hepatobiliary Duct D Pancreatic Duct Duct of Wirsung G Pancreas	X External	Ø Drainage Device Y Other Device	Z No Qualifier

Non-OR All body part, approach, device, and qualifier values

Ø Medical and Surgical
F Hepatobiliary System and Pancreas
5 Destruction Definition: Physical eradication of all or a portion of a body part by the direct use of energy, force, or a destructive agent

Explanation: None of the body part is physically taken out

Body Part Character 4	Approach Character 5	Device Character 6	Qualifier Character 7
Ø Liver Quadrate lobe 1 Liver, Right Lobe 2 Liver, Left Lobe	Ø Open 3 Percutaneous 4 Percutaneous Endoscopic	Z No Device	3 Laser Interstitial Thermal Therapy F Irreversible Electroporation Z No Qualifier
4 Gallbladder	Ø Open 3 Percutaneous 4 Percutaneous Endoscopic	Z No Device	3 Laser Interstitial Thermal Therapy Z No Qualifier
4 Gallbladder	8 Via Natural or Artificial Opening Endoscopic	Z No Device	Z No Qualifier
5 Hepatic Duct, Right 6 Hepatic Duct, Left 7 Hepatic Duct, Common 8 Cystic Duct 9 Common Bile Duct C Ampulla of Vater Duodenal ampulla Hepatopancreatic ampulla D Pancreatic Duct Duct of Wirsung F Pancreatic Duct, Accessory Duct of Santorini	Ø Open 3 Percutaneous 4 Percutaneous Endoscopic	Z No Device	3 Laser Interstitial Thermal Therapy Z No Qualifier
5 Hepatic Duct, Right 6 Hepatic Duct, Left 7 Hepatic Duct, Common 8 Cystic Duct 9 Common Bile Duct C Ampulla of Vater Duodenal ampulla Hepatopancreatic ampulla D Pancreatic Duct Duct of Wirsung F Pancreatic Duct, Accessory Duct of Santorini	7 Via Natural or Artificial Opening 8 Via Natural or Artificial Opening Endoscopic	Z No Device	Z No Qualifier
G Pancreas	Ø Open 3 Percutaneous 4 Percutaneous Endoscopic	Z No Device	3 Laser Interstitial Thermal Therapy F Irreversible Electroporation Z No Qualifier
G Pancreas	8 Via Natural or Artificial Opening Endoscopic	Z No Device	Z No Qualifier

DRG Non-OR ØF5[5,6,7,8,9,C,D,F]4Z3
DRG Non-OR ØF5G4Z3
Non-OR ØF5[5,6,7,8,9,C,D,F]4ZZ
Non-OR ØF5[5,6,7,8,9,C,D,F]8ZZ
Non-OR ØF5G4Z[F,Z]
Non-OR ØF5G8ZZ

Ø Medical and Surgical
F Hepatobiliary System and Pancreas
7 Dilation Definition: Expanding an orifice or the lumen of a tubular body part

Explanation: The orifice can be a natural orifice or an artificially created orifice. Accomplished by stretching a tubular body part using intraluminal pressure or by cutting part of the orifice or wall of the tubular body part.

Body Part Character 4	Approach Character 5	Device Character 6	Qualifier Character 7
5 Hepatic Duct, Right 6 Hepatic Duct, Left 7 Hepatic Duct, Common 8 Cystic Duct 9 Common Bile Duct C Ampulla of Vater Duodenal ampulla Hepatopancreatic ampulla D Pancreatic Duct Duct of Wirsung F Pancreatic Duct, Accessory Duct of Santorini	Ø Open 3 Percutaneous 4 Percutaneous Endoscopic 7 Via Natural or Artificial Opening 8 Via Natural or Artificial Opening Endoscopic	D Intraluminal Device Z No Device	Z No Qualifier

Non-OR ØF7[5,6,7,8,9][3,4,8][D,Z]Z
Non-OR ØF7[5,6,7,8,9,D]]7DZ
Non-OR ØF7C8[D,Z]Z
Non-OR ØF7[D,F][4,8][D,Z]Z

Ø Medical and Surgical
F Hepatobiliary System and Pancreas
8 Division

Definition: Cutting into a body part, without draining fluids and/or gases from the body part, in order to separate or transect a body part

Explanation: All or a portion of the body part is separated into two or more portions

Body Part Character 4	Approach Character 5	Device Character 6	Qualifier Character 7
Ø Liver 1 Liver, Right Lobe 2 Liver, Left Lobe G Pancreas	Ø Open 3 Percutaneous 4 Percutaneous Endoscopic	Z No Device	Z No Qualifier

Non-OR ØF8[Ø,1,2]3ZZ

Ø Medical and Surgical
F Hepatobiliary System and Pancreas
9 Drainage

Definition: Taking or letting out fluids and/or gases from a body part

Explanation: The qualifier DIAGNOSTIC is used to identify drainage procedures that are biopsies

Body Part Character 4	Approach Character 5	Device Character 6	Qualifier Character 7
Ø Liver Quadrate lobe 1 Liver, Right Lobe 2 Liver, Left Lobe	Ø Open 3 Percutaneous 4 Percutaneous Endoscopic	Ø Drainage Device	Z No Qualifier
Ø Liver Quadrate lobe 1 Liver, Right Lobe 2 Liver, Left Lobe	Ø Open 3 Percutaneous 4 Percutaneous Endoscopic	Z No Device	X Diagnostic Z No Qualifier
4 Gallbladder G Pancreas	Ø Open 3 Percutaneous 4 Percutaneous Endoscopic 8 Via Natural or Artificial Opening Endoscopic	Ø Drainage Device	Z No Qualifier
4 Gallbladder G Pancreas	Ø Open 3 Percutaneous 4 Percutaneous Endoscopic 8 Via Natural or Artificial Opening Endoscopic	Z No Device	X Diagnostic Z No Qualifier
5 Hepatic Duct, Right 6 Hepatic Duct, Left 7 Hepatic Duct, Common 8 Cystic Duct 9 Common Bile Duct C Ampulla of Vater Duodenal ampulla Hepatopancreatic ampulla D Pancreatic Duct Duct of Wirsung F Pancreatic Duct, Accessory Duct of Santorini	Ø Open 3 Percutaneous 4 Percutaneous Endoscopic 7 Via Natural or Artificial Opening 8 Via Natural or Artificial Opening Endoscopic	Ø Drainage Device	Z No Qualifier
5 Hepatic Duct, Right 6 Hepatic Duct, Left 7 Hepatic Duct, Common 8 Cystic Duct 9 Common Bile Duct C Ampulla of Vater Duodenal ampulla Hepatopancreatic ampulla D Pancreatic Duct Duct of Wirsung F Pancreatic Duct, Accessory Duct of Santorini	Ø Open 3 Percutaneous 4 Percutaneous Endoscopic 7 Via Natural or Artificial Opening 8 Via Natural or Artificial Opening Endoscopic	Z No Device	X Diagnostic Z No Qualifier

Non-OR ØF9[Ø,1,2][3,4]ØZ
Non-OR ØF9[Ø,1,2][3,4]Z[X,Z]
Non-OR ØF9[4,G]8ØZ
Non-OR ØF9G3ØZ
Non-OR ØF9[4,G]8Z[X,Z]
Non-OR ØF9G3Z[XZ]
Non-OR ØF9G4ZX
Non-OR ØF9[5,6,8][3,8]ØZ
Non-OR ØF97[3,4,7,8]ØZ
Non-OR ØF99[3,8]ØZ
Non-OR ØF9C[3,4,8]ØZ
Non-OR ØF9[D,F][3,8]ØZ
Non-OR ØF9[5,6,8,9,C,D,F]3Z[X,Z]
Non-OR ØF9[5,6,8,9,C,D,F][4,7,8]ZX
Non-OR ØF9[5,6,8,D,F]8ZZ
Non-OR ØF97[3,4,7,8]Z[X,Z]
Non-OR ØF99[4,7,8]ZZ
Non-OR ØF9C[4,8]ZZ

Ø Medical and Surgical
F Hepatobiliary System and Pancreas
B Excision Definition: Cutting out or off, without replacement, a portion of a body part
Explanation: The qualifier DIAGNOSTIC is used to identify excision procedures that are biopsies

Body Part Character 4	Approach Character 5	Device Character 6	Qualifier Character 7
Ø Liver Quadrate lobe **1** Liver, Right Lobe **2** Liver, Left Lobe	**Ø** Open **3** Percutaneous **4** Percutaneous Endoscopic	**Z** No Device	**X** Diagnostic **Z** No Qualifier
4 Gallbladder **G** Pancreas	**Ø** Open **3** Percutaneous **4** Percutaneous Endoscopic **8** Via Natural or Artificial Opening Endoscopic	**Z** No Device	**X** Diagnostic **Z** No Qualifier
5 Hepatic Duct, Right **6** Hepatic Duct, Left **7** Hepatic Duct, Common **8** Cystic Duct **9** Common Bile Duct **C** Ampulla of Vater Duodenal ampulla Hepatopancreatic ampulla **D** Pancreatic Duct Duct of Wirsung **F** Pancreatic Duct, Accessory Duct of Santorini	**Ø** Open **3** Percutaneous **4** Percutaneous Endoscopic **7** Via Natural or Artificial Opening **8** Via Natural or Artificial Opening Endoscopic	**Z** No Device	**X** Diagnostic **Z** No Qualifier

Non-OR ØFB[Ø,1,2]3ZX
Non-OR ØFB[4,G][3,4,8]ZX
Non-OR ØFB[5,6,7,8,9,C,D,F][3,4,7,8]ZX
Non-OR ØFB[5,6,7,8,9,C,D,F][4,8]ZZ

Ø Medical and Surgical
F Hepatobiliary System and Pancreas
C Extirpation Definition: Taking or cutting out solid matter from a body part
Explanation: The solid matter may be an abnormal byproduct of a biological function or a foreign body; it may be imbedded in a body part or in the lumen of a tubular body part. The solid matter may or may not have been previously broken into pieces.

Body Part Character 4	Approach Character 5	Device Character 6	Qualifier Character 7
Ø Liver Quadrate lobe **1** Liver, Right Lobe **2** Liver, Left Lobe	**Ø** Open **3** Percutaneous **4** Percutaneous Endoscopic	**Z** No Device	**Z** No Qualifier
4 Gallbladder **G** Pancreas	**Ø** Open **3** Percutaneous **4** Percutaneous Endoscopic **8** Via Natural or Artificial Opening Endoscopic	**Z** No Device	**Z** No Qualifier
5 Hepatic Duct, Right **6** Hepatic Duct, Left **7** Hepatic Duct, Common **8** Cystic Duct **9** Common Bile Duct **C** Ampulla of Vater Duodenal ampulla Hepatopancreatic ampulla **D** Pancreatic Duct Duct of Wirsung **F** Pancreatic Duct, Accessory Duct of Santorini	**Ø** Open **3** Percutaneous **4** Percutaneous Endoscopic **7** Via Natural or Artificial Opening **8** Via Natural or Artificial Opening Endoscopic	**Z** No Device	**Z** No Qualifier

Non-OR ØFC[5,6,7,8][3,4,7,8]ZZ
Non-OR ØFC9[3,7,8]ZZ
Non-OR ØFCC[4,8]ZZ
Non-OR ØFC[D,F][3,4,8]ZZ

Ø Medical and Surgical
F Hepatobiliary System and Pancreas
D Extraction Definition: Pulling or stripping out or off all or a portion of a body part by the use of force

Explanation: The qualifier DIAGNOSTIC is used to identify extraction procedures that are biopsies

Body Part Character 4	Approach Character 5	Device Character 6	Qualifier Character 7
Ø Liver Quadrate lobe 1 Liver, Right Lobe 2 Liver, Left Lobe	3 Percutaneous 4 Percutaneous Endoscopic	Z No Device	X Diagnostic
4 Gallbladder 5 Hepatic Duct, Right 6 Hepatic Duct, Left 7 Hepatic Duct, Common 8 Cystic Duct 9 Common Bile Duct C Ampulla of Vater Duodenal ampulla Hepatopancreatic ampulla D Pancreatic Duct Duct of Wirsung F Pancreatic Duct, Accessory Duct of Santorini G Pancreas	3 Percutaneous 4 Percutaneous Endoscopic 8 Via Natural or Artificial Opening Endoscopic	Z No Device	X Diagnostic

Non-OR ØFD[Ø,1,2]3ZX
Non-OR ØFD[4,5,6,7,8,9,C,D,F,G][3,4,8]ZX

Ø Medical and Surgical
F Hepatobiliary System and Pancreas
F Fragmentation Definition: Breaking solid matter in a body part into pieces

Explanation: Physical force (e.g., manual, ultrasonic) applied directly or indirectly is used to break the solid matter into pieces. The solid matter may be an abnormal byproduct of a biological function or a foreign body. The pieces of solid matter are not taken out.

Body Part Character 4	Approach Character 5	Device Character 6	Qualifier Character 7
4 Gallbladder NC 5 Hepatic Duct, Right NC 6 Hepatic Duct, Left NC 7 Hepatic Duct, Common 8 Cystic Duct NC 9 Common Bile Duct NC C Ampulla of Vater NC Duodenal ampulla Hepatopancreatic ampulla D Pancreatic Duct NC Duct of Wirsung F Pancreatic Duct, Accessory NC Duct of Santorini	Ø Open 3 Percutaneous 4 Percutaneous Endoscopic 7 Via Natural or Artificial Opening 8 Via Natural or Artificial Opening Endoscopic X External	Z No Device	Z No Qualifier

Non-OR ØFF[4,5,6,7,8,9,C,D,F][8,X]ZZ
NC ØFF[4,5,6,8,9,C,D,F]XZZ

Ø Medical and Surgical
F Hepatobiliary System and Pancreas
H Insertion Definition: Putting in a nonbiological appliance that monitors, assists, performs, or prevents a physiological function but does not physically take the place of a body part

Explanation: None

Body Part Character 4	Approach Character 5	Device Character 6	Qualifier Character 7
Ø Liver Quadrate lobe 4 Gallbladder G Pancreas	Ø Open 3 Percutaneous 4 Percutaneous Endoscopic	1 Radioactive Element 2 Monitoring Device 3 Infusion Device Y Other Device	Z No Qualifier
1 Liver, Right Lobe 2 Liver, Left Lobe	Ø Open 3 Percutaneous 4 Percutaneous Endoscopic	2 Monitoring Device 3 Infusion Device	Z No Qualifier
B Hepatobiliary Duct ⊞ D Pancreatic Duct Duct of Wirsung	Ø Open 3 Percutaneous 4 Percutaneous Endoscopic 7 Via Natural or Artificial Opening 8 Via Natural or Artificial Opening Endoscopic	1 Radioactive Element 2 Monitoring Device 3 Infusion Device D Intraluminal Device Y Other Device	Z No Qualifier

Non-OR ØFH[Ø,4,G]31Z
Non-OR ØFH[Ø,4,G][Ø,3,4]3Z
Non-OR ØFH[Ø,4,G][3,4]YZ
Non-OR ØFH[1,2][Ø,3,4]3Z
Non-OR ØFH[B,D][Ø,3,4]3Z
Non-OR ØFH[B,D][4,8]DZ
Non-OR ØFH[B,D][7,8][2,3]Z
Non-OR ØFH[B,D][3,4,7,8]YZ

See Appendix L for Procedure Combinations
⊞ ØFHB7DZ

Ø Medical and Surgical
F Hepatobiliary System and Pancreas
J Inspection Definition: Visually and/or manually exploring a body part

Explanation: Visual exploration may be performed with or without optical instrumentation. Manual exploration may be performed directly or through intervening body layers.

Body Part Character 4	Approach Character 5	Device Character 6	Qualifier Character 7
Ø Liver Quadrate lobe	**Ø Open** **3 Percutaneous** **4 Percutaneous Endoscopic** **X External**	**Z No Device**	**Z No Qualifier**
4 Gallbladder **G Pancreas**	**Ø Open** **3 Percutaneous** **4 Percutaneous Endoscopic** **8 Via Natural or Artificial Opening Endoscopic** **X External**	**Z No Device**	**Z No Qualifier**
B Hepatobiliary Duct **D Pancreatic Duct** Duct of Wirsung	**Ø Open** **3 Percutaneous** **4 Percutaneous Endoscopic** **7 Via Natural or Artificial Opening** **8 Via Natural or Artificial Opening Endoscopic**	**Z No Device**	**Z No Qualifier**

Non-OR ØFJØ[3,X]ZZ
Non-OR ØFJ[4,G][3,8,X]ZZ
Non-OR ØFJ[B,D][3,7,8]ZZ

Ø Medical and Surgical
F Hepatobiliary System and Pancreas
L Occlusion Definition: Completely closing an orifice or the lumen of a tubular body part

Explanation: The orifice can be a natural orifice or an artificially created orifice

Body Part Character 4	Approach Character 5	Device Character 6	Qualifier Character 7
5 Hepatic Duct, Right **6 Hepatic Duct, Left** **7 Hepatic Duct, Common** **8 Cystic Duct** **9 Common Bile Duct** **C Ampulla of Vater** Duodenal ampulla Hepatopancreatic ampulla **D Pancreatic Duct** Duct of Wirsung **F Pancreatic Duct, Accessory** Duct of Santorini	**Ø Open** **3 Percutaneous** **4 Percutaneous Endoscopic**	**C Extraluminal Device** **D Intraluminal Device** **Z No Device**	**Z No Qualifier**
5 Hepatic Duct, Right **6 Hepatic Duct, Left** **7 Hepatic Duct, Common** **8 Cystic Duct** **9 Common Bile Duct** **C Ampulla of Vater** Duodenal ampulla Hepatopancreatic ampulla **D Pancreatic Duct** Duct of Wirsung **F Pancreatic Duct, Accessory** Duct of Santorini	**7 Via Natural or Artificial Opening** **8 Via Natural or Artificial Opening Endoscopic**	**D Intraluminal Device** **Z No Device**	**Z No Qualifier**

Non-OR ØFL[5,6,7,8,9][3,4][C,D,Z]Z
Non-OR ØFL[5,6,7,8,9][7,8][D,Z]Z

Ø Medical and Surgical
F Hepatobiliary System and Pancreas
M Reattachment Definition: Putting back in or on all or a portion of a separated body part to its normal location or other suitable location
Explanation: Vascular circulation and nervous pathways may or may not be reestablished

Body Part Character 4	Approach Character 5	Device Character 6	Qualifier Character 7
Ø Liver Quadrate lobe **1 Liver, Right Lobe** **2 Liver, Left Lobe** **4 Gallbladder** **5 Hepatic Duct, Right** **6 Hepatic Duct, Left** **7 Hepatic Duct, Common** **8 Cystic Duct** **9 Common Bile Duct** **C Ampulla of Vater** Duodenal ampulla Hepatopancreatic ampulla **D Pancreatic Duct** Duct of Wirsung **F Pancreatic Duct, Accessory** Duct of Santorini **G Pancreas**	**Ø Open** **4 Percutaneous Endoscopic**	**Z No Device**	**Z No Qualifier**

Non-OR ØFM[4,5,6,7,8,9]4ZZ

Ø Medical and Surgical
F Hepatobiliary System and Pancreas
N Release Definition: Freeing a body part from an abnormal physical constraint by cutting or by the use of force
Explanation: Some of the restraining tissue may be taken out but none of the body part is taken out

Body Part Character 4	Approach Character 5	Device Character 6	Qualifier Character 7
Ø Liver Quadrate lobe **1 Liver, Right Lobe** **2 Liver, Left Lobe**	**Ø Open** **3 Percutaneous** **4 Percutaneous Endoscopic**	**Z No Device**	**Z No Qualifier**
4 Gallbladder **G Pancreas**	**Ø Open** **3 Percutaneous** **4 Percutaneous Endoscopic** **8 Via Natural or Artificial Opening Endoscopic**	**Z No Device**	**Z No Qualifier**
5 Hepatic Duct, Right **6 Hepatic Duct, Left** **7 Hepatic Duct, Common** **8 Cystic Duct** **9 Common Bile Duct** **C Ampulla of Vater** Duodenal ampulla Hepatopancreatic ampulla **D Pancreatic Duct** Duct of Wirsung **F Pancreatic Duct, Accessory** Duct of Santorini	**Ø Open** **3 Percutaneous** **4 Percutaneous Endoscopic** **7 Via Natural or Artificial Opening** **8 Via Natural or Artificial Opening Endoscopic**	**Z No Device**	**Z No Qualifier**

Ø Medical and Surgical
F Hepatobiliary System and Pancreas
P Removal Definition: Taking out or off a device from a body part

Explanation: If a device is taken out and a similar device put in without cutting or puncturing the skin or mucous membrane, the procedure is coded to the root operation CHANGE. Otherwise, the procedure for taking out a device is coded to the root operation REMOVAL.

Body Part Character 4	Approach Character 5	Device Character 6	Qualifier Character 7
Ø Liver Quadrate lobe	Ø Open 3 Percutaneous 4 Percutaneous Endoscopic	Ø Drainage Device 2 Monitoring Device 3 Infusion Device Y Other Device	Z No Qualifier
Ø Liver Quadrate lobe	X External	Ø Drainage Device 2 Monitoring Device 3 Infusion Device	Z No Qualifier
4 Gallbladder G Pancreas	Ø Open 3 Percutaneous 4 Percutaneous Endoscopic	Ø Drainage Device 2 Monitoring Device 3 Infusion Device D Intraluminal Device Y Other Device	Z No Qualifier
4 Gallbladder G Pancreas	X External	Ø Drainage Device 2 Monitoring Device 3 Infusion Device D Intraluminal Device	Z No Qualifier
B Hepatobiliary Duct D Pancreatic Duct Duct of Wirsung	Ø Open 3 Percutaneous 4 Percutaneous Endoscopic 7 Via Natural or Artificial Opening 8 Via Natural or Artificial Opening Endoscopic	Ø Drainage Device 1 Radioactive Element 2 Monitoring Device 3 Infusion Device 7 Autologous Tissue Substitute C Extraluminal Device D Intraluminal Device J Synthetic Substitute K Nonautologous Tissue Substitute Y Other Device	Z No Qualifier
B Hepatobiliary Duct D Pancreatic Duct Duct of Wirsung	X External	Ø Drainage Device 1 Radioactive Element 2 Monitoring Device 3 Infusion Device D Intraluminal Device	Z No Qualifier

Non-OR ØFPØ[3,4]YZ
Non-OR ØFPØX[Ø,2,3]Z
Non-OR ØFPG3ØZ
Non-OR ØFP[4,G][3,4]YZ
Non-OR ØFP4X[Ø,2,3,D]Z
Non-OR ØFPGX[Ø,2,3]Z
Non-OR ØFP[B,D][3,4]YZ
Non-OR ØFP[B,D][7,8][Ø,2,3,D,Y]Z
Non-OR ØFP[B,D]X[Ø,1,2,3,D]Z

See Appendix L for Procedure Combinations
Combo-only ØFP[B,D][7,8]DZ
Combo-only ØFP[B,D]XDZ

Ø Medical and Surgical
F Hepatobiliary System and Pancreas
Q Repair Definition: Restoring, to the extent possible, a body part to its normal anatomic structure and function
Explanation: Used only when the method to accomplish the repair is not one of the other root operations

Body Part Character 4	Approach Character 5	Device Character 6	Qualifier Character 7
Ø Liver Quadrate lobe 1 Liver, Right Lobe 2 Liver, Left Lobe	Ø Open 3 Percutaneous 4 Percutaneous Endoscopic	Z No Device	Z No Qualifier
4 Gallbladder G Pancreas	Ø Open 3 Percutaneous 4 Percutaneous Endoscopic 8 Via Natural or Artificial Opening Endoscopic	Z No Device	Z No Qualifier
5 Hepatic Duct, Right 6 Hepatic Duct, Left 7 Hepatic Duct, Common 8 Cystic Duct 9 Common Bile Duct C Ampulla of Vater Duodenal ampulla Hepatopancreatic ampulla D Pancreatic Duct Duct of Wirsung F Pancreatic Duct, Accessory Duct of Santorini	Ø Open 3 Percutaneous 4 Percutaneous Endoscopic 7 Via Natural or Artificial Opening 8 Via Natural or Artificial Opening Endoscopic	Z No Device	Z No Qualifier

Ø Medical and Surgical
F Hepatobiliary System and Pancreas
R Replacement Definition: Putting in or on biological or synthetic material that physically takes the place and/or function of all or a portion of a body part
Explanation: The body part may have been taken out or replaced, or may be taken out, physically eradicated, or rendered nonfunctional during the REPLACEMENT procedure. A REMOVAL procedure is coded for taking out the device used in a previous replacement procedure.

Body Part Character 4	Approach Character 5	Device Character 6	Qualifier Character 7
5 Hepatic Duct, Right 6 Hepatic Duct, Left 7 Hepatic Duct, Common 8 Cystic Duct 9 Common Bile Duct C Ampulla of Vater Duodenal ampulla Hepatopancreatic ampulla D Pancreatic Duct Duct of Wirsung F Pancreatic Duct, Accessory Duct of Santorini	Ø Open 4 Percutaneous Endoscopic 8 Via Natural or Artificial Opening Endoscopic	7 Autologous Tissue Substitute J Synthetic Substitute K Nonautologous Tissue Substitute	Z No Qualifier

Ø Medical and Surgical
F Hepatobiliary System and Pancreas
S Reposition Definition: Moving to its normal location, or other suitable location, all or a portion of a body part
Explanation: The body part is moved to a new location from an abnormal location, or from a normal location where it is not functioning correctly. The body part may or may not be cut out or off to be moved to the new location.

Body Part Character 4	Approach Character 5	Device Character 6	Qualifier Character 7
Ø Liver Quadrate lobe 4 Gallbladder 5 Hepatic Duct, Right 6 Hepatic Duct, Left 7 Hepatic Duct, Common 8 Cystic Duct 9 Common Bile Duct C Ampulla of Vater Duodenal ampulla Hepatopancreatic ampulla D Pancreatic Duct Duct of Wirsung F Pancreatic Duct, Accessory Duct of Santorini G Pancreas	Ø Open 4 Percutaneous Endoscopic	Z No Device	Z No Qualifier

Ø Medical and Surgical
F Hepatobiliary System and Pancreas
T Resection Definition: Cutting out or off, without replacement, all of a body part

Explanation: None

Body Part Character 4	Approach Character 5	Device Character 6	Qualifier Character 7
Ø Liver Quadrate lobe **1** Liver, Right Lobe **2** Liver, Left Lobe **4** Gallbladder **G** Pancreas ⊞	**Ø** Open **4** Percutaneous Endoscopic	**Z** No Device	**Z** No Qualifier
5 Hepatic Duct, Right **6** Hepatic Duct, Left **7** Hepatic Duct, Common **8** Cystic Duct **9** Common Bile Duct **C** Ampulla of Vater Duodenal ampulla Hepatopancreatic ampulla **D** Pancreatic Duct Duct of Wirsung **F** Pancreatic Duct, Accessory Duct of Santorini	**Ø** Open **4** Percutaneous Endoscopic **7** Via Natural or Artificial Opening **8** Via Natural or Artificial Opening Endoscopic	**Z** No Device	**Z** No Qualifier

Non-OR ØFT[D,F][4,8]ZZ

See Appendix L for Procedure Combinations
⊞ ØFTGØZZ

Ø Medical and Surgical
F Hepatobiliary System and Pancreas
U Supplement Definition: Putting in or on biological or synthetic material that physically reinforces and/or augments the function of a portion of a body part

Explanation: The biological material is non-living, or is living and from the same individual. The body part may have been previously replaced, and the SUPPLEMENT procedure is performed to physically reinforce and/or augment the function of the replaced body part.

Body Part Character 4	Approach Character 5	Device Character 6	Qualifier Character 7
5 Hepatic Duct, Right **6** Hepatic Duct, Left **7** Hepatic Duct, Common **8** Cystic Duct **9** Common Bile Duct **C** Ampulla of Vater Duodenal ampulla Hepatopancreatic ampulla **D** Pancreatic Duct Duct of Wirsung **F** Pancreatic Duct, Accessory Duct of Santorini	**Ø** Open **3** Percutaneous **4** Percutaneous Endoscopic **8** Via Natural or Artificial Opening Endoscopic	**7** Autologous Tissue Substitute **J** Synthetic Substitute **K** Nonautologous Tissue Substitute	**Z** No Qualifier

Ø Medical and Surgical
F Hepatobiliary System and Pancreas
V Restriction Definition: Partially closing an orifice or the lumen of a tubular body part
Explanation: The orifice can be a natural orifice or an artificially created orifice

Body Part Character 4	Approach Character 5	Device Character 6	Qualifier Character 7
5 Hepatic Duct, Right **6 Hepatic Duct, Left** **7 Hepatic Duct, Common** **8 Cystic Duct** **9 Common Bile Duct** **C Ampulla of Vater** Duodenal ampulla Hepatopancreatic ampulla **D Pancreatic Duct** Duct of Wirsung **F Pancreatic Duct, Accessory** Duct of Santorini	**Ø Open** **3 Percutaneous** **4 Percutaneous Endoscopic**	**C Extraluminal Device** **D Intraluminal Device** **Z No Device**	**Z No Qualifier**
5 Hepatic Duct, Right **6 Hepatic Duct, Left** **7 Hepatic Duct, Common** **8 Cystic Duct** **9 Common Bile Duct** **C Ampulla of Vater** Duodenal ampulla Hepatopancreatic ampulla **D Pancreatic Duct** Duct of Wirsung **F Pancreatic Duct, Accessory** Duct of Santorini	**7 Via Natural or Artificial Opening** **8 Via Natural or Artificial Opening Endoscopic**	**D Intraluminal Device** **Z No Device**	**Z No Qualifier**

Non-OR ØFV[5,6,7,8,9][3,4][C,D,Z]Z
Non-OR ØFV[5,6,7,8,9][7,8][D,Z]Z

Hepatobiliary System and Pancreas

Ø Medical and Surgical
F Hepatobiliary System and Pancreas
W Revision Definition: Correcting, to the extent possible, a portion of a malfunctioning device or the position of a displaced device

Explanation: Revision can include correcting a malfunctioning or displaced device by taking out or putting in components of the device such as a screw or pin

Body Part Character 4	Approach Character 5	Device Character 6	Qualifier Character 7
Ø Liver Quadrate lobe	Ø Open 3 Percutaneous 4 Percutaneous Endoscopic	Ø Drainage Device 2 Monitoring Device 3 Infusion Device Y Other Device	Z No Qualifier
Ø Liver Quadrate lobe	X External	Ø Drainage Device 2 Monitoring Device 3 Infusion Device	Z No Qualifier
4 Gallbladder G Pancreas	Ø Open 3 Percutaneous 4 Percutaneous Endoscopic	Ø Drainage Device 2 Monitoring Device 3 Infusion Device D Intraluminal Device Y Other Device	Z No Qualifier
4 Gallbladder G Pancreas	X External	Ø Drainage Device 2 Monitoring Device 3 Infusion Device D Intraluminal Device	Z No Qualifier
B Hepatobiliary Duct D Pancreatic Duct Duct of Wirsung	Ø Open 3 Percutaneous 4 Percutaneous Endoscopic 7 Via Natural or Artificial Opening 8 Via Natural or Artificial Opening Endoscopic	Ø Drainage Device 2 Monitoring Device 3 Infusion Device 7 Autologous Tissue Substitute C Extraluminal Device D Intraluminal Device J Synthetic Substitute K Nonautologous Tissue Substitute Y Other Device	Z No Qualifier
B Hepatobiliary Duct D Pancreatic Duct Duct of Wirsung	X External	Ø Drainage Device 2 Monitoring Device 3 Infusion Device 7 Autologous Tissue Substitute C Extraluminal Device D Intraluminal Device J Synthetic Substitute K Nonautologous Tissue Substitute	Z No Qualifier

Non-OR ØFWØ[3,4]YZ
Non-OR ØFWØX[Ø,2,3]Z
Non-OR ØFW[4,G][3,4]YZ
Non-OR ØFW[4,G]X[Ø,2,3,D]Z
Non-OR ØFW[B,D][3,4,7,8]YZ
Non-OR ØFW[B,D]X[Ø,2,3,7,C,D,J,K]Z

Ø Medical and Surgical
F Hepatobiliary System and Pancreas
Y Transplantation Definition: Putting in or on all or a portion of a living body part taken from another individual or animal to physically take the place and/or function of all or a portion of a similar body part

Explanation: The native body part may or may not be taken out, and the transplanted body part may take over all or a portion of its function

Body Part Character 4	Approach Character 5	Device Character 6	Qualifier Character 7
Ø Liver LC Quadrate lobe G Pancreas LC NC ⊞	Ø Open	Z No Device	Ø Allogeneic 1 Syngeneic 2 Zooplastic

LC ØFYØØZ[Ø,1,2]
LC ØFYGØZ[Ø,1]
NC ØFYGØZ2
NC ØFYGØZ[Ø,1] If reported alone without one of the following procedures ØTYØØZ[Ø,1,2], ØTY1ØZ[Ø,1,2] and without one of the following diagnoses E1Ø.1Ø-E1Ø.9, E89.1

See Appendix L for Procedure Combinations
⊞ ØFYGØZ[Ø,1,2]

Endocrine System ØG2–ØGW

Character Meanings

This Character Meaning table is provided as a guide to assist the user in the identification of character members that may be found in this section of code tables. It **SHOULD NOT** be used to build a PCS code.

Operation–Character 3		Body Part–Character 4		Approach–Character 5		Device–Character 6		Qualifier–Character 7	
2	Change	Ø	Pituitary Gland	Ø	Open	Ø	Drainage Device	3	Laser Interstitial Thermal Therapy
5	Destruction	1	Pineal Body	3	Percutaneous	1	Radioactive Element	X	Diagnostic
8	Division	2	Adrenal Gland, Left	4	Percutaneous Endoscopic	2	Monitoring Device	Z	No Qualifier
9	Drainage	3	Adrenal Gland, Right	X	External	3	Infusion Device		
B	Excision	4	Adrenal Glands, Bilateral			Y	Other Device		
C	Extirpation	5	Adrenal Gland			Z	No Device		
H	Insertion	6	Carotid Body, Left						
J	Inspection	7	Carotid Body, Right						
M	Reattachment	8	Carotid Bodies, Bilateral						
N	Release	9	Para-aortic Body						
P	Removal	B	Coccygeal Glomus						
Q	Repair	C	Glomus Jugulare						
S	Reposition	D	Aortic Body						
T	Resection	F	Paraganglion Extremity						
W	Revision	G	Thyroid Gland Lobe, Left						
		H	Thyroid Gland Lobe, Right						
		J	Thyroid Gland Isthmus						
		K	Thyroid Gland						
		L	Superior Parathyroid Gland, Right						
		M	Superior Parathyroid Gland, Left						
		N	Inferior Parathyroid Gland, Right						
		P	Inferior Parathyroid Gland, Left						
		Q	Parathyroid Glands, Multiple						
		R	Parathyroid Gland						
		S	Endocrine Gland						

AHA Coding Clinic for table ØG5
2022, 4Q, 53-54 Laser interstitial thermal therapy

AHA Coding Clinic for table ØGB
2021, 2Q, 7 Infrarenal para-aortic paraganglioma with excision
2017, 2Q, 20 Near total thyroidectomy
2014, 3Q, 22 Transsphenoidal removal of pituitary tumor and fat graft placement

AHA Coding Clinic for table ØGH
2020, 4Q, 43-44 Insertion of radioactive element

AHA Coding Clinic for table ØGT
2017, 2Q, 20 Near total thyroidectomy

Endocrine System

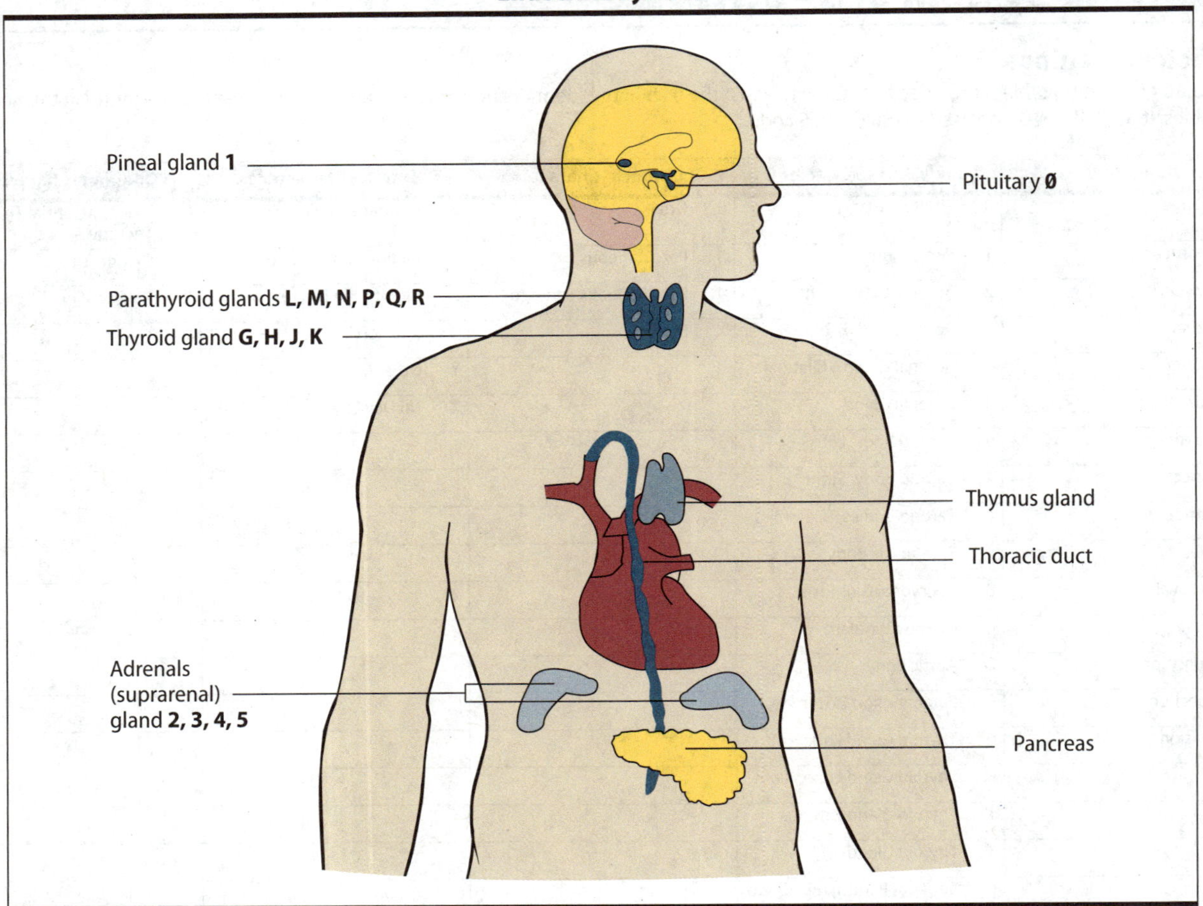

Left Adrenal Gland

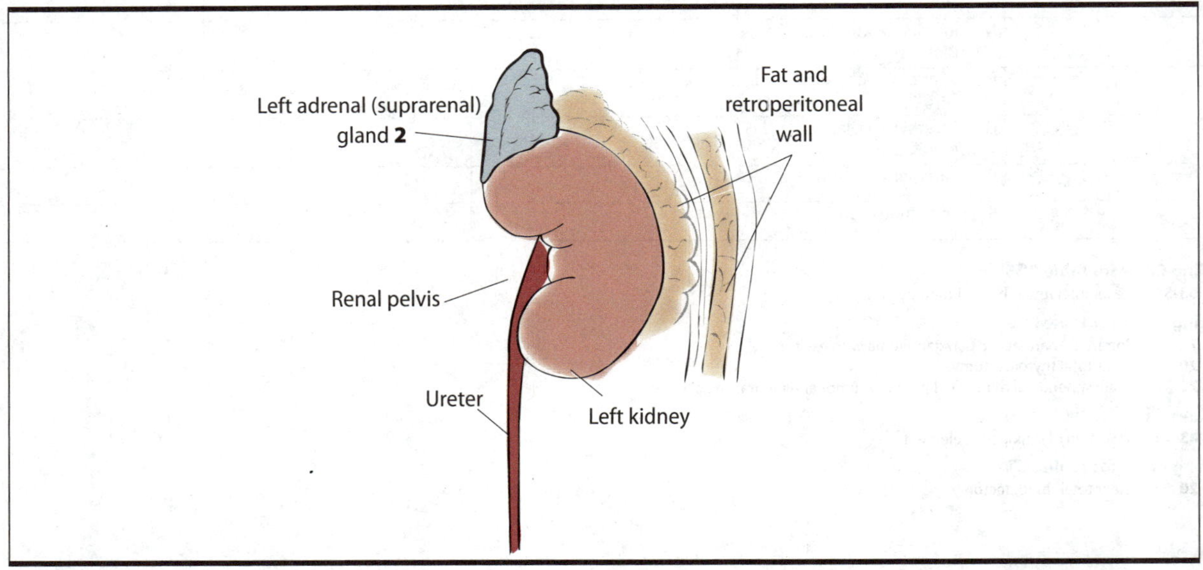

Thyroid

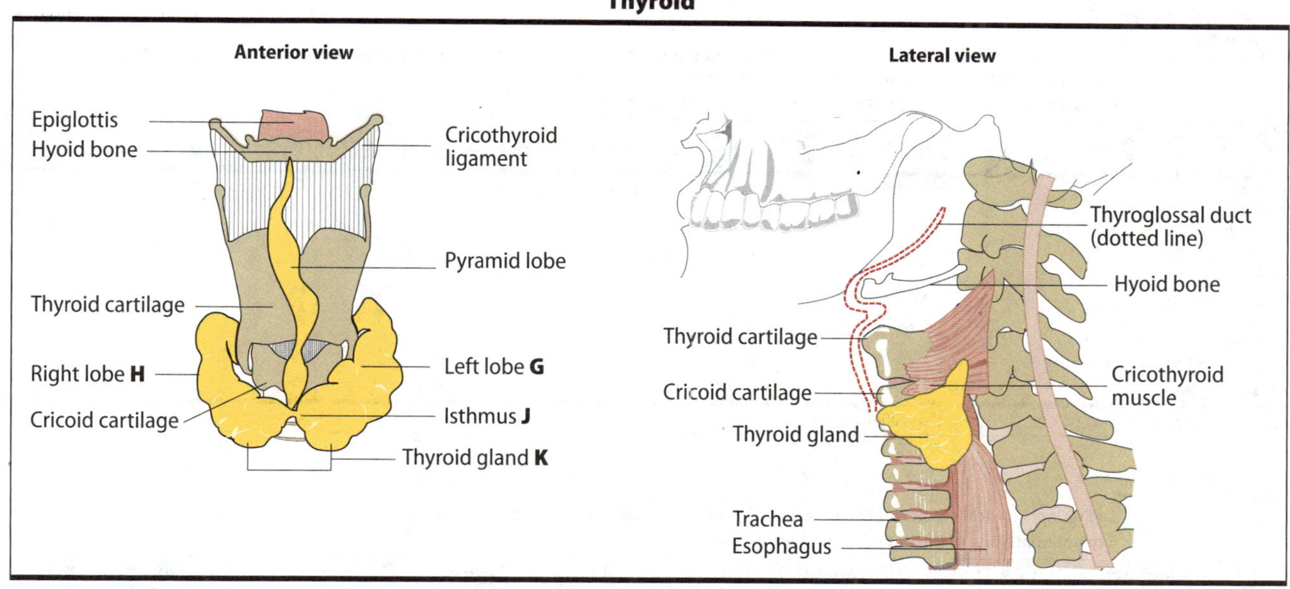

Thyroid and Parathyroid Glands

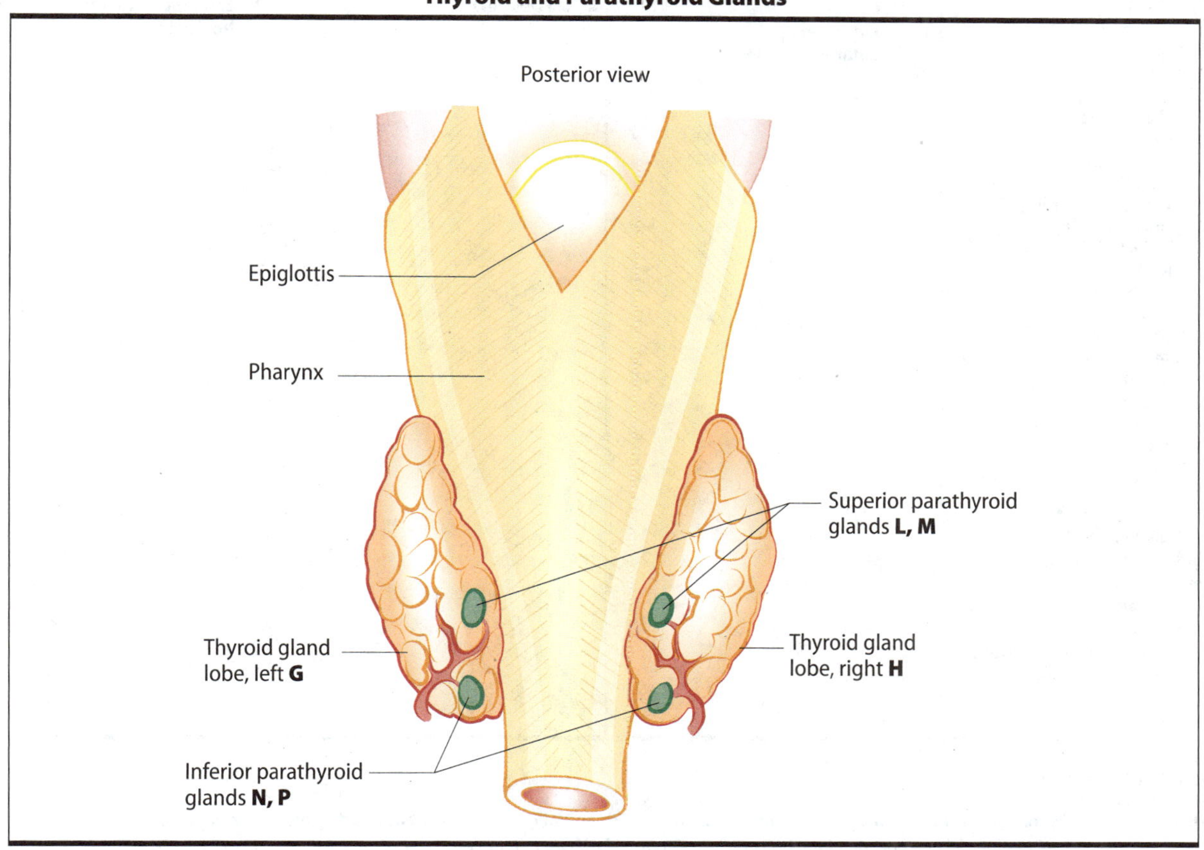

Ø Medical and Surgical
G Endocrine System
2 Change Definition: Taking out or off a device from a body part and putting back an identical or similar device in or on the same body part without cutting or puncturing the skin or a mucous membrane
Explanation: All CHANGE procedures are coded using the approach EXTERNAL

Body Part Character 4	Approach Character 5	Device Character 6	Qualifier Character 7
Ø Pituitary Gland Adenohypophysis Hypophysis Neurohypophysis **1 Pineal Body** **5 Adrenal Gland** Suprarenal gland **K Thyroid Gland** **R Parathyroid Gland** **S Endocrine Gland**	**X External**	**Ø Drainage Device** **Y Other Device**	**Z No Qualifier**

Non-OR All body part, approach, device, and qualifier values

Ø Medical and Surgical
G Endocrine System
5 Destruction Definition: Physical eradication of all or a portion of a body part by the direct use of energy, force, or a destructive agent
Explanation: None of the body part is physically taken out

Body Part Character 4	Approach Character 5	Device Character 6	Qualifier Character 7
Ø Pituitary Gland Adenohypophysis Hypophysis Neurohypophysis **1 Pineal Body** **2 Adrenal Gland, Left** Suprarenal gland **3 Adrenal Gland, Right** *See 2 Adrenal Gland, Left* **4 Adrenal Glands, Bilateral** *See 2 Adrenal Gland, Left* **6 Carotid Body, Left** Carotid glomus **7 Carotid Body, Right** *See 6 Carotid Body, Left* **8 Carotid Bodies, Bilateral** *See 6 Carotid Body, Left* **9 Para-aortic Body** **B Coccygeal Glomus** Coccygeal body **C Glomus Jugulare** Jugular body **D Aortic Body** **F Paraganglion Extremity** **G Thyroid Gland Lobe, Left** **H Thyroid Gland Lobe, Right** **K Thyroid Gland** **L Superior Parathyroid Gland, Right** **M Superior Parathyroid Gland, Left** **N Inferior Parathyroid Gland, Right** **P Inferior Parathyroid Gland, Left** **Q Parathyroid Glands, Multiple** **R Parathyroid Gland**	**Ø Open** **3 Percutaneous** **4 Percutaneous Endoscopic**	**Z No Device**	**3 Laser Interstitial Thermal Therapy** **Z No Qualifier**

Ø Medical and Surgical
G Endocrine System
8 Division Definition: Cutting into a body part, without draining fluids and/or gases from the body part, in order to separate or transect a body part
Explanation: All or a portion of the body part is separated into two or more portions

Body Part Character 4	Approach Character 5	Device Character 6	Qualifier Character 7
Ø Pituitary Gland Adenohypophysis Hypophysis Neurohypophysis **J Thyroid Gland Isthmus**	**Ø Open** **3 Percutaneous** **4 Percutaneous Endoscopic**	**Z No Device**	**Z No Qualifier**

Ø Medical and Surgical
G Endocrine System
9 Drainage Definition: Taking or letting out fluids and/or gases from a body part
Explanation: The qualifier DIAGNOSTIC is used to identify drainage procedures that are biopsies

Body Part Character 4	Approach Character 5	Device Character 6	Qualifier Character 7
Ø Pituitary Gland Adenohypophysis Hypophysis Neurohypophysis **1** Pineal Body **2** Adrenal Gland, Left Suprarenal gland **3** Adrenal Gland, Right *See 2 Adrenal Gland, Left* **4** Adrenal Glands, Bilateral *See 2 Adrenal Gland, Left* **6** Carotid Body, Left Carotid glomus **7** Carotid Body, Right *See 6 Carotid Body, Left* **8** Carotid Bodies, Bilateral *See 6 Carotid Body, Left* **9** Para-aortic Body **B** Coccygeal Glomus Coccygeal body **C** Glomus Jugulare Jugular body **D** Aortic Body **F** Paraganglion Extremity **G** Thyroid Gland Lobe, Left **H** Thyroid Gland Lobe, Right **K** Thyroid Gland **L** Superior Parathyroid Gland, Right **M** Superior Parathyroid Gland, Left **N** Inferior Parathyroid Gland, Right **P** Inferior Parathyroid Gland, Left **Q** Parathyroid Glands, Multiple **R** Parathyroid Gland	**Ø** Open **3** Percutaneous **4** Percutaneous Endoscopic	**Ø** Drainage Device	**Z** No Qualifier
Ø Pituitary Gland Adenohypophysis Hypophysis Neurohypophysis **1** Pineal Body **2** Adrenal Gland, Left Suprarenal gland **3** Adrenal Gland, Right *See 2 Adrenal Gland, Left* **4** Adrenal Glands, Bilateral *See 2 Adrenal Gland, Left* **6** Carotid Body, Left Carotid glomus **7** Carotid Body, Right *See 6 Carotid Body, Left* **8** Carotid Bodies, Bilateral *See 6 Carotid Body, Left* **9** Para-aortic Body **B** Coccygeal Glomus Coccygeal body **C** Glomus Jugulare Jugular body **D** Aortic Body **F** Paraganglion Extremity **G** Thyroid Gland Lobe, Left **H** Thyroid Gland Lobe, Right **K** Thyroid Gland **L** Superior Parathyroid Gland, Right **M** Superior Parathyroid Gland, Left **N** Inferior Parathyroid Gland, Right **P** Inferior Parathyroid Gland, Left **Q** Parathyroid Glands, Multiple **R** Parathyroid Gland	**Ø** Open **3** Percutaneous **4** Percutaneous Endoscopic	**Z** No Device	**X** Diagnostic **Z** No Qualifier

Non-OR ØG9[Ø,1,2,3,4,6,7,8,9,B,C,D,F,G,H,K,L,M,N,P,Q,R]3ØZ
Non-OR ØG9[G,H,K,L,M,N,P,Q,R]4ØZ
Non-OR ØG9[2,3,4,G,H,K][3,4]ZX
Non-OR ØG9[Ø,1,2,3,4,6,7,8,9,B,C,D,F,G,H,K,L,M,N,P,Q,R]3ZZ
Non-OR ØG9[G,H,K,L,M,N,P,Q,R]4ZZ

Ø Medical and Surgical
G Endocrine System
B Excision

Definition: Cutting out or off, without replacement, a portion of a body part
Explanation: The qualifier DIAGNOSTIC is used to identify excision procedures that are biopsies

Body Part Character 4	Approach Character 5	Device Character 6	Qualifier Character 7
Ø Pituitary Gland Adenohypophysis Hypophysis Neurohypophysis **1 Pineal Body** **2 Adrenal Gland, Left** Suprarenal gland **3 Adrenal Gland, Right** *See 2 Adrenal Gland, Left* **4 Adrenal Glands, Bilateral** *See 2 Adrenal Gland, Left* **6 Carotid Body, Left** Carotid glomus **7 Carotid Body, Right** *See 6 Carotid Body, Left* **8 Carotid Bodies, Bilateral** *See 6 Carotid Body, Left* **9 Para-aortic Body** **B Coccygeal Glomus** Coccygeal body **C Glomus Jugulare** Jugular body **D Aortic Body** **F Paraganglion Extremity** **G Thyroid Gland Lobe, Left** **H Thyroid Gland Lobe, Right** **J Thyroid Gland Isthmus** **L Superior Parathyroid Gland, Right** **M Superior Parathyroid Gland, Left** **N Inferior Parathyroid Gland, Right** **P Inferior Parathyroid Gland, Left** **Q Parathyroid Glands, Multiple** **R Parathyroid Gland**	**Ø Open** **3 Percutaneous** **4 Percutaneous Endoscopic**	**Z No Device**	**X Diagnostic** **Z No Qualifier**

Non-OR ØGB[2,3,4,G,H,J][3,4]ZX

Ø Medical and Surgical
G Endocrine System
C Extirpation Definition: Taking or cutting out solid matter from a body part

Explanation: The solid matter may be an abnormal byproduct of a biological function or a foreign body; it may be imbedded in a body part or in the lumen of a tubular body part. The solid matter may or may not have been previously broken into pieces.

Body Part Character 4	Approach Character 5	Device Character 6	Qualifier Character 7
Ø Pituitary Gland Adenohypophysis Hypophysis Neurohypophysis **1 Pineal Body** **2 Adrenal Gland, Left** Suprarenal gland **3 Adrenal Gland, Right** *See 2 Adrenal Gland, Left* **4 Adrenal Glands, Bilateral** *See 2 Adrenal Gland, Left* **6 Carotid Body, Left** Carotid glomus **7 Carotid Body, Right** *See 6 Carotid Body, Left* **8 Carotid Bodies, Bilateral** *See 6 Carotid Body, Left* **9 Para-aortic Body** **B Coccygeal Glomus** Coccygeal body **C Glomus Jugulare** Jugular body **D Aortic Body** **F Paraganglion Extremity** **G Thyroid Gland Lobe, Left** **H Thyroid Gland Lobe, Right** **K Thyroid Gland** **L Superior Parathyroid Gland, Right** **M Superior Parathyroid Gland, Left** **N Inferior Parathyroid Gland, Right** **P Inferior Parathyroid Gland, Left** **Q Parathyroid Glands, Multiple** **R Parathyroid Gland**	Ø Open 3 Percutaneous 4 Percutaneous Endoscopic	Z No Device	Z No Qualifier

Ø Medical and Surgical
G Endocrine System
H Insertion Definition: Putting in a nonbiological appliance that monitors, assists, performs, or prevents a physiological function but does not physically take the place of a body part

Explanation: None

Body Part Character 4	Approach Character 5	Device Character 6	Qualifier Character 7
S Endocrine Gland	Ø Open 3 Percutaneous 4 Percutaneous Endoscopic	1 Radioactive Element 2 Monitoring Device 3 Infusion Device Y Other Device	Z No Qualifier

Non-OR ØGHS31Z
Non-OR ØGHS[3,4]YZ

Ø Medical and Surgical
G Endocrine System
J Inspection Definition: Visually and/or manually exploring a body part

Explanation: Visual exploration may be performed with or without optical instrumentation. Manual exploration may be performed directly or through intervening body layers.

Body Part Character 4	Approach Character 5	Device Character 6	Qualifier Character 7
Ø Pituitary Gland Adenohypophysis Hypophysis Neurohypophysis 1 Pineal Body 5 Adrenal Gland Suprarenal gland K Thyroid Gland R Parathyroid Gland S Endocrine Gland	Ø Open 3 Percutaneous 4 Percutaneous Endoscopic	Z No Device	Z No Qualifier

Non-OR ØGJ[Ø,1,5,K,R,S]3ZZ

Ø Medical and Surgical
G Endocrine System
M Reattachment Definition: Putting back in or on all or a portion of a separated body part to its normal location or other suitable location
Explanation: Vascular circulation and nervous pathways may or may not be reestablished

Body Part Character 4	Approach Character 5	Device Character 6	Qualifier Character 7
2 Adrenal Gland, Left Suprarenal gland **3 Adrenal Gland, Right** *See 2 Adrenal Gland, Left* **G Thyroid Gland Lobe, Left** **H Thyroid Gland Lobe, Right** **L Superior Parathyroid Gland, Right** **M Superior Parathyroid Gland, Left** **N Inferior Parathyroid Gland, Right** **P Inferior Parathyroid Gland, Left** **Q Parathyroid Glands, Multiple** **R Parathyroid Gland**	**Ø Open** **4 Percutaneous Endoscopic**	**Z No Device**	**Z No Qualifier**

Ø Medical and Surgical
G Endocrine System
N Release Definition: Freeing a body part from an abnormal physical constraint by cutting or by the use of force
Explanation: Some of the restraining tissue may be taken out but none of the body part is taken out

Body Part Character 4	Approach Character 5	Device Character 6	Qualifier Character 7
Ø Pituitary Gland Adenohypophysis Hypophysis Neurohypophysis **1 Pineal Body** **2 Adrenal Gland, Left** Suprarenal gland **3 Adrenal Gland, Right** *See 2 Adrenal Gland, Left* **4 Adrenal Glands, Bilateral** *See 2 Adrenal Gland, Left* **6 Carotid Body, Left** Carotid glomus **7 Carotid Body, Right** *See 6 Carotid Body, Left* **8 Carotid Bodies, Bilateral** *See 6 Carotid Body, Left* **9 Para-aortic Body** **B Coccygeal Glomus** Coccygeal body **C Glomus Jugulare** Jugular body **D Aortic Body** **F Paraganglion Extremity** **G Thyroid Gland Lobe, Left** **H Thyroid Gland Lobe, Right** **K Thyroid Gland** **L Superior Parathyroid Gland, Right** **M Superior Parathyroid Gland, Left** **N Inferior Parathyroid Gland, Right** **P Inferior Parathyroid Gland, Left** **Q Parathyroid Glands, Multiple** **R Parathyroid Gland**	**Ø Open** **3 Percutaneous** **4 Percutaneous Endoscopic**	**Z No Device**	**Z No Qualifier**

Non-OR ØGN[6,7,8,9,B,C,D,F][Ø,3,4]ZZ

Ø Medical and Surgical
G Endocrine System
P Removal Definition: Taking out or off a device from a body part

Explanation: If a device is taken out and a similar device put in without cutting or puncturing the skin or mucous membrane, the procedure is coded to the root operation CHANGE. Otherwise, the procedure for taking out a device is coded to the root operation REMOVAL.

Body Part Character 4	Approach Character 5	Device Character 6	Qualifier Character 7
Ø Pituitary Gland Adenohypophysis Hypophysis Neurohypophysis **1 Pineal Body** **5 Adrenal Gland** Suprarenal gland **K Thyroid Gland** **R Parathyroid Gland**	**Ø** Open **3** Percutaneous **4** Percutaneous Endoscopic **X** External	**Ø** Drainage Device	**Z** No Qualifier
S Endocrine Gland	**Ø** Open **3** Percutaneous **4** Percutaneous Endoscopic	**Ø** Drainage Device **2** Monitoring Device **3** Infusion Device **Y** Other Device	**Z** No Qualifier
S Endocrine Gland	**X** External	**Ø** Drainage Device **2** Monitoring Device **3** Infusion Device	**Z** No Qualifier

Non-OR ØGP[Ø,1,5,K,R]XØZ
Non-OR ØGPS[3,4]YZ
Non-OR ØGPSX[Ø,2,3]Z

Ø Medical and Surgical
G Endocrine System
Q Repair Definition: Restoring, to the extent possible, a body part to its normal anatomic structure and function

Explanation: Used only when the method to accomplish the repair is not one of the other root operations

Body Part Character 4	Approach Character 5	Device Character 6	Qualifier Character 7
Ø Pituitary Gland Adenohypophysis Hypophysis Neurohypophysis **1 Pineal Body** **2 Adrenal Gland, Left** Suprarenal gland **3 Adrenal Gland, Right** *See 2 Adrenal Gland, Left* **4 Adrenal Glands, Bilateral** *See 2 Adrenal Gland, Left* **6 Carotid Body, Left** Carotid glomus **7 Carotid Body, Right** *See 6 Carotid Body, Left* **8 Carotid Bodies, Bilateral** *See 6 Carotid Body, Left* **9 Para-aortic Body** **B Coccygeal Glomus** Coccygeal body **C Glomus Jugulare** Jugular body **D Aortic Body** **F Paraganglion Extremity** **G Thyroid Gland Lobe, Left** **H Thyroid Gland Lobe, Right** **J Thyroid Gland Isthmus** **K Thyroid Gland** **L Superior Parathyroid Gland, Right** **M Superior Parathyroid Gland, Left** **N Inferior Parathyroid Gland, Right** **P Inferior Parathyroid Gland, Left** **Q Parathyroid Glands, Multiple** **R Parathyroid Gland**	**Ø** Open **3** Percutaneous **4** Percutaneous Endoscopic	**Z** No Device	**Z** No Qualifier

Ø Medical and Surgical
G Endocrine System
S Reposition Definition: Moving to its normal location, or other suitable location, all or a portion of a body part

Explanation: The body part is moved to a new location from an abnormal location, or from a normal location where it is not functioning correctly. The body part may or may not be cut out or off to be moved to the new location.

Body Part Character 4	Approach Character 5	Device Character 6	Qualifier Character 7
2 Adrenal Gland, Left Suprarenal gland **3 Adrenal Gland, Right** *See 2 Adrenal Gland, Left* **G Thyroid Gland Lobe, Left** **H Thyroid Gland Lobe, Right** **L Superior Parathyroid Gland, Right** **M Superior Parathyroid Gland, Left** **N Inferior Parathyroid Gland, Right** **P Inferior Parathyroid Gland, Left** **Q Parathyroid Glands, Multiple** **R Parathyroid Gland**	**Ø Open** **4 Percutaneous Endoscopic**	**Z No Device**	**Z No Qualifier**

Ø Medical and Surgical
G Endocrine System
T Resection Definition: Cutting out or off, without replacement, all of a body part

Explanation: None

Body Part Character 4	Approach Character 5	Device Character 6	Qualifier Character 7
Ø Pituitary Gland Adenohypophysis Hypophysis Neurohypophysis **1 Pineal Body** **2 Adrenal Gland, Left** Suprarenal gland **3 Adrenal Gland, Right** *See 2 Adrenal Gland, Left* **4 Adrenal Glands, Bilateral** *See 2 Adrenal Gland, Left* **6 Carotid Body, Left** Carotid glomus **7 Carotid Body, Right** *See 6 Carotid Body, Left* **8 Carotid Bodies, Bilateral** *See 6 Carotid Body, Left* **9 Para-aortic Body** **B Coccygeal Glomus** Coccygeal body **C Glomus Jugulare** Jugular body **D Aortic Body** **F Paraganglion Extremity** **G Thyroid Gland Lobe, Left** **H Thyroid Gland Lobe, Right** **J Thyroid Gland Isthmus** **K Thyroid Gland** **L Superior Parathyroid Gland, Right** **M Superior Parathyroid Gland, Left** **N Inferior Parathyroid Gland, Right** **P Inferior Parathyroid Gland, Left** **Q Parathyroid Glands, Multiple** **R Parathyroid Gland**	**Ø Open** **4 Percutaneous Endoscopic**	**Z No Device**	**Z No Qualifier**

Non-OR ØGT[6,7,8,9,B,C,D,F][Ø,4]ZZ

Ø Medical and Surgical
G Endocrine System
W Revision

Definition: Correcting, to the extent possible, a portion of a malfunctioning device or the position of a displaced device

Explanation: Revision can include correcting a malfunctioning or displaced device by taking out or putting in components of the device such as a screw or pin

Body Part Character 4	Approach Character 5	Device Character 6	Qualifier Character 7
Ø Pituitary Gland Adenohypophysis Hypophysis Neurohypophysis **1** Pineal Body **5** Adrenal Gland Suprarenal gland **K** Thyroid Gland **R** Parathyroid Gland	**Ø** Open **3** Percutaneous **4** Percutaneous Endoscopic **X** External	**Ø** Drainage Device	**Z** No Qualifier
S Endocrine Gland	**Ø** Open **3** Percutaneous **4** Percutaneous Endoscopic	**Ø** Drainage Device **2** Monitoring Device **3** Infusion Device **Y** Other Device	**Z** No Qualifier
S Endocrine Gland	**X** External	**Ø** Drainage Device **2** Monitoring Device **3** Infusion Device	**Z** No Qualifier

Non-OR ØGW[Ø,1,5,K,R]XØZ
Non-OR ØGWS[3,4]YZ
Non-OR ØGWSX[Ø,2,3]Z

Skin and Breast ØHØ–ØHX

Character Meanings*

This Character Meaning table is provided as a guide to assist the user in the identification of character members that may be found in this section of code tables. It **SHOULD NOT** be used to build a PCS code.

Operation–Character 3		Body Part–Character 4		Approach–Character 5		Device–Character 6		Qualifier–Character 7	
Ø	Alteration	Ø	Skin, Scalp	Ø	Open	Ø	Drainage Device	2	Cell Suspension Technique
2	Change	1	Skin, Face	3	Percutaneous	1	Radioactive Element	3	Full Thickness OR Laser Interstitial Thermal Therapy
5	Destruction	2	Skin, Right Ear	7	Via Natural or Artificial Opening	7	Autologous Tissue Substitute	4	Partial Thickness
8	Division	3	Skin, Left Ear	8	Via Natural or Artificial Opening Endoscopic	J	Synthetic Substitute	5	Latissimus Dorsi Myocutaneous Flap
9	Drainage	4	Skin, Neck	X	External	K	Nonautologous Tissue Substitute	6	Transverse Rectus Abdominis Myocutaneous Flap
B	Excision	5	Skin, Chest			N	Tissue Expander	7	Deep Inferior Epigastric Artery Perforator Flap
C	Extirpation	6	Skin, Back			Y	Other Device	8	Superficial Inferior Epigastric Artery Flap
D	Extraction	7	Skin, Abdomen			Z	No Device	9	Gluteal Artery Perforator Flap
H	Insertion	8	Skin, Buttock					D	Multiple
J	Inspection	9	Skin, Perineum					X	Diagnostic
M	Reattachment	A	Skin, Inguinal					Z	No Qualifier
N	Release	B	Skin, Right Upper Arm						
P	Removal	C	Skin, Left Upper Arm						
Q	Repair	D	Skin, Right Lower Arm						
R	Replacement	E	Skin, Left Lower Arm						
S	Reposition	F	Skin, Right Hand						
T	Resection	G	Skin, Left Hand						
U	Supplement	H	Skin, Right Upper Leg						
W	Revision	J	Skin, Left Upper Leg						
X	Transfer	K	Skin, Right Lower Leg						
		L	Skin, Left Lower Leg						
		M	Skin, Right Foot						
		N	Skin, Left Foot						
		P	Skin						
		Q	Finger Nail						
		R	Toe Nail						
		S	Hair						
		T	Breast, Right						
		U	Breast, Left						
		V	Breast, Bilateral						
		W	Nipple, Right						
		X	Nipple, Left						
		Y	Supernumerary Breast						

* Includes skin and breast glands and ducts.

AHA Coding Clinic for table ØHØ
2022, 1Q, 14 Reduction mammoplasty for breast symmetry
2022, 1Q, 15 Nipple reconstruction and breast reduction
2019, 4Q, 30-31 Breast procedures

AHA Coding Clinic for table ØH5
2022, 4Q, 53-54 Laser interstitial thermal therapy
2019, 4Q, 30-31 Breast procedures

AHA Coding Clinic for table ØH9
2019, 4Q, 30-31 Breast procedures

AHA Coding Clinic for table ØHB
2022, 1Q, 14 Reduction mammoplasty for breast symmetry
2020, 1Q, 31 Repair of buried penis
2019, 4Q, 30-31 Breast procedures
2018, 1Q, 14 Excisional debridement of breast tissue and skin
2016, 3Q, 29 Closure of bilateral alveolar clefts
2015, 3Q, 3-8 Excisional and nonexcisional debridement

AHA Coding Clinic for table ØHC
2019, 4Q, 30-31 Breast procedures

AHA Coding Clinic for table ØHD
2019, 4Q, 30-31 Breast procedures
2016, 1Q, 40 Nonexcisional debridement of skin and subcutaneous tissue
2015, 3Q, 3-8 Excisional and nonexcisional debridement

AHA Coding Clinic for table ØHH
2019, 4Q, 30-31 Breast procedures
2017, 4Q, 67 New qualifier values - Pedicle flap procedures
2014, 2Q, 12 Pedicle latissimus myocutaneous flap with placement of breast tissue expanders
2013, 4Q, 107 Breast tissue expander placement using acellular dermal matrix

AHA Coding Clinic for table ØHJ
2019, 4Q, 30-31 Breast procedures

AHA Coding Clinic for table ØHN
2019, 4Q, 30-31 Breast procedures

AHA Coding Clinic for table ØHP
2022, 3Q, 20 Bilateral breast capsulectomy and tissue expander removal
2019, 4Q, 30-31 Breast procedures
2018, 3Q, 13 Deep inferior epigastric artery perforator flap breast reconstruction
2016, 2Q, 27 Removal of nonviable transverse rectus abdominis myocutaneous (TRAM) flaps

AHA Coding Clinic for table ØHQ
2019, 4Q, 30-31 Breast procedures
2018, 2Q, 25 Third and fourth degree obstetric lacerations
2016, 1Q, 7 Obstetrical perineal laceration repair
2014, 4Q, 31 Delayed wound closure following fracture treatment

AHA Coding Clinic for table ØHR
2023, 2Q, 30 Inframammary fold adjacent tissue transfer and deep inferior epigastric perforator flap breast reconstruction
2022, 1Q, 15 Nipple reconstruction and breast reduction
2020, 1Q, 27 Delayed reconstruction following mastectomy using gracilis musculocutaneous free flap
2020, 1Q, 28 Free flap microvascular breast reconstruction
2020, 1Q, 30 Polarity Skin TE™ application
2019, 4Q, 30-31 Breast procedures
2019, 4Q, 32 Cell suspension epithelial autograft
2019, 3Q, 32 Breast reconstruction with neurotization
2018, 3Q, 13 Deep inferior epigastric artery perforator flap breast reconstruction
2017, 1Q, 35 Epifix® allograft
2014, 3Q, 14 Application of TheraSkin® and excisional debridement

AHA Coding Clinic for table ØHT
2021, 2Q, 16 Goldilocks breast reconstruction
2018, 3Q, 13 Deep inferior epigastric artery perforator flap breast reconstruction
2014, 4Q, 34 Skin-sparing mastectomy

AHA Coding Clinic for table ØHU
2019, 4Q, 30-31 Breast procedures

AHA Coding Clinic for table ØHW
2019, 4Q, 30-31 Breast procedures

AHA Coding Clinic for table ØHX
2023, 2Q, 23 V-Y anoplasty and excision of mucosal ectropion
2023, 2Q, 30 Inframammary fold adjacent tissue transfer and deep inferior epigastric perforator flap breast reconstruction
2022, 3Q, 13 Repair of prolapsed neovaginal graft

Integumentary Anatomy

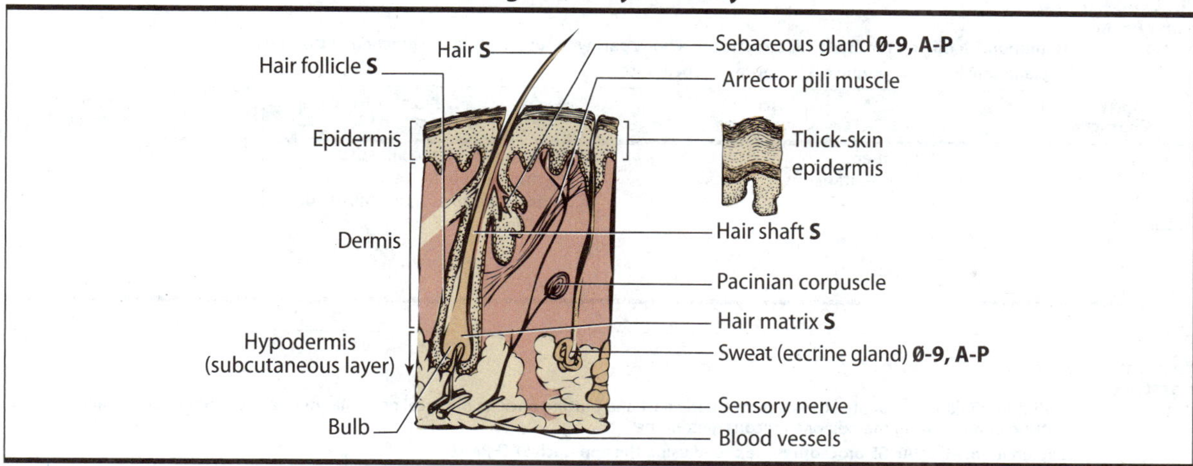

Nail Anatomy

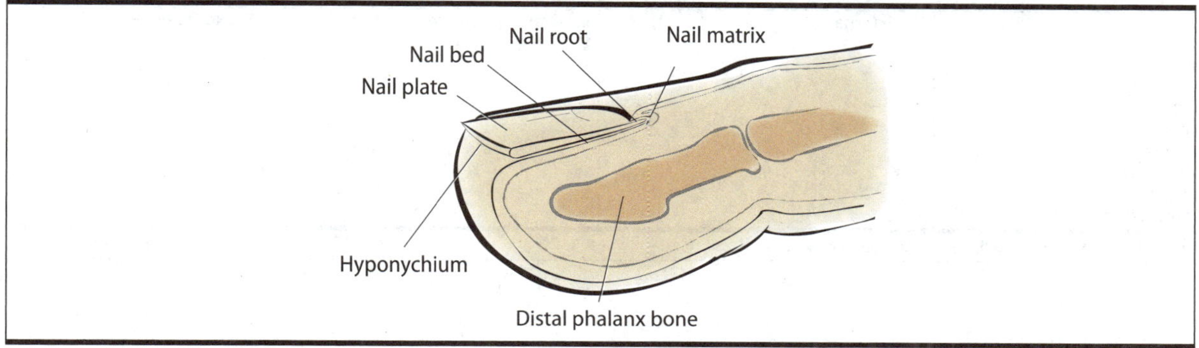

Breast

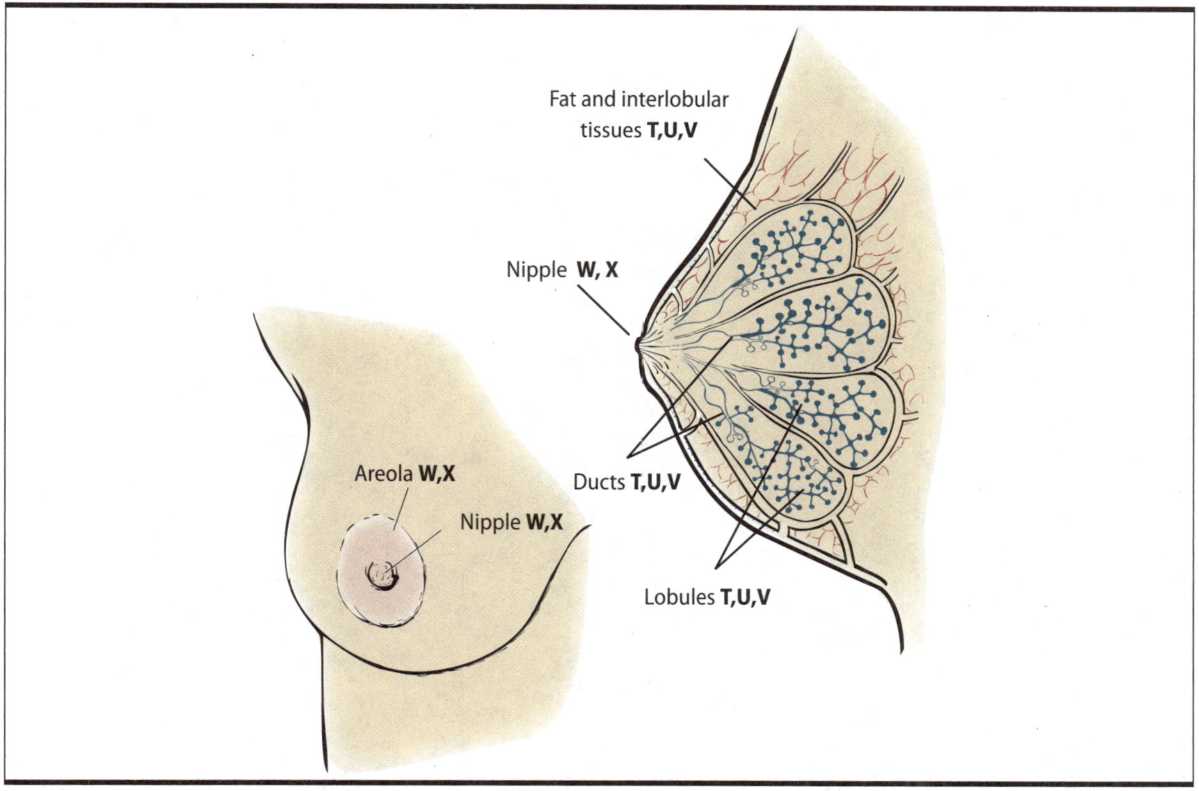

Ø Medical and Surgical
H Skin and Breast
Ø Alteration

Definition: Modifying the anatomic structure of a body part without affecting the function of the body part

Explanation: Principal purpose is to improve appearance

Body Part Character 4	Approach Character 5	Device Character 6	Qualifier Character 7
T Breast, Right Mammary duct Mammary gland **U Breast, Left** *See T Breast, Right* **V Breast, Bilateral** *See T Breast, Right*	**Ø** Open **3** Percutaneous	**7** Autologous Tissue Substitute **J** Synthetic Substitute **K** Nonautologous Tissue Substitute **Z** No Device	**Z** No Qualifier

Non-OR ØHØ[T,U,V]3JZ

Ø Medical and Surgical
H Skin and Breast
2 Change

Definition: Taking out or off a device from a body part and putting back an identical or similar device in or on the same body part without cutting or puncturing the skin or a mucous membrane

Explanation: All CHANGE procedures are coded using the approach EXTERNAL

Body Part Character 4	Approach Character 5	Device Character 6	Qualifier Character 7
P Skin Dermis Epidermis Sebaceous gland Sweat gland **T Breast, Right** Mammary duct Mammary gland **U Breast, Left** *See T Breast, Right*	**X** External	**Ø** Drainage Device **Y** Other Device	**Z** No Qualifier

Non-OR All body part, approach, device, and qualifier values

Ø Medical and Surgical
H Skin and Breast
5 Destruction

Definition: Physical eradication of all or a portion of a body part by the direct use of energy, force, or a destructive agent
Explanation: None of the body part is physically taken out

Body Part Character 4	Approach Character 5	Device Character 6	Qualifier Character 7
Ø Skin, Scalp **1** Skin, Face **2** Skin, Right Ear **3** Skin, Left Ear **4** Skin, Neck **5** Skin, Chest Breast procedures, skin only **6** Skin, Back **7** Skin, Abdomen **8** Skin, Buttock **9** Skin, Perineum Perianal skin **A** Skin, Inguinal **B** Skin, Right Upper Arm **C** Skin, Left Upper Arm **D** Skin, Right Lower Arm **E** Skin, Left Lower Arm **F** Skin, Right Hand **G** Skin, Left Hand **H** Skin, Right Upper Leg **J** Skin, Left Upper Leg **K** Skin, Right Lower Leg **L** Skin, Left Lower Leg **M** Skin, Right Foot **N** Skin, Left Foot	**X** External	**Z** No Device	**D** Multiple **Z** No Qualifier
Q Finger Nail Nail bed Nail plate **R** Toe Nail *See Q Finger Nail*	**X** External	**Z** No Device	**Z** No Qualifier
T Breast, Right Mammary duct Mammary gland **U** Breast, Left *See T Breast, Right* **V** Breast, Bilateral *See T Breast, Right*	**Ø** Open **3** Percutaneous	**Z** No Device	**3** Laser Interstitial Thermal Therapy **Z** No Qualifier
T Breast, Right Mammary duct Mammary gland **U** Breast, Left *See T Breast, Right* **V** Breast, Bilateral *See T Breast, Right*	**7** Via Natural or Artificial Opening **8** Via Natural or Artificial Opening Endoscopic	**Z** No Device	**Z** No Qualifier
W Nipple, Right Areola **X** Nipple, Left *See W Nipple, Right*	**Ø** Open **3** Percutaneous **7** Via Natural or Artificial Opening **8** Via Natural or Artificial Opening Endoscopic **X** External	**Z** No Device	**Z** No Qualifier

DRG Non-OR ØH5[Ø,1,4,5,6,7,8,9,A,B,C,D,E,F,G,H,J,K,L,M,N]XZ[D,Z]
DRG Non-OR ØH5[Q,R]XZZ
Non-OR ØH5[2,3]XZ[D,Z]

Ø Medical and Surgical
H Skin and Breast
8 Division

Definition: Cutting into a body part, without draining fluids and/or gases from the body part, in order to separate or transect a body part

Explanation: All or a portion of the body part is separated into two or more portions

Body Part Character 4	Approach Character 5	Device Character 6	Qualifier Character 7
Ø Skin, Scalp 1 Skin, Face 2 Skin, Right Ear 3 Skin, Left Ear 4 Skin, Neck 5 Skin, Chest Breast procedures, skin only 6 Skin, Back 7 Skin, Abdomen 8 Skin, Buttock 9 Skin, Perineum Perianal skin A Skin, Inguinal B Skin, Right Upper Arm C Skin, Left Upper Arm D Skin, Right Lower Arm E Skin, Left Lower Arm F Skin, Right Hand G Skin, Left Hand H Skin, Right Upper Leg J Skin, Left Upper Leg K Skin, Right Lower Leg L Skin, Left Lower Leg M Skin, Right Foot N Skin, Left Foot	X External	Z No Device	Z No Qualifier

Non-OR All body part, approach, device, and qualifier values

Ø Medical and Surgical
H Skin and Breast
9 Drainage

Definition: Taking or letting out fluids and/or gases from a body part

Explanation: The qualifier DIAGNOSTIC is used to identify drainage procedures that are biopsies

Body Part Character 4	Approach Character 5	Device Character 6	Qualifier Character 7
Ø Skin, Scalp **1** Skin, Face **2** Skin, Right Ear **3** Skin, Left Ear **4** Skin, Neck **5** Skin, Chest Breast procedures, skin only **6** Skin, Back **7** Skin, Abdomen **8** Skin, Buttock **9** Skin, Perineum Perianal skin **A** Skin, Inguinal **B** Skin, Right Upper Arm **C** Skin, Left Upper Arm **D** Skin, Right Lower Arm **E** Skin, Left Lower Arm **F** Skin, Right Hand **G** Skin, Left Hand **H** Skin, Right Upper Leg **J** Skin, Left Upper Leg **K** Skin, Right Lower Leg **L** Skin, Left Lower Leg **M** Skin, Right Foot **N** Skin, Left Foot **Q** Finger Nail Nail bed Nail plate **R** Toe Nail *See Q Finger Nail*	**X** External	**Ø** Drainage Device	**Z** No Qualifier
Ø Skin, Scalp **1** Skin, Face **2** Skin, Right Ear **3** Skin, Left Ear **4** Skin, Neck **5** Skin, Chest Breast procedures, skin only **6** Skin, Back **7** Skin, Abdomen **8** Skin, Buttock **9** Skin, Perineum Perianal skin **A** Skin, Inguinal **B** Skin, Right Upper Arm **C** Skin, Left Upper Arm **D** Skin, Right Lower Arm **E** Skin, Left Lower Arm **F** Skin, Right Hand **G** Skin, Left Hand **H** Skin, Right Upper Leg **J** Skin, Left Upper Leg **K** Skin, Right Lower Leg **L** Skin, Left Lower Leg **M** Skin, Right Foot **N** Skin, Left Foot **Q** Finger Nail Nail bed Nail plate **R** Toe Nail *See Q Finger Nail*	**X** External	**Z** No Device	**X** Diagnostic **Z** No Qualifier
T Breast, Right Mammary duct Mammary gland **U** Breast, Left *See T Breast, Right* **V** Breast, Bilateral *See T Breast, Right*	**Ø** Open **3** Percutaneous **7** Via Natural or Artificial Opening **8** Via Natural or Artificial Opening Endoscopic	**Ø** Drainage Device	**Z** No Qualifier
T Breast, Right Mammary duct Mammary gland **U** Breast, Left *See T Breast, Right* **V** Breast, Bilateral *See T Breast, Right*	**Ø** Open **3** Percutaneous **7** Via Natural or Artificial Opening **8** Via Natural or Artificial Opening Endoscopic	**Z** No Device	**X** Diagnostic **Z** No Qualifier
W Nipple, Right Areola **X** Nipple, Left *See W Nipple, Right*	**Ø** Open **3** Percutaneous **7** Via Natural or Artificial Opening **8** Via Natural or Artificial Opening Endoscopic **X** External	**Ø** Drainage Device	**Z** No Qualifier
W Nipple, Right Areola **X** Nipple, Left *See W Nipple, Right*	**Ø** Open **3** Percutaneous **7** Via Natural or Artificial Opening **8** Via Natural or Artificial Opening Endoscopic **X** External	**Z** No Device	**X** Diagnostic **Z** No Qualifier

Non-OR ØH9[Ø,1,2,3,4,5,6,7,8,A,B,C,D,E,F,G,H,J,K,L,M,N,Q,R]XØZ
Non-OR ØH9[Ø,1,2,3,4,5,6,7,8,A,B,C,D,E,F,G,H,J,K,L,M,N,Q,R]XZ[X,Z]
Non-OR ØH99XZX
Non-OR ØH9[T,U,V][Ø,3,7,8]ØZ
Non-OR ØH9[T,U,V][3,7,8]Z[X,Z]
Non-OR ØH9[W,X][Ø,3,7,8,X]ØZ
Non-OR ØH9[W,X][3,7,8,X]Z[X,Z]

Ø Medical and Surgical
H Skin and Breast
B Excision Definition: Cutting out or off, without replacement, a portion of a body part
Explanation: The qualifier DIAGNOSTIC is used to identify excision procedures that are biopsies

Body Part Character 4	Approach Character 5	Device Character 6	Qualifier Character 7
Ø Skin, Scalp **1 Skin, Face** **2 Skin, Right Ear** **3 Skin, Left Ear** **4 Skin, Neck** **5 Skin, Chest** Breast procedures, skin only **6 Skin, Back** **7 Skin, Abdomen** **8 Skin, Buttock** **9 Skin, Perineum** Perianal skin **A Skin, Inguinal** **B Skin, Right Upper Arm** **C Skin, Left Upper Arm** **D Skin, Right Lower Arm** **E Skin, Left Lower Arm** **F Skin, Right Hand** **G Skin, Left Hand** **H Skin, Right Upper Leg** **J Skin, Left Upper Leg** **K Skin, Right Lower Leg** **L Skin, Left Lower Leg** **M Skin, Right Foot** **N Skin, Left Foot** **Q Finger Nail** Nail bed Nail plate **R Toe Nail** *See Q Finger Nail*	**X External**	**Z No Device**	**X Diagnostic** **Z No Qualifier**
T Breast, Right Mammary duct Mammary gland **U Breast, Left** *See T Breast, Right* **V Breast, Bilateral** *See T Breast, Right* **Y Supernumerary Breast**	**Ø Open** **3 Percutaneous** **7 Via Natural or Artificial Opening** **8 Via Natural or Artificial Opening Endoscopic**	**Z No Device**	**X Diagnostic** **Z No Qualifier**
W Nipple, Right Areola **X Nipple, Left** *See W Nipple, Right*	**Ø Open** **3 Percutaneous** **7 Via Natural or Artificial Opening** **8 Via Natural or Artificial Opening Endoscopic** **X External**	**Z No Device**	**X Diagnostic** **Z No Qualifier**

DRG Non-OR	ØHB9XZZ
Non-OR	ØHB[Ø,1,2,3,4,5,6,7,8,A,B,C,D,E,F,G,H,J,K,L,M,N,Q,R]XZ[X,Z]
Non-OR	ØHB9XZX
Non-OR	ØHB[T,U,V,Y][3,7,8]ZX
Non-OR	ØHB[W,X][3,7,8,X]ZX

Ø Medical and Surgical
H Skin and Breast
C Extirpation

Definition: Taking or cutting out solid matter from a body part

Explanation: The solid matter may be an abnormal byproduct of a biological function or a foreign body; it may be imbedded in a body part or in the lumen of a tubular body part. The solid matter may or may not have been previously broken into pieces.

Body Part Character 4	Approach Character 5	Device Character 6	Qualifier Character 7
Ø Skin, Scalp **1** Skin, Face **2** Skin, Right Ear **3** Skin, Left Ear **4** Skin, Neck **5** Skin, Chest Breast procedures, skin only **6** Skin, Back **7** Skin, Abdomen **8** Skin, Buttock **9** Skin, Perineum Perianal skin **A** Skin, Inguinal **B** Skin, Right Upper Arm **C** Skin, Left Upper Arm **D** Skin, Right Lower Arm **E** Skin, Left Lower Arm **F** Skin, Right Hand **G** Skin, Left Hand **H** Skin, Right Upper Leg **J** Skin, Left Upper Leg **K** Skin, Right Lower Leg **L** Skin, Left Lower Leg **M** Skin, Right Foot **N** Skin, Left Foot **Q** Finger Nail Nail bed Nail plate **R** Toe Nail *See Q Finger Nail*	**X** External	**Z** No Device	**Z** No Qualifier
T Breast, Right Mammary duct Mammary gland **U** Breast, Left *See T Breast, Right* **V** Breast, Bilateral *See T Breast, Right*	**Ø** Open **3** Percutaneous **7** Via Natural or Artificial Opening **8** Via Natural or Artificial Opening Endoscopic	**Z** No Device	**Z** No Qualifier
W Nipple, Right Areola **X** Nipple, Left *See W Nipple, Right*	**Ø** Open **3** Percutaneous **7** Via Natural or Artificial Opening **8** Via Natural or Artificial Opening Endoscopic **X** External	**Z** No Device	**Z** No Qualifier

Non-OR ØHC[Ø,1,2,3,4,5,6,7,8,9,A,B,C,D,E,F,G,H,J,K,L,M,N,Q,R]XZZ
Non-OR ØHC[T,U,V][3,7,8]ZZ
Non-OR ØHC[W,X][3,7,8,X]ZZ

Ø Medical and Surgical
H Skin and Breast
D Extraction

Definition: Pulling or stripping out or off all or a portion of a body part by the use of force
Explanation: The qualifier DIAGNOSTIC is used to identify extraction procedures that are biopsies

Body Part Character 4	Approach Character 5	Device Character 6	Qualifier Character 7
Ø Skin, Scalp 1 Skin, Face 2 Skin, Right Ear 3 Skin, Left Ear 4 Skin, Neck 5 Skin, Chest Breast procedures, skin only 6 Skin, Back 7 Skin, Abdomen 8 Skin, Buttock 9 Skin, Perineum Perianal skin A Skin, Inguinal B Skin, Right Upper Arm C Skin, Left Upper Arm D Skin, Right Lower Arm E Skin, Left Lower Arm F Skin, Right Hand G Skin, Left Hand H Skin, Right Upper Leg J Skin, Left Upper Leg K Skin, Right Lower Leg L Skin, Left Lower Leg M Skin, Right Foot N Skin, Left Foot Q Finger Nail Nail bed Nail plate R Toe Nail *See* *Q Finger Nail* S Hair	X External	Z No Device	Z No Qualifier
T Breast, Right Mammary duct Mammary gland U Breast, Left *See* *T Breast, Right* V Breast, Bilateral *See* *T Breast, Right* Y Supernumerary Breast	Ø Open	Z No Device	Z No Qualifier

Non-OR All body part, approach, device, and qualifier values

Ø Medical and Surgical
H Skin and Breast
H Insertion

Definition: Putting in a nonbiological appliance that monitors, assists, performs, or prevents a physiological function but does not physically take the place of a body part

Explanation: None

Body Part Character 4	Approach Character 5	Device Character 6	Qualifier Character 7
P Skin	X External	Y Other Device	Z No Qualifier
T Breast, Right Mammary duct Mammary gland U Breast, Left *See T Breast, Right*	Ø Open 3 Percutaneous 7 Via Natural or Artificial Opening 8 Via Natural or Artificial Opening Endoscopic	1 Radioactive Element N Tissue Expander Y Other Device	Z No Qualifier
V Breast, Bilateral Mammary duct Mammary gland	Ø Open 3 Percutaneous 7 Via Natural or Artificial Opening 8 Via Natural or Artificial Opening Endoscopic	1 Radioactive Element N Tissue Expander	Z No Qualifier
W Nipple, Right Areola X Nipple, Left *See W Nipple, Right*	Ø Open 3 Percutaneous 7 Via Natural or Artificial Opening 8 Via Natural or Artificial Opening Endoscopic	1 Radioactive Element N Tissue Expander	Z No Qualifier
W Nipple, Right Areola X Nipple, Left *See W Nipple, Right*	X External	1 Radioactive Element	Z No Qualifier

Non-OR ØHHPXYZ
Non-OR ØHH[T,U][3,7,8]YZ

Ø Medical and Surgical
H Skin and Breast
J Inspection

Definition: Visually and/or manually exploring a body part

Explanation: Visual exploration may be performed with or without optical instrumentation. Manual exploration may be performed directly or through intervening body layers.

Body Part Character 4	Approach Character 5	Device Character 6	Qualifier Character 7
P Skin Dermis Epidermis Sebaceous gland Sweat gland Q Finger Nail Nail bed Nail plate R Toe Nail *See Q Finger Nail*	X External	Z No Device	Z No Qualifier
T Breast, Right Mammary duct Mammary gland U Breast, Left *See T Breast, Right*	Ø Open 3 Percutaneous 7 Via Natural or Artificial Opening 8 Via Natural or Artificial Opening Endoscopic	Z No Device	Z No Qualifier

Non-OR All body part, approach, device and qualifier values

Ø Medical and Surgical
H Skin and Breast
M Reattachment

Definition: Putting back in or on all or a portion of a separated body part to its normal location or other suitable location

Explanation: Vascular circulation and nervous pathways may or may not be reestablished

Body Part Character 4	Approach Character 5	Device Character 6	Qualifier Character 7
Ø Skin, Scalp **1 Skin, Face** **2 Skin, Right Ear** **3 Skin, Left Ear** **4 Skin, Neck** **5 Skin, Chest** Breast procedures, skin only **6 Skin, Back** **7 Skin, Abdomen** **8 Skin, Buttock** **9 Skin, Perineum** Perianal skin **A Skin, Inguinal** **B Skin, Right Upper Arm** **C Skin, Left Upper Arm** **D Skin, Right Lower Arm** **E Skin, Left Lower Arm** **F Skin, Right Hand** **G Skin, Left Hand** **H Skin, Right Upper Leg** **J Skin, Left Upper Leg** **K Skin, Right Lower Leg** **L Skin, Left Lower Leg** **M Skin, Right Foot** **N Skin, Left Foot** **T Breast, Right** Mammary duct Mammary gland **U Breast, Left** *See T Breast, Right* **V Breast, Bilateral** *See T Breast, Right* **W Nipple, Right** Areola **X Nipple, Left** *See W Nipple, Right*	**X External**	**Z No Device**	**Z No Qualifier**

Non-OR ØHMØXZZ

Ø Medical and Surgical
H Skin and Breast
N Release Definition: Freeing a body part from an abnormal physical constraint by cutting or by the use of force
Explanation: Some of the restraining tissue may be taken out but none of the body part is taken out

Body Part Character 4	Approach Character 5	Device Character 6	Qualifier Character 7
Ø Skin, Scalp **1** Skin, Face **2** Skin, Right Ear **3** Skin, Left Ear **4** Skin, Neck **5** Skin, Chest Breast procedures, skin only **6** Skin, Back **7** Skin, Abdomen **8** Skin, Buttock **9** Skin, Perineum Perianal skin **A** Skin, Inguinal **B** Skin, Right Upper Arm **C** Skin, Left Upper Arm **D** Skin, Right Lower Arm **E** Skin, Left Lower Arm **F** Skin, Right Hand **G** Skin, Left Hand **H** Skin, Right Upper Leg **J** Skin, Left Upper Leg **K** Skin, Right Lower Leg **L** Skin, Left Lower Leg **M** Skin, Right Foot **N** Skin, Left Foot **Q** Finger Nail Nail bed Nail plate **R** Toe Nail *See Q Finger Nail*	**X** External	**Z** No Device	**Z** No Qualifier
T Breast, Right Mammary duct Mammary gland **U** Breast, Left *See T Breast, Right* **V** Breast, Bilateral *See T Breast, Right*	**Ø** Open **3** Percutaneous **7** Via Natural or Artificial Opening **8** Via Natural or Artificial Opening Endoscopic	**Z** No Device	**Z** No Qualifier
W Nipple, Right Areola **X** Nipple, Left *See W Nipple, Right*	**Ø** Open **3** Percutaneous **7** Via Natural or Artificial Opening **8** Via Natural or Artificial Opening Endoscopic **X** External	**Z** No Device	**Z** No Qualifier

Ø Medical and Surgical
H Skin and Breast
P Removal

Definition: Taking out or off a device from a body part

Explanation: If a device is taken out and a similar device put in without cutting or puncturing the skin or mucous membrane, the procedure is coded to the root operation CHANGE. Otherwise, the procedure for taking out a device is coded to the root operation REMOVAL.

Body Part Character 4	Approach Character 5	Device Character 6	Qualifier Character 7
P Skin Dermis Epidermis Sebaceous gland Sweat gland	**X External**	**Ø Drainage Device** **7 Autologous Tissue Substitute** **J Synthetic Substitute** **K Nonautologous Tissue Substitute** **Y Other Device**	**Z No Qualifier**
Q Finger Nail Nail bed Nail plate **R Toe Nail** *See Q Finger Nail*	**X External**	**Ø Drainage Device** **7 Autologous Tissue Substitute** **J Synthetic Substitute** **K Nonautologous Tissue Substitute**	**Z No Qualifier**
S Hair	**X External**	**7 Autologous Tissue Substitute** **J Synthetic Substitute** **K Nonautologous Tissue Substitute**	**Z No Qualifier**
T Breast, Right Mammary duct Mammary gland **U Breast, Left** *See T Breast, Right*	**Ø Open** **3 Percutaneous** **7 Via Natural or Artificial Opening** **8 Via Natural or Artificial Opening Endoscopic**	**Ø Drainage Device** **1 Radioactive Element** **7 Autologous Tissue Substitute** **J Synthetic Substitute** **K Nonautologous Tissue Substitute** **N Tissue Expander** **Y Other Device**	**Z No Qualifier**

Non-OR ØHPPX[Ø,7,J,K,Y]Z
Non-OR ØHP[Q,R]X[Ø,7,J,K]Z
Non-OR ØHPSX[7,J,K]Z
Non-OR ØHP[T,U]Ø[Ø,1,7,K]Z
Non-OR ØHP[T,U]3[Ø,1,7,K,Y]Z
Non-OR ØHP[T,U][7,8][Ø,1,7,J,K,N,Y]Z

Ø Medical and Surgical
H Skin and Breast
Q Repair Definition: Restoring, to the extent possible, a body part to its normal anatomic structure and function
Explanation: Used only when the method to accomplish the repair is not one of the other root operations

Body Part Character 4	Approach Character 5	Device Character 6	Qualifier Character 7
Ø Skin, Scalp **1** Skin, Face **2** Skin, Right Ear **3** Skin, Left Ear **4** Skin, Neck **5** Skin, Chest Breast procedures, skin only **6** Skin, Back **7** Skin, Abdomen **8** Skin, Buttock **9** Skin, Perineum Perianal skin **A** Skin, Inguinal **B** Skin, Right Upper Arm **C** Skin, Left Upper Arm **D** Skin, Right Lower Arm **E** Skin, Left Lower Arm **F** Skin, Right Hand **G** Skin, Left Hand **H** Skin, Right Upper Leg **J** Skin, Left Upper Leg **K** Skin, Right Lower Leg **L** Skin, Left Lower Leg **M** Skin, Right Foot **N** Skin, Left Foot **Q** Finger Nail Nail bed Nail plate **R** Toe Nail *See Q Finger Nail*	**X** External	**Z** No Device	**Z** No Qualifier
T Breast, Right Mammary duct Mammary gland **U** Breast, Left *See T Breast, Right* **V** Breast, Bilateral *See T Breast, Right* **Y** Supernumerary Breast	**Ø** Open **3** Percutaneous **7** Via Natural or Artificial Opening **8** Via Natural or Artificial Opening Endoscopic	**Z** No Device	**Z** No Qualifier
W Nipple, Right Areola **X** Nipple, Left *See W Nipple, Right*	**Ø** Open **3** Percutaneous **7** Via Natural or Artificial Opening **8** Via Natural or Artificial Opening Endoscopic **X** External	**Z** No Device	**Z** No Qualifier

DRG Non-OR ØHQ9XZZ
Non-OR ØHQ[Ø,1,2,3,4,5,6,7,8,A,B,C,D,E,F,G,H,J,K,L,M,N]XZZ

Ø Medical and Surgical
H Skin and Breast
R Replacement

Definition: Putting in or on biological or synthetic material that physically takes the place and/or function of all or a portion of a body part

Explanation: The body part may have been taken out or replaced, or may be taken out, physically eradicated, or rendered nonfunctional during the REPLACEMENT procedure. A REMOVAL procedure is coded for taking out the device used in a previous replacement procedure.

Body Part Character 4		Approach Character 5	Device Character 6	Qualifier Character 7
Ø Skin, Scalp **1 Skin, Face** **2 Skin, Right Ear** **3 Skin, Left Ear** **4 Skin, Neck** **5 Skin, Chest** Breast procedures, skin only **6 Skin, Back** **7 Skin, Abdomen** **8 Skin, Buttock** **9 Skin, Perineum** Perianal skin **A Skin, Inguinal**	**B Skin, Right Upper Arm** **C Skin, Left Upper Arm** **D Skin, Right Lower Arm** **E Skin, Left Lower Arm** **F Skin, Right Hand** **G Skin, Left Hand** **H Skin, Right Upper Leg** **J Skin, Left Upper Leg** **K Skin, Right Lower Leg** **L Skin, Left Lower Leg** **M Skin, Right Foot** **N Skin, Left Foot**	**X External**	**7 Autologous Tissue Substitute**	**2 Cell Suspension Technique** **3 Full Thickness** **4 Partial Thickness**
Ø Skin, Scalp **1 Skin, Face** **2 Skin, Right Ear** **3 Skin, Left Ear** **4 Skin, Neck** **5 Skin, Chest** Breast procedures, skin only **6 Skin, Back** **7 Skin, Abdomen** **8 Skin, Buttock** **9 Skin, Perineum** Perianal skin **A Skin, Inguinal**	**B Skin, Right Upper Arm** **C Skin, Left Upper Arm** **D Skin, Right Lower Arm** **E Skin, Left Lower Arm** **F Skin, Right Hand** **G Skin, Left Hand** **H Skin, Right Upper Leg** **J Skin, Left Upper Leg** **K Skin, Right Lower Leg** **L Skin, Left Lower Leg** **M Skin, Right Foot** **N Skin, Left Foot**	**X External**	**J Synthetic Substitute**	**3 Full Thickness** **4 Partial Thickness** **Z No Qualifier**
Ø Skin, Scalp **1 Skin, Face** **2 Skin, Right Ear** **3 Skin, Left Ear** **4 Skin, Neck** **5 Skin, Chest** Breast procedures, skin only **6 Skin, Back** **7 Skin, Abdomen** **8 Skin Buttock** **9 Skin, Perineum** Perianal skin **A Skin, Inguinal**	**B Skin, Right Upper Arm** **C Skin, Left Upper Arm** **D Skin, Right Lower Arm** **E Skin, Left Lower Arm** **F Skin, Right Hand** **G Skin, Left Hand** **H Skin, Right Upper Leg** **J Skin, Left Upper Leg** **K Skin, Right Lower Leg** **L Skin, Left Lower Leg** **M Skin, Right Foot** **N Skin, Left Foot**	**X External**	**K Nonautologous Tissue Substitute**	**3 Full Thickness** **4 Partial Thickness**
Q Finger Nail Nail bed Nail plate	**R Toe Nail** *See Q Finger Nail* **S Hair**	**X External**	**7 Autologous Tissue Substitute** **J Synthetic Substitute** **K Nonautologous Tissue Substitute**	**Z No Qualifier**
T Breast, Right Mammary duct Mammary gland	**U Breast, Left** *See T Breast, Right* **V Breast, Bilateral** *See T Breast, Right*	**Ø Open**	**7 Autologous Tissue Substitute**	**5 Latissimus Dorsi Myocutaneous Flap** **6 Transverse Rectus Abdominis Myocutaneous Flap** **7 Deep Inferior Epigastric Artery Perforator Flap** **8 Superficial Inferior Epigastric Artery Flap** **9 Gluteal Artery Perforator Flap** **Z No Qualifier**
T Breast, Right Mammary duct Mammary gland	**U Breast, Left** *See T Breast, Right* **V Breast, Bilateral** *See T Breast, Right*	**Ø Open**	**J Synthetic Substitute** **K Nonautologous Tissue Substitute**	**Z No Qualifier**
T Breast, Right ⊞ Mammary duct Mammary gland **U Breast, Left** ⊞ *See T Breast, Right*	**V Breast, Bilateral** ⊞ *See T Breast, Right*	**3 Percutaneous**	**7 Autologous Tissue Substitute** **J Synthetic Substitute** **K Nonautologous Tissue Substitute**	**Z No Qualifier**
W Nipple, Right Areola	**X Nipple, Left** *See W Nipple, Right*	**Ø Open** **3 Percutaneous** **X External**	**7 Autologous Tissue Substitute** **J Synthetic Substitute** **K Nonautologous Tissue Substitute**	**Z No Qualifier**

Non-OR ØHRSX7Z

See Appendix L for Procedure Combinations
⊞ ØHR[T,U,V]37Z

Ø Medical and Surgical
H Skin and Breast
S Reposition

Definition: Moving to its normal location, or other suitable location, all or a portion of a body part

Explanation: The body part is moved to a new location from an abnormal location, or from a normal location where it is not functioning correctly. The body part may or may not be cut out or off to be moved to the new location.

Body Part Character 4	Approach Character 5	Device Character 6	Qualifier Character 7
S Hair **W** Nipple, Right Areola **X** Nipple, Left *See W Nipple, Right*	**X** External	**Z** No Device	**Z** No Qualifier
T Breast, Right Mammary duct Mammary gland **U** Breast, Left *See T Breast, Right* **V** Breast, Bilateral *See T Breast, Right*	**Ø** Open	**Z** No Device	**Z** No Qualifier

Non-OR ØHSSXZZ

Ø Medical and Surgical
H Skin and Breast
T Resection

Definition: Cutting out or off, without replacement, all of a body part

Explanation: None

Body Part Character 4	Approach Character 5	Device Character 6	Qualifier Character 7
Q Finger Nail Nail bed Nail plate **R** Toe Nail *See Q Finger Nail* **W** Nipple, Right Areola **X** Nipple, Left *See W Nipple, Right*	**X** External	**Z** No Device	**Z** No Qualifier
T Breast, Right ⊞ Mammary duct Mammary gland **U** Breast, Left ⊞ *See T Breast, Right* **V** Breast, Bilateral ⊞ *See T Breast, Right* **Y** Supernumerary Breast	**Ø** Open	**Z** No Device	**Z** No Qualifier

Non-OR ØHT[Q,R]XZZ

See Appendix L for Procedure Combinations
⊞ ØHT[T,U,V]ØZZ

Ø Medical and Surgical
H Skin and Breast
U Supplement

Definition: Putting in or on biological or synthetic material that physically reinforces and/or augments the function of a portion of a body part

Explanation: The biological material is non-living, or is living and from the same individual. The body part may have been previously replaced, and the SUPPLEMENT procedure is performed to physically reinforce and/or augment the function of the replaced body part.

Body Part Character 4	Approach Character 5	Device Character 6	Qualifier Character 7
T Breast, Right Mammary duct Mammary gland **U** Breast, Left *See T Breast, Right* **V** Breast, Bilateral *See T Breast, Right*	**Ø** Open **3** Percutaneous **7** Via Natural or Artificial Opening **8** Via Natural or Artificial Opening Endoscopic	**7** Autologous Tissue Substitute **J** Synthetic Substitute **K** Nonautologous Tissue Substitute	**Z** No Qualifier
W Nipple, Right Areola **X** Nipple, Left *See W Nipple, Right*	**Ø** Open **3** Percutaneous **7** Via Natural or Artificial Opening **8** Via Natural or Artificial Opening Endoscopic **X** External	**7** Autologous Tissue Substitute **J** Synthetic Substitute **K** Nonautologous Tissue Substitute	**Z** No Qualifier

Non-OR ØHU[T,U,V]3JZ

Ø Medical and Surgical
H Skin and Breast
W Revision

Definition: Correcting, to the extent possible, a portion of a malfunctioning device or the position of a displaced device

Explanation: Revision can include correcting a malfunctioning or displaced device by taking out or putting in components of the device such as a screw or pin

Body Part Character 4	Approach Character 5	Device Character 6	Qualifier Character 7
P Skin Dermis Epidermis Sebaceous gland Sweat gland	**X External**	**Ø Drainage Device** **7 Autologous Tissue Substitute** **J Synthetic Substitute** **K Nonautologous Tissue Substitute** **Y Other Device**	**Z No Qualifier**
Q Finger Nail Nail bed Nail plate **R Toe Nail** *See Q Finger Nail*	**X External**	**Ø Drainage Device** **7 Autologous Tissue Substitute** **J Synthetic Substitute** **K Nonautologous Tissue Substitute**	**Z No Qualifier**
S Hair	**X External**	**7 Autologous Tissue Substitute** **J Synthetic Substitute** **K Nonautologous Tissue Substitute**	**Z No Qualifier**
T Breast, Right Mammary duct Mammary gland **U Breast, Left** *See T Breast, Right*	**Ø Open** **3 Percutaneous** **7 Via Natural or Artificial Opening** **8 Via Natural or Artificial Opening Endoscopic**	**Ø Drainage Device** **7 Autologous Tissue Substitute** **J Synthetic Substitute** **K Nonautologous Tissue Substitute** **N Tissue Expander** **Y Other Device**	**Z No Qualifier**

Non-OR ØHWPX[Ø,7,J,K,Y]Z
Non-OR ØHW[Q,R]X[Ø,7,J,K]Z
Non-OR ØHWSX[7,J,K]Z
Non-OR ØHW[T,U]Ø[Ø,7,K,N]Z
Non-OR ØHW[T,U]3[Ø,7,K,N,Y]Z
Non-OR ØHW[T,U][7,8][Ø,7,J,K,N,Y]Z

Ø Medical and Surgical
H Skin and Breast
X Transfer

Definition: Moving, without taking out, all or a portion of a body part to another location to take over the function of all or a portion of a body part

Explanation: The body part transferred remains connected to its vascular and nervous supply

Body Part Character 4	Approach Character 5	Device Character 6	Qualifier Character 7
Ø Skin, Scalp **1 Skin, Face** **2 Skin, Right Ear** **3 Skin, Left Ear** **4 Skin, Neck** **5 Skin, Chest** Breast procedures, skin only **6 Skin, Back** **7 Skin, Abdomen** **8 Skin, Buttock** **9 Skin, Perineum** Perianal skin **A Skin, Inguinal** **B Skin, Right Upper Arm** **C Skin, Left Upper Arm** **D Skin, Right Lower Arm** **E Skin, Left Lower Arm** **F Skin, Right Hand** **G Skin, Left Hand** **H Skin, Right Upper Leg** **J Skin, Left Upper Leg** **K Skin, Right Lower Leg** **L Skin, Left Lower Leg** **M Skin, Right Foot** **N Skin, Left Foot**	**X External**	**Z No Device**	**Z No Qualifier**

Subcutaneous Tissue and Fascia ØJØ–ØJX

Character Meanings

This Character Meaning table is provided as a guide to assist the user in the identification of character members that may be found in this section of code tables. It **SHOULD NOT** be used to build a PCS code.

Operation–Character 3	Body Part–Character 4	Approach–Character 5	Device–Character 6	Qualifier–Character 7
Ø Alteration	Ø Subcutaneous Tissue and Fascia, Scalp	Ø Open	Ø Drainage Device OR Monitoring Device, Hemodynamic	B Skin and Subcutaneous Tissue
2 Change	1 Subcutaneous Tissue and Fascia, Face	3 Percutaneous	1 Radioactive Element	C Skin, Subcutaneous Tissue and Fascia
5 Destruction	4 Subcutaneous Tissue and Fascia, Right Neck	X External	2 Monitoring Device	X Diagnostic
8 Division	5 Subcutaneous Tissue and Fascia, Left Neck		3 Infusion Device	Z No Qualifier
9 Drainage	6 Subcutaneous Tissue and Fascia, Chest		4 Pacemaker, Single Chamber	
B Excision	7 Subcutaneous Tissue and Fascia, Back		5 Pacemaker, Single Chamber Rate Responsive	
C Extirpation	8 Subcutaneous Tissue and Fascia, Abdomen		6 Pacemaker, Dual Chamber	
D Extraction	9 Subcutaneous Tissue and Fascia, Buttock		7 Autologous Tissue Substitute OR Cardiac Resynchronization Pacemaker Pulse Generator	
H Insertion	B Subcutaneous Tissue and Fascia, Perineum		8 Defibrillator Generator	
J Inspection	C Subcutaneous Tissue and Fascia, Pelvic Region		9 Cardiac Resynchronization Defibrillator Pulse Generator	
N Release	D Subcutaneous Tissue and Fascia, Right Upper Arm		A Contractility Modulation Device	
P Removal	F Subcutaneous Tissue and Fascia, Left Upper Arm		B Stimulator Generator, Single Array	
Q Repair	G Subcutaneous Tissue and Fascia, Right Lower Arm		C Stimulator Generator, Single Array Rechargeable	
R Replacement	H Subcutaneous Tissue and Fascia, Left Lower Arm		D Stimulator Generator, Multiple Array	
U Supplement	J Subcutaneous Tissue and Fascia, Right Hand		E Stimulator Generator, Multiple Array Rechargeable	
W Revision	K Subcutaneous Tissue and Fascia, Left Hand		F Subcutaneous Defibrillator Lead	
X Transfer	L Subcutaneous Tissue and Fascia, Right Upper Leg		H Contraceptive Device	
	M Subcutaneous Tissue and Fascia, Left Upper Leg		J Synthetic Substitute	
	N Subcutaneous Tissue and Fascia, Right Lower Leg		K Nonautologous Tissue Substitute	
	P Subcutaneous Tissue and Fascia, Left Lower Leg		M Stimulator Generator	
	Q Subcutaneous Tissue and Fascia, Right Foot		N Tissue Expander	
	R Subcutaneous Tissue and Fascia, Left Foot		P Cardiac Rhythm Related Device	
	S Subcutaneous Tissue and Fascia, Head and Neck		V Infusion Device, Pump	
	T Subcutaneous Tissue and Fascia, Trunk		W Vascular Access Device, Totally Implantable	
	V Subcutaneous Tissue and Fascia, Upper Extremity		X Vascular Access Device, Tunneled	
	W Subcutaneous Tissue and Fascia, Lower Extremity		Y Other Device	
			Z No Device	

AHA Coding Clinic for table ØJ2
2018, 3Q, 10 Disruption of perma-catheter fibrin sheath via angioplasty of superior vena cava
2017, 2Q, 26 Exchange of tunneled catheter

AHA Coding Clinic for table ØJ5
2019, 3Q, 25 Endoscopic removal of pilonidal sinus and cyst

AHA Coding Clinic for table ØJ8
2017, 3Q, 11 Bilateral escharotomy of leg, thigh and foot

AHA Coding Clinic for table ØJ9
2018, 3Q, 16 Incision and drainage of submandibular space
2018, 3Q, 16 Incision and drainage of neck abscess
2015, 3Q, 23 Incision and drainage of multiple abscess cavities using vessel loop

AHA Coding Clinic for table ØJB
2023, 2Q, 30 Excisional debridement and non-excisional debridement at deeper layer same site
2022, 3Q, 11 Ulceration and soft tissue redundancy at amputation site due to osteo-integrated implant
2020, 1Q, 31 Repair of buried penis
2019, 3Q, 25 Endoscopic removal of pilonidal sinus and cyst
2018, 3Q, 17 Excisional debridement of periosteum
2018, 1Q, 7 Placement of fat graft following lumbar decompression surgery
2015, 3Q, 3-8 Excisional and nonexcisional debridement
2015, 2Q, 13 Transfer of free flap to reconstruct orbital defect
2015, 1Q, 29 Fistulectomy with placement of seton
2014, 4Q, 38 Abdominoplasty and abdominal wall plication for hernia repair
2014, 3Q, 22 Transsphenoidal removal of pituitary tumor and fat graft placement

AHA Coding Clinic for table ØJC
2017, 3Q, 22 Replacement of native skull bone flap

AHA Coding Clinic for table ØJD
2023, 2Q, 30 Excisional debridement and non-excisional debridement at deeper layer same site
2023, 1Q, 36 Maggot therapy
2016, 3Q, 20 VersaJet™ nonexcisional debridement of leg muscle
2016, 3Q, 21 Nonexcisional debridement of infected lumbar wound
2016, 3Q, 21 Nonexcisional pulsed lavage debridement
2016, 3Q, 22 Debridement of bone and tendon using Tenex ultrasound device
2016, 1Q, 40 Nonexcisional debridement of skin and subcutaneous tissue
2015, 3Q, 3-8 Excisional and nonexcisional debridement
2015, 1Q, 23 Non-Excisional debridement with lavage of wound

AHA Coding Clinic for table ØJH
2020, 4Q, 54 Insertion of other device into subcutaneous tissue and fascia
2020, 4Q, 55 Insertion of subcutaneous pump system for ascites drainage
2020, 2Q, 15 Ommaya reservoir with ventricular catheter placement
2020, 2Q, 16 Ommaya reservoir placement for cerebrospinal fluid infusion therapy
2019, 4Q, 33 Subcutaneous implantable cardioverter defibrillator lead
2017, 4Q, 63-64 Added and revised device values - Vascular access reservoir
2017, 2Q, 24 Tunneled catheter versus totally implantable catheter
2017, 2Q, 26 Exchange of tunneled catheter
2016, 4Q, 97-98 Phrenic neurostimulator
2016, 2Q, 14 Insertion of peritoneal totally implantable venous access device
2016, 2Q, 15 Removal and replacement of tunneled internal jugular catheter
2015, 4Q, 14 New Section X codes—New Technology procedures
2015, 4Q, 30-31 Vascular access devices
2015, 2Q, 33 Totally implantable central venous access device (Port-a-Cath)
2014, 3Q, 19 End of life replacement of Baclofen pump
2013, 4Q, 116 Device character for Port-A-Cath placement
2012, 4Q, 104 Placement of subcutaneous implantable cardioverter defibrillator

AHA Coding Clinic for table ØJN
2017, 3Q, 11 Bilateral escharotomy of leg, thigh and foot

AHA Coding Clinic for table ØJP
2019, 4Q, 33 Subcutaneous implantable cardioverter defibrillator lead
2018, 4Q, 86 Placement of lumboatrial shunt
2018, 3Q, 29 Decommissioning of left ventricular assist device with exploration of mediastinum
2016, 2Q, 15 Removal and replacement of tunneled internal jugular catheter
2015, 4Q, 31 Vascular access devices
2014, 3Q, 19 End of life replacement of Baclofen pump
2013, 4Q, 109 Separating conjoined twins
2012, 4Q, 104 Placement of subcutaneous implantable cardioverter defibrillator

AHA Coding Clinic for table ØJQ
2022, 3Q, 24 Leakage of cerebrospinal fluid with revision of intrathecal baclofen system
2017, 3Q, 19 Anterior repair of cystocele
2014, 4Q, 44 Posterior colporrhaphy/rectocele repair

AHA Coding Clinic for table ØJR
2015, 2Q, 13 Transfer of free flap to reconstruct orbital defect

AHA Coding Clinic for table ØJU
2018, 2Q, 20 Prelaminated free flap graft using Alloderm™
2018, 1Q, 7 Placement of fat graft following lumbar decompression surgery

AHA Coding Clinic for table ØJW
2022, 3Q, 24 Leakage of cerebrospinal fluid with revision of intrathecal baclofen system
2019, 4Q, 33 Subcutaneous implantable cardioverter defibrillator lead
2018, 1Q, 8 Ventricular peritoneal shunt ligation
2015, 4Q, 33 Externalization of peritoneal dialysis catheter
2015, 2Q, 9 Revision of ventriculoperitoneal (VP) shunt
2012, 4Q, 104 Placement of subcutaneous implantable cardioverter defibrillator

AHA Coding Clinic for table ØJX
2022, 3Q, 11 Ulceration and soft tissue redundancy at amputation site due to osteo-integrated implant
2022, 1Q, 48 Repair of facial fractures of frontal sinus and orbital roof
2021, 3Q, 19 Elbow amputation and targeted muscle reinnervation
2021, 2Q, 16 Goldilocks breast reconstruction
2018, 1Q, 10 Complex wound closure using pericranial flap
2014, 3Q, 18 Placement of reverse sural fasciocutaneous pedicle flap
2013, 4Q, 109 Separating conjoined twins

Ø Medical and Surgical
J Subcutaneous Tissue and Fascia
Ø Alteration Definition: Modifying the anatomic structure of a body part without affecting the function of the body part

Explanation: Principal purpose is to improve appearance

Body Part Character 4		Approach Character 5	Device Character 6	Qualifier Character 7
1 Subcutaneous Tissue and Fascia, Face Chin Masseteric fascia Orbital fascia Submandibular space **4 Subcutaneous Tissue and Fascia, Right Neck** Deep cervical fascia Pretracheal fascia Prevertebral fascia **5 Subcutaneous Tissue and Fascia, Left Neck** *See 4 Subcutaneous Tissue and Fascia, Right Neck* **6 Subcutaneous Tissue and Fascia, Chest** Pectoral fascia **7 Subcutaneous Tissue and Fascia, Back** **8 Subcutaneous Tissue and Fascia, Abdomen** **9 Subcutaneous Tissue and Fascia, Buttock** **D Subcutaneous Tissue and Fascia, Right Upper Arm** Axillary fascia Deltoid fascia Infraspinatus fascia Subscapular aponeurosis Supraspinatus fascia	**F Subcutaneous Tissue and Fascia, Left Upper Arm** *See D Subcutaneous Tissue and Fascia, Right Upper Arm* **G Subcutaneous Tissue and Fascia, Right Lower Arm** Antebrachial fascia Bicipital aponeurosis **H Subcutaneous Tissue and Fascia, Left Lower Arm** *See G Subcutaneous Tissue and Fascia, Right Lower Arm* **L Subcutaneous Tissue and Fascia, Right Upper Leg** Crural fascia Fascia lata Iliac fascia Iliotibial tract (band) **M Subcutaneous Tissue and Fascia, Left Upper Leg** *See L Subcutaneous Tissue and Fascia, Right Upper Leg* **N Subcutaneous Tissue and Fascia, Right Lower Leg** **P Subcutaneous Tissue and Fascia, Left Lower Leg**	**Ø Open** **3 Percutaneous**	**Z No Device**	**Z No Qualifier**

Ø Medical and Surgical
J Subcutaneous Tissue and Fascia
2 Change Definition: Taking out or off a device from a body part and putting back an identical or similar device in or on the same body part without cutting or puncturing the skin or a mucous membrane

Explanation: All CHANGE procedures are coded using the approach EXTERNAL

Body Part Character 4	Approach Character 5	Device Character 6	Qualifier Character 7
S Subcutaneous Tissue and Fascia, Head and Neck **T Subcutaneous Tissue and Fascia, Trunk** External oblique aponeurosis Transversalis fascia **V Subcutaneous Tissue and Fascia, Upper Extremity** **W Subcutaneous Tissue and Fascia, Lower Extremity**	**X External**	**Ø Drainage Device** **Y Other Device**	**Z No Qualifier**

Non-OR All body part, approach, device, and qualifier values

Ø Medical and Surgical
J Subcutaneous Tissue and Fascia
5 Destruction Definition: Physical eradication of all or a portion of a body part by the direct use of energy, force, or a destructive agent
Explanation: None of the body part is physically taken out

Body Part Character 4	Approach Character 5	Device Character 6	Qualifier Character 7
Ø Subcutaneous Tissue and Fascia, Scalp Galea aponeurotica **1** Subcutaneous Tissue and Fascia, Face Chin Masseteric fascia Orbital fascia Submandibular space **4** Subcutaneous Tissue and Fascia, Right Neck Deep cervical fascia Pretracheal fascia Prevertebral fascia **5** Subcutaneous Tissue and Fascia, Left Neck *See 4 Subcutaneous Tissue and Fascia, Right Neck* **6** Subcutaneous Tissue and Fascia, Chest Pectoral fascia **7** Subcutaneous Tissue and Fascia, Back **8** Subcutaneous Tissue and Fascia, Abdomen **9** Subcutaneous Tissue and Fascia, Buttock **B** Subcutaneous Tissue and Fascia, Perineum **C** Subcutaneous Tissue and Fascia, Pelvic Region **D** Subcutaneous Tissue and Fascia, Right Upper Arm Axillary fascia Deltoid fascia Infraspinatus fascia Subscapular aponeurosis Supraspinatus fascia **F** Subcutaneous Tissue and Fascia, Left Upper Arm *See D Subcutaneous Tissue and Fascia, Right Upper Arm* **G** Subcutaneous Tissue and Fascia, Right Lower Arm Antebrachial fascia Bicipital aponeurosis **H** Subcutaneous Tissue and Fascia, Left Lower Arm *See G Subcutaneous Tissue and Fascia, Right Lower Arm* **J** Subcutaneous Tissue and Fascia, Right Hand Palmar fascia (aponeurosis) **K** Subcutaneous Tissue and Fascia, Left Hand *See J Subcutaneous Tissue and Fascia, Right Hand* **L** Subcutaneous Tissue and Fascia, Right Upper Leg Crural fascia Fascia lata Iliac fascia Iliotibial tract (band) **M** Subcutaneous Tissue and Fascia, Left Upper Leg *See L Subcutaneous Tissue and Fascia, Right Upper Leg* **N** Subcutaneous Tissue and Fascia, Right Lower Leg **P** Subcutaneous Tissue and Fascia, Left Lower Leg **Q** Subcutaneous Tissue and Fascia, Right Foot Plantar fascia (aponeurosis) **R** Subcutaneous Tissue and Fascia, Left Foot *See Q Subcutaneous Tissue and Fascia, Right Foot*	**Ø** Open **3** Percutaneous	**Z** No Device	**Z** No Qualifier

DRG Non-OR All body part, approach, device, and qualifier values

Ø Medical and Surgical
J Subcutaneous Tissue and Fascia
8 Division Definition: Cutting into a body part, without draining fluids and/or gases from the body part, in order to separate or transect a body part
Explanation: All or a portion of the body part is separated into two or more portions

Body Part Character 4	Approach Character 5	Device Character 6	Qualifier Character 7
Ø Subcutaneous Tissue and Fascia, Scalp Galea aponeurotica **1 Subcutaneous Tissue and Fascia, Face** Chin Masseteric fascia Orbital fascia Submandibular space **4 Subcutaneous Tissue and Fascia, Right Neck** Deep cervical fascia Pretracheal fascia Prevertebral fascia **5 Subcutaneous Tissue and Fascia, Left Neck** *See 4 Subcutaneous Tissue and Fascia, Right Neck* **6 Subcutaneous Tissue and Fascia, Chest** Pectoral fascia **7 Subcutaneous Tissue and Fascia, Back** **8 Subcutaneous Tissue and Fascia, Abdomen** **9 Subcutaneous Tissue and Fascia, Buttock** **B Subcutaneous Tissue and Fascia, Perineum** **C Subcutaneous Tissue and Fascia, Pelvic Region** **D Subcutaneous Tissue and Fascia, Right Upper Arm** Axillary fascia Deltoid fascia Infraspinatus fascia Subscapular aponeurosis Supraspinatus fascia **F Subcutaneous Tissue and Fascia, Left Upper Arm** *See D Subcutaneous Tissue and Fascia, Right Upper Arm* **G Subcutaneous Tissue and Fascia, Right Lower Arm** Antebrachial fascia Bicipital aponeurosis **H Subcutaneous Tissue and Fascia, Left Lower Arm** *See G Subcutaneous Tissue and Fascia, Right Lower Arm* **J Subcutaneous Tissue and Fascia, Right Hand** Palmar fascia (aponeurosis) **K Subcutaneous Tissue and Fascia, Left Hand** *See J Subcutaneous Tissue and Fascia, Right Hand* **L Subcutaneous Tissue and Fascia, Right Upper Leg** Crural fascia Fascia lata Iliac fascia Iliotibial tract (band) **M Subcutaneous Tissue and Fascia, Left Upper Leg** *See L Subcutaneous Tissue and Fascia, Right Upper Leg* **N Subcutaneous Tissue and Fascia, Right Lower Leg** **P Subcutaneous Tissue and Fascia, Left Lower Leg** **Q Subcutaneous Tissue and Fascia, Right Foot** Plantar fascia (aponeurosis) **R Subcutaneous Tissue and Fascia, Left Foot** *See Q Subcutaneous Tissue and Fascia, Right Foot* **S Subcutaneous Tissue and Fascia, Head and Neck** **T Subcutaneous Tissue and Fascia, Trunk** External oblique aponeurosis Transversalis fascia **V Subcutaneous Tissue and Fascia, Upper Extremity** **W Subcutaneous Tissue and Fascia, Lower Extremity**	**Ø Open** **3 Percutaneous**	**Z No Device**	**Z No Qualifier**

Ø Medical and Surgical
J Subcutaneous Tissue and Fascia
9 Drainage Definition: Taking or letting out fluids and/or gases from a body part
Explanation: The qualifier DIAGNOSTIC is used to identify drainage procedures that are biopsies

Body Part Character 4		Approach Character 5	Device Character 6	Qualifier Character 7
Ø Subcutaneous Tissue and Fascia, Scalp Galea aponeurotica **1 Subcutaneous Tissue and Fascia, Face** Chin Masseteric fascia Orbital fascia Submandibular space **4 Subcutaneous Tissue and Fascia, Right Neck** Deep cervical fascia Pretracheal fascia Prevertebral fascia **5 Subcutaneous Tissue and Fascia, Left Neck** *See 4 Subcutaneous Tissue and Fascia, Right Neck* **6 Subcutaneous Tissue and Fascia, Chest** Pectoral fascia **7 Subcutaneous Tissue and Fascia, Back** **8 Subcutaneous Tissue and Fascia, Abdomen** **9 Subcutaneous Tissue and Fascia, Buttock** **B Subcutaneous Tissue and Fascia, Perineum** **C Subcutaneous Tissue and Fascia, Pelvic Region** **D Subcutaneous Tissue and Fascia, Right Upper Arm** Axillary fascia Deltoid fascia Infraspinatus fascia Subscapular aponeurosis Supraspinatus fascia **F Subcutaneous Tissue and Fascia, Left Upper Arm** *See D Subcutaneous Tissue and Fascia, Right Upper Arm*	**G Subcutaneous Tissue and Fascia, Right Lower Arm** Antebrachial fascia Bicipital aponeurosis **H Subcutaneous Tissue and Fascia, Left Lower Arm** *See G Subcutaneous Tissue and Fascia, Right Lower Arm* **J Subcutaneous Tissue and Fascia, Right Hand** Palmar fascia (aponeurosis) **K Subcutaneous Tissue and Fascia, Left Hand** *See J Subcutaneous Tissue and Fascia, Right Hand* **L Subcutaneous Tissue and Fascia, Right Upper Leg** Crural fascia Fascia lata Iliac fascia Iliotibial tract (band) **M Subcutaneous Tissue and Fascia, Left Upper Leg** *See L Subcutaneous Tissue and Fascia, Right Upper Leg* **N Subcutaneous Tissue and Fascia, Right Lower Leg** **P Subcutaneous Tissue and Fascia, Left Lower Leg** **Q Subcutaneous Tissue and Fascia, Right Foot** Plantar fascia (aponeurosis) **R Subcutaneous Tissue and Fascia, Left Foot** *See Q Subcutaneous Tissue and Fascia, Right Foot*	Ø Open 3 Percutaneous	Ø Drainage Device	Z No Qualifier

Non-OR All body part, approach, device, and qualifier values

ØJ9 Continued on next page

Ø Medical and Surgical
J Subcutaneous Tissue and Fascia
9 Drainage Definition: Taking or letting out fluids and/or gases from a body part
Explanation: The qualifier DIAGNOSTIC is used to identify drainage procedures that are biopsies

ØJ9 Continued

Body Part Character 4	Approach Character 5	Device Character 6	Qualifier Character 7
Ø **Subcutaneous Tissue and Fascia, Scalp** Galea aponeurotica 1 **Subcutaneous Tissue and Fascia, Face** Chin Masseteric fascia Orbital fascia Submandibular space 4 **Subcutaneous Tissue and Fascia, Right Neck** Deep cervical fascia Pretracheal fascia Prevertebral fascia 5 **Subcutaneous Tissue and Fascia, Left Neck** **See** *4 Subcutaneous Tissue and Fascia, Right Neck* 6 **Subcutaneous Tissue and Fascia, Chest** Pectoral fascia 7 **Subcutaneous Tissue and Fascia, Back** 8 **Subcutaneous Tissue and Fascia, Abdomen** 9 **Subcutaneous Tissue and Fascia, Buttock** B **Subcutaneous Tissue and Fascia, Perineum** C **Subcutaneous Tissue and Fascia, Pelvic Region** D **Subcutaneous Tissue and Fascia, Right Upper Arm** Axillary fascia Deltoid fascia Infraspinatus fascia Subscapular aponeurosis Supraspinatus fascia F **Subcutaneous Tissue and Fascia, Left Upper Arm** **See** *D Subcutaneous Tissue and Fascia, Right Upper Arm* G **Subcutaneous Tissue and Fascia, Right Lower Arm** Antebrachial fascia Bicipital aponeurosis H **Subcutaneous Tissue and Fascia, Left Lower Arm** **See** *G Subcutaneous Tissue and Fascia, Right Lower Arm* J **Subcutaneous Tissue and Fascia, Right Hand** Palmar fascia (aponeurosis) K **Subcutaneous Tissue and Fascia, Left Hand** **See** *J Subcutaneous Tissue and Fascia, Right Hand* L **Subcutaneous Tissue and Fascia, Right Upper Leg** Crural fascia Fascia lata Iliac fascia Iliotibial tract (band) M **Subcutaneous Tissue and Fascia, Left Upper Leg** **See** *L Subcutaneous Tissue and Fascia, Right Upper Leg* N **Subcutaneous Tissue and Fascia, Right Lower Leg** P **Subcutaneous Tissue and Fascia, Left Lower Leg** Q **Subcutaneous Tissue and Fascia, Right Foot** Plantar fascia (aponeurosis) R **Subcutaneous Tissue and Fascia, Left Foot** **See** *Q Subcutaneous Tissue and Fascia, Right Foot*	Ø Open 3 Percutaneous	Z No Device	X Diagnostic Z No Qualifier

Non-OR All body part, approach, device, and qualifier values

Ø Medical and Surgical
J Subcutaneous Tissue and Fascia
B Excision Definition: Cutting out or off, without replacement, a portion of a body part
Explanation: The qualifier DIAGNOSTIC is used to identify excision procedures that are biopsies

Body Part Character 4	Approach Character 5	Device Character 6	Qualifier Character 7
Ø Subcutaneous Tissue and Fascia, Scalp Galea aponeurotica 1 Subcutaneous Tissue and Fascia, Face Chin Masseteric fascia Orbital fascia Submandibular space 4 Subcutaneous Tissue and Fascia, Right Neck Deep cervical fascia Pretracheal fascia Prevertebral fascia 5 Subcutaneous Tissue and Fascia, Left Neck *See 4 Subcutaneous Tissue and Fascia, Right Neck* 6 Subcutaneous Tissue and Fascia, Chest Pectoral fascia 7 Subcutaneous Tissue and Fascia, Back 8 Subcutaneous Tissue and Fascia, Abdomen 9 Subcutaneous Tissue and Fascia, Buttock B Subcutaneous Tissue and Fascia, Perineum C Subcutaneous Tissue and Fascia, Pelvic Region D Subcutaneous Tissue and Fascia, Right Upper Arm Axillary fascia Deltoid fascia Infraspinatus fascia Subscapular aponeurosis Supraspinatus fascia F Subcutaneous Tissue and Fascia, Left Upper Arm *See D Subcutaneous Tissue and Fascia, Right Upper Arm* G Subcutaneous Tissue and Fascia, Right Lower Arm Antebrachial fascia Bicipital aponeurosis H Subcutaneous Tissue and Fascia, Left Lower Arm *See G Subcutaneous Tissue and Fascia, Right Lower Arm* J Subcutaneous Tissue and Fascia, Right Hand Palmar fascia (aponeurosis) K Subcutaneous Tissue and Fascia, Left Hand *See J Subcutaneous Tissue and Fascia, Right Hand* L Subcutaneous Tissue and Fascia, Right Upper Leg Crural fascia Fascia lata Iliac fascia Iliotibial tract (band) M Subcutaneous Tissue and Fascia, Left Upper Leg *See L Subcutaneous Tissue and Fascia, Right Upper Leg* N Subcutaneous Tissue and Fascia, Right Lower Leg P Subcutaneous Tissue and Fascia, Left Lower Leg Q Subcutaneous Tissue and Fascia, Right Foot Plantar fascia (aponeurosis) R Subcutaneous Tissue and Fascia, Left Foot *See Q Subcutaneous Tissue and Fascia, Right Foot*	Ø Open 3 Percutaneous	Z No Device	X Diagnostic Z No Qualifier

DRG Non-OR ØJB[Ø,4,5,6,7,8,9,B,C,D,F,G,H,L,M,N,P,Q,R]3ZZ
Non-OR ØJB[Ø,1,4,5,6,7,8,9,B,C,D,F,G,H,J,K,L,M,N,P,Q,R][Ø,3]ZX

Ø Medical and Surgical
J Subcutaneous Tissue and Fascia
C Extirpation Definition: Taking or cutting out solid matter from a body part

Explanation: The solid matter may be an abnormal byproduct of a biological function or a foreign body; it may be imbedded in a body part or in the lumen of a tubular body part. The solid matter may or may not have been previously broken into pieces.

Body Part Character 4	Approach Character 5	Device Character 6	Qualifier Character 7
Ø Subcutaneous Tissue and Fascia, Scalp Galea aponeurotica **1 Subcutaneous Tissue and Fascia, Face** Chin Masseteric fascia Orbital fascia Submandibular space **4 Subcutaneous Tissue and Fascia, Right Neck** Deep cervical fascia Pretracheal fascia Prevertebral fascia **5 Subcutaneous Tissue and Fascia, Left Neck** ***See*** *4 Subcutaneous Tissue and Fascia, Right Neck* **6 Subcutaneous Tissue and Fascia, Chest** Pectoral fascia **7 Subcutaneous Tissue and Fascia, Back** **8 Subcutaneous Tissue and Fascia, Abdomen** **9 Subcutaneous Tissue and Fascia, Buttock** **B Subcutaneous Tissue and Fascia, Perineum** **C Subcutaneous Tissue and Fascia, Pelvic Region** **D Subcutaneous Tissue and Fascia, Right Upper Arm** Axillary fascia Deltoid fascia Infraspinatus fascia Subscapular aponeurosis Supraspinatus fascia **F Subcutaneous Tissue and Fascia, Left Upper Arm** ***See*** *D Subcutaneous Tissue and Fascia, Right Upper Arm* **G Subcutaneous Tissue and Fascia, Right Lower Arm** Antebrachial fascia Bicipital aponeurosis **H Subcutaneous Tissue and Fascia, Left Lower Arm** ***See*** *G Subcutaneous Tissue and Fascia, Right Lower Arm* **J Subcutaneous Tissue and Fascia, Right Hand** Palmar fascia (aponeurosis) **K Subcutaneous Tissue and Fascia, Left Hand** ***See*** *J Subcutaneous Tissue and Fascia, Right Hand* **L Subcutaneous Tissue and Fascia, Right Upper Leg** Crural fascia Fascia lata Iliac fascia Iliotibial tract (band) **M Subcutaneous Tissue and Fascia, Left Upper Leg** ***See*** *L Subcutaneous Tissue and Fascia, Right Upper Leg* **N Subcutaneous Tissue and Fascia, Right Lower Leg** **P Subcutaneous Tissue and Fascia, Left Lower Leg** **Q Subcutaneous Tissue and Fascia, Right Foot** Plantar fascia (aponeurosis) **R Subcutaneous Tissue and Fascia, Left Foot** ***See*** *Q Subcutaneous Tissue and Fascia, Right Foot*	**Ø** Open **3** Percutaneous	**Z** No Device	**Z** No Qualifier

Non-OR ØJC[Ø,1,4,5,6,7,8,9,B,C,D,F,G,H,J,K,L,M,N,P,Q,R]3ZZ

Ø Medical and Surgical
J Subcutaneous Tissue and Fascia
D Extraction Definition: Pulling or stripping out or off all or a portion of a body part by the use of force

Explanation: The qualifier DIAGNOSTIC is used to identify extraction procedures that are biopsies

Body Part Character 4		Approach Character 5	Device Character 6	Qualifier Character 7
Ø Subcutaneous Tissue and Fascia, Scalp Galea aponeurotica **1 Subcutaneous Tissue and Fascia, Face** Chin Masseteric fascia Orbital fascia Submandibular space **4 Subcutaneous Tissue and Fascia, Right Neck** Deep cervical fascia Pretracheal fascia Prevertebral fascia **5 Subcutaneous Tissue and Fascia, Left Neck** *See 4 Subcutaneous Tissue and Fascia, Right Neck* **6 Subcutaneous Tissue and Fascia, Chest** Pectoral fascia **7 Subcutaneous Tissue and Fascia, Back** **8 Subcutaneous Tissue and Fascia, Abdomen** **9 Subcutaneous Tissue and Fascia, Buttock** **B Subcutaneous Tissue and Fascia, Perineum** **C Subcutaneous Tissue and Fascia, Pelvic Region** **D Subcutaneous Tissue and Fascia, Right Upper Arm** Axillary fascia Deltoid fascia Infraspinatus fascia Subscapular aponeurosis Supraspinatus fascia **F Subcutaneous Tissue and Fascia, Left Upper Arm** *See D Subcutaneous Tissue and Fascia, Right Upper Arm*	**G Subcutaneous Tissue and Fascia, Right Lower Arm** Antebrachial fascia Bicipital aponeurosis **H Subcutaneous Tissue and Fascia, Left Lower Arm** *See G Subcutaneous Tissue and Fascia, Right Lower Arm* **J Subcutaneous Tissue and Fascia, Right Hand** Palmar fascia (aponeurosis) **K Subcutaneous Tissue and Fascia, Left Hand** *See J Subcutaneous Tissue and Fascia, Right Hand* **L Subcutaneous Tissue and Fascia, Right Upper Leg** Crural fascia Fascia lata Iliac fascia Iliotibial tract (band) **M Subcutaneous Tissue and Fascia, Left Upper Leg** *See L Subcutaneous Tissue and Fascia, Right Upper Leg* **N Subcutaneous Tissue and Fascia, Right Lower Leg** **P Subcutaneous Tissue and Fascia, Left Lower Leg** **Q Subcutaneous Tissue and Fascia, Right Foot** Plantar fascia (aponeurosis) **R Subcutaneous Tissue and Fascia, Left Foot** *See Q Subcutaneous Tissue and Fascia, Right Foot*	Ø Open 3 Percutaneous	Z No Device	Z No Qualifier

Non-OR ØJD[Ø,1,4,5,B,C,D,F,G,H,J,K,N,P,Q,R]3ZZ

See Appendix L for Procedure Combinations

Combo-only ØJD[6,7,8,9,L,M]3ZZ

Ø Medical and Surgical
J Subcutaneous Tissue and Fascia
H Insertion Definition: Putting in a nonbiological appliance that monitors, assists, performs, or prevents a physiological function but does not physically take the place of a body part

Explanation: None

Body Part Character 4	Approach Character 5	Device Character 6	Qualifier Character 7
Ø Subcutaneous Tissue and Fascia, Scalp Galea aponeurotica **1 Subcutaneous Tissue and Fascia, Face** Chin; Masseteric fascia; Orbital fascia; Submandibular space **4 Subcutaneous Tissue and Fascia, Right Neck** Deep cervical fascia; Pretracheal fascia; Prevertebral fascia **5 Subcutaneous Tissue and Fascia, Left Neck** *See 4 Subcutaneous Tissue and Fascia, Right Neck* **9 Subcutaneous Tissue and Fascia, Buttock** **B Subcutaneous Tissue and Fascia, Perineum** **C Subcutaneous Tissue and Fascia, Pelvic Region** **J Subcutaneous Tissue and Fascia, Right Hand** Palmar fascia (aponeurosis) **K Subcutaneous Tissue and Fascia, Left Hand** *See J Subcutaneous Tissue and Fascia, Right Hand* **Q Subcutaneous Tissue and Fascia, Right Foot** Plantar fascia (aponeurosis) **R Subcutaneous Tissue and Fascia, Left Foot** *See Q Subcutaneous Tissue and Fascia, Right Foot*	**Ø Open** **3 Percutaneous**	**N Tissue Expander**	**Z No Qualifier**
6 Subcutaneous Tissue and Fascia, Chest [Combination Member] Pectoral fascia	**Ø Open** **3 Percutaneous**	**Ø Monitoring Device, Hemodynamic** **2 Monitoring Device** **4 Pacemaker, Single Chamber** **5 Pacemaker, Single Chamber Rate Responsive** **6 Pacemaker, Dual Chamber** **7 Cardiac Resynchronization Pacemaker Pulse Generator** **8 Defibrillator Generator** **9 Cardiac Resynchronization Defibrillator Pulse Generator** **A Contractility Modulation Device** **B Stimulator Generator, Single Array** **C Stimulator Generator, Single Array Rechargeable** **D Stimulator Generator, Multiple Array** **E Stimulator Generator, Multiple Array Rechargeable** **F Subcutaneous Defibrillator Lead** **H Contraceptive Device** **M Stimulator Generator** **N Tissue Expander** **P Cardiac Rhythm Related Device** **V Infusion Device, Pump** **W Vascular Access Device, Totally Implantable** **X Vascular Access Device, Tunneled** **Y Other Device**	**Z No Qualifier**
7 Subcutaneous Tissue and Fascia, Back [NC] [Combination Member]	**Ø Open** **3 Percutaneous**	**B Stimulator Generator, Single Array** **C Stimulator Generator, Single Array Rechargeable** **D Stimulator Generator, Multiple Array** **E Stimulator Generator, Multiple Array Rechargeable** **M Stimulator Generator** **N Tissue Expander** **V Infusion Device, Pump** **Y Other Device**	**Z No Qualifier**

DRG Non-OR ØJH6[Ø,3][4,5,6,7,H,P,X]Z
DRG Non-OR ØJH63WX
Non-OR ØJH63YZ
Non-OR ØJH73YZ
HAC ØJH6[Ø,3][4,5,6,7,8,9,P]Z when reported with SDx K68.11 or T81.4Ø-T81.49, T82.7 with 7th character A
HAC ØJH63XZ when reported with SDx J95.811

NC ØJH7[Ø,3]MZ

See Appendix L for Procedure Combinations
[Combination Member] ØJH6[Ø,3][4,5,6,7,8,9,A,B,C,D,E,F,M,P]Z
[Combination Member] ØJH7[Ø,3][B,C,D,E,M]Z

ØJH Continued on next page

Subcutaneous Tissue and Fascia

ØJH Continued

Ø Medical and Surgical
J Subcutaneous Tissue and Fascia
H Insertion Definition: Putting in a nonbiological appliance that monitors, assists, performs, or prevents a physiological function but does not physically take the place of a body part

Explanation: None

Body Part Character 4	Approach Character 5	Device Character 6	Qualifier Character 7
8 Subcutaneous Tissue and Fascia, Abdomen NC	Ø Open 3 Percutaneous	Ø Monitoring Device, Hemodynamic 2 Monitoring Device 4 Pacemaker, Single Chamber 5 Pacemaker, Single Chamber Rate Responsive 6 Pacemaker, Dual Chamber 7 Cardiac Resynchronization Pacemaker Pulse Generator 8 Defibrillator Generator 9 Cardiac Resynchronization Defibrillator Pulse Generator A Contractility Modulation Device B Stimulator Generator, Single Array C Stimulator Generator, Single Array Rechargeable D Stimulator Generator, Multiple Array E Stimulator Generator, Multiple Array Rechargeable H Contraceptive Device M Stimulator Generator N Tissue Expander P Cardiac Rhythm Related Device V Infusion Device, Pump W Vascular Access Device, Totally Implantable X Vascular Access Device, Tunneled Y Other Device	Z No Qualifier
D Subcutaneous Tissue and Fascia, Right Upper Arm Axillary fascia Deltoid fascia Infraspinatus fascia Subscapular aponeurosis Supraspinatus fascia F Subcutaneous Tissue and Fascia, Left Upper Arm *See D Subcutaneous Tissue and Fascia, Right Upper Arm* G Subcutaneous Tissue and Fascia, Right Lower Arm Antebrachial fascia Bicipital aponeurosis H Subcutaneous Tissue and Fascia, Left Lower Arm *See G Subcutaneous Tissue and Fascia, Right Lower Arm* L Subcutaneous Tissue and Fascia, Right Upper Leg Crural fascia Fascia lata Iliac fascia Iliotibial tract (band) M Subcutaneous Tissue and Fascia, Left Upper Leg *See L Subcutaneous Tissue and Fascia, Right Upper Leg* N Subcutaneous Tissue and Fascia, Right Lower Leg P Subcutaneous Tissue and Fascia, Left Lower Leg	Ø Open 3 Percutaneous	H Contraceptive Device N Tissue Expander V Infusion Device, Pump W Vascular Access Device, Totally Implantable X Vascular Access Device, Tunneled	Z No Qualifier
S Subcutaneous Tissue and Fascia, Head and Neck V Subcutaneous Tissue and Fascia, Upper Extremity W Subcutaneous Tissue and Fascia, Lower Extremity	Ø Open 3 Percutaneous	1 Radioactive Element 3 Infusion Device Y Other Device	Z No Qualifier
T Subcutaneous Tissue and Fascia, Trunk External oblique aponeurosis Transversalis fascia	Ø Open 3 Percutaneous	1 Radioactive Element 3 Infusion Device V Infusion Device, Pump Y Other Device	Z No Qualifier

DRG Non-OR ØJH8[Ø,3][2,4,5,6,7,H,P,X]Z
DRG Non-OR ØJH83WX
DRG Non-OR ØJH[D,F,G,H,L,M,N,P]ØXZ
DRG Non-OR ØJH[D,F,G,H,L,M,N,P]3[W,X]Z
DRG Non-OR ØJHN3HZ
DRG Non-OR ØJHP[Ø,3]HZ

Non-OR ØJH83YZ
Non-OR ØJH[D,F,G,H,L,M][Ø,3]HZ
Non-OR ØJHNØHZ
Non-OR ØJH[S,V,W]Ø3Z
Non-OR ØJH[S,V,W]3[3,Y]Z
Non-OR ØJHTØ3Z
Non-OR ØJHT3[3,Y]Z

HAC ØJH8[Ø,3][4,5,6,7,8,9,P]Z when reported with SDx K68.11 or T81.4Ø-T81.49, T82.7 with 7th character A

NC ØJH8[Ø,3]MZ

See Appendix L for Procedure Combinations

ØJH8[Ø,3][4,5,6,7,8,9,A,B,C,D,E,M,P]Z

Non-OR Procedure | DRG Non-OR Procedure | Valid OR Procedure | HAC Associated Procedure | Combination Only | New/Revised April | New/Revised October

Ø Medical and Surgical
J Subcutaneous Tissue and Fascia
J Inspection Definition: Visually and/or manually exploring a body part

Explanation: Visual exploration may be performed with or without optical instrumentation. Manual exploration may be performed directly or through intervening body layers.

Body Part Character 4	Approach Character 5	Device Character 6	Qualifier Character 7
S Subcutaneous Tissue and Fascia, Head and Neck **T** Subcutaneous Tissue and Fascia, Trunk External oblique aponeurosis Transversalis fascia **V** Subcutaneous Tissue and Fascia, Upper Extremity **W** Subcutaneous Tissue and Fascia, Lower Extremity	**Ø** Open **3** Percutaneous **X** External	**Z** No Device	**Z** No Qualifier

Non-OR All body part, approach, device, and qualifier values

Ø Medical and Surgical
J Subcutaneous Tissue and Fascia
N Release Definition: Freeing a body part from an abnormal physical constraint by cutting or by the use of force

Explanation: Some of the restraining tissue may be taken out but none of the body part is taken out

Body Part Character 4	Approach Character 5	Device Character 6	Qualifier Character 7
Ø Subcutaneous Tissue and Fascia, Scalp Galea aponeurotica **1** Subcutaneous Tissue and Fascia, Face Chin Masseteric fascia Orbital fascia Submandibular space **4** Subcutaneous Tissue and Fascia, Right Neck Deep cervical fascia Pretracheal fascia Prevertebral fascia **5** Subcutaneous Tissue and Fascia, Left Neck *See 4 Subcutaneous Tissue and Fascia, Right Neck* **6** Subcutaneous Tissue and Fascia, Chest Pectoral fascia **7** Subcutaneous Tissue and Fascia, Back **8** Subcutaneous Tissue and Fascia, Abdomen **9** Subcutaneous Tissue and Fascia, Buttock **B** Subcutaneous Tissue and Fascia, Perineum **C** Subcutaneous Tissue and Fascia, Pelvic Region **D** Subcutaneous Tissue and Fascia, Right Upper Arm Axillary fascia Deltoid fascia Infraspinatus fascia Subscapular aponeurosis Supraspinatus fascia **F** Subcutaneous Tissue and Fascia, Left Upper Arm *See D Subcutaneous Tissue and Fascia, Right Upper Arm* **G** Subcutaneous Tissue and Fascia, Right Lower Arm Antebrachial fascia Bicipital aponeurosis **H** Subcutaneous Tissue and Fascia, Left Lower Arm *See G Subcutaneous Tissue and Fascia, Right Lower Arm* **J** Subcutaneous Tissue and Fascia, Right Hand Palmar fascia (aponeurosis) **K** Subcutaneous Tissue and Fascia, Left Hand *See J Subcutaneous Tissue and Fascia, Right Hand* **L** Subcutaneous Tissue and Fascia, Right Upper Leg Crural fascia Fascia lata Iliac fascia Iliotibial tract (band) **M** Subcutaneous Tissue and Fascia, Left Upper Leg *See L Subcutaneous Tissue and Fascia, Right Upper Leg* **N** Subcutaneous Tissue and Fascia, Right Lower Leg **P** Subcutaneous Tissue and Fascia, Left Lower Leg **Q** Subcutaneous Tissue and Fascia, Right Foot Plantar fascia (aponeurosis) **R** Subcutaneous Tissue and Fascia, Left Foot *See Q Subcutaneous Tissue and Fascia, Right Foot*	**Ø** Open **3** Percutaneous **X** External	**Z** No Device	**Z** No Qualifier

Non-OR ØJN[Ø,1,4,5,6,7,8,9,B,C,D,F,G,H,J,K,L,M,N,P,Q,R]XZZ

Ø Medical and Surgical
J Subcutaneous Tissue and Fascia
P Removal Definition: Taking out or off a device from a body part

Explanation: If a device is taken out and a similar device put in without cutting or puncturing the skin or mucous membrane, the procedure is coded to the root operation CHANGE. Otherwise, the procedure for taking out a device is coded to the root operation REMOVAL.

Body Part Character 4	Approach Character 5	Device Character 6	Qualifier Character 7
S Subcutaneous Tissue and Fascia, Head and Neck	**Ø** Open **3** Percutaneous	**Ø** Drainage Device **1** Radioactive Element **3** Infusion Device **7** Autologous Tissue Substitute **J** Synthetic Substitute **K** Nonautologous Tissue Substitute **N** Tissue Expander **Y** Other Device	**Z** No Qualifier
S Subcutaneous Tissue and Fascia, Head and Neck	**X** External	**Ø** Drainage Device **1** Radioactive Element **3** Infusion Device	**Z** No Qualifier
T Subcutaneous Tissue and Fascia, Trunk External oblique aponeurosis Transversalis fascia	**Ø** Open **3** Percutaneous	**Ø** Drainage Device **1** Radioactive Element **2** Monitoring Device **3** Infusion Device **7** Autologous Tissue Substitute **F** Subcutaneous Defibrillator Lead **H** Contraceptive Device **J** Synthetic Substitute **K** Nonautologous Tissue Substitute **M** Stimulator Generator **N** Tissue Expander **P** Cardiac Rhythm Related Device **V** Infusion Device, Pump **W** Vascular Access Device, Totally Implantable **X** Vascular Access Device, Tunneled **Y** Other Device	**Z** No Qualifier
T Subcutaneous Tissue and Fascia, Trunk External oblique aponeurosis Transversalis fascia	**X** External	**Ø** Drainage Device **1** Radioactive Element **2** Monitoring Device **3** Infusion Device **H** Contraceptive Device **V** Infusion Device, Pump **X** Vascular Access Device, Tunneled	**Z** No Qualifier
V Subcutaneous Tissue and Fascia, Upper Extremity **W** Subcutaneous Tissue and Fascia, Lower Extremity	**Ø** Open **3** Percutaneous	**Ø** Drainage Device **1** Radioactive Element **3** Infusion Device **7** Autologous Tissue Substitute **H** Contraceptive Device **J** Synthetic Substitute **K** Nonautologous Tissue Substitute **N** Tissue Expander **V** Infusion Device, Pump **W** Vascular Access Device, Totally Implantable **X** Vascular Access Device, Tunneled **Y** Other Device	**Z** No Qualifier
V Subcutaneous Tissue and Fascia, Upper Extremity **W** Subcutaneous Tissue and Fascia, Lower Extremity	**X** External	**Ø** Drainage Device **1** Radioactive Element **3** Infusion Device **H** Contraceptive Device **V** Infusion Device, Pump **X** Vascular Access Device, Tunneled	**Z** No Qualifier

Non-OR ØJPS[Ø,3][Ø,1,3,7,J,K,N,Y]Z
Non-OR ØJPSX[Ø,1,3]Z
Non-OR ØJPT[Ø,3][Ø,1,2,3,7,H,J,K,M,N,V,W,X,Y]Z
Non-OR ØJPTX[Ø,1,2,3,H,V,X]Z
Non-OR ØJP[V,W][Ø,3][Ø,1,3,7,H,J,K,N,V,W,X,Y]Z
Non-OR ØJP[V,W]X[Ø,1,3,H,V,X]Z
HAC ØJPT[Ø,3][F,P]Z when reported with SDx K68.11 or T81.4Ø-T81.49, T82.7 with 7th character A

Ø Medical and Surgical
J Subcutaneous Tissue and Fascia
Q Repair Definition: Restoring, to the extent possible, a body part to its normal anatomic structure and function
Explanation: Used only when the method to accomplish the repair is not one of the other root operations

Body Part Character 4	Approach Character 5	Device Character 6	Qualifier Character 7
Ø Subcutaneous Tissue and Fascia, Scalp Galea aponeurotica **1 Subcutaneous Tissue and Fascia, Face** Chin Masseteric fascia Orbital fascia Submandibular space **4 Subcutaneous Tissue and Fascia, Right Neck** Deep cervical fascia Pretracheal fascia Prevertebral fascia **5 Subcutaneous Tissue and Fascia, Left Neck** **See** *4 Subcutaneous Tissue and Fascia, Right Neck* **6 Subcutaneous Tissue and Fascia, Chest** Pectoral fascia **7 Subcutaneous Tissue and Fascia, Back** **8 Subcutaneous Tissue and Fascia, Abdomen** **9 Subcutaneous Tissue and Fascia, Buttock** **B Subcutaneous Tissue and Fascia, Perineum** **C Subcutaneous Tissue and Fascia, Pelvic Region** **D Subcutaneous Tissue and Fascia, Right Upper Arm** Axillary fascia Deltoid fascia Infraspinatus fascia Subscapular aponeurosis Supraspinatus fascia **F Subcutaneous Tissue and Fascia, Left Upper Arm** **See** *D Subcutaneous Tissue and Fascia, Right Upper Arm* **G Subcutaneous Tissue and Fascia, Right Lower Arm** Antebrachial fascia Bicipital aponeurosis **H Subcutaneous Tissue and Fascia, Left Lower Arm** **See** *G Subcutaneous Tissue and Fascia, Right Lower Arm* **J Subcutaneous Tissue and Fascia, Right Hand** Palmar fascia (aponeurosis) **K Subcutaneous Tissue and Fascia, Left Hand** **See** *J Subcutaneous Tissue and Fascia, Right Hand* **L Subcutaneous Tissue and Fascia, Right Upper Leg** Crural fascia Fascia lata Iliac fascia Iliotibial tract (band) **M Subcutaneous Tissue and Fascia, Left Upper Leg** **See** *L Subcutaneous Tissue and Fascia, Right Upper Leg* **N Subcutaneous Tissue and Fascia, Right Lower Leg** **P Subcutaneous Tissue and Fascia, Left Lower Leg** **Q Subcutaneous Tissue and Fascia, Right Foot** Plantar fascia (aponeurosis) **R Subcutaneous Tissue and Fascia, Left Foot** **See** *Q Subcutaneous Tissue and Fascia, Right Foot*	Ø Open 3 Percutaneous	Z No Device	Z No Qualifier

Non-OR ØJQ[Ø,1,4,5,6,7,8,9,B,C,D,F,G,H,J,K,L,M,N,P,Q,R]3ZZ

Ø Medical and Surgical
J Subcutaneous Tissue and Fascia
R Replacement Definition: Putting in or on biological or synthetic material that physically takes the place and/or function of all or a portion of a body part

Explanation: The body part may have been taken out or replaced, or may be taken out, physically eradicated, or rendered nonfunctional during the REPLACEMENT procedure. A REMOVAL procedure is coded for taking out the device used in a previous replacement procedure.

Body Part Character 4		Approach Character 5	Device Character 6	Qualifier Character 7
Ø Subcutaneous Tissue and Fascia, Scalp Galea aponeurotica **1 Subcutaneous Tissue and Fascia, Face** Chin Masseteric fascia Orbital fascia Submandibular space **4 Subcutaneous Tissue and Fascia, Right Neck** Deep cervical fascia Pretracheal fascia Prevertebral fascia **5 Subcutaneous Tissue and Fascia, Left Neck** *See 4 Subcutaneous Tissue and Fascia, Right Neck* **6 Subcutaneous Tissue and Fascia, Chest** Pectoral fascia **7 Subcutaneous Tissue and Fascia, Back** **8 Subcutaneous Tissue and Fascia, Abdomen** **9 Subcutaneous Tissue and Fascia, Buttock** **B Subcutaneous Tissue and Fascia, Perineum** **C Subcutaneous Tissue and Fascia, Pelvic Region** **D Subcutaneous Tissue and Fascia, Right Upper Arm** Axillary fascia Deltoid fascia Infraspinatus fascia Subscapular aponeurosis Supraspinatus fascia **F Subcutaneous Tissue and Fascia, Left Upper Arm** *See D Subcutaneous Tissue and Fascia, Right Upper Arm*	**G Subcutaneous Tissue and Fascia, Right Lower Arm** Antebrachial fascia Bicipital aponeurosis **H Subcutaneous Tissue and Fascia, Left Lower Arm** *See G Subcutaneous Tissue and Fascia, Right Lower Arm* **J Subcutaneous Tissue and Fascia, Right Hand** Palmar fascia (aponeurosis) **K Subcutaneous Tissue and Fascia, Left Hand** *See J Subcutaneous Tissue and Fascia, Right Hand* **L Subcutaneous Tissue and Fascia, Right Upper Leg** Crural fascia Fascia lata Iliac fascia Iliotibial tract (band) **M Subcutaneous Tissue and Fascia, Left Upper Leg** *See L Subcutaneous Tissue and Fascia, Right Upper Leg* **N Subcutaneous Tissue and Fascia, Right Lower Leg** **P Subcutaneous Tissue and Fascia, Left Lower Leg** **Q Subcutaneous Tissue and Fascia, Right Foot** Plantar fascia (aponeurosis) **R Subcutaneous Tissue and Fascia, Left Foot** *See Q Subcutaneous Tissue and Fascia, Right Foot*	**Ø Open** **3 Percutaneous**	**7 Autologous Tissue Substitute** **J Synthetic Substitute** **K Nonautologous Tissue Substitute**	**Z No Qualifier**

Ø Medical and Surgical
J Subcutaneous Tissue and Fascia
U Supplement: Definition: Putting in or on biological or synthetic material that physically reinforces and/or augments the function of a portion of a body part
Explanation: The biological material is non-living, or is living and from the same individual. The body part may have been previously replaced, and the SUPPLEMENT procedure is performed to physically reinforce and/or augment the function of the replaced body part.

Body Part Character 4	Approach Character 5	Device Character 6	Qualifier Character 7
Ø Subcutaneous Tissue and Fascia, Scalp Galea aponeurotica **1 Subcutaneous Tissue and Fascia, Face** Chin Masseteric fascia Orbital fascia Submandibular space **4 Subcutaneous Tissue and Fascia, Right Neck** Deep cervical fascia Pretracheal fascia Prevertebral fascia **5 Subcutaneous Tissue and Fascia, Left Neck** ***See*** *4 Subcutaneous Tissue and Fascia, Right Neck* **6 Subcutaneous Tissue and Fascia, Chest** Pectoral fascia **7 Subcutaneous Tissue and Fascia, Back** **8 Subcutaneous Tissue and Fascia, Abdomen** **9 Subcutaneous Tissue and Fascia, Buttock** **B Subcutaneous Tissue and Fascia, Perineum** **C Subcutaneous Tissue and Fascia, Pelvic Region** **D Subcutaneous Tissue and Fascia, Right Upper Arm** Axillary fascia Deltoid fascia Infraspinatus fascia Subscapular aponeurosis Supraspinatus fascia **F Subcutaneous Tissue and Fascia, Left Upper Arm** ***See*** *D Subcutaneous Tissue and Fascia, Right Upper Arm* **G Subcutaneous Tissue and Fascia, Right Lower Arm** Antebrachial fascia Bicipital aponeurosis **H Subcutaneous Tissue and Fascia, Left Lower Arm** ***See*** *G Subcutaneous Tissue and Fascia, Right Lower Arm* **J Subcutaneous Tissue and Fascia, Right Hand** Palmar fascia (aponeurosis) **K Subcutaneous Tissue and Fascia, Left Hand** ***See*** *J Subcutaneous Tissue and Fascia, Right Hand* **L Subcutaneous Tissue and Fascia, Right Upper Leg** Crural fascia Fascia lata Iliac fascia Iliotibial tract (band) **M Subcutaneous Tissue and Fascia, Left Upper Leg** ***See*** *L Subcutaneous Tissue and Fascia, Right Upper Leg* **N Subcutaneous Tissue and Fascia, Right Lower Leg** **P Subcutaneous Tissue and Fascia, Left Lower Leg** **Q Subcutaneous Tissue and Fascia, Right Foot** Plantar fascia (aponeurosis) **R Subcutaneous Tissue and Fascia, Left Foot** ***See*** *Q Subcutaneous Tissue and Fascia, Right Foot*	**Ø Open** **3 Percutaneous**	**7 Autologous Tissue Substitute** **J Synthetic Substitute** **K Nonautologous Tissue Substitute**	**Z No Qualifier**

Ø Medical and Surgical
J Subcutaneous Tissue and Fascia
W Revision

Definition: Correcting, to the extent possible, a portion of a malfunctioning device or the position of a displaced device

Explanation: Revision can include correcting a malfunctioning or displaced device by taking out or putting in components of the device such as a screw or pin

Body Part Character 4	Approach Character 5	Device Character 6	Qualifier Character 7
S Subcutaneous Tissue and Fascia, Head and Neck	**Ø** Open **3** Percutaneous	**Ø** Drainage Device **3** Infusion Device **7** Autologous Tissue Substitute **J** Synthetic Substitute **K** Nonautologous Tissue Substitute **N** Tissue Expander **Y** Other Device	**Z** No Qualifier
S Subcutaneous Tissue and Fascia, Head and Neck	**X** External	**Ø** Drainage Device **3** Infusion Device **7** Autologous Tissue Substitute **J** Synthetic Substitute **K** Nonautologous Tissue Substitute **N** Tissue Expander	**Z** No Qualifier
T Subcutaneous Tissue and Fascia, Trunk External oblique aponeurosis Transversalis fascia	**Ø** Open **3** Percutaneous	**Ø** Drainage Device **2** Monitoring Device **3** Infusion Device **7** Autologous Tissue Substitute **F** Subcutaneous Defibrillator Lead **H** Contraceptive Device **J** Synthetic Substitute **K** Nonautologous Tissue Substitute **M** Stimulator Generator **N** Tissue Expander **P** Cardiac Rhythm Related Device **V** Infusion Device, Pump **W** Vascular Access Device, Totally Implantable **X** Vascular Access Device, Tunneled **Y** Other Device	**Z** No Qualifier
T Subcutaneous Tissue and Fascia, Trunk External oblique aponeurosis Transversalis fascia	**X** External	**Ø** Drainage Device **2** Monitoring Device **3** Infusion Device **7** Autologous Tissue Substitute **F** Subcutaneous Defibrillator Lead **H** Contraceptive Device **J** Synthetic Substitute **K** Nonautologous Tissue Substitute **M** Stimulator Generator **N** Tissue Expander **P** Cardiac Rhythm Related Device **V** Infusion Device, Pump **W** Vascular Access Device, Totally Implantable **X** Vascular Access Device, Tunneled	**Z** No Qualifier
V Subcutaneous Tissue and Fascia, Upper Extremity **W** Subcutaneous Tissue and Fascia, Lower Extremity	**Ø** Open **3** Percutaneous	**Ø** Drainage Device **3** Infusion Device **7** Autologous Tissue Substitute **H** Contraceptive Device **J** Synthetic Substitute **K** Nonautologous Tissue Substitute **N** Tissue Expander **V** Infusion Device, Pump **W** Vascular Access Device, Totally Implantable **X** Vascular Access Device, Tunneled **Y** Other Device	**Z** No Qualifier
V Subcutaneous Tissue and Fascia, Upper Extremity **W** Subcutaneous Tissue and Fascia, Lower Extremity	**X** External	**Ø** Drainage Device **3** Infusion Device **7** Autologous Tissue Substitute **H** Contraceptive Device **J** Synthetic Substitute **K** Nonautologous Tissue Substitute **N** Tissue Expander **V** Infusion Device, Pump **W** Vascular Access Device, Totally Implantable **X** Vascular Access Device, Tunneled	**Z** No Qualifier

DRG Non-OR ØJWS[Ø,3][Ø,3,7,J,K,N,Y]Z
DRG Non-OR ØJWT[Ø,3][Ø,3,7,H,J,K,M,N,V,W,X]Z
DRG Non-OR ØJWTXMZ
DRG Non-OR ØJW[V,W][Ø,3][Ø,3,7,H,J,K,N,V,W,X,Y]Z

Non-OR ØJWSX[Ø,3,7,J,K,N]Z
Non-OR ØJWT3YZ
Non-OR ØJWTX[Ø,2,3,7,F,H,J,K,N,P,V,W,X]Z
Non-OR ØJW[V,W]X[Ø,3,7,H,J,K,N,V,W,X]Z

HAC ØJWT[Ø,3][F,P]Z when reported with SDx K68.11 or T81.4Ø-T81.49, T82.7 with 7th character A

Ø Medical and Surgical
J Subcutaneous Tissue and Fascia
X Transfer Definition: Moving, without taking out, all or a portion of a body part to another location to take over the function of all or a portion of a body part

Explanation: The body part transferred remains connected to its vascular and nervous supply

Body Part Character 4		Approach Character 5	Device Character 6	Qualifier Character 7
Ø Subcutaneous Tissue and Fascia, Scalp Galea aponeurotica **1 Subcutaneous Tissue and Fascia, Face** Chin Masseteric fascia Orbital fascia Submandibular space **4 Subcutaneous Tissue and Fascia, Right Neck** Deep cervical fascia Pretracheal fascia Prevertebral fascia **5 Subcutaneous Tissue and Fascia, Left Neck** ***See*** *4 Subcutaneous Tissue and Fascia, Right Neck* **6 Subcutaneous Tissue and Fascia, Chest** Pectoral fascia **7 Subcutaneous Tissue and Fascia, Back** **8 Subcutaneous Tissue and Fascia, Abdomen** **9 Subcutaneous Tissue and Fascia, Buttock** **B Subcutaneous Tissue and Fascia, Perineum** **C Subcutaneous Tissue and Fascia, Pelvic Region** **D Subcutaneous Tissue and Fascia, Right Upper Arm** Axillary fascia Deltoid fascia Infraspinatus fascia Subscapular aponeurosis Supraspinatus fascia **F Subcutaneous Tissue and Fascia, Left Upper Arm** ***See*** *D Subcutaneous Tissue and Fascia, Right Upper Arm*	**G Subcutaneous Tissue and Fascia, Right Lower Arm** Antebrachial fascia Bicipital aponeurosis **H Subcutaneous Tissue and Fascia, Left Lower Arm** ***See*** *G Subcutaneous Tissue and Fascia, Right Lower Arm* **J Subcutaneous Tissue and Fascia, Right Hand** Palmar fascia (aponeurosis) **K Subcutaneous Tissue and Fascia, Left Hand** ***See*** *J Subcutaneous Tissue and Fascia, Right Hand* **L Subcutaneous Tissue and Fascia, Right Upper Leg** Crural fascia Fascia lata Iliac fascia Iliotibial tract (band) **M Subcutaneous Tissue and Fascia, Left Upper Leg** ***See*** *L Subcutaneous Tissue and Fascia, Right Upper Leg* **N Subcutaneous Tissue and Fascia, Right Lower Leg** **P Subcutaneous Tissue and Fascia, Left Lower Leg** **Q Subcutaneous Tissue and Fascia, Right Foot** Plantar fascia (aponeurosis) **R Subcutaneous Tissue and Fascia, Left Foot** ***See*** *Q Subcutaneous Tissue and Fascia, Right Foot*	**Ø Open** **3 Percutaneous**	**Z No Device**	**B Skin and Subcutaneous Tissue** **C Skin, Subcutaneous Tissue and Fascia** **Z No Qualifier**

Muscles ØK2–ØKX

Character Meanings

This Character Meaning table is provided as a guide to assist the user in the identification of character members that may be found in this section of code tables. It **SHOULD NOT** be used to build a PCS code.

Operation–Character 3	Body Part–Character 4	Approach–Character 5	Device–Character 6	Qualifier–Character 7
2 Change	Ø Head Muscle	Ø Open	Ø Drainage Device	Ø Skin
5 Destruction	1 Facial Muscle	3 Percutaneous	7 Autologous Tissue Substitute	1 Subcutaneous Tissue
8 Division	2 Neck Muscle, Right	4 Percutaneous Endoscopic	J Synthetic Substitute	2 Skin and Subcutaneous Tissue
9 Drainage	3 Neck Muscle, Left	7 Via Natural or Artificial Opening	K Nonautologous Tissue Substitute	5 Latissimus Dorsi Myocutaneous Flap
B Excision	4 Tongue, Palate, Pharynx Muscle	8 Via Natural or Artificial Opening Endoscopic	M Stimulator Lead	6 Transverse Rectus Abdominis Myocutaneous Flap
C Extirpation	5 Shoulder Muscle, Right	X External	Y Other Device	7 Deep Inferior Epigastric Artery Perforator Flap
D Extraction	6 Shoulder Muscle, Left		Z No Device	8 Superficial Inferior Epigastric Artery Flap
H Insertion	7 Upper Arm Muscle, Right			9 Gluteal Artery Perforator Flap
J Inspection	8 Upper Arm Muscle, Left			X Diagnostic
M Reattachment	9 Lower Arm and Wrist Muscle, Right			Z No Qualifier
N Release	B Lower Arm and Wrist Muscle, Left			
P Removal	C Hand Muscle, Right			
Q Repair	D Hand Muscle, Left			
R Replacement	F Trunk Muscle, Right			
S Reposition	G Trunk Muscle, Left			
T Resection	H Thorax Muscle, Right			
U Supplement	J Thorax Muscle, Left			
W Revision	K Abdomen Muscle, Right			
X Transfer	L Abdomen Muscle, Left			
	M Perineum Muscle			
	N Hip Muscle, Right			
	P Hip Muscle, Left			
	Q Upper Leg Muscle, Right			
	R Upper Leg Muscle, Left			
	S Lower Leg Muscle, Right			
	T Lower Leg Muscle, Left			
	V Foot Muscle, Right			
	W Foot Muscle, Left			
	X Upper Muscle			
	Y Lower Muscle			

AHA Coding Clinic for table ØK8

2021, 4Q, 50 Endoscopic division of tongue, palate and pharynx muscle
2020, 2Q, 25 Endoscopic stapling of Zenker's diverticulum

AHA Coding Clinic for table ØKB

2023, 2Q, 30 Excisional debridement and non-excisional debridement at deeper layer same site
2023, 1Q, 32 Zenker's diverticulectomy
2020, 1Q, 27 Delayed reconstruction following mastectomy using gracilis musculocutaneous free flap
2016, 3Q, 20 Excisional debridement of sacrum
2015, 3Q, 3-8 Excisional and nonexcisional debridement

AHA Coding Clinic for table ØKD

2023, 2Q, 30 Excisional debridement and non-excisional debridement at deeper layer same site
2017, 4Q, 41-42 Extraction procedures

AHA Coding Clinic for table ØKH

2020, 4Q, 63 Intercompartmental pressure measurement

AHA Coding Clinic for table ØKN

2017, 2Q, 12 Compartment syndrome and fasciotomy of foot
2017, 2Q, 13 Compartment syndrome and fasciotomy of leg
2015, 2Q, 22 Arthroscopic subacromial decompression
2014, 4Q, 39 Abdominal component release with placement of mesh for hernia repair

AHA Coding Clinic for table ØKQ

2022, 3Q, 13 Repair of prolapsed neovaginal graft
2018, 2Q, 25 Third and fourth degree obstetric lacerations

AHA Coding Clinic for table ØKQ (Continued)

2016, 2Q, 34 Assisted vaginal delivery
2016, 1Q, 7 Obstetrical perineal laceration repair
2014, 4Q, 43 Second degree obstetric perineal laceration
2013, 4Q, 120 Repair of second degree perineum obstetric laceration

AHA Coding Clinic for table ØKS

2022, 3Q, 11 Ulceration and soft tissue redundancy at amputation site due to osteo-integrated implant
2017, 1Q, 41 Manual reduction of hernia

AHA Coding Clinic for table ØKT

2016, 2Q, 12 Resection of malignant neoplasm of infratemporal fossa
2015, 1Q, 38 Abdominoperineal resection with flap closure of the perineum and colostomy

AHA Coding Clinic for table ØKX

2023, 1Q, 34 Repair of Stage 4 pressure ulcer and application of Amniofill®
2022, 3Q, 11 Ulceration and soft tissue redundancy at amputation site due to osteo-integrated implant
2018, 2Q, 18 Transverse rectus abdominis myocutaneous (TRAM) delay
2017, 4Q, 67 New qualifier values - Pedicle flap procedures
2016, 3Q, 30 Resection of femur with interposition arthroplasty
2015, 3Q, 33 Cleft lip repair using Millard rotation advancement
2015, 2Q, 26 Pharyngeal flap to soft palate
2014, 4Q, 41 Abdominoperineal resection (APR) with flap closure of perineum and colostomy
2014, 2Q, 10 Transverse abdominomyocutaneous (TRAM) breast reconstruction
2014, 2Q, 12 Pedicle latissimus myocutaneous flap with placement of breast tissue expanders

Muscles

Frontalis Ø
Temporalis Ø
Orbicularis oculi 1
Orbicularis oris 1
Masseter Ø
Zygomaticus major 1
Depressor labii inferioris 1
Mentalis 1
Splenius 2, 3
Sternocleidomastoid (clavicular head) 2, 3
Sternocleidomastoid (sternal head) 2, 3
Levator scapulae 2, 3
Platysma 2, 3
Deltoid 5, 6
Pectoralis major H, J
Latissimus dorsi F, G
Serratus anterior H, J
Coracobrachialis
Biceps brachii (short head)
Biceps brachii (long head)
Triceps
Brachialis
Upper arm muscles 7, 8
Rectus abdominis K, L
External oblique K, L
Brachioradialis
Extensor carpi radialis longus
Flexor carpi radialis
Palmaris longus
Flexor carpi ulnaris
Flexor digitorum superficialis
Lower arm and wrist muscles 9, B
Pronator teres
Flexor carpi radialis
Extensor carpi radialis longus
Extensor carpi radialis brevis
Extensor digitorum
Extensor digiti minimi
Lower arm and wrist muscles 9, B
Tensor fascia latae N, P
Iliopsoas
Pectineus
Adductor longus
Sartorius
Gracilis
Rectus femoris
Vastus lateralis
Vastus medialis
Upper leg muscles Q, R
Gastrocnemius
Tibialis anterior
Soleus
Peroneus longus
Extensor digitorum longus
Lower leg muscles S, T

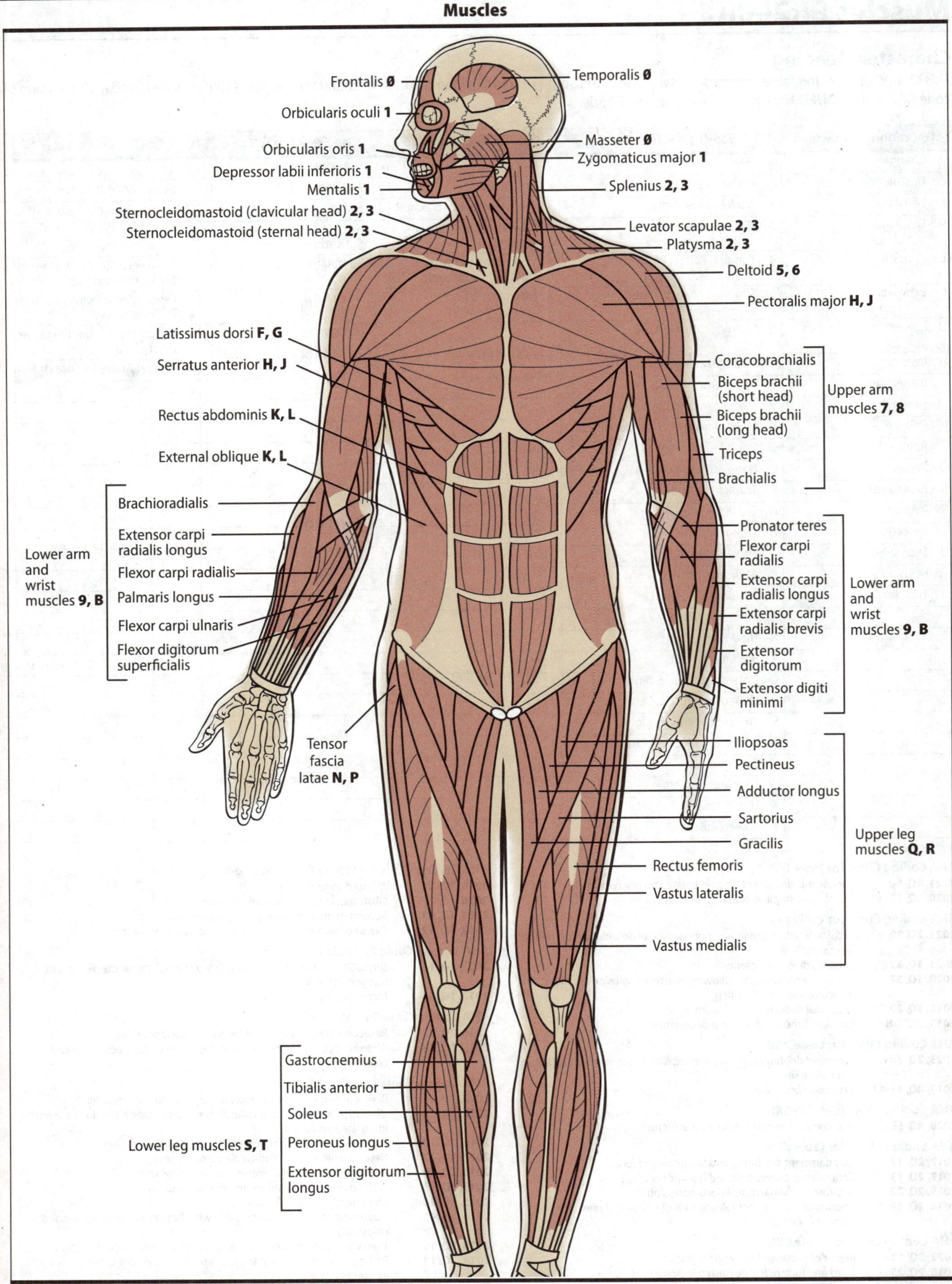

Ø Medical and Surgical
K Muscles
2 Change

Definition: Taking out or off a device from a body part and putting back an identical or similar device in or on the same body part without cutting or puncturing the skin or a mucous membrane

Explanation: All CHANGE procedures are coded using the approach EXTERNAL

Body Part Character 4	Approach Character 5	Device Character 6	Qualifier Character 7
X Upper Muscle Y Lower Muscle	X External	Ø Drainage Device Y Other Device	Z No Qualifier

Non-OR All body part, approach, device, and qualifier values

Ø Medical and Surgical
K Muscles
5 Destruction

Definition: Physical eradication of all or a portion of a body part by the direct use of energy, force, or a destructive agent

Explanation: None of the body part is physically taken out

Body Part Character 4	Approach Character 5	Device Character 6	Qualifier Character 7
Ø Head Muscle Auricularis muscle Masseter muscle Pterygoid muscle Splenius capitis muscle Temporalis muscle Temporoparietalis muscle **1 Facial Muscle** Buccinator muscle Corrugator supercilii muscle Depressor anguli oris muscle Depressor labii inferioris muscle Depressor septi nasi muscle Depressor supercilii muscle Levator anguli oris muscle Levator labii superioris alaeque nasi muscle Levator labii superioris muscle Mentalis muscle Nasalis muscle Occipitofrontalis muscle Orbicularis oris muscle Procerus muscle Risorius muscle Zygomaticus muscle **2 Neck Muscle, Right** Anterior vertebral muscle Arytenoid muscle Cricothyroid muscle Infrahyoid muscle Levator scapulae muscle Platysma muscle Scalene muscle Splenius cervicis muscle Sternocleidomastoid muscle Suprahyoid muscle Thyroarytenoid muscle **3 Neck Muscle, Left** *See 2 Neck Muscle, Right* **4 Tongue, Palate, Pharynx Muscle** Chondroglossus muscle Genioglossus muscle Hyoglossus muscle Inferior longitudinal muscle Levator veli palatini muscle Palatoglossal muscle Palatopharyngeal muscle Pharyngeal constrictor muscle Salpingopharyngeus muscle Styloglossus muscle Stylopharyngeus muscle Superior longitudinal muscle Tensor veli palatini muscle **5 Shoulder Muscle, Right** Deltoid muscle Infraspinatus muscle Subscapularis muscle Supraspinatus muscle Teres major muscle Teres minor muscle **6 Shoulder Muscle, Left** *See 5 Shoulder Muscle, Right* **7 Upper Arm Muscle, Right** Biceps brachii muscle Brachialis muscle Coracobrachialis muscle Triceps brachii muscle **8 Upper Arm Muscle, Left** *See 7 Upper Arm Muscle, Right* **9 Lower Arm and Wrist Muscle, Right** Anatomical snuffbox Brachioradialis muscle Extensor carpi radialis muscle Extensor carpi ulnaris muscle Flexor carpi radialis muscle Flexor carpi ulnaris muscle Flexor pollicis longus muscle Palmaris longus muscle Pronator quadratus muscle Pronator teres muscle **B Lower Arm and Wrist Muscle, Left** *See 9 Lower Arm and Wrist Muscle, Right* **C Hand Muscle, Right** Hypothenar muscle Palmar interosseous muscle Thenar muscle **D Hand Muscle, Left** *See C Hand Muscle, Right* **F Trunk Muscle, Right** Coccygeus muscle Erector spinae muscle Interspinalis muscle Intertransversarius muscle Latissimus dorsi muscle Quadratus lumborum muscle Rhomboid major muscle Rhomboid minor muscle Serratus posterior muscle Transversospinalis muscle Trapezius muscle **G Trunk Muscle, Left** *See F Trunk Muscle, Right* **H Thorax Muscle, Right** Intercostal muscle Levatores costarum muscle Pectoralis major muscle Pectoralis minor muscle Serratus anterior muscle Subclavius muscle Subcostal muscle Transverse thoracis muscle **J Thorax Muscle, Left** *See H Thorax Muscle, Right* **K Abdomen Muscle, Right** External oblique muscle Internal oblique muscle Pyramidalis muscle Rectus abdominis muscle Transversus abdominis muscle **L Abdomen Muscle, Left** *See K Abdomen Muscle, Right* **M Perineum Muscle** Bulbospongiosus muscle Cremaster muscle Deep transverse perineal muscle Ischiocavernosus muscle Levator ani muscle Superficial transverse perineal muscle **N Hip Muscle, Right** Gemellus muscle Gluteus maximus muscle Gluteus medius muscle Gluteus minimus muscle Iliacus muscle Obturator muscle Piriformis muscle Psoas muscle Quadratus femoris muscle Tensor fasciae latae muscle **P Hip Muscle, Left** *See N Hip Muscle, Right* **Q Upper Leg Muscle, Right** Adductor brevis muscle Adductor longus muscle Adductor magnus muscle Biceps femoris muscle Gracilis muscle Pectineus muscle Quadriceps (femoris) Rectus femoris muscle Sartorius muscle Semimembranosus muscle Semitendinosus muscle Vastus intermedius muscle Vastus lateralis muscle Vastus medialis muscle **R Upper Leg Muscle, Left** *See Q Upper Leg Muscle, Right* **S Lower Leg Muscle, Right** Extensor digitorum longus muscle Extensor hallucis longus muscle Fibularis brevis muscle Fibularis longus muscle Flexor digitorum longus muscle Flexor hallucis longus muscle Gastrocnemius muscle Peroneus brevis muscle Peroneus longus muscle Popliteus muscle Soleus muscle Tibialis anterior muscle Tibialis posterior muscle **T Lower Leg Muscle, Left** *See S Lower Leg Muscle, Right* **V Foot Muscle, Right** Abductor hallucis muscle Adductor hallucis muscle Extensor digitorum brevis muscle Extensor hallucis brevis muscle Flexor digitorum brevis muscle Flexor hallucis brevis muscle Quadratus plantae muscle **W Foot Muscle, Left** *See V Foot Muscle, Right*	Ø Open 3 Percutaneous 4 Percutaneous Endoscopic	Z No Device	Z No Qualifier

Ø Medical and Surgical
K Muscles
8 Division

Definition: Cutting into a body part, without draining fluids and/or gases from the body part, in order to separate or transect a body part

Explanation: All or a portion of the body part is separated into two or more portions

Body Part Character 4	Approach Character 5	Device Character 6	Qualifier Character 7
Ø Head Muscle Auricularis muscle Masseter muscle Pterygoid muscle Splenius capitis muscle Temporalis muscle Temporoparietalis muscle **1 Facial Muscle** Buccinator muscle Corrugator supercilii muscle Depressor anguli oris muscle Depressor labii inferioris muscle Depressor septi nasi muscle Depressor supercilii muscle Levator anguli oris muscle Levator labii superioris alaeque nasi muscle Levator labii superioris muscle Mentalis muscle Nasalis muscle Occipitofrontalis muscle Orbicularis oris muscle Procerus muscle Risorius muscle Zygomaticus muscle **2 Neck Muscle, Right** Anterior vertebral muscle Arytenoid muscle Cricothyroid muscle Infrahyoid muscle Levator scapulae muscle Platysma muscle Scalene muscle Splenius cervicis muscle Sternocleidomastoid muscle Suprahyoid muscle Thyroarytenoid muscle **3 Neck Muscle, Left** *See 2 Neck Muscle, Right* Tensor veli palatini muscle **5 Shoulder Muscle, Right** Deltoid muscle Infraspinatus muscle Subscapularis muscle Supraspinatus muscle Teres major muscle Teres minor muscle **6 Shoulder Muscle, Left** *See 5 Shoulder Muscle, Right* **7 Upper Arm Muscle, Right** Biceps brachii muscle Brachialis muscle Coracobrachialis muscle Triceps brachii muscle **8 Upper Arm Muscle, Left** *See 7 Upper Arm Muscle, Right* **9 Lower Arm and Wrist Muscle, Right** Anatomical snuffbox Brachioradialis muscle Extensor carpi radialis muscle Extensor carpi ulnaris muscle Flexor carpi radialis muscle Flexor carpi ulnaris muscle Flexor pollicis longus muscle Palmaris longus muscle Pronator quadratus muscle Pronator teres muscle **B Lower Arm and Wrist Muscle, Left** *See 9 Lower Arm and Wrist Muscle, Right* **C Hand Muscle, Right** Hypothenar muscle Palmar interosseous muscle Thenar muscle **D Hand Muscle, Left** *See C Hand Muscle, Right* **F Trunk Muscle, Right** Coccygeus muscle Erector spinae muscle Interspinalis muscle Intertransversarius muscle Latissimus dorsi muscle Quadratus lumborum muscle Rhomboid major muscle Rhomboid minor muscle Serratus posterior muscle Transversospinalis muscle Trapezius muscle **G Trunk Muscle, Left** *See F Trunk Muscle, Right* **H Thorax Muscle, Right** Intercostal muscle Levatores costarum muscle Pectoralis major muscle Pectoralis minor muscle Serratus anterior muscle Subclavius muscle Subcostal muscle Transverse thoracis muscle **J Thorax Muscle, Left** *See H Thorax Muscle, Right* **K Abdomen Muscle, Right** External oblique muscle Internal oblique muscle Pyramidalis muscle Rectus abdominis muscle Transversus abdominis muscle **L Abdomen Muscle, Left** *See K Abdomen Muscle, Right* **M Perineum Muscle** Bulbospongiosus muscle Cremaster muscle Deep transverse perineal muscle Ischiocavernosus muscle Levator ani muscle Superficial transverse perineal muscle **N Hip Muscle, Right** Gemellus muscle Gluteus maximus muscle Gluteus medius muscle Gluteus minimus muscle Iliacus muscle Obturator muscle Piriformis muscle Psoas muscle Quadratus femoris muscle Tensor fasciae latae muscle **P Hip Muscle, Left** *See N Hip Muscle, Right* **Q Upper Leg Muscle, Right** Adductor brevis muscle Adductor longus muscle Adductor magnus muscle Biceps femoris muscle Gracilis muscle Pectineus muscle Quadriceps (femoris) Rectus femoris muscle Sartorius muscle Semimembranosus muscle Semitendinosus muscle Vastus intermedius muscle Vastus lateralis muscle Vastus medialis muscle **R Upper Leg Muscle, Left** *See Q Upper Leg Muscle, Right* **S Lower Leg Muscle, Right** Extensor digitorum longus muscle Extensor hallucis longus muscle Fibularis brevis muscle Fibularis longus muscle Flexor digitorum longus muscle Flexor hallucis longus muscle Gastrocnemius muscle Peroneus brevis muscle Peroneus longus muscle Popliteus muscle Soleus muscle Tibialis anterior muscle Tibialis posterior muscle **T Lower Leg Muscle, Left** *See S Lower Leg Muscle, Right* **V Foot Muscle, Right** Abductor hallucis muscle Adductor hallucis muscle Extensor digitorum brevis muscle Extensor hallucis brevis muscle Flexor digitorum brevis muscle Flexor hallucis brevis muscle Quadratus plantae muscle **W Foot Muscle, Left** *See V Foot Muscle, Right*	**Ø Open** **3 Percutaneous** **4 Percutaneous Endoscopic**	**Z No Device**	**Z No Qualifier**
4 Tongue, Palate, Pharynx Muscle Chondroglossus muscle Genioglossus muscle Hyoglossus muscle Inferior longitudinal muscle Levator veli palatini muscle Palatoglossal muscle Palatopharyngeal muscle Pharyngeal constrictor muscle Salpingopharyngeus muscle Styloglossus muscle Stylopharyngeus muscle Superior longitudinal muscle Tensor veli palatini muscle	**Ø Open** **3 Percutaneous** **4 Percutaneous Endoscopic** **7 Via Natural or Artificial Opening** **8 Via Natural or Artificial Opening Endoscopic**	**Z No Device**	**Z No Qualifier**

Ø Medical and Surgical
K Muscles
9 Drainage

Definition: Taking or letting out fluids and/or gases from a body part
Explanation: The qualifier DIAGNOSTIC is used to identify drainage procedures that are biopsies

Body Part Character 4	Approach Character 5	Device Character 6	Qualifier Character 7
Ø Head Muscle Auricularis muscle Masseter muscle Pterygoid muscle Splenius capitis muscle Temporalis muscle Temporoparietalis muscle **1 Facial Muscle** Buccinator muscle Corrugator supercilii muscle Depressor anguli oris muscle Depressor labii inferioris muscle Depressor septi nasi muscle Depressor supercilii muscle Levator anguli oris muscle Levator labii superioris alaeque nasi muscle Levator labii superioris muscle Mentalis muscle Nasalis muscle Occipitofrontalis muscle Orbicularis oris muscle Procerus muscle Risorius muscle Zygomaticus muscle **2 Neck Muscle, Right** Anterior vertebral muscle Arytenoid muscle Cricothyroid muscle Infrahyoid muscle Levator scapulae muscle Platysma muscle Scalene muscle Splenius cervicis muscle Sternocleidomastoid muscle Suprahyoid muscle Thyroarytenoid muscle **3 Neck Muscle, Left** *See 2 Neck Muscle, Right* **4 Tongue, Palate, Pharynx Muscle** Chondroglossus muscle Genioglossus muscle Hyoglossus muscle Inferior longitudinal muscle Levator veli palatini muscle Palatoglossal muscle Palatopharyngeal muscle Pharyngeal constrictor muscle Salpingopharyngeus muscle Styloglossus muscle Stylopharyngeus muscle Superior longitudinal muscle Tensor veli palatini muscle **5 Shoulder Muscle, Right** Deltoid muscle Infraspinatus muscle Subscapularis muscle Supraspinatus muscle Teres major muscle Teres minor muscle **6 Shoulder Muscle, Left** *See 5 Shoulder Muscle, Right* **7 Upper Arm Muscle, Right** Biceps brachii muscle Brachialis muscle Coracobrachialis muscle Triceps brachii muscle **8 Upper Arm Muscle, Left** *See 7 Upper Arm Muscle, Right* **9 Lower Arm and Wrist Muscle, Right** Anatomical snuffbox Brachioradialis muscle Extensor carpi radialis muscle Extensor carpi ulnaris muscle Flexor carpi radialis muscle Flexor carpi ulnaris muscle Flexor pollicis longus muscle Palmaris longus muscle Pronator quadratus muscle Pronator teres muscle **B Lower Arm and Wrist Muscle, Left** *See 9 Lower Arm and Wrist Muscle, Right* **C Hand Muscle, Right** Hypothenar muscle Palmar interosseous muscle Thenar muscle **D Hand Muscle, Left** *See C Hand Muscle, Right* **F Trunk Muscle, Right** Coccygeus muscle Erector spinae muscle Interspinalis muscle Intertransversarius muscle Latissimus dorsi muscle Quadratus lumborum muscle Rhomboid major muscle Rhomboid minor muscle Serratus posterior muscle Transversospinalis muscle Trapezius muscle **G Trunk Muscle, Left** *See F Trunk Muscle, Right* **H Thorax Muscle, Right** Intercostal muscle Levatores costarum muscle Pectoralis major muscle Pectoralis minor muscle Serratus anterior muscle Subclavius muscle Subcostal muscle Transverse thoracis muscle **J Thorax Muscle, Left** *See H Thorax Muscle, Right* **K Abdomen Muscle, Right** External oblique muscle Internal oblique muscle Pyramidalis muscle Rectus abdominis muscle Transversus abdominis muscle **L Abdomen Muscle, Left** *See K Abdomen Muscle, Right* **M Perineum Muscle** Bulbospongiosus muscle Cremaster muscle Deep transverse perineal muscle Ischiocavernosus muscle Levator ani muscle Superficial transverse perineal muscle **N Hip Muscle, Right** Gemellus muscle Gluteus maximus muscle Gluteus medius muscle Gluteus minimus muscle Iliacus muscle Obturator muscle Piriformis muscle Psoas muscle Quadratus femoris muscle Tensor fasciae latae muscle **P Hip Muscle, Left** *See N Hip Muscle, Right* **Q Upper Leg Muscle, Right** Adductor brevis muscle Adductor longus muscle Adductor magnus muscle Biceps femoris muscle Gracilis muscle Pectineus muscle Quadriceps (femoris) Rectus femoris muscle Sartorius muscle Semimembranosus muscle Semitendinosus muscle Vastus intermedius muscle Vastus lateralis muscle Vastus medialis muscle **R Upper Leg Muscle, Left** *See Q Upper Leg Muscle, Right* **S Lower Leg Muscle, Right** Extensor digitorum longus muscle Extensor hallucis longus muscle Fibularis brevis muscle Fibularis longus muscle Flexor digitorum longus muscle Flexor hallucis longus muscle Gastrocnemius muscle Peroneus brevis muscle Peroneus longus muscle Popliteus muscle Soleus muscle Tibialis anterior muscle Tibialis posterior muscle **T Lower Leg Muscle, Left** *See S Lower Leg Muscle, Right* **V Foot Muscle, Right** Abductor hallucis muscle Adductor hallucis muscle Extensor digitorum brevis muscle Extensor hallucis brevis muscle Flexor digitorum brevis muscle Flexor hallucis brevis muscle Quadratus plantae muscle **W Foot Muscle, Left** *See V Foot Muscle, Right*	**Ø Open** **3 Percutaneous** **4 Percutaneous Endoscopic**	**Ø Drainage Device**	**Z No Qualifier**

Non-OR ØK9[Ø,1,2,3,4,5,6,7,8,9,B,C,D,F,G,H,J,K,L,M,N,P,Q,R,S,T,V,W]3ØZ

ØK9 Continued on next page

NC Noncovered Procedure LC Limited Coverage QA Questionable OB Admit NT New Tech Add-on Combination Member ♂ Male ♀ Female

ØK9 Continued

Ø Medical and Surgical
K Muscles
9 Drainage

Definition: Taking or letting out fluids and/or gases from a body part
Explanation: The qualifier DIAGNOSTIC is used to identify drainage procedures that are biopsies

Body Part Character 4	Approach Character 5	Device Character 6	Qualifier Character 7
Ø Head Muscle Auricularis muscle Masseter muscle Pterygoid muscle Splenius capitis muscle Temporalis muscle Temporoparietalis muscle	**Ø Open**	**Z No Device**	**X Diagnostic**
1 Facial Muscle Buccinator muscle Corrugator supercilii muscle Depressor anguli oris muscle Depressor labii inferioris muscle Depressor septi nasi muscle Depressor supercilii muscle Levator anguli oris muscle Levator labii superioris alaeque nasi muscle Levator labii superioris muscle Mentalis muscle Nasalis muscle Occipitofrontalis muscle Orbicularis oris muscle Procerus muscle Risorius muscle Zygomaticus muscle	**3 Percutaneous**		**Z No Qualifier**
2 Neck Muscle, Right Anterior vertebral muscle Arytenoid muscle Cricothyroid muscle Infrahyoid muscle Levator scapulae muscle Platysma muscle Scalene muscle Splenius cervicis muscle Sternocleidomastoid muscle Suprahyoid muscle Thyroarytenoid muscle	**4 Percutaneous Endoscopic**		
3 Neck Muscle, Left *See 2 Neck Muscle, Right*			
4 Tongue, Palate, Pharynx Muscle Chondroglossus muscle Genioglossus muscle Hyoglossus muscle Inferior longitudinal muscle Levator veli palatini muscle Palatoglossal muscle Palatopharyngeal muscle Pharyngeal constrictor muscle Salpingopharyngeus muscle Styloglossus muscle Stylopharyngeus muscle Superior longitudinal muscle Tensor veli palatini muscle			
5 Shoulder Muscle, Right Deltoid muscle Infraspinatus muscle Subscapularis muscle Supraspinatus muscle Teres major muscle Teres minor muscle			
6 Shoulder Muscle, Left *See 5 Shoulder Muscle, Right*			
7 Upper Arm Muscle, Right Biceps brachii muscle Brachialis muscle Coracobrachialis muscle Triceps brachii muscle			
8 Upper Arm Muscle, Left *See 7 Upper Arm Muscle, Right*			
9 Lower Arm and Wrist Muscle, Right Anatomical snuffbox Brachioradialis muscle Extensor carpi radialis muscle Extensor carpi ulnaris muscle Flexor carpi radialis muscle Flexor carpi ulnaris muscle Flexor pollicis longus muscle Palmaris longus muscle Pronator quadratus muscle Pronator teres muscle			
B Lower Arm and Wrist Muscle, Left *See 9 Lower Arm and Wrist Muscle, Right*			
C Hand Muscle, Right Hypothenar muscle Palmar interosseous muscle Thenar muscle			
D Hand Muscle, Left *See C Hand Muscle, Right*			
F Trunk Muscle, Right Coccygeus muscle Erector spinae muscle Interspinalis muscle Intertransversarius muscle Latissimus dorsi muscle Quadratus lumborum muscle Rhomboid major muscle Rhomboid minor muscle Serratus posterior muscle Transversospinalis muscle Trapezius muscle			
G Trunk Muscle, Left *See F Trunk Muscle, Right*			
H Thorax Muscle, Right Intercostal muscle Levatores costarum muscle Pectoralis major muscle Pectoralis minor muscle Serratus anterior muscle Subclavius muscle Subcostal muscle Transverse thoracis muscle			
J Thorax Muscle, Left *See H Thorax Muscle, Right*			
K Abdomen Muscle, Right External oblique muscle Internal oblique muscle Pyramidalis muscle Rectus abdominis muscle Transversus abdominis muscle			
L Abdomen Muscle, Left *See K Abdomen Muscle, Right*			
M Perineum Muscle Bulbospongiosus muscle Cremaster muscle Deep transverse perineal muscle Ischiocavernosus muscle Levator ani muscle Superficial transverse perineal muscle			
N Hip Muscle, Right Gemellus muscle Gluteus maximus muscle Gluteus medius muscle Gluteus minimus muscle Iliacus muscle Obturator muscle Piriformis muscle Psoas muscle Quadratus femoris muscle Tensor fasciae latae muscle			
P Hip Muscle, Left *See N Hip Muscle, Right*			
Q Upper Leg Muscle, Right Adductor brevis muscle Adductor longus muscle Adductor magnus muscle Biceps femoris muscle Gracilis muscle Pectineus muscle Quadriceps (femoris) Rectus femoris muscle Sartorius muscle Semimembranosus muscle Semitendinosus muscle Vastus intermedius muscle Vastus lateralis muscle Vastus medialis muscle			
R Upper Leg Muscle, Left *See Q Upper Leg Muscle, Right*			
S Lower Leg Muscle, Right Extensor digitorum longus muscle Extensor hallucis longus muscle Fibularis brevis muscle Fibularis longus muscle Flexor digitorum longus muscle Flexor hallucis longus muscle Gastrocnemius muscle Peroneus brevis muscle Peroneus longus muscle Popliteus muscle Soleus muscle Tibialis anterior muscle Tibialis posterior muscle			
T Lower Leg Muscle, Left *See S Lower Leg Muscle, Right*			
V Foot Muscle, Right Abductor hallucis muscle Adductor hallucis muscle Extensor digitorum brevis muscle Extensor hallucis brevis muscle Flexor digitorum brevis muscle Flexor hallucis brevis muscle Quadratus plantae muscle			
W Foot Muscle, Left *See V Foot Muscle, Right*			

Non-OR ØK9[Ø,1,2,3,4,5,6,7,8,9,B,F,G,H,J,K,L,M,N,P,Q,R,S,T,V,W]3ZZ
Non-OR ØK9[C,D][3,4]ZZ

Non-OR Procedure DRG Non-OR Procedure Valid OR Procedure HAC Associated Procedure Combination Only New/Revised April New/Revised October

Ø Medical and Surgical
K Muscles
B Excision

Definition: Cutting out or off, without replacement, a portion of a body part
Explanation: The qualifier DIAGNOSTIC is used to identify excision procedures that are biopsies

Body Part Character 4	Approach Character 5	Device Character 6	Qualifier Character 7
Ø Head Muscle Auricularis muscle; Masseter muscle; Pterygoid muscle; Splenius capitis muscle; Temporalis muscle; Temporoparietalis muscle **1 Facial Muscle** Buccinator muscle; Corrugator supercilii muscle; Depressor anguli oris muscle; Depressor labii inferioris muscle; Depressor septi nasi muscle; Depressor supercilii muscle; Levator anguli oris muscle; Levator labii superioris alaeque nasi muscle; Levator labii superioris muscle; Mentalis muscle; Nasalis muscle; Occipitofrontalis muscle; Orbicularis oris muscle; Procerus muscle; Risorius muscle; Zygomaticus muscle **2 Neck Muscle, Right** Anterior vertebral muscle; Arytenoid muscle; Cricothyroid muscle; Infrahyoid muscle; Levator scapulae muscle; Platysma muscle; Scalene muscle; Splenius cervicis muscle; Sternocleidomastoid muscle; Suprahyoid muscle; Thyroarytenoid muscle **3 Neck Muscle, Left** *See 2 Neck Muscle, Right* **4 Tongue, Palate, Pharynx Muscle** Chondroglossus muscle; Genioglossus muscle; Hyoglossus muscle; Inferior longitudinal muscle; Levator veli palatini muscle; Palatoglossal muscle; Palatopharyngeal muscle; Pharyngeal constrictor muscle; Salpingopharyngeus muscle; Styloglossus muscle; Stylopharyngeus muscle; Superior longitudinal muscle; Tensor veli palatini muscle **5 Shoulder Muscle, Right** Deltoid muscle; Infraspinatus muscle; Subscapularis muscle; Supraspinatus muscle; Teres major muscle; Teres minor muscle **6 Shoulder Muscle, Left** *See 5 Shoulder Muscle, Right* **7 Upper Arm Muscle, Right** Biceps brachii muscle; Brachialis muscle; Coracobrachialis muscle; Triceps brachii muscle **8 Upper Arm Muscle, Left** *See 7 Upper Arm Muscle, Right* **9 Lower Arm and Wrist Muscle, Right** Anatomical snuffbox; Brachioradialis muscle; Extensor carpi radialis muscle; Extensor carpi ulnaris muscle; Flexor carpi radialis muscle; Flexor carpi ulnaris muscle; Flexor pollicis longus muscle; Palmaris longus muscle; Pronator quadratus muscle; Pronator teres muscle **B Lower Arm and Wrist Muscle, Left** *See 9 Lower Arm and Wrist Muscle, Right* **C Hand Muscle, Right** Hypothenar muscle; Palmar interosseous muscle; Thenar muscle **D Hand Muscle, Left** *See C Hand Muscle, Right* **F Trunk Muscle, Right** Coccygeus muscle; Erector spinae muscle; Interspinalis muscle; Intertransversarius muscle; Latissimus dorsi muscle; Quadratus lumborum muscle; Rhomboid major muscle; Rhomboid minor muscle; Serratus posterior muscle; Transversospinalis muscle; Trapezius muscle **G Trunk Muscle, Left** *See F Trunk Muscle, Right* **H Thorax Muscle, Right** Intercostal muscle; Levatores costarum muscle; Pectoralis major muscle; Pectoralis minor muscle; Serratus anterior muscle; Subclavius muscle; Subcostal muscle; Transverse thoracis muscle **J Thorax Muscle, Left** *See H Thorax Muscle, Right* **K Abdomen Muscle, Right** External oblique muscle; Internal oblique muscle; Pyramidalis muscle; Rectus abdominis muscle; Transversus abdominis muscle **L Abdomen Muscle, Left** *See K Abdomen Muscle, Right* **M Perineum Muscle** Bulbospongiosus muscle; Cremaster muscle; Deep transverse perineal muscle; Ischiocavernosus muscle; Levator ani muscle; Superficial transverse perineal muscle **N Hip Muscle, Right** Gemellus muscle; Gluteus maximus muscle; Gluteus medius muscle; Gluteus minimus muscle; Iliacus muscle; Obturator muscle; Piriformis muscle; Psoas muscle; Quadratus femoris muscle; Tensor fasciae latae muscle **P Hip Muscle, Left** *See N Hip Muscle, Right* **Q Upper Leg Muscle, Right** Adductor brevis muscle; Adductor longus muscle; Adductor magnus muscle; Biceps femoris muscle; Gracilis muscle; Pectineus muscle; Quadriceps (femoris); Rectus femoris muscle; Sartorius muscle; Semimembranosus muscle; Semitendinosus muscle; Vastus intermedius muscle; Vastus lateralis muscle; Vastus medialis muscle **R Upper Leg Muscle, Left** *See Q Upper Leg Muscle, Right* **S Lower Leg Muscle, Right** Extensor digitorum longus muscle; Extensor hallucis longus muscle; Fibularis brevis muscle; Fibularis longus muscle; Flexor digitorum longus muscle; Flexor hallucis longus muscle; Gastrocnemius muscle; Peroneus brevis muscle; Peroneus longus muscle; Popliteus muscle; Soleus muscle; Tibialis anterior muscle; Tibialis posterior muscle **T Lower Leg Muscle, Left** *See S Lower Leg Muscle, Right* **V Foot Muscle, Right** Abductor hallucis muscle; Adductor hallucis muscle; Extensor digitorum brevis muscle; Extensor hallucis brevis muscle; Flexor digitorum brevis muscle; Flexor hallucis brevis muscle; Quadratus plantae muscle **W Foot Muscle, Left** *See V Foot Muscle, Right*	**Ø** Open **3** Percutaneous **4** Percutaneous Endoscopic	**Z** No Device	**X** Diagnostic **Z** No Qualifier

Non-OR ØKB[N,P]3Z[X,Z]

Ø Medical and Surgical
K Muscles
C Extirpation

Definition: Taking or cutting out solid matter from a body part

Explanation: The solid matter may be an abnormal byproduct of a biological function or a foreign body; it may be imbedded in a body part or in the lumen of a tubular body part. The solid matter may or may not have been previously broken into pieces.

Body Part Character 4	Approach Character 5	Device Character 6	Qualifier Character 7
Ø Head Muscle Auricularis muscle Masseter muscle Pterygoid muscle Splenius capitis muscle Temporalis muscle Temporoparietalis muscle **1 Facial Muscle** Buccinator muscle Corrugator supercilii muscle Depressor anguli oris muscle Depressor labii inferioris muscle Depressor septi nasi muscle Depressor supercilii muscle Levator anguli oris muscle Levator labii superioris alaeque nasi muscle Levator labii superioris muscle Mentalis muscle Nasalis muscle Occipitofrontalis muscle Orbicularis oris muscle Procerus muscle Risorius muscle Zygomaticus muscle **2 Neck Muscle, Right** Anterior vertebral muscle Arytenoid muscle Cricothyroid muscle Infrahyoid muscle Levator scapulae muscle Platysma muscle Scalene muscle Splenius cervicis muscle Sternocleidomastoid muscle Suprahyoid muscle Thyroarytenoid muscle **3 Neck Muscle, Left** *See 2 Neck Muscle, Right* **4 Tongue, Palate, Pharynx Muscle** Chondroglossus muscle Genioglossus muscle Hyoglossus muscle Inferior longitudinal muscle Levator veli palatini muscle Palatoglossal muscle Palatopharyngeal muscle Pharyngeal constrictor muscle Salpingopharyngeus muscle Styloglossus muscle Stylopharyngeus muscle Superior longitudinal muscle Tensor veli palatini muscle **5 Shoulder Muscle, Right** Deltoid muscle Infraspinatus muscle Subscapularis muscle Supraspinatus muscle Teres major muscle Teres minor muscle **6 Shoulder Muscle, Left** *See 5 Shoulder Muscle, Right* **7 Upper Arm Muscle, Right** Biceps brachii muscle Brachialis muscle Coracobrachialis muscle Triceps brachii muscle **8 Upper Arm Muscle, Left** *See 7 Upper Arm Muscle, Right* **9 Lower Arm and Wrist Muscle, Right** Anatomical snuffbox Brachioradialis muscle Extensor carpi radialis muscle Extensor carpi ulnaris muscle Flexor carpi radialis muscle Flexor carpi ulnaris muscle Flexor pollicis longus muscle Palmaris longus muscle Pronator quadratus muscle Pronator teres muscle **B Lower Arm and Wrist Muscle, Left** *See 9 Lower Arm and Wrist Muscle, Right* **C Hand Muscle, Right** Hypothenar muscle Palmar interosseous muscle Thenar muscle **D Hand Muscle, Left** *See C Hand Muscle, Right* **F Trunk Muscle, Right** Coccygeus muscle Erector spinae muscle Interspinalis muscle Intertransversarius muscle Latissimus dorsi muscle Quadratus lumborum muscle Rhomboid major muscle Rhomboid minor muscle Serratus posterior muscle Transversospinalis muscle Trapezius muscle **G Trunk Muscle, Left** *See F Trunk Muscle, Right* **H Thorax Muscle, Right** Intercostal muscle Levatores costarum muscle Pectoralis major muscle Pectoralis minor muscle Serratus anterior muscle Subclavius muscle Subcostal muscle Transverse thoracis muscle **J Thorax Muscle, Left** *See H Thorax Muscle, Right* **K Abdomen Muscle, Right** External oblique muscle Internal oblique muscle Pyramidalis muscle Rectus abdominis muscle Transversus abdominis muscle **L Abdomen Muscle, Left** *See K Abdomen Muscle, Right* **M Perineum Muscle** Bulbospongiosus muscle Cremaster muscle Deep transverse perineal muscle Ischiocavernosus muscle Levator ani muscle Superficial transverse perineal muscle **N Hip Muscle, Right** Gemellus muscle Gluteus maximus muscle Gluteus medius muscle Gluteus minimus muscle Iliacus muscle Obturator muscle Piriformis muscle Psoas muscle Quadratus femoris muscle Tensor fasciae latae muscle **P Hip Muscle, Left** *See N Hip Muscle, Right* **Q Upper Leg Muscle, Right** Adductor brevis muscle Adductor longus muscle Adductor magnus muscle Biceps femoris muscle Gracilis muscle Pectineus muscle Quadriceps (femoris) Rectus femoris muscle Sartorius muscle Semimembranosus muscle Semitendinosus muscle Vastus intermedius muscle Vastus lateralis muscle Vastus medialis muscle **R Upper Leg Muscle, Left** *See Q Upper Leg Muscle, Right* **S Lower Leg Muscle, Right** Extensor digitorum longus muscle Extensor hallucis longus muscle Fibularis brevis muscle Fibularis longus muscle Flexor digitorum longus muscle Flexor hallucis longus muscle Gastrocnemius muscle Peroneus brevis muscle Peroneus longus muscle Popliteus muscle Soleus muscle Tibialis anterior muscle Tibialis posterior muscle **T Lower Leg Muscle, Left** *See S Lower Leg Muscle, Right* **V Foot Muscle, Right** Abductor hallucis muscle Adductor hallucis muscle Extensor digitorum brevis muscle Extensor hallucis brevis muscle Flexor digitorum brevis muscle Flexor hallucis brevis muscle Quadratus plantae muscle **W Foot Muscle, Left** *See V Foot Muscle, Right*	**Ø Open** **3 Percutaneous** **4 Percutaneous Endoscopic**	**Z No Device**	**Z No Qualifier**

Ø Medical and Surgical
K Muscles
D Extraction

Definition: Pulling or stripping out or off all or a portion of a body part by the use of force
Explanation: The qualifier DIAGNOSTIC is used to identify extraction procedures that are biopsies

Body Part Character 4	Approach Character 5	Device Character 6	Qualifier Character 7
Ø Head Muscle Auricularis muscle Masseter muscle Pterygoid muscle Splenius capitis muscle Temporalis muscle Temporoparietalis muscle **1 Facial Muscle** Buccinator muscle Corrugator supercilii muscle Depressor anguli oris muscle Depressor labii inferioris muscle Depressor septi nasi muscle Depressor supercilii muscle Levator anguli oris muscle Levator labii superioris alaeque nasi muscle Levator labii superioris muscle Mentalis muscle Nasalis muscle Occipitofrontalis muscle Orbicularis oris muscle Procerus muscle Risorius muscle Zygomaticus muscle **2 Neck Muscle, Right** Anterior vertebral muscle Arytenoid muscle Cricothyroid muscle Infrahyoid muscle Levator scapulae muscle Platysma muscle Scalene muscle Splenius cervicis muscle Sternocleidomastoid muscle Suprahyoid muscle Thyroarytenoid muscle **3 Neck Muscle, Left** *See 2 Neck Muscle, Right* **4 Tongue, Palate, Pharynx Muscle** Chondroglossus muscle Genioglossus muscle Hyoglossus muscle Inferior longitudinal muscle Levator veli palatini muscle Palatoglossal muscle Palatopharyngeal muscle Pharyngeal constrictor muscle Salpingopharyngeus muscle Styloglossus muscle Stylopharyngeus muscle Superior longitudinal muscle Tensor veli palatini muscle **5 Shoulder Muscle, Right** Deltoid muscle Infraspinatus muscle Subscapularis muscle Supraspinatus muscle Teres major muscle Teres minor muscle **6 Shoulder Muscle, Left** *See 5 Shoulder Muscle, Right* **7 Upper Arm Muscle, Right** Biceps brachii muscle Brachialis muscle Coracobrachialis muscle Triceps brachii muscle **8 Upper Arm Muscle, Left** *See 7 Upper Arm Muscle, Right* **9 Lower Arm and Wrist Muscle, Right** Anatomical snuffbox Brachioradialis muscle Extensor carpi radialis muscle Extensor carpi ulnaris muscle Flexor carpi radialis muscle Flexor carpi ulnaris muscle Flexor pollicis longus muscle Palmaris longus muscle Pronator quadratus muscle Pronator teres muscle **B Lower Arm and Wrist Muscle, Left** *See 9 Lower Arm and Wrist Muscle, Right* **C Hand Muscle, Right** Hypothenar muscle Palmar interosseous muscle Thenar muscle **D Hand Muscle, Left** *See C Hand Muscle, Right* **F Trunk Muscle, Right** Coccygeus muscle Erector spinae muscle Interspinalis muscle Intertransversarius muscle Latissimus dorsi muscle Quadratus lumborum muscle Rhomboid major muscle Rhomboid minor muscle Serratus posterior muscle Transversospinalis muscle Trapezius muscle **G Trunk Muscle, Left** *See F Trunk Muscle, Right* **H Thorax Muscle, Right** Intercostal muscle Levatores costarum muscle Pectoralis major muscle Pectoralis minor muscle Serratus anterior muscle Subclavius muscle Subcostal muscle Transverse thoracis muscle **J Thorax Muscle, Left** *See H Thorax Muscle, Right* **K Abdomen Muscle, Right** External oblique muscle Internal oblique muscle Pyramidalis muscle Rectus abdominis muscle Transversus abdominis muscle **L Abdomen Muscle, Left** *See K Abdomen Muscle, Right* **M Perineum Muscle** Bulbospongiosus muscle Cremaster muscle Deep transverse perineal muscle Ischiocavernosus muscle Levator ani muscle Superficial transverse perineal muscle **N Hip Muscle, Right** Gemellus muscle Gluteus maximus muscle Gluteus medius muscle Gluteus minimus muscle Iliacus muscle Obturator muscle Piriformis muscle Psoas muscle Quadratus femoris muscle Tensor fasciae latae muscle **P Hip Muscle, Left** *See N Hip Muscle, Right* **Q Upper Leg Muscle, Right** Adductor brevis muscle Adductor longus muscle Adductor magnus muscle Biceps femoris muscle Gracilis muscle Pectineus muscle Quadriceps (femoris) Rectus femoris muscle Sartorius muscle Semimembranosus muscle Semitendinosus muscle Vastus intermedius muscle Vastus lateralis muscle Vastus medialis muscle **R Upper Leg Muscle, Left** *See Q Upper Leg Muscle, Right* **S Lower Leg Muscle, Right** Extensor digitorum longus muscle Extensor hallucis longus muscle Fibularis brevis muscle Fibularis longus muscle Flexor digitorum longus muscle Flexor hallucis longus muscle Gastrocnemius muscle Peroneus brevis muscle Peroneus longus muscle Popliteus muscle Soleus muscle Tibialis anterior muscle Tibialis posterior muscle **T Lower Leg Muscle, Left** *See S Lower Leg Muscle, Right* **V Foot Muscle, Right** Abductor hallucis muscle Adductor hallucis muscle Extensor digitorum brevis muscle Extensor hallucis brevis muscle Flexor digitorum brevis muscle Flexor hallucis brevis muscle Quadratus plantae muscle **W Foot Muscle, Left** *See V Foot Muscle, Right*	Ø Open	Z No Device	Z No Qualifier

Ø Medical and Surgical
K Muscles
H Insertion

Definition: Putting in a nonbiological appliance that monitors, assists, performs, or prevents a physiological function but does not physically take the place of a body part

Explanation: None

Body Part Character 4	Approach Character 5	Device Character 6	Qualifier Character 7
X Upper Muscle Y Lower Muscle	Ø Open 3 Percutaneous 4 Percutaneous Endoscopic	M Stimulator Lead Y Other Device	Z No Qualifier

Non-OR ØKH[X,Y][3,4]YZ

Ø Medical and Surgical
K Muscles
J Inspection

Definition: Visually and/or manually exploring a body part

Explanation: Visual exploration may be performed with or without optical instrumentation. Manual exploration may be performed directly or through intervening body layers.

Body Part Character 4	Approach Character 5	Device Character 6	Qualifier Character 7
X Upper Muscle Y Lower Muscle	Ø Open 3 Percutaneous 4 Percutaneous Endoscopic X External	Z No Device	Z No Qualifier

Non-OR ØKJ[X,Y][3,X]ZZ

Ø Medical and Surgical
K Muscles
M Reattachment Definition: Putting back in or on all or a portion of a separated body part to its normal location or other suitable location
Explanation: Vascular circulation and nervous pathways may or may not be reestablished

Body Part Character 4	Approach Character 5	Device Character 6	Qualifier Character 7
Ø Head Muscle Auricularis muscle Masseter muscle Pterygoid muscle Splenius capitis muscle Temporalis muscle Temporoparietalis muscle **1 Facial Muscle** Buccinator muscle Corrugator supercilii muscle Depressor anguli oris muscle Depressor labii inferioris muscle Depressor septi nasi muscle Depressor supercilii muscle Levator anguli oris muscle Levator labii superioris alaeque nasi muscle Levator labii superioris muscle Mentalis muscle Nasalis muscle Occipitofrontalis muscle Orbicularis oris muscle Procerus muscle Risorius muscle Zygomaticus muscle **2 Neck Muscle, Right** Anterior vertebral muscle Arytenoid muscle Cricothyroid muscle Infrahyoid muscle Levator scapulae muscle Platysma muscle Scalene muscle Splenius cervicis muscle Sternocleidomastoid muscle Suprahyoid muscle Thyroarytenoid muscle **3 Neck Muscle, Left** *See 2 Neck Muscle, Right* **4 Tongue, Palate, Pharynx Muscle** Chondroglossus muscle Genioglossus muscle Hyoglossus muscle Inferior longitudinal muscle Levator veli palatini muscle Palatoglossal muscle Palatopharyngeal muscle Pharyngeal constrictor muscle Salpingopharyngeus muscle Styloglossus muscle Stylopharyngeus muscle Superior longitudinal muscle Tensor veli palatini muscle **5 Shoulder Muscle, Right** Deltoid muscle Infraspinatus muscle Subscapularis muscle Supraspinatus muscle Teres major muscle Teres minor muscle **6 Shoulder Muscle, Left** *See 5 Shoulder Muscle, Right* **7 Upper Arm Muscle, Right** Biceps brachii muscle Brachialis muscle Coracobrachialis muscle Triceps brachii muscle **8 Upper Arm Muscle, Left** *See 7 Upper Arm Muscle, Right* **9 Lower Arm and Wrist Muscle, Right** Anatomical snuffbox Brachioradialis muscle Extensor carpi radialis muscle Extensor carpi ulnaris muscle Flexor carpi radialis muscle Flexor carpi ulnaris muscle Flexor pollicis longus muscle Palmaris longus muscle Pronator quadratus muscle Pronator teres muscle **B Lower Arm and Wrist Muscle, Left** *See 9 Lower Arm and Wrist Muscle, Right* **C Hand Muscle, Right** Hypothenar muscle Palmar interosseous muscle Thenar muscle **D Hand Muscle, Left** *See C Hand Muscle, Right* **F Trunk Muscle, Right** Coccygeus muscle Erector spinae muscle Interspinalis muscle Intertransversarius muscle Latissimus dorsi muscle Quadratus lumborum muscle Rhomboid major muscle Rhomboid minor muscle Serratus posterior muscle Transversospinalis muscle Trapezius muscle **G Trunk Muscle, Left** *See F Trunk Muscle, Right* **H Thorax Muscle, Right** Intercostal muscle Levatores costarum muscle Pectoralis major muscle Pectoralis minor muscle Serratus anterior muscle Subclavius muscle Subcostal muscle Transverse thoracis muscle **J Thorax Muscle, Left** *See H Thorax Muscle, Right* **K Abdomen Muscle, Right** External oblique muscle Internal oblique muscle Pyramidalis muscle Rectus abdominis muscle Transversus abdominis muscle **L Abdomen Muscle, Left** *See K Abdomen Muscle, Right* **M Perineum Muscle** Bulbospongiosus muscle Cremaster muscle Deep transverse perineal muscle Ischiocavernosus muscle Levator ani muscle Superficial transverse perineal muscle **N Hip Muscle, Right** Gemellus muscle Gluteus maximus muscle Gluteus medius muscle Gluteus minimus muscle Iliacus muscle Obturator muscle Piriformis muscle Psoas muscle Quadratus femoris muscle Tensor fasciae latae muscle **P Hip Muscle, Left** *See N Hip Muscle, Right* **Q Upper Leg Muscle, Right** Adductor brevis muscle Adductor longus muscle Adductor magnus muscle Biceps femoris muscle Gracilis muscle Pectineus muscle Quadriceps (femoris) Rectus femoris muscle Sartorius muscle Semimembranosus muscle Semitendinosus muscle Vastus intermedius muscle Vastus lateralis muscle Vastus medialis muscle **R Upper Leg Muscle, Left** *See Q Upper Leg Muscle, Right* **S Lower Leg Muscle, Right** Extensor digitorum longus muscle Extensor hallucis longus muscle Fibularis brevis muscle Fibularis longus muscle Flexor digitorum longus muscle Flexor hallucis longus muscle Gastrocnemius muscle Peroneus brevis muscle Peroneus longus muscle Popliteus muscle Soleus muscle Tibialis anterior muscle Tibialis posterior muscle **T Lower Leg Muscle, Left** *See S Lower Leg Muscle, Right* **V Foot Muscle, Right** Abductor hallucis muscle Adductor hallucis muscle Extensor digitorum brevis muscle Extensor hallucis brevis muscle Flexor digitorum brevis muscle Flexor hallucis brevis muscle Quadratus plantae muscle **W Foot Muscle, Left** *See V Foot Muscle, Right*	**Ø Open** **4 Percutaneous Endoscopic**	**Z No Device**	**Z No Qualifier**

Ø Medical and Surgical
K Muscles
N Release

Definition: Freeing a body part from an abnormal physical constraint by cutting or by the use of force
Explanation: Some of the restraining tissue may be taken out but none of the body part is taken out

Body Part Character 4	Approach Character 5	Device Character 6	Qualifier Character 7
Ø Head Muscle Auricularis muscle Masseter muscle Pterygoid muscle Splenius capitis muscle Temporalis muscle Temporoparietalis muscle 1 Facial Muscle Buccinator muscle Corrugator supercilii muscle Depressor anguli oris muscle Depressor labii inferioris muscle Depressor septi nasi muscle Depressor supercilii muscle Levator anguli oris muscle Levator labii superioris alaeque nasi muscle Levator labii superioris muscle Mentalis muscle Nasalis muscle Occipitofrontalis muscle Orbicularis oris muscle Procerus muscle Risorius muscle Zygomaticus muscle 2 Neck Muscle, Right Anterior vertebral muscle Arytenoid muscle Cricothyroid muscle Infrahyoid muscle Levator scapulae muscle Platysma muscle Scalene muscle Splenius cervicis muscle Sternocleidomastoid muscle Suprahyoid muscle Thyroarytenoid muscle 3 Neck Muscle, Left *See 2 Neck Muscle, Right* 4 Tongue, Palate, Pharynx Muscle Chondroglossus muscle Genioglossus muscle Hyoglossus muscle Inferior longitudinal muscle Levator veli palatini muscle Palatoglossal muscle Palatopharyngeal muscle Pharyngeal constrictor muscle Salpingopharyngeus muscle Styloglossus muscle Stylopharyngeus muscle Superior longitudinal muscle Tensor veli palatini muscle 5 Shoulder Muscle, Right Deltoid muscle Infraspinatus muscle Subscapularis muscle Supraspinatus muscle Teres major muscle Teres minor muscle 6 Shoulder Muscle, Left *See 5 Shoulder Muscle, Right* 7 Upper Arm Muscle, Right Biceps brachii muscle Brachialis muscle Coracobrachialis muscle Triceps brachii muscle 8 Upper Arm Muscle, Left *See 7 Upper Arm Muscle, Right* 9 Lower Arm and Wrist Muscle, Right Anatomical snuffbox Brachioradialis muscle Extensor carpi radialis muscle Extensor carpi ulnaris muscle Flexor carpi radialis muscle Flexor carpi ulnaris muscle Flexor pollicis longus muscle Palmaris longus muscle Pronator quadratus muscle Pronator teres muscle B Lower Arm and Wrist Muscle, Left *See 9 Lower Arm and Wrist Muscle, Right* C Hand Muscle, Right Hypothenar muscle Palmar interosseous muscle Thenar muscle D Hand Muscle, Left *See C Hand Muscle, Right* F Trunk Muscle, Right Coccygeus muscle Erector spinae muscle Interspinalis muscle Intertransversarius muscle Latissimus dorsi muscle Quadratus lumborum muscle Rhomboid major muscle Rhomboid minor muscle Serratus posterior muscle Transversospinalis muscle Trapezius muscle G Trunk Muscle, Left *See F Trunk Muscle, Right* H Thorax Muscle, Right Intercostal muscle Levatores costarum muscle Pectoralis major muscle Pectoralis minor muscle Serratus anterior muscle Subclavius muscle Subcostal muscle Transverse thoracis muscle J Thorax Muscle, Left *See H Thorax Muscle, Right* K Abdomen Muscle, Right External oblique muscle Internal oblique muscle Pyramidalis muscle Rectus abdominis muscle Transversus abdominis muscle L Abdomen Muscle, Left *See K Abdomen Muscle, Right* M Perineum Muscle Bulbospongiosus muscle Cremaster muscle Deep transverse perineal muscle Ischiocavernosus muscle Levator ani muscle Superficial transverse perineal muscle N Hip Muscle, Right Gemellus muscle Gluteus maximus muscle Gluteus medius muscle Gluteus minimus muscle Iliacus muscle Obturator muscle Piriformis muscle Psoas muscle Quadratus femoris muscle Tensor fasciae latae muscle P Hip Muscle, Left *See N Hip Muscle, Right* Q Upper Leg Muscle, Right Adductor brevis muscle Adductor longus muscle Adductor magnus muscle Biceps femoris muscle Gracilis muscle Pectineus muscle Quadriceps (femoris) Rectus femoris muscle Sartorius muscle Semimembranosus muscle Semitendinosus muscle Vastus intermedius muscle Vastus lateralis muscle Vastus medialis muscle R Upper Leg Muscle, Left *See Q Upper Leg Muscle, Right* S Lower Leg Muscle, Right Extensor digitorum longus muscle Extensor hallucis longus muscle Fibularis brevis muscle Fibularis longus muscle Flexor digitorum longus muscle Flexor hallucis longus muscle Gastrocnemius muscle Peroneus brevis muscle Peroneus longus muscle Popliteus muscle Soleus muscle Tibialis anterior muscle Tibialis posterior muscle T Lower Leg Muscle, Left *See S Lower Leg Muscle, Right* V Foot Muscle, Right Abductor hallucis muscle Adductor hallucis muscle Extensor digitorum brevis muscle Extensor hallucis brevis muscle Flexor digitorum brevis muscle Flexor hallucis brevis muscle Quadratus plantae muscle W Foot Muscle, Left *See V Foot Muscle, Right*	Ø Open 3 Percutaneous 4 Percutaneous Endoscopic X External	Z No Device	Z No Qualifier

Non-OR ØKN[Ø,1,2,3,4,5,6,7,8,9,B,C,D,F,G,H,J,K,L,M,N,P,Q,R,S,T,V,W]XZZ

Ø Medical and Surgical
K Muscles
P Removal

Definition: Taking out or off a device from a body part

Explanation: If a device is taken out and a similar device put in without cutting or puncturing the skin or mucous membrane, the procedure is coded to the root operation CHANGE. Otherwise, the procedure for taking out a device is coded to the root operation REMOVAL.

Body Part Character 4	Approach Character 5	Device Character 6	Qualifier Character 7
X Upper Muscle Y Lower Muscle	Ø Open 3 Percutaneous 4 Percutaneous Endoscopic	Ø Drainage Device 7 Autologous Tissue Substitute J Synthetic Substitute K Nonautologous Tissue Substitute M Stimulator Lead Y Other Device	Z No Qualifier
X Upper Muscle Y Lower Muscle	X External	Ø Drainage Device M Stimulator Lead	Z No Qualifier

Non-OR ØKP[X,Y][3,4]YZ
Non-OR ØKP[X,Y]X[Ø,M]Z

Ø Medical and Surgical
K Muscles
Q Repair

Definition: Restoring, to the extent possible, a body part to its normal anatomic structure and function
Explanation: Used only when the method to accomplish the repair is not one of the other root operations

Body Part Character 4	Approach Character 5	Device Character 6	Qualifier Character 7
Ø Head Muscle Auricularis muscle Masseter muscle Pterygoid muscle Splenius capitis muscle Temporalis muscle Temporoparietalis muscle **1 Facial Muscle** Buccinator muscle Corrugator supercilii muscle Depressor anguli oris muscle Depressor labii inferioris muscle Depressor septi nasi muscle Depressor supercilii muscle Levator anguli oris muscle Levator labii superioris alaeque nasi muscle Levator labii superioris muscle Mentalis muscle Nasalis muscle Occipitofrontalis muscle Orbicularis oris muscle Procerus muscle Risorius muscle Zygomaticus muscle **2 Neck Muscle, Right** Anterior vertebral muscle Arytenoid muscle Cricothyroid muscle Infrahyoid muscle Levator scapulae muscle Platysma muscle Scalene muscle Splenius cervicis muscle Sternocleidomastoid muscle Suprahyoid muscle Thyroarytenoid muscle **3 Neck Muscle, Left** ***See*** *2 Neck Muscle, Right* **4 Tongue, Palate, Pharynx Muscle** Chondroglossus muscle Genioglossus muscle Hyoglossus muscle Inferior longitudinal muscle Levator veli palatini muscle Palatoglossal muscle Palatopharyngeal muscle Pharyngeal constrictor muscle Salpingopharyngeus muscle Styloglossus muscle Stylopharyngeus muscle Superior longitudinal muscle Tensor veli palatini muscle **5 Shoulder Muscle, Right** Deltoid muscle Infraspinatus muscle Subscapularis muscle Supraspinatus muscle Teres major muscle Teres minor muscle **6 Shoulder Muscle, Left** ***See*** *5 Shoulder Muscle, Right* **7 Upper Arm Muscle, Right** Biceps brachii muscle Brachialis muscle Coracobrachialis muscle Triceps brachii muscle **8 Upper Arm Muscle, Left** ***See*** *7 Upper Arm Muscle, Right* **9 Lower Arm and Wrist Muscle, Right** Anatomical snuffbox Brachioradialis muscle Extensor carpi radialis muscle Extensor carpi ulnaris muscle Flexor carpi radialis muscle Flexor carpi ulnaris muscle Flexor pollicis longus muscle Palmaris longus muscle Pronator quadratus muscle Pronator teres muscle **B Lower Arm and Wrist Muscle, Left** ***See*** *9 Lower Arm and Wrist Muscle, Right* **C Hand Muscle, Right** Hypothenar muscle Palmar interosseous muscle Thenar muscle **D Hand Muscle, Left** ***See*** *C Hand Muscle, Right* **F Trunk Muscle, Right** Coccygeus muscle Erector spinae muscle Interspinalis muscle Intertransversarius muscle Latissimus dorsi muscle Quadratus lumborum muscle Rhomboid major muscle Rhomboid minor muscle Serratus posterior muscle Transversospinalis muscle Trapezius muscle **G Trunk Muscle, Left** ***See*** *F Trunk Muscle, Right* **H Thorax Muscle, Right** Intercostal muscle Levatores costarum muscle Pectoralis major muscle Pectoralis minor muscle Serratus anterior muscle Subclavius muscle Subcostal muscle Transverse thoracis muscle **J Thorax Muscle, Left** ***See*** *H Thorax Muscle, Right* **K Abdomen Muscle, Right** External oblique muscle Internal oblique muscle Pyramidalis muscle Rectus abdominis muscle Transversus abdominis muscle **L Abdomen Muscle, Left** ***See*** *K Abdomen Muscle, Right* **M Perineum Muscle** Bulbospongiosus muscle Cremaster muscle Deep transverse perineal muscle Ischiocavernosus muscle Levator ani muscle Superficial transverse perineal muscle **N Hip Muscle, Right** Gemellus muscle Gluteus maximus muscle Gluteus medius muscle Gluteus minimus muscle Iliacus muscle Obturator muscle Piriformis muscle Psoas muscle Quadratus femoris muscle Tensor fasciae latae muscle **P Hip Muscle, Left** ***See*** *N Hip Muscle, Right* **Q Upper Leg Muscle, Right** Adductor brevis muscle Adductor longus muscle Adductor magnus muscle Biceps femoris muscle Gracilis muscle Pectineus muscle Quadriceps (femoris) Rectus femoris muscle Sartorius muscle Semimembranosus muscle Semitendinosus muscle Vastus intermedius muscle Vastus lateralis muscle Vastus medialis muscle **R Upper Leg Muscle, Left** ***See*** *Q Upper Leg Muscle, Right* **S Lower Leg Muscle, Right** Extensor digitorum longus muscle Extensor hallucis longus muscle Fibularis brevis muscle Fibularis longus muscle Flexor digitorum longus muscle Flexor hallucis longus muscle Gastrocnemius muscle Peroneus brevis muscle Peroneus longus muscle Popliteus muscle Soleus muscle Tibialis anterior muscle Tibialis posterior muscle **T Lower Leg Muscle, Left** ***See*** *S Lower Leg Muscle, Right* **V Foot Muscle, Right** Abductor hallucis muscle Adductor hallucis muscle Extensor digitorum brevis muscle Extensor hallucis brevis muscle Flexor digitorum brevis muscle Flexor hallucis brevis muscle Quadratus plantae muscle **W Foot Muscle, Left** ***See*** *V Foot Muscle, Right*	**Ø Open** **3 Percutaneous** **4 Percutaneous Endoscopic**	**Z No Device**	**Z No Qualifier**

Non-OR Procedure | DRG Non-OR Procedure | Valid OR Procedure | HAC Associated Procedure | Combination Only | New/Revised April | New/Revised October

Ø Medical and Surgical
K Muscles
R Replacement

Definition: Putting in or on biological or synthetic material that physically takes the place and/or function of all or a portion of a body part

Explanation: The body part may have been taken out or replaced, or may be taken out, physically eradicated, or rendered nonfunctional during the REPLACEMENT procedure. A REMOVAL procedure is coded for taking out the device used in a previous replacement procedure.

Body Part Character 4	Approach Character 5	Device Character 6	Qualifier Character 7
Ø Head Muscle Auricularis muscle Masseter muscle Pterygoid muscle Splenius capitis muscle Temporalis muscle Temporoparietalis muscle **1 Facial Muscle** Buccinator muscle Corrugator supercilii muscle Depressor anguli oris muscle Depressor labii inferioris muscle Depressor septi nasi muscle Depressor supercilii muscle Levator anguli oris muscle Levator labii superioris alaeque nasi muscle Levator labii superioris muscle Mentalis muscle Nasalis muscle Occipitofrontalis muscle Orbicularis oris muscle Procerus muscle Risorius muscle Zygomaticus muscle **2 Neck Muscle, Right** Anterior vertebral muscle Arytenoid muscle Cricothyroid muscle Infrahyoid muscle Levator scapulae muscle Platysma muscle Scalene muscle Splenius cervicis muscle Sternocleidomastoid muscle Suprahyoid muscle Thyroarytenoid muscle **3 Neck Muscle, Left** *See 2 Neck Muscle, Right* **4 Tongue, Palate, Pharynx Muscle** Chondroglossus muscle Genioglossus muscle Hyoglossus muscle Inferior longitudinal muscle Levator veli palatini muscle Palatoglossal muscle Palatopharyngeal muscle Pharyngeal constrictor muscle Salpingopharyngeus muscle Styloglossus muscle Stylopharyngeus muscle Superior longitudinal muscle Tensor veli palatini muscle **5 Shoulder Muscle, Right** Deltoid muscle Infraspinatus muscle Subscapularis muscle Supraspinatus muscle Teres major muscle Teres minor muscle **6 Shoulder Muscle, Left** *See 5 Shoulder Muscle, Right* **7 Upper Arm Muscle, Right** Biceps brachii muscle Brachialis muscle Coracobrachialis muscle Triceps brachii muscle **8 Upper Arm Muscle, Left** *See 7 Upper Arm Muscle, Right* **9 Lower Arm and Wrist Muscle, Right** Anatomical snuffbox Brachioradialis muscle Extensor carpi radialis muscle Extensor carpi ulnaris muscle Flexor carpi radialis muscle Flexor carpi ulnaris muscle Flexor pollicis longus muscle Palmaris longus muscle Pronator quadratus muscle Pronator teres muscle **B Lower Arm and Wrist Muscle, Left** *See 9 Lower Arm and Wrist Muscle, Right* **C Hand Muscle, Right** Hypothenar muscle Palmar interosseous muscle Thenar muscle **D Hand Muscle, Left** *See C Hand Muscle, Right* **F Trunk Muscle, Right** Coccygeus muscle Erector spinae muscle Interspinalis muscle Intertransversarius muscle Latissimus dorsi muscle Quadratus lumborum muscle Rhomboid major muscle Rhomboid minor muscle Serratus posterior muscle Transversospinalis muscle Trapezius muscle **G Trunk Muscle, Left** *See F Trunk Muscle, Right* **H Thorax Muscle, Right** Intercostal muscle Levatores costarum muscle Pectoralis major muscle Pectoralis minor muscle Serratus anterior muscle Subclavius muscle Subcostal muscle Transverse thoracis muscle **J Thorax Muscle, Left** *See H Thorax Muscle, Right* **K Abdomen Muscle, Right** External oblique muscle Internal oblique muscle Pyramidalis muscle Rectus abdominis muscle Transversus abdominis muscle **L Abdomen Muscle, Left** *See K Abdomen Muscle, Right* **M Perineum Muscle** Bulbospongiosus muscle Cremaster muscle Deep transverse perineal muscle Ischiocavernosus muscle Levator ani muscle Superficial transverse perineal muscle **N Hip Muscle, Right** Gemellus muscle Gluteus maximus muscle Gluteus medius muscle Gluteus minimus muscle Iliacus muscle Obturator muscle Piriformis muscle Psoas muscle Quadratus femoris muscle Tensor fasciae latae muscle **P Hip Muscle, Left** *See N Hip Muscle, Right* **Q Upper Leg Muscle, Right** Adductor brevis muscle Adductor longus muscle Adductor magnus muscle Biceps femoris muscle Gracilis muscle Pectineus muscle Quadriceps (femoris) Rectus femoris muscle Sartorius muscle Semimembranosus muscle Semitendinosus muscle Vastus intermedius muscle Vastus lateralis muscle Vastus medialis muscle **R Upper Leg Muscle, Left** *See Q Upper Leg Muscle, Right* **S Lower Leg Muscle, Right** Extensor digitorum longus muscle Extensor hallucis longus muscle Fibularis brevis muscle Fibularis longus muscle Flexor digitorum longus muscle Flexor hallucis longus muscle Gastrocnemius muscle Peroneus brevis muscle Peroneus longus muscle Popliteus muscle Soleus muscle Tibialis anterior muscle Tibialis posterior muscle **T Lower Leg Muscle, Left** *See S Lower Leg Muscle, Right* **V Foot Muscle, Right** Abductor hallucis muscle Adductor hallucis muscle Extensor digitorum brevis muscle Extensor hallucis brevis muscle Flexor digitorum brevis muscle Flexor hallucis brevis muscle Quadratus plantae muscle **W Foot Muscle, Left** *See V Foot Muscle, Right*	**Ø Open** **4 Percutaneous Endoscopic**	**7 Autologous Tissue Substitute** **J Synthetic Substitute** **K Nonautologous Tissue Substitute**	**Z No Qualifier**

Ø Medical and Surgical
K Muscles
S Reposition

Definition: Moving to its normal location, or other suitable location, all or a portion of a body part

Explanation: The body part is moved to a new location from an abnormal location, or from a normal location where it is not functioning correctly. The body part may or may not be cut out or off to be moved to the new location.

Body Part Character 4	Approach Character 5	Device Character 6	Qualifier Character 7
Ø Head Muscle Auricularis muscle Masseter muscle Pterygoid muscle Splenius capitis muscle Temporalis muscle Temporoparietalis muscle	**Ø Open** **4 Percutaneous Endoscopic**	**Z No Device**	**Z No Qualifier**
1 Facial Muscle Buccinator muscle Corrugator supercilii muscle Depressor anguli oris muscle Depressor labii inferioris muscle Depressor septi nasi muscle Depressor supercilii muscle Levator anguli oris muscle Levator labii superioris alaeque nasi muscle Levator labii superioris muscle Mentalis muscle Nasalis muscle Occipitofrontalis muscle Orbicularis oris muscle Procerus muscle Risorius muscle Zygomaticus muscle			
2 Neck Muscle, Right Anterior vertebral muscle Arytenoid muscle Cricothyroid muscle Infrahyoid muscle Levator scapulae muscle Platysma muscle Scalene muscle Splenius cervicis muscle Sternocleidomastoid muscle Suprahyoid muscle Thyroarytenoid muscle			
3 Neck Muscle, Left ***See*** *2 Neck Muscle, Right*			
4 Tongue, Palate, Pharynx Muscle Chondroglossus muscle Genioglossus muscle Hyoglossus muscle Inferior longitudinal muscle Levator veli palatini muscle Palatoglossal muscle Palatopharyngeal muscle Pharyngeal constrictor muscle Salpingopharyngeus muscle Styloglossus muscle Stylopharyngeus muscle Superior longitudinal muscle Tensor veli palatini muscle			
5 Shoulder Muscle, Right Deltoid muscle Infraspinatus muscle Subscapularis muscle Supraspinatus muscle Teres major muscle Teres minor muscle			
6 Shoulder Muscle, Left ***See*** *5 Shoulder Muscle, Right*			
7 Upper Arm Muscle, Right Biceps brachii muscle Brachialis muscle Coracobrachialis muscle Triceps brachii muscle			
8 Upper Arm Muscle, Left ***See*** *7 Upper Arm Muscle, Right*			
9 Lower Arm and Wrist Muscle, Right Anatomical snuffbox Brachioradialis muscle Extensor carpi radialis muscle Extensor carpi ulnaris muscle Flexor carpi radialis muscle Flexor carpi ulnaris muscle Flexor pollicis longus muscle Palmaris longus muscle Pronator quadratus muscle Pronator teres muscle			
B Lower Arm and Wrist Muscle, Left ***See*** *9 Lower Arm and Wrist Muscle, Right*			
C Hand Muscle, Right Hypothenar muscle Palmar interosseous muscle Thenar muscle			
D Hand Muscle, Left ***See*** *C Hand Muscle, Right*			
F Trunk Muscle, Right Coccygeus muscle Erector spinae muscle Interspinalis muscle Intertransversarius muscle Latissimus dorsi muscle Quadratus lumborum muscle Rhomboid major muscle Rhomboid minor muscle Serratus posterior muscle Transversospinalis muscle Trapezius muscle			
G Trunk Muscle, Left ***See*** *F Trunk Muscle, Right*			
H Thorax Muscle, Right Intercostal muscle Levatores costarum muscle Pectoralis major muscle Pectoralis minor muscle Serratus anterior muscle Subclavius muscle Subcostal muscle Transverse thoracis muscle			
J Thorax Muscle, Left ***See*** *H Thorax Muscle, Right*			
K Abdomen Muscle, Right External oblique muscle Internal oblique muscle Pyramidalis muscle Rectus abdominis muscle Transversus abdominis muscle			
L Abdomen Muscle, Left ***See*** *K Abdomen Muscle, Right*			
M Perineum Muscle Bulbospongiosus muscle Cremaster muscle Deep transverse perineal muscle Ischiocavernosus muscle Levator ani muscle Superficial transverse perineal muscle			
N Hip Muscle, Right Gemellus muscle Gluteus maximus muscle Gluteus medius muscle Gluteus minimus muscle Iliacus muscle Obturator muscle Piriformis muscle Psoas muscle Quadratus femoris muscle Tensor fasciae latae muscle			
P Hip Muscle, Left ***See*** *N Hip Muscle, Right*			
Q Upper Leg Muscle, Right Adductor brevis muscle Adductor longus muscle Adductor magnus muscle Biceps femoris muscle Gracilis muscle Pectineus muscle Quadriceps (femoris) Rectus femoris muscle Sartorius muscle Semimembranosus muscle Semitendinosus muscle Vastus intermedius muscle Vastus lateralis muscle Vastus medialis muscle			
R Upper Leg Muscle, Left ***See*** *Q Upper Leg Muscle, Right*			
S Lower Leg Muscle, Right Extensor digitorum longus muscle Extensor hallucis longus muscle Fibularis brevis muscle Fibularis longus muscle Flexor digitorum longus muscle Flexor hallucis longus muscle Gastrocnemius muscle Peroneus brevis muscle Peroneus longus muscle Popliteus muscle Soleus muscle Tibialis anterior muscle Tibialis posterior muscle			
T Lower Leg Muscle, Left ***See*** *S Lower Leg Muscle, Right*			
V Foot Muscle, Right Abductor hallucis muscle Adductor hallucis muscle Extensor digitorum brevis muscle Extensor hallucis brevis muscle Flexor digitorum brevis muscle Flexor hallucis brevis muscle Quadratus plantae muscle			
W Foot Muscle, Left ***See*** *V Foot Muscle, Right*			

Ø Medical and Surgical
K Muscles
T Resection

Definition: Cutting out or off, without replacement, all of a body part
Explanation: None

Body Part Character 4	Approach Character 5	Device Character 6	Qualifier Character 7
Ø Head Muscle Auricularis muscle Masseter muscle Pterygoid muscle Splenius capitis muscle Temporalis muscle Temporoparietalis muscle **1 Facial Muscle** Buccinator muscle Corrugator supercilii muscle Depressor anguli oris muscle Depressor labii inferioris muscle Depressor septi nasi muscle Depressor supercilii muscle Levator anguli oris muscle Levator labii superioris alaeque nasi muscle Levator labii superioris muscle Mentalis muscle Nasalis muscle Occipitofrontalis muscle Orbicularis oris muscle Procerus muscle Risorius muscle Zygomaticus muscle **2 Neck Muscle, Right** Anterior vertebral muscle Arytenoid muscle Cricothyroid muscle Infrahyoid muscle Levator scapulae muscle Platysma muscle Scalene muscle Splenius cervicis muscle Sternocleidomastoid muscle Suprahyoid muscle Thyroarytenoid muscle **3 Neck Muscle, Left** *See 2 Neck Muscle, Right* **4 Tongue, Palate, Pharynx Muscle** Chondroglossus muscle Genioglossus muscle Hyoglossus muscle Inferior longitudinal muscle Levator veli palatini muscle Palatoglossal muscle Palatopharyngeal muscle Pharyngeal constrictor muscle Salpingopharyngeus muscle Styloglossus muscle Stylopharyngeus muscle Superior longitudinal muscle Tensor veli palatini muscle **5 Shoulder Muscle, Right** Deltoid muscle Infraspinatus muscle Subscapularis muscle Supraspinatus muscle Teres major muscle Teres minor muscle **6 Shoulder Muscle, Left** *See 5 Shoulder Muscle, Right* **7 Upper Arm Muscle, Right** Biceps brachii muscle Brachialis muscle Coracobrachialis muscle Triceps brachii muscle **8 Upper Arm Muscle, Left** *See 7 Upper Arm Muscle, Right* **9 Lower Arm and Wrist Muscle, Right** Anatomical snuffbox Brachioradialis muscle Extensor carpi radialis muscle Extensor carpi ulnaris muscle Flexor carpi radialis muscle Flexor carpi ulnaris muscle Flexor pollicis longus muscle Palmaris longus muscle Pronator quadratus muscle Pronator teres muscle **B Lower Arm and Wrist Muscle, Left** *See 9 Lower Arm and Wrist Muscle, Right* **C Hand Muscle, Right** Hypothenar muscle Palmar interosseous muscle Thenar muscle **D Hand Muscle, Left** *See C Hand Muscle, Right* **F Trunk Muscle, Right** Coccygeus muscle Erector spinae muscle Interspinalis muscle Intertransversarius muscle Latissimus dorsi muscle Quadratus lumborum muscle Rhomboid major muscle Rhomboid minor muscle Serratus posterior muscle Transversospinalis muscle Trapezius muscle **G Trunk Muscle, Left** *See F Trunk Muscle, Right* **H Thorax Muscle, Right** ⊞ Intercostal muscle Levatores costarum muscle Pectoralis major muscle Pectoralis minor muscle Serratus anterior muscle Subclavius muscle Subcostal muscle Transverse thoracis muscle **J Thorax Muscle, Left** ⊞ *See H Thorax Muscle, Right* **K Abdomen Muscle, Right** External oblique muscle Internal oblique muscle Pyramidalis muscle Rectus abdominis muscle Transversus abdominis muscle **L Abdomen Muscle, Left** *See K Abdomen Muscle, Right* **M Perineum Muscle** Bulbospongiosus muscle Cremaster muscle Deep transverse perineal muscle Ischiocavernosus muscle Levator ani muscle Superficial transverse perineal muscle **N Hip Muscle, Right** Gemellus muscle Gluteus maximus muscle Gluteus medius muscle Gluteus minimus muscle Iliacus muscle Obturator muscle Piriformis muscle Psoas muscle Quadratus femoris muscle Tensor fasciae latae muscle **P Hip Muscle, Left** *See N Hip Muscle, Right* **Q Upper Leg Muscle, Right** Adductor brevis muscle Adductor longus muscle Adductor magnus muscle Biceps femoris muscle Gracilis muscle Pectineus muscle Quadriceps (femoris) Rectus femoris muscle Sartorius muscle Semimembranosus muscle Semitendinosus muscle Vastus intermedius muscle Vastus lateralis muscle Vastus medialis muscle **R Upper Leg Muscle, Left** *See Q Upper Leg Muscle, Right* **S Lower Leg Muscle, Right** Extensor digitorum longus muscle Extensor hallucis longus muscle Fibularis brevis muscle Fibularis longus muscle Flexor digitorum longus muscle Flexor hallucis longus muscle Gastrocnemius muscle Peroneus brevis muscle Peroneus longus muscle Popliteus muscle Soleus muscle Tibialis anterior muscle Tibialis posterior muscle **T Lower Leg Muscle, Left** *See S Lower Leg Muscle, Right* **V Foot Muscle, Right** Abductor hallucis muscle Adductor hallucis muscle Extensor digitorum brevis muscle Extensor hallucis brevis muscle Flexor digitorum brevis muscle Flexor hallucis brevis muscle Quadratus plantae muscle **W Foot Muscle, Left** *See V Foot Muscle, Right*	**Ø Open** **4 Percutaneous Endoscopic**	**Z No Device**	**Z No Qualifier**

See Appendix L for Procedure Combinations
⊞ ØKT[H,J]ØZZ

Ø Medical and Surgical
K Muscles
U Supplement

Definition: Putting in or on biological or synthetic material that physically reinforces and/or augments the function of a portion of a body part

Explanation: The biological material is non-living, or is living and from the same individual. The body part may have been previously replaced, and the SUPPLEMENT procedure is performed to physically reinforce and/or augment the function of the replaced body part.

Body Part Character 4	Approach Character 5	Device Character 6	Qualifier Character 7
Ø Head Muscle Auricularis muscle Masseter muscle Pterygoid muscle Splenius capitis muscle Temporalis muscle Temporoparietalis muscle **1 Facial Muscle** Buccinator muscle Corrugator supercilii muscle Depressor anguli oris muscle Depressor labii inferioris muscle Depressor septi nasi muscle Depressor supercilii muscle Levator anguli oris muscle Levator labii superioris alaeque nasi muscle Levator labii superioris muscle Mentalis muscle Nasalis muscle Occipitofrontalis muscle Orbicularis oris muscle Procerus muscle Risorius muscle Zygomaticus muscle **2 Neck Muscle, Right** Anterior vertebral muscle Arytenoid muscle Cricothyroid muscle Infrahyoid muscle Levator scapulae muscle Platysma muscle Scalene muscle Splenius cervicis muscle Sternocleidomastoid muscle Suprahyoid muscle Thyroarytenoid muscle **3 Neck Muscle, Left** *See 2 Neck Muscle, Right* **4 Tongue, Palate, Pharynx Muscle** Chondroglossus muscle Genioglossus muscle Hyoglossus muscle Inferior longitudinal muscle Levator veli palatini muscle Palatoglossal muscle Palatopharyngeal muscle Pharyngeal constrictor muscle Salpingopharyngeus muscle Styloglossus muscle Stylopharyngeus muscle Superior longitudinal muscle Tensor veli palatini muscle **5 Shoulder Muscle, Right** Deltoid muscle Infraspinatus muscle Subscapularis muscle Supraspinatus muscle Teres major muscle Teres minor muscle **6 Shoulder Muscle, Left** *See 5 Shoulder Muscle, Right* **7 Upper Arm Muscle, Right** Biceps brachii muscle Brachialis muscle Coracobrachialis muscle Triceps brachii muscle **8 Upper Arm Muscle, Left** *See 7 Upper Arm Muscle, Right* **9 Lower Arm and Wrist Muscle, Right** Anatomical snuffbox Brachioradialis muscle Extensor carpi radialis muscle Extensor carpi ulnaris muscle Flexor carpi radialis muscle Flexor carpi ulnaris muscle Flexor pollicis longus muscle Palmaris longus muscle Pronator quadratus muscle Pronator teres muscle **B Lower Arm and Wrist Muscle, Left** *See 9 Lower Arm and Wrist Muscle, Right* **C Hand Muscle, Right** Hypothenar muscle Palmar interosseous muscle Thenar muscle **D Hand Muscle, Left** *See C Hand Muscle, Right* **F Trunk Muscle, Right** Coccygeus muscle Erector spinae muscle Interspinalis muscle Intertransversarius muscle Latissimus dorsi muscle Quadratus lumborum muscle Rhomboid major muscle Rhomboid minor muscle Serratus posterior muscle Transversospinalis muscle Trapezius muscle **G Trunk Muscle, Left** *See F Trunk Muscle, Right* **H Thorax Muscle, Right** Intercostal muscle Levatores costarum muscle Pectoralis major muscle Pectoralis minor muscle Serratus anterior muscle Subclavius muscle Subcostal muscle Transverse thoracis muscle **J Thorax Muscle, Left** *See H Thorax Muscle, Right* **K Abdomen Muscle, Right** External oblique muscle Internal oblique muscle Pyramidalis muscle Rectus abdominis muscle Transversus abdominis muscle **L Abdomen Muscle, Left** *See K Abdomen Muscle, Right* **M Perineum Muscle** Bulbospongiosus muscle Cremaster muscle Deep transverse perineal muscle Ischiocavernosus muscle Levator ani muscle Superficial transverse perineal muscle **N Hip Muscle, Right** Gemellus muscle Gluteus maximus muscle Gluteus medius muscle Gluteus minimus muscle Iliacus muscle Obturator muscle Piriformis muscle Psoas muscle Quadratus femoris muscle Tensor fasciae latae muscle **P Hip Muscle, Left** *See N Hip Muscle, Right* **Q Upper Leg Muscle, Right** Adductor brevis muscle Adductor longus muscle Adductor magnus muscle Biceps femoris muscle Gracilis muscle Pectineus muscle Quadriceps (femoris) Rectus femoris muscle Sartorius muscle Semimembranosus muscle Semitendinosus muscle Vastus intermedius muscle Vastus lateralis muscle Vastus medialis muscle **R Upper Leg Muscle, Left** *See Q Upper Leg Muscle, Right* **S Lower Leg Muscle, Right** Extensor digitorum longus muscle Extensor hallucis longus muscle Fibularis brevis muscle Fibularis longus muscle Flexor digitorum longus muscle Flexor hallucis longus muscle Gastrocnemius muscle Peroneus brevis muscle Peroneus longus muscle Popliteus muscle Soleus muscle Tibialis anterior muscle Tibialis posterior muscle **T Lower Leg Muscle, Left** *See S Lower Leg Muscle, Right* **V Foot Muscle, Right** Abductor hallucis muscle Adductor hallucis muscle Extensor digitorum brevis muscle Extensor hallucis brevis muscle Flexor digitorum brevis muscle Flexor hallucis brevis muscle Quadratus plantae muscle **W Foot Muscle, Left** *See V Foot Muscle, Right*	**Ø Open** **4 Percutaneous Endoscopic**	**7 Autologous Tissue Substitute** **J Synthetic Substitute** **K Nonautologous Tissue Substitute**	**Z No Qualifier**

Ø Medical and Surgical
K Muscles
W Revision

Definition: Correcting, to the extent possible, a portion of a malfunctioning device or the position of a displaced device

Explanation: Revision can include correcting a malfunctioning or displaced device by taking out or putting in components of the device such as a screw or pin

Body Part Character 4	Approach Character 5	Device Character 6	Qualifier Character 7
X Upper Muscle Y Lower Muscle	Ø Open 3 Percutaneous 4 Percutaneous Endoscopic	Ø Drainage Device 7 Autologous Tissue Substitute J Synthetic Substitute K Nonautologous Tissue Substitute M Stimulator Lead Y Other Device	Z No Qualifier
X Upper Muscle Y Lower Muscle	X External	Ø Drainage Device 7 Autologous Tissue Substitute J Synthetic Substitute K Nonautologous Tissue Substitute M Stimulator Lead	Z No Qualifier

Non-OR ØKW[X,Y][3,4]YZ
Non-OR ØKW[X,Y]X[Ø,7,J,K,M]Z

Ø Medical and Surgical
K Muscles
X Transfer

Definition: Moving, without taking out, all or a portion of a body part to another location to take over the function of all or a portion of a body part

Explanation: The body part transferred remains connected to its vascular and nervous supply

Body Part Character 4	Approach Character 5	Device Character 6	Qualifier Character 7
Ø Head Muscle Auricularis muscle Masseter muscle Pterygoid muscle Splenius capitis muscle Temporalis muscle Temporoparietalis muscle **1 Facial Muscle** Buccinator muscle Corrugator supercilii muscle Depressor anguli oris muscle Depressor labii inferioris muscle Depressor septi nasi muscle Depressor supercilii muscle Levator anguli oris muscle Levator labii superioris alaeque nasi muscle Levator labii superioris muscle Mentalis muscle Nasalis muscle Occipitofrontalis muscle Orbicularis oris muscle Procerus muscle Risorius muscle Zygomaticus muscle **2 Neck Muscle, Right** Anterior vertebral muscle Arytenoid muscle Cricothyroid muscle Infrahyoid muscle Levator scapulae muscle Platysma muscle Scalene muscle Splenius cervicis muscle Sternocleidomastoid muscle Suprahyoid muscle Thyroarytenoid muscle **3 Neck Muscle, Left** ***See*** *2 Neck Muscle, Right* **4 Tongue, Palate, Pharynx Muscle** Chondroglossus muscle Genioglossus muscle Hyoglossus muscle Inferior longitudinal muscle Levator veli palatini muscle Palatoglossal muscle Palatopharyngeal muscle Pharyngeal constrictor muscle Salpingopharyngeus muscle Styloglossus muscle Stylopharyngeus muscle Superior longitudinal muscle Tensor veli palatini muscle **5 Shoulder Muscle, Right** Deltoid muscle Infraspinatus muscle Subscapularis muscle Supraspinatus muscle Teres major muscle Teres minor muscle **6 Shoulder Muscle, Left** ***See*** *5 Shoulder Muscle, Right* **7 Upper Arm Muscle, Right** Biceps brachii muscle Brachialis muscle Coracobrachialis muscle Triceps brachii muscle **8 Upper Arm Muscle, Left** ***See*** *7 Upper Arm Muscle, Right* **9 Lower Arm and Wrist Muscle, Right** Anatomical snuffbox Brachioradialis muscle Extensor carpi radialis muscle Extensor carpi ulnaris muscle Flexor carpi radialis muscle Flexor carpi ulnaris muscle Flexor pollicis longus muscle Palmaris longus muscle Pronator quadratus muscle Pronator teres muscle **B Lower Arm and Wrist Muscle, Left** ***See*** *9 Lower Arm and Wrist Muscle, Right* **C Hand Muscle, Right** Hypothenar muscle Palmar interosseous muscle Thenar muscle **D Hand Muscle, Left** ***See*** *C Hand Muscle, Right* **H Thorax Muscle, Right** Intercostal muscle Levatores costarum muscle Pectoralis major muscle Pectoralis minor muscle Serratus anterior muscle Subclavius muscle Subcostal muscle Transverse thoracis muscle **J Thorax Muscle, Left** ***See*** *H Thorax Muscle, Right* **M Perineum Muscle** Bulbospongiosus muscle Cremaster muscle Deep transverse perineal muscle Ischiocavernosus muscle Levator ani muscle Superficial transverse perineal muscle **N Hip Muscle, Right** Gemellus muscle Gluteus maximus muscle Gluteus medius muscle Gluteus minimus muscle Iliacus muscle Obturator muscle Piriformis muscle Psoas muscle Quadratus femoris muscle Tensor fasciae latae muscle **P Hip Muscle, Left** ***See*** *N Hip Muscle, Right* **Q Upper Leg Muscle, Right** Adductor brevis muscle Adductor longus muscle Adductor magnus muscle Biceps femoris muscle Gracilis muscle Pectineus muscle Quadriceps (femoris) Rectus femoris muscle Sartorius muscle Semimembranosus muscle Semitendinosus muscle Vastus intermedius muscle Vastus lateralis muscle Vastus medialis muscle **R Upper Leg Muscle, Left** ***See*** *Q Upper Leg Muscle, Right* **S Lower Leg Muscle, Right** Extensor digitorum longus muscle Extensor hallucis longus muscle Fibularis brevis muscle Fibularis longus muscle Flexor digitorum longus muscle Flexor hallucis longus muscle Gastrocnemius muscle Peroneus brevis muscle Peroneus longus muscle Popliteus muscle Soleus muscle Tibialis anterior muscle Tibialis posterior muscle **T Lower Leg Muscle, Left** ***See*** *S Lower Leg Muscle, Right* **V Foot Muscle, Right** Abductor hallucis muscle Adductor hallucis muscle Extensor digitorum brevis muscle Extensor hallucis brevis muscle Flexor digitorum brevis muscle Flexor hallucis brevis muscle Quadratus plantae muscle **W Foot Muscle, Left** ***See*** *V Foot Muscle, Right*	**Ø Open** **4 Percutaneous Endoscopic**	**Z No Device**	**Ø Skin** **1 Subcutaneous Tissue** **2 Skin and Subcutaneous Tissue** **Z No Qualifier**

ØKX Continued on next page

Ø Medical and Surgical
K Muscles
X Transfer

Definition: Moving, without taking out, all or a portion of a body part to another location to take over the function of all or a portion of a body part

Explanation: The body part transferred remains connected to its vascular and nervous supply

ØKX Continued

Body Part Character 4	Approach Character 5	Device Character 6	Qualifier Character 7
F Trunk Muscle, Right Coccygeus muscle Erector spinae muscle Interspinalis muscle Intertransversarius muscle Latissimus dorsi muscle Quadratus lumborum muscle Rhomboid major muscle Rhomboid minor muscle Serratus posterior muscle Transversospinalis muscle Trapezius muscle **G Trunk Muscle, Left** *See F Trunk Muscle, Right*	**Ø Open** **4 Percutaneous Endoscopic**	**Z No Device**	**Ø Skin** **1 Subcutaneous Tissue** **2 Skin and Subcutaneous Tissue** **5 Latissimus Dorsi Myocutaneous Flap** **7 Deep Inferior Epigastric Artery Perforator Flap** **8 Superficial Inferior Epigastric Artery Flap** **9 Gluteal Artery Perforator Flap** **Z No Qualifier**
K Abdomen Muscle, Right External oblique muscle Internal oblique muscle Pyramidalis muscle Rectus abdominis muscle Transversus abdominis muscle **L Abdomen Muscle, Left** *See K Abdomen Muscle, Right*	**Ø Open** **4 Percutaneous Endoscopic**	**Z No Device**	**Ø Skin** **1 Subcutaneous Tissue** **2 Skin and Subcutaneous Tissue** **6 Transverse Rectus Abdominis Myocutaneous Flap** **Z No Qualifier**

Tendons ØL2–ØLX

Character Meanings*

This Character Meaning table is provided as a guide to assist the user in the identification of character members that may be found in this section of code tables. It **SHOULD NOT** be used to build a PCS code.

Operation–Character 3	Body Part–Character 4	Approach–Character 5	Device–Character 6	Qualifier–Character 7
2 Change	Ø Head and Neck Tendon	Ø Open	Ø Drainage Device	X Diagnostic
5 Destruction	1 Shoulder Tendon, Right	3 Percutaneous	7 Autologous Tissue Substitute	Z No Qualifier
8 Division	2 Shoulder Tendon, Left	4 Percutaneous Endoscopic	J Synthetic Substitute	
9 Drainage	3 Upper Arm Tendon, Right	X External	K Nonautologous Tissue Substitute	
B Excision	4 Upper Arm Tendon, Left		Y Other Device	
C Extirpation	5 Lower Arm and Wrist Tendon, Right		Z No Device	
D Extraction	6 Lower Arm and Wrist Tendon, Left			
H Insertion	7 Hand Tendon, Right			
J Inspection	8 Hand Tendon, Left			
M Reattachment	9 Trunk Tendon, Right			
N Release	B Trunk Tendon, Left			
P Removal	C Thorax Tendon, Right			
Q Repair	D Thorax Tendon, Left			
R Replacement	F Abdomen Tendon, Right			
S Reposition	G Abdomen Tendon, Left			
T Resection	H Perineum Tendon			
U Supplement	J Hip Tendon, Right			
W Revision	K Hip Tendon, Left			
X Transfer	L Upper Leg Tendon, Right			
	M Upper Leg Tendon, Left			
	N Lower Leg Tendon, Right			
	P Lower Leg Tendon, Left			
	Q Knee Tendon, Right			
	R Knee Tendon, Left			
	S Ankle Tendon, Right			
	T Ankle Tendon, Left			
	V Foot Tendon, Right			
	W Foot Tendon, Left			
	X Upper Tendon			
	Y Lower Tendon			

* Includes synovial membrane.

AHA Coding Clinic for table ØL8
2016, 3Q, 30 Resection of femur with interposition arthroplasty

AHA Coding Clinic for table ØLB
2017, 2Q, 21 Arthroscopic anterior cruciate ligament revision using autograft with anterolateral ligament reconstruction
2015, 3Q, 26 Thumb arthroplasty with resection of trapezium
2014, 3Q, 14 Application of TheraSkin® and excisional debridement
2014, 3Q, 18 Placement of reverse sural fasciocutaneous pedicle flap

AHA Coding Clinic for table ØLD
2017, 4Q, 41 Extraction procedures

AHA Coding Clinic for table ØLQ
2016, 3Q, 32 Rotator cuff repair, tenodesis, decompression, acromioplasty and coracoplasty
2015, 2Q, 11 Repair of patellar and quadriceps tendons with allograft
2013, 3Q, 20 Superior labrum anterior posterior (SLAP) repair and subacromial decompression

AHA Coding Clinic for table ØLS
2016, 3Q, 32 Rotator cuff repair, tenodesis, decompression, acromioplasty and coracoplasty
2015, 3Q, 14 Endoprosthetic replacement of humerus and tendon reattachment

AHA Coding Clinic for table ØLU
2015, 2Q, 11 Repair of patellar and quadriceps tendons with allograft

Foot Tendons

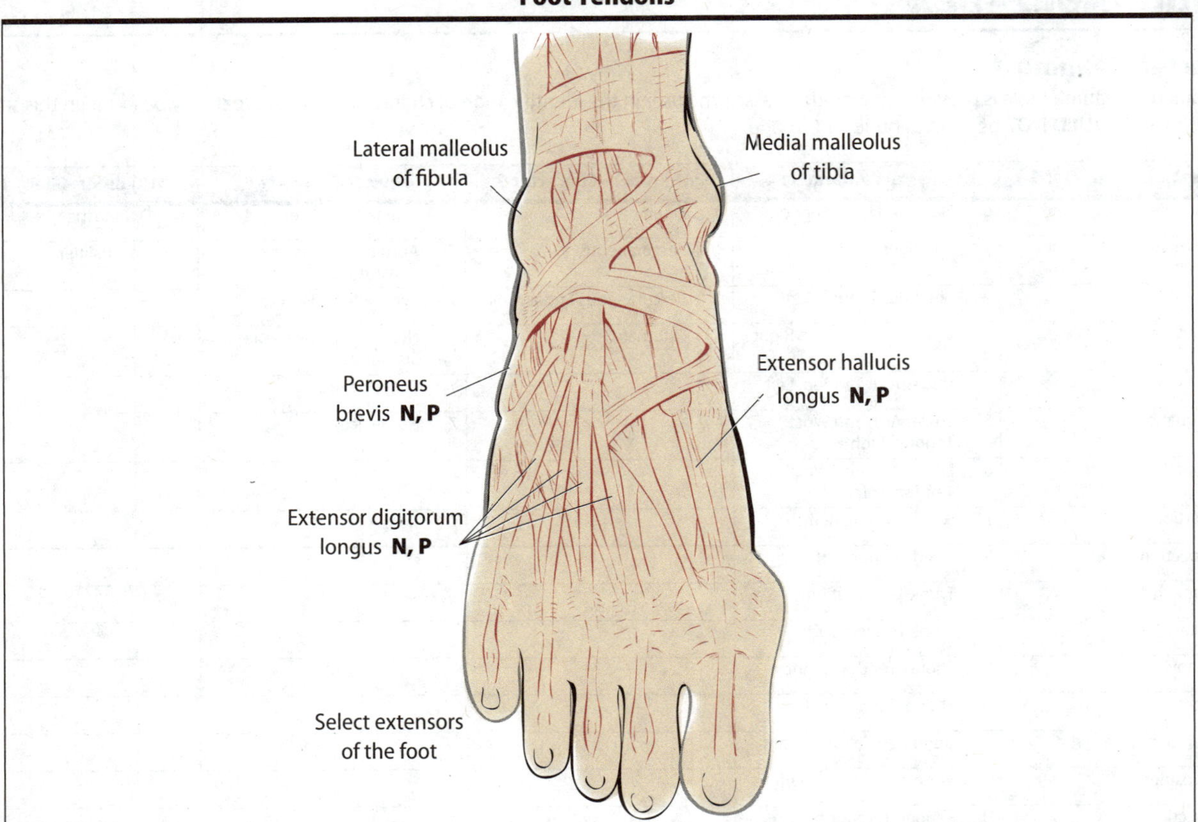

Shoulder Tendons

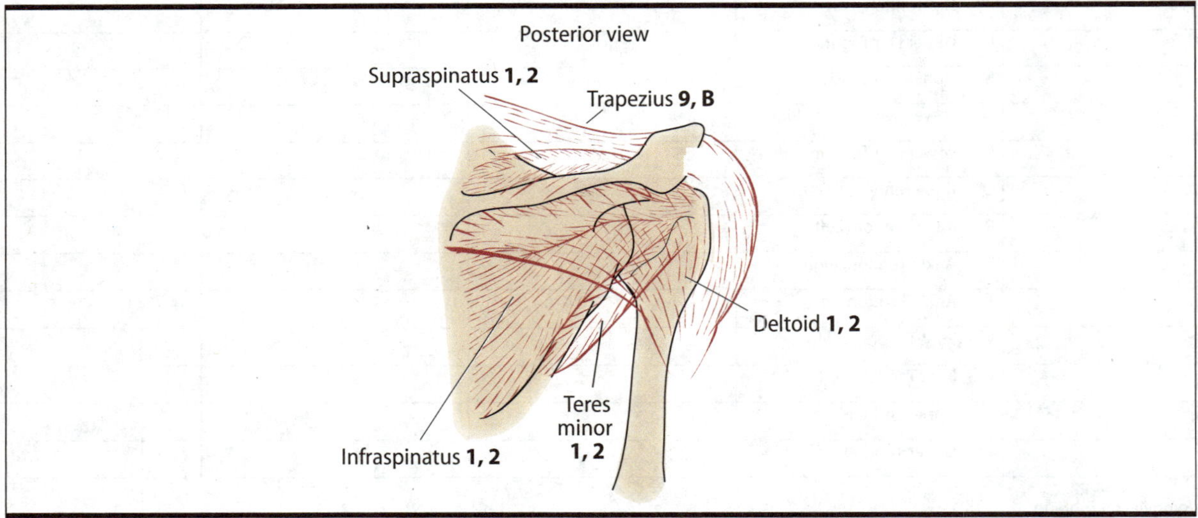

Tendons of Wrist and Hand

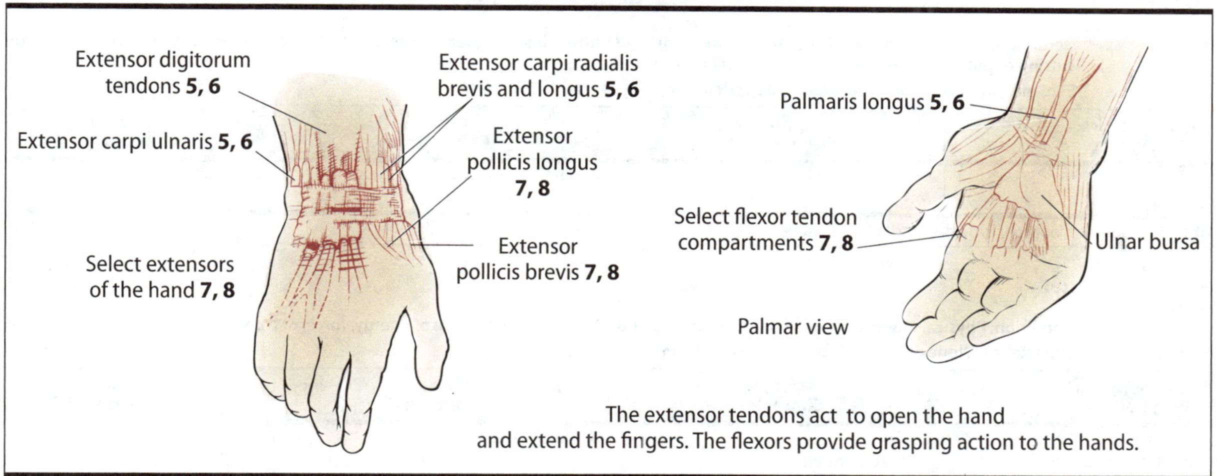

The extensor tendons act to open the hand and extend the fingers. The flexors provide grasping action to the hands.

Leg Muscles and Tendons

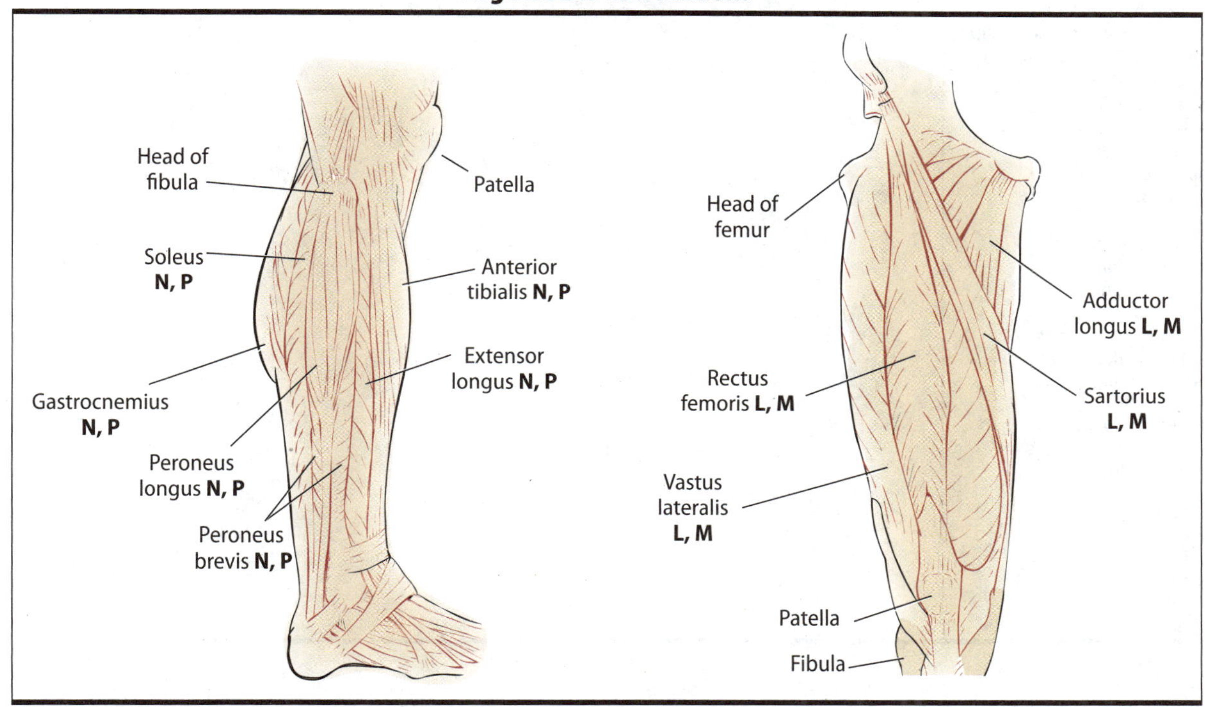

Ø Medical and Surgical
L Tendons
2 Change

Definition: Taking out or off a device from a body part and putting back an identical or similar device in or on the same body part without cutting or puncturing the skin or a mucous membrane

Explanation: All CHANGE procedures are coded using the approach EXTERNAL

Body Part Character 4	Approach Character 5	Device Character 6	Qualifier Character 7
X Upper Tendon Y Lower Tendon	X External	Ø Drainage Device Y Other Device	Z No Qualifier

Non-OR All body part, approach, device, and qualifier values

Ø Medical and Surgical
L Tendons
5 Destruction

Definition: Physical eradication of all or a portion of a body part by the direct use of energy, force, or a destructive agent

Explanation: None of the body part is physically taken out

Body Part Character 4	Approach Character 5	Device Character 6	Qualifier Character 7
Ø Head and Neck Tendon 1 Shoulder Tendon, Right 2 Shoulder Tendon, Left 3 Upper Arm Tendon, Right 4 Upper Arm Tendon, Left 5 Lower Arm and Wrist Tendon, Right 6 Lower Arm and Wrist Tendon, Left 7 Hand Tendon, Right 8 Hand Tendon, Left 9 Trunk Tendon, Right B Trunk Tendon, Left C Thorax Tendon, Right D Thorax Tendon, Left F Abdomen Tendon, Right G Abdomen Tendon, Left H Perineum Tendon J Hip Tendon, Right K Hip Tendon, Left L Upper Leg Tendon, Right M Upper Leg Tendon, Left N Lower Leg Tendon, Right Achilles tendon P Lower Leg Tendon, Left *See N Lower Leg Tendon, Right* Q Knee Tendon, Right Patellar tendon R Knee Tendon, Left *See Q Knee Tendon, Right* S Ankle Tendon, Right T Ankle Tendon, Left V Foot Tendon, Right W Foot Tendon, Left	Ø Open 3 Percutaneous 4 Percutaneous Endoscopic	Z No Device	Z No Qualifier

Ø Medical and Surgical
L Tendons
8 Division

Definition: Cutting into a body part, without draining fluids and/or gases from the body part, in order to separate or transect a body part
Explanation: All or a portion of the body part is separated into two or more portions

Body Part Character 4	Approach Character 5	Device Character 6	Qualifier Character 7
Ø Head and Neck Tendon 1 Shoulder Tendon, Right 2 Shoulder Tendon, Left 3 Upper Arm Tendon, Right 4 Upper Arm Tendon, Left 5 Lower Arm and Wrist Tendon, Right 6 Lower Arm and Wrist Tendon, Left 7 Hand Tendon, Right 8 Hand Tendon, Left 9 Trunk Tendon, Right B Trunk Tendon, Left C Thorax Tendon, Right D Thorax Tendon, Left F Abdomen Tendon, Right G Abdomen Tendon, Left H Perineum Tendon J Hip Tendon, Right K Hip Tendon, Left L Upper Leg Tendon, Right M Upper Leg Tendon, Left N Lower Leg Tendon, Right Achilles tendon P Lower Leg Tendon, Left *See N Lower Leg Tendon, Right* Q Knee Tendon, Right Patellar tendon R Knee Tendon, Left *See Q Knee Tendon, Right* S Ankle Tendon, Right T Ankle Tendon, Left V Foot Tendon, Right W Foot Tendon, Left	Ø Open 3 Percutaneous 4 Percutaneous Endoscopic	Z No Device	Z No Qualifier

Ø Medical and Surgical
L Tendons
9 Drainage

Definition: Taking or letting out fluids and/or gases from a body part

Explanation: The qualifier DIAGNOSTIC is used to identify drainage procedures that are biopsies

Body Part Character 4	Approach Character 5	Device Character 6	Qualifier Character 7
Ø Head and Neck Tendon **1** Shoulder Tendon, Right **2** Shoulder Tendon, Left **3** Upper Arm Tendon, Right **4** Upper Arm Tendon, Left **5** Lower Arm and Wrist Tendon, Right **6** Lower Arm and Wrist Tendon, Left **7** Hand Tendon, Right **8** Hand Tendon, Left **9** Trunk Tendon, Right **B** Trunk Tendon, Left **C** Thorax Tendon, Right **D** Thorax Tendon, Left **F** Abdomen Tendon, Right **G** Abdomen Tendon, Left **H** Perineum Tendon **J** Hip Tendon, Right **K** Hip Tendon, Left **L** Upper Leg Tendon, Right **M** Upper Leg Tendon, Left **N** Lower Leg Tendon, Right Achilles tendon **P** Lower Leg Tendon, Left *See N Lower Leg Tendon, Right* **Q** Knee Tendon, Right Patellar tendon **R** Knee Tendon, Left *See Q Knee Tendon, Right* **S** Ankle Tendon, Right **T** Ankle Tendon, Left **V** Foot Tendon, Right **W** Foot Tendon, Left	**Ø** Open **3** Percutaneous **4** Percutaneous Endoscopic	**Ø** Drainage Device	**Z** No Qualifier
Ø Head and Neck Tendon **1** Shoulder Tendon, Right **2** Shoulder Tendon, Left **3** Upper Arm Tendon, Right **4** Upper Arm Tendon, Left **5** Lower Arm and Wrist Tendon, Right **6** Lower Arm and Wrist Tendon, Left **7** Hand Tendon, Right **8** Hand Tendon, Left **9** Trunk Tendon, Right **B** Trunk Tendon, Left **C** Thorax Tendon, Right **D** Thorax Tendon, Left **F** Abdomen Tendon, Right **G** Abdomen Tendon, Left **H** Perineum Tendon **J** Hip Tendon, Right **K** Hip Tendon, Left **L** Upper Leg Tendon, Right **M** Upper Leg Tendon, Left **N** Lower Leg Tendon, Right Achilles tendon **P** Lower Leg Tendon, Left *See N Lower Leg Tendon, Right* **Q** Knee Tendon, Right Patellar tendon **R** Knee Tendon, Left *See Q Knee Tendon, Right* **S** Ankle Tendon, Right **T** Ankle Tendon, Left **V** Foot Tendon, Right **W** Foot Tendon, Left	**Ø** Open **3** Percutaneous **4** Percutaneous Endoscopic	**Z** No Device	**X** Diagnostic **Z** No Qualifier

Non-OR ØL9[Ø,1,2,3,4,5,6,7,8,9,B,C,D,F,G,H,J,K,L,M,N,P,Q,R,S,T,V,W]3ØZ
Non-OR ØL9[Ø,1,2,3,4,5,6,7,8,9,B,C,D,F,G,H,J,K,L,M,N,P,Q,R,S,T,V,W]3ZZ
Non-OR ØL9[7,8]4ZZ

Ø Medical and Surgical
L Tendons
B Excision

Definition: Cutting out or off, without replacement, a portion of a body part
Explanation: The qualifier DIAGNOSTIC is used to identify excision procedures that are biopsies

Body Part Character 4	Approach Character 5	Device Character 6	Qualifier Character 7
Ø Head and Neck Tendon **1** Shoulder Tendon, Right **2** Shoulder Tendon, Left **3** Upper Arm Tendon, Right **4** Upper Arm Tendon, Left **5** Lower Arm and Wrist Tendon, Right **6** Lower Arm and Wrist Tendon, Left **7** Hand Tendon, Right **8** Hand Tendon, Left **9** Trunk Tendon, Right **B** Trunk Tendon, Left **C** Thorax Tendon, Right **D** Thorax Tendon, Left **F** Abdomen Tendon, Right **G** Abdomen Tendon, Left **H** Perineum Tendon **J** Hip Tendon, Right **K** Hip Tendon, Left **L** Upper Leg Tendon, Right **M** Upper Leg Tendon, Left **N** Lower Leg Tendon, Right Achilles tendon **P** Lower Leg Tendon, Left *See N Lower Leg Tendon, Right* **Q** Knee Tendon, Right Patellar tendon **R** Knee Tendon, Left *See Q Knee Tendon, Right* **S** Ankle Tendon, Right **T** Ankle Tendon, Left **V** Foot Tendon, Right **W** Foot Tendon, Left	**Ø** Open **3** Percutaneous **4** Percutaneous Endoscopic	**Z** No Device	**X** Diagnostic **Z** No Qualifier

Ø Medical and Surgical
L Tendons
C Extirpation

Definition: Taking or cutting out solid matter from a body part

Explanation: The solid matter may be an abnormal byproduct of a biological function or a foreign body; it may be imbedded in a body part or in the lumen of a tubular body part. The solid matter may or may not have been previously broken into pieces.

Body Part Character 4	Approach Character 5	Device Character 6	Qualifier Character 7
Ø Head and Neck Tendon 1 Shoulder Tendon, Right 2 Shoulder Tendon, Left 3 Upper Arm Tendon, Right 4 Upper Arm Tendon, Left 5 Lower Arm and Wrist Tendon, Right 6 Lower Arm and Wrist Tendon, Left 7 Hand Tendon, Right 8 Hand Tendon, Left 9 Trunk Tendon, Right B Trunk Tendon, Left C Thorax Tendon, Right D Thorax Tendon, Left F Abdomen Tendon, Right G Abdomen Tendon, Left H Perineum Tendon J Hip Tendon, Right K Hip Tendon, Left L Upper Leg Tendon, Right M Upper Leg Tendon, Left N Lower Leg Tendon, Right Achilles tendon P Lower Leg Tendon, Left *See N Lower Leg Tendon, Right* Q Knee Tendon, Right Patellar tendon R Knee Tendon, Left *See Q Knee Tendon, Right* S Ankle Tendon, Right T Ankle Tendon, Left V Foot Tendon, Right W Foot Tendon, Left	Ø Open 3 Percutaneous 4 Percutaneous Endoscopic	Z No Device	Z No Qualifier

Ø Medical and Surgical
L Tendons
D Extraction

Definition: Pulling or stripping out or off all or a portion of a body part by the use of force

Explanation: The qualifier DIAGNOSTIC is used to identify extraction procedures that are biopsies

Body Part Character 4	Approach Character 5	Device Character 6	Qualifier Character 7
Ø Head and Neck Tendon 1 Shoulder Tendon, Right 2 Shoulder Tendon, Left 3 Upper Arm Tendon, Right 4 Upper Arm Tendon, Left 5 Lower Arm and Wrist Tendon, Right 6 Lower Arm and Wrist Tendon, Left 7 Hand Tendon, Right 8 Hand Tendon, Left 9 Trunk Tendon, Right B Trunk Tendon, Left C Thorax Tendon, Right D Thorax Tendon, Left F Abdomen Tendon, Right G Abdomen Tendon, Left H Perineum Tendon J Hip Tendon, Right K Hip Tendon, Left L Upper Leg Tendon, Right M Upper Leg Tendon, Left N Lower Leg Tendon, Right Achilles tendon P Lower Leg Tendon, Left *See N Lower Leg Tendon, Right* Q Knee Tendon, Right Patellar tendon R Knee Tendon, Left *See Q Knee Tendon, Right* S Ankle Tendon, Right T Ankle Tendon, Left V Foot Tendon, Right W Foot Tendon, Left	Ø Open	Z No Device	Z No Qualifier

Ø Medical and Surgical
L Tendons
H Insertion

Definition: Putting in a nonbiological appliance that monitors, assists, performs, or prevents a physiological function but does not physically take the place of a body part

Explanation: None

Body Part Character 4	Approach Character 5	Device Character 6	Qualifier Character 7
X Upper Tendon Y Lower Tendon	Ø Open 3 Percutaneous 4 Percutaneous Endoscopic	Y Other Device	Z No Qualifier

Non-OR ØLH[X,Y][3,4]YZ

Ø Medical and Surgical
L Tendons
J Inspection

Definition: Visually and/or manually exploring a body part

Explanation: Visual exploration may be performed with or without optical instrumentation. Manual exploration may be performed directly or through intervening body layers.

Body Part Character 4	Approach Character 5	Device Character 6	Qualifier Character 7
X Upper Tendon Y Lower Tendon	Ø Open 3 Percutaneous 4 Percutaneous Endoscopic X External	Z No Device	Z No Qualifier

Non-OR ØLJ[X,Y][3,X]ZZ

Ø Medical and Surgical
L Tendons
M Reattachment Definition: Putting back in or on all or a portion of a separated body part to its normal location or other suitable location
Explanation: Vascular circulation and nervous pathways may or may not be reestablished

Body Part Character 4	Approach Character 5	Device Character 6	Qualifier Character 7
Ø Head and Neck Tendon 1 Shoulder Tendon, Right 2 Shoulder Tendon, Left 3 Upper Arm Tendon, Right 4 Upper Arm Tendon, Left 5 Lower Arm and Wrist Tendon, Right 6 Lower Arm and Wrist Tendon, Left 7 Hand Tendon, Right 8 Hand Tendon, Left 9 Trunk Tendon, Right B Trunk Tendon, Left C Thorax Tendon, Right D Thorax Tendon, Left F Abdomen Tendon, Right G Abdomen Tendon, Left H Perineum Tendon J Hip Tendon, Right K Hip Tendon, Left L Upper Leg Tendon, Right M Upper Leg Tendon, Left N Lower Leg Tendon, Right Achilles tendon P Lower Leg Tendon, Left *See N Lower Leg Tendon, Right* Q Knee Tendon, Right Patellar tendon R Knee Tendon, Left *See Q Knee Tendon, Right* S Ankle Tendon, Right T Ankle Tendon, Left V Foot Tendon, Right W Foot Tendon, Left	Ø Open 4 Percutaneous Endoscopic	Z No Device	Z No Qualifier

Ø Medical and Surgical
L Tendons
N Release Definition: Freeing a body part from an abnormal physical constraint by cutting or by the use of force
Explanation: Some of the restraining tissue may be taken out but none of the body part is taken out

Body Part Character 4	Approach Character 5	Device Character 6	Qualifier Character 7
Ø Head and Neck Tendon 1 Shoulder Tendon, Right 2 Shoulder Tendon, Left 3 Upper Arm Tendon, Right 4 Upper Arm Tendon, Left 5 Lower Arm and Wrist Tendon, Right 6 Lower Arm and Wrist Tendon, Left 7 Hand Tendon, Right 8 Hand Tendon, Left 9 Trunk Tendon, Right B Trunk Tendon, Left C Thorax Tendon, Right D Thorax Tendon, Left F Abdomen Tendon, Right G Abdomen Tendon, Left H Perineum Tendon J Hip Tendon, Right K Hip Tendon, Left L Upper Leg Tendon, Right M Upper Leg Tendon, Left N Lower Leg Tendon, Right Achilles tendon P Lower Leg Tendon, Left *See N Lower Leg Tendon, Right* Q Knee Tendon, Right Patellar tendon R Knee Tendon, Left *See Q Knee Tendon, Right* S Ankle Tendon, Right T Ankle Tendon, Left V Foot Tendon, Right W Foot Tendon, Left	Ø Open 3 Percutaneous 4 Percutaneous Endoscopic X External	Z No Device	Z No Qualifier

Non-OR ØLN[Ø,1,2,3,4,5,6,7,8,9,B,C,D,F,G,H,J,K,L,M,N,P,Q,R,S,T,V,W]XZZ

Ø Medical and Surgical
L Tendons
P Removal

Definition: Taking out or off a device from a body part

Explanation: If a device is taken out and a similar device put in without cutting or puncturing the skin or mucous membrane, the procedure is coded to the root operation CHANGE. Otherwise, the procedure for taking out a device is coded to the root operation REMOVAL.

Body Part Character 4	Approach Character 5	Device Character 6	Qualifier Character 7
X Upper Tendon Y Lower Tendon	Ø Open 3 Percutaneous 4 Percutaneous Endoscopic	Ø Drainage Device 7 Autologous Tissue Substitute J Synthetic Substitute K Nonautologous Tissue Substitute Y Other Device	Z No Qualifier
X Upper Tendon Y Lower Tendon	X External	Ø Drainage Device	Z No Qualifier

Non-OR ØLP[X,Y]3ØZ
Non-OR ØLP[X,Y][3,4]YZ
Non-OR ØLP[X,Y]XØZ

Ø Medical and Surgical
L Tendons
Q Repair

Definition: Restoring, to the extent possible, a body part to its normal anatomic structure and function

Explanation: Used only when the method to accomplish the repair is not one of the other root operations

Body Part Character 4	Approach Character 5	Device Character 6	Qualifier Character 7
Ø Head and Neck Tendon 1 Shoulder Tendon, Right 2 Shoulder Tendon, Left 3 Upper Arm Tendon, Right 4 Upper Arm Tendon, Left 5 Lower Arm and Wrist Tendon, Right 6 Lower Arm and Wrist Tendon, Left 7 Hand Tendon, Right 8 Hand Tendon, Left 9 Trunk Tendon, Right B Trunk Tendon, Left C Thorax Tendon, Right D Thorax Tendon, Left F Abdomen Tendon, Right G Abdomen Tendon, Left H Perineum Tendon J Hip Tendon, Right K Hip Tendon, Left L Upper Leg Tendon, Right M Upper Leg Tendon, Left N Lower Leg Tendon, Right Achilles tendon P Lower Leg Tendon, Left *See N Lower Leg Tendon, Right* Q Knee Tendon, Right Patellar tendon R Knee Tendon, Left *See Q Knee Tendon, Right* S Ankle Tendon, Right T Ankle Tendon, Left V Foot Tendon, Right W Foot Tendon, Left	Ø Open 3 Percutaneous 4 Percutaneous Endoscopic	Z No Device	Z No Qualifier

Ø Medical and Surgical
L Tendons
R Replacement

Definition: Putting in or on biological or synthetic material that physically takes the place and/or function of all or a portion of a body part

Explanation: The body part may have been taken out or replaced, or may be taken out, physically eradicated, or rendered nonfunctional during the REPLACEMENT procedure. A REMOVAL procedure is coded for taking out the device used in a previous replacement procedure.

Body Part Character 4	Approach Character 5	Device Character 6	Qualifier Character 7
Ø Head and Neck Tendon 1 Shoulder Tendon, Right 2 Shoulder Tendon, Left 3 Upper Arm Tendon, Right 4 Upper Arm Tendon, Left 5 Lower Arm and Wrist Tendon, Right 6 Lower Arm and Wrist Tendon, Left 7 Hand Tendon, Right 8 Hand Tendon, Left 9 Trunk Tendon, Right B Trunk Tendon, Left C Thorax Tendon, Right D Thorax Tendon, Left F Abdomen Tendon, Right G Abdomen Tendon, Left H Perineum Tendon J Hip Tendon, Right K Hip Tendon, Left L Upper Leg Tendon, Right M Upper Leg Tendon, Left N Lower Leg Tendon, Right Achilles tendon P Lower Leg Tendon, Left *See N Lower Leg Tendon, Right* Q Knee Tendon, Right Patellar tendon R Knee Tendon, Left *See Q Knee Tendon, Right* S Ankle Tendon, Right T Ankle Tendon, Left V Foot Tendon, Right W Foot Tendon, Left	Ø Open 4 Percutaneous Endoscopic	7 Autologous Tissue Substitute J Synthetic Substitute K Nonautologous Tissue Substitute	Z No Qualifier

Ø Medical and Surgical
L Tendons
S Reposition

Definition: Moving to its normal location, or other suitable location, all or a portion of a body part

Explanation: The body part is moved to a new location from an abnormal location, or from a normal location where it is not functioning correctly. The body part may or may not be cut out or off to be moved to the new location.

Body Part Character 4	Approach Character 5	Device Character 6	Qualifier Character 7
Ø Head and Neck Tendon 1 Shoulder Tendon, Right 2 Shoulder Tendon, Left 3 Upper Arm Tendon, Right 4 Upper Arm Tendon, Left 5 Lower Arm and Wrist Tendon, Right 6 Lower Arm and Wrist Tendon, Left 7 Hand Tendon, Right 8 Hand Tendon, Left 9 Trunk Tendon, Right B Trunk Tendon, Left C Thorax Tendon, Right D Thorax Tendon, Left F Abdomen Tendon, Right G Abdomen Tendon, Left H Perineum Tendon J Hip Tendon, Right K Hip Tendon, Left L Upper Leg Tendon, Right M Upper Leg Tendon, Left N Lower Leg Tendon, Right Achilles tendon P Lower Leg Tendon, Left *See N Lower Leg Tendon, Right* Q Knee Tendon, Right Patellar tendon R Knee Tendon, Left *See Q Knee Tendon, Right* S Ankle Tendon, Right T Ankle Tendon, Left V Foot Tendon, Right W Foot Tendon, Left	Ø Open 4 Percutaneous Endoscopic	Z No Device	Z No Qualifier

Ø Medical and Surgical
L Tendons
T Resection

Definition: Cutting out or off, without replacement, all of a body part
Explanation: None

Body Part Character 4	Approach Character 5	Device Character 6	Qualifier Character 7
Ø Head and Neck Tendon 1 Shoulder Tendon, Right 2 Shoulder Tendon, Left 3 Upper Arm Tendon, Right 4 Upper Arm Tendon, Left 5 Lower Arm and Wrist Tendon, Right 6 Lower Arm and Wrist Tendon, Left 7 Hand Tendon, Right 8 Hand Tendon, Left 9 Trunk Tendon, Right B Trunk Tendon, Left C Thorax Tendon, Right D Thorax Tendon, Left F Abdomen Tendon, Right G Abdomen Tendon, Left H Perineum Tendon J Hip Tendon, Right K Hip Tendon, Left L Upper Leg Tendon, Right M Upper Leg Tendon, Left N Lower Leg Tendon, Right Achilles tendon P Lower Leg Tendon, Left *See* *N Lower Leg Tendon, Right* Q Knee Tendon, Right Patellar tendon R Knee Tendon, Left *See* *Q Knee Tendon, Right* S Ankle Tendon, Right T Ankle Tendon, Left V Foot Tendon, Right W Foot Tendon, Left	Ø Open 4 Percutaneous Endoscopic	Z No Device	Z No Qualifier

Ø Medical and Surgical
L Tendons
U Supplement

Definition: Putting in or on biological or synthetic material that physically reinforces and/or augments the function of a portion of a body part
Explanation: The biological material is non-living, or is living and from the same individual. The body part may have been previously replaced, and the SUPPLEMENT procedure is performed to physically reinforce and/or augment the function of the replaced body part.

Body Part Character 4	Approach Character 5	Device Character 6	Qualifier Character 7
Ø Head and Neck Tendon 1 Shoulder Tendon, Right 2 Shoulder Tendon, Left 3 Upper Arm Tendon, Right 4 Upper Arm Tendon, Left 5 Lower Arm and Wrist Tendon, Right 6 Lower Arm and Wrist Tendon, Left 7 Hand Tendon, Right 8 Hand Tendon, Left 9 Trunk Tendon, Right B Trunk Tendon, Left C Thorax Tendon, Right D Thorax Tendon, Left F Abdomen Tendon, Right G Abdomen Tendon, Left H Perineum Tendon J Hip Tendon, Right K Hip Tendon, Left L Upper Leg Tendon, Right M Upper Leg Tendon, Left N Lower Leg Tendon, Right Achilles tendon P Lower Leg Tendon, Left *See* *N Lower Leg Tendon, Right* Q Knee Tendon, Right Patellar tendon R Knee Tendon, Left *See* *Q Knee Tendon, Right* S Ankle Tendon, Right T Ankle Tendon, Left V Foot Tendon, Right W Foot Tendon, Left	Ø Open 4 Percutaneous Endoscopic	7 Autologous Tissue Substitute J Synthetic Substitute K Nonautologous Tissue Substitute	Z No Qualifier

Ø Medical and Surgical
L Tendons
W Revision

Definition: Correcting, to the extent possible, a portion of a malfunctioning device or the position of a displaced device

Explanation: Revision can include correcting a malfunctioning or displaced device by taking out or putting in components of the device such as a screw or pin

Body Part Character 4	Approach Character 5	Device Character 6	Qualifier Character 7
X Upper Tendon Y Lower Tendon	Ø Open 3 Percutaneous 4 Percutaneous Endoscopic	Ø Drainage Device 7 Autologous Tissue Substitute J Synthetic Substitute K Nonautologous Tissue Substitute Y Other Device	Z No Qualifier
X Upper Tendon Y Lower Tendon	X External	Ø Drainage Device 7 Autologous Tissue Substitute J Synthetic Substitute K Nonautologous Tissue Substitute	Z No Qualifier

Non-OR ØLW[X,Y][3,4]YZ
Non-OR ØLW[X,Y]X[Ø,7,J,K]Z

Ø Medical and Surgical
L Tendons
X Transfer

Definition: Moving, without taking out, all or a portion of a body part to another location to take over the function of all or a portion of a body part

Explanation: The body part transferred remains connected to its vascular and nervous supply

Body Part Character 4	Approach Character 5	Device Character 6	Qualifier Character 7
Ø Head and Neck Tendon 1 Shoulder Tendon, Right 2 Shoulder Tendon, Left 3 Upper Arm Tendon, Right 4 Upper Arm Tendon, Left 5 Lower Arm and Wrist Tendon, Right 6 Lower Arm and Wrist Tendon, Left 7 Hand Tendon, Right 8 Hand Tendon, Left 9 Trunk Tendon, Right B Trunk Tendon, Left C Thorax Tendon, Right D Thorax Tendon, Left F Abdomen Tendon, Right G Abdomen Tendon, Left H Perineum Tendon J Hip Tendon, Right K Hip Tendon, Left L Upper Leg Tendon, Right M Upper Leg Tendon, Left N Lower Leg Tendon, Right Achilles tendon P Lower Leg Tendon, Left *See N Lower Leg Tendon, Right* Q Knee Tendon, Right Patellar tendon R Knee Tendon, Left *See Q Knee Tendon, Right* S Ankle Tendon, Right T Ankle Tendon, Left V Foot Tendon, Right W Foot Tendon, Left	Ø Open 4 Percutaneous Endoscopic	Z No Device	Z No Qualifier

Bursae and Ligaments ØM2–ØMX

Character Meanings*

This Character Meaning table is provided as a guide to assist the user in the identification of character members that may be found in this section of code tables. It **SHOULD NOT** be used to build a PCS code.

Operation–Character 3		Body Part–Character 4		Approach–Character 5		Device–Character 6		Qualifier–Character 7	
2	Change	Ø	Head and Neck Bursa and Ligament	Ø	Open	Ø	Drainage Device	X	Diagnostic
5	Destruction	1	Shoulder Bursa and Ligament, Right	3	Percutaneous	7	Autologous Tissue Substitute	Z	No Qualifier
8	Division	2	Shoulder Bursa and Ligament, Left	4	Percutaneous Endoscopic	J	Synthetic Substitute		
9	Drainage	3	Elbow Bursa and Ligament, Right	X	External	K	Nonautologous Tissue Substitute		
B	Excision	4	Elbow Bursa and Ligament, Left			Y	Other Device		
C	Extirpation	5	Wrist Bursa and Ligament, Right			Z	No Device		
D	Extraction	6	Wrist Bursa and Ligament, Left						
H	Insertion	7	Hand Bursa and Ligament, Right						
J	Inspection	8	Hand Bursa and Ligament, Left						
M	Reattachment	9	Upper Extremity Bursa and Ligament, Right						
N	Release	B	Upper Extremity Bursa and Ligament, Left						
P	Removal	C	Upper Spine Bursa and Ligament						
Q	Repair	D	Lower Spine Bursa and Ligament						
R	Replacement	F	Sternum Bursa and Ligament						
S	Reposition	G	Rib(s) Bursa and Ligament						
T	Resection	H	Abdomen Bursa and Ligament, Right						
U	Supplement	J	Abdomen Bursa and Ligament, Left						
W	Revision	K	Perineum Bursa and Ligament						
X	Transfer	L	Hip Bursa and Ligament, Right						
		M	Hip Bursa and Ligament, Left						
		N	Knee Bursa and Ligament, Right						
		P	Knee Bursa and Ligament, Left						
		Q	Ankle Bursa and Ligament, Right						
		R	Ankle Bursa and Ligament, Left						
		S	Foot Bursa and Ligament, Right						
		T	Foot Bursa and Ligament, Left						
		V	Lower Extremity Bursa and Ligament, Right						
		W	Lower Extremity Bursa and Ligament, Left						
		X	Upper Bursa and Ligament						
		Y	Lower Bursa and Ligament						

* Includes synovial membrane.

AHA Coding Clinic for table ØMB
2018, 3Q, 17 Excisional debridement of periosteum

AHA Coding Clinic for table ØMM
2013, 3Q, 20 Superior labrum anterior posterior (SLAP) repair and subacromial decompression

AHA Coding Clinic for table ØMQ
2014, 3Q, 9 Interspinous ligamentoplasty

AHA Coding Clinic for table ØMT
2017, 2Q, 21 Arthroscopic anterior cruciate ligament revision using autograft with anterolateral ligament reconstruction

AHA Coding Clinic for table ØMU
2017, 2Q, 21 Arthroscopic anterior cruciate ligament revision using autograft with anterolateral ligament reconstruction

Shoulder Ligaments

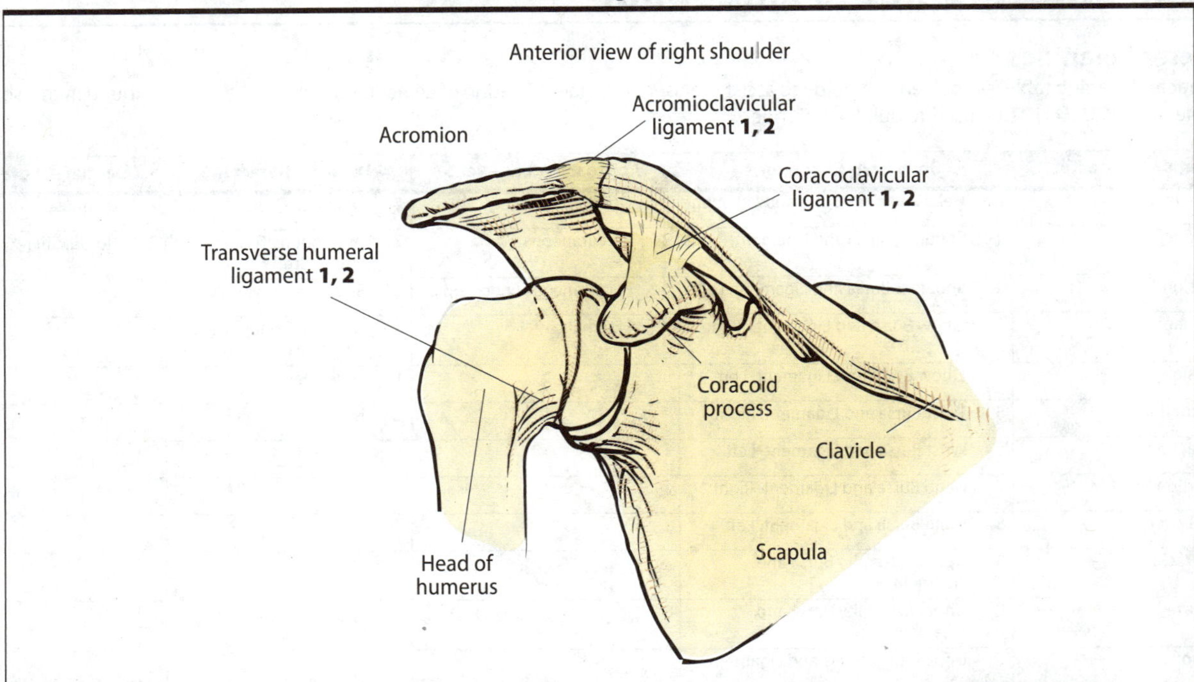

Knee Bursae

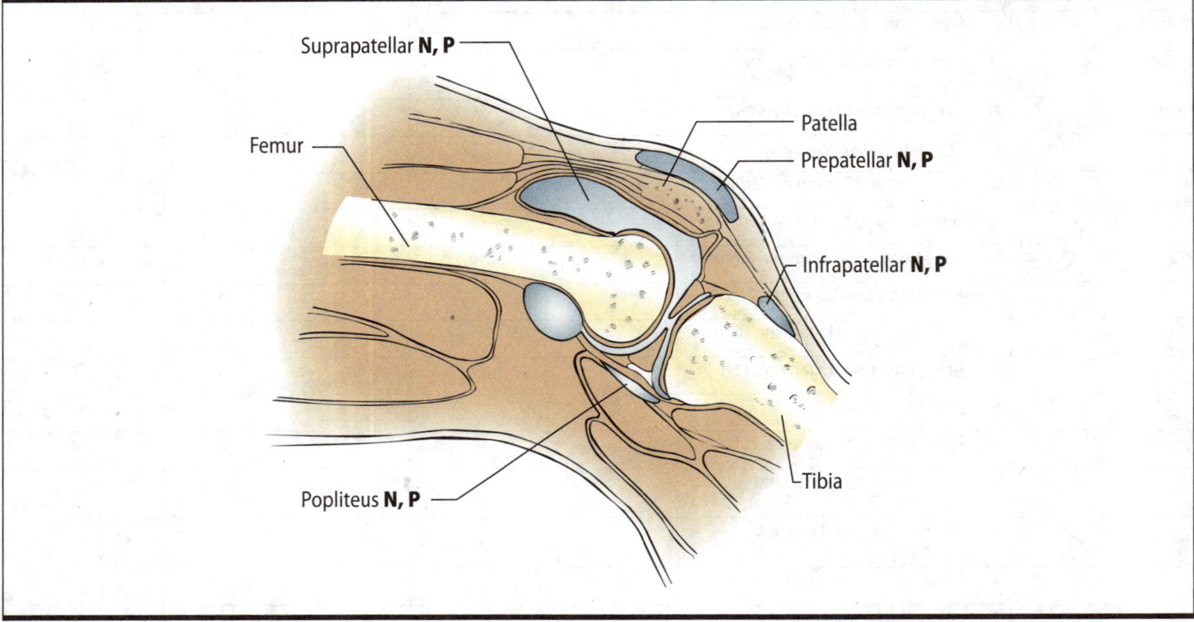

Knee Ligaments

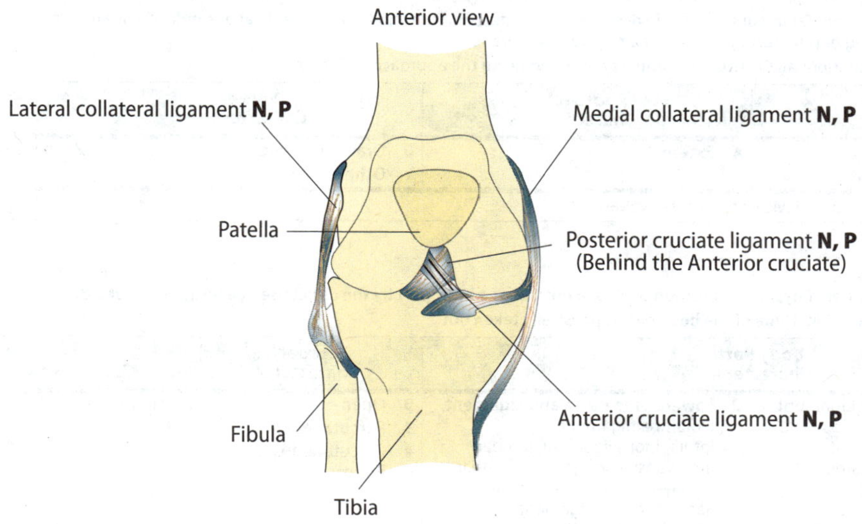

Anterior view
Lateral collateral ligament **N, P**
Medial collateral ligament **N, P**
Patella
Posterior cruciate ligament **N, P**
(Behind the Anterior cruciate)
Fibula
Anterior cruciate ligament **N, P**
Tibia

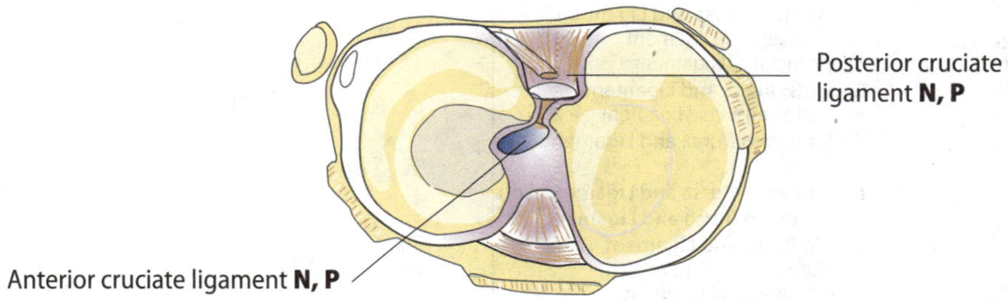

Posterior cruciate ligament **N, P**
Anterior cruciate ligament **N, P**

Wrist Ligaments

Palmar view
5
4
3
2
1
Flexor carpi ulnaris **5, 6**
Radial collateral carpal **5, 6**
Ulnar collateral carpal **5, 6**
Palmar radiocarpal **5, 6**

Dorsal view
1
2
3
4
5
Radial collateral carpal **5, 6**
Ulnar collateral carpal **5, 6**
Dorsal radiocarpal **5, 6**
Ulnocarpal **5, 6**

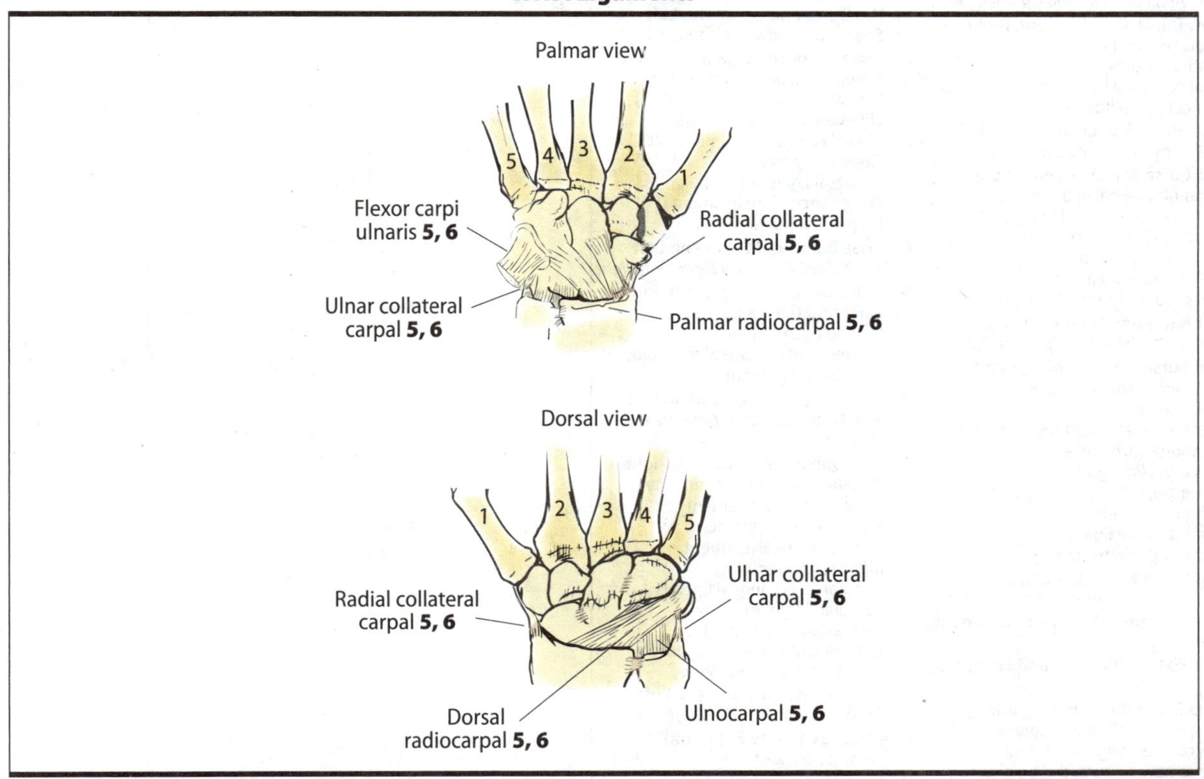

Ø Medical and Surgical
M Bursae and Ligaments
2 Change

Definition: Taking out or off a device from a body part and putting back an identical or similar device in or on the same body part without cutting or puncturing the skin or a mucous membrane

Explanation: All CHANGE procedures are coded using the approach EXTERNAL

Body Part Character 4	Approach Character 5	Device Character 6	Qualifier Character 7
X Upper Bursa and Ligament Y Lower Bursa and Ligament	X External	Ø Drainage Device Y Other Device	Z No Qualifier

Non-OR All body part, approach, device, and qualifier values

Ø Medical and Surgical
M Bursae and Ligaments
5 Destruction

Definition: Physical eradication of all or a portion of a body part by the direct use of energy, force, or a destructive agent

Explanation: None of the body part is physically taken out

Body Part Character 4	Approach Character 5	Device Character 6	Qualifier Character 7
Ø Head and Neck Bursa and Ligament Alar ligament of axis Cervical interspinous ligament Cervical intertransverse ligament Cervical ligamentum flavum Interspinous ligament, cervical Intertransverse ligament, cervical Lateral temporomandibular ligament Ligamentum flavum, cervical Sphenomandibular ligament Stylomandibular ligament Transverse ligament of atlas **1 Shoulder Bursa and Ligament, Right** Acromioclavicular ligament Coracoacromial ligament Coracoclavicular ligament Coracohumeral ligament Costoclavicular ligament Glenohumeral ligament Interclavicular ligament Sternoclavicular ligament Subacromial bursa Transverse humeral ligament Transverse scapular ligament **2 Shoulder Bursa and Ligament, Left** *See 1 Shoulder Bursa and Ligament, Right* **3 Elbow Bursa and Ligament, Right** Annular ligament Olecranon bursa Radial collateral ligament Ulnar collateral ligament **4 Elbow Bursa and Ligament, Left** *See 3 Elbow Bursa and Ligament, Right* **5 Wrist Bursa and Ligament, Right** Palmar ulnocarpal ligament Radial collateral carpal ligament Radiocarpal ligament Radioulnar ligament Scapholunate ligament Ulnar collateral carpal ligament **6 Wrist Bursa and Ligament, Left** *See 5 Wrist Bursa and Ligament, Right* **7 Hand Bursa and Ligament, Right** Carpometacarpal ligament Intercarpal ligament Interphalangeal ligament Lunotriquetral ligament Metacarpal ligament Metacarpophalangeal ligament Pisohamate ligament Pisometacarpal ligament Scaphotrapezium ligament **8 Hand Bursa and Ligament, Left** *See 7 Hand Bursa and Ligament, Right* **9 Upper Extremity Bursa and Ligament, Right** **B Upper Extremity Bursa and Ligament, Left** **C Upper Spine Bursa and Ligament** Interspinous ligament, thoracic Intertransverse ligament, thoracic Ligamentum flavum, thoracic Supraspinous ligament **D Lower Spine Bursa and Ligament** Iliolumbar ligament Interspinous ligament, lumbar Intertransverse ligament, lumbar Ligamentum flavum, lumbar Sacrococcygeal ligament Sacroiliac ligament Sacrospinous ligament Sacrotuberous ligament Supraspinous ligament **F Sternum Bursa and Ligament** Costoxiphoid ligament Sternocostal ligament **G Rib(s) Bursa and Ligament** Costotransverse ligament **H Abdomen Bursa and Ligament, Right** **J Abdomen Bursa and Ligament, Left** **K Perineum Bursa and Ligament** **L Hip Bursa and Ligament, Right** Iliofemoral ligament Ischiofemoral ligament Pubofemoral ligament Transverse acetabular ligament Trochanteric bursa **M Hip Bursa and Ligament, Left** *See L Hip Bursa and Ligament, Right* **N Knee Bursa and Ligament, Right** Anterior cruciate ligament (ACL) Lateral collateral ligament (LCL) Ligament of head of fibula Medial collateral ligament (MCL) Patellar ligament Popliteal ligament Posterior cruciate ligament (PCL) Prepatellar bursa **P Knee Bursa and Ligament, Left** *See N Knee Bursa and Ligament, Right* **Q Ankle Bursa and Ligament, Right** Calcaneofibular ligament Deltoid ligament Ligament of the lateral malleolus Talofibular ligament **R Ankle Bursa and Ligament, Left** *See Q Ankle Bursa and Ligament, Right* **S Foot Bursa and Ligament, Right** Calcaneocuboid ligament Cuneonavicular ligament Intercuneiform ligament Interphalangeal ligament Metatarsal ligament Metatarsophalangeal ligament Subtalar ligament Talocalcaneal ligament Talocalcaneonavicular ligament Tarsometatarsal ligament **T Foot Bursa and Ligament, Left** *See S Foot Bursa and Ligament, Right* **V Lower Extremity Bursa and Ligament, Right** **W Lower Extremity Bursa and Ligament, Left**	Ø Open 3 Percutaneous 4 Percutaneous Endoscopic	Z No Device	Z No Qualifier

Non-OR Procedure DRG Non-OR Procedure Valid OR Procedure HAC Associated Procedure Combination Only New/Revised April New/Revised October

Ø Medical and Surgical
M Bursae and Ligaments
8 Division

Definition: Cutting into a body part, without draining fluids and/or gases from the body part, in order to separate or transect a body part
Explanation: All or a portion of the body part is separated into two or more portions

Body Part Character 4	Approach Character 5	Device Character 6	Qualifier Character 7
Ø Head and Neck Bursa and Ligament Alar ligament of axis Cervical interspinous ligament Cervical intertransverse ligament Cervical ligamentum flavum Interspinous ligament, cervical Intertransverse ligament, cervical Lateral temporomandibular ligament Ligamentum flavum, cervical Sphenomandibular ligament Stylomandibular ligament Transverse ligament of atlas **1 Shoulder Bursa and Ligament, Right** Acromioclavicular ligament Coracoacromial ligament Coracoclavicular ligament Coracohumeral ligament Costoclavicular ligament Glenohumeral ligament Interclavicular ligament Sternoclavicular ligament Subacromial bursa Transverse humeral ligament Transverse scapular ligament **2 Shoulder Bursa and Ligament, Left** ***See*** *1 Shoulder Bursa and Ligament, Right* **3 Elbow Bursa and Ligament, Right** Annular ligament Olecranon bursa Radial collateral ligament Ulnar collateral ligament **4 Elbow Bursa and Ligament, Left** ***See*** *3 Elbow Bursa and Ligament, Right* **5 Wrist Bursa and Ligament, Right** Palmar ulnocarpal ligament Radial collateral carpal ligament Radiocarpal ligament Radioulnar ligament Scapholunate ligament Ulnar collateral carpal ligament **6 Wrist Bursa and Ligament, Left** ***See*** *5 Wrist Bursa and Ligament, Right* **7 Hand Bursa and Ligament, Right** Carpometacarpal ligament Intercarpal ligament Interphalangeal ligament Lunotriquetral ligament Metacarpal ligament Metacarpophalangeal ligament Pisohamate ligament Pisometacarpal ligament Scaphotrapezium ligament **8 Hand Bursa and Ligament, Left** ***See*** *7 Hand Bursa and Ligament, Right* **9 Upper Extremity Bursa and Ligament, Right** **B Upper Extremity Bursa and Ligament, Left** **C Upper Spine Bursa and Ligament** Interspinous ligament, thoracic Intertransverse ligament, thoracic Ligamentum flavum, thoracic Supraspinous ligament **D Lower Spine Bursa and Ligament** Iliolumbar ligament Interspinous ligament, lumbar Intertransverse ligament, lumbar Ligamentum flavum, lumbar Sacrococcygeal ligament Sacroiliac ligament Sacrospinous ligament Sacrotuberous ligament Supraspinous ligament **F Sternum Bursa and Ligament** Costoxiphoid ligament Sternocostal ligament **G Rib(s) Bursa and Ligament** Costotransverse ligament **H Abdomen Bursa and Ligament, Right** **J Abdomen Bursa and Ligament, Left** **K Perineum Bursa and Ligament** **L Hip Bursa and Ligament, Right** Iliofemoral ligament Ischiofemoral ligament Pubofemoral ligament Transverse acetabular ligament Trochanteric bursa **M Hip Bursa and Ligament, Left** ***See*** *L Hip Bursa and Ligament, Right* **N Knee Bursa and Ligament, Right** Anterior cruciate ligament (ACL) Lateral collateral ligament (LCL) Ligament of head of fibula Medial collateral ligament (MCL) Patellar ligament Popliteal ligament Posterior cruciate ligament (PCL) Prepatellar bursa **P Knee Bursa and Ligament, Left** ***See*** *N Knee Bursa and Ligament, Right* **Q Ankle Bursa and Ligament, Right** Calcaneofibular ligament Deltoid ligament Ligament of the lateral malleolus Talofibular ligament **R Ankle Bursa and Ligament, Left** ***See*** *Q Ankle Bursa and Ligament, Right* **S Foot Bursa and Ligament, Right** Calcaneocuboid ligament Cuneonavicular ligament Intercuneiform ligament Interphalangeal ligament Metatarsal ligament Metatarsophalangeal ligament Subtalar ligament Talocalcaneal ligament Talocalcaneonavicular ligament Tarsometatarsal ligament **T Foot Bursa and Ligament, Left** ***See*** *S Foot Bursa and Ligament, Right* **V Lower Extremity Bursa and Ligament, Right** **W Lower Extremity Bursa and Ligament, Left**	**Ø** Open **3** Percutaneous **4** Percutaneous Endoscopic	**Z** No Device	**Z** No Qualifier

Ø Medical and Surgical
M Bursae and Ligaments
9 Drainage Definition: Taking or letting out fluids and/or gases from a body part
Explanation: The qualifier DIAGNOSTIC is used to identify drainage procedures that are biopsies

Body Part Character 4		Approach Character 5	Device Character 6	Qualifier Character 7
Ø Head and Neck Bursa and Ligament Alar ligament of axis Cervical interspinous ligament Cervical intertransverse ligament Cervical ligamentum flavum Interspinous ligament, cervical Intertransverse ligament, cervical Lateral temporomandibular ligament Ligamentum flavum, cervical Sphenomandibular ligament Stylomandibular ligament Transverse ligament of atlas **1 Shoulder Bursa and Ligament, Right** Acromioclavicular ligament Coracoacromial ligament Coracoclavicular ligament Coracohumeral ligament Costoclavicular ligament Glenohumeral ligament Interclavicular ligament Sternoclavicular ligament Subacromial bursa Transverse humeral ligament Transverse scapular ligament **2 Shoulder Bursa and Ligament, Left** ***See*** *1 Shoulder Bursa and Ligament, Right* **3 Elbow Bursa and Ligament, Right** Annular ligament Olecranon bursa Radial collateral ligament Ulnar collateral ligament **4 Elbow Bursa and Ligament, Left** ***See*** *3 Elbow Bursa and Ligament, Right* **5 Wrist Bursa and Ligament, Right** Palmar ulnocarpal ligament Radial collateral carpal ligament Radiocarpal ligament Radioulnar ligament Scapholunate ligament Ulnar collateral carpal ligament **6 Wrist Bursa and Ligament, Left** ***See*** *5 Wrist Bursa and Ligament, Right* **7 Hand Bursa and Ligament, Right** Carpometacarpal ligament Intercarpal ligament Interphalangeal ligament Lunotriquetral ligament Metacarpal ligament Metacarpophalangeal ligament Pisohamate ligament Pisometacarpal ligament Scaphotrapezium ligament **8 Hand Bursa and Ligament, Left** ***See*** *7 Hand Bursa and Ligament, Right* **9 Upper Extremity Bursa and Ligament, Right** **B Upper Extremity Bursa and Ligament, Left** **C Upper Spine Bursa and Ligament** Interspinous ligament, thoracic Intertransverse ligament, thoracic Ligamentum flavum, thoracic Supraspinous ligament	**D Lower Spine Bursa and Ligament** Iliolumbar ligament Interspinous ligament, lumbar Intertransverse ligament, lumbar Ligamentum flavum, lumbar Sacrococcygeal ligament Sacroiliac ligament Sacrospinous ligament Sacrotuberous ligament Supraspinous ligament **F Sternum Bursa and Ligament** Costoxiphoid ligament Sternocostal ligament **G Rib(s) Bursa and Ligament** Costotransverse ligament **H Abdomen Bursa and Ligament, Right** **J Abdomen Bursa and Ligament, Left** **K Perineum Bursa and Ligament** **L Hip Bursa and Ligament, Right** Iliofemoral ligament Ischiofemoral ligament Pubofemoral ligament Transverse acetabular ligament Trochanteric bursa **M Hip Bursa and Ligament, Left** ***See*** *L Hip Bursa and Ligament, Right* **N Knee Bursa and Ligament, Right** Anterior cruciate ligament (ACL) Lateral collateral ligament (LCL) Ligament of head of fibula Medial collateral ligament (MCL) Patellar ligament Popliteal ligament Posterior cruciate ligament (PCL) Prepatellar bursa **P Knee Bursa and Ligament, Left** ***See*** *N Knee Bursa and Ligament, Right* **Q Ankle Bursa and Ligament, Right** Calcaneofibular ligament Deltoid ligament Ligament of the lateral malleolus Talofibular ligament **R Ankle Bursa and Ligament, Left** ***See*** *Q Ankle Bursa and Ligament, Right* **S Foot Bursa and Ligament, Right** Calcaneocuboid ligament Cuneonavicular ligament Intercuneiform ligament Interphalangeal ligament Metatarsal ligament Metatarsophalangeal ligament Subtalar ligament Talocalcaneal ligament Talocalcaneonavicular ligament Tarsometatarsal ligament **T Foot Bursa and Ligament, Left** ***See*** *S Foot Bursa and Ligament, Right* **V Lower Extremity Bursa and Ligament, Right** **W Lower Extremity Bursa and Ligament, Left**	**Ø Open** **3 Percutaneous** **4 Percutaneous Endoscopic**	**Ø Drainage Device**	**Z No Qualifier**

Non-OR ØM9[Ø,1,2,3,4,5,6,7,8,9,B,C,D,F,G,H,J,K,L,M,N,P,Q,R,S,T,V,W]3ØZ
Non-OR ØM9[1,2,3,4,7,8,9,B,C,D,F,G,H,J,K,L,M,V,W]4ØZ

ØM9 Continued on next page

Ø Medical and Surgical
M Bursae and Ligaments
9 Drainage Definition: Taking or letting out fluids and/or gases from a body part
Explanation: The qualifier DIAGNOSTIC is used to identify drainage procedures that are biopsies

ØM9 Continued

Body Part Character 4	Approach Character 5	Device Character 6	Qualifier Character 7
Ø Head and Neck Bursa and Ligament Alar ligament of axis Cervical interspinous ligament Cervical intertransverse ligament Cervical ligamentum flavum Interspinous ligament, cervical Intertransverse ligament, cervical Lateral temporomandibular ligament Ligamentum flavum, cervical Sphenomandibular ligament Stylomandibular ligament Transverse ligament of atlas **1 Shoulder Bursa and Ligament, Right** Acromioclavicular ligament Coracoacromial ligament Coracoclavicular ligament Coracohumeral ligament Costoclavicular ligament Glenohumeral ligament Interclavicular ligament Sternoclavicular ligament Subacromial bursa Transverse humeral ligament Transverse scapular ligament **2 Shoulder Bursa and Ligament, Left** **See** *1 Shoulder Bursa and Ligament, Right* **3 Elbow Bursa and Ligament, Right** Annular ligament Olecranon bursa Radial collateral ligament Ulnar collateral ligament **4 Elbow Bursa and Ligament, Left** **See** *3 Elbow Bursa and Ligament, Right* **5 Wrist Bursa and Ligament, Right** Palmar ulnocarpal ligament Radial collateral carpal ligament Radiocarpal ligament Radioulnar ligament Scapholunate ligament Ulnar collateral carpal ligament **6 Wrist Bursa and Ligament, Left** **See** *5 Wrist Bursa and Ligament, Right* **7 Hand Bursa and Ligament, Right** Carpometacarpal ligament Intercarpal ligament Interphalangeal ligament Lunotriquetral ligament Metacarpal ligament Metacarpophalangeal ligament Pisohamate ligament Pisometacarpal ligament Scaphotrapezium ligament **8 Hand Bursa and Ligament, Left** **See** *7 Hand Bursa and Ligament, Right* **9 Upper Extremity Bursa and Ligament, Right** **B Upper Extremity Bursa and Ligament, Left** **C Upper Spine Bursa and Ligament** Interspinous ligament, thoracic Intertransverse ligament, thoracic Ligamentum flavum, thoracic Supraspinous ligament **D Lower Spine Bursa and Ligament** Iliolumbar ligament Interspinous ligament, lumbar Intertransverse ligament, lumbar Ligamentum flavum, lumbar Sacrococcygeal ligament Sacroiliac ligament Sacrospinous ligament Sacrotuberous ligament Supraspinous ligament **F Sternum Bursa and Ligament** Costoxiphoid ligament Sternocostal ligament **G Rib(s) Bursa and Ligament** Costotransverse ligament **H Abdomen Bursa and Ligament, Right** **J Abdomen Bursa and Ligament, Left** **K Perineum Bursa and Ligament** **L Hip Bursa and Ligament, Right** Iliofemoral ligament Ischiofemoral ligament Pubofemoral ligament Transverse acetabular ligament Trochanteric bursa **M Hip Bursa and Ligament, Left** **See** *L Hip Bursa and Ligament, Right* **N Knee Bursa and Ligament, Right** Anterior cruciate ligament (ACL) Lateral collateral ligament (LCL) Ligament of head of fibula Medial collateral ligament (MCL) Patellar ligament Popliteal ligament Posterior cruciate ligament (PCL) Prepatellar bursa **P Knee Bursa and Ligament, Left** **See** *N Knee Bursa and Ligament, Right* **Q Ankle Bursa and Ligament, Right** Calcaneofibular ligament Deltoid ligament Ligament of the lateral malleolus Talofibular ligament **R Ankle Bursa and Ligament, Left** **See** *Q Ankle Bursa and Ligament, Right* **S Foot Bursa and Ligament, Right** Calcaneocuboid ligament Cuneonavicular ligament Intercuneiform ligament Interphalangeal ligament Metatarsal ligament Metatarsophalangeal ligament Subtalar ligament Talocalcaneal ligament Talocalcaneonavicular ligament Tarsometatarsal ligament **T Foot Bursa and Ligament, Left** **See** *S Foot Bursa and Ligament, Right* **V Lower Extremity Bursa and Ligament, Right** **W Lower Extremity Bursa and Ligament, Left**	**Ø Open** **3 Percutaneous** **4 Percutaneous Endoscopic**	**Z No Device**	**X Diagnostic** **Z No Qualifier**

Non-OR ØM9[Ø,1,2,3,4,5,6,7,8,C,D,F,G,L,M,N,P,Q,R,S,T][Ø,3,4]ZX
Non-OR ØM9[Ø,1,2,3,4,5,6,7,8,9,B,C,D,F,G,H,J,K,L,M,N,P,Q,R,S,T,V,W]3ZZ
Non-OR ØM9[Ø,5,6,7,8,9,B,C,D,F,G,H,J,K,N,P,Q,R,S,T,V,W]4ZZ

Ø Medical and Surgical
M Bursae and Ligaments
B Excision Definition: Cutting out or off, without replacement, a portion of a body part
Explanation: The qualifier DIAGNOSTIC is used to identify excision procedures that are biopsies

Body Part Character 4		Approach Character 5	Device Character 6	Qualifier Character 7
Ø Head and Neck Bursa and Ligament Alar ligament of axis Cervical interspinous ligament Cervical intertransverse ligament Cervical ligamentum flavum Interspinous ligament, cervical Intertransverse ligament, cervical Lateral temporomandibular ligament Ligamentum flavum, cervical Sphenomandibular ligament Stylomandibular ligament Transverse ligament of atlas **1 Shoulder Bursa and Ligament, Right** Acromioclavicular ligament Coracoacromial ligament Coracoclavicular ligament Coracohumeral ligament Costoclavicular ligament Glenohumeral ligament Interclavicular ligament Sternoclavicular ligament Subacromial bursa Transverse humeral ligament Transverse scapular ligament **2 Shoulder Bursa and Ligament, Left** **See** *1 Shoulder Bursa and Ligament, Right* **3 Elbow Bursa and Ligament, Right** Annular ligament Olecranon bursa Radial collateral ligament Ulnar collateral ligament **4 Elbow Bursa and Ligament, Left** **See** *3 Elbow Bursa and Ligament, Right* **5 Wrist Bursa and Ligament, Right** Palmar ulnocarpal ligament Radial collateral carpal ligament Radiocarpal ligament Radioulnar ligament Scapholunate ligament Ulnar collateral carpal ligament **6 Wrist Bursa and Ligament, Left** **See** *5 Wrist Bursa and Ligament, Right* **7 Hand Bursa and Ligament, Right** Carpometacarpal ligament Intercarpal ligament Interphalangeal ligament Lunotriquetral ligament Metacarpal ligament Metacarpophalangeal ligament Pisohamate ligament Pisometacarpal ligament Scaphotrapezium ligament **8 Hand Bursa and Ligament, Left** **See** *7 Hand Bursa and Ligament, Right* **9 Upper Extremity Bursa and Ligament, Right** **B Upper Extremity Bursa and Ligament, Left** **C Upper Spine Bursa and Ligament** Interspinous ligament, thoracic Intertransverse ligament, thoracic Ligamentum flavum, thoracic Supraspinous ligament	**D Lower Spine Bursa and Ligament** Iliolumbar ligament Interspinous ligament, lumbar Intertransverse ligament, lumbar Ligamentum flavum, lumbar Sacrococcygeal ligament Sacroiliac ligament Sacrospinous ligament Sacrotuberous ligament Supraspinous ligament **F Sternum Bursa and Ligament** Costoxiphoid ligament Sternocostal ligament **G Rib(s) Bursa and Ligament** Costotransverse ligament **H Abdomen Bursa and Ligament, Right** **J Abdomen Bursa and Ligament, Left** **K Perineum Bursa and Ligament** **L Hip Bursa and Ligament, Right** Iliofemoral ligament Ischiofemoral ligament Pubofemoral ligament Transverse acetabular ligament Trochanteric bursa **M Hip Bursa and Ligament, Left** **See** *L Hip Bursa and Ligament, Right* **N Knee Bursa and Ligament, Right** Anterior cruciate ligament (ACL) Lateral collateral ligament (LCL) Ligament of head of fibula Medial collateral ligament (MCL) Patellar ligament Popliteal ligament Posterior cruciate ligament (PCL) Prepatellar bursa **P Knee Bursa and Ligament, Left** **See** *N Knee Bursa and Ligament, Right* **Q Ankle Bursa and Ligament, Right** Calcaneofibular ligament Deltoid ligament Ligament of the lateral malleolus Talofibular ligament **R Ankle Bursa and Ligament, Left** **See** *Q Ankle Bursa and Ligament, Right* **S Foot Bursa and Ligament, Right** Calcaneocuboid ligament Cuneonavicular ligament Intercuneiform ligament Interphalangeal ligament Metatarsal ligament Metatarsophalangeal ligament Subtalar ligament Talocalcaneal ligament Talocalcaneonavicular ligament Tarsometatarsal ligament **T Foot Bursa and Ligament, Left** **See** *S Foot Bursa and Ligament, Right* **V Lower Extremity Bursa and Ligament, Right** **W Lower Extremity Bursa and Ligament, Left**	**Ø Open** **3 Percutaneous** **4 Percutaneous Endoscopic**	**Z No Device**	**X Diagnostic** **Z No Qualifier**

Non-OR ØMB[Ø,1,2,3,4,5,6,7,8,B,C,D,F,G,L,M,N,P,Q,R,S,T][Ø,3,4]ZX
Non-OR ØMB94ZX

Ø Medical and Surgical
M Bursae and Ligaments
C Extirpation Definition: Taking or cutting out solid matter from a body part

Explanation: The solid matter may be an abnormal byproduct of a biological function or a foreign body; it may be imbedded in a body part or in the lumen of a tubular body part. The solid matter may or may not have been previously broken into pieces.

Body Part Character 4	Approach Character 5	Device Character 6	Qualifier Character 7
Ø Head and Neck Bursa and Ligament Alar ligament of axis Cervical interspinous ligament Cervical intertransverse ligament Cervical ligamentum flavum Interspinous ligament, cervical Intertransverse ligament, cervical Lateral temporomandibular ligament Ligamentum flavum, cervical Sphenomandibular ligament Stylomandibular ligament Transverse ligament of atlas **1 Shoulder Bursa and Ligament, Right** Acromioclavicular ligament Coracoacromial ligament Coracoclavicular ligament Coracohumeral ligament Costoclavicular ligament Glenohumeral ligament Interclavicular ligament Sternoclavicular ligament Subacromial bursa Transverse humeral ligament Transverse scapular ligament **2 Shoulder Bursa and Ligament, Left** *See 1 Shoulder Bursa and Ligament, Right* **3 Elbow Bursa and Ligament, Right** Annular ligament Olecranon bursa Radial collateral ligament Ulnar collateral ligament **4 Elbow Bursa and Ligament, Left** *See 3 Elbow Bursa and Ligament, Right* **5 Wrist Bursa and Ligament, Right** Palmar ulnocarpal ligament Radial collateral carpal ligament Radiocarpal ligament Radioulnar ligament Scapholunate ligament Ulnar collateral carpal ligament **6 Wrist Bursa and Ligament, Left** *See 5 Wrist Bursa and Ligament, Right* **7 Hand Bursa and Ligament, Right** Carpometacarpal ligament Intercarpal ligament Interphalangeal ligament Lunotriquetral ligament Metacarpal ligament Metacarpophalangeal ligament Pisohamate ligament Pisometacarpal ligament Scaphotrapezium ligament **8 Hand Bursa and Ligament, Left** *See 7 Hand Bursa and Ligament, Right* **9 Upper Extremity Bursa and Ligament, Right** **B Upper Extremity Bursa and Ligament, Left** **C Upper Spine Bursa and Ligament** Interspinous ligament, thoracic Intertransverse ligament, thoracic Ligamentum flavum, thoracic Supraspinous ligament **D Lower Spine Bursa and Ligament** Iliolumbar ligament Interspinous ligament, lumbar Intertransverse ligament, lumbar Ligamentum flavum, lumbar Sacrococcygeal ligament Sacroiliac ligament Sacrospinous ligament Sacrotuberous ligament Supraspinous ligament **F Sternum Bursa and Ligament** Costoxiphoid ligament Sternocostal ligament **G Rib(s) Bursa and Ligament** Costotransverse ligament **H Abdomen Bursa and Ligament, Right** **J Abdomen Bursa and Ligament, Left** **K Perineum Bursa and Ligament** **L Hip Bursa and Ligament, Right** Iliofemoral ligament Ischiofemoral ligament Pubofemoral ligament Transverse acetabular ligament Trochanteric bursa **M Hip Bursa and Ligament, Left** *See L Hip Bursa and Ligament, Right* **N Knee Bursa and Ligament, Right** Anterior cruciate ligament (ACL) Lateral collateral ligament (LCL) Ligament of head of fibula Medial collateral ligament (MCL) Patellar ligament Popliteal ligament Posterior cruciate ligament (PCL) Prepatellar bursa **P Knee Bursa and Ligament, Left** *See N Knee Bursa and Ligament, Right* **Q Ankle Bursa and Ligament, Right** Calcaneofibular ligament Deltoid ligament Ligament of the lateral malleolus Talofibular ligament **R Ankle Bursa and Ligament, Left** *See Q Ankle Bursa and Ligament, Right* **S Foot Bursa and Ligament, Right** Calcaneocuboid ligament Cuneonavicular ligament Intercuneiform ligament Interphalangeal ligament Metatarsal ligament Metatarsophalangeal ligament Subtalar ligament Talocalcaneal ligament Talocalcaneonavicular ligament Tarsometatarsal ligament **T Foot Bursa and Ligament, Left** *See S Foot Bursa and Ligament, Right* **V Lower Extremity Bursa and Ligament, Right** **W Lower Extremity Bursa and Ligament, Left**	**Ø Open** **3 Percutaneous** **4 Percutaneous Endoscopic**	**Z No Device**	**Z No Qualifier**

Ø Medical and Surgical
M Bursae and Ligaments
D Extraction Definition: Pulling or stripping out or off all or a portion of a body part by the use of force
Explanation: The qualifier DIAGNOSTIC is used to identify extraction procedures that are biopsies

Body Part Character 4	Body Part Character 4	Approach Character 5	Device Character 6	Qualifier Character 7
Ø Head and Neck Bursa and Ligament Alar ligament of axis Cervical interspinous ligament Cervical intertransverse ligament Cervical ligamentum flavum Interspinous ligament, cervical Intertransverse ligament, cervical Lateral temporomandibular ligament Ligamentum flavum, cervical Sphenomandibular ligament Stylomandibular ligament Transverse ligament of atlas **1 Shoulder Bursa and Ligament, Right** Acromioclavicular ligament Coracoacromial ligament Coracoclavicular ligament Coracohumeral ligament Costoclavicular ligament Glenohumeral ligament Interclavicular ligament Sternoclavicular ligament Subacromial bursa Transverse humeral ligament Transverse scapular ligament **2 Shoulder Bursa and Ligament, Left** ***See*** *1 Shoulder Bursa and Ligament, Right* **3 Elbow Bursa and Ligament, Right** Annular ligament Olecranon bursa Radial collateral ligament Ulnar collateral ligament **4 Elbow Bursa and Ligament, Left** ***See*** *3 Elbow Bursa and Ligament, Right* **5 Wrist Bursa and Ligament, Right** Palmar ulnocarpal ligament Radial collateral carpal ligament Radiocarpal ligament Radioulnar ligament Scapholunate ligament Ulnar collateral carpal ligament **6 Wrist Bursa and Ligament, Left** ***See*** *5 Wrist Bursa and Ligament, Right* **7 Hand Bursa and Ligament, Right** Carpometacarpal ligament Intercarpal ligament Interphalangeal ligament Lunotriquetral ligament Metacarpal ligament Metacarpophalangeal ligament Pisohamate ligament Pisometacarpal ligament Scaphotrapezium ligament **8 Hand Bursa and Ligament, Left** ***See*** *7 Hand Bursa and Ligament, Right* **9 Upper Extremity Bursa and Ligament, Right** **B Upper Extremity Bursa and Ligament, Left** **C Upper Spine Bursa and Ligament** Interspinous ligament, thoracic Intertransverse ligament, thoracic Ligamentum flavum, thoracic Supraspinous ligament	**D Lower Spine Bursa and Ligament** Iliolumbar ligament Interspinous ligament, lumbar Intertransverse ligament, lumbar Ligamentum flavum, lumbar Sacrococcygeal ligament Sacroiliac ligament Sacrospinous ligament Sacrotuberous ligament Supraspinous ligament **F Sternum Bursa and Ligament** Costoxiphoid ligament Sternocostal ligament **G Rib(s) Bursa and Ligament** Costotransverse ligament **H Abdomen Bursa and Ligament, Right** **J Abdomen Bursa and Ligament, Left** **K Perineum Bursa and Ligament** **L Hip Bursa and Ligament, Right** Iliofemoral ligament Ischiofemoral ligament Pubofemoral ligament Transverse acetabular ligament Trochanteric bursa **M Hip Bursa and Ligament, Left** ***See*** *L Hip Bursa and Ligament, Right* **N Knee Bursa and Ligament, Right** Anterior cruciate ligament (ACL) Lateral collateral ligament (LCL) Ligament of head of fibula Medial collateral ligament (MCL) Patellar ligament Popliteal ligament Posterior cruciate ligament (PCL) Prepatellar bursa **P Knee Bursa and Ligament, Left** ***See*** *N Knee Bursa and Ligament, Right* **Q Ankle Bursa and Ligament, Right** Calcaneofibular ligament Deltoid ligament Ligament of the lateral malleolus Talofibular ligament **R Ankle Bursa and Ligament, Left** ***See*** *Q Ankle Bursa and Ligament, Right* **S Foot Bursa and Ligament, Right** Calcaneocuboid ligament Cuneonavicular ligament Intercuneiform ligament Interphalangeal ligament Metatarsal ligament Metatarsophalangeal ligament Subtalar ligament Talocalcaneal ligament Talocalcaneonavicular ligament Tarsometatarsal ligament **T Foot Bursa and Ligament, Left** ***See*** *S Foot Bursa and Ligament, Right* **V Lower Extremity Bursa and Ligament, Right** **W Lower Extremity Bursa and Ligament, Left**	**Ø Open** **3 Percutaneous** **4 Percutaneous Endoscopic**	**Z No Device**	**Z No Qualifier**

Ø Medical and Surgical
M Bursae and Ligaments
H Insertion Definition: Putting in a nonbiological appliance that monitors, assists, performs, or prevents a physiological function but does not physically take the place of a body part

Explanation: None

Body Part Character 4	Approach Character 5	Device Character 6	Qualifier Character 7
X Upper Bursa and Ligament Y Lower Bursa and Ligament	Ø Open 3 Percutaneous 4 Percutaneous Endoscopic	Y Other Device	Z No Qualifier

Non-OR ØMH[X,Y][3,4]YZ

Ø Medical and Surgical
M Bursae and Ligaments
J Inspection Definition: Visually and/or manually exploring a body part

Explanation: Visual exploration may be performed with or without optical instrumentation. Manual exploration may be performed directly or through intervening body layers.

Body Part Character 4	Approach Character 5	Device Character 6	Qualifier Character 7
X Upper Bursa and Ligament Y Lower Bursa and Ligament	Ø Open 3 Percutaneous 4 Percutaneous Endoscopic X External	Z No Device	Z No Qualifier

Non-OR ØMJ[X,Y][3,X]ZZ

Ø Medical and Surgical
M Bursae and Ligaments
M Reattachment Definition: Putting back in or on all or a portion of a separated body part to its normal location or other suitable location
Explanation: Vascular circulation and nervous pathways may or may not be reestablished

Body Part Character 4	Approach Character 5	Device Character 6	Qualifier Character 7
Ø Head and Neck Bursa and Ligament Alar ligament of axis Cervical interspinous ligament Cervical intertransverse ligament Cervical ligamentum flavum Interspinous ligament, cervical Intertransverse ligament, cervical Lateral temporomandibular ligament Ligamentum flavum, cervical Sphenomandibular ligament Stylomandibular ligament Transverse ligament of atlas **1 Shoulder Bursa and Ligament, Right** Acromioclavicular ligament Coracoacromial ligament Coracoclavicular ligament Coracohumeral ligament Costoclavicular ligament Glenohumeral ligament Interclavicular ligament Sternoclavicular ligament Subacromial bursa Transverse humeral ligament Transverse scapular ligament **2 Shoulder Bursa and Ligament, Left** ***See*** *1 Shoulder Bursa and Ligament, Right* **3 Elbow Bursa and Ligament, Right** Annular ligament Olecranon bursa Radial collateral ligament Ulnar collateral ligament **4 Elbow Bursa and Ligament, Left** ***See*** *3 Elbow Bursa and Ligament, Right* **5 Wrist Bursa and Ligament, Right** Palmar ulnocarpal ligament Radial collateral carpal ligament Radiocarpal ligament Radioulnar ligament Scapholunate ligament Ulnar collateral carpal ligament **6 Wrist Bursa and Ligament, Left** ***See*** *5 Wrist Bursa and Ligament, Right* **7 Hand Bursa and Ligament, Right** Carpometacarpal ligament Intercarpal ligament Interphalangeal ligament Lunotriquetral ligament Metacarpal ligament Metacarpophalangeal ligament Pisohamate ligament Pisometacarpal ligament Scaphotrapezium ligament **8 Hand Bursa and Ligament, Left** ***See*** *7 Hand Bursa and Ligament, Right* **9 Upper Extremity Bursa and Ligament, Right** **B Upper Extremity Bursa and Ligament, Left** **C Upper Spine Bursa and Ligament** Interspinous ligament, thoracic Intertransverse ligament, thoracic Ligamentum flavum, thoracic Supraspinous ligament **D Lower Spine Bursa and Ligament** Iliolumbar ligament Interspinous ligament, lumbar Intertransverse ligament, lumbar Ligamentum flavum, lumbar Sacrococcygeal ligament Sacroiliac ligament Sacrospinous ligament Sacrotuberous ligament Supraspinous ligament **F Sternum Bursa and Ligament** Costoxiphoid ligament Sternocostal ligament **G Rib(s) Bursa and Ligament** Costotransverse ligament **H Abdomen Bursa and Ligament, Right** **J Abdomen Bursa and Ligament, Left** **K Perineum Bursa and Ligament** **L Hip Bursa and Ligament, Right** Iliofemoral ligament Ischiofemoral ligament Pubofemoral ligament Transverse acetabular ligament Trochanteric bursa **M Hip Bursa and Ligament, Left** ***See*** *L Hip Bursa and Ligament, Right* **N Knee Bursa and Ligament, Right** Anterior cruciate ligament (ACL) Lateral collateral ligament (LCL) Ligament of head of fibula Medial collateral ligament (MCL) Patellar ligament Popliteal ligament Posterior cruciate ligament (PCL) Prepatellar bursa **P Knee Bursa and Ligament, Left** ***See*** *N Knee Bursa and Ligament, Right* **Q Ankle Bursa and Ligament, Right** Calcaneofibular ligament Deltoid ligament Ligament of the lateral malleolus Talofibular ligament **R Ankle Bursa and Ligament, Left** ***See*** *Q Ankle Bursa and Ligament, Right* **S Foot Bursa and Ligament, Right** Calcaneocuboid ligament Cuneonavicular ligament Intercuneiform ligament Interphalangeal ligament Metatarsal ligament Metatarsophalangeal ligament Subtalar ligament Talocalcaneal ligament Talocalcaneonavicular ligament Tarsometatarsal ligament **T Foot Bursa and Ligament, Left** ***See*** *S Foot Bursa and Ligament, Right* **V Lower Extremity Bursa and Ligament, Right** **W Lower Extremity Bursa and Ligament, Left**	**Ø Open** **4 Percutaneous Endoscopic**	**Z No Device**	**Z No Qualifier**

Ø Medical and Surgical
M Bursae and Ligaments
N Release Definition: Freeing a body part from an abnormal physical constraint by cutting or by the use of force

Explanation: Some of the restraining tissue may be taken out but none of the body part is taken out

Body Part Character 4	Approach Character 5	Device Character 6	Qualifier Character 7
Ø Head and Neck Bursa and Ligament Alar ligament of axis Cervical interspinous ligament Cervical intertransverse ligament Cervical ligamentum flavum Interspinous ligament, cervical Intertransverse ligament, cervical Lateral temporomandibular ligament Ligamentum flavum, cervical Sphenomandibular ligament Stylomandibular ligament Transverse ligament of atlas **1 Shoulder Bursa and Ligament, Right** Acromioclavicular ligament Coracoacromial ligament Coracoclavicular ligament Coracohumeral ligament Costoclavicular ligament Glenohumeral ligament Interclavicular ligament Sternoclavicular ligament Subacromial bursa Transverse humeral ligament Transverse scapular ligament **2 Shoulder Bursa and Ligament, Left** **See** *1 Shoulder Bursa and Ligament, Right* **3 Elbow Bursa and Ligament, Right** Annular ligament Olecranon bursa Radial collateral ligament Ulnar collateral ligament **4 Elbow Bursa and Ligament, Left** **See** *3 Elbow Bursa and Ligament, Right* **5 Wrist Bursa and Ligament, Right** Palmar ulnocarpal ligament Radial collateral carpal ligament Radiocarpal ligament Radioulnar ligament Scapholunate ligament Ulnar collateral carpal ligament **6 Wrist Bursa and Ligament, Left** **See** *5 Wrist Bursa and Ligament, Right* **7 Hand Bursa and Ligament, Right** Carpometacarpal ligament Intercarpal ligament Interphalangeal ligament Lunotriquetral ligament Metacarpal ligament Metacarpophalangeal ligament Pisohamate ligament Pisometacarpal ligament Scaphotrapezium ligament **8 Hand Bursa and Ligament, Left** **See** *7 Hand Bursa and Ligament, Right* **9 Upper Extremity Bursa and Ligament, Right** **B Upper Extremity Bursa and Ligament, Left** **C Upper Spine Bursa and Ligament** Interspinous ligament, thoracic Intertransverse ligament, thoracic Ligamentum flavum, thoracic Supraspinous ligament **D Lower Spine Bursa and Ligament** Iliolumbar ligament Interspinous ligament, lumbar Intertransverse ligament, lumbar Ligamentum flavum, lumbar Sacrococcygeal ligament Sacroiliac ligament Sacrospinous ligament Sacrotuberous ligament Supraspinous ligament **F Sternum Bursa and Ligament** Costoxiphoid ligament Sternocostal ligament **G Rib(s) Bursa and Ligament** Costotransverse ligament **H Abdomen Bursa and Ligament, Right** **J Abdomen Bursa and Ligament, Left** **K Perineum Bursa and Ligament** **L Hip Bursa and Ligament, Right** Iliofemoral ligament Ischiofemoral ligament Pubofemoral ligament Transverse acetabular ligament Trochanteric bursa **M Hip Bursa and Ligament, Left** **See** *L Hip Bursa and Ligament, Right* **N Knee Bursa and Ligament, Right** Anterior cruciate ligament (ACL) Lateral collateral ligament (LCL) Ligament of head of fibula Medial collateral ligament (MCL) Patellar ligament Popliteal ligament Posterior cruciate ligament (PCL) Prepatellar bursa **P Knee Bursa and Ligament, Left** **See** *N Knee Bursa and Ligament, Right* **Q Ankle Bursa and Ligament, Right** Calcaneofibular ligament Deltoid ligament Ligament of the lateral malleolus Talofibular ligament **R Ankle Bursa and Ligament, Left** **See** *Q Ankle Bursa and Ligament, Right* **S Foot Bursa and Ligament, Right** Calcaneocuboid ligament Cuneonavicular ligament Intercuneiform ligament Interphalangeal ligament Metatarsal ligament Metatarsophalangeal ligament Subtalar ligament Talocalcaneal ligament Talocalcaneonavicular ligament Tarsometatarsal ligament **T Foot Bursa and Ligament, Left** **See** *S Foot Bursa and Ligament, Right* **V Lower Extremity Bursa and Ligament, Right** **W Lower Extremity Bursa and Ligament, Left**	**Ø Open** **3 Percutaneous** **4 Percutaneous Endoscopic** **X External**	**Z No Device**	**Z No Qualifier**

Non-OR ØMN[Ø,1,2,3,4,5,6,7,8,9,B,C,D,F,G,H,J,K,L,M,N,P,Q,R,S,T,V,W]XZZ

Ø Medical and Surgical
M Bursae and Ligaments
P Removal

Definition: Taking out or off a device from a body part

Explanation: If a device is taken out and a similar device put in without cutting or puncturing the skin or mucous membrane, the procedure is coded to the root operation CHANGE. Otherwise, the procedure for taking out a device is coded to the root operation REMOVAL.

Body Part Character 4	Approach Character 5	Device Character 6	Qualifier Character 7
X Upper Bursa and Ligament Y Lower Bursa and Ligament	Ø Open 3 Percutaneous 4 Percutaneous Endoscopic	Ø Drainage Device 7 Autologous Tissue Substitute J Synthetic Substitute K Nonautologous Tissue Substitute Y Other Device	Z No Qualifier
X Upper Bursa and Ligament Y Lower Bursa and Ligament	X External	Ø Drainage Device	Z No Qualifier

Non-OR ØMP[X,Y]3ØZ
Non-OR ØMP[X,Y][3,4]YZ
Non-OR ØMP[X,Y]XØZ

Ø Medical and Surgical
M Bursae and Ligaments
Q Repair Definition: Restoring, to the extent possible, a body part to its normal anatomic structure and function
Explanation: Used only when the method to accomplish the repair is not one of the other root operations

Body Part Character 4	Approach Character 5	Device Character 6	Qualifier Character 7
Ø Head and Neck Bursa and Ligament Alar ligament of axis Cervical interspinous ligament Cervical intertransverse ligament Cervical ligamentum flavum Interspinous ligament, cervical Intertransverse ligament, cervical Lateral temporomandibular ligament Ligamentum flavum, cervical Sphenomandibular ligament Stylomandibular ligament Transverse ligament of atlas **1 Shoulder Bursa and Ligament, Right** Acromioclavicular ligament Coracoacromial ligament Coracoclavicular ligament Coracohumeral ligament Costoclavicular ligament Glenohumeral ligament Interclavicular ligament Sternoclavicular ligament Subacromial bursa Transverse humeral ligament Transverse scapular ligament **2 Shoulder Bursa and Ligament, Left** *See 1 Shoulder Bursa and Ligament, Right* **3 Elbow Bursa and Ligament, Right** Annular ligament Olecranon bursa Radial collateral ligament Ulnar collateral ligament **4 Elbow Bursa and Ligament, Left** *See 3 Elbow Bursa and Ligament, Right* **5 Wrist Bursa and Ligament, Right** Palmar ulnocarpal ligament Radial collateral carpal ligament Radiocarpal ligament Radioulnar ligament Scapholunate ligament Ulnar collateral carpal ligament **6 Wrist Bursa and Ligament, Left** *See 5 Wrist Bursa and Ligament, Right* **7 Hand Bursa and Ligament, Right** Carpometacarpal ligament Intercarpal ligament Interphalangeal ligament Lunotriquetral ligament Metacarpal ligament Metacarpophalangeal ligament Pisohamate ligament Pisometacarpal ligament Scaphotrapezium ligament **8 Hand Bursa and Ligament, Left** *See 7 Hand Bursa and Ligament, Right* **9 Upper Extremity Bursa and Ligament, Right** **B Upper Extremity Bursa and Ligament, Left** **C Upper Spine Bursa and Ligament** Interspinous ligament, thoracic Intertransverse ligament, thoracic Ligamentum flavum, thoracic Supraspinous ligament **D Lower Spine Bursa and Ligament** Iliolumbar ligament Interspinous ligament, lumbar Intertransverse ligament, lumbar Ligamentum flavum, lumbar Sacrococcygeal ligament Sacroiliac ligament Sacrospinous ligament Sacrotuberous ligament Supraspinous ligament **F Sternum Bursa and Ligament** Costoxiphoid ligament Sternocostal ligament **G Rib(s) Bursa and Ligament** Costotransverse ligament **H Abdomen Bursa and Ligament, Right** **J Abdomen Bursa and Ligament, Left** **K Perineum Bursa and Ligament** **L Hip Bursa and Ligament, Right** Iliofemoral ligament Ischiofemoral ligament Pubofemoral ligament Transverse acetabular ligament Trochanteric bursa **M Hip Bursa and Ligament, Left** *See L Hip Bursa and Ligament, Right* **N Knee Bursa and Ligament, Right** Anterior cruciate ligament (ACL) Lateral collateral ligament (LCL) Ligament of head of fibula Medial collateral ligament (MCL) Patellar ligament Popliteal ligament Posterior cruciate ligament (PCL) Prepatellar bursa **P Knee Bursa and Ligament, Left** *See N Knee Bursa and Ligament, Right* **Q Ankle Bursa and Ligament, Right** Calcaneofibular ligament Deltoid ligament Ligament of the lateral malleolus Talofibular ligament **R Ankle Bursa and Ligament, Left** *See Q Ankle Bursa and Ligament, Right* **S Foot Bursa and Ligament, Right** Calcaneocuboid ligament Cuneonavicular ligament Intercuneiform ligament Interphalangeal ligament Metatarsal ligament Metatarsophalangeal ligament Subtalar ligament Talocalcaneal ligament Talocalcaneonavicular ligament Tarsometatarsal ligament **T Foot Bursa and Ligament, Left** *See S Foot Bursa and Ligament, Right* **V Lower Extremity Bursa and Ligament, Right** **W Lower Extremity Bursa and Ligament, Left**	**Ø Open** **3 Percutaneous** **4 Percutaneous Endoscopic**	**Z No Device**	**Z No Qualifier**

Bursae and Ligaments

ØMQ–ØMQ

Ø Medical and Surgical
M Bursae and Ligaments
R Replacement Definition: Putting in or on biological or synthetic material that physically takes the place and/or function of all or a portion of a body part

Explanation: The body part may have been taken out or replaced, or may be taken out, physically eradicated, or rendered nonfunctional during the REPLACEMENT procedure. A REMOVAL procedure is coded for taking out the device used in a previous replacement procedure.

Body Part Character 4	Approach Character 5	Device Character 6	Qualifier Character 7
Ø Head and Neck Bursa and Ligament Alar ligament of axis Cervical interspinous ligament Cervical intertransverse ligament Cervical ligamentum flavum Interspinous ligament, cervical Intertransverse ligament, cervical Lateral temporomandibular ligament Ligamentum flavum, cervical Sphenomandibular ligament Stylomandibular ligament Transverse ligament of atlas **1 Shoulder Bursa and Ligament, Right** Acromioclavicular ligament Coracoacromial ligament Coracoclavicular ligament Coracohumeral ligament Costoclavicular ligament Glenohumeral ligament Interclavicular ligament Sternoclavicular ligament Subacromial bursa Transverse humeral ligament Transverse scapular ligament **2 Shoulder Bursa and Ligament, Left** **See** *1 Shoulder Bursa and Ligament, Right* **3 Elbow Bursa and Ligament, Right** Annular ligament Olecranon bursa Radial collateral ligament Ulnar collateral ligament **4 Elbow Bursa and Ligament, Left** **See** *3 Elbow Bursa and Ligament, Right* **5 Wrist Bursa and Ligament, Right** Palmar ulnocarpal ligament Radial collateral carpal ligament Radiocarpal ligament Radioulnar ligament Scapholunate ligament Ulnar collateral carpal ligament **6 Wrist Bursa and Ligament, Left** **See** *5 Wrist Bursa and Ligament, Right* **7 Hand Bursa and Ligament, Right** Carpometacarpal ligament Intercarpal ligament Interphalangeal ligament Lunotriquetral ligament Metacarpal ligament Metacarpophalangeal ligament Pisohamate ligament Pisometacarpal ligament Scaphotrapezium ligament **8 Hand Bursa and Ligament, Left** **See** *7 Hand Bursa and Ligament, Right* **9 Upper Extremity Bursa and Ligament, Right** **B Upper Extremity Bursa and Ligament, Left** **C Upper Spine Bursa and Ligament** Interspinous ligament, thoracic Intertransverse ligament, thoracic Ligamentum flavum, thoracic Supraspinous ligament **D Lower Spine Bursa and Ligament** Iliolumbar ligament Interspinous ligament, lumbar Intertransverse ligament, lumbar Ligamentum flavum, lumbar Sacrococcygeal ligament Sacroiliac ligament Sacrospinous ligament Sacrotuberous ligament Supraspinous ligament **F Sternum Bursa and Ligament** Costoxiphoid ligament Sternocostal ligament **G Rib(s) Bursa and Ligament** Costotransverse ligament **H Abdomen Bursa and Ligament, Right** **J Abdomen Bursa and Ligament, Left** **K Perineum Bursa and Ligament** **L Hip Bursa and Ligament, Right** Iliofemoral ligament Ischiofemoral ligament Pubofemoral ligament Transverse acetabular ligament Trochanteric bursa **M Hip Bursa and Ligament, Left** **See** *L Hip Bursa and Ligament, Right* **N Knee Bursa and Ligament, Right** Anterior cruciate ligament (ACL) Lateral collateral ligament (LCL) Ligament of head of fibula Medial collateral ligament (MCL) Patellar ligament Popliteal ligament Posterior cruciate ligament (PCL) Prepatellar bursa **P Knee Bursa and Ligament, Left** **See** *N Knee Bursa and Ligament, Right* **Q Ankle Bursa and Ligament, Right** Calcaneofibular ligament Deltoid ligament Ligament of the lateral malleolus Talofibular ligament **R Ankle Bursa and Ligament, Left** **See** *Q Ankle Bursa and Ligament, Right* **S Foot Bursa and Ligament, Right** Calcaneocuboid ligament Cuneonavicular ligament Intercuneiform ligament Interphalangeal ligament Metatarsal ligament Metatarsophalangeal ligament Subtalar ligament Talocalcaneal ligament Talocalcaneonavicular ligament Tarsometatarsal ligament **T Foot Bursa and Ligament, Left** **See** *S Foot Bursa and Ligament, Right* **V Lower Extremity Bursa and Ligament, Right** **W Lower Extremity Bursa and Ligament, Left**	**Ø Open** **4 Percutaneous Endoscopic**	**7 Autologous Tissue Substitute** **J Synthetic Substitute** **K Nonautologous Tissue Substitute**	**Z No Qualifier**

Ø Medical and Surgical
M Bursae and Ligaments
S Reposition Definition: Moving to its normal location, or other suitable location, all or a portion of a body part

Explanation: The body part is moved to a new location from an abnormal location, or from a normal location where it is not functioning correctly. The body part may or may not be cut out or off to be moved to the new location.

Body Part Character 4	Approach Character 5	Device Character 6	Qualifier Character 7
Ø Head and Neck Bursa and Ligament Alar ligament of axis Cervical interspinous ligament Cervical intertransverse ligament Cervical ligamentum flavum Interspinous ligament, cervical Intertransverse ligament, cervical Lateral temporomandibular ligament Ligamentum flavum, cervical Sphenomandibular ligament Stylomandibular ligament Transverse ligament of atlas **1 Shoulder Bursa and Ligament, Right** Acromioclavicular ligament Coracoacromial ligament Coracoclavicular ligament Coracohumeral ligament Costoclavicular ligament Glenohumeral ligament Interclavicular ligament Sternoclavicular ligament Subacromial bursa Transverse humeral ligament Transverse scapular ligament **2 Shoulder Bursa and Ligament, Left** *See 1 Shoulder Bursa and Ligament, Right* **3 Elbow Bursa and Ligament, Right** Annular ligament Olecranon bursa Radial collateral ligament Ulnar collateral ligament **4 Elbow Bursa and Ligament, Left** *See 3 Elbow Bursa and Ligament, Right* **5 Wrist Bursa and Ligament, Right** Palmar ulnocarpal ligament Radial collateral carpal ligament Radiocarpal ligament Radioulnar ligament Scapholunate ligament Ulnar collateral carpal ligament **6 Wrist Bursa and Ligament, Left** *See 5 Wrist Bursa and Ligament, Right* **7 Hand Bursa and Ligament, Right** Carpometacarpal ligament Intercarpal ligament Interphalangeal ligament Lunotriquetral ligament Metacarpal ligament Metacarpophalangeal ligament Pisohamate ligament Pisometacarpal ligament Scaphotrapezium ligament **8 Hand Bursa and Ligament, Left** *See 7 Hand Bursa and Ligament, Right* **9 Upper Extremity Bursa and Ligament, Right** **B Upper Extremity Bursa and Ligament, Left** **C Upper Spine Bursa and Ligament** Interspinous ligament, thoracic Intertransverse ligament, thoracic Ligamentum flavum, thoracic Supraspinous ligament **D Lower Spine Bursa and Ligament** Iliolumbar ligament Interspinous ligament, lumbar Intertransverse ligament, lumbar Ligamentum flavum, lumbar Sacrococcygeal ligament Sacroiliac ligament Sacrospinous ligament Sacrotuberous ligament Supraspinous ligament **F Sternum Bursa and Ligament** Costoxiphoid ligament Sternocostal ligament **G Rib(s) Bursa and Ligament** Costotransverse ligament **H Abdomen Bursa and Ligament, Right** **J Abdomen Bursa and Ligament, Left** **K Perineum Bursa and Ligament** **L Hip Bursa and Ligament, Right** Iliofemoral ligament Ischiofemoral ligament Pubofemoral ligament Transverse acetabular ligament Trochanteric bursa **M Hip Bursa and Ligament, Left** *See L Hip Bursa and Ligament, Right* **N Knee Bursa and Ligament, Right** Anterior cruciate ligament (ACL) Lateral collateral ligament (LCL) Ligament of head of fibula Medial collateral ligament (MCL) Patellar ligament Popliteal ligament Posterior cruciate ligament (PCL) Prepatellar bursa **P Knee Bursa and Ligament, Left** *See N Knee Bursa and Ligament, Right* **Q Ankle Bursa and Ligament, Right** Calcaneofibular ligament Deltoid ligament Ligament of the lateral malleolus Talofibular ligament **R Ankle Bursa and Ligament, Left** *See Q Ankle Bursa and Ligament, Right* **S Foot Bursa and Ligament, Right** Calcaneocuboid ligament Cuneonavicular ligament Intercuneiform ligament Interphalangeal ligament Metatarsal ligament Metatarsophalangeal ligament Subtalar ligament Talocalcaneal ligament Talocalcaneonavicular ligament Tarsometatarsal ligament **T Foot Bursa and Ligament, Left** *See S Foot Bursa and Ligament, Right* **V Lower Extremity Bursa and Ligament, Right** **W Lower Extremity Bursa and Ligament, Left**	Ø Open 4 Percutaneous Endoscopic	Z No Device	Z No Qualifier

Ø Medical and Surgical
M Bursae and Ligaments
T Resection Definition: Cutting out or off, without replacement, all of a body part
Explanation: None

Body Part Character 4	Approach Character 5	Device Character 6	Qualifier Character 7
Ø Head and Neck Bursa and Ligament Alar ligament of axis Cervical interspinous ligament Cervical intertransverse ligament Cervical ligamentum flavum Interspinous ligament, cervical Intertransverse ligament, cervical Lateral temporomandibular ligament Ligamentum flavum, cervical Sphenomandibular ligament Stylomandibular ligament Transverse ligament of atlas **1 Shoulder Bursa and Ligament, Right** Acromioclavicular ligament Coracoacromial ligament Coracoclavicular ligament Coracohumeral ligament Costoclavicular ligament Glenohumeral ligament Interclavicular ligament Sternoclavicular ligament Subacromial bursa Transverse humeral ligament Transverse scapular ligament **2 Shoulder Bursa and Ligament, Left** **See** *1 Shoulder Bursa and Ligament, Right* **3 Elbow Bursa and Ligament, Right** Annular ligament Olecranon bursa Radial collateral ligament Ulnar collateral ligament **4 Elbow Bursa and Ligament, Left** **See** *3 Elbow Bursa and Ligament, Right* **5 Wrist Bursa and Ligament, Right** Palmar ulnocarpal ligament Radial collateral carpal ligament Radiocarpal ligament Radioulnar ligament Scapholunate ligament Ulnar collateral carpal ligament **6 Wrist Bursa and Ligament, Left** **See** *5 Wrist Bursa and Ligament, Right* **7 Hand Bursa and Ligament, Right** Carpometacarpal ligament Intercarpal ligament Interphalangeal ligament Lunotriquetral ligament Metacarpal ligament Metacarpophalangeal ligament Pisohamate ligament Pisometacarpal ligament Scaphotrapezium ligament **8 Hand Bursa and Ligament, Left** **See** *7 Hand Bursa and Ligament, Right* **9 Upper Extremity Bursa and Ligament, Right** **B Upper Extremity Bursa and Ligament, Left** **C Upper Spine Bursa and Ligament** Interspinous ligament, thoracic Intertransverse ligament, thoracic Ligamentum flavum, thoracic Supraspinous ligament **D Lower Spine Bursa and Ligament** Iliolumbar ligament Interspinous ligament, lumbar Intertransverse ligament, lumbar Ligamentum flavum, lumbar Sacrococcygeal ligament Sacroiliac ligament Sacrospinous ligament Sacrotuberous ligament Supraspinous ligament **F Sternum Bursa and Ligament** Costoxiphoid ligament Sternocostal ligament **G Rib(s) Bursa and Ligament** Costotransverse ligament **H Abdomen Bursa and Ligament, Right** **J Abdomen Bursa and Ligament, Left** **K Perineum Bursa and Ligament** **L Hip Bursa and Ligament, Right** Iliofemoral ligament Ischiofemoral ligament Pubofemoral ligament Transverse acetabular ligament Trochanteric bursa **M Hip Bursa and Ligament, Left** **See** *L Hip Bursa and Ligament, Right* **N Knee Bursa and Ligament, Right** Anterior cruciate ligament (ACL) Lateral collateral ligament (LCL) Ligament of head of fibula Medial collateral ligament (MCL) Patellar ligament Popliteal ligament Posterior cruciate ligament (PCL) Prepatellar bursa **P Knee Bursa and Ligament, Left** **See** *N Knee Bursa and Ligament, Right* **Q Ankle Bursa and Ligament, Right** Calcaneofibular ligament Deltoid ligament Ligament of the lateral malleolus Talofibular ligament **R Ankle Bursa and Ligament, Left** **See** *Q Ankle Bursa and Ligament, Right* **S Foot Bursa and Ligament, Right** Calcaneocuboid ligament Cuneonavicular ligament Intercuneiform ligament Interphalangeal ligament Metatarsal ligament Metatarsophalangeal ligament Subtalar ligament Talocalcaneal ligament Talocalcaneonavicular ligament Tarsometatarsal ligament **T Foot Bursa and Ligament, Left** **See** *S Foot Bursa and Ligament, Right* **V Lower Extremity Bursa and Ligament, Right** **W Lower Extremity Bursa and Ligament, Left**	**Ø Open** **4 Percutaneous Endoscopic**	**Z No Device**	**Z No Qualifier**

Ø Medical and Surgical
M Bursae and Ligaments
U Supplement

Definition: Putting in or on biological or synthetic material that physically reinforces and/or augments the function of a portion of a body part

Explanation: The biological material is non-living, or is living and from the same individual. The body part may have been previously replaced, and the SUPPLEMENT procedure is performed to physically reinforce and/or augment the function of the replaced body part.

Body Part Character 4	Approach Character 5	Device Character 6	Qualifier Character 7
Ø Head and Neck Bursa and Ligament Alar ligament of axis Cervical interspinous ligament Cervical intertransverse ligament Cervical ligamentum flavum Interspinous ligament, cervical Intertransverse ligament, cervical Lateral temporomandibular ligament Ligamentum flavum, cervical Sphenomandibular ligament Stylomandibular ligament Transverse ligament of atlas **1 Shoulder Bursa and Ligament, Right** Acromioclavicular ligament Coracoacromial ligament Coracoclavicular ligament Coracohumeral ligament Costoclavicular ligament Glenohumeral ligament Interclavicular ligament Sternoclavicular ligament Subacromial bursa Transverse humeral ligament Transverse scapular ligament **2 Shoulder Bursa and Ligament, Left** **See** *1 Shoulder Bursa and Ligament, Right* **3 Elbow Bursa and Ligament, Right** Annular ligament Olecranon bursa Radial collateral ligament Ulnar collateral ligament **4 Elbow Bursa and Ligament, Left** **See** *3 Elbow Bursa and Ligament, Right* **5 Wrist Bursa and Ligament, Right** Palmar ulnocarpal ligament Radial collateral carpal ligament Radiocarpal ligament Radioulnar ligament Scapholunate ligament Ulnar collateral carpal ligament **6 Wrist Bursa and Ligament, Left** **See** *5 Wrist Bursa and Ligament, Right* **7 Hand Bursa and Ligament, Right** Carpometacarpal ligament Intercarpal ligament Interphalangeal ligament Lunotriquetral ligament Metacarpal ligament Metacarpophalangeal ligament Pisohamate ligament Pisometacarpal ligament Scaphotrapezium ligament **8 Hand Bursa and Ligament, Left** **See** *7 Hand Bursa and Ligament, Right* **9 Upper Extremity Bursa and Ligament, Right** **B Upper Extremity Bursa and Ligament, Left** **C Upper Spine Bursa and Ligament** Interspinous ligament, thoracic Intertransverse ligament, thoracic Ligamentum flavum, thoracic Supraspinous ligament **D Lower Spine Bursa and Ligament** Iliolumbar ligament Interspinous ligament, lumbar Intertransverse ligament, lumbar Ligamentum flavum, lumbar Sacrococcygeal ligament Sacroiliac ligament Sacrospinous ligament Sacrotuberous ligament Supraspinous ligament **F Sternum Bursa and Ligament** Costoxiphoid ligament Sternocostal ligament **G Rib(s) Bursa and Ligament** Costotransverse ligament **H Abdomen Bursa and Ligament, Right** **J Abdomen Bursa and Ligament, Left** **K Perineum Bursa and Ligament** **L Hip Bursa and Ligament, Right** Iliofemoral ligament Ischiofemoral ligament Pubofemoral ligament Transverse acetabular ligament Trochanteric bursa **M Hip Bursa and Ligament, Left** **See** *L Hip Bursa and Ligament, Right* **N Knee Bursa and Ligament, Right** Anterior cruciate ligament (ACL) Lateral collateral ligament (LCL) Ligament of head of fibula Medial collateral ligament (MCL) Patellar ligament Popliteal ligament Posterior cruciate ligament (PCL) Prepatellar bursa **P Knee Bursa and Ligament, Left** **See** *N Knee Bursa and Ligament, Right* **Q Ankle Bursa and Ligament, Right** Calcaneofibular ligament Deltoid ligament Ligament of the lateral malleolus Talofibular ligament **R Ankle Bursa and Ligament, Left** **See** *Q Ankle Bursa and Ligament, Right* **S Foot Bursa and Ligament, Right** Calcaneocuboid ligament Cuneonavicular ligament Intercuneiform ligament Interphalangeal ligament Metatarsal ligament Metatarsophalangeal ligament Subtalar ligament Talocalcaneal ligament Talocalcaneonavicular ligament Tarsometatarsal ligament **T Foot Bursa and Ligament, Left** **See** *S Foot Bursa and Ligament, Right* **V Lower Extremity Bursa and Ligament, Right** **W Lower Extremity Bursa and Ligament, Left**	**Ø Open** **4 Percutaneous Endoscopic**	**7 Autologous Tissue Substitute** **J Synthetic Substitute** **K Nonautologous Tissue Substitute**	**Z No Qualifier**

Bursae and Ligaments
ØMU–ØMU

Ø Medical and Surgical
M Bursae and Ligaments
W Revision

Definition: Correcting, to the extent possible, a portion of a malfunctioning device or the position of a displaced device

Explanation: Revision can include correcting a malfunctioning or displaced device by taking out or putting in components of the device such as a screw or pin

Body Part Character 4	Approach Character 5	Device Character 6	Qualifier Character 7
X Upper Bursa and Ligament Y Lower Bursa and Ligament	Ø Open 3 Percutaneous 4 Percutaneous Endoscopic	Ø Drainage Device 7 Autologous Tissue Substitute J Synthetic Substitute K Nonautologous Tissue Substitute Y Other Device	Z No Qualifier
X Upper Bursa and Ligament Y Lower Bursa and Ligament	X External	Ø Drainage Device 7 Autologous Tissue Substitute J Synthetic Substitute K Nonautologous Tissue Substitute	Z No Qualifier

Non-OR ØMW[X,Y][3,4]YZ
Non-OR ØMW[X,Y]X[Ø,7,J,K]Z

Ø Medical and Surgical
M Bursae and Ligaments
X Transfer Definition: Moving, without taking out, all or a portion of a body part to another location to take over the function of all or a portion of a body part

Explanation: The body part transferred remains connected to its vascular and nervous supply

Body Part Character 4	Approach Character 5	Device Character 6	Qualifier Character 7
Ø Head and Neck Bursa and Ligament Alar ligament of axis Cervical interspinous ligament Cervical intertransverse ligament Cervical ligamentum flavum Interspinous ligament, cervical Intertransverse ligament, cervical Lateral temporomandibular ligament Ligamentum flavum, cervical Sphenomandibular ligament Stylomandibular ligament Transverse ligament of atlas **1 Shoulder Bursa and Ligament, Right** Acromioclavicular ligament Coracoacromial ligament Coracoclavicular ligament Coracohumeral ligament Costoclavicular ligament Glenohumeral ligament Interclavicular ligament Sternoclavicular ligament Subacromial bursa Transverse humeral ligament Transverse scapular ligament **2 Shoulder Bursa and Ligament, Left** *See 1 Shoulder Bursa and Ligament, Right* **3 Elbow Bursa and Ligament, Right** Annular ligament Olecranon bursa Radial collateral ligament Ulnar collateral ligament **4 Elbow Bursa and Ligament, Left** *See 3 Elbow Bursa and Ligament, Right* **5 Wrist Bursa and Ligament, Right** Palmar ulnocarpal ligament Radial collateral carpal ligament Radiocarpal ligament Radioulnar ligament Scapholunate ligament Ulnar collateral carpal ligament **6 Wrist Bursa and Ligament, Left** *See 5 Wrist Bursa and Ligament, Right* **7 Hand Bursa and Ligament, Right** Carpometacarpal ligament Intercarpal ligament Interphalangeal ligament Lunotriquetral ligament Metacarpal ligament Metacarpophalangeal ligament Pisohamate ligament Pisometacarpal ligament Scaphotrapezium ligament **8 Hand Bursa and Ligament, Left** *See 7 Hand Bursa and Ligament, Right* **9 Upper Extremity Bursa and Ligament, Right** **B Upper Extremity Bursa and Ligament, Left** **C Upper Spine Bursa and Ligament** Interspinous ligament, thoracic Intertransverse ligament, thoracic Ligamentum flavum, thoracic Supraspinous ligament **D Lower Spine Bursa and Ligament** Iliolumbar ligament Interspinous ligament, lumbar Intertransverse ligament, lumbar Ligamentum flavum, lumbar Sacrococcygeal ligament Sacroiliac ligament Sacrospinous ligament Sacrotuberous ligament Supraspinous ligament **F Sternum Bursa and Ligament** Costoxiphoid ligament Sternocostal ligament **G Rib(s) Bursa and Ligament** Costotransverse ligament **H Abdomen Bursa and Ligament, Right** **J Abdomen Bursa and Ligament, Left** **K Perineum Bursa and Ligament** **L Hip Bursa and Ligament, Right** Iliofemoral ligament Ischiofemoral ligament Pubofemoral ligament Transverse acetabular ligament Trochanteric bursa **M Hip Bursa and Ligament, Left** *See L Hip Bursa and Ligament, Right* **N Knee Bursa and Ligament, Right** Anterior cruciate ligament (ACL) Lateral collateral ligament (LCL) Ligament of head of fibula Medial collateral ligament (MCL) Patellar ligament Popliteal ligament Posterior cruciate ligament (PCL) Prepatellar bursa **P Knee Bursa and Ligament, Left** *See N Knee Bursa and Ligament, Right* **Q Ankle Bursa and Ligament, Right** Calcaneofibular ligament Deltoid ligament Ligament of the lateral malleolus Talofibular ligament **R Ankle Bursa and Ligament, Left** *See Q Ankle Bursa and Ligament, Right* **S Foot Bursa and Ligament, Right** Calcaneocuboid ligament Cuneonavicular ligament Intercuneiform ligament Interphalangeal ligament Metatarsal ligament Metatarsophalangeal ligament Subtalar ligament Talocalcaneal ligament Talocalcaneonavicular ligament Tarsometatarsal ligament **T Foot Bursa and Ligament, Left** *See S Foot Bursa and Ligament, Right* **V Lower Extremity Bursa and Ligament, Right** **W Lower Extremity Bursa and Ligament, Left**	**Ø Open** **4 Percutaneous Endoscopic**	**Z No Device**	**Z No Qualifier**

Head and Facial Bones ØN2–ØNW

Character Meanings

This Character Meaning table is provided as a guide to assist the user in the identification of character members that may be found in this section of code tables. It **SHOULD NOT** be used to build a PCS code.

Operation–Character 3		Body Part–Character 4		Approach–Character 5		Device–Character 6		Qualifier–Character 7	
2	Change	Ø	Skull	Ø	Open	Ø	Drainage Device	X	Diagnostic
5	Destruction	1	Frontal Bone	3	Percutaneous	3	Infusion Device	Z	No Qualifier
8	Division	3	Parietal Bone, Right	4	Percutaneous Endoscopic	4	Internal Fixation Device		
9	Drainage	4	Parietal Bone, Left	X	External	5	External Fixation Device		
B	Excision	5	Temporal Bone, Right			7	Autologous Tissue Substitute		
C	Extirpation	6	Temporal Bone, Left			J	Synthetic Substitute		
D	Extraction	7	Occipital Bone			K	Nonautologous Tissue Substitute		
H	Insertion	B	Nasal Bone			M	Bone Growth Stimulator		
J	Inspection	C	Sphenoid Bone			N	Neurostimulator Generator		
N	Release	F	Ethmoid Bone, Right			S	Hearing Device		
P	Removal	G	Ethmoid Bone, Left			Y	Other Device		
Q	Repair	H	Lacrimal Bone, Right			Z	No Device		
R	Replacement	J	Lacrimal Bone, Left						
S	Reposition	K	Palatine Bone, Right						
T	Resection	L	Palatine Bone, Left						
U	Supplement	M	Zygomatic Bone, Right						
W	Revision	N	Zygomatic Bone, Left						
		P	Orbit, Right						
		Q	Orbit, Left						
		R	Maxilla						
		T	Mandible, Right						
		V	Mandible, Left						
		W	Facial Bone						
		X	Hyoid Bone						

AHA Coding Clinic for table ØNB

2022, 2Q, 17 Congenital nasal pyriform aperture stenosis and repair
2021, 3Q, 21 Excision of thyroglossal duct cyst
2021, 1Q, 21 Maxillectomy with reconstruction of maxilla
2017, 1Q, 20 Preparatory nasal adhesion repair before definitive cleft palate repair
2015, 3Q, 3-8 Excisional and nonexcisional debridement
2015, 2Q, 12 Orbital exenteration

AHA Coding Clinic for table ØND

2017, 4Q, 41 Extraction procedures

AHA Coding Clinic for table ØNH

2021, 4Q, 51 Insertion of infusion device in skull
2015, 3Q, 13 Nonexcisional debridement of cranial wound with removal and replacement of hardware

AHA Coding Clinic for table ØNP

2023, 1Q, 31 Removal of autologous bone flap due to bone resorption
2022, 4Q, 58-59 Infusion device in head and facial bones
2015, 3Q, 13 Nonexcisional debridement of cranial wound with removal and replacement of hardware

AHA Coding Clinic for table ØNQ

2016, 3Q, 29 Closure of bilateral alveolar clefts

AHA Coding Clinic for table ØNR

2021, 3Q, 29 Repair of superior semicircular canal dehiscence
2021, 1Q, 21 Maxillectomy with reconstruction of maxilla
2017, 3Q, 17 Resection of schwannoma and placement of DuraGen and Lorenz cranial plating system
2017, 3Q, 22 Replacement of native skull bone flap
2017, 1Q, 23 Reconstruction of mandible using titanium and bone
2014, 3Q, 7 Hemi-cranioplasty for repair of cranial defect

AHA Coding Clinic for table ØNS

2022, 1Q, 48 Repair of facial fractures of frontal sinus and orbital roof
2017, 3Q, 22 Replacement of native skull bone flap
2017, 1Q, 20 Preparatory nasal adhesion repair before definitive cleft palate repair
2016, 2Q, 30 Clipping (occlusion) of cerebral artery, decompressive craniectomy and storage of bone flap in abdominal wall
2015, 3Q, 17 Craniosynostosis with cranial vault reconstruction
2015, 3Q, 27 Moyamoya disease and hemispheric pial synangiosis with craniotomy
2014, 3Q, 23 Le Fort I osteotomy
2013, 3Q, 24 Distraction osteogenesis
2013, 3Q, 25 Fracture of frontal bone with repair and coagulation for hemostasis

AHA Coding Clinic for table ØNU

2023, 2Q, 19 Sigmoid sinus dehiscence with mastoidectomy with resurfacing
2021, 3Q, 29 Repair of superior semicircular canal dehiscence
2016, 3Q, 29 Closure of bilateral alveolar clefts
2013, 3Q, 24 Distraction osteogenesis

AHA Coding Clinic for table ØNW

2022, 4Q, 58-59 Infusion device in head and facial bones

Head and Facial Bones

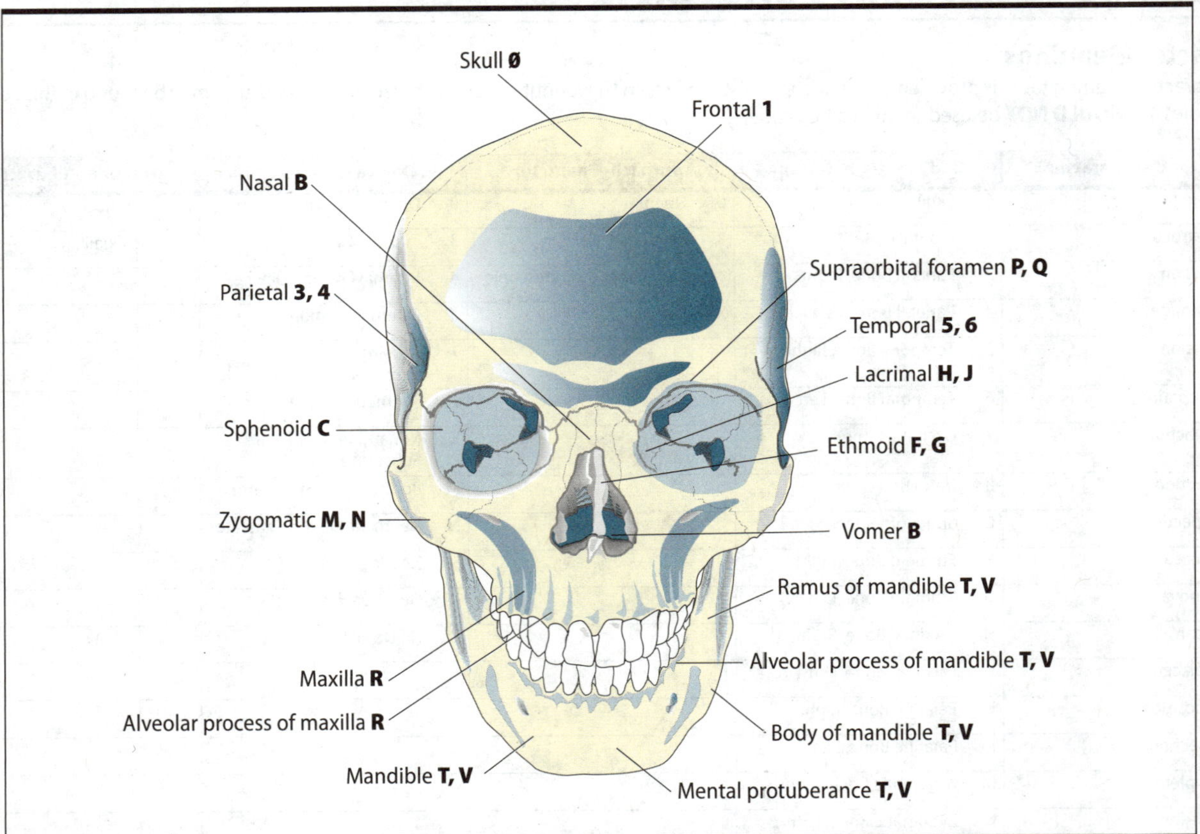

Skull Bones

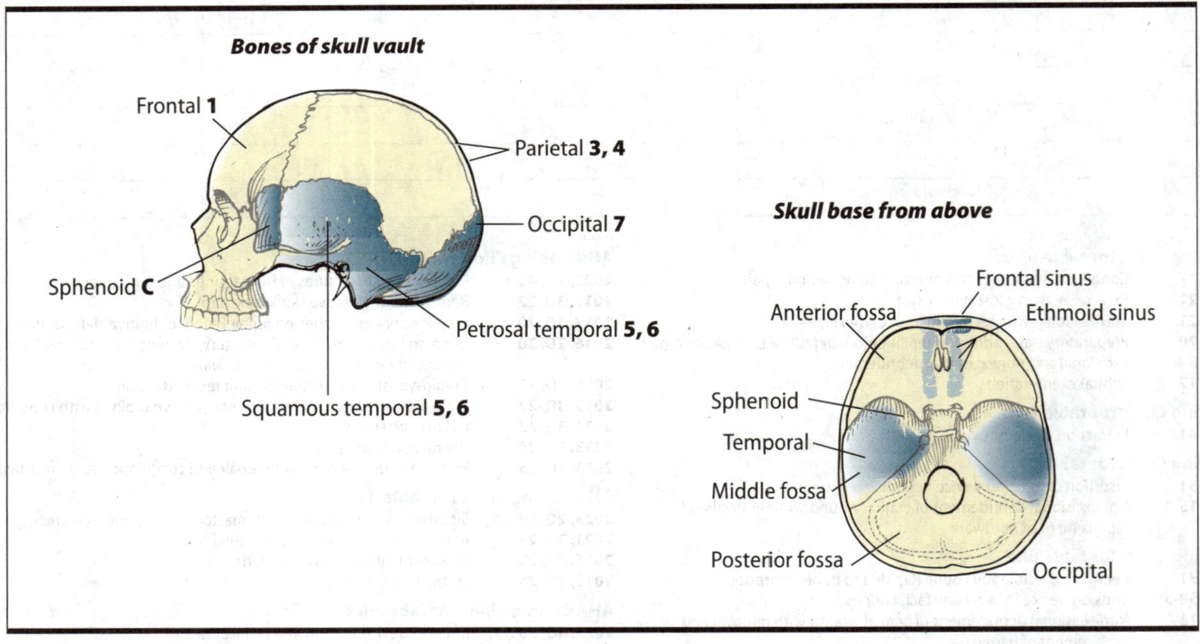

Ø Medical and Surgical
N Head and Facial Bones
2 Change Definition: Taking out or off a device from a body part and putting back an identical or similar device in or on the same body part without cutting or puncturing the skin or a mucous membrane

Explanation: All CHANGE procedures are coded using the approach EXTERNAL

Body Part Character 4	Approach Character 5	Device Character 6	Qualifier Character 7
Ø Skull **B Nasal Bone** Vomer of nasal septum **W Facial Bone**	**X External**	**Ø Drainage Device** **Y Other Device**	**Z No Qualifier**
Non-OR All body part, approach, device, and qualifier values			

Ø Medical and Surgical
N Head and Facial Bones
5 Destruction Definition: Physical eradication of all or a portion of a body part by the direct use of energy, force, or a destructive agent

Explanation: None of the body part is physically taken out

Body Part Character 4	Approach Character 5	Device Character 6	Qualifier Character 7
Ø Skull **1 Frontal Bone** Zygomatic process of frontal bone **3 Parietal Bone, Right** **4 Parietal Bone, Left** **5 Temporal Bone, Right** Mastoid process Petrous part of temporal bone Tympanic part of temporal bone Zygomatic process of temporal bone **6 Temporal Bone, Left** *See 5 Temporal Bone, Right* **7 Occipital Bone** Foramen magnum **B Nasal Bone** Vomer of nasal septum **C Sphenoid Bone** Greater wing Lesser wing Optic foramen Pterygoid process Sella turcica **F Ethmoid Bone, Right** Cribriform plate **G Ethmoid Bone, Left** *See F Ethmoid Bone, Right* **H Lacrimal Bone, Right** **J Lacrimal Bone, Left** **K Palatine Bone, Right** **L Palatine Bone, Left** **M Zygomatic Bone, Right** **N Zygomatic Bone, Left** **P Orbit, Right** Bony orbit Orbital portion of ethmoid bone Orbital portion of frontal bone Orbital portion of lacrimal bone Orbital portion of maxilla Orbital portion of palatine bone Orbital portion of sphenoid bone Orbital portion of zygomatic bone **Q Orbit, Left** *See P Orbit, Right* **R Maxilla** Alveolar process of maxilla **T Mandible, Right** Alveolar process of mandible Condyloid process Mandibular notch Mental foramen **V Mandible, Left** *See T Mandible, Right* **X Hyoid Bone**	**Ø Open** **3 Percutaneous** **4 Percutaneous Endoscopic**	**Z No Device**	**Z No Qualifier**

Ø Medical and Surgical
N Head and Facial Bones
8 Division Definition: Cutting into a body part, without draining fluids and/or gases from the body part, in order to separate or transect a body part
Explanation: All or a portion of the body part is separated into two or more portions

Body Part Character 4	Approach Character 5	Device Character 6	Qualifier Character 7
Ø Skull **1 Frontal Bone** Zygomatic process of frontal bone **3 Parietal Bone, Right** **4 Parietal Bone, Left** **5 Temporal Bone, Right** Mastoid process Petrous part of temporal bone Tympanic part of temporal bone Zygomatic process of temporal bone **6 Temporal Bone, Left** *See 5 Temporal Bone, Right* **7 Occipital Bone** Foramen magnum **B Nasal Bone** Vomer of nasal septum **C Sphenoid Bone** Greater wing Lesser wing Optic foramen Pterygoid process Sella turcica **F Ethmoid Bone, Right** Cribriform plate **G Ethmoid Bone, Left** *See F Ethmoid Bone, Right* **H Lacrimal Bone, Right** **J Lacrimal Bone, Left** **K Palatine Bone, Right** **L Palatine Bone, Left** **M Zygomatic Bone, Right** **N Zygomatic Bone, Left** **P Orbit, Right** Bony orbit Orbital portion of ethmoid bone Orbital portion of frontal bone Orbital portion of lacrimal bone Orbital portion of maxilla Orbital portion of palatine bone Orbital portion of sphenoid bone Orbital portion of zygomatic bone **Q Orbit, Left** *See P Orbit, Right* **R Maxilla** Alveolar process of maxilla **T Mandible, Right** Alveolar process of mandible Condyloid process Mandibular notch Mental foramen **V Mandible, Left** *See T Mandible, Right* **X Hyoid Bone**	**Ø Open** **3 Percutaneous** **4 Percutaneous Endoscopic**	**Z No Device**	**Z No Qualifier**

Non-OR ØN8B[Ø,3,4]ZZ

Ø Medical and Surgical
N Head and Facial Bones
9 Drainage

Definition: Taking or letting out fluids and/or gases from a body part

Explanation: The qualifier DIAGNOSTIC is used to identify drainage procedures that are biopsies

Body Part Character 4	Approach Character 5	Device Character 6	Qualifier Character 7
Ø Skull **1** Frontal Bone Zygomatic process of frontal bone **3** Parietal Bone, Right **4** Parietal Bone, Left **5** Temporal Bone, Right Mastoid process Petrous part of temporal bone Tympanic part of temporal bone Zygomatic process of temporal bone **6** Temporal Bone, Left *See 5 Temporal Bone, Right* **7** Occipital Bone Foramen magnum **B** Nasal Bone Vomer of nasal septum **C** Sphenoid Bone Greater wing Lesser wing Optic foramen Pterygoid process Sella turcica **F** Ethmoid Bone, Right Cribriform plate **G** Ethmoid Bone, Left *See F Ethmoid Bone, Right* **H** Lacrimal Bone, Right **J** Lacrimal Bone, Left **K** Palatine Bone, Right **L** Palatine Bone, Left **M** Zygomatic Bone, Right **N** Zygomatic Bone, Left **P** Orbit, Right Bony orbit Orbital portion of ethmoid bone Orbital portion of frontal bone Orbital portion of lacrimal bone Orbital portion of maxilla Orbital portion of palatine bone Orbital portion of sphenoid bone Orbital portion of zygomatic bone **Q** Orbit, Left *See P Orbit, Right* **R** Maxilla Alveolar process of maxilla **T** Mandible, Right Alveolar process of mandible Condyloid process Mandibular notch Mental foramen **V** Mandible, Left *See T Mandible, Right* **X** Hyoid Bone	**Ø** Open **3** Percutaneous **4** Percutaneous Endoscopic	**Ø** Drainage Device	**Z** No Qualifier

Non-OR ØN9[Ø,1,3,4,5,6,7,C,F,G,H,J,K,L,M,N,P,Q,X]3ØZ
Non-OR ØN9[B,R,T,V][Ø,3,4]ØZ

ØN9 Continued on next page

ØN9 Continued

Ø Medical and Surgical
N Head and Facial Bones
9 Drainage Definition: Taking or letting out fluids and/or gases from a body part
Explanation: The qualifier DIAGNOSTIC is used to identify drainage procedures that are biopsies

Body Part Character 4	Approach Character 5	Device Character 6	Qualifier Character 7
Ø Skull 1 Frontal Bone Zygomatic process of frontal bone 3 Parietal Bone, Right 4 Parietal Bone, Left 5 Temporal Bone, Right Mastoid process Petrous part of temporal bone Tympanic part of temporal bone Zygomatic process of temporal bone 6 Temporal Bone, Left *See 5 Temporal Bone, Right* 7 Occipital Bone Foramen magnum B Nasal Bone Vomer of nasal septum C Sphenoid Bone Greater wing Lesser wing Optic foramen Pterygoid process Sella turcica F Ethmoid Bone, Right Cribriform plate G Ethmoid Bone, Left *See F Ethmoid Bone, Right* H Lacrimal Bone, Right J Lacrimal Bone, Left K Palatine Bone, Right L Palatine Bone, Left M Zygomatic Bone, Right N Zygomatic Bone, Left P Orbit, Right Bony orbit Orbital portion of ethmoid bone Orbital portion of frontal bone Orbital portion of lacrimal bone Orbital portion of maxilla Orbital portion of palatine bone Orbital portion of sphenoid bone Orbital portion of zygomatic bone Q Orbit, Left *See P Orbit, Right* R Maxilla Alveolar process of maxilla T Mandible, Right Alveolar process of mandible Condyloid process Mandibular notch Mental foramen V Mandible, Left *See T Mandible, Right* X Hyoid Bone	Ø Open 3 Percutaneous 4 Percutaneous Endoscopic	Z No Device	X Diagnostic Z No Qualifier

Non-OR ØN9[Ø,1,3,4,5,6,7,C,F,G,H,J,K,L,M,N,P,Q,X]3ZZ
Non-OR ØN9B[Ø,3,4]Z[X,Z]
Non-OR ØN9[R,T,V][Ø,3,4]ZZ

Ø Medical and Surgical
N Head and Facial Bones
B Excision Definition: Cutting out or off, without replacement, a portion of a body part
Explanation: The qualifier DIAGNOSTIC is used to identify excision procedures that are biopsies

Body Part Character 4	Approach Character 5	Device Character 6	Qualifier Character 7
Ø Skull **1 Frontal Bone** Zygomatic process of frontal bone **3 Parietal Bone, Right** **4 Parietal Bone, Left** **5 Temporal Bone, Right** Mastoid process Petrous part of temporal bone Tympanic part of temporal bone Zygomatic process of temporal bone **6 Temporal Bone, Left** *See 5 Temporal Bone, Right* **7 Occipital Bone** Foramen magnum **B Nasal Bone** Vomer of nasal septum **C Sphenoid Bone** Greater wing Lesser wing Optic foramen Pterygoid process Sella turcica **F Ethmoid Bone, Right** Cribriform plate **G Ethmoid Bone, Left** *See F Ethmoid Bone, Right* **H Lacrimal Bone, Right** **J Lacrimal Bone, Left** **K Palatine Bone, Right** **L Palatine Bone, Left** **M Zygomatic Bone, Right** **N Zygomatic Bone, Left** **P Orbit, Right** Bony orbit Orbital portion of ethmoid bone Orbital portion of frontal bone Orbital portion of lacrimal bone Orbital portion of maxilla Orbital portion of palatine bone Orbital portion of sphenoid bone Orbital portion of zygomatic bone **Q Orbit, Left** *See P Orbit, Right* **R Maxilla** Alveolar process of maxilla **T Mandible, Right** Alveolar process of mandible Condyloid process Mandibular notch Mental foramen **V Mandible, Left** *See T Mandible, Right* **X Hyoid Bone**	**Ø Open** **3 Percutaneous** **4 Percutaneous Endoscopic**	**Z No Device**	**X Diagnostic** **Z No Qualifier**

Non-OR ØNB[B,R,T,V][Ø,3,4]ZX

Ø Medical and Surgical
N Head and Facial Bones
C Extirpation Definition: Taking or cutting out solid matter from a body part

Explanation: The solid matter may be an abnormal byproduct of a biological function or a foreign body; it may be imbedded in a body part or in the lumen of a tubular body part. The solid matter may or may not have been previously broken into pieces.

Body Part Character 4	Approach Character 5	Device Character 6	Qualifier Character 7
1 Frontal Bone Zygomatic process of frontal bone **3 Parietal Bone, Right** **4 Parietal Bone, Left** **5 Temporal Bone, Right** Mastoid process Petrous part of temporal bone Tympanic part of temporal bone Zygomatic process of temporal bone **6 Temporal Bone, Left** *See 5 Temporal Bone, Right* **7 Occipital Bone** Foramen magnum **B Nasal Bone** Vomer of nasal septum **C Sphenoid Bone** Greater wing Lesser wing Optic foramen Pterygoid process Sella turcica **F Ethmoid Bone, Right** Cribriform plate **G Ethmoid Bone, Left** *See F Ethmoid Bone, Right* **H Lacrimal Bone, Right** **J Lacrimal Bone, Left** **K Palatine Bone, Right** **L Palatine Bone, Left** **M Zygomatic Bone, Right** **N Zygomatic Bone, Left** **P Orbit, Right** Bony orbit Orbital portion of ethmoid bone Orbital portion of frontal bone Orbital portion of lacrimal bone Orbital portion of maxilla Orbital portion of palatine bone Orbital portion of sphenoid bone Orbital portion of zygomatic bone **Q Orbit, Left** *See P Orbit, Right* **R Maxilla** Alveolar process of maxilla **T Mandible, Right** Alveolar process of mandible Condyloid process Mandibular notch Mental foramen **V Mandible, Left** *See T Mandible, Right* **X Hyoid Bone**	**Ø Open** **3 Percutaneous** **4 Percutaneous Endoscopic**	**Z No Device**	**Z No Qualifier**

Non-OR ØNC[B,R,T,V][Ø,3,4]ZZ

Ø Medical and Surgical
N Head and Facial Bones
D Extraction Definition: Pulling or stripping out or off all or a portion of a body part by the use of force
Explanation: The qualifier DIAGNOSTIC is used to identify extraction procedures that are biopsies

Body Part Character 4	Approach Character 5	Device Character 6	Qualifier Character 7
Ø Skull **1 Frontal Bone** Zygomatic process of frontal bone **3 Parietal Bone, Right** **4 Parietal Bone, Left** **5 Temporal Bone, Right** Mastoid process Petrous part of temporal bone Tympanic part of temporal bone Zygomatic process of temporal bone **6 Temporal Bone, Left** *See 5 Temporal Bone, Right* **7 Occipital Bone** Foramen magnum **B Nasal Bone** Vomer of nasal septum **C Sphenoid Bone** Greater wing Lesser wing Optic foramen Pterygoid process Sella turcica **F Ethmoid Bone, Right** Cribriform plate **G Ethmoid Bone, Left** *See F Ethmoid Bone, Right* **H Lacrimal Bone, Right** **J Lacrimal Bone, Left** **K Palatine Bone, Right** **L Palatine Bone, Left** **M Zygomatic Bone, Right** **N Zygomatic Bone, Left** **P Orbit, Right** Bony orbit Orbital portion of ethmoid bone Orbital portion of frontal bone Orbital portion of lacrimal bone Orbital portion of maxilla Orbital portion of palatine bone Orbital portion of sphenoid bone Orbital portion of zygomatic bone **Q Orbit, Left** *See P Orbit, Right* **R Maxilla** Alveolar process of maxilla **T Mandible, Right** Alveolar process of mandible Condyloid process Mandibular notch Mental foramen **V Mandible, Left** *See T Mandible, Right* **X Hyoid Bone**	**Ø Open**	**Z No Device**	**Z No Qualifier**

Ø Medical and Surgical
N Head and Facial Bones
H Insertion Definition: Putting in a nonbiological appliance that monitors, assists, performs, or prevents a physiological function but does not physically take the place of a body part

Explanation: None

Body Part Character 4	Approach Character 5	Device Character 6	Qualifier Character 7
Ø Skull	**Ø Open**	**3 Infusion Device** **4 Internal Fixation Device** **5 External Fixation Device** **M Bone Growth Stimulator** **N Neurostimulator Generator**	**Z No Qualifier**
Ø Skull	**3 Percutaneous** **4 Percutaneous Endoscopic**	**3 Infusion Device** **4 Internal Fixation Device** **5 External Fixation Device** **M Bone Growth Stimulator**	**Z No Qualifier**
1 Frontal Bone Zygomatic process of frontal bone **3 Parietal Bone, Right** **4 Parietal Bone, Left** **7 Occipital Bone** Foramen magnum **C Sphenoid Bone** Greater wing Lesser wing Optic foramen Pterygoid process Sella turcica **F Ethmoid Bone, Right** Cribriform plate **G Ethmoid Bone, Left** *See F Ethmoid Bone, Right* **H Lacrimal Bone, Right** **J Lacrimal Bone, Left** **K Palatine Bone, Right** **L Palatine Bone, Left** **M Zygomatic Bone, Right** **N Zygomatic Bone, Left** **P Orbit, Right** Bony orbit Orbital portion of ethmoid bone Orbital portion of frontal bone Orbital portion of lacrimal bone Orbital portion of maxilla Orbital portion of palatine bone Orbital portion of sphenoid bone Orbital portion of zygomatic bone **Q Orbit, Left** *See P Orbit, Right* **X Hyoid Bone**	**Ø Open** **3 Percutaneous** **4 Percutaneous Endoscopic**	**4 Internal Fixation Device**	**Z No Qualifier**
5 Temporal Bone, Right Mastoid process Petrous part of temporal bone Tympanic part of temporal bone Zygomatic process of temporal bone **6 Temporal Bone, Left** *See 5 Temporal Bone, Right*	**Ø Open** **3 Percutaneous** **4 Percutaneous Endoscopic**	**4 Internal Fixation Device** **S Hearing Device**	**Z No Qualifier**
B Nasal Bone Vomer of nasal septum	**Ø Open** **3 Percutaneous** **4 Percutaneous Endoscopic**	**4 Internal Fixation Device** **M Bone Growth Stimulator**	**Z No Qualifier**
R Maxilla Alveolar process of maxilla **T Mandible, Right** Alveolar process of mandible Condyloid process Mandibular notch Mental foramen **V Mandible, Left** *See T Mandible, Right*	**Ø Open** **3 Percutaneous** **4 Percutaneous Endoscopic**	**4 Internal Fixation Device** **5 External Fixation Device**	**Z No Qualifier**
W Facial Bone	**Ø Open** **3 Percutaneous** **4 Percutaneous Endoscopic**	**M Bone Growth Stimulator**	**Z No Qualifier**

Non-OR ØNHØØ5Z
Non-OR ØNHØ[3,4]5Z
Non-OR ØNHB[Ø,3,4][4,M]Z

See Appendix L for Procedure Combinations
ØNHØØNZ

Ø Medical and Surgical
N Head and Facial Bones
J Inspection Definition: Visually and/or manually exploring a body part

Explanation: Visual exploration may be performed with or without optical instrumentation. Manual exploration may be performed directly or through intervening body layers.

Body Part Character 4	Approach Character 5	Device Character 6	Qualifier Character 7
Ø Skull B Nasal Bone Vomer of nasal septum W Facial Bone	Ø Open 3 Percutaneous 4 Percutaneous Endoscopic X External	Z No Device	Z No Qualifier

Non-OR ØNJ[Ø,B,W][3,X]ZZ

Ø Medical and Surgical
N Head and Facial Bones
N Release Definition: Freeing a body part from an abnormal physical constraint by cutting or by the use of force

Explanation: Some of the restraining tissue may be taken out but none of the body part is taken out

Body Part Character 4	Approach Character 5	Device Character 6	Qualifier Character 7
1 Frontal Bone Zygomatic process of frontal bone 3 Parietal Bone, Right 4 Parietal Bone, Left 5 Temporal Bone, Right Mastoid process Petrous part of temporal bone Tympanic part of temporal bone Zygomatic process of temporal bone 6 Temporal Bone, Left *See 5 Temporal Bone, Right* 7 Occipital Bone Foramen magnum B Nasal Bone Vomer of nasal septum C Sphenoid Bone Greater wing Lesser wing Optic foramen Pterygoid process Sella turcica F Ethmoid Bone, Right Cribriform plate G Ethmoid Bone, Left *See F Ethmoid Bone, Right* H Lacrimal Bone, Right J Lacrimal Bone, Left K Palatine Bone, Right L Palatine Bone, Left M Zygomatic Bone, Right N Zygomatic Bone, Left P Orbit, Right Bony orbit Orbital portion of ethmoid bone Orbital portion of frontal bone Orbital portion of lacrimal bone Orbital portion of maxilla Orbital portion of palatine bone Orbital portion of sphenoid bone Orbital portion of zygomatic bone Q Orbit, Left *See P Orbit, Right* R Maxilla Alveolar process of maxilla T Mandible, Right Alveolar process of mandible Condyloid process Mandibular notch Mental foramen V Mandible, Left *See T Mandible, Right* X Hyoid Bone	Ø Open 3 Percutaneous 4 Percutaneous Endoscopic	Z No Device	Z No Qualifier

Non-OR ØNNB[Ø,3,4]ZZ

Ø Medical and Surgical
N Head and Facial Bones
P Removal

Definition: Taking out or off a device from a body part

Explanation: If a device is taken out and a similar device put in without cutting or puncturing the skin or mucous membrane, the procedure is coded to the root operation CHANGE. Otherwise, the procedure for taking out a device is coded to the root operation REMOVAL.

Body Part Character 4	Approach Character 5	Device Character 6	Qualifier Character 7
Ø Skull	Ø Open	Ø Drainage Device 3 Infusion Device 4 Internal Fixation Device 5 External Fixation Device 7 Autologous Tissue Substitute J Synthetic Substitute K Nonautologous Tissue Substitute M Bone Growth Stimulator N Neurostimulator Generator S Hearing Device	Z No Qualifier
Ø Skull	3 Percutaneous 4 Percutaneous Endoscopic	Ø Drainage Device 3 Infusion Device 4 Internal Fixation Device 5 External Fixation Device 7 Autologous Tissue Substitute J Synthetic Substitute K Nonautologous Tissue Substitute M Bone Growth Stimulator S Hearing Device	Z No Qualifier
Ø Skull	X External	Ø Drainage Device 3 Infusion Device 4 Internal Fixation Device 5 External Fixation Device M Bone Growth Stimulator S Hearing Device	Z No Qualifier
B Nasal Bone Vomer of nasal septum W Facial Bone	Ø Open 3 Percutaneous 4 Percutaneous Endoscopic	Ø Drainage Device 4 Internal Fixation Device 7 Autologous Tissue Substitute J Synthetic Substitute K Nonautologous Tissue Substitute M Bone Growth Stimulator	Z No Qualifier
B Nasal Bone Vomer of nasal septum W Facial Bone	X External	Ø Drainage Device 4 Internal Fixation Device M Bone Growth Stimulator	Z No Qualifier

Non-OR ØNPØ[3,4]5Z
Non-OR ØNPØX[Ø,3,5]Z
Non-OR ØNPB[Ø,3,4][Ø,4,7,J,K,M]Z
Non-OR ØNPBX[Ø,4,M]Z
Non-OR ØNPWX[Ø,M]Z

Ø Medical and Surgical
N Head and Facial Bones
Q Repair Definition: Restoring, to the extent possible, a body part to its normal anatomic structure and function
Explanation: Used only when the method to accomplish the repair is not one of the other root operations

Body Part Character 4	Approach Character 5	Device Character 6	Qualifier Character 7
Ø Skull 1 Frontal Bone Zygomatic process of frontal bone 3 Parietal Bone, Right 4 Parietal Bone, Left 5 Temporal Bone, Right Mastoid process Petrous part of temporal bone Tympanic part of temporal bone Zygomatic process of temporal bone 6 Temporal Bone, Left *See 5 Temporal Bone, Right* 7 Occipital Bone Foramen magnum B Nasal Bone Vomer of nasal septum C Sphenoid Bone Greater wing Lesser wing Optic foramen Pterygoid process Sella turcica F Ethmoid Bone, Right Cribriform plate G Ethmoid Bone, Left *See F Ethmoid Bone, Right* H Lacrimal Bone, Right J Lacrimal Bone, Left K Palatine Bone, Right L Palatine Bone, Left M Zygomatic Bone, Right N Zygomatic Bone, Left P Orbit, Right Bony orbit Orbital portion of ethmoid bone Orbital portion of frontal bone Orbital portion of lacrimal bone Orbital portion of maxilla Orbital portion of palatine bone Orbital portion of sphenoid bone Orbital portion of zygomatic bone Q Orbit, Left *See P Orbit, Right* R Maxilla Alveolar process of maxilla T Mandible, Right Alveolar process of mandible Condyloid process Mandibular notch Mental foramen V Mandible, Left *See T Mandible, Right* X Hyoid Bone	Ø Open 3 Percutaneous 4 Percutaneous Endoscopic X External	Z No Device	Z No Qualifier

Non-OR ØNQ[Ø,1,3,4,5,6,7,B,C,F,G,H,J,K,L,M,N,P,Q,R,T,V,X]XZZ

Ø Medical and Surgical
N Head and Facial Bones
R Replacement Definition: Putting in or on biological or synthetic material that physically takes the place and/or function of all or a portion of a body part

Explanation: The body part may have been taken out or replaced, or may be taken out, physically eradicated, or rendered nonfunctional during the REPLACEMENT procedure. A REMOVAL procedure is coded for taking out the device used in a previous replacement procedure.

Body Part Character 4	Approach Character 5	Device Character 6	Qualifier Character 7
Ø Skull **1 Frontal Bone** Zygomatic process of frontal bone **3 Parietal Bone, Right** **4 Parietal Bone, Left** **5 Temporal Bone, Right** Mastoid process Petrous part of temporal bone Tympanic part of temporal bone Zygomatic process of temporal bone **6 Temporal Bone, Left** *See 5 Temporal Bone, Right* **7 Occipital Bone** Foramen magnum **B Nasal Bone** Vomer of nasal septum **C Sphenoid Bone** Greater wing Lesser wing Optic foramen Pterygoid process Sella turcica **F Ethmoid Bone, Right** Cribriform plate **G Ethmoid Bone, Left** *See F Ethmoid Bone, Right* **H Lacrimal Bone, Right** **J Lacrimal Bone, Left** **K Palatine Bone, Right** **L Palatine Bone, Left** **M Zygomatic Bone, Right** **N Zygomatic Bone, Left** **P Orbit, Right** Bony orbit Orbital portion of ethmoid bone Orbital portion of frontal bone Orbital portion of lacrimal bone Orbital portion of maxilla Orbital portion of palatine bone Orbital portion of sphenoid bone Orbital portion of zygomatic bone **Q Orbit, Left** *See P Orbit, Right* **R Maxilla** Alveolar process of maxilla **T Mandible, Right** Alveolar process of mandible Condyloid process Mandibular notch Mental foramen **V Mandible, Left** *See T Mandible, Right* **X Hyoid Bone**	**Ø Open** **3 Percutaneous** **4 Percutaneous Endoscopic**	**7 Autologous Tissue Substitute** **J Synthetic Substitute** **K Nonautologous Tissue Substitute**	**Z No Qualifier**

Ø Medical and Surgical
N Head and Facial Bones
S Reposition Definition: Moving to its normal location, or other suitable location, all or a portion of a body part

Explanation: The body part is moved to a new location from an abnormal location, or from a normal location where it is not functioning correctly. The body part may or may not be cut out or off to be moved to the new location.

Body Part Character 4	Approach Character 5	Device Character 6	Qualifier Character 7
Ø Skull **R** Maxilla Alveolar process of maxilla **T** Mandible, Right Alveolar process of mandible Condyloid process Mandibular notch Mental foramen **V** Mandible, Left *See T Mandible, Right*	**Ø** Open **3** Percutaneous **4** Percutaneous Endoscopic	**4** Internal Fixation Device **5** External Fixation Device **Z** No Device	**Z** No Qualifier
Ø Skull **R** Maxilla Alveolar process of maxilla **T** Mandible, Right Alveolar process of mandible Condyloid process Mandibular notch Mental foramen **V** Mandible, Left *See T Mandible, Right*	**X** External	**Z** No Device	**Z** No Qualifier
1 Frontal Bone Zygomatic process of frontal bone **3** Parietal Bone, Right **4** Parietal Bone, Left **5** Temporal Bone, Right Mastoid process Petrous part of temporal bone Tympanic part of temporal bone Zygomatic process of temporal bone **6** Temporal Bone, Left *See 5 Temporal Bone, Right* **7** Occipital Bone Foramen magnum **B** Nasal Bone Vomer of nasal septum **C** Sphenoid Bone Greater wing Lesser wing Optic foramen Pterygoid process Sella turcica **F** Ethmoid Bone, Right Cribriform plate **G** Ethmoid Bone, Left *See F Ethmoid Bone, Right* **H** Lacrimal Bone, Right **J** Lacrimal Bone, Left **K** Palatine Bone, Right **L** Palatine Bone, Left **M** Zygomatic Bone, Right **N** Zygomatic Bone, Left **P** Orbit, Right Bony orbit Orbital portion of ethmoid bone Orbital portion of frontal bone Orbital portion of lacrimal bone Orbital portion of maxilla Orbital portion of palatine bone Orbital portion of sphenoid bone Orbital portion of zygomatic bone **Q** Orbit, Left *See P Orbit, Right* **X** Hyoid Bone	**Ø** Open **3** Percutaneous **4** Percutaneous Endoscopic	**4** Internal Fixation Device **Z** No Device	**Z** No Qualifier

Non-OR ØNS[R,T,V][3,4][4,5,Z]Z
Non-OR ØNS[Ø,R,T,V]XZZ
Non-OR ØNS[B,C,F,G,H,J,K,L,M,N,P,Q,X][3,4][4,Z]Z

ØNS Continued on next page

ØNS Continued

Ø Medical and Surgical
N Head and Facial Bones
S Reposition

Definition: Moving to its normal location, or other suitable location, all or a portion of a body part

Explanation: The body part is moved to a new location from an abnormal location, or from a normal location where it is not functioning correctly. The body part may or may not be cut out or off to be moved to the new location.

Body Part Character 4	Approach Character 5	Device Character 6	Qualifier Character 7
1 Frontal Bone Zygomatic process of frontal bone **3 Parietal Bone, Right** **4 Parietal Bone, Left** **5 Temporal Bone, Right** Mastoid process Petrous part of temporal bone Tympanic part of temporal bone Zygomatic process of temporal bone **6 Temporal Bone, Left** *See 5 Temporal Bone, Right* **7 Occipital Bone** Foramen magnum **B Nasal Bone** Vomer of nasal septum **C Sphenoid Bone** Greater wing Lesser wing Optic foramen Pterygoid process Sella turcica **F Ethmoid Bone, Right** Cribriform plate **G Ethmoid Bone, Left** *See F Ethmoid Bone, Right* **H Lacrimal Bone, Right** **J Lacrimal Bone, Left** **K Palatine Bone, Right** **L Palatine Bone, Left** **M Zygomatic Bone, Right** **N Zygomatic Bone, Left** **P Orbit, Right** Bony orbit Orbital portion of ethmoid bone Orbital portion of frontal bone Orbital portion of lacrimal bone Orbital portion of maxilla Orbital portion of palatine bone Orbital portion of sphenoid bone Orbital portion of zygomatic bone **Q Orbit, Left** *See P Orbit, Right* **X Hyoid Bone**	**X External**	**Z No Device**	**Z No Qualifier**

Non-OR ØNS[1,3,4,5,6,7,B,C,F,G,H,J,K,L,M,N,P,Q,X]XZZ

Ø Medical and Surgical
N Head and Facial Bones
T Resection Definition: Cutting out or off, without replacement, all of a body part
Explanation: None

Body Part Character 4	Approach Character 5	Device Character 6	Qualifier Character 7
1 Frontal Bone Zygomatic process of frontal bone **3 Parietal Bone, Right** **4 Parietal Bone, Left** **5 Temporal Bone, Right** Mastoid process Petrous part of temporal bone Tympanic part of temporal bone Zygomatic process of temporal bone **6 Temporal Bone, Left** *See 5 Temporal Bone, Right* **7 Occipital Bone** Foramen magnum **B Nasal Bone** Vomer of nasal septum **C Sphenoid Bone** Greater wing Lesser wing Optic foramen Pterygoid process Sella turcica **F Ethmoid Bone, Right** Cribriform plate **G Ethmoid Bone, Left** *See F Ethmoid Bone, Right* **H Lacrimal Bone, Right** **J Lacrimal Bone, Left** **K Palatine Bone, Right** **L Palatine Bone, Left** **M Zygomatic Bone, Right** **N Zygomatic Bone, Left** **P Orbit, Right** Bony orbit Orbital portion of ethmoid bone Orbital portion of frontal bone Orbital portion of lacrimal bone Orbital portion of maxilla Orbital portion of palatine bone Orbital portion of sphenoid bone Orbital portion of zygomatic bone **Q Orbit, Left** *See P Orbit, Right* **R Maxilla** Alveolar process of maxilla **T Mandible, Right** Alveolar process of mandible Condyloid process Mandibular notch Mental foramen **V Mandible, Left** *See T Mandible, Right* **X Hyoid Bone**	**Ø Open**	**Z No Device**	**Z No Qualifier**

Ø Medical and Surgical
N Head and Facial Bones
U Supplement Definition: Putting in or on biological or synthetic material that physically reinforces and/or augments the function of a portion of a body part

Explanation: The biological material is non-living, or is living and from the same individual. The body part may have been previously replaced, and the SUPPLEMENT procedure is performed to physically reinforce and/or augment the function of the replaced body part.

Body Part Character 4	Approach Character 5	Device Character 6	Qualifier Character 7
Ø Skull **1 Frontal Bone** Zygomatic process of frontal bone **3 Parietal Bone, Right** **4 Parietal Bone, Left** **5 Temporal Bone, Right** Mastoid process Petrous part of temporal bone Tympanic part of temporal bone Zygomatic process of temporal bone **6 Temporal Bone, Left** *See 5 Temporal Bone, Right* **7 Occipital Bone** Foramen magnum **B Nasal Bone** Vomer of nasal septum **C Sphenoid Bone** Greater wing Lesser wing Optic foramen Pterygoid process Sella turcica **F Ethmoid Bone, Right** Cribriform plate **G Ethmoid Bone, Left** *See F Ethmoid Bone, Right* **H Lacrimal Bone, Right** **J Lacrimal Bone, Left** **K Palatine Bone, Right** **L Palatine Bone, Left** **M Zygomatic Bone, Right** **N Zygomatic Bone, Left** **P Orbit, Right** Bony orbit Orbital portion of ethmoid bone Orbital portion of frontal bone Orbital portion of lacrimal bone Orbital portion of maxilla Orbital portion of palatine bone Orbital portion of sphenoid bone Orbital portion of zygomatic bone **Q Orbit, Left** *See P Orbit, Right* **R Maxilla** Alveolar process of maxilla **T Mandible, Right** Alveolar process of mandible Condyloid process Mandibular notch Mental foramen **V Mandible, Left** *See T Mandible, Right* **X Hyoid Bone**	**Ø Open** **3 Percutaneous** **4 Percutaneous Endoscopic**	**7 Autologous Tissue Substitute** **J Synthetic Substitute** **K Nonautologous Tissue Substitute**	**Z No Qualifier**

Ø Medical and Surgical
N Head and Facial Bones
W Revision

Definition: Correcting, to the extent possible, a portion of a malfunctioning device or the position of a displaced device

Explanation: Revision can include correcting a malfunctioning or displaced device by taking out or putting in components of the device such as a screw or pin

Body Part Character 4	Approach Character 5	Device Character 6	Qualifier Character 7
Ø Skull	Ø Open	Ø Drainage Device 3 Infusion Device 4 Internal Fixation Device 5 External Fixation Device 7 Autologous Tissue Substitute J Synthetic Substitute K Nonautologous Tissue Substitute M Bone Growth Stimulator N Neurostimulator Generator S Hearing Device	Z No Qualifier
Ø Skull	3 Percutaneous 4 Percutaneous Endoscopic X External	Ø Drainage Device 3 Infusion Device 4 Internal Fixation Device 5 External Fixation Device 7 Autologous Tissue Substitute J Synthetic Substitute K Nonautologous Tissue Substitute M Bone Growth Stimulator S Hearing Device	Z No Qualifier
B Nasal Bone Vomer of nasal septum W Facial Bone	Ø Open 3 Percutaneous 4 Percutaneous Endoscopic X External	Ø Drainage Device 4 Internal Fixation Device 7 Autologous Tissue Substitute J Synthetic Substitute K Nonautologous Tissue Substitute M Bone Growth Stimulator	Z No Qualifier

Non-OR ØNWØX[Ø,3,4,5,7,J,K,M,S]Z
Non-OR ØNWB[Ø,3,4,X][Ø,4,7,J,K,M]Z
Non-OR ØNWWX[Ø,4,7,J,K,M]Z

Upper Bones ØP2–ØPW

Character Meanings

This Character Meaning table is provided as a guide to assist the user in the identification of character members that may be found in this section of code tables. It **SHOULD NOT** be used to build a PCS code.

Operation–Character 3	Body Part–Character 4	Approach–Character 5	Device–Character 6	Qualifier–Character 7
2 Change	Ø Sternum	Ø Open	Ø Drainage Device OR Internal Fixation Device, Rigid Plate	3 Laser Interstitial Thermal Therapy
5 Destruction	1 Ribs, 1 to 2	3 Percutaneous	3 Spinal Stabilization Device, Vertebral Body Tether	X Diagnostic
8 Division	2 Ribs, 3 or more	4 Percutaneous Endoscopic	4 Internal Fixation Device	Z No Qualifier
9 Drainage	3 Cervical Vertebra	X External	5 External Fixation Device	
B Excision	4 Thoracic Vertebra		6 Internal Fixation Device, Intramedullary	
C Extirpation	5 Scapula, Right		7 Autologous Tissue Substitute OR Internal Fixation Device, Intramedullary Limb Lengthening	
D Extraction	6 Scapula, Left		8 External Fixation Device, Limb Lengthening	
H Insertion	7 Glenoid Cavity, Right		B External Fixation Device, Monoplanar	
J Inspection	8 Glenoid Cavity, Left		C External Fixation Device, Ring	
N Release	9 Clavicle, Right		D External Fixation Device, Hybrid	
P Removal	B Clavicle, Left		J Synthetic Substitute	
Q Repair	C Humeral Head, Right		K Nonautologous Tissue Substitute	
R Replacement	D Humeral Head, Left		M Bone Growth Stimulator	
S Reposition	F Humeral Shaft, Right		Y Other Device	
T Resection	G Humeral Shaft, Left		Z No Device	
U Supplement	H Radius, Right			
W Revision	J Radius, Left			
	K Ulna, Right			
	L Ulna, Left			
	M Carpal, Right			
	N Carpal, Left			
	P Metacarpal, Right			
	Q Metacarpal, Left			
	R Thumb Phalanx, Right			
	S Thumb Phalanx, Left			
	T Finger Phalanx, Right			
	V Finger Phalanx, Left			
	Y Upper Bone			

AHA Coding Clinic for table ØP5
2023, 1Q, 10 Laser interstitial thermal therapy

AHA Coding Clinic for table ØPB
2023, 2Q, 30 Excisional debridement and non-excisional debridement at deeper layer same site
2015, 3Q, 3-8 Excisional and nonexcisional debridement
2015, 2Q, 34 Decompressive laminectomy
2013, 4Q, 109 Separating conjoined twins
2013, 4Q, 116 Spinal decompression
2013, 3Q, 20 Superior labrum anterior posterior (SLAP) repair and subacromial decompression
2012, 4Q, 101 Rib resection with reconstruction of anterior chest wall
2012, 2Q, 19 Multiple decompressive cervical laminectomies

AHA Coding Clinic for table ØPC
2021, 3Q, 15 Curettage of bilateral humeral head and bone graft placement
2019, 3Q, 19 Removal of sternal wire

AHA Coding Clinic for table ØPD
2023, 2Q, 30 Excisional debridement and non-excisional debridement at deeper layer same site
2017, 4Q, 41 Extraction procedures

AHA Coding Clinic for table ØPH
2020, 1Q, 29 Repair of sternal dehiscence using Sternal Talon® device
2019, 4Q, 34 Intramedullary limb lengthening internal fixation device
2019, 2Q, 40 Decompression of spinal cord and placement of instrumentation
2018, 3Q, 26 Anterior vertebral tethering using Dynesys Tethering System
2017, 2Q, 20 Exchange of intramedullary antibiotic impregnated spacer
2016, 4Q, 117 Placement of magnetic growth rods
2014, 4Q, 28 Removal and replacement of displaced growing rods

AHA Coding Clinic for table ØPP
2019, 3Q, 19 Removal of sternal wire
2017, 2Q, 20 Exchange of intramedullary antibiotic impregnated spacer
2016, 4Q, 117 Placement of magnetic growth rods
2014, 4Q, 28 Removal and replacement of displaced growing rods

AHA Coding Clinic for table ØPR
2018, 4Q, 92 Radial head arthroplasty

AHA Coding Clinic for table ØPS
2021, 4Q, 51-52 Vertebral body tethering
2020, 1Q, 33 Spinal fusion without use of bone graft
2018, 3Q, 26 Anterior vertebral tethering using Dynesys Tethering System
2017, 4Q, 53 New and revised body part values - Ribs
2016, 1Q, 21 Elongation derotation flexion casting
2015, 4Q, 33 Ravitch operation
2015, 2Q, 35 Application of tongs to reduce and stabilize cervical fracture
2014, 4Q, 26 Placement of vertical expandable prosthetic titanium rib (VEPTR)
2014, 4Q, 32 Open reduction internal fixation of fracture with debridement
2014, 3Q, 33 Radial fracture treatment with open reduction internal fixation, and release of carpal ligament

AHA Coding Clinic for table ØPT
2015, 3Q, 26 Thumb arthroplasty with resection of trapezium

AHA Coding Clinic for table ØPU
2023, 2Q, 24 Remplissage of subscapularis tendon
2021, 3Q, 15 Curettage of bilateral humeral head and bone graft placement
2015, 2Q, 20 Cervical laminoplasty
2013, 4Q, 109 Separating conjoined twins

AHA Coding Clinic for table ØPW
2014, 4Q, 26 Adjustment of VEPTR lengthening mechanism
2014, 4Q, 27 Bilateral lengthening of growing rods

Upper Bones

Cervical vertebra 3
Clavicle 9, B
Sternum Ø
Scapula 5, 6
Rib 1, 2
Humerus C, D, F, G
Thoracic vertebra 4
Ulna K, L
Radius H, J
Carpal M, N
Metacarpal P, Q
Thumb phalanx R, S
Finger phalanx T, V

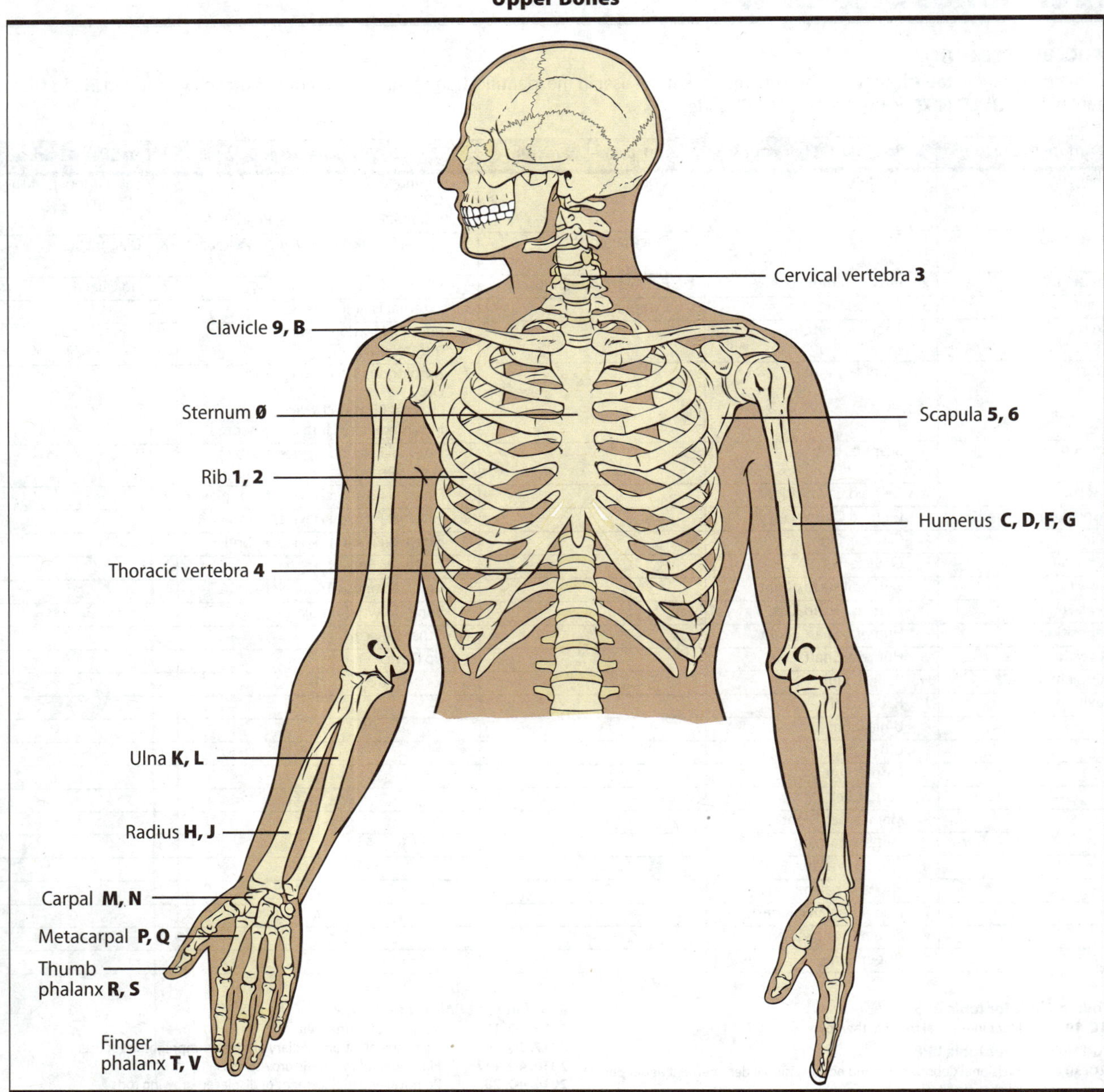

Humerus and Scapula

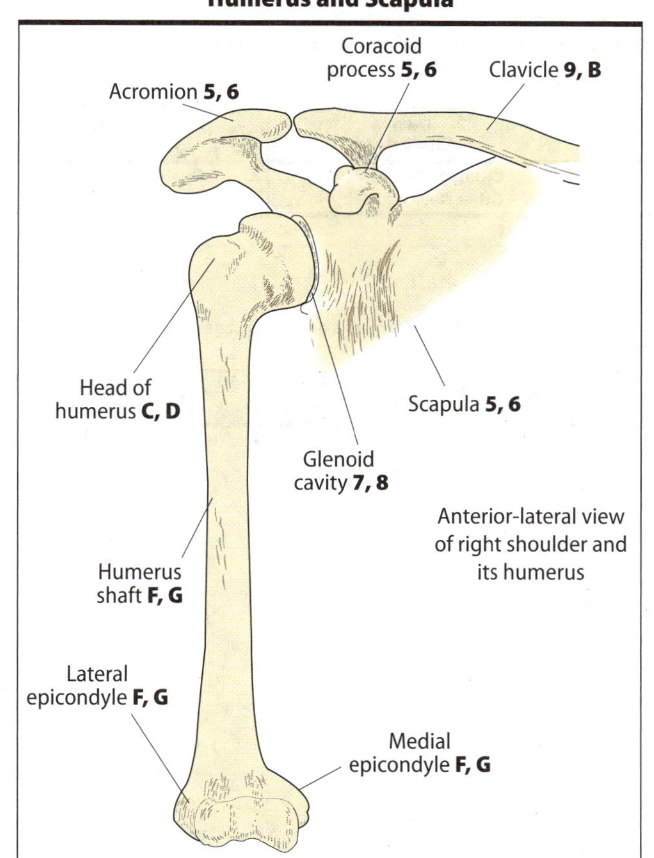

Radius and Ulna

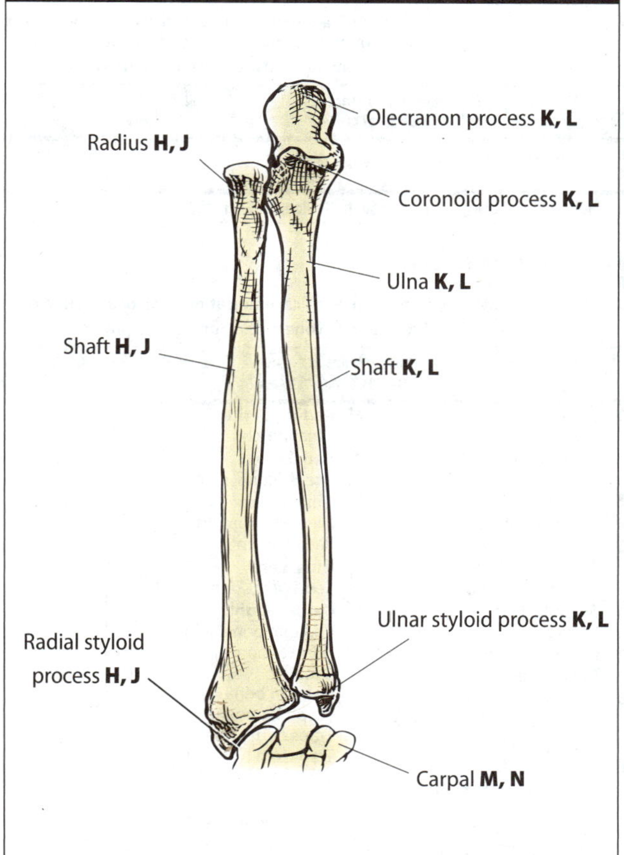

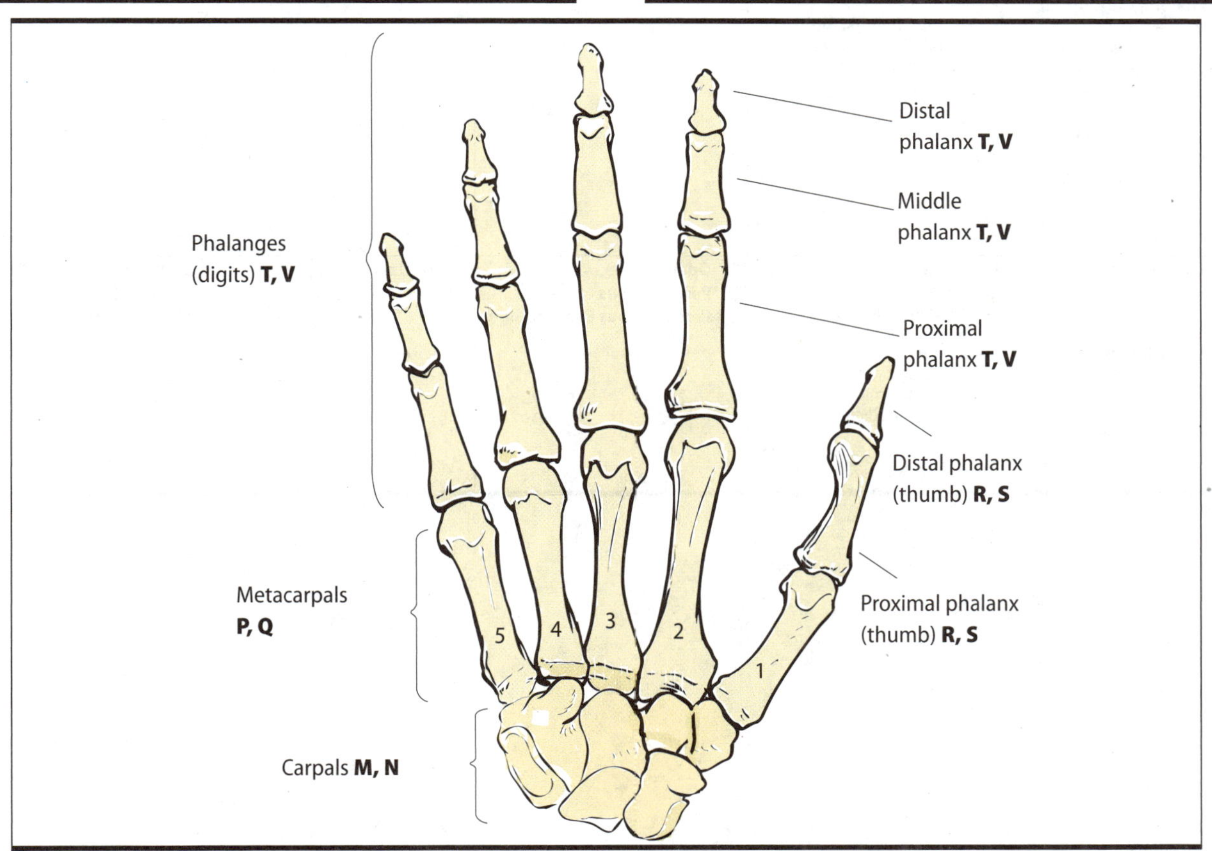

Ø Medical and Surgical
P Upper Bones
2 Change

Definition: Taking out or off a device from a body part and putting back an identical or similar device in or on the same body part without cutting or puncturing the skin or a mucous membrane

Explanation: All CHANGE procedures are coded using the approach EXTERNAL

Body Part Character 4	Approach Character 5	Device Character 6	Qualifier Character 7
Y Upper Bone	X External	Ø Drainage Device Y Other Device	Z No Qualifier

Non-OR All body part, approach, device, and qualifier values

Ø Medical and Surgical
P Upper Bones
5 Destruction

Definition: Physical eradication of all or a portion of a body part by the direct use of energy, force, or a destructive agent

Explanation: None of the body part is physically taken out

Body Part Character 4	Body Part Character 4 (cont.)	Approach Character 5	Device Character 6	Qualifier Character 7
Ø Sternum Manubrium Suprasternal notch Xiphoid process **1 Ribs, 1 to 2** **2 Ribs, 3 or More** **5 Scapula, Right** Acromion (process) Coracoid process **6 Scapula, Left** *See 5 Scapula, Right* **7 Glenoid Cavity, Right** Glenoid fossa (of scapula) **8 Glenoid Cavity, Left** *See 7 Glenoid Cavity, Right* **9 Clavicle, Right** **B Clavicle, Left** **C Humeral Head, Right** Greater tuberosity Lesser tuberosity Neck of humerus (anatomical)(surgical) **D Humeral Head, Left** *See C Humeral Head, Right* **F Humeral Shaft, Right** Distal humerus Humerus, distal Lateral epicondyle of humerus Medial epicondyle of humerus **G Humeral Shaft, Left** *See F Humeral Shaft, Right*	**H Radius, Right** Ulnar notch **J Radius, Left** *See H Radius, Right* **K Ulna, Right** Olecranon process Radial notch **L Ulna, Left** *See K Ulna, Right* **M Carpal, Right** Capitate bone Hamate bone Lunate bone Pisiform bone Scaphoid bone Trapezium bone Trapezoid bone Triquetral bone **N Carpal, Left** *See M Carpal, Right* **P Metacarpal, Right** **Q Metacarpal, Left** **R Thumb Phalanx, Right** **S Thumb Phalanx, Left** **T Finger Phalanx, Right** **V Finger Phalanx, Left**	Ø Open 3 Percutaneous 4 Percutaneous Endoscopic	Z No Device	Z No Qualifier
3 Cervical Vertebra Dens Odontoid process Spinous process Transverse foramen Transverse process Vertebral arch Vertebral body Vertebral foramen Vertebral lamina Vertebral pedicle	**4 Thoracic Vertebra** Spinous process Transverse process Vertebral arch Vertebral body Vertebral foramen Vertebral lamina Vertebral pedicle	Ø Open 3 Percutaneous 4 Percutaneous Endoscopic	Z No Device	3 Laser Interstitial Thermal Therapy Z No Qualifier

Ø Medical and Surgical
P Upper Bones
8 Division

Definition: Cutting into a body part, without draining fluids and/or gases from the body part, in order to separate or transect a body part
Explanation: All or a portion of the body part is separated into two or more portions

Body Part Character 4	Approach Character 5	Device Character 6	Qualifier Character 7
Ø Sternum Manubrium Suprasternal notch Xiphoid process **1 Ribs, 1 to 2** **2 Ribs, 3 or More** **3 Cervical Vertebra** Dens Odontoid process Spinous process Transverse foramen Transverse process Vertebral arch Vertebral body Vertebral foramen Vertebral lamina Vertebral pedicle **4 Thoracic Vertebra** Spinous process Transverse process Vertebral arch Vertebral body Vertebral foramen Vertebral lamina Vertebral pedicle **5 Scapula, Right** Acromion (process) Coracoid process **6 Scapula, Left** *See 5 Scapula, Right* **7 Glenoid Cavity, Right** Glenoid fossa (of scapula) **8 Glenoid Cavity, Left** *See 7 Glenoid Cavity, Right* **9 Clavicle, Right** **B Clavicle, Left** **C Humeral Head, Right** Greater tuberosity Lesser tuberosity Neck of humerus (anatomical)(surgical) **D Humeral Head, Left** *See C Humeral Head, Right* **F Humeral Shaft, Right** Distal humerus Humerus, distal Lateral epicondyle of humerus Medial epicondyle of humerus **G Humeral Shaft, Left** *See F Humeral Shaft, Right* **H Radius, Right** Ulnar notch **J Radius, Left** *See H Radius, Right* **K Ulna, Right** Olecranon process Radial notch **L Ulna, Left** *See K Ulna, Right* **M Carpal, Right** Capitate bone Hamate bone Lunate bone Pisiform bone Scaphoid bone Trapezium bone Trapezoid bone Triquetral bone **N Carpal, Left** *See M Carpal, Right* **P Metacarpal, Right** **Q Metacarpal, Left** **R Thumb Phalanx, Right** **S Thumb Phalanx, Left** **T Finger Phalanx, Right** **V Finger Phalanx, Left**	**Ø Open** **3 Percutaneous** **4 Percutaneous Endoscopic**	**Z No Device**	**Z No Qualifier**

Ø Medical and Surgical
P Upper Bones
9 Drainage

Definition: Taking or letting out fluids and/or gases from a body part
Explanation: The qualifier DIAGNOSTIC is used to identify drainage procedures that are biopsies

Body Part Character 4		Approach Character 5	Device Character 6	Qualifier Character 7
Ø Sternum Manubrium Suprasternal notch Xiphoid process **1 Ribs, 1 to 2** **2 Ribs, 3 or More** **3 Cervical Vertebra** Dens Odontoid process Spinous process Transverse foramen Transverse process Vertebral arch Vertebral body Vertebral foramen Vertebral lamina Vertebral pedicle **4 Thoracic Vertebra** Spinous process Transverse process Vertebral arch Vertebral body Vertebral foramen Vertebral lamina Vertebral pedicle **5 Scapula, Right** Acromion (process) Coracoid process **6 Scapula, Left** *See 5 Scapula, Right* **7 Glenoid Cavity, Right** Glenoid fossa (of scapula) **8 Glenoid Cavity, Left** *See 7 Glenoid Cavity, Right* **9 Clavicle, Right** **B Clavicle, Left** **C Humeral Head, Right** Greater tuberosity Lesser tuberosity Neck of humerus (anatomical)(surgical)	**D Humeral Head, Left** *See C Humeral Head, Right* **F Humeral Shaft, Right** Distal humerus Humerus, distal Lateral epicondyle of humerus Medial epicondyle of humerus **G Humeral Shaft, Left** *See F Humeral Shaft, Right* **H Radius, Right** Ulnar notch **J Radius, Left** *See H Radius, Right* **K Ulna, Right** Olecranon process Radial notch **L Ulna, Left** *See K Ulna, Right* **M Carpal, Right** Capitate bone Hamate bone Lunate bone Pisiform bone Scaphoid bone Trapezium bone Trapezoid bone Triquetral bone **N Carpal, Left** *See M Carpal, Right* **P Metacarpal, Right** **Q Metacarpal, Left** **R Thumb Phalanx, Right** **S Thumb Phalanx, Left** **T Finger Phalanx, Right** **V Finger Phalanx, Left**	**Ø Open** **3 Percutaneous** **4 Percutaneous Endoscopic**	**Ø Drainage Device**	**Z No Qualifier**

Non-OR ØP9[Ø,1,2,3,4,5,6,7,8,9,B,C,D,F,G,H,J,K,L,M,N,P,Q,R,S,T,V]3ØZ

ØP9 Continued on next page

Ø Medical and Surgical
P Upper Bones
9 Drainage

ØP9 Continued

Definition: Taking or letting out fluids and/or gases from a body part
Explanation: The qualifier DIAGNOSTIC is used to identify drainage procedures that are biopsies

Body Part Character 4	Approach Character 5	Device Character 6	Qualifier Character 7
Ø Sternum Manubrium Suprasternal notch Xiphoid process **1 Ribs, 1 to 2** **2 Ribs, 3 or More** **3 Cervical Vertebra** Dens Odontoid process Spinous process Transverse foramen Transverse process Vertebral arch Vertebral body Vertebral foramen Vertebral lamina Vertebral pedicle **4 Thoracic Vertebra** Spinous process Transverse process Vertebral arch Vertebral body Vertebral foramen Vertebral lamina Vertebral pedicle **5 Scapula, Right** Acromion (process) Coracoid process **6 Scapula, Left** *See 5 Scapula, Right* **7 Glenoid Cavity, Right** Glenoid fossa (of scapula) **8 Glenoid Cavity, Left** *See 7 Glenoid Cavity, Right* **9 Clavicle, Right** **B Clavicle, Left** **C Humeral Head, Right** Greater tuberosity Lesser tuberosity Neck of humerus (anatomical)(surgical) **D Humeral Head, Left** *See C Humeral Head, Right* **F Humeral Shaft, Right** Distal humerus Humerus, distal Lateral epicondyle of humerus Medial epicondyle of humerus **G Humeral Shaft, Left** *See F Humeral Shaft, Right* **H Radius, Right** Ulnar notch **J Radius, Left** *See H Radius, Right* **K Ulna, Right** Olecranon process Radial notch **L Ulna, Left** *See K Ulna, Right* **M Carpal, Right** Capitate bone Hamate bone Lunate bone Pisiform bone Scaphoid bone Trapezium bone Trapezoid bone Triquetral bone **N Carpal, Left** *See M Carpal, Right* **P Metacarpal, Right** **Q Metacarpal, Left** **R Thumb Phalanx, Right** **S Thumb Phalanx, Left** **T Finger Phalanx, Right** **V Finger Phalanx, Left**	**Ø Open** **3 Percutaneous** **4 Percutaneous Endoscopic**	**Z No Device**	**X Diagnostic** **Z No Qualifier**

Non-OR ØP9[Ø,1,2,3,4,5,6,7,8,9,B,C,D,F,G,H,J,K,L,M,N,P,Q,R,S,T,V]3ZZ

Ø Medical and Surgical
P Upper Bones
B Excision

Definition: Cutting out or off, without replacement, a portion of a body part
Explanation: The qualifier DIAGNOSTIC is used to identify excision procedures that are biopsies

Body Part Character 4	Approach Character 5	Device Character 6	Qualifier Character 7
Ø Sternum Manubrium Suprasternal notch Xiphoid process **1 Ribs, 1 to 2** **2 Ribs, 3 or More** **3 Cervical Vertebra** Dens Odontoid process Spinous process Transverse foramen Transverse process Vertebral arch Vertebral body Vertebral foramen Vertebral lamina Vertebral pedicle **4 Thoracic Vertebra** Spinous process Transverse process Vertebral arch Vertebral body Vertebral foramen Vertebral lamina Vertebral pedicle **5 Scapula, Right** Acromion (process) Coracoid process **6 Scapula, Left** *See 5 Scapula, Right* **7 Glenoid Cavity, Right** Glenoid fossa (of scapula) **8 Glenoid Cavity, Left** *See 7 Glenoid Cavity, Right* **9 Clavicle, Right** **B Clavicle, Left** **C Humeral Head, Right** Greater tuberosity Lesser tuberosity Neck of humerus (anatomical)(surgical) **D Humeral Head, Left** *See C Humeral Head, Right* **F Humeral Shaft, Right** Distal humerus Humerus, distal Lateral epicondyle of humerus Medial epicondyle of humerus **G Humeral Shaft, Left** *See F Humeral Shaft, Right* **H Radius, Right** Ulnar notch **J Radius, Left** *See H Radius, Right* **K Ulna, Right** Olecranon process Radial notch **L Ulna, Left** *See K Ulna, Right* **M Carpal, Right** Capitate bone Hamate bone Lunate bone Pisiform bone Scaphoid bone Trapezium bone Trapezoid bone Triquetral bone **N Carpal, Left** *See M Carpal, Right* **P Metacarpal, Right** **Q Metacarpal, Left** **R Thumb Phalanx, Right** **S Thumb Phalanx, Left** **T Finger Phalanx, Right** **V Finger Phalanx, Left**	**Ø Open** **3 Percutaneous** **4 Percutaneous Endoscopic**	**Z No Device**	**X Diagnostic** **Z No Qualifier**

Ø Medical and Surgical
P Upper Bones
C Extirpation

Definition: Taking or cutting out solid matter from a body part

Explanation: The solid matter may be an abnormal byproduct of a biological function or a foreign body; it may be imbedded in a body part or in the lumen of a tubular body part. The solid matter may or may not have been previously broken into pieces.

Body Part Character 4	Approach Character 5	Device Character 6	Qualifier Character 7
Ø Sternum Manubrium Suprasternal notch Xiphoid process **1 Ribs, 1 to 2** **2 Ribs, 3 or More** **3 Cervical Vertebra** Dens Odontoid process Spinous process Transverse foramen Transverse process Vertebral arch Vertebral body Vertebral foramen Vertebral lamina Vertebral pedicle **4 Thoracic Vertebra** Spinous process Transverse process Vertebral arch Vertebral body Vertebral foramen Vertebral lamina Vertebral pedicle **5 Scapula, Right** Acromion (process) Coracoid process **6 Scapula, Left** ***See*** *5 Scapula, Right* **7 Glenoid Cavity, Right** Glenoid fossa (of scapula) **8 Glenoid Cavity, Left** ***See*** *7 Glenoid Cavity, Right* **9 Clavicle, Right** **B Clavicle, Left** **C Humeral Head, Right** Greater tuberosity Lesser tuberosity Neck of humerus (anatomical)(surgical) **D Humeral Head, Left** ***See*** *C Humeral Head, Right* **F Humeral Shaft, Right** Distal humerus Humerus, distal Lateral epicondyle of humerus Medial epicondyle of humerus **G Humeral Shaft, Left** ***See*** *F Humeral Shaft, Right* **H Radius, Right** Ulnar notch **J Radius, Left** ***See*** *H Radius, Right* **K Ulna, Right** Olecranon process Radial notch **L Ulna, Left** ***See*** *K Ulna, Right* **M Carpal, Right** Capitate bone Hamate bone Lunate bone Pisiform bone Scaphoid bone Trapezium bone Trapezoid bone Triquetral bone **N Carpal, Left** ***See*** *M Carpal, Right* **P Metacarpal, Right** **Q Metacarpal, Left** **R Thumb Phalanx, Right** **S Thumb Phalanx, Left** **T Finger Phalanx, Right** **V Finger Phalanx, Left**	**Ø Open** **3 Percutaneous** **4 Percutaneous Endoscopic**	**Z No Device**	**Z No Qualifier**

Ø Medical and Surgical
P Upper Bones
D Extraction Definition: Pulling or stripping out or off all or a portion of a body part by the use of force
Explanation: The qualifier DIAGNOSTIC is used to identify extraction procedures that are biopsies

Body Part Character 4	Approach Character 5	Device Character 6	Qualifier Character 7
Ø Sternum Manubrium Suprasternal notch Xiphoid process **1 Ribs, 1 to 2** **2 Ribs, 3 or More** **3 Cervical Vertebra** Dens Odontoid process Spinous process Transverse foramen Transverse process Vertebral arch Vertebral body Vertebral foramen Vertebral lamina Vertebral pedicle **4 Thoracic Vertebra** Spinous process Transverse process Vertebral arch Vertebral body Vertebral foramen Vertebral lamina Vertebral pedicle **5 Scapula, Right** Acromion (process) Coracoid process **6 Scapula, Left** ***See** 5 Scapula, Right* **7 Glenoid Cavity, Right** Glenoid fossa (of scapula) **8 Glenoid Cavity, Left** ***See** 7 Glenoid Cavity, Right* **9 Clavicle, Right** **B Clavicle, Left** **C Humeral Head, Right** Greater tuberosity Lesser tuberosity Neck of humerus (anatomical)(surgical) **D Humeral Head, Left** ***See** C Humeral Head, Right* **F Humeral Shaft, Right** Distal humerus Humerus, distal Lateral epicondyle of humerus Medial epicondyle of humerus **G Humeral Shaft, Left** ***See** F Humeral Shaft, Right* **H Radius, Right** Ulnar notch **J Radius, Left** ***See** H Radius, Right* **K Ulna, Right** Olecranon process Radial notch **L Ulna, Left** ***See** K Ulna, Right* **M Carpal, Right** Capitate bone Hamate bone Lunate bone Pisiform bone Scaphoid bone Trapezium bone Trapezoid bone Triquetral bone **N Carpal, Left** ***See** M Carpal, Right* **P Metacarpal, Right** **Q Metacarpal, Left** **R Thumb Phalanx, Right** **S Thumb Phalanx, Left** **T Finger Phalanx, Right** **V Finger Phalanx, Left**	**Ø** Open	**Z** No Device	**Z** No Qualifier

Ø Medical and Surgical
P Upper Bones
H Insertion

Definition: Putting in a nonbiological appliance that monitors, assists, performs, or prevents a physiological function but does not physically take the place of a body part

Explanation: None

Body Part Character 4	Approach Character 5	Device Character 6	Qualifier Character 7
Ø Sternum Manubrium Suprasternal notch Xiphoid process	**Ø** Open **3** Percutaneous **4** Percutaneous Endoscopic	**Ø** Internal Fixation Device, Rigid Plate **4** Internal Fixation Device	**Z** No Qualifier
1 Ribs, 1 to 2 **2 Ribs, 3 or More** **3 Cervical Vertebra** Dens Odontoid process Spinous process Transverse foramen Transverse process Vertebral arch Vertebral body Vertebral foramen Vertebral lamina Vertebral pedicle **4 Thoracic Vertebra** Spinous process Transverse process Vertebral arch Vertebral body Vertebral foramen Vertebral lamina Vertebral pedicle **5 Scapula, Right** Acromion (process) Coracoid process **6 Scapula, Left** *See 5 Scapula, Right* **7 Glenoid Cavity, Right** Glenoid fossa (of scapula) **8 Glenoid Cavity, Left** *See 7 Glenoid Cavity, Right* **9 Clavicle, Right** **B Clavicle, Left**	**Ø** Open **3** Percutaneous **4** Percutaneous Endoscopic	**4** Internal Fixation Device	**Z** No Qualifier
C Humeral Head, Right Greater tuberosity Lesser tuberosity Neck of humerus (anatomical)(surgical) **D Humeral Head, Left** *See C Humeral Head, Right* **H Radius, Right** Ulnar notch **J Radius, Left** *See H Radius, Right* **K Ulna, Right** Olecranon process Radial notch **L Ulna, Left** *See K Ulna, Right*	**Ø** Open **3** Percutaneous **4** Percutaneous Endoscopic	**4** Internal Fixation Device **5** External Fixation Device **6** Internal Fixation Device, Intramedullary **8** External Fixation Device, Limb Lengthening **B** External Fixation Device, Monoplanar **C** External Fixation Device, Ring **D** External Fixation Device, Hybrid	**Z** No Qualifier
F Humeral Shaft, Right Distal humerus Humerus, distal Lateral epicondyle of humerus Medial epicondyle of humerus **G Humeral Shaft, Left** *See F Humeral Shaft, Right*	**Ø** Open **3** Percutaneous **4** Percutaneous Endoscopic	**4** Internal Fixation Device **5** External Fixation Device **6** Internal Fixation Device, Intramedullary **7** Internal Fixation Device, Intramedullary Limb Lengthening **8** External Fixation Device, Limb Lengthening **B** External Fixation Device, Monoplanar **C** External Fixation Device, Ring **D** External Fixation Device, Hybrid	**Z** No Qualifier
M Carpal, Right Capitate bone Hamate bone Lunate bone Pisiform bone Scaphoid bone Trapezium bone Trapezoid bone Triquetral bone **N Carpal, Left** *See M Carpal, Right* **P Metacarpal, Right** **Q Metacarpal, Left** **R Thumb Phalanx, Right** **S Thumb Phalanx, Left** **T Finger Phalanx, Right** **V Finger Phalanx, Left**	**Ø** Open **3** Percutaneous **4** Percutaneous Endoscopic	**4** Internal Fixation Device **5** External Fixation Device	**Z** No Qualifier
Y Upper Bone	**Ø** Open **3** Percutaneous **4** Percutaneous Endoscopic	**M** Bone Growth Stimulator	**Z** No Qualifier

Non-OR ØPH[C,D,H,J,K,L][Ø,3,4]8Z
Non-OR ØPH[F,G][Ø,3,4]8Z

Ø Medical and Surgical
P Upper Bones
J Inspection

Definition: Visually and/or manually exploring a body part

Explanation: Visual exploration may be performed with or without optical instrumentation. Manual exploration may be performed directly or through intervening body layers.

Body Part Character 4	Approach Character 5	Device Character 6	Qualifier Character 7
Y Upper Bone	**Ø Open** **3 Percutaneous** **4 Percutaneous Endoscopic** **X External**	**Z No Device**	**Z No Qualifier**

Non-OR ØPJY[3,X]ZZ

Ø Medical and Surgical
P Upper Bones
N Release

Definition: Freeing a body part from an abnormal physical constraint by cutting or by the use of force

Explanation: Some of the restraining tissue may be taken out but none of the body part is taken out

Body Part Character 4	Approach Character 5	Device Character 6	Qualifier Character 7
Ø Sternum Manubrium Suprasternal notch Xiphoid process **1 Ribs, 1 to 2** **2 Ribs, 3 or More** **3 Cervical Vertebra** Dens Odontoid process Spinous process Transverse foramen Transverse process Vertebral arch Vertebral body Vertebral foramen Vertebral lamina Vertebral pedicle **4 Thoracic Vertebra** Spinous process Transverse process Vertebral arch Vertebral body Vertebral foramen Vertebral lamina Vertebral pedicle **5 Scapula, Right** Acromion (process) Coracoid process **6 Scapula, Left** *See 5 Scapula, Right* **7 Glenoid Cavity, Right** Glenoid fossa (of scapula) **8 Glenoid Cavity, Left** *See 7 Glenoid Cavity, Right* **9 Clavicle, Right** **B Clavicle, Left** **C Humeral Head, Right** Greater tuberosity Lesser tuberosity Neck of humerus (anatomical) (surgical) **D Humeral Head, Left** *See C Humeral Head, Right* **F Humeral Shaft, Right** Distal humerus Humerus, distal Lateral epicondyle of humerus Medial epicondyle of humerus **G Humeral Shaft, Left** *See F Humeral Shaft, Right* **H Radius, Right** Ulnar notch **J Radius, Left** *See H Radius, Right* **K Ulna, Right** Olecranon process Radial notch **L Ulna, Left** *See K Ulna, Right* **M Carpal, Right** Capitate bone Hamate bone Lunate bone Pisiform bone Scaphoid bone Trapezium bone Trapezoid bone Triquetral bone **N Carpal, Left** *See M Carpal, Right* **P Metacarpal, Right** **Q Metacarpal, Left** **R Thumb Phalanx, Right** **S Thumb Phalanx, Left** **T Finger Phalanx, Right** **V Finger Phalanx, Left**	**Ø Open** **3 Percutaneous** **4 Percutaneous Endoscopic**	**Z No Device**	**Z No Qualifier**

Ø Medical and Surgical
P Upper Bones
P Removal

Definition: Taking out or off a device from a body part

Explanation: If a device is taken out and a similar device put in without cutting or puncturing the skin or mucous membrane, the procedure is coded to the root operation CHANGE. Otherwise, the procedure for taking out a device is coded to the root operation REMOVAL.

Body Part Character 4		Approach Character 5	Device Character 6	Qualifier Character 7
Ø Sternum Manubrium Suprasternal notch Xiphoid process **1 Ribs, 1 to 2** **2 Ribs, 3 or More** **3 Cervical Vertebra** Dens Odontoid process Spinous process Transverse foramen Transverse process Vertebral arch Vertebral body Vertebral foramen Vertebral lamina Vertebral pedicle	**4 Thoracic Vertebra** Spinous process Transverse process Vertebral arch Vertebral body Vertebral foramen Vertebral lamina Vertebral pedicle **5 Scapula, Right** Acromion (process) Coracoid process **6 Scapula, Left** *See 5 Scapula, Right* **7 Glenoid Cavity, Right** Glenoid fossa (of scapula) **8 Glenoid Cavity, Left** *See 7 Glenoid Cavity, Right* **9 Clavicle, Right** **B Clavicle, Left**	**Ø Open** **3 Percutaneous** **4 Percutaneous Endoscopic**	**4 Internal Fixation Device** **7 Autologous Tissue Substitute** **J Synthetic Substitute** **K Nonautologous Tissue Substitute**	**Z No Qualifier**
Ø Sternum Manubrium Suprasternal notch Xiphoid process **1 Ribs, 1 to 2** **2 Ribs, 3 or More** **3 Cervical Vertebra** Dens Odontoid process Spinous process Transverse foramen Transverse process Vertebral arch Vertebral body Vertebral foramen Vertebral lamina Vertebral pedicle	**4 Thoracic Vertebra** Spinous process Transverse process Vertebral arch Vertebral body Vertebral foramen Vertebral lamina Vertebral pedicle **5 Scapula, Right** Acromion (process) Coracoid process **6 Scapula, Left** *See 5 Scapula, Right* **7 Glenoid Cavity, Right** Glenoid fossa (of scapula) **8 Glenoid Cavity, Left** *See 7 Glenoid Cavity, Right* **9 Clavicle, Right** **B Clavicle, Left**	**X External**	**4 Internal Fixation Device**	**Z No Qualifier**
C Humeral Head, Right Greater tuberosity Lesser tuberosity Neck of humerus (anatomical) (surgical) **D Humeral Head, Left** *See C Humeral Head, Right* **F Humeral Shaft, Right** Distal humerus Humerus, distal Lateral epicondyle of humerus Medial epicondyle of humerus **G Humeral Shaft, Left** *See F Humeral Shaft, Right* **H Radius, Right** Ulnar notch **J Radius, Left** *See H Radius, Right* **K Ulna, Right** Olecranon process Radial notch	**L Ulna, Left** *See K Ulna, Right* **M Carpal, Right** Capitate bone Hamate bone Lunate bone Pisiform bone Scaphoid bone Trapezium bone Trapezoid bone Triquetral bone **N Carpal, Left** *See M Carpal, Right* **P Metacarpal, Right** **Q Metacarpal, Left** **R Thumb Phalanx, Right** **S Thumb Phalanx, Left** **T Finger Phalanx, Right** **V Finger Phalanx, Left**	**Ø Open** **3 Percutaneous** **4 Percutaneous Endoscopic**	**4 Internal Fixation Device** **5 External Fixation Device** **7 Autologous Tissue Substitute** **J Synthetic Substitute** **K Nonautologous Tissue Substitute**	**Z No Qualifier**

Non-OR ØPP[Ø,1,2,3,4,5,6,7,8,9,B]X4Z

ØPP Continued on next page

Upper Bones

ØPP Continued

Ø Medical and Surgical
P Upper Bones
P Removal

Definition: Taking out or off a device from a body part

Explanation: If a device is taken out and a similar device put in without cutting or puncturing the skin or mucous membrane, the procedure is coded to the root operation CHANGE. Otherwise, the procedure for taking out a device is coded to the root operation REMOVAL.

Body Part Character 4	Approach Character 5	Device Character 6	Qualifier Character 7
C Humeral Head, Right Greater tuberosity; Lesser tuberosity; Neck of humerus (anatomical) (surgical) **D Humeral Head, Left** *See C Humeral Head, Right* **F Humeral Shaft, Right** Distal humerus; Humerus, distal; Lateral epicondyle of humerus; Medial epicondyle of humerus **G Humeral Shaft, Left** *See F Humeral Shaft, Right* **H Radius, Right** Ulnar notch **J Radius, Left** *See H Radius, Right* **K Ulna, Right** Olecranon process; Radial notch **L Ulna, Left** *See K Ulna, Right* **M Carpal, Right** Capitate bone; Hamate bone; Lunate bone; Pisiform bone; Scaphoid bone; Trapezium bone; Trapezoid bone; Triquetral bone **N Carpal, Left** *See M Carpal, Right* **P Metacarpal, Right** **Q Metacarpal, Left** **R Thumb Phalanx, Right** **S Thumb Phalanx, Left** **T Finger Phalanx, Right** **V Finger Phalanx, Left**	X External	4 Internal Fixation Device 5 External Fixation Device	Z No Qualifier
Y Upper Bone	Ø Open 3 Percutaneous 4 Percutaneous Endoscopic X External	Ø Drainage Device M Bone Growth Stimulator	Z No Qualifier

Non-OR ØPP[C,D,F,G,H,J,K,L,M,N,P,Q,R,S,T,V]X[4,5]Z
Non-OR ØPPY3ØZ
Non-OR ØPPYX[Ø,M]Z

Ø Medical and Surgical
P Upper Bones
Q Repair

Definition: Restoring, to the extent possible, a body part to its normal anatomic structure and function
Explanation: Used only when the method to accomplish the repair is not one of the other root operations

Body Part Character 4	Approach Character 5	Device Character 6	Qualifier Character 7
Ø Sternum Manubrium Suprasternal notch Xiphoid process **1 Ribs, 1 to 2** **2 Ribs, 3 or More** **3 Cervical Vertebra** Dens Odontoid process Spinous process Transverse foramen Transverse process Vertebral arch Vertebral body Vertebral foramen Vertebral lamina Vertebral pedicle **4 Thoracic Vertebra** Spinous process Transverse process Vertebral arch Vertebral body Vertebral foramen Vertebral lamina Vertebral pedicle **5 Scapula, Right** Acromion (process) Coracoid process **6 Scapula, Left** *See 5 Scapula, Right* **7 Glenoid Cavity, Right** Glenoid fossa (of scapula) **8 Glenoid Cavity, Left** *See 7 Glenoid Cavity, Right* **9 Clavicle, Right** **B Clavicle, Left** **C Humeral Head, Right** Greater tuberosity Lesser tuberosity Neck of humerus (anatomical)(surgical) **D Humeral Head, Left** *See C Humeral Head, Right* **F Humeral Shaft, Right** Distal humerus Humerus, distal Lateral epicondyle of humerus Medial epicondyle of humerus **G Humeral Shaft, Left** *See F Humeral Shaft, Right* **H Radius, Right** Ulnar notch **J Radius, Left** *See H Radius, Right* **K Ulna, Right** Olecranon process Radial notch **L Ulna, Left** *See K Ulna, Right* **M Carpal, Right** Capitate bone Hamate bone Lunate bone Pisiform bone Scaphoid bone Trapezium bone Trapezoid bone Triquetral bone **N Carpal, Left** *See M Carpal, Right* **P Metacarpal, Right** **Q Metacarpal, Left** **R Thumb Phalanx, Right** **S Thumb Phalanx, Left** **T Finger Phalanx, Right** **V Finger Phalanx, Left**	**Ø Open** **3 Percutaneous** **4 Percutaneous Endoscopic** **X External**	**Z No Device**	**Z No Qualifier**

Non-OR ØPQ[Ø,1,2,3,4,5,6,7,8,9,B,C,D,F,G,H,J,K,L,M,N,P,Q,R,S,T,V]XZZ

Ø Medical and Surgical
P Upper Bones
R Replacement

Definition: Putting in or on biological or synthetic material that physically takes the place and/or function of all or a portion of a body part

Explanation: The body part may have been taken out or replaced, or may be taken out, physically eradicated, or rendered nonfunctional during the REPLACEMENT procedure. A REMOVAL procedure is coded for taking out the device used in a previous replacement procedure.

Body Part Character 4		Approach Character 5	Device Character 6	Qualifier Character 7
Ø Sternum Manubrium Suprasternal notch Xiphoid process **1 Ribs, 1 to 2** **2 Ribs, 3 or More** **3 Cervical Vertebra** Dens Odontoid process Spinous process Transverse foramen Transverse process Vertebral arch Vertebral body Vertebral foramen Vertebral lamina Vertebral pedicle **4 Thoracic Vertebra** Spinous process Transverse process Vertebral arch Vertebral body Vertebral foramen Vertebral lamina Vertebral pedicle **5 Scapula, Right** Acromion (process) Coracoid process **6 Scapula, Left** *See 5 Scapula, Right* **7 Glenoid Cavity, Right** Glenoid fossa (of scapula) **8 Glenoid Cavity, Left** *See 7 Glenoid Cavity, Right* **9 Clavicle, Right** **B Clavicle, Left** **C Humeral Head, Right** Greater tuberosity Lesser tuberosity Neck of humerus (anatomical)(surgical) **D Humeral Head, Left** *See C Humeral Head, Right*	**F Humeral Shaft, Right** Distal humerus Humerus, distal Lateral epicondyle of humerus Medial epicondyle of humerus **G Humeral Shaft, Left** *See F Humeral Shaft, Right* **H Radius, Right** Ulnar notch **J Radius, Left** *See H Radius, Right* **K Ulna, Right** Olecranon process Radial notch **L Ulna, Left** *See K Ulna, Right* **M Carpal, Right** Capitate bone Hamate bone Lunate bone Pisiform bone Scaphoid bone Trapezium bone Trapezoid bone Triquetral bone **N Carpal, Left** *See M Carpal, Right* **P Metacarpal, Right** **Q Metacarpal, Left** **R Thumb Phalanx, Right** **S Thumb Phalanx, Left** **T Finger Phalanx, Right** **V Finger Phalanx, Left**	**Ø Open** **3 Percutaneous** **4 Percutaneous Endoscopic**	**7 Autologous Tissue Substitute** **J Synthetic Substitute** **K Nonautologous Tissue Substitute**	**Z No Qualifier**

Ø Medical and Surgical
P Upper Bones
S Reposition

Definition: Moving to its normal location, or other suitable location, all or a portion of a body part

Explanation: The body part is moved to a new location from an abnormal location, or from a normal location where it is not functioning correctly. The body part may or may not be cut out or off to be moved to the new location.

Body Part Character 4		Approach Character 5	Device Character 6	Qualifier Character 7
Ø Sternum Manubrium Suprasternal notch Xiphoid process		Ø Open 3 Percutaneous 4 Percutaneous Endoscopic	Ø Internal Fixation Device, Rigid Plate 4 Internal Fixation Device Z No Device	Z No Qualifier
Ø Sternum Manubrium Suprasternal notch Xiphoid process		X External	Z No Device	Z No Qualifier
1 Ribs, 1 to 2 2 Ribs, 3 or More 3 Cervical Vertebra ⊞ Dens Odontoid process Spinous process Transverse foramen Transverse process Vertebral arch Vertebral body Vertebral foramen Vertebral lamina Vertebral pedicle	5 Scapula, Right Acromion (process) Coracoid process 6 Scapula, Left *See 5 Scapula, Right* 7 Glenoid Cavity, Right Glenoid fossa (of scapula) 8 Glenoid Cavity, Left *See 7 Glenoid Cavity, Right* 9 Clavicle, Right B Clavicle, Left	Ø Open 3 Percutaneous 4 Percutaneous Endoscopic	4 Internal Fixation Device Z No Device	Z No Qualifier
1 Ribs, 1 to 2 2 Ribs, 3 or More 3 Cervical Vertebra Dens Odontoid process Spinous process Transverse foramen Transverse process Vertebral arch Vertebral body Vertebral foramen Vertebral lamina Vertebral pedicle	5 Scapula, Right Acromion (process) Coracoid process 6 Scapula, Left *See 5 Scapula, Right* 7 Glenoid Cavity, Right Glenoid fossa (of scapula) 8 Glenoid Cavity, Left *See 7 Glenoid Cavity, Right* 9 Clavicle, Right B Clavicle, Left	X External	Z No Device	Z No Qualifier
4 Thoracic Vertebra Spinous process Transverse process Vertebral arch Vertebral body Vertebral foramen Vertebral lamina Vertebral pedicle		Ø Open 4 Percutaneous Endoscopic	3 Spinal Stabilization Device, Vertebral Body Tether 4 Internal Fixation Device Z No Device	Z No Qualifier
4 Thoracic Vertebra ⊞ Spinous process Transverse process Vertebral arch Vertebral body Vertebral foramen Vertebral lamina Vertebral pedicle		3 Percutaneous	4 Internal Fixation Device Z No Device	Z No Qualifier
4 Thoracic Vertebra Spinous process Transverse process Vertebral arch Vertebral body Vertebral foramen Vertebral lamina Vertebral pedicle		X External	Z No Device	Z No Qualifier
C Humeral Head, Right Greater tuberosity Lesser tuberosity Neck of humerus (anatomical)(surgical) D Humeral Head, Left *See C Humeral Head, Right* F Humeral Shaft, Right Distal humerus Humerus, distal Lateral epicondyle of humerus Medial epicondyle of humerus	G Humeral Shaft, Left *See F Humeral Shaft, Right* H Radius, Right Ulnar notch J Radius, Left *See H Radius, Right* K Ulna, Right Olecranon process Radial notch L Ulna, Left *See K Ulna, Right*	Ø Open 3 Percutaneous 4 Percutaneous Endoscopic	4 Internal Fixation Device 5 External Fixation Device 6 Internal Fixation Device, Intramedullary B External Fixation Device, Monoplanar C External Fixation Device, Ring D External Fixation Device, Hybrid Z No Device	Z No Qualifier

Non-OR ØPSØ[3,4]ZZ
Non-OR ØPSØXZZ
Non-OR ØPS[1,2,5,6,7,8,9,B][3,4]ZZ
Non-OR ØPS[1,2,3,5,6,7,8,9,B]XZZ
Non-OR ØPS4XZZ
Non-OR ØPS[C,D,F,G,H,J,K,L][3,4]ZZ

See Appendix L for Procedure Combinations
⊞ ØPS33ZZ
⊞ ØPS43ZZ

ØPS Continued on next page

Ø Medical and Surgical
P Upper Bones
S Reposition

ØPS Continued

Definition: Moving to its normal location, or other suitable location, all or a portion of a body part

Explanation: The body part is moved to a new location from an abnormal location, or from a normal location where it is not functioning correctly. The body part may or may not be cut out or off to be moved to the new location.

Body Part Character 4		Approach Character 5	Device Character 6	Qualifier Character 7
C Humeral Head, Right Greater tuberosity Lesser tuberosity Neck of humerus (anatomical)(surgical) **D Humeral Head, Left** *See C Humeral Head, Right* **F Humeral Shaft, Right** Distal humerus Humerus, distal Lateral epicondyle of humerus Medial epicondyle of humerus	**G Humeral Shaft, Left** *See F Humeral Shaft, Right* **H Radius, Right** Ulnar notch **J Radius, Left** *See H Radius, Right* **K Ulna, Right** Olecranon process Radial notch **L Ulna, Left** *See K Ulna, Right*	X External	Z No Device	Z No Qualifier
M Carpal, Right Capitate bone Hamate bone Lunate bone Pisiform bone Scaphoid bone Trapezium bone Trapezoid bone Triquetral bone	**N Carpal, Left** *See M Carpal, Right* **P Metacarpal, Right** **Q Metacarpal, Left** **R Thumb Phalanx, Right** **S Thumb Phalanx, Left** **T Finger Phalanx, Right** **V Finger Phalanx, Left**	Ø Open 3 Percutaneous 4 Percutaneous Endoscopic	4 Internal Fixation Device 5 External Fixation Device Z No Device	Z No Qualifier
M Carpal, Right Capitate bone Hamate bone Lunate bone Pisiform bone Scaphoid bone Trapezium bone Trapezoid bone Triquetral bone	**N Carpal, Left** *See M Carpal, Right* **P Metacarpal, Right** **Q Metacarpal, Left** **R Thumb Phalanx, Right** **S Thumb Phalanx, Left** **T Finger Phalanx, Right** **V Finger Phalanx, Left**	X External	Z No Device	Z No Qualifier

Non-OR ØPS[C,D,F,G,H,J,K,L]XZZ
Non-OR ØPS[M,N,P,Q,R,S,T,V][3,4]ZZ
Non-OR ØPS[M,N,P,Q,R,S,T,V]XZZ

Ø Medical and Surgical
P Upper Bones
T Resection

Definition: Cutting out or off, without replacement, all of a body part

Explanation: None

Body Part Character 4		Approach Character 5	Device Character 6	Qualifier Character 7
Ø Sternum Manubrium Suprasternal notch Xiphoid process **1 Ribs, 1 to 2** **2 Ribs, 3 or More** **5 Scapula, Right** Acromion (process) Coracoid process **6 Scapula, Left** *See 5 Scapula, Right* **7 Glenoid Cavity, Right** Glenoid fossa (of scapula) **8 Glenoid Cavity, Left** *See 7 Glenoid Cavity, Right* **9 Clavicle, Right** **B Clavicle, Left** **C Humeral Head, Right** Greater tuberosity Lesser tuberosity Neck of humerus (anatomical) (surgical) **D Humeral Head, Left** *See C Humeral Head, Right* **F Humeral Shaft, Right** Distal humerus Humerus, distal Lateral epicondyle of humerus Medial epicondyle of humerus	**G Humeral Shaft, Left** *See F Humeral Shaft, Right* **H Radius, Right** Ulnar notch **J Radius, Left** *See H Radius, Right* **K Ulna, Right** Olecranon process Radial notch **L Ulna, Left** *See K Ulna, Right* **M Carpal, Right** Capitate bone Hamate bone Lunate bone Pisiform bone Scaphoid bone Trapezium bone Trapezoid bone Triquetral bone **N Carpal, Left** *See M Carpal, Right* **P Metacarpal, Right** **Q Metacarpal, Left** **R Thumb Phalanx, Right** **S Thumb Phalanx, Left** **T Finger Phalanx, Right** **V Finger Phalanx, Left**	Ø Open	Z No Device	Z No Qualifier

Ø Medical and Surgical
P Upper Bones
U Supplement

Definition: Putting in or on biological or synthetic material that physically reinforces and/or augments the function of a portion of a body part

Explanation: The biological material is non-living, or is living and from the same individual. The body part may have been previously replaced, and the SUPPLEMENT procedure is performed to physically reinforce and/or augment the function of the replaced body part.

Body Part Character 4	Approach Character 5	Device Character 6	Qualifier Character 7
Ø Sternum Manubrium Suprasternal notch Xiphoid process **1 Ribs, 1 to 2** **2 Ribs, 3 or More** **3 Cervical Vertebra** ⊞ Dens Odontoid process Spinous process Transverse foramen Transverse process Vertebral arch Vertebral body Vertebral foramen Vertebral lamina Vertebral pedicle **4 Thoracic Vertebra** ⊞ Spinous process Transverse process Vertebral arch Vertebral body Vertebral foramen Vertebral lamina Vertebral pedicle **5 Scapula, Right** Acromion (process) Coracoid process **6 Scapula, Left** *See 5 Scapula, Right* **7 Glenoid Cavity, Right** Glenoid fossa (of scapula) **8 Glenoid Cavity, Left** *See 7 Glenoid Cavity, Right* **9 Clavicle, Right** **B Clavicle, Left** **C Humeral Head, Right** Greater tuberosity Lesser tuberosity Neck of humerus (anatomical) (surgical) **D Humeral Head, Left** *See C Humeral Head, Right* **F Humeral Shaft, Right** Distal humerus Humerus, distal Lateral epicondyle of humerus Medial epicondyle of humerus **G Humeral Shaft, Left** *See F Humeral Shaft, Right* **H Radius, Right** Ulnar notch **J Radius, Left** *See H Radius, Right* **K Ulna, Right** Olecranon process Radial notch **L Ulna, Left** *See K Ulna, Right* **M Carpal, Right** Capitate bone Hamate bone Lunate bone Pisiform bone Scaphoid bone Trapezium bone Trapezoid bone Triquetral bone **N Carpal, Left** *See M Carpal, Right* **P Metacarpal, Right** **Q Metacarpal, Left** **R Thumb Phalanx, Right** **S Thumb Phalanx, Left** **T Finger Phalanx, Right** **V Finger Phalanx, Left**	**Ø Open** **3 Percutaneous** **4 Percutaneous Endoscopic**	**7 Autologous Tissue Substitute** **J Synthetic Substitute** **K Nonautologous Tissue Substitute**	**Z No Qualifier**

See Appendix L for Procedure Combinations

⊞ ØPU[3,4]3JZ

Ø Medical and Surgical
P Upper Bones
W Revision

Definition: Correcting, to the extent possible, a portion of a malfunctioning device or the position of a displaced device

Explanation: Revision can include correcting a malfunctioning or displaced device by taking out or putting in components of the device such as a screw or pin

Body Part Character 4	Approach Character 5	Device Character 6	Qualifier Character 7
Ø Sternum Manubrium Suprasternal notch Xiphoid process **1 Ribs, 1 to 2** **2 Ribs, 3 or More** **3 Cervical Vertebra** Dens Odontoid process Spinous process Transverse foramen Transverse process Vertebral arch Vertebral body Vertebral foramen Vertebral lamina Vertebral pedicle **4 Thoracic Vertebra** Spinous process Transverse process Vertebral arch Vertebral body Vertebral foramen Vertebral lamina Vertebral pedicle **5 Scapula, Right** Acromion (process) Coracoid process **6 Scapula, Left** *See 5 Scapula, Right* **7 Glenoid Cavity, Right** Glenoid fossa (of scapula) **8 Glenoid Cavity, Left** *See 7 Glenoid Cavity, Right* **9 Clavicle, Right** **B Clavicle, Left**	**Ø Open** **3 Percutaneous** **4 Percutaneous Endoscopic** **X External**	**4 Internal Fixation Device** **7 Autologous Tissue Substitute** **J Synthetic Substitute** **K Nonautologous Tissue Substitute**	**Z No Qualifier**
C Humeral Head, Right Greater tuberosity Lesser tuberosity Neck of humerus (anatomical)(surgical) **D Humeral Head, Left** *See C Humeral Head, Right* **F Humeral Shaft, Right** Distal humerus Humerus, distal Lateral epicondyle of humerus Medial epicondyle of humerus **G Humeral Shaft, Left** *See F Humeral Shaft, Right* **H Radius, Right** Ulnar notch **J Radius, Left** *See H Radius, Right* **K Ulna, Right** Olecranon process Radial notch **L Ulna, Left** *See K Ulna, Right* **M Carpal, Right** Capitate bone Hamate bone Lunate bone Pisiform bone Scaphoid bone Trapezium bone Trapezoid bone Triquetral bone **N Carpal, Left** *See M Carpal, Right* **P Metacarpal, Right** **Q Metacarpal, Left** **R Thumb Phalanx, Right** **S Thumb Phalanx, Left** **T Finger Phalanx, Right** **V Finger Phalanx, Left**	**Ø Open** **3 Percutaneous** **4 Percutaneous Endoscopic** **X External**	**4 Internal Fixation Device** **5 External Fixation Device** **7 Autologous Tissue Substitute** **J Synthetic Substitute** **K Nonautologous Tissue Substitute**	**Z No Qualifier**
Y Upper Bone	**Ø Open** **3 Percutaneous** **4 Percutaneous Endoscopic** **X External**	**Ø Drainage Device** **M Bone Growth Stimulator**	**Z No Qualifier**

Non-OR ØPW[Ø,1,2,3,4,5,6,7,8,9,B]X[4,7,J,K]Z
Non-OR ØPW[C,D,F,G,H,J,K,L,M,N,P,Q,R,S,T,V]X[4,5,7,J,K]Z
Non-OR ØPWYX[Ø,M]Z

Lower Bones ØQ2–ØQW

Character Meanings

This Character Meaning table is provided as a guide to assist the user in the identification of character members that may be found in this section of code tables. It **SHOULD NOT** be used to build a PCS code.

Operation–Character 3	Body Part–Character 4	Approach–Character 5	Device–Character 6	Qualifier–Character 7
2 Change	Ø Lumbar Vertebra	Ø Open	Ø Drainage Device	2 Sesamoid Bone(s) 1st Toe
5 Destruction	1 Sacrum	3 Percutaneous	3 Spinal Stabilization Device, Vertebral Body Tether	3 Laser Interstitial Thermal Therapy
8 Division	2 Pelvic Bone, Right	4 Percutaneous Endoscopic	4 Internal Fixation Device	X Diagnostic
9 Drainage	3 Pelvic Bone, Left	X External	5 External Fixation Device	Z No Qualifier
B Excision	4 Acetabulum, Right		6 Internal Fixation Device, Intramedullary	
C Extirpation	5 Acetabulum, Left		7 Autologous Tissue Substitute OR Internal Fixation Device, Intramedullary Limb Lengthening	
D Extraction	6 Upper Femur, Right		8 External Fixation Device, Limb Lengthening	
H Insertion	7 Upper Femur, Left		B External Fixation Device, Monoplanar	
J Inspection	8 Femoral Shaft, Right		C External Fixation Device, Ring	
N Release	9 Femoral Shaft, Left		D External Fixation Device, Hybrid	
P Removal	B Lower Femur, Right		J Synthetic Substitute	
Q Repair	C Lower Femur, Left		K Nonautologous Tissue Substitute	
R Replacement	D Patella, Right		M Bone Growth Stimulator	
S Reposition	F Patella, Left		Y Other Device	
T Resection	G Tibia, Right		Z No Device	
U Supplement	H Tibia, Left			
W Revision	J Fibula, Right			
	K Fibula, Left			
	L Tarsal, Right			
	M Tarsal, Left			
	N Metatarsal, Right			
	P Metatarsal, Left			
	Q Toe Phalanx, Right			
	R Toe Phalanx, Left			
	S Coccyx			
	Y Lower Bone			

AHA Coding Clinic for table ØQ5
2023, 1Q, 10 Laser interstitial thermal therapy

AHA Coding Clinic for table ØQ8
2018, 1Q, 25 Periacetabular osteotomy for repair of congenital hip dysplasia
2016, 2Q, 31 Periacetabular ostectomy for repair of congenital hip dysplasia

AHA Coding Clinic for table ØQ9
2022, 1Q, 31 Septic arthritis/osteomyelitis of pubic symphysis and aspiration biopsy

AHA Coding Clinic for table ØQB
2023, 2Q, 30 Excisional debridement and non-excisional debridement at deeper layer same site
2021, 4Q, 52-53 Sesamoidectomy of great toe
2021, 2Q, 18 Excision of tibial sesamoid
2020, 2Q, 26 Sacral pressure ulcer with excisional and nonexcisional debridement of same site
2019, 2Q, 19 Cervical spinal fusion, decompression and placement of interfacet stabilization device
2018, 3Q, 17 Excisional debridement of periosteum
2017, 1Q, 23 Reconstruction of mandible using titanium and bone
2016, 3Q, 30 Resection of femur with interposition arthroplasty
2015, 3Q, 3-8 Excisional and nonexcisional debridement
2015, 3Q, 26 Femoral head resection
2015, 2Q, 34 Decompressive laminectomy
2014, 4Q, 25 Femoroacetabular impingement and labral tear with repair
2014, 2Q, 6 Posterior lumbar fusion with discectomy
2013, 4Q, 116 Spinal decompression
2013, 2Q, 39 Ankle fusion, osteotomy, and removal of hardware
2012, 2Q, 19 Multiple decompressive cervical laminectomies

AHA Coding Clinic for table ØQD
2023, 2Q, 30 Excisional debridement and non-excisional debridement at deeper layer same site
2017, 4Q, 41 Extraction procedures

AHA Coding Clinic for table ØQH
2022, 2Q, 19 Limb lengthening surgery
2019, 4Q, 34 Intramedullary limb lengthening internal fixation device
2017, 1Q, 21 Staged scoliosis surgery with iliac fixation and spinal fusion
2016, 3Q, 34 Tibial/fibula epiphysiodesis

AHA Coding Clinic for table ØQP
2023, 1Q, 33 Removal of S2-Alar-Iliac screws
2020, 4Q, 56 Removal of external fixation device
2017, 4Q, 74-75 Magnetic growth rods
2015, 2Q, 6 Planned implant break

AHA Coding Clinic for table ØQQ
2018, 1Q, 15 Pubic symphysis fusion
2014, 3Q, 24 Repair of lipomyelomeningocele and tethered cord

AHA Coding Clinic for table ØQR
2017, 1Q, 22 Total knee replacement and patellar component
2016, 3Q, 30 Resection of femur with interposition arthroplasty

AHA Coding Clinic for table ØQS
2022, 2Q, 19 Limb lengthening surgery
2021, 4Q, 51-52 Vertebral body tethering
2020, 1Q, 33 Spinal fusion without use of bone graft
2019, 3Q, 26 Open reduction with internal fixation and placement of strut allograft
2018, 1Q, 13 Bilateral cuboid osteotomy for repair of congenital talipes equinovarus
2018, 1Q, 25 Periacetabular osteotomy for repair of congenital hip dysplasia
2016, 3Q, 34 Tibial/fibula epiphysiodesis
2014, 4Q, 29 Rotational osteosynthesis
2014, 4Q, 31 Reposition of femur for correction of valgus and recurvatum deformities

AHA Coding Clinic for table ØQT
2017, 1Q, 22 Chopart amputation of foot
2016, 3Q, 30 Resection of femur with interposition arthroplasty
2015, 3Q, 26 Femoral head resection
2014, 4Q, 29 Rotational osteosynthesis

AHA Coding Clinic for table ØQU
2019, 3Q, 26 Open reduction with internal fixation and placement of strut allograft
2019, 2Q, 35 Kiva® kyphoplasty
2015, 3Q, 18 Total hip replacement with acetabular reconstruction
2014, 4Q, 31 Reposition of femur for correction of valgus and recurvatum deformities
2014, 2Q, 12 Percutaneous vertebroplasty using cement
2013, 2Q, 35 Use of bone void filler in grafting

AHA Coding Clinic for table ØQW
2017, 4Q, 74-75 Magnetic growth rods

Lower Bones

Lumbar vertebra **Ø**
Pelvic **2, 3**
Sacrum **1**
Coccyx **S**
Acetabulum **4, 5**
Femur **6, 7, 8, 9, B, C**
Patella **D, F**
Tibia **G, H**
Fibula **J, K**
Metatarsal **N, P**
Tarsal **L, M**
Toe phalanx **Q, R**

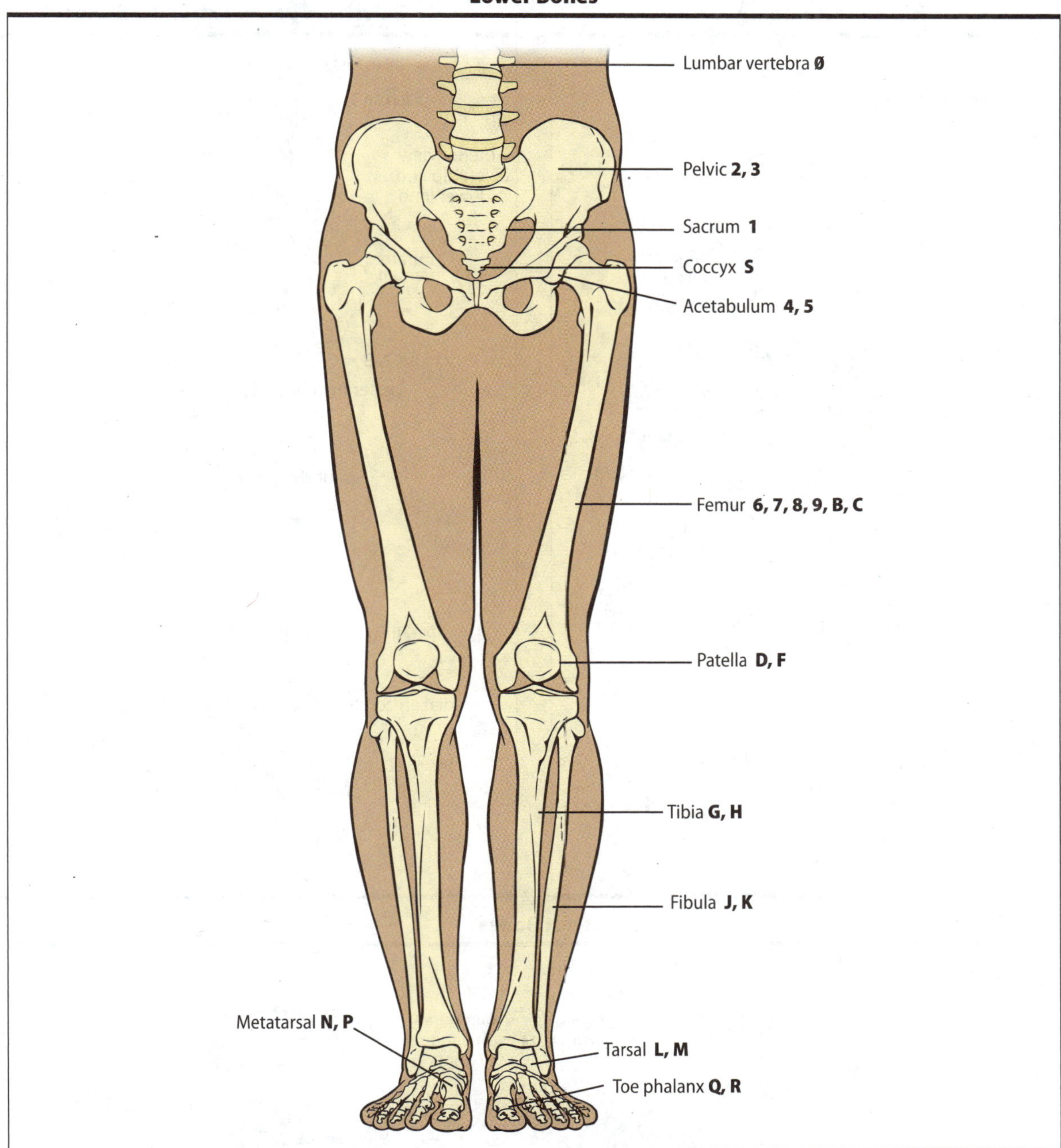

Hip Bone Anatomy

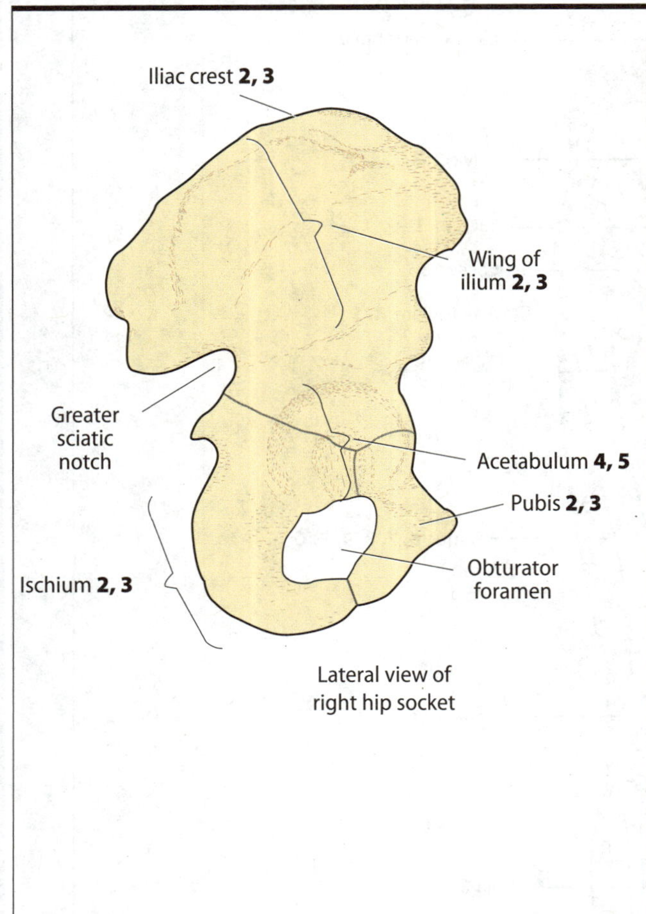

Pelvic and Lower Extremity Bones

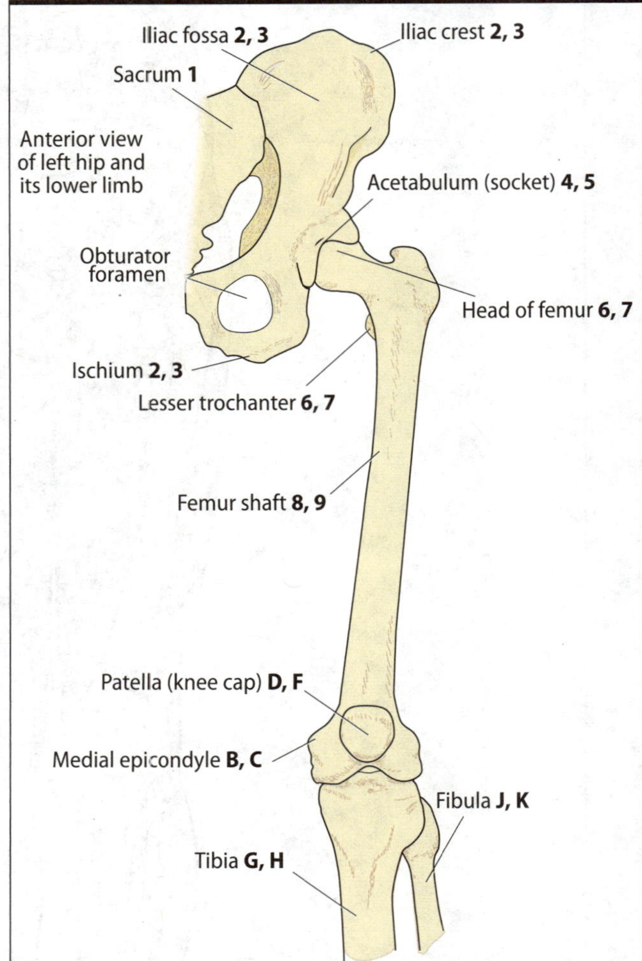

Foot Bones

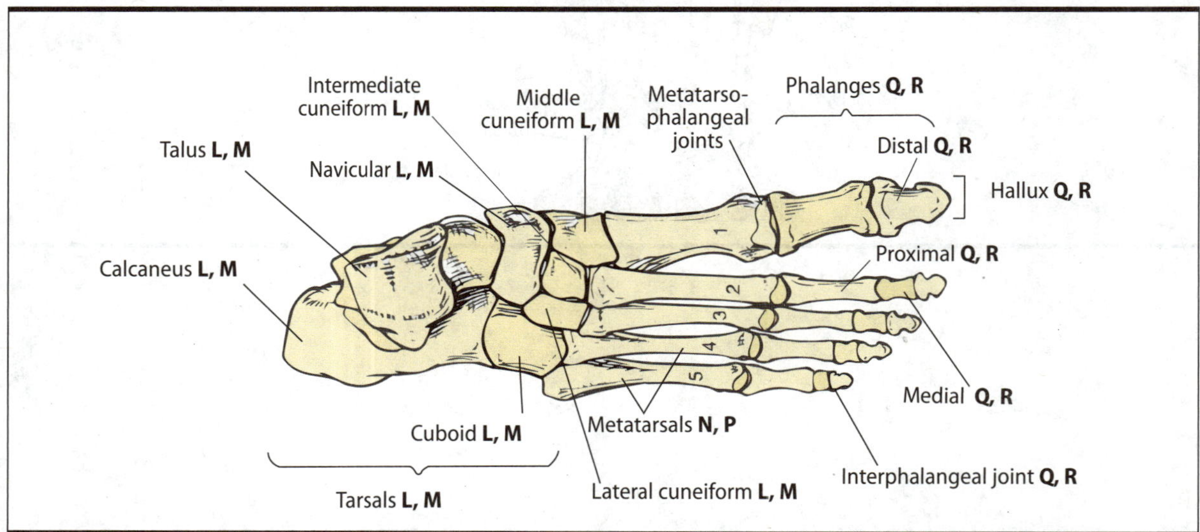

Ø Medical and Surgical
Q Lower Bones
2 Change

Definition: Taking out or off a device from a body part and putting back an identical or similar device in or on the same body part without cutting or puncturing the skin or a mucous membrane

Explanation: All CHANGE procedures are coded using the approach EXTERNAL

Body Part Character 4	Approach Character 5	Device Character 6	Qualifier Character 7
Y Lower Bone	X External	Ø Drainage Device Y Other Device	Z No Qualifier

Non-OR All body part, approach, device, and qualifier values

Ø Medical and Surgical
Q Lower Bones
5 Destruction

Definition: Physical eradication of all or a portion of a body part by the direct use of energy, force, or a destructive agent

Explanation: None of the body part is physically taken out

Body Part Character 4	Approach Character 5	Device Character 6	Qualifier Character 7
Ø Lumbar Vertebra Spinous process Transverse process Vertebral arch Vertebral body Vertebral foramen Vertebral lamina Vertebral pedicle **1 Sacrum**	Ø Open 3 Percutaneous 4 Percutaneous Endoscopic	Z No Device	3 Laser Interstitial Thermal Therapy Z No Qualifier
2 Pelvic Bone, Right Iliac crest Ilium Ischium Pubis **3 Pelvic Bone, Left** *See 2 Pelvic Bone, Right* **4 Acetabulum, Right** **5 Acetabulum, Left** **6 Upper Femur, Right** Femoral head Greater trochanter Lesser trochanter Neck of femur **7 Upper Femur, Left** *See 6 Upper Femur, Right* **8 Femoral Shaft, Right** Body of femur **9 Femoral Shaft, Left** *See 8 Femoral Shaft, Right* **B Lower Femur, Right** Lateral condyle of femur Lateral epicondyle of femur Medial condyle of femur Medial epicondyle of femur **C Lower Femur, Left** *See B Lower Femur, Right* **D Patella, Right** **F Patella, Left** **G Tibia, Right** Lateral condyle of tibia Medial condyle of tibia Medial malleolus **H Tibia, Left** *See G Tibia, Right* **J Fibula, Right** Body of fibula Head of fibula Lateral malleolus **K Fibula, Left** *See J Fibula, Right* **L Tarsal, Right** Calcaneus Cuboid bone Intermediate cuneiform bone Lateral cuneiform bone Medial cuneiform bone Navicular bone Talus bone **M Tarsal, Left** *See L Tarsal, Right* **N Metatarsal, Right** Fibular sesamoid Tibial sesamoid **P Metatarsal, Left** *See N Metatarsal, Right* **Q Toe Phalanx, Right** **R Toe Phalanx, Left** **S Coccyx**	Ø Open 3 Percutaneous 4 Percutaneous Endoscopic	Z No Device	Z No Qualifier

Ø Medical and Surgical
Q Lower Bones
8 Division

Definition: Cutting into a body part, without draining fluids and/or gases from the body part, in order to separate or transect a body part
Explanation: All or a portion of the body part is separated into two or more portions

Body Part Character 4	Approach Character 5	Device Character 6	Qualifier Character 7
Ø Lumbar Vertebra Spinous process Transverse process Vertebral arch Vertebral body Vertebral foramen Vertebral lamina Vertebral pedicle **1 Sacrum** **2 Pelvic Bone, Right** Iliac crest Ilium Ischium Pubis **3 Pelvic Bone, Left** *See 2 Pelvic Bone, Right* **4 Acetabulum, Right** **5 Acetabulum, Left** **6 Upper Femur, Right** Femoral head Greater trochanter Lesser trochanter Neck of femur **7 Upper Femur, Left** *See 6 Upper Femur, Right* **8 Femoral Shaft, Right** Body of femur **9 Femoral Shaft, Left** *See 8 Femoral Shaft, Right* **B Lower Femur, Right** Lateral condyle of femur Lateral epicondyle of femur Medial condyle of femur Medial epicondyle of femur **C Lower Femur, Left** *See B Lower Femur, Right* **D Patella, Right** **F Patella, Left** **G Tibia, Right** Lateral condyle of tibia Medial condyle of tibia Medial malleolus **H Tibia, Left** *See G Tibia, Right* **J Fibula, Right** Body of fibula Head of fibula Lateral malleolus **K Fibula, Left** *See J Fibula, Right* **L Tarsal, Right** Calcaneus Cuboid bone Intermediate cuneiform bone Lateral cuneiform bone Medial cuneiform bone Navicular bone Talus bone **M Tarsal, Left** *See L Tarsal, Right* **N Metatarsal, Right** Fibular sesamoid Tibial sesamoid **P Metatarsal, Left** *See N Metatarsal, Right* **Q Toe Phalanx, Right** **R Toe Phalanx, Left** **S Coccyx**	**Ø Open** **3 Percutaneous** **4 Percutaneous Endoscopic**	**Z No Device**	**Z No Qualifier**

Ø Medical and Surgical
Q Lower Bones
9 Drainage

Definition: Taking or letting out fluids and/or gases from a body part

Explanation: The qualifier DIAGNOSTIC is used to identify drainage procedures that are biopsies

Body Part Character 4	Approach Character 5	Device Character 6	Qualifier Character 7
Ø Lumbar Vertebra Spinous process Transverse process Vertebral arch Vertebral body Vertebral foramen Vertebral lamina Vertebral pedicle **1 Sacrum** **2 Pelvic Bone, Right** Iliac crest Ilium Ischium Pubis **3 Pelvic Bone, Left** *See 2 Pelvic Bone, Right* **4 Acetabulum, Right** **5 Acetabulum, Left** **6 Upper Femur, Right** Femoral head Greater trochanter Lesser trochanter Neck of femur **7 Upper Femur, Left** *See 6 Upper Femur, Right* **8 Femoral Shaft, Right** Body of femur **9 Femoral Shaft, Left** *See 8 Femoral Shaft, Right* **B Lower Femur, Right** Lateral condyle of femur Lateral epicondyle of femur Medial condyle of femur Medial epicondyle of femur **C Lower Femur, Left** *See B Lower Femur, Right* **D Patella, Right** **F Patella, Left** **G Tibia, Right** Lateral condyle of tibia Medial condyle of tibia Medial malleolus **H Tibia, Left** *See G Tibia, Right* **J Fibula, Right** Body of fibula Head of fibula Lateral malleolus **K Fibula, Left** *See J Fibula, Right* **L Tarsal, Right** Calcaneus Cuboid bone Intermediate cuneiform bone Lateral cuneiform bone Medial cuneiform bone Navicular bone Talus bone **M Tarsal, Left** *See L Tarsal, Right* **N Metatarsal, Right** Fibular sesamoid Tibial sesamoid **P Metatarsal, Left** *See N Metatarsal, Right* **Q Toe Phalanx, Right** **R Toe Phalanx, Left** **S Coccyx**	Ø Open 3 Percutaneous 4 Percutaneous Endoscopic	Ø Drainage Device	Z No Qualifier
Ø Lumbar Vertebra Spinous process Transverse process Vertebral arch Vertebral body Vertebral foramen Vertebral lamina Vertebral pedicle **1 Sacrum** **2 Pelvic Bone, Right** Iliac crest Ilium Ischium Pubis **3 Pelvic Bone, Left** *See 2 Pelvic Bone, Right* **4 Acetabulum, Right** **5 Acetabulum, Left** **6 Upper Femur, Right** Femoral head Greater trochanter Lesser trochanter Neck of femur **7 Upper Femur, Left** *See 6 Upper Femur, Right* **8 Femoral Shaft, Right** Body of femur **9 Femoral Shaft, Left** *See 8 Femoral Shaft, Right* **B Lower Femur, Right** Lateral condyle of femur Lateral epicondyle of femur Medial condyle of femur Medial epicondyle of femur **C Lower Femur, Left** *See B Lower Femur, Right* **D Patella, Right** **F Patella, Left** **G Tibia, Right** Lateral condyle of tibia Medial condyle of tibia Medial malleolus **H Tibia, Left** *See G Tibia, Right* **J Fibula, Right** Body of fibula Head of fibula Lateral malleolus **K Fibula, Left** *See J Fibula, Right* **L Tarsal, Right** Calcaneus Cuboid bone Intermediate cuneiform bone Lateral cuneiform bone Medial cuneiform bone Navicular bone Talus bone **M Tarsal, Left** *See L Tarsal, Right* **N Metatarsal, Right** Fibular sesamoid Tibial sesamoid **P Metatarsal, Left** *See N Metatarsal, Right* **Q Toe Phalanx, Right** **R Toe Phalanx, Left** **S Coccyx**	Ø Open 3 Percutaneous 4 Percutaneous Endoscopic	Z No Device	X Diagnostic Z No Qualifier

Non-OR ØQ9[Ø,1,2,3,4,5,6,7,8,9,B,C,D,F,G,H,J,K,L,M,P,Q,R,S]3ØZ
Non-OR ØQ9[Ø,1,2,3,4,5,6,7,8,9,B,C,D,F,G,H,J,K,L,M,P,Q,R,S]3ZZ

Ø Medical and Surgical
Q Lower Bones
B Excision

Definition: Cutting out or off, without replacement, a portion of a body part
Explanation: The qualifier DIAGNOSTIC is used to identify excision procedures that are biopsies

Body Part Character 4	Approach Character 5	Device Character 6	Qualifier Character 7
Ø Lumbar Vertebra Spinous process Transverse process Vertebral arch Vertebral body Vertebral foramen Vertebral lamina Vertebral pedicle **1 Sacrum** **2 Pelvic Bone, Right** Iliac crest Ilium Ischium Pubis **3 Pelvic Bone, Left** *See 2 Pelvic Bone, Right* **4 Acetabulum, Right** **5 Acetabulum, Left** **6 Upper Femur, Right** Femoral head Greater trochanter Lesser trochanter Neck of femur **7 Upper Femur, Left** *See 6 Upper Femur, Right* **8 Femoral Shaft, Right** Body of femur **9 Femoral Shaft, Left** *See 8 Femoral Shaft, Right* **B Lower Femur, Right** Lateral condyle of femur Lateral epicondyle of femur Medial condyle of femur Medial epicondyle of femur **C Lower Femur, Left** *See B Lower Femur, Right* **D Patella, Right** **F Patella, Left** **G Tibia, Right** Lateral condyle of tibia Medial condyle of tibia Medial malleolus **H Tibia, Left** *See G Tibia, Right* **J Fibula, Right** Body of fibula Head of fibula Lateral malleolus **K Fibula, Left** *See J Fibula, Right* **L Tarsal, Right** Calcaneus Cuboid bone Intermediate cuneiform bone Lateral cuneiform bone Medial cuneiform bone Navicular bone Talus bone **M Tarsal, Left** *See L Tarsal, Right* **Q Toe Phalanx, Right** **R Toe Phalanx, Left** **S Coccyx**	**Ø Open** **3 Percutaneous** **4 Percutaneous Endoscopic**	**Z No Device**	**X Diagnostic** **Z No Qualifier**
N Metatarsal, Right Fibular sesamoid Tibial sesamoid **P Metatarsal, Left** *See N Metatarsal, Right*	**Ø Open** **3 Percutaneous** **4 Percutaneous Endoscopic**	**Z No Device**	**2 Sesamoid Bone(s) 1st Toe** **X Diagnostic** **Z No Qualifier**

Ø Medical and Surgical
Q Lower Bones
C Extirpation

Definition: Taking or cutting out solid matter from a body part

Explanation: The solid matter may be an abnormal byproduct of a biological function or a foreign body; it may be imbedded in a body part or in the lumen of a tubular body part. The solid matter may or may not have been previously broken into pieces.

Body Part Character 4	Approach Character 5	Device Character 6	Qualifier Character 7
Ø Lumbar Vertebra Spinous process Transverse process Vertebral arch Vertebral body Vertebral foramen Vertebral lamina Vertebral pedicle **1 Sacrum** **2 Pelvic Bone, Right** Iliac crest Ilium Ischium Pubis **3 Pelvic Bone, Left** **See** *2 Pelvic Bone, Right* **4 Acetabulum, Right** **5 Acetabulum, Left** **6 Upper Femur, Right** Femoral head Greater trochanter Lesser trochanter Neck of femur **7 Upper Femur, Left** **See** *6 Upper Femur, Right* **8 Femoral Shaft, Right** Body of femur **9 Femoral Shaft, Left** **See** *8 Femoral Shaft, Right* **B Lower Femur, Right** Lateral condyle of femur Lateral epicondyle of femur Medial condyle of femur Medial epicondyle of femur **C Lower Femur, Left** **See** *B Lower Femur, Right* **D Patella, Right** **F Patella, Left** **G Tibia, Right** Lateral condyle of tibia Medial condyle of tibia Medial malleolus **H Tibia, Left** **See** *G Tibia, Right* **J Fibula, Right** Body of fibula Head of fibula Lateral malleolus **K Fibula, Left** **See** *J Fibula, Right* **L Tarsal, Right** Calcaneus Cuboid bone Intermediate cuneiform bone Lateral cuneiform bone Medial cuneiform bone Navicular bone Talus bone **M Tarsal, Left** **See** *L Tarsal, Right* **N Metatarsal, Right** Fibular sesamoid Tibial sesamoid **P Metatarsal, Left** **See** *N Metatarsal, Right* **Q Toe Phalanx, Right** **R Toe Phalanx, Left** **S Coccyx**	**Ø Open** **3 Percutaneous** **4 Percutaneous Endoscopic**	**Z No Device**	**Z No Qualifier**

Ø Medical and Surgical
Q Lower Bones
D Extraction

Definition: Pulling or stripping out or off all or a portion of a body part by the use of force
Explanation: The qualifier DIAGNOSTIC is used to identify extraction procedures that are biopsies

Body Part Character 4	Approach Character 5	Device Character 6	Qualifier Character 7
Ø Lumbar Vertebra Spinous process Transverse process Vertebral arch Vertebral body Vertebral foramen Vertebral lamina Vertebral pedicle **1 Sacrum** **2 Pelvic Bone, Right** Iliac crest Ilium Ischium Pubis **3 Pelvic Bone, Left** *See 2 Pelvic Bone, Right* **4 Acetabulum, Right** **5 Acetabulum, Left** **6 Upper Femur, Right** Femoral head Greater trochanter Lesser trochanter Neck of femur **7 Upper Femur, Left** *See 6 Upper Femur, Right* **8 Femoral Shaft, Right** Body of femur **9 Femoral Shaft, Left** *See 8 Femoral Shaft, Right* **B Lower Femur, Right** Lateral condyle of femur Lateral epicondyle of femur Medial condyle of femur Medial epicondyle of femur **C Lower Femur, Left** *See B Lower Femur, Right* **D Patella, Right** **F Patella, Left** **G Tibia, Right** Lateral condyle of tibia Medial condyle of tibia Medial malleolus **H Tibia, Left** *See G Tibia, Right* **J Fibula, Right** Body of fibula Head of fibula Lateral malleolus **K Fibula, Left** *See J Fibula, Right* **L Tarsal, Right** Calcaneus Cuboid bone Intermediate cuneiform bone Lateral cuneiform bone Medial cuneiform bone Navicular bone Talus bone **M Tarsal, Left** *See L Tarsal, Right* **N Metatarsal, Right** Fibular sesamoid Tibial sesamoid **P Metatarsal, Left** *See N Metatarsal, Right* **Q Toe Phalanx, Right** **R Toe Phalanx, Left** **S Coccyx**	**Ø Open**	**Z No Device**	**Z No Qualifier**

Ø Medical and Surgical
Q Lower Bones
H Insertion

Definition: Putting in a nonbiological appliance that monitors, assists, performs, or prevents a physiological function but does not physically take the place of a body part

Explanation: None

Body Part Character 4		Approach Character 5	Device Character 6	Qualifier Character 7
Ø Lumbar Vertebra Spinous process Transverse process Vertebral arch Vertebral body Vertebral foramen Vertebral lamina Vertebral pedicle **1 Sacrum** **2 Pelvic Bone, Right** Iliac crest Ilium Ischium Pubis **3 Pelvic Bone, Left** *See 2 Pelvic Bone, Right* **4 Acetabulum, Right** **5 Acetabulum, Left**	**D Patella, Right** **F Patella, Left** **L Tarsal, Right** Calcaneus Cuboid bone Intermediate cuneiform bone Lateral cuneiform bone Medial cuneiform bone Navicular bone Talus bone **M Tarsal, Left** *See L Tarsal, Right* **N Metatarsal, Right** Fibular sesamoid Tibial sesamoid **P Metatarsal, Left** *See N Metatarsal, Right* **Q Toe Phalanx, Right** **R Toe Phalanx, Left** **S Coccyx**	**Ø** Open **3** Percutaneous **4** Percutaneous Endoscopic	**4** Internal Fixation Device **5** External Fixation Device	**Z** No Qualifier
6 Upper Femur, Right Femoral head Greater trochanter Lesser trochanter Neck of femur **7 Upper Femur, Left** *See 6 Upper Femur, Right* **B Lower Femur, Right** Lateral condyle of femur Lateral epicondyle of femur Medial condyle of femur Medial epicondyle of femur	**C Lower Femur, Left** *See B Lower Femur, Right* **J Fibula, Right** Body of fibula Head of fibula Lateral malleolus **K Fibula, Left** *See J Fibula, Right*	**Ø** Open **3** Percutaneous **4** Percutaneous Endoscopic	**4** Internal Fixation Device **5** External Fixation Device **6** Internal Fixation Device, Intramedullary **8** External Fixation Device, Limb Lengthening **B** External Fixation Device, Monoplanar **C** External Fixation Device, Ring **D** External Fixation Device, Hybrid	**Z** No Qualifier
8 Femoral Shaft, Right Body of femur **9 Femoral Shaft, Left** *See 8 Femoral Shaft, Right*	**G Tibia, Right** Lateral condyle of tibia Medial condyle of tibia Medial malleolus **H Tibia, Left** *See G Tibia, Right*	**Ø** Open **3** Percutaneous **4** Percutaneous Endoscopic	**4** Internal Fixation Device **5** External Fixation Device **6** Internal Fixation Device, Intramedullary **7** Internal Fixation Device, Intramedullary Limb Lengthening **8** External Fixation Device, Limb Lengthening **B** External Fixation Device, Monoplanar **C** External Fixation Device, Ring **D** External Fixation Device, Hybrid	**Z** No Qualifier
Y Lower Bone		**Ø** Open **3** Percutaneous **4** Percutaneous Endoscopic	**M** Bone Growth Stimulator	**Z** No Qualifier

Non-OR ØQH[6,7,B,C,J,K][Ø,3,4]8Z
Non-OR ØQH[8,9,G,H][Ø,3,4]8Z

Ø Medical and Surgical
Q Lower Bones
J Inspection

Definition: Visually and/or manually exploring a body part

Explanation: Visual exploration may be performed with or without optical instrumentation. Manual exploration may be performed directly or through intervening body layers.

Body Part Character 4	Approach Character 5	Device Character 6	Qualifier Character 7
Y Lower Bone	**Ø** Open **3** Percutaneous **4** Percutaneous Endoscopic **X** External	**Z** No Device	**Z** No Qualifier

Non-OR ØQJY[3,X]ZZ

Ø Medical and Surgical
Q Lower Bones
N Release Definition: Freeing a body part from an abnormal physical constraint by cutting or by the use of force
Explanation: Some of the restraining tissue may be taken out but none of the body part is taken out

Body Part Character 4	Approach Character 5	Device Character 6	Qualifier Character 7
Ø Lumbar Vertebra Spinous process Transverse process Vertebral arch Vertebral body Vertebral foramen Vertebral lamina Vertebral pedicle **1 Sacrum** **2 Pelvic Bone, Right** Iliac crest Ilium Ischium Pubis **3 Pelvic Bone, Left** *See 2 Pelvic Bone, Right* **4 Acetabulum, Right** **5 Acetabulum, Left** **6 Upper Femur, Right** Femoral head Greater trochanter Lesser trochanter Neck of femur **7 Upper Femur, Left** *See 6 Upper Femur, Right* **8 Femoral Shaft, Right** Body of femur **9 Femoral Shaft, Left** *See 8 Femoral Shaft, Right* **B Lower Femur, Right** Lateral condyle of femur Lateral epicondyle of femur Medial condyle of femur Medial epicondyle of femur **C Lower Femur, Left** *See B Lower Femur, Right* **D Patella, Right** **F Patella, Left** **G Tibia, Right** Lateral condyle of tibia Medial condyle of tibia Medial malleolus **H Tibia, Left** *See G Tibia, Right* **J Fibula, Right** Body of fibula Head of fibula Lateral malleolus **K Fibula, Left** *See J Fibula, Right* **L Tarsal, Right** Calcaneus Cuboid bone Intermediate cuneiform bone Lateral cuneiform bone Medial cuneiform bone Navicular bone Talus bone **M Tarsal, Left** *See L Tarsal, Right* **N Metatarsal, Right** Fibular sesamoid Tibial sesamoid **P Metatarsal, Left** *See N Metatarsal, Right* **Q Toe Phalanx, Right** **R Toe Phalanx, Left** **S Coccyx**	**Ø Open** **3 Percutaneous** **4 Percutaneous Endoscopic**	**Z No Device**	**Z No Qualifier**

Ø Medical and Surgical
Q Lower Bones
P Removal

Definition: Taking out or off a device from a body part

Explanation: If a device is taken out and a similar device put in without cutting or puncturing the skin or mucous membrane, the procedure is coded to the root operation CHANGE. Otherwise, the procedure for taking out a device is coded to the root operation REMOVAL.

Body Part Character 4		Approach Character 5	Device Character 6	Qualifier Character 7
Ø Lumbar Vertebra Spinous process Transverse process Vertebral arch Vertebral body Vertebral foramen Vertebral lamina Vertebral pedicle **1 Sacrum** **2 Pelvic Bone, Right** Iliac crest Ilium Ischium Pubis **3 Pelvic Bone, Left** *See 2 Pelvic Bone, Right* **4 Acetabulum, Right** **5 Acetabulum, Left** **6 Upper Femur, Right** Femoral head Greater trochanter Lesser trochanter Neck of femur **7 Upper Femur, Left** *See 6 Upper Femur, Right* **8 Femoral Shaft, Right** Body of femur **9 Femoral Shaft, Left** *See 8 Femoral Shaft, Right* **B Lower Femur, Right** Lateral condyle of femur Lateral epicondyle of femur Medial condyle of femur Medial epicondyle of femur	**C Lower Femur, Left** *See B Lower Femur, Right* **D Patella, Right** **F Patella, Left** **G Tibia, Right** Lateral condyle of tibia Medial condyle of tibia Medial malleolus **H Tibia, Left** *See G Tibia, Right* **J Fibula, Right** Body of fibula Head of fibula Lateral malleolus **K Fibula, Left** *See J Fibula, Right* **L Tarsal, Right** Calcaneus Cuboid bone Intermediate cuneiform bone Lateral cuneiform bone Medial cuneiform bone Navicular bone Talus bone **M Tarsal, Left** *See L Tarsal, Right* **N Metatarsal, Right** Fibular sesamoid Tibial sesamoid **P Metatarsal, Left** *See N Metatarsal, Right* **Q Toe Phalanx, Right** **R Toe Phalanx, Left** **S Coccyx**	**Ø Open** **3 Percutaneous** **4 Percutaneous Endoscopic**	**4 Internal Fixation Device** **5 External Fixation Device** **7 Autologous Tissue Substitute** **J Synthetic Substitute** **K Nonautologous Tissue Substitute**	**Z No Qualifier**
Ø Lumbar Vertebra Spinous process Transverse process Vertebral arch Vertebral body Vertebral foramen Vertebral lamina Vertebral pedicle **1 Sacrum** **2 Pelvic Bone, Right** Iliac crest Ilium Ischium Pubis **3 Pelvic Bone, Left** *See 2 Pelvic Bone, Right* **4 Acetabulum, Right** **5 Acetabulum, Left** **6 Upper Femur, Right** Femoral head Greater trochanter Lesser trochanter Neck of femur **7 Upper Femur, Left** *See 6 Upper Femur, Right* **8 Femoral Shaft, Right** Body of femur **9 Femoral Shaft, Left** *See 8 Femoral Shaft, Right* **B Lower Femur, Right** Lateral condyle of femur Lateral epicondyle of femur Medial condyle of femur Medial epicondyle of femur	**C Lower Femur, Left** *See B Lower Femur, Right* **D Patella, Right** **F Patella, Left** **G Tibia, Right** Lateral condyle of tibia Medial condyle of tibia Medial malleolus **H Tibia, Left** *See G Tibia, Right* **J Fibula, Right** Body of fibula Head of fibula Lateral malleolus **K Fibula, Left** *See J Fibula, Right* **L Tarsal, Right** Calcaneus Cuboid bone Intermediate cuneiform bone Lateral cuneiform bone Medial cuneiform bone Navicular bone Talus bone **M Tarsal, Left** *See L Tarsal, Right* **N Metatarsal, Right** Fibular sesamoid Tibial sesamoid **P Metatarsal, Left** *See N Metatarsal, Right* **Q Toe Phalanx, Right** **R Toe Phalanx, Left** **S Coccyx**	**X External**	**4 Internal Fixation Device** **5 External Fixation Device**	**Z No Qualifier**
Y Lower Bone		**Ø Open** **3 Percutaneous** **4 Percutaneous Endoscopic** **X External**	**Ø Drainage Device** **M Bone Growth Stimulator**	**Z No Qualifier**

Non-OR ØQPYX[Ø,M]Z Non-OR ØQPY3ØZ Non-OR ØQP[Ø,1,2,3,4,5,6,7,8,9,B,C,D,F,G,H,J,K,L,M,N,P,Q,R,S]X[4,5]Z

NC Noncovered Procedure LC Limited Coverage QA Questionable OB Admit NT New Tech Add-on Combination Member ♂ Male ♀ Female

Ø Medical and Surgical
Q Lower Bones
Q Repair

Definition: Restoring, to the extent possible, a body part to its normal anatomic structure and function

Explanation: Used only when the method to accomplish the repair is not one of the other root operations

Body Part Character 4	Approach Character 5	Device Character 6	Qualifier Character 7
Ø Lumbar Vertebra Spinous process Transverse process Vertebral arch Vertebral body Vertebral foramen Vertebral lamina Vertebral pedicle **1 Sacrum** **2 Pelvic Bone, Right** Iliac crest Ilium Ischium Pubis **3 Pelvic Bone, Left** *See 2 Pelvic Bone, Right* **4 Acetabulum, Right** **5 Acetabulum, Left** **6 Upper Femur, Right** Femoral head Greater trochanter Lesser trochanter Neck of femur **7 Upper Femur, Left** *See 6 Upper Femur, Right* **8 Femoral Shaft, Right** Body of femur **9 Femoral Shaft, Left** *See 8 Femoral Shaft, Right* **B Lower Femur, Right** Lateral condyle of femur Lateral epicondyle of femur Medial condyle of femur Medial epicondyle of femur **C Lower Femur, Left** *See B Lower Femur, Right* **D Patella, Right** **F Patella, Left** **G Tibia, Right** Lateral condyle of tibia Medial condyle of tibia Medial malleolus **H Tibia, Left** *See G Tibia, Right* **J Fibula, Right** Body of fibula Head of fibula Lateral malleolus **K Fibula, Left** *See J Fibula, Right* **L Tarsal, Right** Calcaneus Cuboid bone Intermediate cuneiform bone Lateral cuneiform bone Medial cuneiform bone Navicular bone Talus bone **M Tarsal, Left** *See L Tarsal, Right* **N Metatarsal, Right** Fibular sesamoid Tibial sesamoid **P Metatarsal, Left** *See N Metatarsal, Right* **Q Toe Phalanx, Right** **R Toe Phalanx, Left** **S Coccyx**	**Ø Open** **3 Percutaneous** **4 Percutaneous Endoscopic** **X External**	**Z No Device**	**Z No Qualifier**

Non-OR ØQQ[Ø,1,2,3,4,5,6,7,8,9,B,C,D,F,G,H,J,K,L,M,N,P,Q,R,S]XZZ

Ø Medical and Surgical
Q Lower Bones
R Replacement

Definition: Putting in or on biological or synthetic material that physically takes the place and/or function of all or a portion of a body part

Explanation: The body part may have been taken out or replaced, or may be taken out, physically eradicated, or rendered nonfunctional during the REPLACEMENT procedure. A REMOVAL procedure is coded for taking out the device used in a previous replacement procedure.

Body Part Character 4	Approach Character 5	Device Character 6	Qualifier Character 7
Ø Lumbar Vertebra Spinous process Transverse process Vertebral arch Vertebral body Vertebral foramen Vertebral lamina Vertebral pedicle **1 Sacrum** **2 Pelvic Bone, Right** Iliac crest Ilium Ischium Pubis **3 Pelvic Bone, Left** *See 2 Pelvic Bone, Right* **4 Acetabulum, Right** **5 Acetabulum, Left** **6 Upper Femur, Right** Femoral head Greater trochanter Lesser trochanter Neck of femur **7 Upper Femur, Left** *See 6 Upper Femur, Right* **8 Femoral Shaft, Right** Body of femur **9 Femoral Shaft, Left** *See 8 Femoral Shaft, Right* **B Lower Femur, Right** Lateral condyle of femur Lateral epicondyle of femur Medial condyle of femur Medial epicondyle of femur **C Lower Femur, Left** *See B Lower Femur, Right* **D Patella, Right** **F Patella, Left** **G Tibia, Right** Lateral condyle of tibia Medial condyle of tibia Medial malleolus **H Tibia, Left** *See G Tibia, Right* **J Fibula, Right** Body of fibula Head of fibula Lateral malleolus **K Fibula, Left** *See J Fibula, Right* **L Tarsal, Right** Calcaneus Cuboid bone Intermediate cuneiform bone Lateral cuneiform bone Medial cuneiform bone Navicular bone Talus bone **M Tarsal, Left** *See L Tarsal, Right* **N Metatarsal, Right** Fibular sesamoid Tibial sesamoid **P Metatarsal, Left** *See N Metatarsal, Right* **Q Toe Phalanx, Right** **R Toe Phalanx, Left** **S Coccyx**	**Ø Open** **3 Percutaneous** **4 Percutaneous Endoscopic**	**7 Autologous Tissue Substitute** **J Synthetic Substitute** **K Nonautologous Tissue Substitute**	**Z No Qualifier**

Ø Medical and Surgical
Q Lower Bones
S Reposition

Definition: Moving to its normal location, or other suitable location, all or a portion of a body part

Explanation: The body part is moved to a new location from an abnormal location, or from a normal location where it is not functioning correctly. The body part may or may not be cut out or off to be moved to the new location.

Body Part Character 4	Approach Character 5	Device Character 6	Qualifier Character 7
Ø Lumbar Vertebra Spinous process Transverse process Vertebral arch Vertebral body Vertebral foramen Vertebral lamina Vertebral pedicle	**Ø Open** **4 Percutaneous Endoscopic**	**3 Spinal Stabilization Device, Vertebral Body Tether** **4 Internal Fixation Device** **Z No Device**	**Z No Qualifier**
Ø Lumbar Vertebra ⊞ Spinous process Transverse process Vertebral arch Vertebral body Vertebral foramen Vertebral lamina Vertebral pedicle	**3 Percutaneous**	**4 Internal Fixation Device** **Z No Device**	**Z No Qualifier**
Ø Lumbar Vertebra Spinous process Transverse process Vertebral arch Vertebral body Vertebral foramen Vertebral lamina Vertebral pedicle	**X External**	**Z No Device**	**Z No Qualifier**
1 Sacrum ⊞ **4 Acetabulum, Right** **5 Acetabulum, Left** **S Coccyx** ⊞	**Ø Open** **3 Percutaneous** **4 Percutaneous Endoscopic**	**4 Internal Fixation Device** **Z No Device**	**Z No Qualifier**
1 Sacrum **4 Acetabulum, Right** **5 Acetabulum, Left** **S Coccyx**	**X External**	**Z No Device**	**Z No Qualifier**
2 Pelvic Bone, Right Iliac crest Ilium Ischium Pubis **3 Pelvic Bone, Left** *See 2 Pelvic Bone, Right* **D Patella, Right** **F Patella, Left** **L Tarsal, Right** Calcaneus Cuboid bone Intermediate cuneiform bone Lateral cuneiform bone Medial cuneiform bone Navicular bone Talus bone **M Tarsal, Left** *See L Tarsal, Right* **Q Toe Phalanx, Right** **R Toe Phalanx, Left**	**Ø Open** **3 Percutaneous** **4 Percutaneous Endoscopic**	**4 Internal Fixation Device** **5 External Fixation Device** **Z No Device**	**Z No Qualifier**
2 Pelvic Bone, Right Iliac crest Ilium Ischium Pubis **3 Pelvic Bone, Left** *See 2 Pelvic Bone, Right* **D Patella, Right** **F Patella, Left** **L Tarsal, Right** Calcaneus Cuboid bone Intermediate cuneiform bone Lateral cuneiform bone Medial cuneiform bone Navicular bone Talus bone **M Tarsal, Left** *See L Tarsal, Right* **Q Toe Phalanx, Right** **R Toe Phalanx, Left**	**X External**	**Z No Device**	**Z No Qualifier**

Non-OR ØQSØXZZ
Non-OR ØQS[4,5][3,4]ZZ
Non-OR ØQS[1,4,5,S]XZZ
Non-OR ØQS[2,3,D,F,L,M,Q,R][3,4]ZZ
Non-OR ØQS[2,3,D,F,L,M,Q,R]XZZ

See Appendix L for Procedure Combinations
⊞ ØQSØ3ZZ
⊞ ØQS[1,S]3ZZ

ØQS Continued on next page

Non-OR Procedure | DRG Non-OR Procedure | Valid OR Procedure | HAC Associated Procedure | Combination Only | New/Revised April | New/Revised October

Ø Medical and Surgical
Q Lower Bones
S Reposition

ØQS Continued

Definition: Moving to its normal location, or other suitable location, all or a portion of a body part

Explanation: The body part is moved to a new location from an abnormal location, or from a normal location where it is not functioning correctly. The body part may or may not be cut out or off to be moved to the new location.

Body Part Character 4	Approach Character 5	Device Character 6	Qualifier Character 7
6 Upper Femur, Right Femoral head Greater trochanter Lesser trochanter Neck of femur **7 Upper Femur, Left** ***See*** *6 Upper Femur, Right* **8 Femoral Shaft, Right** Body of femur **9 Femoral Shaft, Left** ***See*** *8 Femoral Shaft, Right* **B Lower Femur, Right** Lateral condyle of femur Lateral epicondyle of femur Medial condyle of femur Medial epicondyle of femur **C Lower Femur, Left** ***See*** *B Lower Femur, Right* **G Tibia, Right** Lateral condyle of tibia Medial condyle of tibia Medial malleolus **H Tibia, Left** ***See*** *G Tibia, Right* **J Fibula, Right** Body of fibula Head of fibula Lateral malleolus **K Fibula, Left** ***See*** *J Fibula, Right*	**Ø Open** **3 Percutaneous** **4 Percutaneous Endoscopic**	**4 Internal Fixation Device** **5 External Fixation Device** **6 Internal Fixation Device, Intramedullary** **B External Fixation Device, Monoplanar** **C External Fixation Device, Ring** **D External Fixation Device, Hybrid** **Z No Device**	**Z No Qualifier**
6 Upper Femur, Right Femoral head Greater trochanter Lesser trochanter Neck of femur **7 Upper Femur, Left** ***See*** *6 Upper Femur, Right* **8 Femoral Shaft, Right** Body of femur **9 Femoral Shaft, Left** ***See*** *8 Femoral Shaft, Right* **B Lower Femur, Right** Lateral condyle of femur Lateral epicondyle of femur Medial condyle of femur Medial epicondyle of femur **C Lower Femur, Left** ***See*** *B Lower Femur, Right* **G Tibia, Right** Lateral condyle of tibia Medial condyle of tibia Medial malleolus **H Tibia, Left** ***See*** *G Tibia, Right* **J Fibula, Right** Body of fibula Head of fibula Lateral malleolus **K Fibula, Left** ***See*** *J Fibula, Right*	**X External**	**Z No Device**	**Z No Qualifier**
N Metatarsal, Right Fibular sesamoid Tibial sesamoid **P Metatarsal, Left** ***See*** *N Metatarsal, Right*	**Ø Open** **3 Percutaneous** **4 Percutaneous Endoscopic**	**4 Internal Fixation Device** **5 External Fixation Device** **Z No Device**	**2 Sesamoid Bone(s) 1st Toe** **Z No Qualifier**
N Metatarsal, Right Fibular sesamoid Tibial sesamoid **P Metatarsal, Left** ***See*** *N Metatarsal, Right*	**X External**	**Z No Device**	**2 Sesamoid Bone(s) 1st Toe** **Z No Qualifier**

Non-OR ØQS[6,7,8,9,B,C,G,H,J,K][3,4]ZZ
Non-OR ØQS[6,7,8,9,B,C,G,H,J,K]XZZ
Non-OR ØQS[N,P][3,4]Z[2,Z]
Non-OR ØQS[N,P]XZ[2,Z]

NC Noncovered Procedure 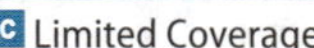 LC Limited Coverage 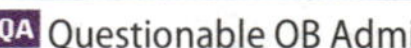 QA Questionable OB Admit 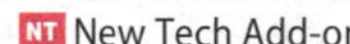 NT New Tech Add-on ✚ Combination Member ♂ Male ♀ Female

Ø Medical and Surgical
Q Lower Bones
T Resection

Definition: Cutting out or off, without replacement, all of a body part

Explanation: None

Body Part Character 4		Approach Character 5	Device Character 6	Qualifier Character 7
2 Pelvic Bone, Right Iliac crest Ilium Ischium Pubis **3 Pelvic Bone, Left** *See 2 Pelvic Bone, Right* **4 Acetabulum, Right** **5 Acetabulum, Left** **6 Upper Femur, Right** Femoral head Greater trochanter Lesser trochanter Neck of femur **7 Upper Femur, Left** *See 6 Upper Femur, Right* **8 Femoral Shaft, Right** Body of femur **9 Femoral Shaft, Left** *See 8 Femoral Shaft, Right* **B Lower Femur, Right** Lateral condyle of femur Lateral epicondyle of femur Medial condyle of femur Medial epicondyle of femur **C Lower Femur, Left** *See B Lower Femur, Right* **D Patella, Right**	**F Patella, Left** **G Tibia, Right** Lateral condyle of tibia Medial condyle of tibia Medial malleolus **H Tibia, Left** *See G Tibia, Right* **J Fibula, Right** Body of fibula Head of fibula Lateral malleolus **K Fibula, Left** *See J Fibula, Right* **L Tarsal, Right** Calcaneus Cuboid bone Intermediate cuneiform bone Lateral cuneiform bone Medial cuneiform bone Navicular bone Talus bone **M Tarsal, Left** *See L Tarsal, Right* **N Metatarsal, Right** Fibular sesamoid Tibial sesamoid **P Metatarsal, Left** *See N Metatarsal, Right* **Q Toe Phalanx, Right** **R Toe Phalanx, Left** **S Coccyx**	**Ø Open**	**Z No Device**	**Z No Qualifier**

Ø Medical and Surgical
Q Lower Bones
U Supplement

Definition: Putting in or on biological or synthetic material that physically reinforces and/or augments the function of a portion of a body part

Explanation: The biological material is non-living, or is living and from the same individual. The body part may have been previously replaced, and the SUPPLEMENT procedure is performed to physically reinforce and/or augment the function of the replaced body part.

Body Part Character 4		Approach Character 5	Device Character 6	Qualifier Character 7
Ø Lumbar Vertebra ⊞ Spinous process Transverse process Vertebral arch Vertebral body Vertebral foramen Vertebral lamina Vertebral pedicle **1 Sacrum** ⊞ **2 Pelvic Bone, Right** Iliac crest Ilium Ischium Pubis **3 Pelvic Bone, Left** *See 2 Pelvic Bone, Right* **4 Acetabulum, Right** **5 Acetabulum, Left** **6 Upper Femur, Right** Femoral head Greater trochanter Lesser trochanter Neck of femur **7 Upper Femur, Left** *See 6 Upper Femur, Right* **8 Femoral Shaft, Right** Body of femur **9 Femoral Shaft, Left** *See 8 Femoral Shaft, Right* **B Lower Femur, Right** Lateral condyle of femur Lateral epicondyle of femur Medial condyle of femur Medial epicondyle of femur	**C Lower Femur, Left** *See B Lower Femur, Right* **D Patella, Right** **F Patella, Left** **G Tibia, Right** Lateral condyle of tibia Medial condyle of tibia Medial malleolus **H Tibia, Left** *See G Tibia, Right* **J Fibula, Right** Body of fibula Head of fibula Lateral malleolus **K Fibula, Left** *See J Fibula, Right* **L Tarsal, Right** Calcaneus Cuboid bone Intermediate cuneiform bone Lateral cuneiform bone Medial cuneiform bone Navicular bone Talus bone **M Tarsal, Left** *See L Tarsal, Right* **N Metatarsal, Right** Fibular sesamoid Tibial sesamoid **P Metatarsal, Left** *See N Metatarsal, Right* **Q Toe Phalanx, Right** **R Toe Phalanx, Left** **S Coccyx** ⊞	**Ø Open** **3 Percutaneous** **4 Percutaneous Endoscopic**	**7 Autologous Tissue Substitute** **J Synthetic Substitute** **K Nonautologous Tissue Substitute**	**Z No Qualifier**

See Appendix L for Procedure Combinations

⊞ ØQU[Ø,1,S]3JZ

Ø Medical and Surgical
Q Lower Bones
W Revision

Definition: Correcting, to the extent possible, a portion of a malfunctioning device or the position of a displaced device

Explanation: Revision can include correcting a malfunctioning or displaced device by taking out or putting in components of the device such as a screw or pin

Body Part Character 4	Approach Character 5	Device Character 6	Qualifier Character 7
Ø Lumbar Vertebra Spinous process Transverse process Vertebral arch Vertebral body Vertebral foramen Vertebral lamina Vertebral pedicle **1 Sacrum** **4 Acetabulum, Right** **5 Acetabulum, Left** **S Coccyx**	**Ø** Open **3** Percutaneous **4** Percutaneous Endoscopic **X** External	**4** Internal Fixation Device **7** Autologous Tissue Substitute **J** Synthetic Substitute **K** Nonautologous Tissue Substitute	**Z** No Qualifier
2 Pelvic Bone, Right Iliac crest Ilium Ischium Pubis **3 Pelvic Bone, Left** *See 2 Pelvic Bone, Right* **6 Upper Femur, Right** Femoral head Greater trochanter Lesser trochanter Neck of femur **7 Upper Femur, Left** *See 6 Upper Femur, Right* **8 Femoral Shaft, Right** Body of femur **9 Femoral Shaft, Left** *See 8 Femoral Shaft, Right* **B Lower Femur, Right** Lateral condyle of femur Lateral epicondyle of femur Medial condyle of femur Medial epicondyle of femur **C Lower Femur, Left** *See B Lower Femur, Right* **D Patella, Right** **F Patella, Left** **G Tibia, Right** Lateral condyle of tibia Medial condyle of tibia Medial malleolus **H Tibia, Left** *See G Tibia, Right* **J Fibula, Right** Body of fibula Head of fibula Lateral malleolus **K Fibula, Left** *See J Fibula, Right* **L Tarsal, Right** Calcaneus Cuboid bone Intermediate cuneiform bone Lateral cuneiform bone Medial cuneiform bone Navicular bone Talus bone **M Tarsal, Left** *See L Tarsal, Right* **N Metatarsal, Right** Fibular sesamoid Tibial sesamoid **P Metatarsal, Left** *See N Metatarsal, Right* **Q Toe Phalanx, Right** **R Toe Phalanx, Left**	**Ø** Open **3** Percutaneous **4** Percutaneous Endoscopic **X** External	**4** Internal Fixation Device **5** External Fixation Device **7** Autologous Tissue Substitute **J** Synthetic Substitute **K** Nonautologous Tissue Substitute	**Z** No Qualifier
Y Lower Bone	**Ø** Open **3** Percutaneous **4** Percutaneous Endoscopic **X** External	**Ø** Drainage Device **M** Bone Growth Stimulator	**Z** No Qualifier

Non-OR ØQW[Ø,1,4,5,S]X[4,7,J,K]Z
Non-OR ØQW[2,3,6,7,8,9,B,C,D,F,G,H,J,K,L,M,N,P,Q,R]X[4,5,7,J,K]Z
Non-OR ØQWYX[Ø,M]Z

Upper Joints ØR2–ØRW

Character Meanings*

This Character Meaning table is provided as a guide to assist the user in the identification of character members that may be found in this section of code tables. It **SHOULD NOT** be used to build a PCS code.

Operation–Character 3	Body Part–Character 4	Approach–Character 5	Device–Character 6	Qualifier–Character 7
2 Change	Ø Occipital-cervical Joint	Ø Open	Ø Drainage Device OR Synthetic Substitute, Reverse Ball and Socket	Ø Anterior Approach, Anterior Column
5 Destruction	1 Cervical Vertebral Joint	3 Percutaneous	3 Infusion Device OR Internal Fixation Device, Sustained Compression	1 Posterior Approach, Posterior Column
9 Drainage	2 Cervical Vertebral Joint, 2 or more	4 Percutaneous Endoscopic	4 Internal Fixation Device	6 Humeral Surface
B Excision	3 Cervical Vertebral Disc	X External	5 External Fixation Device	7 Glenoid Surface
C Extirpation	4 Cervicothoracic Vertebral Joint		7 Autologous Tissue Substitute	J Posterior Approach, Anterior Column
G Fusion	5 Cervicothoracic Vertebral Disc		8 Spacer	X Diagnostic
H Insertion	6 Thoracic Vertebral Joint		A Interbody Fusion Device	Z No Qualifier
J Inspection	7 Thoracic Vertebral Joint, 2 to 7		B Spinal Stabilization Device, Interspinous Process	
N Release	8 Thoracic Vertebral Joint, 8 or more		C Spinal Stabilization Device, Pedicle-Based	
P Removal	9 Thoracic Vertebral Disc		D Spinal Stabilization Device, Facet Replacement	
Q Repair	A Thoracolumbar Vertebral Joint		J Synthetic Substitute	
R Replacement	B Thoracolumbar Vertebral Disc		K Nonautologous Tissue Substitute	
S Reposition	C Temporomandibular Joint, Right		Y Other Device	
T Resection	D Temporomandibular Joint, Left		Z No Device	
U Supplement	E Sternoclavicular Joint, Right			
W Revision	F Sternoclavicular Joint, Left			
	G Acromioclavicular Joint, Right			
	H Acromioclavicular Joint, Left			
	J Shoulder Joint, Right			
	K Shoulder Joint, Left			
	L Elbow Joint, Right			
	M Elbow Joint, Left			
	N Wrist Joint, Right			
	P Wrist Joint, Left			
	Q Carpal Joint, Right			
	R Carpal Joint, Left			
	S Carpometacarpal Joint, Right			
	T Carpometacarpal Joint, Left			
	U Metacarpophalangeal Joint, Right			
	V Metacarpophalangeal Joint, Left			
	W Finger Phalangeal Joint, Right			
	X Finger Phalangeal Joint, Left			
	Y Upper Joint			

* Includes synovial membrane.

AHA Coding Clinic for table ØRB
2019, 3Q, 26 Acromioclavicular joint reconstruction using allograft

AHA Coding Clinic for table ØRG
2023, 2Q, 25 Spinal fusion using allograft bone graft and bone marrow aspirate
2022, 3Q, 21 Breakage of intervertebral cage during surgery
2021, 4Q, 67 Posterior dynamic distraction
2021, 1Q, 18 Placement of interspinous distraction device (spacer) for decompression
2021, 1Q, 53 Official guidelines for coding and reporting for interbody fusion device B3.10c
2020, 4Q, 56-58 Intramedullary sustained compression joint fusion
2020, 2Q, 27 Spinal fusion with NuVasive® VersaTie®
2020, 1Q, 33 Spinal fusion without use of bone graft
2019, 3Q, 28 Use of VERTE-STACK™ implant with fusion
2019, 3Q, 35 Fusion procedures of the spine (guideline B3.10c)
2019, 2Q, 19 Cervical spinal fusion, decompression and placement of interfacet stabilization device
2019, 1Q, 30 Spinal fusion performed at same level as decompressive laminectomy
2018, 4Q, 43 Joint fusion device value
2018, 1Q, 22 Spinal fusion procedures without bone graft
2017, 4Q, 62 Added and revised device values - Nerve substitutes
2017, 4Q, 76 Radiolucent porous interbody fusion device
2017, 2Q, 23 Decompression of spinal cord and placement of instrumentation
2014, 3Q, 30 Spinal fusion and fixation instrumentation
2014, 2Q, 7 Anterior cervical thoracic fusion with total discectomy
2013, 1Q, 21-23 Spinal fusion of thoracic and lumbar vertebrae
2013, 1Q, 29 Cervical and thoracic spinal fusion

AHA Coding Clinic for table ØRH
2021, 1Q, 18 Placement of interspinous distraction device (spacer) for decompression
2019, 2Q, 40 Decompression of spinal cord and placement of instrumentation
2018, 3Q, 26 Anterior vertebral tethering using Dynesys Tethering System
2017, 2Q, 23 Decompression of spinal cord and placement of instrumentation
2016, 3Q, 32 Rotator cuff repair, tenodesis, decompression, acromioplasty and coracoplasty

AHA Coding Clinic for table ØRN
2019, 1Q, 30 Spinal fusion performed at same level as decompressive laminectomy
2016, 3Q, 32 Rotator cuff repair, tenodesis, decompression, acromioplasty and coracoplasty
2015, 2Q, 22 Arthroscopic subacromial decompression
2015, 2Q, 23 Arthroscopic release of shoulder joint

AHA Coding Clinic for table ØRP
2022, 3Q, 21 Breakage of intervertebral cage during surgery
2021, 4Q, 53 Shoulder hemiarthroplasty
2017, 4Q, 107 Total ankle replacement versus revision

AHA Coding Clinic for table ØRQ
2016, 1Q, 30 Thermal capsulorrhaphy of shoulder

AHA Coding Clinic for table ØRR
2018, 4Q, 92 Radial head arthroplasty
2017, 4Q, 107 Total ankle replacement versus revision
2015, 3Q, 14 Endoprosthetic replacement of humerus and tendon reattachment
2015, 1Q, 27 Reverse total shoulder arthroplasty

AHA Coding Clinic for table ØRS
2019, 3Q, 26 Acromioclavicular joint reconstruction using allograft
2018, 3Q, 26 Anterior vertebral tethering using Dynesys Tethering System
2015, 2Q, 35 Application of tongs to reduce and stabilize cervical fracture
2014, 4Q, 32 Open reduction internal fixation of fracture with debridement
2014, 3Q, 33 Radial fracture treatment with open reduction internal fixation, and release of carpal ligament
2013, 2Q, 39 Application of cervical tongs for reduction of cervical fracture

AHA Coding Clinic for table ØRT
2019, 3Q, 26 Acromioclavicular joint reconstruction using allograft
2014, 2Q, 7 Anterior cervical thoracic fusion with total discectomy

AHA Coding Clinic for table ØRU
2019, 3Q, 26 Acromioclavicular joint reconstruction using allograft
2015, 3Q, 26 Thumb arthroplasty with resection of trapezium

AHA Coding Clinic for table ØRW
2021, 4Q, 53 Shoulder hemiarthroplasty
2017, 4Q, 107 Total ankle replacement versus revision

Upper Joints

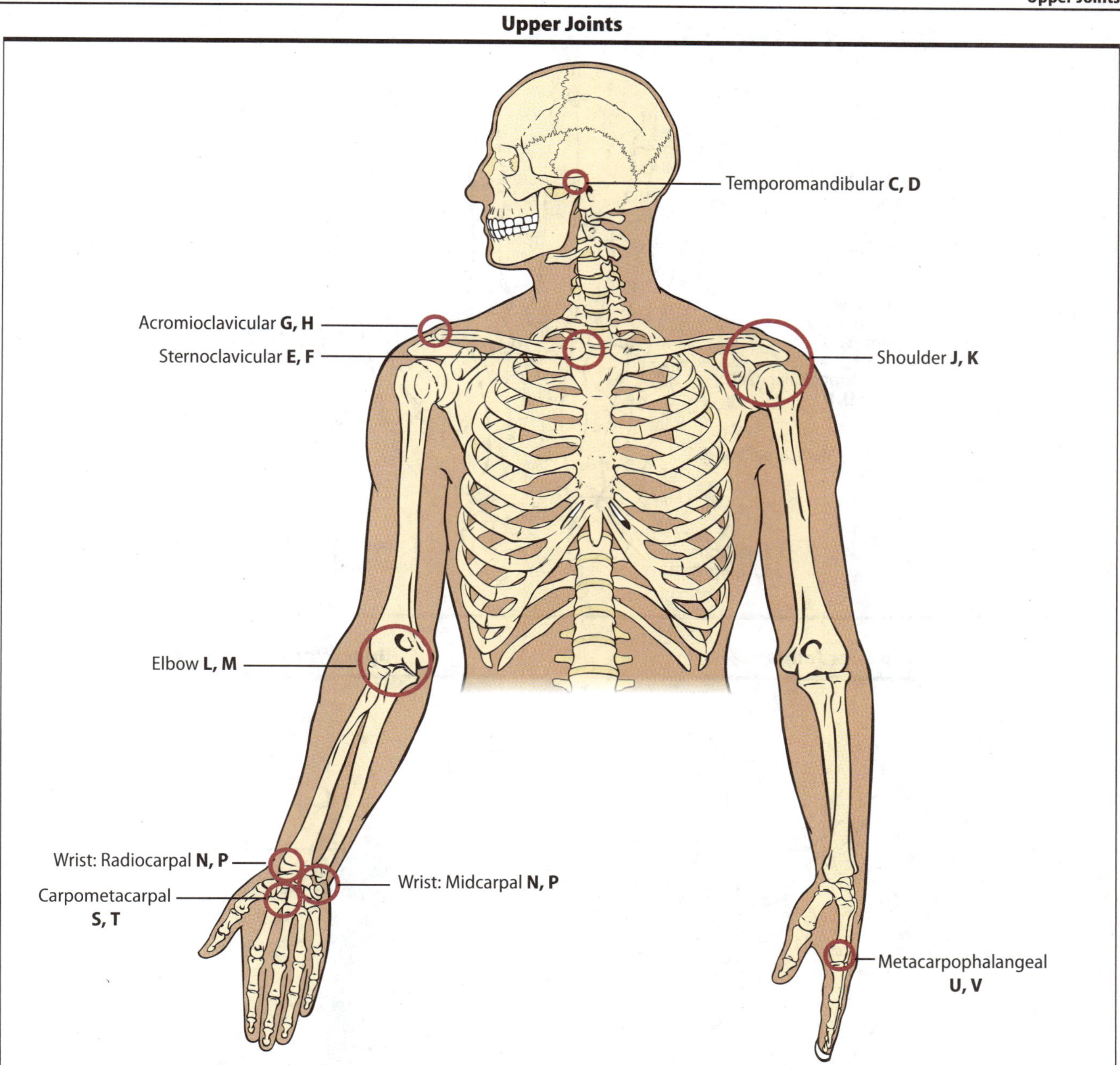

Hand Joints

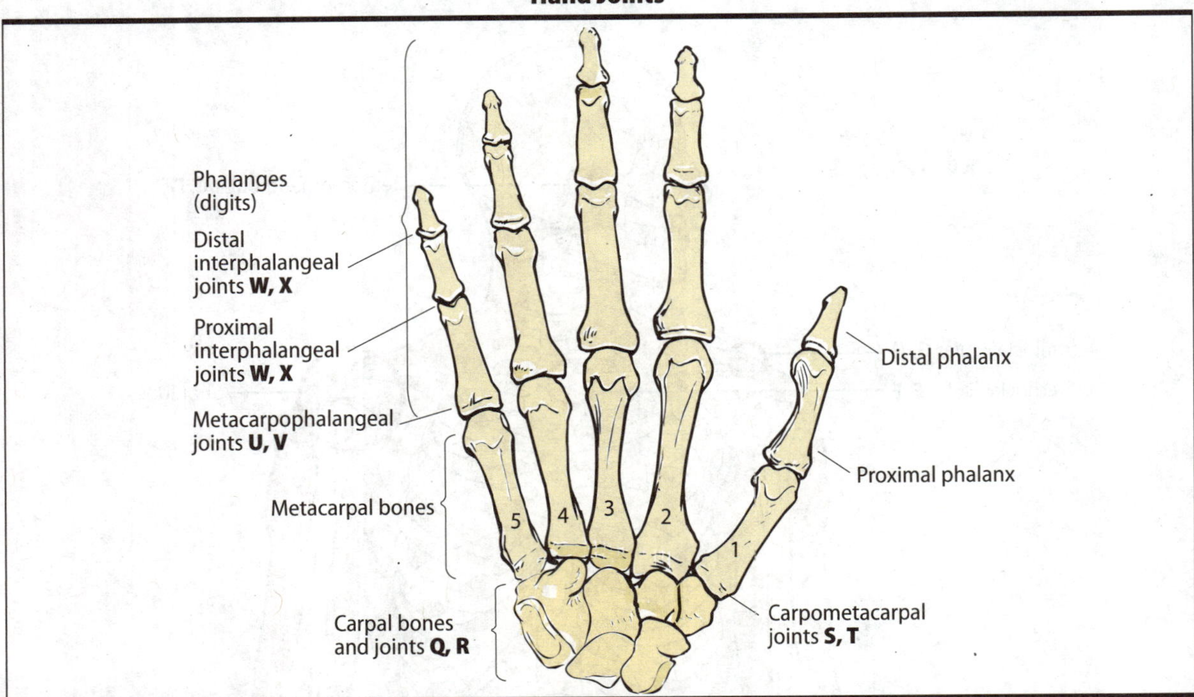

Shoulder Joints

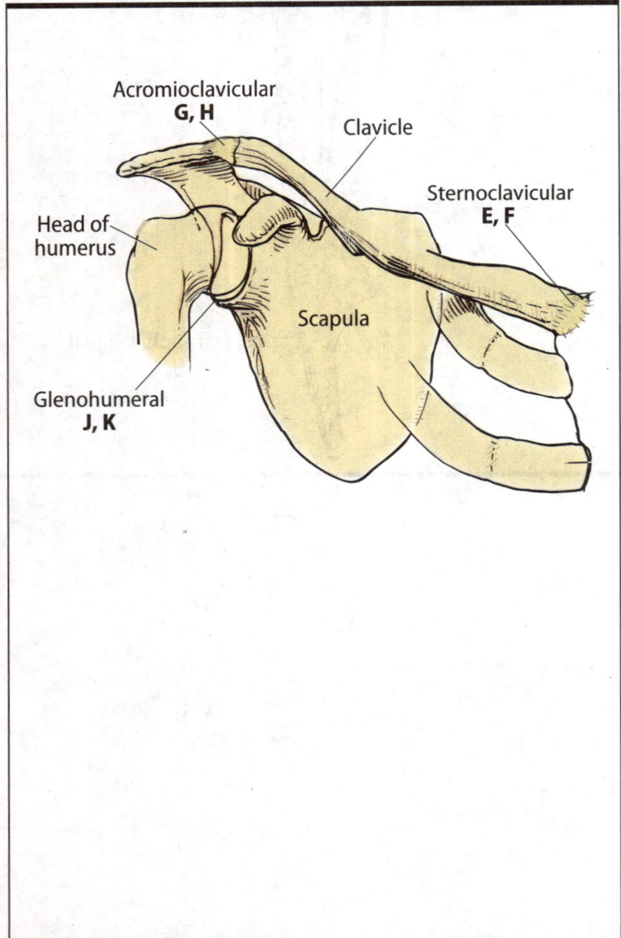

Upper Vertebral Joints

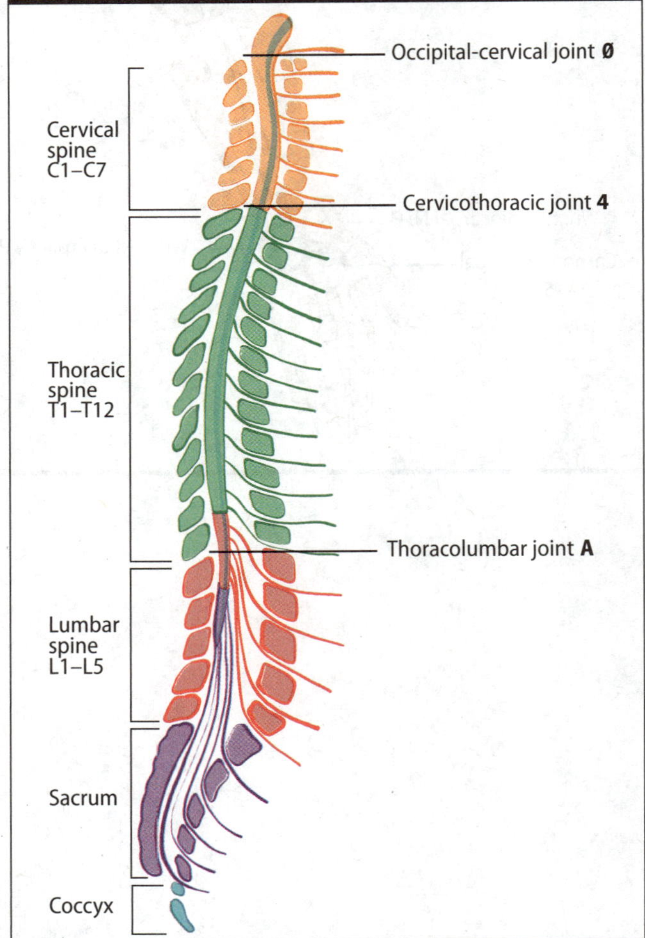

Ø Medical and Surgical
R Upper Joints
2 Change

Definition: Taking out or off a device from a body part and putting back an identical or similar device in or on the same body part without cutting or puncturing the skin or a mucous membrane

Explanation: All CHANGE procedures are coded using the approach EXTERNAL

Body Part Character 4	Approach Character 5	Device Character 6	Qualifier Character 7
Y Upper Joint	X External	Ø Drainage Device Y Other Device	Z No Qualifier

Non-OR All body part, approach, device, and qualifier values

Ø Medical and Surgical
R Upper Joints
5 Destruction

Definition: Physical eradication of all or a portion of a body part by the direct use of energy, force, or a destructive agent

Explanation: None of the body part is physically taken out

Body Part Character 4	Approach Character 5	Device Character 6	Qualifier Character 7
Ø Occipital-cervical Joint 1 Cervical Vertebral Joint Atlantoaxial joint Cervical facet joint 3 Cervical Vertebral Disc 4 Cervicothoracic Vertebral Joint Cervicothoracic facet joint 5 Cervicothoracic Vertebral Disc 6 Thoracic Vertebral Joint Costotransverse joint Costovertebral joint Thoracic facet joint 9 Thoracic Vertebral Disc A Thoracolumbar Vertebral Joint Thoracolumbar facet joint B Thoracolumbar Vertebral Disc C Temporomandibular Joint, Right D Temporomandibular Joint, Left E Sternoclavicular Joint, Right F Sternoclavicular Joint, Left G Acromioclavicular Joint, Right H Acromioclavicular Joint, Left J Shoulder Joint, Right Glenohumeral joint Glenoid ligament (labrum) K Shoulder Joint, Left *See J Shoulder Joint, Right* L Elbow Joint, Right Distal humerus, involving joint Humeroradial joint Humeroulnar joint Proximal radioulnar joint M Elbow Joint, Left *See L Elbow Joint, Right* N Wrist Joint, Right Distal radioulnar joint Radiocarpal joint P Wrist Joint, Left *See N Wrist Joint, Right* Q Carpal Joint, Right Intercarpal joint Midcarpal joint R Carpal Joint, Left *See Q Carpal Joint, Right* S Carpometacarpal Joint, Right T Carpometacarpal Joint, Left U Metacarpophalangeal Joint, Right V Metacarpophalangeal Joint, Left W Finger Phalangeal Joint, Right Interphalangeal (IP) joint X Finger Phalangeal Joint, Left *See W Finger Phalangeal Joint, Right*	Ø Open 3 Percutaneous 4 Percutaneous Endoscopic	Z No Device	Z No Qualifier

Non-OR ØR5[3,5,9,B][3,4]ZZ

Ø Medical and Surgical
R Upper Joints
9 Drainage Definition: Taking or letting out fluids and/or gases from a body part
Explanation: The qualifier DIAGNOSTIC is used to identify drainage procedures that are biopsies

Body Part Character 4	Approach Character 5	Device Character 6	Qualifier Character 7
Ø Occipital-cervical Joint **1 Cervical Vertebral Joint** Atlantoaxial joint Cervical facet joint **3 Cervical Vertebral Disc** **4 Cervicothoracic Vertebral Joint** Cervicothoracic facet joint **5 Cervicothoracic Vertebral Disc** **6 Thoracic Vertebral Joint** Costotransverse joint Costovertebral joint Thoracic facet joint **9 Thoracic Vertebral Disc** **A Thoracolumbar Vertebral Joint** Thoracolumbar facet joint **B Thoracolumbar Vertebral Disc** **C Temporomandibular Joint, Right** **D Temporomandibular Joint, Left** **E Sternoclavicular Joint, Right** **F Sternoclavicular Joint, Left** **G Acromioclavicular Joint, Right** **H Acromioclavicular Joint, Left** **J Shoulder Joint, Right** Glenohumeral joint Glenoid ligament (labrum) **K Shoulder Joint, Left** *See J Shoulder Joint, Right* **L Elbow Joint, Right** Distal humerus, involving joint Humeroradial joint Humeroulnar joint Proximal radioulnar joint **M Elbow Joint, Left** *See L Elbow Joint, Right* **N Wrist Joint, Right** Distal radioulnar joint Radiocarpal joint **P Wrist Joint, Left** *See N Wrist Joint, Right* **Q Carpal Joint, Right** Intercarpal joint Midcarpal joint **R Carpal Joint, Left** *See Q Carpal Joint, Right* **S Carpometacarpal Joint, Right** **T Carpometacarpal Joint, Left** **U Metacarpophalangeal Joint, Right** **V Metacarpophalangeal Joint, Left** **W Finger Phalangeal Joint, Right** Interphalangeal (IP) joint **X Finger Phalangeal Joint, Left** *See W Finger Phalangeal Joint, Right*	**Ø** Open **3** Percutaneous **4** Percutaneous Endoscopic	**Ø** Drainage Device	**Z** No Qualifier
Ø Occipital-cervical Joint **1 Cervical Vertebral Joint** Atlantoaxial joint Cervical facet joint **3 Cervical Vertebral Disc** **4 Cervicothoracic Vertebral Joint** Cervicothoracic facet joint **5 Cervicothoracic Vertebral Disc** **6 Thoracic Vertebral Joint** Costotransverse joint Costovertebral joint Thoracic facet joint **9 Thoracic Vertebral Disc** **A Thoracolumbar Vertebral Joint** Thoracolumbar facet joint **B Thoracolumbar Vertebral Disc** **C Temporomandibular Joint, Right** **D Temporomandibular Joint, Left** **E Sternoclavicular Joint, Right** **F Sternoclavicular Joint, Left** **G Acromioclavicular Joint, Right** **H Acromioclavicular Joint, Left** **J Shoulder Joint, Right** Glenohumeral joint Glenoid ligament (labrum) **K Shoulder Joint, Left** *See J Shoulder Joint, Right* **L Elbow Joint, Right** Distal humerus, involving joint Humeroradial joint Humeroulnar joint Proximal radioulnar joint **M Elbow Joint, Left** *See L Elbow Joint, Right* **N Wrist Joint, Right** Distal radioulnar joint Radiocarpal joint **P Wrist Joint, Left** *See N Wrist Joint, Right* **Q Carpal Joint, Right** Intercarpal joint Midcarpal joint **R Carpal Joint, Left** *See Q Carpal Joint, Right* **S Carpometacarpal Joint, Right** **T Carpometacarpal Joint, Left** **U Metacarpophalangeal Joint, Right** **V Metacarpophalangeal Joint, Left** **W Finger Phalangeal Joint, Right** Interphalangeal (IP) joint **X Finger Phalangeal Joint, Left** *See W Finger Phalangeal Joint, Right*	**Ø** Open **3** Percutaneous **4** Percutaneous Endoscopic	**Z** No Device	**X** Diagnostic **Z** No Qualifier

Non-OR ØR9[Ø,1,3,4,5,6,9,A,B,E,F,G,H,J,K,L,M,N,P,Q,R,S,T,U,V,W,X][3,4]ØZ
Non-OR ØR9[C,D]3ØZ
Non-OR ØR9[Ø,1,3,4,5,6,9,A,B,E,F,G,H,J,K,L,M,N,P,Q,R,S,T,U,V,W,X][Ø,3,4]ZX
Non-OR ØR9[Ø,1,3,4,5,6,9,A,B,E,F,G,H,J,K,L,M,N,P,Q,R,S,T,U,V,W,X][3,4]ZZ
Non-OR ØR9[C,D]3ZZ

Ø Medical and Surgical
R Upper Joints
B Excision

Definition: Cutting out or off, without replacement, a portion of a body part

Explanation: The qualifier DIAGNOSTIC is used to identify excision procedures that are biopsies

Body Part Character 4	Approach Character 5	Device Character 6	Qualifier Character 7
Ø Occipital-cervical Joint **1 Cervical Vertebral Joint** Atlantoaxial joint Cervical facet joint **3 Cervical Vertebral Disc** **4 Cervicothoracic Vertebral Joint** Cervicothoracic facet joint **5 Cervicothoracic Vertebral Disc** **6 Thoracic Vertebral Joint** Costotransverse joint Costovertebral joint Thoracic facet joint **9 Thoracic Vertebral Disc** **A Thoracolumbar Vertebral Joint** Thoracolumbar facet joint **B Thoracolumbar Vertebral Disc** **C Temporomandibular Joint, Right** **D Temporomandibular Joint, Left** **E Sternoclavicular Joint, Right** **F Sternoclavicular Joint, Left** **G Acromioclavicular Joint, Right** **H Acromioclavicular Joint, Left** **J Shoulder Joint, Right** Glenohumeral joint Glenoid ligament (labrum) **K Shoulder Joint, Left** *See J Shoulder Joint, Right* **L Elbow Joint, Right** Distal humerus, involving joint Humeroradial joint Humeroulnar joint Proximal radioulnar joint **M Elbow Joint, Left** *See L Elbow Joint, Right* **N Wrist Joint, Right** Distal radioulnar joint Radiocarpal joint **P Wrist Joint, Left** *See N Wrist Joint, Right* **Q Carpal Joint, Right** Intercarpal joint Midcarpal joint **R Carpal Joint, Left** *See Q Carpal Joint, Right* **S Carpometacarpal Joint, Right** **T Carpometacarpal Joint, Left** **U Metacarpophalangeal Joint, Right** **V Metacarpophalangeal Joint, Left** **W Finger Phalangeal Joint, Right** Interphalangeal (IP) joint **X Finger Phalangeal Joint, Left** *See W Finger Phalangeal Joint, Right*	**Ø** Open **3** Percutaneous **4** Percutaneous Endoscopic	**Z** No Device	**X** Diagnostic **Z** No Qualifier

Non-OR ØRB[Ø,1,3,4,5,6,9,A,B,E,F,G,H,J,K,L,M,N,P,Q,R,S,T,U,V,W,X][Ø,3,4]ZX

Ø Medical and Surgical
R Upper Joints
C Extirpation

Definition: Taking or cutting out solid matter from a body part

Explanation: The solid matter may be an abnormal byproduct of a biological function or a foreign body; it may be imbedded in a body part or in the lumen of a tubular body part. The solid matter may or may not have been previously broken into pieces.

Body Part Character 4	Approach Character 5	Device Character 6	Qualifier Character 7
Ø Occipital-cervical Joint **1 Cervical Vertebral Joint** Atlantoaxial joint Cervical facet joint **3 Cervical Vertebral Disc** **4 Cervicothoracic Vertebral Joint** Cervicothoracic facet joint **5 Cervicothoracic Vertebral Disc** **6 Thoracic Vertebral Joint** Costotransverse joint Costovertebral joint Thoracic facet joint **9 Thoracic Vertebral Disc** **A Thoracolumbar Vertebral Joint** Thoracolumbar facet joint **B Thoracolumbar Vertebral Disc** **C Temporomandibular Joint, Right** **D Temporomandibular Joint, Left** **E Sternoclavicular Joint, Right** **F Sternoclavicular Joint, Left** **G Acromioclavicular Joint, Right** **H Acromioclavicular Joint, Left** **J Shoulder Joint, Right** Glenohumeral joint Glenoid ligament (labrum) **K Shoulder Joint, Left** *See J Shoulder Joint, Right* **L Elbow Joint, Right** Distal humerus, involving joint Humeroradial joint Humeroulnar joint Proximal radioulnar joint **M Elbow Joint, Left** *See L Elbow Joint, Right* **N Wrist Joint, Right** Distal radioulnar joint Radiocarpal joint **P Wrist Joint, Left** *See N Wrist Joint, Right* **Q Carpal Joint, Right** Intercarpal joint Midcarpal joint **R Carpal Joint, Left** *See Q Carpal Joint, Right* **S Carpometacarpal Joint, Right** **T Carpometacarpal Joint, Left** **U Metacarpophalangeal Joint, Right** **V Metacarpophalangeal Joint, Left** **W Finger Phalangeal Joint, Right** Interphalangeal (IP) joint **X Finger Phalangeal Joint, Left** *See W Finger Phalangeal Joint, Right*	**Ø Open** **3 Percutaneous** **4 Percutaneous Endoscopic**	**Z No Device**	**Z No Qualifier**

Ø Medical and Surgical
R Upper Joints
G Fusion

Definition: Joining together portions of an articular body part rendering the articular body part immobile
Explanation: The body part is joined together by fixation device, bone graft, or other means

Body Part Character 4	Approach Character 5	Device Character 6	Qualifier Character 7
Ø Occipital-cervical Joint **1 Cervical Vertebral Joint** Atlantoaxial joint Cervical facet joint **2 Cervical Vertebral Joints, 2 or more** Cervical facet joint **4 Cervicothoracic Vertebral Joint** Cervicothoracic facet joint **6 Thoracic Vertebral Joint** Costotransverse joint Costovertebral joint Thoracic facet joint **7 Thoracic Vertebral Joints, 2 to 7** [Combination Member] **8 Thoracic Vertebral Joints, 8 or more** **A Thoracolumbar Vertebral Joint** Thoracolumbar facet joint	**Ø Open** **3 Percutaneous** **4 Percutaneous Endoscopic**	**7 Autologous Tissue Substitute** **J Synthetic Substitute** **K Nonautologous Tissue Substitute**	**Ø Anterior Approach, Anterior Column** **1 Posterior Approach, Posterior Column** **J Posterior Approach, Anterior Column**
Ø Occipital-cervical Joint **1 Cervical Vertebral Joint** Atlantoaxial joint Cervical facet joint **2 Cervical Vertebral Joints, 2 or more** Cervical facet joint **4 Cervicothoracic Vertebral Joint** Cervicothoracic facet joint **6 Thoracic Vertebral Joint** Costotransverse joint Costovertebral joint Thoracic facet joint **7 Thoracic Vertebral Joints, 2 to 7** [Combination Member] **8 Thoracic Vertebral Joints, 8 or more** **A Thoracolumbar Vertebral Joint** Thoracolumbar facet joint	**Ø Open** **3 Percutaneous** **4 Percutaneous Endoscopic**	**A Interbody Fusion Device**	**Ø Anterior Approach, Anterior Column** **J Posterior Approach, Anterior Column**
C Temporomandibular Joint, Right **D Temporomandibular Joint, Left** **E Sternoclavicular Joint, Right** **F Sternoclavicular Joint, Left** **G Acromioclavicular Joint, Right** **H Acromioclavicular Joint, Left** **J Shoulder Joint, Right** Glenohumeral joint Glenoid ligament (labrum) **K Shoulder Joint, Left** *See J Shoulder Joint, Right*	**Ø Open** **3 Percutaneous** **4 Percutaneous Endoscopic**	**4 Internal Fixation Device** **7 Autologous Tissue Substitute** **J Synthetic Substitute** **K Nonautologous Tissue Substitute**	**Z No Qualifier**
L Elbow Joint, Right Distal humerus, involving joint Humeroradial joint Humeroulnar joint Proximal radioulnar joint **M Elbow Joint, Left** *See L Elbow Joint, Right* **N Wrist Joint, Right** Distal radioulnar joint Radiocarpal joint **P Wrist Joint, Left** *See N Wrist Joint, Right* **Q Carpal Joint, Right** Intercarpal joint Midcarpal joint **R Carpal Joint, Left** *See Q Carpal Joint, Right* **S Carpometacarpal Joint, Right** **T Carpometacarpal Joint, Left** **U Metacarpophalangeal Joint, Right** **V Metacarpophalangeal Joint, Left** **W Finger Phalangeal Joint, Right** Interphalangeal (IP) joint **X Finger Phalangeal Joint, Left** *See W Finger Phalangeal Joint, Right*	**Ø Open** **3 Percutaneous** **4 Percutaneous Endoscopic**	**3 Internal Fixation Device, Sustained Compression** **4 Internal Fixation Device** **5 External Fixation Device** **7 Autologous Tissue Substitute** **J Synthetic Substitute** **K Nonautologous Tissue Substitute**	**Z No Qualifier**

HAC ØRG[Ø,1,2,4,6,7,8,A][Ø,3,4][7,J,K][Ø,1,J] when reported with SDx K68.11 or T81.4Ø–T81.49, T84.6Ø-T84.619, T84.63-T84.7 with 7th character A

HAC ØRG[Ø,1,2,4,6,7,8,A][Ø,3,4]A[Ø,J] when reported with SDx K68.11 or T81.4Ø–T81.49, T84.6Ø-T84.619, T84.63-T84.7 with 7th character A

HAC ØRG[E,F,G,H,J,K][Ø,3,4][4,7,J,K]Z when reported with SDx K68.11 or T81.4Ø–T81.49, T84.6Ø-T84.619, T84.63-T84.7 with 7th character A

HAC ØRG[L,M][Ø,3,4][3,4,5,7,J,K]Z when reported with SDx K68.11 or T81.4Ø–T81.49, T84.6Ø-T84.619, T84.63-T84.7 with 7th character A

See Appendix L for Procedure Combinations
[Combination Member] ØRG7[Ø,3,4][7,J,K][Ø,1,J]
[Combination Member] ØRG7[Ø,3,4]A[Ø,J]

Ø Medical and Surgical
R Upper Joints
H Insertion

Definition: Putting in a nonbiological appliance that monitors, assists, performs, or prevents a physiological function but does not physically take the place of a body part

Explanation: None

Body Part Character 4	Approach Character 5	Device Character 6	Qualifier Character 7
Ø Occipital-cervical Joint **1 Cervical Vertebral Joint** Atlantoaxial joint Cervical facet joint **4 Cervicothoracic Vertebral Joint** Cervicothoracic facet joint **6 Thoracic Vertebral Joint** Costotransverse joint Costovertebral joint Thoracic facet joint **A Thoracolumbar Vertebral Joint** Thoracolumbar facet joint	**Ø Open** **3 Percutaneous** **4 Percutaneous Endoscopic**	**3 Infusion Device** **4 Internal Fixation Device** **8 Spacer** **B Spinal Stabilization Device, Interspinous Process** **C Spinal Stabilization Device, Pedicle-Based** **D Spinal Stabilization Device, Facet Replacement**	**Z No Qualifier**
3 Cervical Vertebral Disc **5 Cervicothoracic Vertebral Disc** **9 Thoracic Vertebral Disc** **B Thoracolumbar Vertebral Disc**	**Ø Open** **3 Percutaneous** **4 Percutaneous Endoscopic**	**3 Infusion Device**	**Z No Qualifier**
C Temporomandibular Joint, Right **D Temporomandibular Joint, Left** **E Sternoclavicular Joint, Right** **F Sternoclavicular Joint, Left** **G Acromioclavicular Joint, Right** **H Acromioclavicular Joint, Left** **J Shoulder Joint, Right** Glenohumeral joint Glenoid ligament (labrum) **K Shoulder Joint, Left** *See J Shoulder Joint, Right*	**Ø Open** **3 Percutaneous** **4 Percutaneous Endoscopic**	**3 Infusion Device** **4 Internal Fixation Device** **8 Spacer**	**Z No Qualifier**
L Elbow Joint, Right Distal humerus, involving joint Humeroradial joint Humeroulnar joint Proximal radioulnar joint **M Elbow Joint, Left** *See L Elbow Joint, Right* **N Wrist Joint, Right** Distal radioulnar joint Radiocarpal joint **P Wrist Joint, Left** *See N Wrist Joint, Right* **Q Carpal Joint, Right** Intercarpal joint Midcarpal joint **R Carpal Joint, Left** *See Q Carpal Joint, Right* **S Carpometacarpal Joint, Right** **T Carpometacarpal Joint, Left** **U Metacarpophalangeal Joint, Right** **V Metacarpophalangeal Joint, Left** **W Finger Phalangeal Joint, Right** Interphalangeal (IP) joint **X Finger Phalangeal Joint, Left** *See W Finger Phalangeal Joint, Right*	**Ø Open** **3 Percutaneous** **4 Percutaneous Endoscopic**	**3 Infusion Device** **4 Internal Fixation Device** **5 External Fixation Device** **8 Spacer**	**Z No Qualifier**

Non-OR ØRH[Ø,1,4,6,A][Ø,3,4][3,8]Z
Non-OR ØRH[3,5,9,B][Ø,3,4]3Z
Non-OR ØRH[C,D][Ø,4]8Z
Non-OR ØRH[C,D]3[3,8]Z
Non-OR ØRH[E,F,G,H][Ø,3,4][3,8]Z
Non-OR ØRH[J,K][Ø,3,4]3Z
Non-OR ØRH[J,K]38Z
Non-OR ØRH[L,M,N,P,Q,R,S,T,U,V,W,X][Ø,3,4][3,8]Z

Ø Medical and Surgical
R Upper Joints
J Inspection

Definition: Visually and/or manually exploring a body part

Explanation: Visual exploration may be performed with or without optical instrumentation. Manual exploration may be performed directly or through intervening body layers.

Body Part Character 4	Approach Character 5	Device Character 6	Qualifier Character 7
Ø Occipital-cervical Joint **1 Cervical Vertebral Joint** Atlantoaxial joint Cervical facet joint **3 Cervical Vertebral Disc** **4 Cervicothoracic Vertebral Joint** Cervicothoracic facet joint **5 Cervicothoracic Vertebral Disc** **6 Thoracic Vertebral Joint** Costotransverse joint Costovertebral joint Thoracic facet joint **9 Thoracic Vertebral Disc** **A Thoracolumbar Vertebral Joint** Thoracolumbar facet joint **B Thoracolumbar Vertebral Disc** **C Temporomandibular Joint, Right** **D Temporomandibular Joint, Left** **E Sternoclavicular Joint, Right** **F Sternoclavicular Joint, Left** **G Acromioclavicular Joint, Right** **H Acromioclavicular Joint, Left** **J Shoulder Joint, Right** Glenohumeral joint Glenoid ligament (labrum) **K Shoulder Joint, Left** *See J Shoulder Joint, Right* **L Elbow Joint, Right** Distal humerus, involving joint Humeroradial joint Humeroulnar joint Proximal radioulnar joint **M Elbow Joint, Left** *See L Elbow Joint, Right* **N Wrist Joint, Right** Distal radioulnar joint Radiocarpal joint **P Wrist Joint, Left** *See N Wrist Joint, Right* **Q Carpal Joint, Right** Intercarpal joint Midcarpal joint **R Carpal Joint, Left** *See Q Carpal Joint, Right* **S Carpometacarpal Joint, Right** **T Carpometacarpal Joint, Left** **U Metacarpophalangeal Joint, Right** **V Metacarpophalangeal Joint, Left** **W Finger Phalangeal Joint, Right** Interphalangeal (IP) joint **X Finger Phalangeal Joint, Left** *See W Finger Phalangeal Joint, Right*	**Ø Open** **3 Percutaneous** **4 Percutaneous Endoscopic** **X External**	**Z No Device**	**Z No Qualifier**

Non-OR ØRJ[Ø,1,3,4,5,6,9,A,B,C,D,E,F,G,H,J,K,L,M,N,P,Q,R,S,T,U,V,W,X][3,X]ZZ

Ø Medical and Surgical
R Upper Joints
N Release

Definition: Freeing a body part from an abnormal physical constraint by cutting or by the use of force

Explanation: Some of the restraining tissue may be taken out but none of the body part is taken out

Body Part Character 4	Approach Character 5	Device Character 6	Qualifier Character 7
Ø Occipital-cervical Joint **1 Cervical Vertebral Joint** Atlantoaxial joint Cervical facet joint **3 Cervical Vertebral Disc** **4 Cervicothoracic Vertebral Joint** Cervicothoracic facet joint **5 Cervicothoracic Vertebral Disc** **6 Thoracic Vertebral Joint** Costotransverse joint Costovertebral joint Thoracic facet joint **9 Thoracic Vertebral Disc** **A Thoracolumbar Vertebral Joint** Thoracolumbar facet joint **B Thoracolumbar Vertebral Disc** **C Temporomandibular Joint, Right** **D Temporomandibular Joint, Left** **E Sternoclavicular Joint, Right** **F Sternoclavicular Joint, Left** **G Acromioclavicular Joint, Right** **H Acromioclavicular Joint, Left** **J Shoulder Joint, Right** Glenohumeral joint Glenoid ligament (labrum) **K Shoulder Joint, Left** *See J Shoulder Joint, Right* **L Elbow Joint, Right** Distal humerus, involving joint Humeroradial joint Humeroulnar joint Proximal radioulnar joint **M Elbow Joint, Left** *See L Elbow Joint, Right* **N Wrist Joint, Right** Distal radioulnar joint Radiocarpal joint **P Wrist Joint, Left** *See N Wrist Joint, Right* **Q Carpal Joint, Right** Intercarpal joint Midcarpal joint **R Carpal Joint, Left** *See Q Carpal Joint, Right* **S Carpometacarpal Joint, Right** **T Carpometacarpal Joint, Left** **U Metacarpophalangeal Joint, Right** **V Metacarpophalangeal Joint, Left** **W Finger Phalangeal Joint, Right** Interphalangeal (IP) joint **X Finger Phalangeal Joint, Left** *See W Finger Phalangeal Joint, Right*	**Ø Open** **3 Percutaneous** **4 Percutaneous Endoscopic** **X External**	**Z No Device**	**Z No Qualifier**

Non-OR ØRN[Ø,1,3,4,5,6,9,A,B,C,D,E,F,G,H,J,K,L,M,N,P,Q,R,S,T,U,V,W,X]XZZ

Ø Medical and Surgical
R Upper Joints
P Removal Definition: Taking out or off a device from a body part

Explanation: If a device is taken out and a similar device put in without cutting or puncturing the skin or mucous membrane, the procedure is coded to the root operation CHANGE. Otherwise, the procedure for taking out the device is coded to the root operation REMOVAL.

Body Part Character 4	Approach Character 5	Device Character 6	Qualifier Character 7
Ø Occipital-cervical Joint **1 Cervical Vertebral Joint** Atlantoaxial joint Cervical facet joint **4 Cervicothoracic Vertebral Joint** Cervicothoracic facet joint **6 Thoracic Vertebral Joint** Costotransverse joint Costovertebral joint Thoracic facet joint **A Thoracolumbar Vertebral Joint** Thoracolumbar facet joint	Ø Open 3 Percutaneous 4 Percutaneous Endoscopic	Ø Drainage Device 3 Infusion Device 4 Internal Fixation Device 7 Autologous Tissue Substitute 8 Spacer A Interbody Fusion Device J Synthetic Substitute K Nonautologous Tissue Substitute	Z No Qualifier
Ø Occipital-cervical Joint **1 Cervical Vertebral Joint** Atlantoaxial joint Cervical facet joint **4 Cervicothoracic Vertebral Joint** Cervicothoracic facet joint **6 Thoracic Vertebral Joint** Costotransverse joint Costovertebral joint Thoracic facet joint **A Thoracolumbar Vertebral Joint** Thoracolumbar facet joint	X External	Ø Drainage Device 3 Infusion Device 4 Internal Fixation Device	Z No Qualifier
3 Cervical Vertebral Disc **5 Cervicothoracic Vertebral Disc** **9 Thoracic Vertebral Disc** **B Thoracolumbar Vertebral Disc**	Ø Open 3 Percutaneous 4 Percutaneous Endoscopic	Ø Drainage Device 3 Infusion Device 7 Autologous Tissue Substitute J Synthetic Substitute K Nonautologous Tissue Substitute	Z No Qualifier
3 Cervical Vertebral Disc **5 Cervicothoracic Vertebral Disc** **9 Thoracic Vertebral Disc** **B Thoracolumbar Vertebral Disc**	X External	Ø Drainage Device 3 Infusion Device	Z No Qualifier
C Temporomandibular Joint, Right **D Temporomandibular Joint, Left** **E Sternoclavicular Joint, Right** **F Sternoclavicular Joint, Left** **G Acromioclavicular Joint, Right** **H Acromioclavicular Joint, Left**	Ø Open 3 Percutaneous 4 Percutaneous Endoscopic	Ø Drainage Device 3 Infusion Device 4 Internal Fixation Device 7 Autologous Tissue Substitute 8 Spacer J Synthetic Substitute K Nonautologous Tissue Substitute	Z No Qualifier
C Temporomandibular Joint, Right **D Temporomandibular Joint, Left** **E Sternoclavicular Joint, Right** **F Sternoclavicular Joint, Left** **G Acromioclavicular Joint, Right** **H Acromioclavicular Joint, Left**	X External	Ø Drainage Device 3 Infusion Device 4 Internal Fixation Device	Z No Qualifier
J Shoulder Joint, Right Glenohumeral joint Glenoid ligament (labrum) **K Shoulder Joint, Left** *See J Shoulder Joint, Right*	Ø Open 3 Percutaneous 4 Percutaneous Endoscopic	Ø Drainage Device 3 Infusion Device 4 Internal Fixation Device 7 Autologous Tissue Substitute 8 Spacer K Nonautologous Tissue Substitute	Z No Qualifier
J Shoulder Joint, Right Glenohumeral joint Glenoid ligament (labrum) **K Shoulder Joint, Left** *See J Shoulder Joint, Right*	Ø Open 3 Percutaneous 4 Percutaneous Endoscopic	J Synthetic Substitute	6 Humeral Surface 7 Glenoid Surface Z No Qualifier
J Shoulder Joint, Right Glenohumeral joint Glenoid ligament (labrum) **K Shoulder Joint, Left** *See J Shoulder Joint, Right*	X External	Ø Drainage Device 3 Infusion Device 4 Internal Fixation Device	Z No Qualifier

Non-OR ØRP[Ø,1,4,6,A]3[Ø,3,8]Z
Non-OR ØRP[Ø,1,4,6,A][Ø,4]8Z
Non-OR ØRP[Ø,1,4,6,A]X[Ø,3,4]Z
Non-OR ØRP[3,5,9,B]3[Ø,3]Z
Non-OR ØRP[3,5,9,B]X[Ø,3]Z
Non-OR ØRP[C,D,E,F,G,H]3[Ø,3,8]Z
Non-OR ØRP[C,D,E,F,G,H][Ø,4]8Z
Non-OR ØRP[C,D]X[Ø,3]Z
Non-OR ØRP[E,F,G,H,J,K]X[Ø,3,4]Z
Non-OR ØRP[J,K]3[Ø,3,8]Z
Non-OR ØRP[J,K]X[Ø,3,4]Z

ØRP Continued on next page

ØRP Continued

Ø Medical and Surgical
R Upper Joints
P Removal

Definition: Taking out or off a device from a body part

Explanation: If a device is taken out and a similar device put in without cutting or puncturing the skin or mucous membrane, the procedure is coded to the root operation CHANGE. Otherwise, the procedure for taking out the device is coded to the root operation REMOVAL.

Body Part Character 4	Approach Character 5	Device Character 6	Qualifier Character 7
L Elbow Joint, Right Distal humerus, involving joint Humeroradial joint Humeroulnar joint Proximal radioulnar joint **M Elbow Joint, Left** *See L Elbow Joint, Right* **N Wrist Joint, Right** Distal radioulnar joint Radiocarpal joint **P Wrist Joint, Left** *See N Wrist Joint, Right* **Q Carpal Joint, Right** Intercarpal joint Midcarpal joint **R Carpal Joint, Left** *See Q Carpal Joint, Right* **S Carpometacarpal Joint, Right** **T Carpometacarpal Joint, Left** **U Metacarpophalangeal Joint, Right** **V Metacarpophalangeal Joint, Left** **W Finger Phalangeal Joint, Right** Interphalangeal (IP) joint **X Finger Phalangeal Joint, Left** *See W Finger Phalangeal Joint, Right*	**Ø Open** **3 Percutaneous** **4 Percutaneous Endoscopic**	**Ø Drainage Device** **3 Infusion Device** **4 Internal Fixation Device** **5 External Fixation Device** **7 Autologous Tissue Substitute** **8 Spacer** **J Synthetic Substitute** **K Nonautologous Tissue Substitute**	**Z No Qualifier**
L Elbow Joint, Right Distal humerus, involving joint Humeroradial joint Humeroulnar joint Proximal radioulnar joint **M Elbow Joint, Left** *See L Elbow Joint, Right* **N Wrist Joint, Right** Distal radioulnar joint Radiocarpal joint **P Wrist Joint, Left** *See N Wrist Joint, Right* **Q Carpal Joint, Right** Intercarpal joint Midcarpal joint **R Carpal Joint, Left** *See Q Carpal Joint, Right* **S Carpometacarpal Joint, Right** **T Carpometacarpal Joint, Left** **U Metacarpophalangeal Joint, Right** **V Metacarpophalangeal Joint, Left** **W Finger Phalangeal Joint, Right** Interphalangeal (IP) joint **X Finger Phalangeal Joint, Left** *See W Finger Phalangeal Joint, Right*	**X External**	**Ø Drainage Device** **3 Infusion Device** **4 Internal Fixation Device** **5 External Fixation Device**	**Z No Qualifier**

Non-OR ØRP[L,M,N,P,Q,R,S,T,U,V,W,X]3[Ø,3,8]Z
Non-OR ØRP[L,M,N,P,Q,R,S,T,U,V,W,X][Ø,4]8Z
Non-OR ØRP[L,M,N,P,Q,R,S,T,U,V,W,X]X[Ø,3,4,5]Z

Ø Medical and Surgical
R Upper Joints
Q Repair Definition: Restoring, to the extent possible, a body part to its normal anatomic structure and function
Explanation: Used only when the method to accomplish the repair is not one of the other root operations

Body Part Character 4	Approach Character 5	Device Character 6	Qualifier Character 7
Ø Occipital-cervical Joint 1 Cervical Vertebral Joint Atlantoaxial joint Cervical facet joint 3 Cervical Vertebral Disc 4 Cervicothoracic Vertebral Joint Cervicothoracic facet joint 5 Cervicothoracic Vertebral Disc 6 Thoracic Vertebral Joint Costotransverse joint Costovertebral joint Thoracic facet joint 9 Thoracic Vertebral Disc A Thoracolumbar Vertebral Joint Thoracolumbar facet joint B Thoracolumbar Vertebral Disc C Temporomandibular Joint, Right D Temporomandibular Joint, Left E Sternoclavicular Joint, Right F Sternoclavicular Joint, Left G Acromioclavicular Joint, Right H Acromioclavicular Joint, Left J Shoulder Joint, Right Glenohumeral joint Glenoid ligament (labrum) K Shoulder Joint, Left *See J Shoulder Joint, Right* L Elbow Joint, Right Distal humerus, involving joint Humeroradial joint Humeroulnar joint Proximal radioulnar joint M Elbow Joint, Left *See L Elbow Joint, Right* N Wrist Joint, Right Distal radioulnar joint Radiocarpal joint P Wrist Joint, Left *See N Wrist Joint, Right* Q Carpal Joint, Right Intercarpal joint Midcarpal joint R Carpal Joint, Left *See Q Carpal Joint, Right* S Carpometacarpal Joint, Right T Carpometacarpal Joint, Left U Metacarpophalangeal Joint, Right V Metacarpophalangeal Joint, Left W Finger Phalangeal Joint, Right Interphalangeal (IP) joint X Finger Phalangeal Joint, Left *See W Finger Phalangeal Joint, Right*	Ø Open 3 Percutaneous 4 Percutaneous Endoscopic X External	Z No Device	Z No Qualifier

Non-OR ØRQ[Ø,1,3,4,5,6,9,A,B,C,D,E,F,G,H,J,K,L,M,N,P,Q,R,S,T,U,V,W,X]XZZ
HAC ØRQ[E,F,G,H,J,K,L,M][Ø,3,4]ZZ when reported with SDx K68.11 or T81.4Ø–T81.49, T84.6Ø-T84.619, T84.63-T84.7 with 7th character A

Ø Medical and Surgical
R Upper Joints
R Replacement

Definition: Putting in or on biological or synthetic material that physically takes the place and/or function of all or a portion of a body part

Explanation: The body part may have been taken out or replaced, or may be taken out, physically eradicated, or rendered nonfunctional during the REPLACEMENT procedure. A REMOVAL procedure is coded for taking out the device used in a previous replacement procedure.

Body Part Character 4	Approach Character 5	Device Character 6	Qualifier Character 7
Ø Occipital-cervical Joint **1 Cervical Vertebral Joint** Atlantoaxial joint Cervical facet joint **3 Cervical Vertebral Disc** **4 Cervicothoracic Vertebral Joint** Cervicothoracic facet joint **5 Cervicothoracic Vertebral Disc** **6 Thoracic Vertebral Joint** Costotransverse joint Costovertebral joint Thoracic facet joint **9 Thoracic Vertebral Disc** **A Thoracolumbar Vertebral Joint** Thoracolumbar facet joint **B Thoracolumbar Vertebral Disc** **C Temporomandibular Joint, Right** **D Temporomandibular Joint, Left** **E Sternoclavicular Joint, Right** **F Sternoclavicular Joint, Left** **G Acromioclavicular Joint, Right** **H Acromioclavicular Joint, Left** **L Elbow Joint, Right** Distal humerus, involving joint Humeroradial joint Humeroulnar joint Proximal radioulnar joint **M Elbow Joint, Left** *See L Elbow Joint, Right* **N Wrist Joint, Right** Distal radioulnar joint Radiocarpal joint **P Wrist Joint, Left** *See N Wrist Joint, Right* **Q Carpal Joint, Right** Intercarpal joint Midcarpal joint **R Carpal Joint, Left** *See Q Carpal Joint, Right* **S Carpometacarpal Joint, Right** **T Carpometacarpal Joint, Left** **U Metacarpophalangeal Joint, Right** **V Metacarpophalangeal Joint, Left** **W Finger Phalangeal Joint, Right** Interphalangeal (IP) joint **X Finger Phalangeal Joint, Left** *See W Finger Phalangeal Joint, Right*	**Ø Open**	**7 Autologous Tissue Substitute** **J Synthetic Substitute** **K Nonautologous Tissue Substitute**	**Z No Qualifier**
J Shoulder Joint, Right Glenohumeral joint Glenoid ligament (labrum) **K Shoulder Joint, Left** *See J Shoulder Joint, Right*	**Ø Open**	**Ø Synthetic Substitute, Reverse Ball and Socket** **7 Autologous Tissue Substitute** **K Nonautologous Tissue Substitute**	**Z No Qualifier**
J Shoulder Joint, Right Glenohumeral joint Glenoid ligament (labrum) **K Shoulder Joint, Left** *See J Shoulder Joint, Right*	**Ø Open**	**J Synthetic Substitute**	**6 Humeral Surface** **7 Glenoid Surface** **Z No Qualifier**

Ø Medical and Surgical
R Upper Joints
S Reposition

Definition: Moving to its normal location, or other suitable location, all or a portion of a body part

Explanation: The body part is moved to a new location from an abnormal location, or from a normal location where it is not functioning correctly. The body part may or may not be cut out or off to be moved to the new location.

Body Part Character 4	Approach Character 5	Device Character 6	Qualifier Character 7
Ø Occipital-cervical Joint **1 Cervical Vertebral Joint** Atlantoaxial joint Cervical facet joint **4 Cervicothoracic Vertebral Joint** Cervicothoracic facet joint **6 Thoracic Vertebral Joint** Costotransverse joint Costovertebral joint Thoracic facet joint **A Thoracolumbar Vertebral Joint** Thoracolumbar facet joint **C Temporomandibular Joint, Right** **D Temporomandibular Joint, Left** **E Sternoclavicular Joint, Right** **F Sternoclavicular Joint, Left** **G Acromioclavicular Joint, Right** **H Acromioclavicular Joint, Left** **J Shoulder Joint, Right** Glenohumeral joint Glenoid ligament (labrum) **K Shoulder Joint, Left** *See J Shoulder Joint, Right*	**Ø** Open **3** Percutaneous **4** Percutaneous Endoscopic **X** External	**4** Internal Fixation Device **Z** No Device	**Z** No Qualifier
L Elbow Joint, Right Distal humerus, involving joint Humeroradial joint Humeroulnar joint Proximal radioulnar joint **M Elbow Joint, Left** *See L Elbow Joint, Right* **N Wrist Joint, Right** Distal radioulnar joint Radiocarpal joint **P Wrist Joint, Left** *See N Wrist Joint, Right* **Q Carpal Joint, Right** Intercarpal joint Midcarpal joint **R Carpal Joint, Left** *See Q Carpal Joint, Right* **S Carpometacarpal Joint, Right** **T Carpometacarpal Joint, Left** **U Metacarpophalangeal Joint, Right** **V Metacarpophalangeal Joint, Left** **W Finger Phalangeal Joint, Right** Interphalangeal (IP) joint **X Finger Phalangeal Joint, Left** *See W Finger Phalangeal Joint, Right*	**Ø** Open **3** Percutaneous **4** Percutaneous Endoscopic **X** External	**4** Internal Fixation Device **5** External Fixation Device **Z** No Device	**Z** No Qualifier

Non-OR ØRS[Ø,1,4,6,A,C,D,E,F,G,H,J,K][3,4,X][4,Z]Z
Non-OR ØRS[L,M,N,P,Q,R,S,T,U,V,W,X][3,4,X][4,5,Z]Z

Ø Medical and Surgical
R Upper Joints
T Resection Definition: Cutting out or off, without replacement, all of a body part

Explanation: None

Body Part Character 4	Approach Character 5	Device Character 6	Qualifier Character 7
3 Cervical Vertebral Disc **4 Cervicothoracic Vertebral Joint** Cervicothoracic facet joint **5 Cervicothoracic Vertebral Disc** **9 Thoracic Vertebral Disc** **B Thoracolumbar Vertebral Disc** **C Temporomandibular Joint, Right** **D Temporomandibular Joint, Left** **E Sternoclavicular Joint, Right** **F Sternoclavicular Joint, Left** **G Acromioclavicular Joint, Right** **H Acromioclavicular Joint, Left** **J Shoulder Joint, Right** Glenohumeral joint Glenoid ligament (labrum) **K Shoulder Joint, Left** *See J Shoulder Joint, Right* **L Elbow Joint, Right** Distal humerus, involving joint Humeroradial joint Humeroulnar joint Proximal radioulnar joint **M Elbow Joint, Left** *See L Elbow Joint, Right* **N Wrist Joint, Right** Distal radioulnar joint Radiocarpal joint **P Wrist Joint, Left** *See N Wrist Joint, Right* **Q Carpal Joint, Right** Intercarpal joint Midcarpal joint **R Carpal Joint, Left** *See Q Carpal Joint, Right* **S Carpometacarpal Joint, Right** **T Carpometacarpal Joint, Left** **U Metacarpophalangeal Joint, Right** **V Metacarpophalangeal Joint, Left** **W Finger Phalangeal Joint, Right** Interphalangeal (IP) joint **X Finger Phalangeal Joint, Left** *See W Finger Phalangeal Joint, Right*	Ø Open	Z No Device	Z No Qualifier

Ø Medical and Surgical
R Upper Joints
U Supplement

Definition: Putting in or on biological or synthetic material that physically reinforces and/or augments the function of a portion of a body part

Explanation: The biological material is non-living, or is living and from the same individual. The body part may have been previously replaced, and the SUPPLEMENT procedure is performed to physically reinforce and/or augment the function of the replaced body part.

Body Part Character 4	Approach Character 5	Device Character 6	Qualifier Character 7
Ø Occipital-cervical Joint **1 Cervical Vertebral Joint** Atlantoaxial joint Cervical facet joint **3 Cervical Vertebral Disc** **4 Cervicothoracic Vertebral Joint** Cervicothoracic facet joint **5 Cervicothoracic Vertebral Disc** **6 Thoracic Vertebral Joint** Costotransverse joint Costovertebral joint Thoracic facet joint **9 Thoracic Vertebral Disc** **A Thoracolumbar Vertebral Joint** Thoracolumbar facet joint **B Thoracolumbar Vertebral Disc** **C Temporomandibular Joint, Right** **D Temporomandibular Joint, Left** **E Sternoclavicular Joint, Right** **F Sternoclavicular Joint, Left** **G Acromioclavicular Joint, Right** **H Acromioclavicular Joint, Left** **J Shoulder Joint, Right** Glenohumeral joint Glenoid ligament (labrum) **K Shoulder Joint, Left** *See J Shoulder Joint, Right* **L Elbow Joint, Right** Distal humerus, involving joint Humeroradial joint Humeroulnar joint Proximal radioulnar joint **M Elbow Joint, Left** *See L Elbow Joint, Right* **N Wrist Joint, Right** Distal radioulnar joint Radiocarpal joint **P Wrist Joint, Left** *See N Wrist Joint, Right* **Q Carpal Joint, Right** Intercarpal joint Midcarpal joint **R Carpal Joint, Left** *See Q Carpal Joint, Right* **S Carpometacarpal Joint, Right** **T Carpometacarpal Joint, Left** **U Metacarpophalangeal Joint, Right** **V Metacarpophalangeal Joint, Left** **W Finger Phalangeal Joint, Right** Interphalangeal (IP) joint **X Finger Phalangeal Joint, Left** *See W Finger Phalangeal Joint, Right*	**Ø Open** **3 Percutaneous** **4 Percutaneous Endoscopic**	**7 Autologous Tissue Substitute** **J Synthetic Substitute** **K Nonautologous Tissue Substitute**	**Z No Qualifier**

HAC ØRU[E,F,G,H,J,K,L,M][Ø,3,4][7,J,K]Z when reported with SDx K68.11 or T81.4Ø–T81.49, T84.6Ø-T84.619, T84.63-T84.7 with 7th character A

Ø Medical and Surgical
R Upper Joints
W Revision

Definition: Correcting, to the extent possible, a portion of a malfunctioning device or the position of a displaced device

Explanation: Revision can include correcting a malfunctioning or displaced device by taking out or putting in components of the device such as a screw or pin

Body Part Character 4	Approach Character 5	Device Character 6	Qualifier Character 7
Ø Occipital-cervical Joint **1 Cervical Vertebral Joint** Atlantoaxial joint Cervical facet joint **4 Cervicothoracic Vertebral Joint** Cervicothoracic facet joint **6 Thoracic Vertebral Joint** Costotransverse joint Costovertebral joint Thoracic facet joint **A Thoracolumbar Vertebral Joint** Thoracolumbar facet joint	**Ø Open** **3 Percutaneous** **4 Percutaneous Endoscopic** **X External**	**Ø Drainage Device** **3 Infusion Device** **4 Internal Fixation Device** **7 Autologous Tissue Substitute** **8 Spacer** **A Interbody Fusion Device** **J Synthetic Substitute** **K Nonautologous Tissue Substitute**	**Z No Qualifier**
3 Cervical Vertebral Disc **5 Cervicothoracic Vertebral Disc** **9 Thoracic Vertebral Disc** **B Thoracolumbar Vertebral Disc**	**Ø Open** **3 Percutaneous** **4 Percutaneous Endoscopic** **X External**	**Ø Drainage Device** **3 Infusion Device** **7 Autologous Tissue Substitute** **J Synthetic Substitute** **K Nonautologous Tissue Substitute**	**Z No Qualifier**
C Temporomandibular Joint, Right **D Temporomandibular Joint, Left** **E Sternoclavicular Joint, Right** **F Sternoclavicular Joint, Left** **G Acromioclavicular Joint, Right** **H Acromioclavicular Joint, Left**	**Ø Open** **3 Percutaneous** **4 Percutaneous Endoscopic** **X External**	**Ø Drainage Device** **3 Infusion Device** **4 Internal Fixation Device** **7 Autologous Tissue Substitute** **8 Spacer** **J Synthetic Substitute** **K Nonautologous Tissue Substitute**	**Z No Qualifier**
J Shoulder Joint, Right Glenohumeral joint Glenoid ligament (labrum) **K Shoulder Joint, Left** *See J Shoulder Joint, Right*	**Ø Open** **3 Percutaneous** **4 Percutaneous Endoscopic** **X External**	**Ø Drainage Device** **3 Infusion Device** **4 Internal Fixation Device** **7 Autologous Tissue Substitute** **8 Spacer** **J Synthetic Substitute** **K Nonautologous Tissue Substitute**	**Z No Qualifier**
J Shoulder Joint, Right Glenohumeral joint Glenoid ligament (labrum) **K Shoulder Joint, Left** *See J Shoulder Joint, Right*	**Ø Open** **3 Percutaneous** **4 Percutaneous Endoscopic** **X External**	**J Synthetic Substitute**	**6 Humeral Surface** **7 Glenoid Surface** **Z No Qualifier**
L Elbow Joint, Right Distal humerus, involving joint Humeroradial joint Humeroulnar joint Proximal radioulnar joint **M Elbow Joint, Left** *See L Elbow Joint, Right* **N Wrist Joint, Right** Distal radioulnar joint Radiocarpal joint **P Wrist Joint, Left** *See N Wrist Joint, Right* **Q Carpal Joint, Right** Intercarpal joint Midcarpal joint **R Carpal Joint, Left** *See Q Carpal Joint, Right* **S Carpometacarpal Joint, Right** **T Carpometacarpal Joint, Left** **U Metacarpophalangeal Joint, Right** **V Metacarpophalangeal Joint, Left** **W Finger Phalangeal Joint, Right** Interphalangeal (IP) joint **X Finger Phalangeal Joint, Left** *See W Finger Phalangeal Joint, Right*	**Ø Open** **3 Percutaneous** **4 Percutaneous Endoscopic** **X External**	**Ø Drainage Device** **3 Infusion Device** **4 Internal Fixation Device** **5 External Fixation Device** **7 Autologous Tissue Substitute** **8 Spacer** **J Synthetic Substitute** **K Nonautologous Tissue Substitute**	**Z No Qualifier**

Non-OR ØRW[Ø,1,4,6,A]X[Ø,3,4,7,8,A,J,K]Z
Non-OR ØRW[3,5,9,B]X[Ø,3,7,J,K]Z
Non-OR ØRW[C,D,E,F,G,H]X[Ø,3,4,7,8,J,K]Z
Non-OR ØRW[J,K]X[Ø,3,4,7,8,J,K]Z
Non-OR ØRW[J,K]XJ[6,7,Z]
Non-OR ØRW[L,M,N,P,Q,R,S,T,U,V,W,X]X[Ø,3,4,5,7,8,J,K]Z

Lower Joints ØS2–ØSW

Character Meanings*

This Character Meaning table is provided as a guide to assist the user in the identification of character members that may be found in this section of code tables. It **SHOULD NOT** be used to build a PCS code.

Operation–Character 3	Body Part–Character 4	Approach–Character 5	Device–Character 6	Qualifier–Character 7
2 Change	Ø Lumbar Vertebral Joint	Ø Open	Ø Drainage Device OR Synthetic Substitute, Polyethylene	Ø Anterior Approach, Anterior Column
5 Destruction	1 Lumbar Vertebral Joint, 2 or more	3 Percutaneous	1 Synthetic Substitute, Metal	1 Posterior Approach, Posterior Column
9 Drainage	2 Lumbar Vertebral Disc	4 Percutaneous Endoscopic	2 Synthetic Substitute, Metal on Polyethylene	9 Cemented
B Excision	3 Lumbosacral Joint	X External	3 Infusion Device OR Internal Fixation Device, Sustained Compression OR Synthetic Substitute, Ceramic	A Uncemented
C Extirpation	4 Lumbosacral Disc		4 Internal Fixation Device OR Synthetic Substitute, Ceramic on Polyethylene	C Patellar Surface
G Fusion	5 Sacrococcygeal Joint		5 External Fixation Device	J Posterior Approach, Anterior Column
H Insertion	6 Coccygeal Joint		6 Synthetic Substitute, Oxidized Zirconium on Polyethylene	X Diagnostic
J Inspection	7 Sacroiliac Joint, Right		7 Autologous Tissue Substitute	Z No Qualifier
N Release	8 Sacroiliac Joint, Left		8 Spacer	
P Removal	9 Hip Joint, Right		9 Liner	
Q Repair	A Hip Joint, Acetabular Surface, Right		A Interbody Fusion Device	
R Replacement	B Hip Joint, Left		B Resurfacing Device OR Spinal Stabilization Device, Interspinous Process	
S Reposition	C Knee Joint, Right		C Spinal Stabilization Device, Pedicle-Based	
T Resection	D Knee Joint, Left		D Spinal Stabilization Device, Facet Replacement	
U Supplement	E Hip Joint, Acetabular Surface, Left		E Articulating Spacer	
W Revision	F Ankle Joint, Right		J Synthetic Substitute	
	G Ankle Joint, Left		K Nonautologous Tissue Substitute	
	H Tarsal Joint, Right		L Synthetic Substitute, Unicondylar Medial	
	J Tarsal Joint, Left		M Synthetic Substitute, Unicondylar Lateral	
	K Tarsometatarsal Joint, Right		N Synthetic Substitute, Patellofemoral	
	L Tarsometatarsal Joint, Left		Y Other Device	
	M Metatarsal-Phalangeal Joint, Right		Z No Device	
	N Metatarsal-Phalangeal Joint, Left			
	P Toe Phalangeal Joint, Right			
	Q Toe Phalangeal Joint, Left			
	R Hip Joint, Femoral Surface, Right			
	S Hip Joint, Femoral Surface, Left			
	T Knee Joint, Femoral Surface, Right			
	U Knee Joint, Femoral Surface, Left			
	V Knee Joint, Tibial Surface, Right			
	W Knee Joint, Tibial Surface, Left			
	Y Lower Joint			

* Includes synovial membrane.

AHA Coding Clinic for table ØS9

2018, 2Q, 17 Arthroscopic drainage of knee and nonexcisional debridement
2017, 1Q, 50 Dry aspiration of ankle joint

AHA Coding Clinic for table ØSB

2017, 4Q, 76 Radiolucent porous interbody fusion device
2016, 2Q, 16 Decompressive laminectomy/foraminotomy and lumbar discectomy
2016, 1Q, 20 Metatarsophalangeal joint resection arthroplasty
2015, 1Q, 34 Arthroscopic meniscectomy with debridement and abrasion chondroplasty
2014, 2Q, 6 Posterior lumbar fusion with discectomy

AHA Coding Clinic for table ØSG

2023, 2Q, 25 Spinal fusion using allograft bone graft and bone marrow aspirate
2022, 3Q, 21 Breakage of intervertebral cage during surgery
2022, 2Q, 23 Sacroiliac joint fusion
2021, 4Q, 67 Posterior dynamic distraction
2021, 3Q, 24 Mid-foot fusion with bone graft
2021, 3Q, 25 Placement of X-Spine Axle Cage
2021, 1Q, 18 Placement of interspinous distraction device (spacer) for decompression
2021, 1Q, 53 Official guidelines for coding and reporting for interbody fusion device B3.10c
2020, 4Q, 56-58 Intramedullary sustained compression joint fusion
2020, 2Q, 27 Spinal fusion with NuVasive® VersaTie®
2020, 1Q, 33 Spinal fusion without use of bone graft
2019, 3Q, 35 Fusion procedures of the spine (guideline B3.10c)
2019, 1Q, 30 Spinal fusion performed at same level as decompressive laminectomy
2018, 4Q, 43 Joint fusion device value
2018, 1Q, 22 Spinal fusion procedures without bone graft
2017, 4Q, 76 Radiolucent porous interbody fusion device
2017, 2Q, 23 Decompression of spinal cord and placement of instrumentation
2014, 3Q, 30 Spinal fusion and fixation instrumentation
2014, 3Q, 36 Lumbar interbody fusion of two vertebral levels
2014, 2Q, 6 Posterior lumbar fusion with discectomy
2013, 3Q, 25 360-degree spinal fusion
2013, 2Q, 39 Ankle fusion, osteotomy, and removal of hardware
2013, 1Q, 21-23 Spinal fusion of thoracic and lumbar vertebrae

AHA Coding Clinic for table ØSH

2021, 3Q, 25 Placement of X-Spine Axle Cage
2021, 1Q, 18 Placement of interspinous distraction device (spacer) for decompression
2017, 2Q, 23 Decompression of spinal cord and placement of instrumentation

AHA Coding Clinic for table ØSJ

2017, 1Q, 50 Dry aspiration of ankle joint

AHA Coding Clinic for table ØSN

2020, 2Q, 26 Arthroscopic manipulation and nonexcisional debridement of knee joint
2019, 1Q, 30 Spinal fusion performed at same level as decompressive laminectomy

AHA Coding Clinic for table ØSP

2022, 3Q, 21 Breakage of intervertebral cage during surgery
2021, 3Q, 25 Revision total knee arthroplasty
2021, 1Q, 17 Revision of ankle arthroplasty with placement of tibial insert
2018, 4Q, 43 Articulating spacer for hip and knee joint
2018, 2Q, 16 Exchange of tibial polyethylene component with stabilizing insert (tibial tray)
2017, 4Q, 107 Total ankle replacement versus revision
2016, 4Q, 110-112 Removal and revision of hip and knee devices
2015, 2Q, 18 Total knee revision
2015, 2Q, 19 Revision of femoral head and acetabular liner
2013, 2Q, 39 Ankle fusion, osteotomy, and removal of hardware

AHA Coding Clinic for table ØSQ

2014, 4Q, 25 Femoroacetabular impingement and labral tear with repair

AHA Coding Clinic for table ØSR

2022, 1Q, 39 Provisional total hip arthroplasty
2021, 3Q, 25 Revision total knee arthroplasty
2021, 1Q, 17 Revision of ankle arthroplasty with placement of tibial insert
2020, 3Q, 33 Total hip arthroplasty using dual mobility components
2018, 4Q, 43 Articulating spacer for hip and knee joint
2018, 2Q, 16 Exchange of tibial polyethylene component with stabilizing insert (tibial tray)
2017, 4Q, 38-39 Oxidized zirconium on polyethylene bearing surface
2017, 4Q, 107 Total ankle replacement versus revision
2017, 1Q, 22 Total knee replacement and patellar component
2016, 4Q, 110-111 Partial (unicondylar) knee replacement
2016, 4Q, 111-112 Removal and revision of hip and knee devices
2016, 3Q, 35 Use of cemented versus uncemented qualifier for joint replacement
2015, 3Q, 18 Total hip replacement with acetabular reconstruction
2015, 2Q, 18 Total knee revision
2015, 2Q, 19 Revision of femoral head and acetabular liner

AHA Coding Clinic for table ØSS

2022, 3Q, 27 Ankle and tarsal joint distraction
2022, 2Q, 22 Ankle distraction procedure
2016, 2Q, 31 Periacetabular ostectomy for repair of congenital hip dysplasia

AHA Coding Clinic for table ØST

2016, 1Q, 20 Metatarsophalangeal joint resection arthroplasty
2014, 4Q, 29 Rotational osteosynthesis

AHA Coding Clinic for table ØSU

2022, 1Q, 47 Matrix-induced autologous chondrocyte implantation
2021, 1Q, 17 Revision of ankle arthroplasty with placement of tibial insert
2018, 2Q, 16 Exchange of tibial polyethylene component with stabilizing insert (tibial tray)
2016, 4Q, 111 Removal and revision of hip and knee devices
2015, 2Q, 19 Revision of femoral head and acetabular liner

AHA Coding Clinic for table ØSW

2017, 4Q, 107 Total ankle replacement versus revision
2016, 4Q, 110-112 Removal and revision of hip and knee devices
2015, 2Q, 18 Total knee revision
2015, 2Q, 19 Revision of femoral head and acetabular liner

Lower Joints

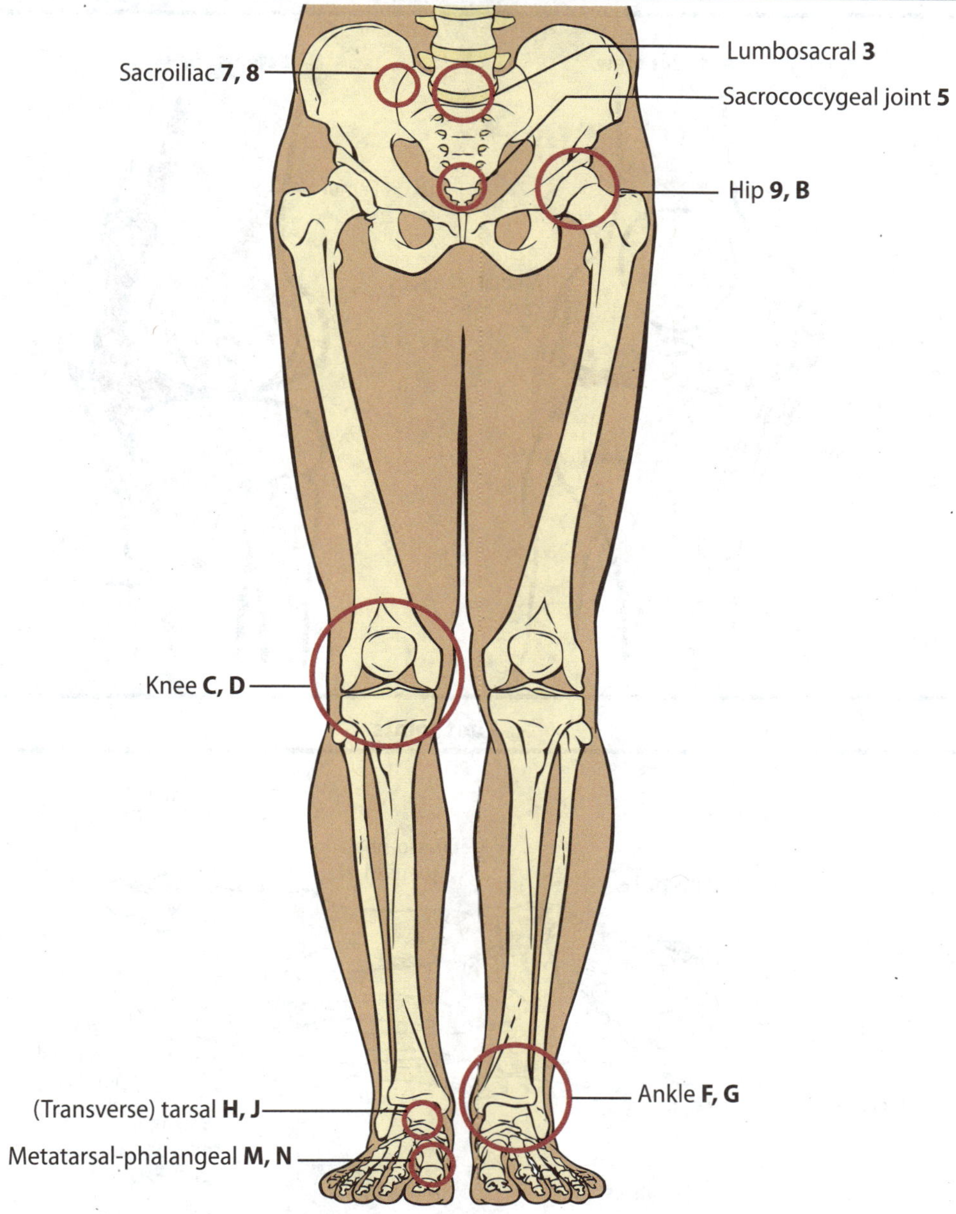

Sacroiliac **7, 8**
Lumbosacral **3**
Sacrococcygeal joint **5**
Hip **9, B**
Knee **C, D**
Ankle **F, G**
(Transverse) tarsal **H, J**
Metatarsal-phalangeal **M, N**

Hip Joint

Ilium
Sacroiliac joint **7, 8**
Sacrum
Acetabulofemoral joint **9, B**
Head of femur
Ischium

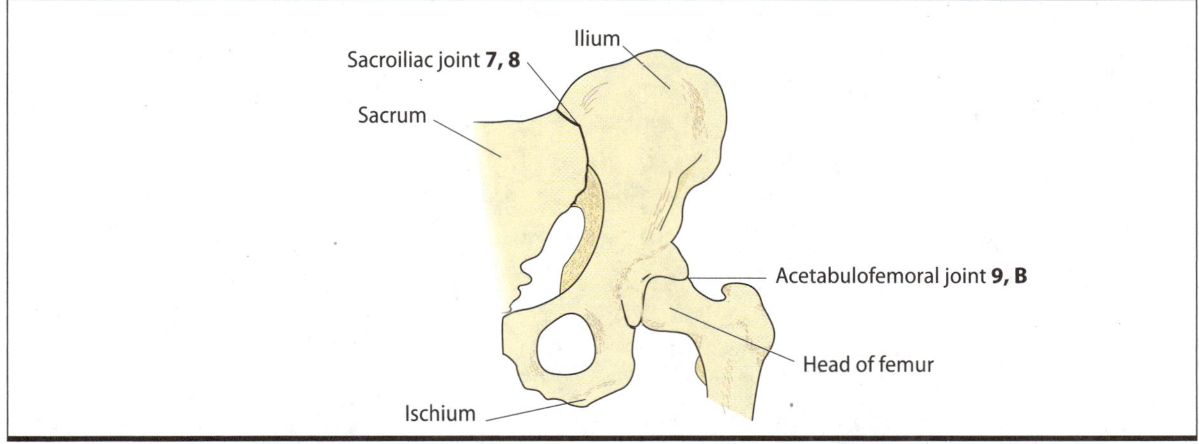

Knee Joint

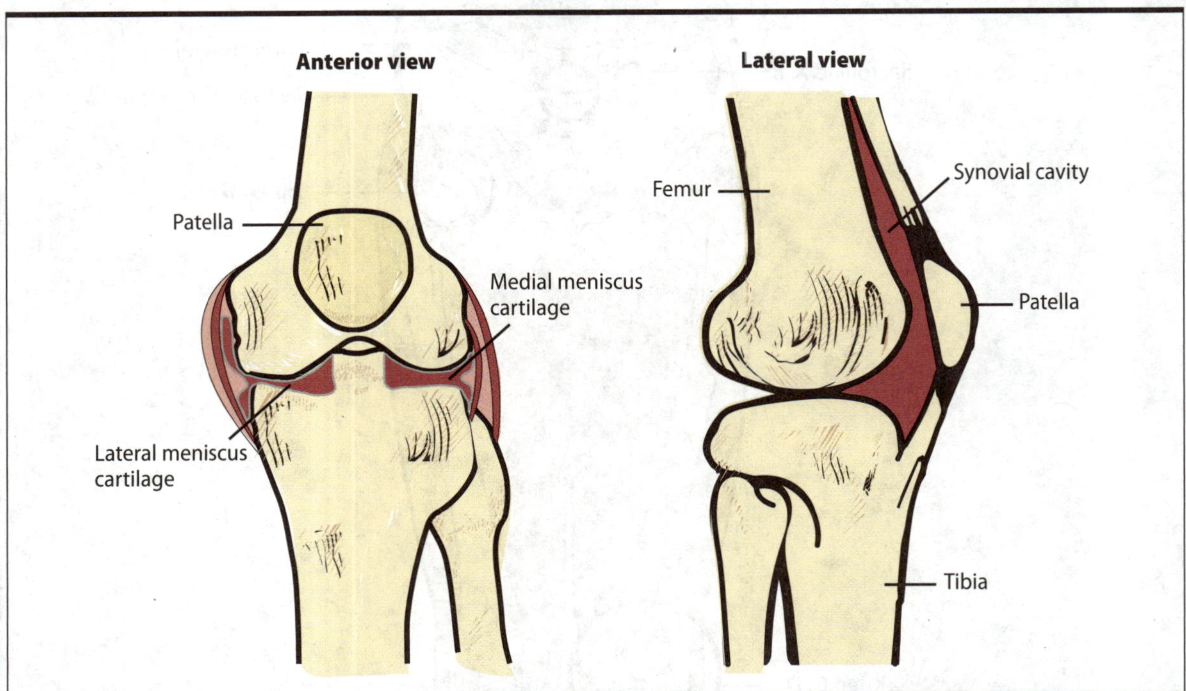

Foot Joints

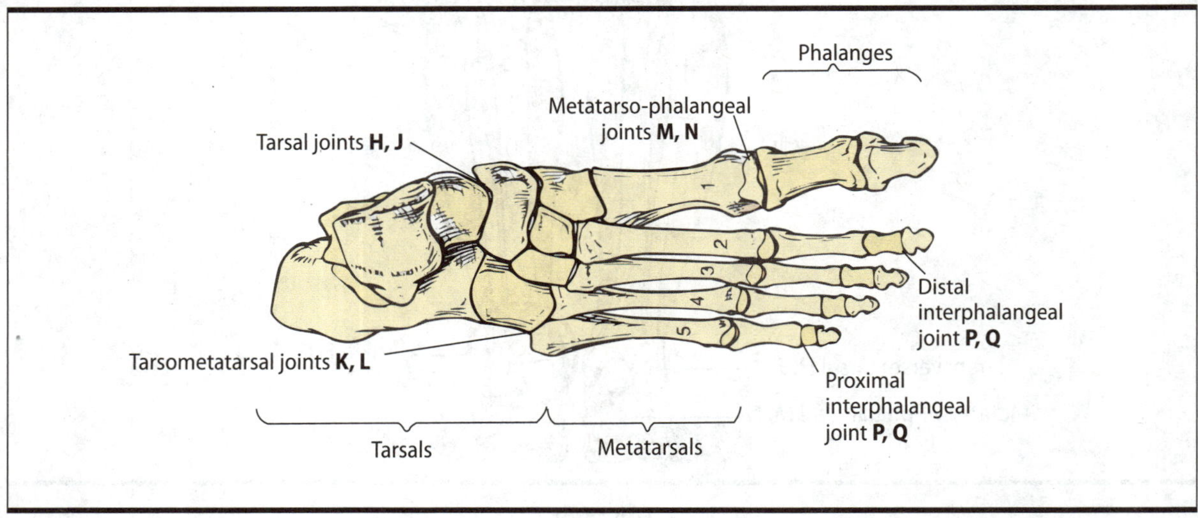

Ø Medical and Surgical
S Lower Joints
2 Change

Definition: Taking out or off a device from a body part and putting back an identical or similar device in or on the same body part without cutting or puncturing the skin or a mucous membrane

Explanation: All CHANGE procedures are coded using the approach EXTERNAL

Body Part Character 4	Approach Character 5	Device Character 6	Qualifier Character 7
Y Lower Joint	**X** External	**Ø** Drainage Device **Y** Other Device	**Z** No Qualifier

Non-OR All body part, approach, device, and qualifier values

Ø Medical and Surgical
S Lower Joints
5 Destruction

Definition: Physical eradication of all or a portion of a body part by the direct use of energy, force, or a destructive agent

Explanation: None of the body part is physically taken out

Body Part Character 4	Approach Character 5	Device Character 6	Qualifier Character 7
Ø **Lumbar Vertebral Joint** Lumbar facet joint **2** **Lumbar Vertebral Disc** **3** **Lumbosacral Joint** Lumbosacral facet joint **4** **Lumbosacral Disc** **5** **Sacrococcygeal Joint** Sacrococcygeal symphysis **6** **Coccygeal Joint** **7** **Sacroiliac Joint, Right** **8** **Sacroiliac Joint, Left** **9** **Hip Joint, Right** Acetabulofemoral joint **B** **Hip Joint, Left** *See 9 Hip Joint, Right* **C** **Knee Joint, Right** Femoropatellar joint Femorotibial joint Lateral meniscus Medial meniscus Patellofemoral joint Tibiofemoral joint **D** **Knee Joint, Left** *See C Knee Joint, Right* **F** **Ankle Joint, Right** Inferior tibiofibular joint Talocrural joint **G** **Ankle Joint, Left** *See F Ankle Joint, Right* **H** **Tarsal Joint, Right** Calcaneocuboid joint Cuboideonavicular joint Cuneonavicular joint Intercuneiform joint Subtalar (talocalcaneal) joint Talocalcaneal (subtalar) joint Talocalcaneonavicular joint **J** **Tarsal Joint, Left** *See H Tarsal Joint, Right* **K** **Tarsometatarsal Joint, Right** **L** **Tarsometatarsal Joint, Left** **M** **Metatarsal-Phalangeal Joint, Right** Metatarsophalangeal (MTP) joint **N** **Metatarsal-Phalangeal Joint, Left** *See M Metatarsal-Phalangeal Joint, Right* **P** **Toe Phalangeal Joint, Right** Interphalangeal (IP) joint **Q** **Toe Phalangeal Joint, Left** *See P Toe Phalangeal Joint, Right*	**Ø** Open **3** Percutaneous **4** Percutaneous Endoscopic	**Z** No Device	**Z** No Qualifier

Ø Medical and Surgical
S Lower Joints
9 Drainage

Definition: Taking or letting out fluids and/or gases from a body part
Explanation: The qualifier DIAGNOSTIC is used to identify drainage procedures that are biopsies

Body Part Character 4		Approach Character 5	Device Character 6	Qualifier Character 7
Ø Lumbar Vertebral Joint Lumbar facet joint **2 Lumbar Vertebral Disc** **3 Lumbosacral Joint** Lumbosacral facet joint **4 Lumbosacral Disc** **5 Sacrococcygeal Joint** Sacrococcygeal symphysis **6 Coccygeal Joint** **7 Sacroiliac Joint, Right** **8 Sacroiliac Joint, Left** **9 Hip Joint, Right** Acetabulofemoral joint **B Hip Joint, Left** *See 9 Hip Joint, Right* **C Knee Joint, Right** Femoropatellar joint Femorotibial joint Lateral meniscus Medial meniscus Patellofemoral joint Tibiofemoral joint **D Knee Joint, Left** *See C Knee Joint, Right* **F Ankle Joint, Right** Inferior tibiofibular joint Talocrural joint **G Ankle Joint, Left** *See F Ankle Joint, Right*	**H Tarsal Joint, Right** Calcaneocuboid joint Cuboideonavicular joint Cuneonavicular joint Intercuneiform joint Subtalar (talocalcaneal) joint Talocalcaneal (subtalar) joint Talocalcaneonavicular joint **J Tarsal Joint, Left** *See H Tarsal Joint, Right* **K Tarsometatarsal Joint, Right** **L Tarsometatarsal Joint, Left** **M Metatarsal-Phalangeal Joint, Right** Metatarsophalangeal (MTP) joint **N Metatarsal-Phalangeal Joint, Left** *See M Metatarsal-Phalangeal Joint, Right* **P Toe Phalangeal Joint, Right** Interphalangeal (IP) joint **Q Toe Phalangeal Joint, Left** *See P Toe Phalangeal Joint, Right*	**Ø Open** **3 Percutaneous** **4 Percutaneous Endoscopic**	**Ø Drainage Device**	**Z No Qualifier**
Ø Lumbar Vertebral Joint Lumbar facet joint **2 Lumbar Vertebral Disc** **3 Lumbosacral Joint** Lumbosacral facet joint **4 Lumbosacral Disc** **5 Sacrococcygeal Joint** Sacrococcygeal symphysis **6 Coccygeal Joint** **7 Sacroiliac Joint, Right** **8 Sacroiliac Joint, Left** **9 Hip Joint, Right** Acetabulofemoral joint **B Hip Joint, Left** *See 9 Hip Joint, Right* **C Knee Joint, Right** Femoropatellar joint Femorotibial joint Lateral meniscus Medial meniscus Patellofemoral joint Tibiofemoral joint **D Knee Joint, Left** *See C Knee Joint, Right* **F Ankle Joint, Right** Inferior tibiofibular joint Talocrural joint **G Ankle Joint, Left** *See F Ankle Joint, Right*	**H Tarsal Joint, Right** Calcaneocuboid joint Cuboideonavicular joint Cuneonavicular joint Intercuneiform joint Subtalar (talocalcaneal) joint Talocalcaneal (subtalar) joint Talocalcaneonavicular joint **J Tarsal Joint, Left** *See H Tarsal Joint, Right* **K Tarsometatarsal Joint, Right** **L Tarsometatarsal Joint, Left** **M Metatarsal-Phalangeal Joint, Right** Metatarsophalangeal (MTP) joint **N Metatarsal-Phalangeal Joint, Left** *See M Metatarsal-Phalangeal Joint, Right* **P Toe Phalangeal Joint, Right** Interphalangeal (IP) joint **Q Toe Phalangeal Joint, Left** *See P Toe Phalangeal Joint, Right*	**Ø Open** **3 Percutaneous** **4 Percutaneous Endoscopic**	**Z No Device**	**X Diagnostic** **Z No Qualifier**

Non-OR ØS9[Ø,2,3,4,5,6,7,8,9,B,C,D,F,G,H,J,K,L,M,N,P,Q][3,4]ØZ
Non-OR ØS9[Ø,2,3,4,5,6,7,8,9,B,C,D,F,G,H,J,K,L,M,N,P,Q][Ø,3,4]ZX
Non-OR ØS9[Ø,2,3,4,5,6,7,8,9,B,C,D,F,G,H,J,K,L,M,N,P,Q][3,4]ZZ

Ø Medical and Surgical
S Lower Joints
B Excision Definition: Cutting out or off, without replacement, a portion of a body part
Explanation: The qualifier DIAGNOSTIC is used to identify excision procedures that are biopsies

Body Part Character 4	Approach Character 5	Device Character 6	Qualifier Character 7
Ø Lumbar Vertebral Joint Lumbar facet joint **2 Lumbar Vertebral Disc** **3 Lumbosacral Joint** Lumbosacral facet joint **4 Lumbosacral Disc** **5 Sacrococcygeal Joint** Sacrococcygeal symphysis **6 Coccygeal Joint** **7 Sacroiliac Joint, Right** **8 Sacroiliac Joint, Left** **9 Hip Joint, Right** Acetabulofemoral joint **B Hip Joint, Left** *See 9 Hip Joint, Right* **C Knee Joint, Right** Femoropatellar joint Femorotibial joint Lateral meniscus Medial meniscus Patellofemoral joint Tibiofemoral joint **D Knee Joint, Left** *See C Knee Joint, Right* **F Ankle Joint, Right** Inferior tibiofibular joint Talocrural joint **G Ankle Joint, Left** *See F Ankle Joint, Right* **H Tarsal Joint, Right** Calcaneocuboid joint Cuboideonavicular joint Cuneonavicular joint Intercuneiform joint Subtalar (talocalcaneal) joint Talocalcaneal (subtalar) joint Talocalcaneonavicular joint **J Tarsal Joint, Left** *See H Tarsal Joint, Right* **K Tarsometatarsal Joint, Right** **L Tarsometatarsal Joint, Left** **M Metatarsal-Phalangeal Joint, Right** Metatarsophalangeal (MTP) joint **N Metatarsal-Phalangeal Joint, Left** *See M Metatarsal-Phalangeal Joint, Right* **P Toe Phalangeal Joint, Right** Interphalangeal (IP) joint **Q Toe Phalangeal Joint, Left** *See P Toe Phalangeal Joint, Right*	**Ø Open** **3 Percutaneous** **4 Percutaneous Endoscopic**	**Z No Device**	**X Diagnostic** **Z No Qualifier**

Non-OR ØSB[Ø,2,3,4,5,6,7,8,9,B,C,D,F,G,H,J,K,L,M,N,P,Q][Ø,3,4]ZX

Ø Medical and Surgical
S Lower Joints
C Extirpation Definition: Taking or cutting out solid matter from a body part

Explanation: The solid matter may be an abnormal byproduct of a biological function or a foreign body; it may be imbedded in a body part or in the lumen of a tubular body part. The solid matter may or may not have been previously broken into pieces.

Body Part Character 4	Approach Character 5	Device Character 6	Qualifier Character 7
Ø Lumbar Vertebral Joint Lumbar facet joint **2 Lumbar Vertebral Disc** **3 Lumbosacral Joint** Lumbosacral facet joint **4 Lumbosacral Disc** **5 Sacrococcygeal Joint** Sacrococcygeal symphysis **6 Coccygeal Joint** **7 Sacroiliac Joint, Right** **8 Sacroiliac Joint, Left** **9 Hip Joint, Right** Acetabulofemoral joint **B Hip Joint, Left** *See 9 Hip Joint, Right* **C Knee Joint, Right** Femoropatellar joint Femorotibial joint Lateral meniscus Medial meniscus Patellofemoral joint Tibiofemoral joint **D Knee Joint, Left** *See C Knee Joint, Right* **F Ankle Joint, Right** Inferior tibiofibular joint Talocrural joint **G Ankle Joint, Left** *See F Ankle Joint, Right* **H Tarsal Joint, Right** Calcaneocuboid joint Cuboideonavicular joint Cuneonavicular joint Intercuneiform joint Subtalar (talocalcaneal) joint Talocalcaneal (subtalar) joint Talocalcaneonavicular joint **J Tarsal Joint, Left** *See H Tarsal Joint, Right* **K Tarsometatarsal Joint, Right** **L Tarsometatarsal Joint, Left** **M Metatarsal-Phalangeal Joint, Right** Metatarsophalangeal (MTP) joint **N Metatarsal-Phalangeal Joint, Left** *See M Metatarsal-Phalangeal Joint, Right* **P Toe Phalangeal Joint, Right** Interphalangeal (IP) joint **Q Toe Phalangeal Joint, Left** *See P Toe Phalangeal Joint, Right*	**Ø Open** **3 Percutaneous** **4 Percutaneous Endoscopic**	**Z No Device**	**Z No Qualifier**

Ø Medical and Surgical
S Lower Joints
G Fusion

Definition: Joining together portions of an articular body part rendering the articular body part immobile
Explanation: The body part is joined together by fixation device, bone graft, or other means

Body Part Character 4	Approach Character 5	Device Character 6	Qualifier Character 7
Ø Lumbar Vertebral Joint Lumbar facet joint **1 Lumbar Vertebral Joints, 2 or more** ⊞ **3 Lumbosacral Joint** Lumbosacral facet joint	**Ø Open** **3 Percutaneous** **4 Percutaneous Endoscopic**	**7 Autologous Tissue Substitute** **J Synthetic Substitute** **K Nonautologous Tissue Substitute**	**Ø Anterior Approach, Anterior Column** **1 Posterior Approach, Posterior Column** **J Posterior Approach, Anterior Column**
Ø Lumbar Vertebral Joint Lumbar facet joint **1 Lumbar Vertebral Joints, 2 or more** ⊞ **3 Lumbosacral Joint** Lumbosacral facet joint	**Ø Open** **3 Percutaneous** **4 Percutaneous Endoscopic**	**A Interbody Fusion Device**	**Ø Anterior Approach, Anterior Column** **J Posterior Approach, Anterior Column**
5 Sacrococcygeal Joint Sacrococcygeal symphysis **6 Coccygeal Joint** **7 Sacroiliac Joint, Right** **8 Sacroiliac Joint, Left**	**Ø Open** **3 Percutaneous** **4 Percutaneous Endoscopic**	**4 Internal Fixation Device** **7 Autologous Tissue Substitute** **J Synthetic Substitute** **K Nonautologous Tissue Substitute**	**Z No Qualifier**
9 Hip Joint, Right Acetabulofemoral joint **B Hip Joint, Left** *See 9 Hip Joint, Right* **C Knee Joint, Right** Femoropatellar joint Femorotibial joint Lateral meniscus Medial meniscus Patellofemoral joint Tibiofemoral joint **D Knee Joint, Left** *See C Knee Joint, Right* **F Ankle Joint, Right** Inferior tibiofibular joint Talocrural joint **G Ankle Joint, Left** *See F Ankle Joint, Right* **H Tarsal Joint, Right** Calcaneocuboid joint Cuboideonavicular joint Cuneonavicular joint Intercuneiform joint Subtalar (talocalcaneal) joint Talocalcaneal (subtalar) joint Talocalcaneonavicular joint **J Tarsal Joint, Left** *See H Tarsal Joint, Right* **K Tarsometatarsal Joint, Right** **L Tarsometatarsal Joint, Left** **M Metatarsal-Phalangeal Joint, Right** Metatarsophalangeal (MTP) joint **N Metatarsal-Phalangeal Joint, Left** *See M Metatarsal-Phalangeal Joint, Right* **P Toe Phalangeal Joint, Right** Interphalangeal (IP) joint **Q Toe Phalangeal Joint, Left** *See P Toe Phalangeal Joint, Right*	**Ø Open** **3 Percutaneous** **4 Percutaneous Endoscopic**	**3 Internal Fixation Device, Sustained Compression** **4 Internal Fixation Device** **5 External Fixation Device** **7 Autologous Tissue Substitute** **J Synthetic Substitute** **K Nonautologous Tissue Substitute**	**Z No Qualifier**

HAC ØSG[Ø,1,3][Ø,3,4][7,J,K][Ø,1,J] when reported with SDx K68.11 or T81.4Ø–T81.49, T84.6Ø-T84.619, T84.63-T84.7 with 7th character A

HAC ØSG[Ø,1,3][Ø,3,4]A[Ø,J] when reported with SDx K68.11 or T81.4Ø–T81.49, T84.6Ø-T84.619, T84.63-T84.7 with 7th character A

HAC ØSG[7,8][Ø,3,4][4,7,J,K]Z when reported with SDx K68.11 or T81.4Ø–T81.49, T84.6Ø-T84.619, T84.63-T84.7 with 7th character A

See Appendix L for Procedure Combinations
⊞ ØSG1[Ø,3,4][7,J,K][Ø,1,J]
⊞ ØSG1[Ø,3,4]A[Ø,J]

Ø Medical and Surgical
S Lower Joints
H Insertion

Definition: Putting in a nonbiological appliance that monitors, assists, performs, or prevents a physiological function but does not physically take the place of a body part

Explanation: None

Body Part Character 4	Approach Character 5	Device Character 6	Qualifier Character 7
Ø Lumbar Vertebral Joint Lumbar facet joint **3 Lumbosacral Joint** Lumbosacral facet joint	**Ø Open** **3 Percutaneous** **4 Percutaneous Endoscopic**	**3 Infusion Device** **4 Internal Fixation Device** **8 Spacer** **B Spinal Stabilization Device, Interspinous Process** **C Spinal Stabilization Device, Pedicle-Based** **D Spinal Stabilization Device, Facet Replacement**	**Z No Qualifier**
2 Lumbar Vertebral Disc **4 Lumbosacral Disc**	**Ø Open** **3 Percutaneous** **4 Percutaneous Endoscopic**	**3 Infusion Device** **8 Spacer**	**Z No Qualifier**
5 Sacrococcygeal Joint Sacrococcygeal symphysis **6 Coccygeal Joint** **7 Sacroiliac Joint, Right** **8 Sacroiliac Joint, Left**	**Ø Open** **3 Percutaneous** **4 Percutaneous Endoscopic**	**3 Infusion Device** **4 Internal Fixation Device** **8 Spacer**	**Z No Qualifier**
9 Hip Joint, Right Acetabulofemoral joint **B Hip Joint, Left** *See 9 Hip Joint, Right* **C Knee Joint, Right** Femoropatellar joint Femorotibial joint Lateral meniscus Medial meniscus Patellofemoral joint Tibiofemoral joint **D Knee Joint, Left** *See C Knee Joint, Right* **F Ankle Joint, Right** Inferior tibiofibular joint Talocrural joint **G Ankle Joint, Left** *See F Ankle Joint, Right* **H Tarsal Joint, Right** Calcaneocuboid joint Cuboideonavicular joint Cuneonavicular joint Intercuneiform joint Subtalar (talocalcaneal) joint Talocalcaneal (subtalar) joint Talocalcaneonavicular joint **J Tarsal Joint, Left** *See H Tarsal Joint, Right* **K Tarsometatarsal Joint, Right** **L Tarsometatarsal Joint, Left** **M Metatarsal-Phalangeal Joint, Right** Metatarsophalangeal (MTP) joint **N Metatarsal-Phalangeal Joint, Left** *See M Metatarsal-Phalangeal Joint, Right* **P Toe Phalangeal Joint, Right** Interphalangeal (IP) joint **Q Toe Phalangeal Joint, Left** *See P Toe Phalangeal Joint, Right*	**Ø Open** **3 Percutaneous** **4 Percutaneous Endoscopic**	**3 Infusion Device** **4 Internal Fixation Device** **5 External Fixation Device** **8 Spacer**	**Z No Qualifier**

Non-OR ØSH[Ø,3][Ø,3,4][3,8]Z
Non-OR ØSH[2,4][Ø,3,4][3,8]Z
Non-OR ØSH[5,6,7,8][Ø,3,4][3,8]Z
Non-OR ØSH[9,B,C,D][Ø,3,4]3Z
Non-OR ØSH[9,B,C,D][3,4]8Z
Non-OR ØSH[F,G,H,J,K,L,M,N,P,Q][Ø,3,4][3,8]Z

Ø Medical and Surgical
S Lower Joints
J Inspection Definition: Visually and/or manually exploring a body part

Explanation: Visual exploration may be performed with or without optical instrumentation. Manual exploration may be performed directly or through intervening body layers.

Body Part Character 4		Approach Character 5	Device Character 6	Qualifier Character 7
Ø Lumbar Vertebral Joint Lumbar facet joint 2 Lumbar Vertebral Disc 3 Lumbosacral Joint Lumbosacral facet joint 4 Lumbosacral Disc 5 Sacrococcygeal Joint Sacrococcygeal symphysis 6 Coccygeal Joint 7 Sacroiliac Joint, Right 8 Sacroiliac Joint, Left 9 Hip Joint, Right Acetabulofemoral joint B Hip Joint, Left *See 9 Hip Joint, Right* C Knee Joint, Right Femoropatellar joint Femorotibial joint Lateral meniscus Medial meniscus Patellofemoral joint Tibiofemoral joint D Knee Joint, Left *See C Knee Joint, Right* F Ankle Joint, Right Inferior tibiofibular joint Talocrural joint G Ankle Joint, Left *See F Ankle Joint, Right*	H Tarsal Joint, Right Calcaneocuboid joint Cuboideonavicular joint Cuneonavicular joint Intercuneiform joint Subtalar (talocalcaneal) joint Talocalcaneal (subtalar) joint Talocalcaneonavicular joint J Tarsal Joint, Left *See H Tarsal Joint, Right* K Tarsometatarsal Joint, Right L Tarsometatarsal Joint, Left M Metatarsal-Phalangeal Joint, Right Metatarsophalangeal (MTP) joint N Metatarsal-Phalangeal Joint, Left *See M Metatarsal-Phalangeal Joint, Right* P Toe Phalangeal Joint, Right Interphalangeal (IP) joint Q Toe Phalangeal Joint, Left *See P Toe Phalangeal Joint, Right*	Ø Open 3 Percutaneous 4 Percutaneous Endoscopic X External	Z No Device	Z No Qualifier

Non-OR ØSJ[Ø,2,3,4,5,6,7,8,9,B,C,D,F,G,H,J,K,L,M,N,P,Q][3,X]ZZ

Ø Medical and Surgical
S Lower Joints
N Release Definition: Freeing a body part from an abnormal physical constraint by cutting or by the use of force

Explanation: Some of the restraining tissue may be taken out but none of the body part is taken out

Body Part Character 4		Approach Character 5	Device Character 6	Qualifier Character 7
Ø Lumbar Vertebral Joint Lumbar facet joint 2 Lumbar Vertebral Disc 3 Lumbosacral Joint Lumbosacral facet joint 4 Lumbosacral Disc 5 Sacrococcygeal Joint Sacrococcygeal symphysis 6 Coccygeal Joint 7 Sacroiliac Joint, Right 8 Sacroiliac Joint, Left 9 Hip Joint, Right Acetabulofemoral joint B Hip Joint, Left *See 9 Hip Joint, Right* C Knee Joint, Right Femoropatellar joint Femorotibial joint Lateral meniscus Medial meniscus Patellofemoral joint Tibiofemoral joint D Knee Joint, Left *See C Knee Joint, Right* F Ankle Joint, Right Inferior tibiofibular joint Talocrural joint G Ankle Joint, Left *See F Ankle Joint, Right*	H Tarsal Joint, Right Calcaneocuboid joint Cuboideonavicular joint Cuneonavicular joint Intercuneiform joint Subtalar (talocalcaneal) joint Talocalcaneal (subtalar) joint Talocalcaneonavicular joint J Tarsal Joint, Left *See H Tarsal Joint, Right* K Tarsometatarsal Joint, Right L Tarsometatarsal Joint, Left M Metatarsal-Phalangeal Joint, Right Metatarsophalangeal (MTP) joint N Metatarsal-Phalangeal Joint, Left *See M Metatarsal-Phalangeal Joint, Right* P Toe Phalangeal Joint, Right Interphalangeal (IP) joint Q Toe Phalangeal Joint, Left *See P Toe Phalangeal Joint, Right*	Ø Open 3 Percutaneous 4 Percutaneous Endoscopic X External	Z No Device	Z No Qualifier

Non-OR ØSN[Ø,2,3,4,5,6,7,8,9,B,C,D,F,G,H,J,K,L,M,N,P,Q]XZZ

Ø Medical and Surgical
S Lower Joints
P Removal

Definition: Taking out or off a device from a body part

Explanation: If a device is taken out and a similar device put in without cutting or puncturing the skin or mucous membrane, the procedure is coded to the root operation CHANGE. Otherwise, the procedure for taking out the device is coded to the root operation REMOVAL.

Body Part Character 4	Approach Character 5	Device Character 6	Qualifier Character 7
Ø Lumbar Vertebral Joint Lumbar facet joint **3 Lumbosacral Joint** Lumbosacral facet joint	**Ø Open** **3 Percutaneous** **4 Percutaneous Endoscopic**	**Ø Drainage Device** **3 Infusion Device** **4 Internal Fixation Device** **7 Autologous Tissue Substitute** **8 Spacer** **A Interbody Fusion Device** **J Synthetic Substitute** **K Nonautologous Tissue Substitute**	**Z No Qualifier**
Ø Lumbar Vertebral Joint Lumbar facet joint **3 Lumbosacral Joint** Lumbosacral facet joint	**X External**	**Ø Drainage Device** **3 Infusion Device** **4 Internal Fixation Device**	**Z No Qualifier**
2 Lumbar Vertebral Disc **4 Lumbosacral Disc**	**Ø Open** **3 Percutaneous** **4 Percutaneous Endoscopic**	**Ø Drainage Device** **3 Infusion Device** **7 Autologous Tissue Substitute** **J Synthetic Substitute** **K Nonautologous Tissue Substitute**	**Z No Qualifier**
2 Lumbar Vertebral Disc **4 Lumbosacral Disc**	**X External**	**Ø Drainage Device** **3 Infusion Device**	**Z No Qualifier**
5 Sacrococcygeal Joint Sacrococcygeal symphysis **6 Coccygeal Joint** **7 Sacroiliac Joint, Right** **8 Sacroiliac Joint, Left**	**Ø Open** **3 Percutaneous** **4 Percutaneous Endoscopic**	**Ø Drainage Device** **3 Infusion Device** **4 Internal Fixation Device** **7 Autologous Tissue Substitute** **8 Spacer** **J Synthetic Substitute** **K Nonautologous Tissue Substitute**	**Z No Qualifier**
5 Sacrococcygeal Joint Sacrococcygeal symphysis **6 Coccygeal Joint** **7 Sacroiliac Joint, Right** **8 Sacroiliac Joint, Left**	**X External**	**Ø Drainage Device** **3 Infusion Device** **4 Internal Fixation Device**	**Z No Qualifier**
9 Hip Joint, Right ⊞ Acetabulofemoral joint **B Hip Joint, Left** ⊞ *See 9 Hip Joint, Right*	**Ø Open**	**Ø Drainage Device** **3 Infusion Device** **4 Internal Fixation Device** **5 External Fixation Device** **7 Autologous Tissue Substitute** **8 Spacer** **9 Liner** **B Resurfacing Device** **E Articulating Spacer** **J Synthetic Substitute** **K Nonautologous Tissue Substitute**	**Z No Qualifier**
9 Hip Joint, Right ⊞ Acetabulofemoral joint **B Hip Joint, Left** ⊞ *See 9 Hip Joint, Right*	**3 Percutaneous** **4 Percutaneous Endoscopic**	**Ø Drainage Device** **3 Infusion Device** **4 Internal Fixation Device** **5 External Fixation Device** **7 Autologous Tissue Substitute** **8 Spacer** **J Synthetic Substitute** **K Nonautologous Tissue Substitute**	**Z No Qualifier**
9 Hip Joint, Right Acetabulofemoral joint **B Hip Joint, Left** *See 9 Hip Joint, Right*	**X External**	**Ø Drainage Device** **3 Infusion Device** **4 Internal Fixation Device** **5 External Fixation Device**	**Z No Qualifier**

Non-OR ØSP[Ø,3][Ø,3,4]8Z
Non-OR ØSP[Ø,3]3[Ø,3]Z
Non-OR ØSP[Ø,3]X[Ø,3,4]Z
Non-OR ØSP[2,4]3[Ø,3]Z
Non-OR ØSP[2,4]X[Ø,3]Z
Non-OR ØSP[5,6,7,8][Ø,3,4]8Z
Non-OR ØSP[5,6,7,8]3[Ø,3]Z
Non-OR ØSP[5,6,7,8]X[Ø,3,4]Z
Non-OR ØSP[9,B]3[Ø,3,8]Z
Non-OR ØSP[9,B]X[Ø,3,4,5]Z

See Appendix L for Procedure Combinations
Combo-only ØSP[9,B]48Z
⊞ ØSP[9,B]Ø[8,9,B,E,J]Z
⊞ ØSP[9,B]4JZ

ØSP Continued on next page

ØSP Continued

Ø Medical and Surgical
S Lower Joints
P Removal

Definition: Taking out or off a device from a body part

Explanation: If a device is taken out and a similar device put in without cutting or puncturing the skin or mucous membrane, the procedure is coded to the root operation CHANGE. Otherwise, the procedure for taking out the device is coded to the root operation REMOVAL.

Body Part Character 4	Approach Character 5	Device Character 6	Qualifier Character 7
A Hip Joint, Acetabular Surface, Right **E** Hip Joint, Acetabular Surface, Left **R** Hip Joint, Femoral Surface, Right **S** Hip Joint, Femoral Surface, Left **T** Knee Joint, Femoral Surface, Right Femoropatellar joint Patellofemoral joint **U** Knee Joint, Femoral Surface, Left *See T Knee Joint, Femoral Surface, Right* **V** Knee Joint, Tibial Surface, Right Femorotibial joint Tibiofemoral joint **W** Knee Joint, Tibial Surface, Left *See V Knee Joint, Tibial Surface, Right*	**Ø** Open **3** Percutaneous **4** Percutaneous Endoscopic	**J** Synthetic Substitute	**Z** No Qualifier
C Knee Joint, Right Femoropatellar joint Femorotibial joint Lateral meniscus Medial meniscus Patellofemoral joint Tibiofemoral joint **D** Knee Joint, Left *See C Knee Joint, Right*	**Ø** Open	**Ø** Drainage Device **3** Infusion Device **4** Internal Fixation Device **5** External Fixation Device **7** Autologous Tissue Substitute **8** Spacer **9** Liner **E** Articulating Spacer **K** Nonautologous Tissue Substitute **L** Synthetic Substitute, Unicondylar Medial **M** Synthetic Substitute, Unicondylar Lateral **N** Synthetic Substitute, Patellofemoral	**Z** No Qualifier
C Knee Joint, Right Femoropatellar joint Femorotibial joint Lateral meniscus Medial meniscus Patellofemoral joint Tibiofemoral joint **D** Knee Joint, Left *See C Knee Joint, Right*	**Ø** Open	**J** Synthetic Substitute	**C** Patellar Surface **Z** No Qualifier
C Knee Joint, Right Femoropatellar joint Femorotibial joint Lateral meniscus Medial meniscus Patellofemoral joint Tibiofemoral joint **D** Knee Joint, Left *See C Knee Joint, Right*	**3** Percutaneous **4** Percutaneous Endoscopic	**Ø** Drainage Device **3** Infusion Device **4** Internal Fixation Device **5** External Fixation Device **7** Autologous Tissue Substitute **8** Spacer **K** Nonautologous Tissue Substitute **L** Synthetic Substitute, Unicondylar Medial **M** Synthetic Substitute, Unicondylar Lateral **N** Synthetic Substitute, Patellofemoral	**Z** No Qualifier
C Knee Joint, Right Femoropatellar joint Femorotibial joint Lateral meniscus Medial meniscus Patellofemoral joint Tibiofemoral joint **D** Knee Joint, Left *See C Knee Joint, Right*	**3** Percutaneous **4** Percutaneous Endoscopic	**J** Synthetic Substitute	**C** Patellar Surface **Z** No Qualifier

Non-OR ØSP[C,D]3[Ø,3]Z

See Appendix L for Procedure Combinations

Combo-only ØSP[C,D][3,4]8Z

ØSP[A,E,R,S,T,U,V,W][Ø,4]JZ
ØSP[C,D]Ø[8,9,E,L,M,N]Z
ØSP[C,D]ØJ[C,Z]
ØSP[C,D]4[L,M,N]Z
ØSP[C,D]4J[C,Z]

ØSP Continued on next page

ØSP Continued

Ø Medical and Surgical
S Lower Joints
P Removal

Definition: Taking out or off a device from a body part

Explanation: If a device is taken out and a similar device put in without cutting or puncturing the skin or mucous membrane, the procedure is coded to the root operation CHANGE. Otherwise, the procedure for taking out the device is coded to the root operation REMOVAL.

Body Part Character 4	Approach Character 5	Device Character 6	Qualifier Character 7
C Knee Joint, Right Femoropatellar joint Femorotibial joint Lateral meniscus Medial meniscus Patellofemoral joint Tibiofemoral joint **D Knee Joint, Left** *See C Knee Joint, Right*	X External	Ø Drainage Device 3 Infusion Device 4 Internal Fixation Device 5 External Fixation Device	Z No Qualifier
F Ankle Joint, Right Inferior tibiofibular joint Talocrural joint **G Ankle Joint, Left** *See F Ankle Joint, Right* **H Tarsal Joint, Right** Calcaneocuboid joint Cuboideonavicular joint Cuneonavicular joint Intercuneiform joint Subtalar (talocalcaneal) joint Talocalcaneal (subtalar) joint Talocalcaneonavicular joint **J Tarsal Joint, Left** *See H Tarsal Joint, Right* **K Tarsometatarsal Joint, Right** **L Tarsometatarsal Joint, Left** **M Metatarsal-Phalangeal Joint, Right** Metatarsophalangeal (MTP) joint **N Metatarsal-Phalangeal Joint, Left** *See M Metatarsal-Phalangeal Joint, Right* **P Toe Phalangeal Joint, Right** Interphalangeal (IP) joint **Q Toe Phalangeal Joint, Left** *See P Toe Phalangeal Joint, Right*	Ø Open 3 Percutaneous 4 Percutaneous Endoscopic	Ø Drainage Device 3 Infusion Device 4 Internal Fixation Device 5 External Fixation Device 7 Autologous Tissue Substitute 8 Spacer J Synthetic Substitute K Nonautologous Tissue Substitute	Z No Qualifier
F Ankle Joint, Right Inferior tibiofibular joint Talocrural joint **G Ankle Joint, Left** *See F Ankle Joint, Right* **H Tarsal Joint, Right** Calcaneocuboid joint Cuboideonavicular joint Cuneonavicular joint Intercuneiform joint Subtalar (talocalcaneal) joint Talocalcaneal (subtalar) joint Talocalcaneonavicular joint **J Tarsal Joint, Left** *See H Tarsal Joint, Right* **K Tarsometatarsal Joint, Right** **L Tarsometatarsal Joint, Left** **M Metatarsal-Phalangeal Joint, Right** Metatarsophalangeal (MTP) joint **N Metatarsal-Phalangeal Joint, Left** *See M Metatarsal-Phalangeal Joint, Right* **P Toe Phalangeal Joint, Right** Interphalangeal (IP) joint **Q Toe Phalangeal Joint, Left** *See P Toe Phalangeal Joint, Right*	X External	Ø Drainage Device 3 Infusion Device 4 Internal Fixation Device 5 External Fixation Device	Z No Qualifier

Non-OR ØSP[C,D]X[Ø,3,4,5]Z
Non-OR ØSP[F,G,H,J,K,L,M,N,P,Q]3[Ø,3,8]Z
Non-OR ØSP[F,G,H,J,K,L,M,N,P,Q][Ø,4]8Z
Non-OR ØSP[F,G,H,J,K,L,M,N,P,Q]X[Ø,3,4,5]Z

Ø Medical and Surgical
S Lower Joints
Q Repair Definition: Restoring, to the extent possible, a body part to its normal anatomic structure and function
Explanation: Used only when the method to accomplish the repair is not one of the other root operations

Body Part Character 4	Approach Character 5	Device Character 6	Qualifier Character 7
Ø Lumbar Vertebral Joint Lumbar facet joint **2 Lumbar Vertebral Disc** **3 Lumbosacral Joint** Lumbosacral facet joint **4 Lumbosacral Disc** **5 Sacrococcygeal Joint** Sacrococcygeal symphysis **6 Coccygeal Joint** **7 Sacroiliac Joint, Right** **8 Sacroiliac Joint, Left** **9 Hip Joint, Right** Acetabulofemoral joint **B Hip Joint, Left** *See 9 Hip Joint, Right* **C Knee Joint, Right** Femoropatellar joint Femorotibial joint Lateral meniscus Medial meniscus Patellofemoral joint Tibiofemoral joint **D Knee Joint, Left** *See C Knee Joint, Right* **F Ankle Joint, Right** Inferior tibiofibular joint Talocrural joint **G Ankle Joint, Left** *See F Ankle Joint, Right* **H Tarsal Joint, Right** Calcaneocuboid joint Cuboideonavicular joint Cuneonavicular joint Intercuneiform joint Subtalar (talocalcaneal) joint Talocalcaneal (subtalar) joint Talocalcaneonavicular joint **J Tarsal Joint, Left** *See H Tarsal Joint, Right* **K Tarsometatarsal Joint, Right** **L Tarsometatarsal Joint, Left** **M Metatarsal-Phalangeal Joint, Right** Metatarsophalangeal (MTP) joint **N Metatarsal-Phalangeal Joint, Left** *See M Metatarsal-Phalangeal Joint, Right* **P Toe Phalangeal Joint, Right** Interphalangeal (IP) joint **Q Toe Phalangeal Joint, Left** *See P Toe Phalangeal Joint, Right*	**Ø Open** **3 Percutaneous** **4 Percutaneous Endoscopic** **X External**	**Z No Device**	**Z No Qualifier**

Non-OR ØSQ[Ø,2,3,4,5,6,7,8,9,B,C,D,F,G,H,J,K,L,M,N,P,Q]XZZ

Ø Medical and Surgical
S Lower Joints
R Replacement

Definition: Putting in or on biological or synthetic material that physically takes the place and/or function of all or a portion of a body part

Explanation: The body part may have been taken out or replaced, or may be taken out, physically eradicated, or rendered nonfunctional during the REPLACEMENT procedure. A REMOVAL procedure is coded for taking out the device used in a previous replacement procedure.

Body Part Character 4	Approach Character 5	Device Character 6	Qualifier Character 7
Ø Lumbar Vertebral Joint Lumbar facet joint **2 Lumbar Vertebral Disc** NC **3 Lumbosacral Joint** Lumbosacral facet joint **4 Lumbosacral Disc** NC **5 Sacrococcygeal Joint** Sacrococcygeal symphysis **6 Coccygeal Joint** **7 Sacroiliac Joint, Right** **8 Sacroiliac Joint, Left** **H Tarsal Joint, Right** Calcaneocuboid joint Cuboideonavicular joint Cuneonavicular joint Intercuneiform joint Subtalar (talocalcaneal) joint Talocalcaneal (subtalar) joint Talocalcaneonavicular joint **J Tarsal Joint, Left** *See H Tarsal Joint, Right* **K Tarsometatarsal Joint, Right** **L Tarsometatarsal Joint, Left** **M Metatarsal-Phalangeal Joint, Right** Metatarsophalangeal (MTP) joint **N Metatarsal-Phalangeal Joint, Left** *See M Metatarsal-Phalangeal Joint, Right* **P Toe Phalangeal Joint, Right** Interphalangeal (IP) joint **Q Toe Phalangeal Joint, Left** *See P Toe Phalangeal Joint, Right*	**Ø Open**	**7 Autologous Tissue Substitute** **J Synthetic Substitute** **K Nonautologous Tissue Substitute**	**Z No Qualifier**
9 Hip Joint, Right ⊞ Acetabulofemoral joint **B Hip Joint, Left** ⊞ *See 9 Hip Joint, Right*	**Ø Open**	**1 Synthetic Substitute, Metal** **2 Synthetic Substitute, Metal on Polyethylene** **3 Synthetic Substitute, Ceramic** **4 Synthetic Substitute, Ceramic on Polyethylene** **6 Synthetic Substitute, Oxidized Zirconium on Polyethylene** **J Synthetic Substitute**	**9 Cemented** **A Uncemented** **Z No Qualifier**
9 Hip Joint, Right ⊞ Acetabulofemoral joint **B Hip Joint, Left** ⊞ *See 9 Hip Joint, Right*	**Ø Open**	**7 Autologous Tissue Substitute** **E Articulating Spacer** **K Nonautologous Tissue Substitute**	**Z No Qualifier**
A Hip Joint, Acetabular Surface, Right ⊞ **E Hip Joint, Acetabular Surface, Left** ⊞	**Ø Open**	**Ø Synthetic Substitute, Polyethylene** **1 Synthetic Substitute, Metal** **3 Synthetic Substitute, Ceramic** **J Synthetic Substitute**	**9 Cemented** **A Uncemented** **Z No Qualifier**
A Hip Joint, Acetabular Surface, Right **E Hip Joint, Acetabular Surface, Left**	**Ø Open**	**7 Autologous Tissue Substitute** **K Nonautologous Tissue Substitute**	**Z No Qualifier**

HAC ØSR[9,B]Ø[1,2,3,4,6,J][9,A,Z] when reported with SDx of I26.Ø2-I26.Ø9, I26.92-I26.99, or I82.4Ø1-I82.4Z9

HAC ØSR[9,B]Ø[7,E,K]Z when reported with SDx of I26.Ø2-I26.Ø9, I26.92-I26.99, or I82.4Ø1-I82.4Z9

HAC ØSR[A,E]Ø[Ø,1,3,J][9,A,Z] when reported with SDx of I26.Ø2-I26.Ø9, I26.92-I26.99, or I82.4Ø1-I82.4Z9

HAC ØSR[A,E]Ø[7,K]Z when reported with SDx of I26.Ø2-I26.Ø9, I26.92-I26.99, or I82.4Ø1-I82.4Z9

NC ØSR[2,4]ØJZ when beneficiary age is over 6Ø

See Appendix L for Procedure Combinations

⊞ ØSR[9,B]Ø[1,2,3,4,6,J][9,A,Z]
⊞ ØSR[9,B]ØEZ
⊞ ØSR[A,E]Ø[Ø,1,3,J][9,A,Z]

ØSR Continued on next page

Ø Medical and Surgical
S Lower Joints
R Replacement

ØSR Continued

Definition: Putting in or on biological or synthetic material that physically takes the place and/or function of all or a portion of a body part

Explanation: The body part may have been taken out or replaced, or may be taken out, physically eradicated, or rendered nonfunctional during the REPLACEMENT procedure. A REMOVAL procedure is coded for taking out the device used in a previous replacement procedure.

Body Part Character 4	Approach Character 5	Device Character 6	Qualifier Character 7
C Knee Joint, Right ⊞ Femoropatellar joint Femorotibial joint Lateral meniscus Medial meniscus Patellofemoral joint Tibiofemoral joint **D Knee Joint, Left** ⊞ *See C Knee Joint, Right*	**Ø Open**	**6 Synthetic Substitute, Oxidized Zirconium on Polyethylene** **J Synthetic Substitute** **L Synthetic Substitute, Unicondylar Medial** **M Synthetic Substitute, Unicondylar Lateral** **N Synthetic Substitute, Patellofemoral**	**9 Cemented** **A Uncemented** **Z No Qualifier**
C Knee Joint, Right ⊞ Femoropatellar joint Femorotibial joint Lateral meniscus Medial meniscus Patellofemoral joint Tibiofemoral joint **D Knee Joint, Left** ⊞ *See C Knee Joint, Right*	**Ø Open**	**7 Autologous Tissue Substitute** **E Articulating Spacer** **K Nonautologous Tissue Substitute**	**Z No Qualifier**
F Ankle Joint, Right Inferior tibiofibular joint Talocrural joint **G Ankle Joint, Left** *See F Ankle Joint, Right* **T Knee Joint, Femoral Surface, Right** Femoropatellar joint Patellofemoral joint **U Knee Joint, Femoral Surface, Left** *See T Knee Joint, Femoral Surface, Right* **V Knee Joint, Tibial Surface, Right** Femorotibial joint Tibiofemoral joint **W Knee Joint, Tibial Surface, Left** *See V Knee Joint, Tibial Surface, Right*	**Ø Open**	**7 Autologous Tissue Substitute** **K Nonautologous Tissue Substitute**	**Z No Qualifier**
F Ankle Joint, Right Inferior tibiofibular joint Talocrural joint **G Ankle Joint, Left** *See F Ankle Joint, Right* **T Knee Joint, Femoral Surface, Right** ⊞ Femoropatellar joint Patellofemoral joint **U Knee Joint, Femoral Surface, Left** ⊞ *See T Knee Joint, Femoral Surface, Right* **V Knee Joint, Tibial Surface, Right** ⊞ Femorotibial joint Tibiofemoral joint **W Knee Joint, Tibial Surface, Left** ⊞ *See V Knee Joint, Tibial Surface, Right*	**Ø Open**	**J Synthetic Substitute**	**9 Cemented** **A Uncemented** **Z No Qualifier**
R Hip Joint, Femoral Surface, Right ⊞ **S Hip Joint, Femoral Surface, Left** ⊞	**Ø Open**	**1 Synthetic Substitute, Metal** **3 Synthetic Substitute, Ceramic** **J Synthetic Substitute**	**9 Cemented** **A Uncemented** **Z No Qualifier**
R Hip Joint, Femoral Surface, Right **S Hip Joint, Femoral Surface, Left**	**Ø Open**	**7 Autologous Tissue Substitute** **K Nonautologous Tissue Substitute**	**Z No Qualifier**

HAC ØSR[C,D]Ø[6,J,L,M,N][9,A,Z] when reported with SDx of I26.Ø2-I26.Ø9, I26.92-I26.99 or I82.4Ø1-I82.4Z9

HAC ØSR[C,D]Ø[7,E,K]Z when reported with SDx of I26.Ø2-I26.Ø9, I26.92-I26.99 or I82.4Ø1-I82.4Z9

HAC ØSR[T,U,V,W]Ø[7,K]Z when reported with SDx of I26.Ø2-I26.Ø9, I26.92-I26.99 or I82.4Ø1-I82.4Z9

HAC ØSR[T,U,V,W]ØJ[9,A,Z] when reported with SDx of I26.Ø2-I26.Ø9, I26.92-I26.99 or I82.4Ø1-I82.4Z9

HAC ØSR[R,S]Ø[1,3,J][9,A,Z] when reported with SDx of I26.Ø2-I26.Ø9, I26.92-I26.99, or I82.4Ø1-I82.4Z9

HAC ØSR[R,S]Ø[7,K]Z when reported with SDx of I26.Ø2-I26.Ø9, I26.92-I26.99, or I82.4Ø1-I82.4Z9

See Appendix L for Procedure Combinations

⊞ ØSR[C,D]Ø[6,J,L,M,N][9,A,Z]
⊞ ØSR[C,D]ØEZ
⊞ ØSR[T,U,V,W]ØJ[9,A,Z]
⊞ ØSR[R,S]Ø[1,3,J][9,A,Z]

Ø Medical and Surgical
S Lower Joints
S Reposition

Definition: Moving to its normal location, or other suitable location, all or a portion of a body part

Explanation: The body part is moved to a new location from an abnormal location, or from a normal location where it is not functioning correctly. The body part may or may not be cut out or off to be moved to the new location.

Body Part Character 4	Approach Character 5	Device Character 6	Qualifier Character 7
Ø Lumbar Vertebral Joint Lumbar facet joint **3 Lumbosacral Joint** Lumbosacral facet joint **5 Sacrococcygeal Joint** Sacrococcygeal symphysis **6 Coccygeal Joint** **7 Sacroiliac Joint, Right** **8 Sacroiliac Joint, Left**	**Ø Open** **3 Percutaneous** **4 Percutaneous Endoscopic** **X External**	**4 Internal Fixation Device** **Z No Device**	**Z No Qualifier**
9 Hip Joint, Right Acetabulofemoral joint **B Hip Joint, Left** *See 9 Hip Joint, Right* **C Knee Joint, Right** Femoropatellar joint Femorotibial joint Lateral meniscus Medial meniscus Patellofemoral joint Tibiofemoral joint **D Knee Joint, Left** *See C Knee Joint, Right* **F Ankle Joint, Right** Inferior tibiofibular joint Talocrural joint **G Ankle Joint, Left** *See F Ankle Joint, Right* **H Tarsal Joint, Right** Calcaneocuboid joint Cuboideonavicular joint Cuneonavicular joint Intercuneiform joint Subtalar (talocalcaneal) joint Talocalcaneal (subtalar) joint Talocalcaneonavicular joint **J Tarsal Joint, Left** *See H Tarsal Joint, Right* **K Tarsometatarsal Joint, Right** **L Tarsometatarsal Joint, Left** **M Metatarsal-Phalangeal Joint, Right** Metatarsophalangeal (MTP) joint **N Metatarsal-Phalangeal Joint, Left** *See M Metatarsal-Phalangeal Joint, Right* **P Toe Phalangeal Joint, Right** Interphalangeal (IP) joint **Q Toe Phalangeal Joint, Left** *See P Toe Phalangeal Joint, Right*	**Ø Open** **3 Percutaneous** **4 Percutaneous Endoscopic** **X External**	**4 Internal Fixation Device** **5 External Fixation Device** **Z No Device**	**Z No Qualifier**

Non-OR ØSS[Ø,3,5,6,][3,4,X][4,Z]Z
Non-OR ØSS[7,8]3ZZ
Non-OR ØSS[7,8][4,X][4,Z]Z
Non-OR ØSS[9,B]3ZZ
Non-OR ØSS[9,B][3,4,X]5Z
Non-OR ØSS[9,B][4,X][4,Z]Z
Non-OR ØSS[C,D,F,G,H,J,K,L,M,N,P,Q][3,4,X][4,5,Z]Z

Ø Medical and Surgical
S Lower Joints
T Resection Definition: Cutting out or off, without replacement, all of a body part

Explanation: None

Body Part Character 4	Approach Character 5	Device Character 6	Qualifier Character 7
2 Lumbar Vertebral Disc **4 Lumbosacral Disc** **5 Sacrococcygeal Joint** Sacrococcygeal symphysis **6 Coccygeal Joint** **7 Sacroiliac Joint, Right** **8 Sacroiliac Joint, Left** **9 Hip Joint, Right** Acetabulofemoral joint **B Hip Joint, Left** *See 9 Hip Joint, Right* **C Knee Joint, Right** Femoropatellar joint Femorotibial joint Lateral meniscus Medial meniscus Patellofemoral joint Tibiofemoral joint **D Knee Joint, Left** *See C Knee Joint, Right* **F Ankle Joint, Right** Inferior tibiofibular joint Talocrural joint **G Ankle Joint, Left** *See F Ankle Joint, Right* **H Tarsal Joint, Right** Calcaneocuboid joint Cuboideonavicular joint Cuneonavicular joint Intercuneiform joint Subtalar (talocalcaneal) joint Talocalcaneal (subtalar) joint Talocalcaneonavicular joint **J Tarsal Joint, Left** *See H Tarsal Joint, Right* **K Tarsometatarsal Joint, Right** **L Tarsometatarsal Joint, Left** **M Metatarsal-Phalangeal Joint, Right** Metatarsophalangeal (MTP) joint **N Metatarsal-Phalangeal Joint, Left** *See M Metatarsal-Phalangeal Joint, Right* **P Toe Phalangeal Joint, Right** Interphalangeal (IP) joint **Q Toe Phalangeal Joint, Left** *See P Toe Phalangeal Joint, Right*	**Ø Open**	**Z No Device**	**Z No Qualifier**

Ø Medical and Surgical
S Lower Joints
U Supplement

Definition: Putting in or on biological or synthetic material that physically reinforces and/or augments the function of a portion of a body part

Explanation: The biological material is non-living, or is living and from the same individual. The body part may have been previously replaced, and the SUPPLEMENT procedure is performed to physically reinforce and/or augment the function of the replaced body part.

Body Part Character 4	Approach Character 5	Device Character 6	Qualifier Character 7
Ø Lumbar Vertebral Joint Lumbar facet joint **2 Lumbar Vertebral Disc** **3 Lumbosacral Joint** Lumbosacral facet joint **4 Lumbosacral Disc** **5 Sacrococcygeal Joint** Sacrococcygeal symphysis **6 Coccygeal Joint** **7 Sacroiliac Joint, Right** **8 Sacroiliac Joint, Left** **F Ankle Joint, Right** Inferior tibiofibular joint Talocrural joint **G Ankle Joint, Left** *See F Ankle Joint, Right* **H Tarsal Joint, Right** Calcaneocuboid joint Cuboideonavicular joint Cuneonavicular joint Intercuneiform joint Subtalar (talocalcaneal) joint Talocalcaneal (subtalar) joint Talocalcaneonavicular joint **J Tarsal Joint, Left** *See H Tarsal Joint, Right* **K Tarsometatarsal Joint, Right** **L Tarsometatarsal Joint, Left** **M Metatarsal-Phalangeal Joint, Right** Metatarsophalangeal (MTP) joint **N Metatarsal-Phalangeal Joint, Left** *See M Metatarsal-Phalangeal Joint, Right* **P Toe Phalangeal Joint, Right** Interphalangeal (IP) joint **Q Toe Phalangeal Joint, Left** *See P Toe Phalangeal Joint, Right*	**Ø Open** **3 Percutaneous** **4 Percutaneous Endoscopic**	**7 Autologous Tissue Substitute** **J Synthetic Substitute** **K Nonautologous Tissue Substitute**	**Z No Qualifier**
9 Hip Joint, Right ⊞ Acetabulofemoral joint **B Hip Joint, Left** ⊞ *See 9 Hip Joint, Right*	**Ø Open**	**7 Autologous Tissue Substitute** **9 Liner** **B Resurfacing Device** **J Synthetic Substitute** **K Nonautologous Tissue Substitute**	**Z No Qualifier**
9 Hip Joint, Right Acetabulofemoral joint **B Hip Joint, Left** *See 9 Hip Joint, Right*	**3 Percutaneous** **4 Percutaneous Endoscopic**	**7 Autologous Tissue Substitute** **J Synthetic Substitute** **K Nonautologous Tissue Substitute**	**Z No Qualifier**
A Hip Joint, Acetabular Surface, Right ⊞ **E Hip Joint, Acetabular Surface, Left** ⊞ **R Hip Joint, Femoral Surface, Right** ⊞ **S Hip Joint, Femoral Surface, Left** ⊞	**Ø Open**	**9 Liner** **B Resurfacing Device**	**Z No Qualifier**
C Knee Joint, Right Femoropatellar joint Femorotibial joint Lateral meniscus Medial meniscus Patellofemoral joint Tibiofemoral joint **D Knee Joint, Left** *See C Knee Joint, Right*	**Ø Open**	**7 Autologous Tissue Substitute** **J Synthetic Substitute** **K Nonautologous Tissue Substitute**	**Z No Qualifier**
C Knee Joint, Right Femoropatellar joint Femorotibial joint Lateral meniscus Medial meniscus Patellofemoral joint Tibiofemoral joint **D Knee Joint, Left** *See C Knee Joint, Right*	**Ø Open**	**9 Liner**	**C Patellar Surface** **Z No Qualifier**

HAC ØSU[9,B]ØBZ when reported with SDx of I26.Ø2-I26.Ø9, I26.92-I26.99, or I82.4Ø1-I82.4Z9

HAC ØSU[A,E,R,S]ØBZ when reported with SDx of I26.Ø2-I26.Ø9, I26.92-I26.99, or I82.4Ø1-I82.4Z9

See Appendix L for Procedure Combinations
⊞ ØSU[9,B]Ø9Z
⊞ ØSU[A,E,R,S]Ø9Z

ØSU Continued on next page

Ø Medical and Surgical
S Lower Joints
U Supplement

ØSU Continued

Definition: Putting in or on biological or synthetic material that physically reinforces and/or augments the function of a portion of a body part

Explanation: The biological material is non-living, or is living and from the same individual. The body part may have been previously replaced, and the SUPPLEMENT procedure is performed to physically reinforce and/or augment the function of the replaced body part.

Body Part Character 4	Approach Character 5	Device Character 6	Qualifier Character 7
C Knee Joint, Right Femoropatellar joint Femorotibial joint Lateral meniscus Medial meniscus Patellofemoral joint Tibiofemoral joint **D Knee Joint, Left** ***See*** *C Knee Joint, Right*	**3 Percutaneous** **4 Percutaneous Endoscopic**	**7 Autologous Tissue Substitute** **J Synthetic Substitute** **K Nonautologous Tissue Substitute**	**Z No Qualifier**
T Knee Joint, Femoral Surface, Right Femoropatellar joint Patellofemoral joint **U Knee Joint, Femoral Surface, Left** ***See*** *T Knee Joint, Femoral Surface, Right* **V Knee Joint, Tibial Surface, Right** ⊞ Femorotibial joint Tibiofemoral joint **W Knee Joint, Tibial Surface, Left** ⊞ ***See*** *V Knee Joint, Tibial Surface, Right*	**Ø Open**	**9 Liner**	**Z No Qualifier**

See Appendix L for Procedure Combinations
⊞ ØSU[V,W]Ø9Z

Ø Medical and Surgical
S Lower Joints
W Revision

Definition: Correcting, to the extent possible, a portion of a malfunctioning device or the position of a displaced device

Explanation: Revision can include correcting a malfunctioning or displaced device by taking out or putting in components of the device such as a screw or pin

Body Part Character 4	Approach Character 5	Device Character 6	Qualifier Character 7
Ø Lumbar Vertebral Joint Lumbar facet joint 3 Lumbosacral Joint Lumbosacral facet joint	Ø Open 3 Percutaneous 4 Percutaneous Endoscopic X External	Ø Drainage Device 3 Infusion Device 4 Internal Fixation Device 7 Autologous Tissue Substitute 8 Spacer A Interbody Fusion Device J Synthetic Substitute K Nonautologous Tissue Substitute	Z No Qualifier
2 Lumbar Vertebral Disc 4 Lumbosacral Disc	Ø Open 3 Percutaneous 4 Percutaneous Endoscopic X External	Ø Drainage Device 3 Infusion Device 7 Autologous Tissue Substitute J Synthetic Substitute K Nonautologous Tissue Substitute	Z No Qualifier
5 Sacrococcygeal Joint Sacrococcygeal symphysis 6 Coccygeal Joint 7 Sacroiliac Joint, Right 8 Sacroiliac Joint, Left	Ø Open 3 Percutaneous 4 Percutaneous Endoscopic X External	Ø Drainage Device 3 Infusion Device 4 Internal Fixation Device 7 Autologous Tissue Substitute 8 Spacer J Synthetic Substitute K Nonautologous Tissue Substitute	Z No Qualifier
9 Hip Joint, Right Acetabulofemoral joint B Hip Joint, Left *See 9 Hip Joint, Right*	Ø Open	Ø Drainage Device 3 Infusion Device 4 Internal Fixation Device 5 External Fixation Device 7 Autologous Tissue Substitute 8 Spacer 9 Liner B Resurfacing Device J Synthetic Substitute K Nonautologous Tissue Substitute	Z No Qualifier
9 Hip Joint, Right Acetabulofemoral joint B Hip Joint, Left *See 9 Hip Joint, Right*	3 Percutaneous 4 Percutaneous Endoscopic X External	Ø Drainage Device 3 Infusion Device 4 Internal Fixation Device 5 External Fixation Device 7 Autologous Tissue Substitute 8 Spacer J Synthetic Substitute K Nonautologous Tissue Substitute	Z No Qualifier
A Hip Joint, Acetabular Surface, Right E Hip Joint, Acetabular Surface, Left R Hip Joint, Femoral Surface, Right S Hip Joint, Femoral Surface, Left T Knee Joint, Femoral Surface, Right Femoropatellar joint Patellofemoral joint U Knee Joint, Femoral Surface, Left *See T Knee Joint, Femoral Surface, Right* V Knee Joint, Tibial Surface, Right Femorotibial joint Tibiofemoral joint W Knee Joint, Tibial Surface, Left *See V Knee Joint, Tibial Surface, Right*	Ø Open 3 Percutaneous 4 Percutaneous Endoscopic X External	J Synthetic Substitute	Z No Qualifier
C Knee Joint, Right Femoropatellar joint Femorotibial joint Lateral meniscus Medial meniscus Patellofemoral joint Tibiofemoral joint D Knee Joint, Left *See C Knee Joint, Right*	Ø Open	Ø Drainage Device 3 Infusion Device 4 Internal Fixation Device 5 External Fixation Device 7 Autologous Tissue Substitute 8 Spacer 9 Liner K Nonautologous Tissue Substitute	Z No Qualifier

Non-OR ØSW[Ø,3]X[Ø,3,4,7,8,A,J,K]Z
Non-OR ØSW[2,4]X[Ø,3,7,J,K]Z
Non-OR ØSW[5,6,7,8]X[Ø,3,4,7,8,J,K]Z
Non-OR ØSW[9,B]X[Ø,3,4,5,7,8,J,K]Z
Non-OR ØSW[A,E,R,S,T,U,V,W]XJZ

ØSW Continued on next page

Ø Medical and Surgical
S Lower Joints
W Revision

ØSW Continued

Definition: Correcting, to the extent possible, a portion of a malfunctioning device or the position of a displaced device

Explanation: Revision can include correcting a malfunctioning or displaced device by taking out or putting in components of the device such as a screw or pin

Body Part Character 4	Approach Character 5	Device Character 6	Qualifier Character 7
C Knee Joint, Right Femoropatellar joint Femorotibial joint Lateral meniscus Medial meniscus Patellofemoral joint Tibiofemoral joint **D Knee Joint, Left** *See C Knee Joint, Right*	**Ø Open**	**J Synthetic Substitute**	**C Patellar Surface** **Z No Qualifier**
C Knee Joint, Right Femoropatellar joint Femorotibial joint Lateral meniscus Medial meniscus Patellofemoral joint Tibiofemoral joint **D Knee Joint, Left** *See C Knee Joint, Right*	**3 Percutaneous** **4 Percutaneous Endoscopic** **X External**	**Ø Drainage Device** **3 Infusion Device** **4 Internal Fixation Device** **5 External Fixation Device** **7 Autologous Tissue Substitute** **8 Spacer** **K Nonautologous Tissue Substitute**	**Z No Qualifier**
C Knee Joint, Right Femoropatellar joint Femorotibial joint Lateral meniscus Medial meniscus Patellofemoral joint Tibiofemoral joint **D Knee Joint, Left** *See C Knee Joint, Right*	**3 Percutaneous** **4 Percutaneous Endoscopic** **X External**	**J Synthetic Substitute**	**C Patellar Surface** **Z No Qualifier**
F Ankle Joint, Right Inferior tibiofibular joint Talocrural joint **G Ankle Joint, Left** *See F Ankle Joint, Right* **H Tarsal Joint, Right** Calcaneocuboid joint Cuboideonavicular joint Cuneonavicular joint Intercuneiform joint Subtalar (talocalcaneal) joint Talocalcaneal (subtalar) joint Talocalcaneonavicular joint **J Tarsal Joint, Left** *See H Tarsal Joint, Right* **K Tarsometatarsal Joint, Right** **L Tarsometatarsal Joint, Left** **M Metatarsal-Phalangeal Joint, Right** Metatarsophalangeal (MTP) joint **N Metatarsal-Phalangeal Joint, Left** *See M Metatarsal-Phalangeal Joint, Right* **P Toe Phalangeal Joint, Right** Interphalangeal (IP) joint **Q Toe Phalangeal Joint, Left** *See P Toe Phalangeal Joint, Right*	**Ø Open** **3 Percutaneous** **4 Percutaneous Endoscopic** **X External**	**Ø Drainage Device** **3 Infusion Device** **4 Internal Fixation Device** **5 External Fixation Device** **7 Autologous Tissue Substitute** **8 Spacer** **J Synthetic Substitute** **K Nonautologous Tissue Substitute**	**Z No Qualifier**

Non-OR ØSW[C,D]X[Ø,3,4,5,7,8,K]Z
Non-OR ØSW[C,D]XJ[C,Z]
Non-OR ØSW[F,G,H,J,K,L,M,N,P,Q]X[Ø,3,4,5,7,8,J,K]Z

Urinary System ØT1–ØTY

Character Meanings

This Character Meaning table is provided as a guide to assist the user in the identification of character members that may be found in this section of code tables. It **SHOULD NOT** be used to build a PCS code.

Operation–Character 3		Body Part–Character 4		Approach–Character 5		Device–Character 6		Qualifier–Character 7	
1	Bypass	Ø	Kidney, Right	Ø	Open	Ø	Drainage Device	Ø	Allogeneic
2	Change	1	Kidney, Left	3	Percutaneous	1	Radioactive Element	1	Syngeneic
5	Destruction	2	Kidneys, Bilateral	4	Percutaneous Endoscopic	2	Monitoring Device	2	Zooplastic
7	Dilation	3	Kidney Pelvis, Right	7	Via Natural or Artificial Opening	3	Infusion Device	3	Kidney Pelvis, Right
8	Division	4	Kidney Pelvis, Left	8	Via Natural or Artificial Opening Endoscopic	7	Autologous Tissue Substitute	4	Kidney Pelvis, Left
9	Drainage	5	Kidney	X	External	C	Extraluminal Device	6	Ureter, Right
B	Excision	6	Ureter, Right			D	Intraluminal Device	7	Ureter, Left
C	Extirpation	7	Ureter, Left			J	Synthetic Substitute	8	Colon
D	Extraction	8	Ureters, Bilateral			K	Nonautologous Tissue Substitute	9	Colocutaneous
F	Fragmentation	9	Ureter			L	Artificial Sphincter	A	Ileum
H	Insertion	B	Bladder			M	Stimulator Lead	B	Bladder
J	Inspection	C	Bladder Neck			Y	Other Device	C	Ileocutaneous
L	Occlusion	D	Urethra			Z	No Device	D	Cutaneous
M	Reattachment							X	Diagnostic
N	Release							Z	No Qualifier
P	Removal								
Q	Repair								
R	Replacement								
S	Reposition								
T	Resection								
U	Supplement								
V	Restriction								
W	Revision								
Y	Transplantation								

AHA Coding Clinic for table ØT1
2017, 3Q, 20 Creation of Indiana pouch
2017, 3Q, 21 Augmentation cystoplasty with Indiana pouch and continent urinary diversion
2017, 1Q, 37 Perineal urethrostomy
2015, 3Q, 34 Redo urinary diversion surgery via left ureteral reimplantation

AHA Coding Clinic for table ØT7
2019, 2Q, 16 Reimplantation of ureters with insertion of tubes
2017, 4Q, 111 Exchange of ureteral stent
2016, 2Q, 27 Exchange of ureteral stents
2015, 2Q, 8 Urinary calculi fragmentation and evacuation
2013, 4Q, 123 Urolift® procedure

AHA Coding Clinic for table ØT9
2017, 3Q, 19 Ureteral stent placement for urinary leakage
2017, 3Q, 20 Creation of Indiana pouch
2017, 3Q, 21 Augmentation cystoplasty with Indiana pouch and continent urinary diversion

AHA Coding Clinic for table ØTB
2016, 1Q, 19 Biopsy of neobladder malignancy
2015, 3Q, 34 Excision of Mitrofanoff polyp
2014, 2Q, 8 Ileoscopy with excision of polyp of Ileal loop urinary diversion

AHA Coding Clinic for table ØTC
2019, 3Q, 4 Evacuation of clots from bladder dome
2016, 3Q, 23 Ureteral stone migrating into bladder
2015, 2Q, 7 Urinary calculi fragmentation and evacuation
2015, 2Q, 8 Urinary calculi fragmentation and evacuation
2013, 4Q, 122 Laser lithotripsy with removal of fragments

AHA Coding Clinic for table ØTF
2015, 2Q, 7 Urinary calculi fragmentation and evacuation
2013, 4Q, 122 Extracorporeal shock wave lithotripsy
2013, 4Q, 122 Laser lithotripsy with removal of fragments

AHA Coding Clinic for table ØTH
2020, 4Q, 43-44 Insertion of radioactive element
2019, 2Q, 16 Reimplantation of ureters with insertion of tubes

AHA Coding Clinic for table ØTP
2017, 4Q, 111 Exchange of ureteral stent
2016, 2Q, 27 Exchange of ureteral stents

AHA Coding Clinic for table ØTQ
2018, 2Q, 27 Dismembered pyeloplasty
2017, 1Q, 37 Perineal urethrostomy

AHA Coding Clinic for table ØTR
2017, 3Q, 20 Creation of Indiana pouch

AHA Coding Clinic for table ØTS
2019, 1Q, 29 Young-Dees-Leadbetter bladder neck reconstruction
2018, 2Q, 27 Dismembered pyeloplasty
2017, 1Q, 36 Dismembered pyeloplasty
2016, 1Q, 15 Pubovaginal sling placement

AHA Coding Clinic for table ØTT
2014, 3Q, 16 Hand-assisted laparoscopy nephroureterectomy

AHA Coding Clinic for table ØTU
2019, 1Q, 29 Young-Dees-Leadbetter bladder neck reconstruction
2017, 3Q, 21 Augmentation cystoplasty with Indiana pouch and continent urinary diversion

AHA Coding Clinic for table ØTV
2015, 2Q, 11 Cystourethroscopic Deflux® injection

AHA Coding Clinic for table ØTY
2023, 2Q, 32 Preparation of donor organ before transplantation

Urinary System

Urinary System

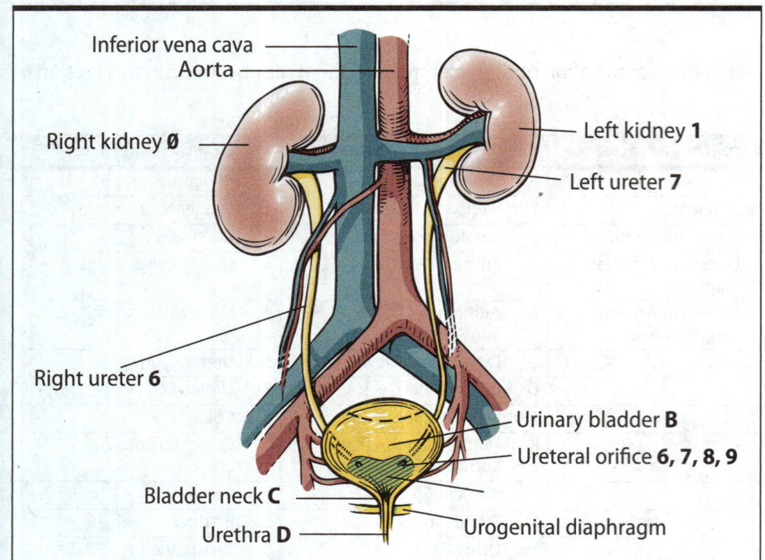

Kidney

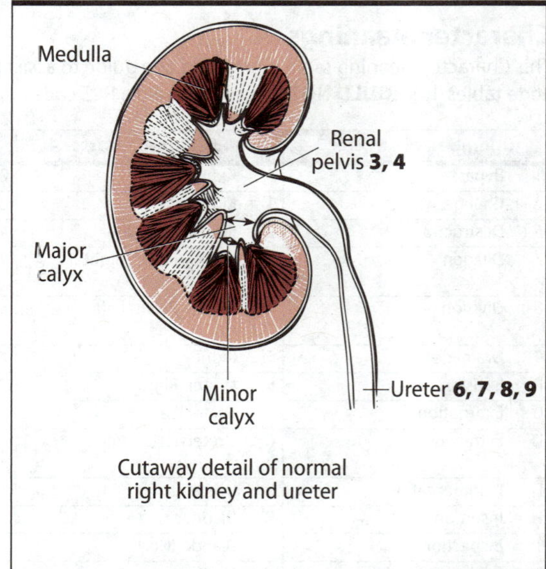

Cutaway detail of normal right kidney and ureter

Bladder

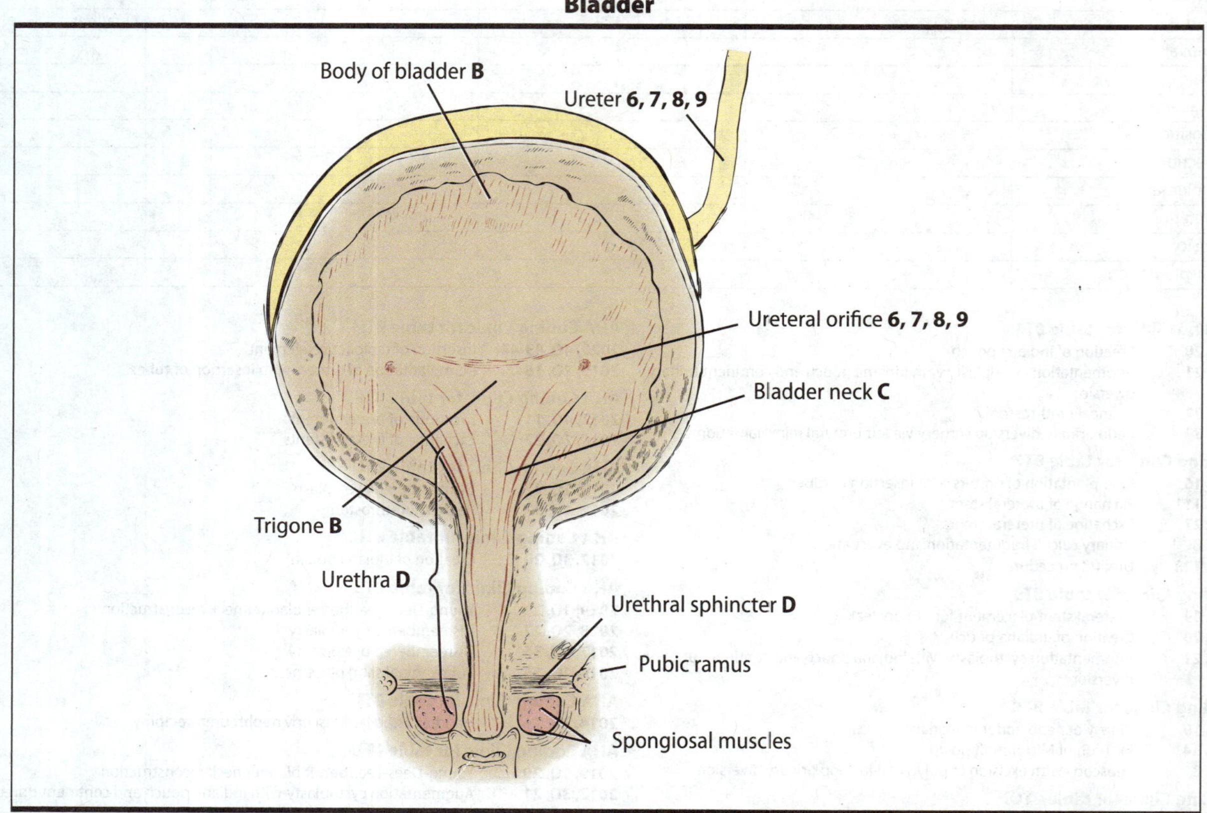

Ø Medical and Surgical
T Urinary System
1 Bypass Definition: Altering the route of passage of the contents of a tubular body part

Explanation: Rerouting contents of a body part to a downstream area of the normal route, to a similar route and body part, or to an abnormal route and dissimilar body part. Includes one or more anastomoses, with or without the use of a device.

Body Part Character 4	Approach Character 5	Device Character 6	Qualifier Character 7
3 Kidney Pelvis, Right Ureteropelvic junction (UPJ) **4 Kidney Pelvis, Left** *See 3 Kidney Pelvis, Right*	**Ø Open** **4 Percutaneous Endoscopic**	**7 Autologous Tissue Substitute** **J Synthetic Substitute** **K Nonautologous Tissue Substitute** **Z No Device**	**3 Kidney Pelvis, Right** **4 Kidney Pelvis, Left** **6 Ureter, Right** **7 Ureter, Left** **8 Colon** **9 Colocutaneous** **A Ileum** **B Bladder** **C Ileocutaneous** **D Cutaneous**
3 Kidney Pelvis, Right Ureteropelvic junction (UPJ) **4 Kidney Pelvis, Left** *See 3 Kidney Pelvis, Right*	**3 Percutaneous**	**J Synthetic Substitute**	**D Cutaneous**
6 Ureter, Right Ureteral orifice Ureterovesical orifice **7 Ureter, Left** *See 6 Ureter, Right* **8 Ureters, Bilateral** *See 6 Ureter, Right*	**Ø Open** **4 Percutaneous Endoscopic**	**7 Autologous Tissue Substitute** **J Synthetic Substitute** **K Nonautologous Tissue Substitute** **Z No Device**	**6 Ureter, Right** **7 Ureter, Left** **8 Colon** **9 Colocutaneous** **A Ileum** **B Bladder** **C Ileocutaneous** **D Cutaneous**
6 Ureter, Right Ureteral orifice Ureterovesical orifice **7 Ureter, Left** *See 6 Ureter, Right* **8 Ureters, Bilateral** *See 6 Ureter, Right*	**3 Percutaneous**	**J Synthetic Substitute**	**D Cutaneous**
B Bladder Trigone of bladder	**Ø Open** **4 Percutaneous Endoscopic**	**7 Autologous Tissue Substitute** **J Synthetic Substitute** **K Nonautologous Tissue Substitute** **Z No Device**	**9 Colocutaneous** **C Ileocutaneous** **D Cutaneous**
B Bladder Trigone of bladder	**3 Percutaneous**	**J Synthetic Substitute**	**D Cutaneous**

Ø Medical and Surgical
T Urinary System
2 Change Definition: Taking out or off a device from a body part and putting back an identical or similar device in or on the same body part without cutting or puncturing the skin or a mucous membrane

Explanation: All CHANGE procedures are coded using the approach EXTERNAL

Body Part Character 4	Approach Character 5	Device Character 6	Qualifier Character 7
5 Kidney Renal calyx Renal capsule Renal cortex Renal segment **9 Ureter** Ureteral orifice Ureterovesical orifice **B Bladder** Trigone of bladder **D Urethra** Bulbourethral (Cowper's) gland Cowper's (bulbourethral) gland External urethral sphincter Internal urethral sphincter Membranous urethra Penile urethra Prostatic urethra	**X External**	**Ø Drainage Device** **Y Other Device**	**Z No Qualifier**

Non-OR All body part, approach, device, and qualifier values

Ø Medical and Surgical
T Urinary System
5 Destruction

Definition: Physical eradication of all or a portion of a body part by the direct use of energy, force, or a destructive agent

Explanation: None of the body part is physically taken out

Body Part Character 4	Approach Character 5	Device Character 6	Qualifier Character 7
Ø Kidney, Right Renal calyx Renal capsule Renal cortex Renal segment **1 Kidney, Left** *See Ø Kidney, Right* **3 Kidney Pelvis, Right** Ureteropelvic junction (UPJ) **4 Kidney Pelvis, Left** *See 3 Kidney Pelvis, Right* **6 Ureter, Right** Ureteral orifice Ureterovesical orifice **7 Ureter, Left** *See 6 Ureter, Right* **B Bladder** Trigone of bladder **C Bladder Neck**	**Ø Open** **3 Percutaneous** **4 Percutaneous Endoscopic** **7 Via Natural or Artificial Opening** **8 Via Natural or Artificial Opening Endoscopic**	**Z No Device**	**Z No Qualifier**
D Urethra Bulbourethral (Cowper's) gland Cowper's (bulbourethral) gland External urethral sphincter Internal urethral sphincter Membranous urethra Penile urethra Prostatic urethra	**Ø Open** **3 Percutaneous** **4 Percutaneous Endoscopic** **7 Via Natural or Artificial Opening** **8 Via Natural or Artificial Opening Endoscopic** **X External**	**Z No Device**	**Z No Qualifier**

Non-OR ØT5D[Ø,3,4,7,8,X]ZZ

Ø Medical and Surgical
T Urinary System
7 Dilation

Definition: Expanding an orifice or the lumen of a tubular body part

Explanation: The orifice can be a natural orifice or an artificially created orifice. Accomplished by stretching a tubular body part using intraluminal pressure or by cutting part of the orifice or wall of the tubular body part.

Body Part Character 4	Approach Character 5	Device Character 6	Qualifier Character 7
3 Kidney Pelvis, Right Ureteropelvic junction (UPJ) **4 Kidney Pelvis, Left** *See 3 Kidney Pelvis, Right* **6 Ureter, Right** Ureteral orifice Ureterovesical orifice **7 Ureter, Left** *See 6 Ureter, Right* **8 Ureters, Bilateral** *See 6 Ureter, Right* **B Bladder** Trigone of bladder **C Bladder Neck** **D Urethra** Bulbourethral (Cowper's) gland Cowper's (bulbourethral) gland External urethral sphincter Internal urethral sphincter Membranous urethra Penile urethra Prostatic urethra	**Ø Open** **3 Percutaneous** **4 Percutaneous Endoscopic** **7 Via Natural or Artificial Opening** **8 Via Natural or Artificial Opening Endoscopic**	**D Intraluminal Device** **Z No Device**	**Z No Qualifier**

Non-OR ØT7[6,7,8][Ø,3,4,7]DZ
Non-OR ØT7[6,7,8]7ZZ
Non-OR ØT788ZZ
Non-OR ØT7B7[D,Z]Z
Non-OR ØT7C[Ø,3,4]ZZ
Non-OR ØT7[C,D][Ø,3,4]DZ
Non-OR ØT7[C,D][7,8][D,Z]Z

Ø Medical and Surgical
T Urinary System
8 Division

Definition: Cutting into a body part, without draining fluids and/or gases from the body part, in order to separate or transect a body part

Explanation: All or a portion of the body part is separated into two or more portions

Body Part Character 4	Approach Character 5	Device Character 6	Qualifier Character 7
2 Kidneys, Bilateral Renal calyx Renal capsule Renal cortex Renal segment **C Bladder Neck**	**Ø Open** **3 Percutaneous** **4 Percutaneous Endoscopic**	**Z No Device**	**Z No Qualifier**

Ø Medical and Surgical
T Urinary System
9 Drainage Definition: Taking or letting out fluids and/or gases from a body part
Explanation: The qualifier DIAGNOSTIC is used to identify drainage procedures that are biopsies

Body Part Character 4	Approach Character 5	Device Character 6	Qualifier Character 7
Ø Kidney, Right Renal calyx Renal capsule Renal cortex Renal segment **1 Kidney, Left** *See Ø Kidney, Right* **3 Kidney Pelvis, Right** Ureteropelvic junction (UPJ) **4 Kidney Pelvis, Left** *See 3 Kidney Pelvis, Right* **6 Ureter, Right** Ureteral orifice Ureterovesical orifice **7 Ureter, Left** *See 6 Ureter, Right* **8 Ureters, Bilateral** *See 6 Ureter, Right* **B Bladder** Trigone of bladder **C Bladder Neck**	**Ø Open** **3 Percutaneous** **4 Percutaneous Endoscopic** **7 Via Natural or Artificial Opening** **8 Via Natural or Artificial Opening Endoscopic**	**Ø Drainage Device**	**Z No Qualifier**
Ø Kidney, Right Renal calyx Renal capsule Renal cortex Renal segment **1 Kidney, Left** *See Ø Kidney, Right* **3 Kidney Pelvis, Right** Ureteropelvic junction (UPJ) **4 Kidney Pelvis, Left** *See 3 Kidney Pelvis, Right* **6 Ureter, Right** Ureteral orifice Ureterovesical orifice **7 Ureter, Left** *See 6 Ureter, Right* **8 Ureters, Bilateral** *See 6 Ureter, Right* **B Bladder** Trigone of bladder **C Bladder Neck**	**Ø Open** **3 Percutaneous** **4 Percutaneous Endoscopic** **7 Via Natural or Artificial Opening** **8 Via Natural or Artificial Opening Endoscopic**	**Z No Device**	**X Diagnostic** **Z No Qualifier**
D Urethra Bulbourethral (Cowper's) gland Cowper's (bulbourethral) gland External urethral sphincter Internal urethral sphincter Membranous urethra Penile urethra Prostatic urethra	**Ø Open** **3 Percutaneous** **4 Percutaneous Endoscopic** **7 Via Natural or Artificial Opening** **8 Via Natural or Artificial Opening Endoscopic** **X External**	**Ø Drainage Device**	**Z No Qualifier**
D Urethra Bulbourethral (Cowper's) gland Cowper's (bulbourethral) gland External urethral sphincter Internal urethral sphincter Membranous urethra Penile urethra Prostatic urethra	**Ø Open** **3 Percutaneous** **4 Percutaneous Endoscopic** **7 Via Natural or Artificial Opening** **8 Via Natural or Artificial Opening Endoscopic** **X External**	**Z No Device**	**X Diagnostic** **Z No Qualifier**

Non-OR ØT9[Ø,1,3,4]3ØZ
Non-OR ØT9[6,7,8][Ø,3,4,7,8]ØZ
Non-OR ØT9[B,C][3,4,7,8]ØZ
Non-OR ØT9[Ø,1,3,4,6,7,8][3,4,7,8]ZX
Non-OR ØT9[Ø,1,3,4][3,4]ZZ
Non-OR ØT9[6,7,8]3ZZ
Non-OR ØT9[B,C][3,4,7,8]ZZ
Non-OR ØT9D3ØZ
Non-OR ØT9D[Ø,3,4,7,8,X]ZX
Non-OR ØT9D3ZZ

Ø Medical and Surgical
T Urinary System
B Excision

Definition: Cutting out or off, without replacement, a portion of a body part

Explanation: The qualifier DIAGNOSTIC is used to identify excision procedures that are biopsies

Body Part Character 4	Approach Character 5	Device Character 6	Qualifier Character 7
Ø Kidney, Right Renal calyx Renal capsule Renal cortex Renal segment **1 Kidney, Left** *See Ø Kidney, Right* **3 Kidney Pelvis, Right** Ureteropelvic junction (UPJ) **4 Kidney Pelvis, Left** *See 3 Kidney Pelvis, Right* **6 Ureter, Right** Ureteral orifice Ureterovesical orifice **7 Ureter, Left** *See 6 Ureter, Right* **B Bladder** Trigone of bladder **C Bladder Neck**	**Ø Open** **3 Percutaneous** **4 Percutaneous Endoscopic** **7 Via Natural or Artificial Opening** **8 Via Natural or Artificial Opening Endoscopic**	**Z No Device**	**X Diagnostic** **Z No Qualifier**
D Urethra Bulbourethral (Cowper's) gland Cowper's (bulbourethral) gland External urethral sphincter Internal urethral sphincter Membranous urethra Penile urethra Prostatic urethra	**Ø Open** **3 Percutaneous** **4 Percutaneous Endoscopic** **7 Via Natural or Artificial Opening** **8 Via Natural or Artificial Opening Endoscopic** **X External**	**Z No Device**	**X Diagnostic** **Z No Qualifier**

Non-OR ØTB[Ø,1,3,4,6,7][3,4,7,8]ZX
Non-OR ØTBD[Ø,3,4,7,8,X]ZX

Ø Medical and Surgical
T Urinary System
C Extirpation

Definition: Taking or cutting out solid matter from a body part

Explanation: The solid matter may be an abnormal byproduct of a biological function or a foreign body; it may be imbedded in a body part or in the lumen of a tubular body part. The solid matter may or may not have been previously broken into pieces.

Body Part Character 4	Approach Character 5	Device Character 6	Qualifier Character 7
Ø Kidney, Right Renal calyx Renal capsule Renal cortex Renal segment **1 Kidney, Left** *See Ø Kidney, Right* **3 Kidney Pelvis, Right** Ureteropelvic junction (UPJ) **4 Kidney Pelvis, Left** *See 3 Kidney Pelvis, Right* **6 Ureter, Right** Ureteral orifice Ureterovesical orifice **7 Ureter, Left** *See 6 Ureter, Right* **B Bladder** Trigone of bladder **C Bladder Neck**	**Ø Open** **3 Percutaneous** **4 Percutaneous Endoscopic** **7 Via Natural or Artificial Opening** **8 Via Natural or Artificial Opening Endoscopic**	**Z No Device**	**Z No Qualifier**
D Urethra Bulbourethral (Cowper's) gland Cowper's (bulbourethral) gland External urethral sphincter Internal urethral sphincter Membranous urethra Penile urethra Prostatic urethra	**Ø Open** **3 Percutaneous** **4 Percutaneous Endoscopic** **7 Via Natural or Artificial Opening** **8 Via Natural or Artificial Opening Endoscopic** **X External**	**Z No Device**	**Z No Qualifier**

Non-OR ØTC[Ø,1,3,4,6,7]8ZZ
Non-OR ØTC[B,C][7,8]ZZ
Non-OR ØTCD[7,8,X]ZZ

Ø Medical and Surgical
T Urinary System
D Extraction Definition: Pulling or stripping out or off all or a portion of a body part by the use of force

Explanation: The qualifier DIAGNOSTIC is used to identify extraction procedures that are biopsies

Body Part Character 4	Approach Character 5	Device Character 6	Qualifier Character 7
Ø Kidney, Right Renal calyx Renal capsule Renal cortex Renal segment **1 Kidney, Left** *See Ø Kidney, Right*	**Ø Open** **3 Percutaneous** **4 Percutaneous Endoscopic**	**Z No Device**	**Z No Qualifier**

Ø Medical and Surgical
T Urinary System
F Fragmentation Definition: Breaking solid matter in a body part into pieces

Explanation: Physical force (e.g., manual, ultrasonic) applied directly or indirectly is used to break the solid matter into pieces. The solid matter may be an abnormal byproduct of a biological function or a foreign body. The pieces of solid matter are not taken out.

Body Part Character 4	Approach Character 5	Device Character 6	Qualifier Character 7
3 Kidney Pelvis, Right Ureteropelvic junction (UPJ) **4 Kidney Pelvis, Left** *See 3 Kidney Pelvis, Right* **6 Ureter, Right** Ureteral orifice Ureterovesical orifice **7 Ureter, Left** *See 6 Ureter, Right* **B Bladder** Trigone of bladder **C Bladder Neck** **D Urethra** NC Bulbourethral (Cowper's) gland Cowper's (bulbourethral) gland External urethral sphincter Internal urethral sphincter Membranous urethra Penile urethra Prostatic urethra	**Ø Open** **3 Percutaneous** **4 Percutaneous Endoscopic** **7 Via Natural or Artificial Opening** **8 Via Natural or Artificial Opening Endoscopic** **X External**	**Z No Device**	**Z No Qualifier**

Non-OR ØTF[3,4][Ø,7,8]ZZ
Non-OR ØTF[6,7,B,C,D][Ø,3,4,7,8]ZZ
Non-OR ØTF[3,4,6,7,B,C,D]XZZ
NC ØTFDXZZ

Ø Medical and Surgical
T Urinary System
H Insertion

Definition: Putting in a nonbiological appliance that monitors, assists, performs, or prevents a physiological function but does not physically take the place of a body part

Explanation: None

Body Part Character 4	Approach Character 5	Device Character 6	Qualifier Character 7
5 Kidney Renal calyx Renal capsule Renal cortex Renal segment	**Ø Open** **3 Percutaneous** **4 Percutaneous Endoscopic** **7 Via Natural or Artificial Opening** **8 Via Natural or Artificial Opening Endoscopic**	**1 Radioactive Element** **2 Monitoring Device** **3 Infusion Device** **Y Other Device**	**Z No Qualifier**
9 Ureter Ureteral orifice Ureterovesical orifice	**Ø Open** **3 Percutaneous** **4 Percutaneous Endoscopic** **7 Via Natural or Artificial Opening** **8 Via Natural or Artificial Opening Endoscopic**	**1 Radioactive Element** **2 Monitoring Device** **3 Infusion Device** **M Stimulator Lead** **Y Other Device**	**Z No Qualifier**
B Bladder NC Trigone of bladder	**Ø Open** **3 Percutaneous** **4 Percutaneous Endoscopic** **7 Via Natural or Artificial Opening** **8 Via Natural or Artificial Opening Endoscopic**	**1 Radioactive Element** **2 Monitoring Device** **3 Infusion Device** **L Artificial Sphincter** **M Stimulator Lead** **Y Other Device**	**Z No Qualifier**
C Bladder Neck	**Ø Open** **3 Percutaneous** **4 Percutaneous Endoscopic** **7 Via Natural or Artificial Opening** **8 Via Natural or Artificial Opening Endoscopic**	**L Artificial Sphincter**	**Z No Qualifier**
D Urethra Bulbourethral (Cowper's) gland Cowper's (bulbourethral) gland External urethral sphincter Internal urethral sphincter Membranous urethra Penile urethra Prostatic urethra	**Ø Open** **3 Percutaneous** **4 Percutaneous Endoscopic** **7 Via Natural or Artificial Opening** **8 Via Natural or Artificial Opening Endoscopic**	**1 Radioactive Element** **2 Monitoring Device** **3 Infusion Device** **L Artificial Sphincter** **Y Other Device**	**Z No Qualifier**
D Urethra Bulbourethral (Cowper's) gland Cowper's (bulbourethral) gland External urethral sphincter Internal urethral sphincter Membranous urethra Penile urethra Prostatic urethra	**X External**	**2 Monitoring Device** **3 Infusion Device** **L Artificial Sphincter**	**Z No Qualifier**

Non-OR ØTH5Ø3Z
Non-OR ØTH53[1,3,Y]Z
Non-OR ØTH54[3,Y]Z
Non-OR ØTH57[1,2,3,Y]Z
Non-OR ØTH58[2,3]Z
Non-OR ØTH9Ø3Z
Non-OR ØTH93[1,3,Y]Z
Non-OR ØTH94[3,Y]Z
Non-OR ØTH97[1,2,3,Y]Z
Non-OR ØTH98[2,3]Z
Non-OR ØTHBØ3Z
Non-OR ØTHB3[1,3,Y]Z
Non-OR ØTHB4[3,Y]Z
Non-OR ØTHB7[1,2,3,Y]Z
Non-OR ØTHB8[2,3]Z
Non-OR ØTHDØ3Z
Non-OR ØTHD3[1,3,Y]Z
Non-OR ØTHD4[3,Y]Z
Non-OR ØTHD7[1,2,3,Y]Z
Non-OR ØTHD8[2,3,Y]Z
Non-OR ØTHDX3Z
NC ØTHB[Ø,3,4,7,8]MZ

Ø Medical and Surgical
T Urinary System
J Inspection

Definition: Visually and/or manually exploring a body part

Explanation: Visual exploration may be performed with or without optical instrumentation. Manual exploration may be performed directly or through intervening body layers.

Body Part Character 4	Approach Character 5	Device Character 6	Qualifier Character 7
5 Kidney Renal calyx Renal capsule Renal cortex Renal segment **9 Ureter** Ureteral orifice Ureterovesical orifice **B Bladder** Trigone of bladder **D Urethra** Bulbourethral (Cowper's) gland Cowper's (bulbourethral) gland External urethral sphincter Internal urethral sphincter Membranous urethra Penile urethra Prostatic urethra	**Ø Open** **3 Percutaneous** **4 Percutaneous Endoscopic** **7 Via Natural or Artificial Opening** **8 Via Natural or Artificial Opening Endoscopic** **X External**	**Z No Device**	**Z No Qualifier**

Non-OR ØTJ[5,9,D][3,4,7,8,X]ZZ
Non-OR ØTJB[3,7,8,X]ZZ

Ø Medical and Surgical
T Urinary System
L Occlusion

Definition: Completely closing an orifice or the lumen of a tubular body part

Explanation: The orifice can be a natural orifice or an artificially created orifice

Body Part Character 4	Approach Character 5	Device Character 6	Qualifier Character 7
3 Kidney Pelvis, Right Ureteropelvic junction (UPJ) **4 Kidney Pelvis, Left** *See 3 Kidney Pelvis, Right* **6 Ureter, Right** Ureteral orifice Ureterovesical orifice **7 Ureter, Left** *See 6 Ureter, Right* **B Bladder** Trigone of bladder **C Bladder Neck**	**Ø Open** **3 Percutaneous** **4 Percutaneous Endoscopic**	**C Extraluminal Device** **D Intraluminal Device** **Z No Device**	**Z No Qualifier**
3 Kidney Pelvis, Right Ureteropelvic junction (UPJ) **4 Kidney Pelvis, Left** *See 3 Kidney Pelvis, Right* **6 Ureter, Right** Ureteral orifice Ureterovesical orifice **7 Ureter, Left** *See 6 Ureter, Right* **B Bladder** Trigone of bladder **C Bladder Neck**	**7 Via Natural or Artificial Opening** **8 Via Natural or Artificial Opening Endoscopic**	**D Intraluminal Device** **Z No Device**	**Z No Qualifier**
D Urethra Bulbourethral (Cowper's) gland Cowper's (bulbourethral) gland External urethral sphincter Internal urethral sphincter Membranous urethra Penile urethra Prostatic urethra	**Ø Open** **3 Percutaneous** **4 Percutaneous Endoscopic** **X External**	**C Extraluminal Device** **D Intraluminal Device** **Z No Device**	**Z No Qualifier**
D Urethra Bulbourethral (Cowper's) gland Cowper's (bulbourethral) gland External urethral sphincter Internal urethral sphincter Membranous urethra Penile urethra Prostatic urethra	**7 Via Natural or Artificial Opening** **8 Via Natural or Artificial Opening Endoscopic**	**D Intraluminal Device** **Z No Device**	**Z No Qualifier**

Ø Medical and Surgical
T Urinary System
M Reattachment Definition: Putting back in or on all or a portion of a separated body part to its normal location or other suitable location

Explanation: Vascular circulation and nervous pathways may or may not be reestablished

Body Part Character 4	Approach Character 5	Device Character 6	Qualifier Character 7
Ø Kidney, Right Renal calyx Renal capsule Renal cortex Renal segment **1 Kidney, Left** *See Ø Kidney, Right* **2 Kidneys, Bilateral** *See Ø Kidney, Right* **3 Kidney Pelvis, Right** Ureteropelvic junction (UPJ) **4 Kidney Pelvis, Left** *See 3 Kidney Pelvis, Right* **6 Ureter, Right** Ureteral orifice Ureterovesical orifice **7 Ureter, Left** *See 6 Ureter, Right* **8 Ureters, Bilateral** *See 6 Ureter, Right* **B Bladder** Trigone of bladder **C Bladder Neck** **D Urethra** Bulbourethral (Cowper's) gland Cowper's (bulbourethral) gland External urethral sphincter Internal urethral sphincter Membranous urethra Penile urethra Prostatic urethra	**Ø Open** **4 Percutaneous Endoscopic**	**Z No Device**	**Z No Qualifier**

Ø Medical and Surgical
T Urinary System
N Release Definition: Freeing a body part from an abnormal physical constraint by cutting or by the use of force

Explanation: Some of the restraining tissue may be taken out but none of the body part is taken out

Body Part Character 4	Approach Character 5	Device Character 6	Qualifier Character 7
Ø Kidney, Right Renal calyx Renal capsule Renal cortex Renal segment **1 Kidney, Left** *See Ø Kidney, Right* **3 Kidney Pelvis, Right** Ureteropelvic junction (UPJ) **4 Kidney Pelvis, Left** *See 3 Kidney Pelvis, Right* **6 Ureter, Right** Ureteral orifice Ureterovesical orifice **7 Ureter, Left** *See 6 Ureter, Right* **B Bladder** Trigone of bladder **C Bladder Neck**	**Ø Open** **3 Percutaneous** **4 Percutaneous Endoscopic** **7 Via Natural or Artificial Opening** **8 Via Natural or Artificial Opening Endoscopic**	**Z No Device**	**Z No Qualifier**
D Urethra Bulbourethral (Cowper's) gland Cowper's (bulbourethral) gland External urethral sphincter Internal urethral sphincter Membranous urethra Penile urethra Prostatic urethra	**Ø Open** **3 Percutaneous** **4 Percutaneous Endoscopic** **7 Via Natural or Artificial Opening** **8 Via Natural or Artificial Opening Endoscopic** **X External**	**Z No Device**	**Z No Qualifier**

Ø Medical and Surgical
T Urinary System
P Removal Definition: Taking out or off a device from a body part

Explanation: If a device is taken out and a similar device put in without cutting or puncturing the skin or mucous membrane, the procedure is coded to the root operation CHANGE. Otherwise, the procedure for taking out the device is coded to the root operation REMOVAL.

Body Part Character 4	Approach Character 5	Device Character 6	Qualifier Character 7
5 Kidney Renal calyx Renal capsule Renal cortex Renal segment	Ø Open 3 Percutaneous 4 Percutaneous Endoscopic 7 Via Natural or Artificial Opening 8 Via Natural or Artificial Opening Endoscopic	Ø Drainage Device 2 Monitoring Device 3 Infusion Device 7 Autologous Tissue Substitute C Extraluminal Device D Intraluminal Device J Synthetic Substitute K Nonautologous Tissue Substitute Y Other Device	Z No Qualifier
5 Kidney Renal calyx Renal capsule Renal cortex Renal segment	X External	Ø Drainage Device 2 Monitoring Device 3 Infusion Device D Intraluminal Device	Z No Qualifier
9 Ureter Ureteral orifice Ureterovesical orifice	Ø Open 3 Percutaneous 4 Percutaneous Endoscopic 7 Via Natural or Artificial Opening 8 Via Natural or Artificial Opening Endoscopic	Ø Drainage Device 2 Monitoring Device 3 Infusion Device 7 Autologous Tissue Substitute C Extraluminal Device D Intraluminal Device J Synthetic Substitute K Nonautologous Tissue Substitute M Stimulator Lead Y Other Device	Z No Qualifier
9 Ureter Ureteral orifice Ureterovesical orifice	X External	Ø Drainage Device 2 Monitoring Device 3 Infusion Device D Intraluminal Device M Stimulator Lead	Z No Qualifier
B Bladder NC Trigone of bladder	Ø Open 3 Percutaneous 4 Percutaneous Endoscopic 7 Via Natural or Artificial Opening 8 Via Natural or Artificial Opening Endoscopic	Ø Drainage Device 2 Monitoring Device 3 Infusion Device 7 Autologous Tissue Substitute C Extraluminal Device D Intraluminal Device J Synthetic Substitute K Nonautologous Tissue Substitute L Artificial Sphincter M Stimulator Lead Y Other Device	Z No Qualifier
B Bladder Trigone of bladder	X External	Ø Drainage Device 2 Monitoring Device 3 Infusion Device D Intraluminal Device L Artificial Sphincter M Stimulator Lead	Z No Qualifier
D Urethra Bulbourethral (Cowper's) gland Cowper's (bulbourethral) gland External urethral sphincter Internal urethral sphincter Membranous urethra Penile urethra Prostatic urethra	Ø Open 3 Percutaneous 4 Percutaneous Endoscopic 7 Via Natural or Artificial Opening 8 Via Natural or Artificial Opening Endoscopic	Ø Drainage Device 2 Monitoring Device 3 Infusion Device 7 Autologous Tissue Substitute C Extraluminal Device D Intraluminal Device J Synthetic Substitute K Nonautologous Tissue Substitute L Artificial Sphincter Y Other Device	Z No Qualifier
D Urethra Bulbourethral (Cowper's) gland Cowper's (bulbourethral) gland External urethral sphincter Internal urethral sphincter Membranous urethra Penile urethra Prostatic urethra	X External	Ø Drainage Device 2 Monitoring Device 3 Infusion Device D Intraluminal Device L Artificial Sphincter	Z No Qualifier

Non-OR ØTP5[3,4,7]YZ
Non-OR ØTP5[7,8][Ø,2,3,D]Z
Non-OR ØTP5X[Ø,2,3,D]Z
Non-OR ØTP9[3,4,7]YZ
Non-OR ØTP9[7,8][Ø,2,3,D]Z
Non-OR ØTP9X[Ø,2,3,D]Z
Non-OR ØTPB[3,4,7]YZ
Non-OR ØTPB[7,8][Ø,2,3,D]Z
Non-OR ØTPBX[Ø,2,3,D,L]Z
Non-OR ØTPD[3,4]YZ
Non-OR ØTPD[7,8][Ø,2,3,D,Y]Z
Non-OR ØTPDX[Ø,2,3,D]Z
NC ØTPB[Ø,3,4,7,8]MZ

Ø Medical and Surgical
T Urinary System
Q Repair Definition: Restoring, to the extent possible, a body part to its normal anatomic structure and function
Explanation: Used only when the method to accomplish the repair is not one of the other root operations

Body Part Character 4	Approach Character 5	Device Character 6	Qualifier Character 7
Ø Kidney, Right Renal calyx Renal capsule Renal cortex Renal segment **1 Kidney, Left** *See Ø Kidney, Right* **3 Kidney Pelvis, Right** Ureteropelvic junction (UPJ) **4 Kidney Pelvis, Left** *See 3 Kidney Pelvis, Right* **6 Ureter, Right** Ureteral orifice Ureterovesical orifice **7 Ureter, Left** *See 6 Ureter, Right* **B Bladder** ⊞ Trigone of bladder **C Bladder Neck**	**Ø Open** **3 Percutaneous** **4 Percutaneous Endoscopic** **7 Via Natural or Artificial Opening** **8 Via Natural or Artificial Opening Endoscopic**	**Z No Device**	**Z No Qualifier**
D Urethra Bulbourethral (Cowper's) gland Cowper's (bulbourethral) gland External urethral sphincter Internal urethral sphincter Membranous urethra Penile urethra Prostatic urethra	**Ø Open** **3 Percutaneous** **4 Percutaneous Endoscopic** **7 Via Natural or Artificial Opening** **8 Via Natural or Artificial Opening Endoscopic** **X External**	**Z No Device**	**Z No Qualifier**

See Appendix L for Procedure Combinations
⊞ ØTQB[Ø,3,4]ZZ

Ø Medical and Surgical
T Urinary System
R Replacement Definition: Putting in or on biological or synthetic material that physically takes the place and/or function of all or a portion of a body part
Explanation: The body part may have been taken out or replaced, or may be taken out, physically eradicated, or rendered nonfunctional during the REPLACEMENT procedure. A REMOVAL procedure is coded for taking out the device used in a previous replacement procedure.

Body Part Character 4	Approach Character 5	Device Character 6	Qualifier Character 7
3 Kidney Pelvis, Right Ureteropelvic junction (UPJ) **4 Kidney Pelvis, Left** *See 3 Kidney Pelvis, Right* **6 Ureter, Right** Ureteral orifice Ureterovesical orifice **7 Ureter, Left** *See 6 Ureter, Right* **B Bladder** Trigone of bladder **C Bladder Neck**	**Ø Open** **4 Percutaneous Endoscopic** **7 Via Natural or Artificial Opening** **8 Via Natural or Artificial Opening Endoscopic**	**7 Autologous Tissue Substitute** **J Synthetic Substitute** **K Nonautologous Tissue Substitute**	**Z No Qualifier**
D Urethra Bulbourethral (Cowper's) gland Cowper's (bulbourethral) gland External urethral sphincter Internal urethral sphincter Membranous urethra Penile urethra Prostatic urethra	**Ø Open** **4 Percutaneous Endoscopic** **7 Via Natural or Artificial Opening** **8 Via Natural or Artificial Opening Endoscopic** **X External**	**7 Autologous Tissue Substitute** **J Synthetic Substitute** **K Nonautologous Tissue Substitute**	**Z No Qualifier**

Ø Medical and Surgical
T Urinary System
S Reposition

Definition: Moving to its normal location, or other suitable location, all or a portion of a body part

Explanation: The body part is moved to a new location from an abnormal location, or from a normal location where it is not functioning correctly. The body part may or may not be cut out or off to be moved to the new location.

Body Part Character 4	Approach Character 5	Device Character 6	Qualifier Character 7
Ø Kidney, Right Renal calyx Renal capsule Renal cortex Renal segment **1 Kidney, Left** *See Ø Kidney, Right* **2 Kidneys, Bilateral** *See Ø Kidney, Right* **3 Kidney Pelvis, Right** Ureteropelvic junction (UPJ) **4 Kidney Pelvis, Left** *See 3 Kidney Pelvis, Right* **6 Ureter, Right** Ureteral orifice Ureterovesical orifice **7 Ureter, Left** *See 6 Ureter, Right* **8 Ureters, Bilateral** *See 6 Ureter, Right* **B Bladder** Trigone of bladder **C Bladder Neck** **D Urethra** Bulbourethral (Cowper's) gland Cowper's (bulbourethral) gland External urethral sphincter Internal urethral sphincter Membranous urethra Penile urethra Prostatic urethra	**Ø Open** **4 Percutaneous Endoscopic**	**Z No Device**	**Z No Qualifier**

Ø Medical and Surgical
T Urinary System
T Resection

Definition: Cutting out or off, without replacement, all of a body part

Explanation: None

Body Part Character 4	Approach Character 5	Device Character 6	Qualifier Character 7
Ø Kidney, Right Renal calyx Renal capsule Renal cortex Renal segment **1 Kidney, Left** *See Ø Kidney, Right* **2 Kidneys, Bilateral** *See Ø Kidney, Right*	**Ø Open** **4 Percutaneous Endoscopic**	**Z No Device**	**Z No Qualifier**
3 Kidney Pelvis, Right Ureteropelvic junction (UPJ) **4 Kidney Pelvis, Left** *See 3 Kidney Pelvis, Right* **6 Ureter, Right** Ureteral orifice Ureterovesical orifice **7 Ureter, Left** *See 6 Ureter, Right* **B Bladder** ⊞ Trigone of bladder **C Bladder Neck** **D Urethra** Bulbourethral (Cowper's) gland Cowper's (bulbourethral) gland External urethral sphincter Internal urethral sphincter Membranous urethra Penile urethra Prostatic urethra	**Ø Open** **4 Percutaneous Endoscopic** **7 Via Natural or Artificial Opening** **8 Via Natural or Artificial Opening Endoscopic**	**Z No Device**	**Z No Qualifier**

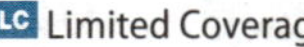 ØTTD[4,7,8]ZZ

See Appendix L for Procedure Combinations

Combo-only ØTTDØZZ

⊞ ØTTBØZZ

NC Noncovered Procedure LC Limited Coverage QA Questionable OB Admit NT New Tech Add-on ⊞ Combination Member ♂ Male ♀ Female

Ø Medical and Surgical
T Urinary System
U Supplement Definition: Putting in or on biological or synthetic material that physically reinforces and/or augments the function of a portion of a body part

Explanation: The biological material is non-living, or is living and from the same individual. The body part may have been previously replaced, and the SUPPLEMENT procedure is performed to physically reinforce and/or augment the function of the replaced body part.

Body Part Character 4	Approach Character 5	Device Character 6	Qualifier Character 7
3 Kidney Pelvis, Right Ureteropelvic junction (UPJ) **4 Kidney Pelvis, Left** *See 3 Kidney Pelvis, Right* **6 Ureter, Right** Ureteral orifice Ureterovesical orifice **7 Ureter, Left** *See 6 Ureter, Right* **B Bladder** Trigone of bladder **C Bladder Neck**	**Ø Open** **4 Percutaneous Endoscopic** **7 Via Natural or Artificial Opening** **8 Via Natural or Artificial Opening Endoscopic**	**7 Autologous Tissue Substitute** **J Synthetic Substitute** **K Nonautologous Tissue Substitute**	**Z No Qualifier**
D Urethra Bulbourethral (Cowper's) gland Cowper's (bulbourethral) gland External urethral sphincter Internal urethral sphincter Membranous urethra Penile urethra Prostatic urethra	**Ø Open** **4 Percutaneous Endoscopic** **7 Via Natural or Artificial Opening** **8 Via Natural or Artificial Opening Endoscopic** **X External**	**7 Autologous Tissue Substitute** **J Synthetic Substitute** **K Nonautologous Tissue Substitute**	**Z No Qualifier**

Ø Medical and Surgical
T Urinary System
V Restriction Definition: Partially closing an orifice or the lumen of a tubular body part

Explanation: The orifice can be a natural orifice or an artificially created orifice

Body Part Character 4	Approach Character 5	Device Character 6	Qualifier Character 7
3 Kidney Pelvis, Right Ureteropelvic junction (UPJ) **4 Kidney Pelvis, Left** *See 3 Kidney Pelvis, Right* **6 Ureter, Right** Ureteral orifice Ureterovesical orifice **7 Ureter, Left** *See 6 Ureter, Right* **B Bladder** Trigone of bladder **C Bladder Neck**	**Ø Open** **3 Percutaneous** **4 Percutaneous Endoscopic**	**C Extraluminal Device** **D Intraluminal Device** **Z No Device**	**Z No Qualifier**
3 Kidney Pelvis, Right Ureteropelvic junction (UPJ) **4 Kidney Pelvis, Left** *See 3 Kidney Pelvis, Right* **6 Ureter, Right** Ureteral orifice Ureterovesical orifice **7 Ureter, Left** *See 6 Ureter, Right* **B Bladder** Trigone of bladder **C Bladder Neck**	**7 Via Natural or Artificial Opening** **8 Via Natural or Artificial Opening Endoscopic**	**D Intraluminal Device** **Z No Device**	**Z No Qualifier**
D Urethra Bulbourethral (Cowper's) gland Cowper's (bulbourethral) gland External urethral sphincter Internal urethral sphincter Membranous urethra Penile urethra Prostatic urethra	**Ø Open** **3 Percutaneous** **4 Percutaneous Endoscopic**	**C Extraluminal Device** **D Intraluminal Device** **Z No Device**	**Z No Qualifier**
D Urethra Bulbourethral (Cowper's) gland Cowper's (bulbourethral) gland External urethral sphincter Internal urethral sphincter Membranous urethra Penile urethra Prostatic urethra	**7 Via Natural or Artificial Opening** **8 Via Natural or Artificial Opening Endoscopic**	**D Intraluminal Device** **Z No Device**	**Z No Qualifier**
D Urethra Bulbourethral (Cowper's) gland Cowper's (bulbourethral) gland External urethral sphincter Internal urethral sphincter Membranous urethra Penile urethra Prostatic urethra	**X External**	**Z No Device**	**Z No Qualifier**

Ø Medical and Surgical
T Urinary System
W Revision

Definition: Correcting, to the extent possible, a portion of a malfunctioning device or the position of a displaced device

Explanation: Revision can include correcting a malfunctioning or displaced device by taking out or putting in components of the device such as a screw or pin

Body Part Character 4	Approach Character 5	Device Character 6	Qualifier Character 7
5 Kidney Renal calyx Renal capsule Renal cortex Renal segment	Ø Open 3 Percutaneous 4 Percutaneous Endoscopic 7 Via Natural or Artificial Opening 8 Via Natural or Artificial Opening Endoscopic	Ø Drainage Device 2 Monitoring Device 3 Infusion Device 7 Autologous Tissue Substitute C Extraluminal Device D Intraluminal Device J Synthetic Substitute K Nonautologous Tissue Substitute Y Other Device	Z No Qualifier
5 Kidney Renal calyx Renal capsule Renal cortex Renal segment	X External	Ø Drainage Device 2 Monitoring Device 3 Infusion Device 7 Autologous Tissue Substitute C Extraluminal Device D Intraluminal Device J Synthetic Substitute K Nonautologous Tissue Substitute	Z No Qualifier
9 Ureter Ureteral orifice Ureterovesical orifice	Ø Open 3 Percutaneous 4 Percutaneous Endoscopic 7 Via Natural or Artificial Opening 8 Via Natural or Artificial Opening Endoscopic	Ø Drainage Device 2 Monitoring Device 3 Infusion Device 7 Autologous Tissue Substitute C Extraluminal Device D Intraluminal Device J Synthetic Substitute K Nonautologous Tissue Substitute M Stimulator Lead Y Other Device	Z No Qualifier
9 Ureter Ureteral orifice Ureterovesical orifice	X External	Ø Drainage Device 2 Monitoring Device 3 Infusion Device 7 Autologous Tissue Substitute C Extraluminal Device D Intraluminal Device J Synthetic Substitute K Nonautologous Tissue Substitute M Stimulator Lead	Z No Qualifier
B Bladder Trigone of bladder	Ø Open 3 Percutaneous 4 Percutaneous Endoscopic 7 Via Natural or Artificial Opening 8 Via Natural or Artificial Opening Endoscopic	Ø Drainage Device 2 Monitoring Device 3 Infusion Device 7 Autologous Tissue Substitute C Extraluminal Device D Intraluminal Device J Synthetic Substitute K Nonautologous Tissue Substitute L Artificial Sphincter M Stimulator Lead Y Other Device	Z No Qualifier
B Bladder Trigone of bladder	X External	Ø Drainage Device 2 Monitoring Device 3 Infusion Device 7 Autologous Tissue Substitute C Extraluminal Device D Intraluminal Device J Synthetic Substitute K Nonautologous Tissue Substitute L Artificial Sphincter M Stimulator Lead	Z No Qualifier

Non-OR ØTW5[3,4,7]YZ
Non-OR ØTW5X[Ø,2,3,7,C,D,J,K]Z
Non-OR ØTW9[3,4,7]YZ
Non-OR ØTW9X[Ø,2,3,7,C,D,J,K,M]Z
Non-OR ØTWB[3,4,7]YZ
Non-OR ØTWBX[Ø,2,3,7,C,D,J,K,L,M]Z

ØTW Continued on next page

Urinary System

ØTW Continued

Ø Medical and Surgical
T Urinary System
W Revision

Definition: Correcting, to the extent possible, a portion of a malfunctioning device or the position of a displaced device

Explanation: Revision can include correcting a malfunctioning or displaced device by taking out or putting in components of the device such as a screw or pin

Body Part Character 4	Approach Character 5	Device Character 6	Qualifier Character 7
D Urethra Bulbourethral (Cowper's) gland Cowper's (bulbourethral) gland External urethral sphincter Internal urethral sphincter Membranous urethra Penile urethra Prostatic urethra	**Ø Open** **3 Percutaneous** **4 Percutaneous Endoscopic** **7 Via Natural or Artificial Opening** **8 Via Natural or Artificial Opening Endoscopic**	**Ø Drainage Device** **2 Monitoring Device** **3 Infusion Device** **7 Autologous Tissue Substitute** **C Extraluminal Device** **D Intraluminal Device** **J Synthetic Substitute** **K Nonautologous Tissue Substitute** **L Artificial Sphincter** **Y Other Device**	**Z No Qualifier**
D Urethra Bulbourethral (Cowper's) gland Cowper's (bulbourethral) gland External urethral sphincter Internal urethral sphincter Membranous urethra Penile urethra Prostatic urethra	**X External**	**Ø Drainage Device** **2 Monitoring Device** **3 Infusion Device** **7 Autologous Tissue Substitute** **C Extraluminal Device** **D Intraluminal Device** **J Synthetic Substitute** **K Nonautologous Tissue Substitute** **L Artificial Sphincter**	**Z No Qualifier**

Non-OR ØTWD[3,4,7,8]YZ
Non-OR ØTWDX[Ø,2,3,7,C,D,J,K,L]Z

Ø Medical and Surgical
T Urinary System
Y Transplantation

Definition: Putting in or on all or a portion of a living body part taken from another individual or animal to physically take the place and/or function of all or a portion of a similar body part

Explanation: The native body part may or may not be taken out, and the transplanted body part may take over all or a portion of its function

Body Part Character 4	Approach Character 5	Device Character 6	Qualifier Character 7
Ø Kidney, Right LC ⊞ Renal calyx Renal capsule Renal cortex Renal segment **1 Kidney, Left** LC ⊞ *See Ø Kidney, Right*	**Ø Open**	**Z No Device**	**Ø Allogeneic** **1 Syngeneic** **2 Zooplastic**

LC ØTY[Ø,1]ØZ[Ø,1,2]

See Appendix L for Procedure Combinations
⊞ ØTY[Ø,1]ØZ[Ø,1,2]

Non-OR Procedure | DRG Non-OR Procedure | Valid OR Procedure | HAC Associated Procedure | Combination Only | New/Revised April | New/Revised October

Female Reproductive System ØU1–ØUY

Character Meanings

This Character Meaning table is provided as a guide to assist the user in the identification of character members that may be found in this section of code tables. It **SHOULD NOT** be used to build a PCS code.

Operation–Character 3		Body Part–Character 4		Approach–Character 5		Device–Character 6		Qualifier–Character 7	
1	Bypass	Ø	Ovary, Right	Ø	Open	Ø	Drainage Device	Ø	Allogeneic
2	Change	1	Ovary, Left	3	Percutaneous	1	Radioactive Element	1	Syngeneic
5	Destruction	2	Ovaries, Bilateral	4	Percutaneous Endoscopic	3	Infusion Device	2	Zooplastic
7	Dilation	3	Ovary	7	Via Natural or Artificial Opening	7	Autologous Tissue Substitute	5	Fallopian Tube, Right
8	Division	4	Uterine Supporting Structure	8	Via Natural or Artificial Opening Endoscopic	C	Extraluminal Device	6	Fallopian Tube, Left
9	Drainage	5	Fallopian Tube, Right	F	Via Natural or Artificial Opening With Percutaneous Endoscopic Assistance	D	Intraluminal Device	9	Uterus
B	Excision	6	Fallopian Tube, Left	X	External	G	Intraluminal Device, Pessary	L	Supracervical
C	Extirpation	7	Fallopian Tubes, Bilateral			H	Contraceptive Device	X	Diagnostic
D	Extraction	8	Fallopian Tube			J	Synthetic Substitute	Z	No Qualifier
F	Fragmentation	9	Uterus			K	Nonautologous Tissue Substitute		
H	Insertion	B	Endometrium			Y	Other Device		
J	Inspection	C	Cervix			Z	No Device		
L	Occlusion	D	Uterus and Cervix						
M	Reattachment	F	Cul-de-sac						
N	Release	G	Vagina						
P	Removal	H	Vagina and Cul-de-sac						
Q	Repair	J	Clitoris						
S	Reposition	K	Hymen						
T	Resection	L	Vestibular Gland						
U	Supplement	M	Vulva						
V	Restriction	N	Ova						
W	Revision								
Y	Transplantation								

AHA Coding Clinic for table ØU5
2015, 3Q, 31 Tubal ligation for sterilization

AHA Coding Clinic for table ØU7
2020, 2Q, 30 Duhrssen cervical incision

AHA Coding Clinic for table ØU9
2016, 4Q, 58 Longitudinal vaginal septum

AHA Coding Clinic for table ØUB
2018, 1Q, 23 Tubal ligation procedure
2015, 3Q, 31 Laparoscopic partial salpingectomy for ectopic pregnancy
2015, 3Q, 31 Tubal ligation for sterilization
2014, 4Q, 16 Excision of multiple uterine fibroids
2014, 3Q, 12 Excision of skin tag from labia majora

AHA Coding Clinic for table ØUC
2015, 3Q, 30 Removal of cervical cerclage
2013, 2Q, 38 Evacuation of clot post-partum

AHA Coding Clinic for table ØUH
2020, 4Q, 43-44 Insertion of radioactive element
2018, 1Q, 25 Intrauterine brachytherapy & placement of tandems & ovoids
2013, 2Q, 34 Placement of intrauterine device via open approach

AHA Coding Clinic for table ØUJ
2015, 1Q, 33 Robotic-assisted laparoscopic hysterectomy converted to open procedure

AHA Coding Clinic for table ØUL
2018, 1Q, 23 Tubal ligation procedure
2015, 3Q, 31 Tubal ligation for sterilization

AHA Coding Clinic for table ØUP
2022, 3Q, 13 Repair of prolapsed neovaginal graft

AHA Coding Clinic for table ØUQ
2020, 4Q, 59-60 Extraction of ectopic products of conception
2014, 4Q, 18 Obstetrical periurethral laceration
2013, 4Q, 120 Repair of clitoral obstetric laceration

AHA Coding Clinic for table ØUS
2016, 1Q, 9 Anteversion of retroverted pregnant uterus

AHA Coding Clinic for table ØUT
2022, 1Q, 21 Gravid hysterectomy due to placenta increta
2017, 4Q, 68 New qualifier values - Supracervical hysterectomy
2015, 1Q, 33 Robotic-assisted laparoscopic hysterectomy converted to open procedure
2013, 3Q, 28 Total hysterectomy
2013, 1Q, 24 Excision versus Resection of remaining ovarian remnant following previous excision

AHA Coding Clinic for table ØUV
2015, 3Q, 30 Insertion of cervical cerclage

AHA Coding Clinic for table ØUY
2023, 2Q, 32 Preparation of donor organ before transplantation
2018, 4Q, 40 Uterus transplant

Female Reproductive System

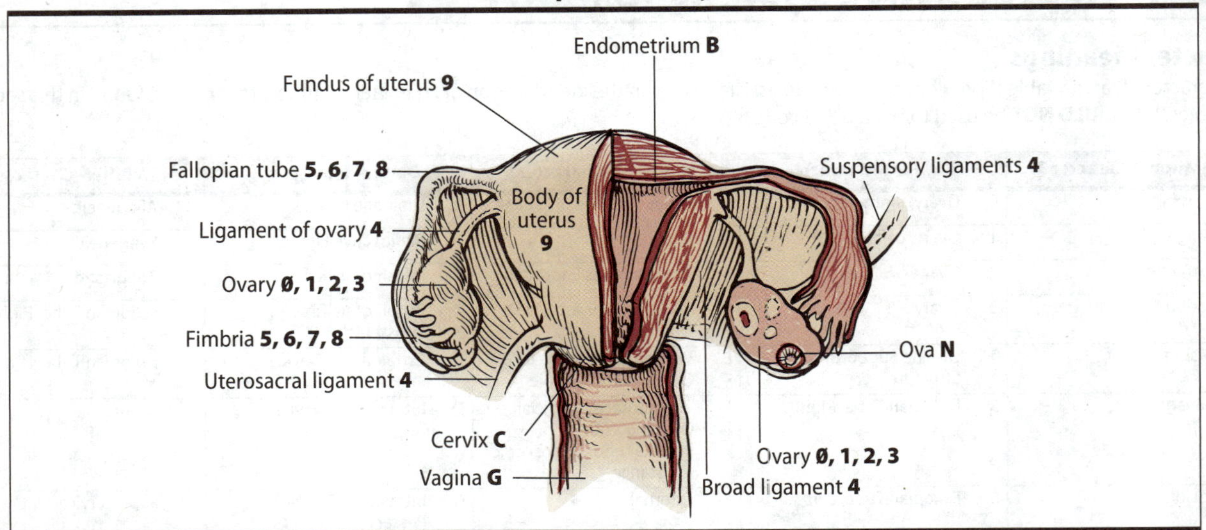

Female Internal/External Structures

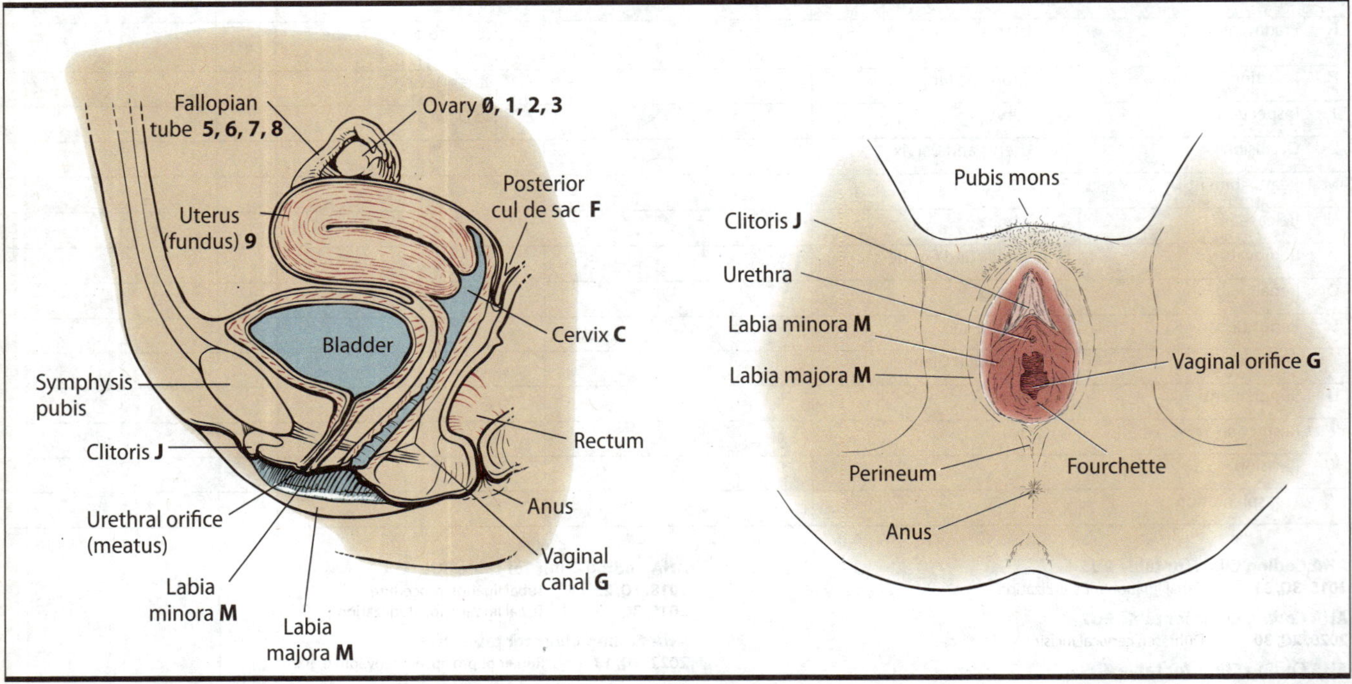

Ø Medical and Surgical
U Female Reproductive System
1 Bypass Definition: Altering the route of passage of the contents of a tubular body part

Explanation: Rerouting contents of a body part to a downstream area of the normal route, to a similar route and body part, or to an abnormal route and dissimilar body part. Includes one or more anastomoses, with or without the use of a device.

Body Part Character 4	Approach Character 5	Device Character 6	Qualifier Character 7
5 Fallopian Tube, Right ♀ Oviduct Salpinx Uterine tube **6 Fallopian Tube, Left** ♀ *See 5 Fallopian Tube, Right*	**Ø Open** **4 Percutaneous Endoscopic**	**7 Autologous Tissue Substitute** **J Synthetic Substitute** **K Nonautologous Tissue Substitute** **Z No Device**	**5 Fallopian Tube, Right** **6 Fallopian Tube, Left** **9 Uterus**

♀ All body part, approach, device, and qualifier values

Ø Medical and Surgical
U Female Reproductive System
2 Change Definition: Taking out or off a device from a body part and putting back an identical or similar device in or on the same body part without cutting or puncturing the skin or a mucous membrane

Explanation: All CHANGE procedures are coded using the approach EXTERNAL

Body Part Character 4	Approach Character 5	Device Character 6	Qualifier Character 7
3 Ovary ♀ **8 Fallopian Tube** ♀ **M Vulva** ♀ Labia majora Labia minora	**X External**	**Ø Drainage Device** **Y Other Device**	**Z No Qualifier**
D Uterus and Cervix ♀	**X External**	**Ø Drainage Device** **H Contraceptive Device** **Y Other Device**	**Z No Qualifier**
H Vagina and Cul-de-sac ♀	**X External**	**Ø Drainage Device** **G Intraluminal Device, Pessary** **Y Other Device**	**Z No Qualifier**

Non-OR All body part, approach, device, and qualifier values
♀ All body part, approach, device, and qualifier values

Ø Medical and Surgical
U Female Reproductive System
5 Destruction Definition: Physical eradication of all or a portion of a body part by the direct use of energy, force, or a destructive agent

Explanation: None of the body part is physically taken out

Body Part Character 4	Approach Character 5	Device Character 6	Qualifier Character 7
Ø Ovary, Right ♀ **1 Ovary, Left** ♀ **2 Ovaries, Bilateral** ♀ **4 Uterine Supporting Structure** ♀ Broad ligament Infundibulopelvic ligament Ovarian ligament Round ligament of uterus	**Ø Open** **3 Percutaneous** **4 Percutaneous Endoscopic** **8 Via Natural or Artificial Opening Endoscopic**	**Z No Device**	**Z No Qualifier**
5 Fallopian Tube, Right ♀ Oviduct Salpinx Uterine tube **6 Fallopian Tube, Left** ♀ *See 5 Fallopian Tube, Right* **7 Fallopian Tubes, Bilateral** NC ♀ **9 Uterus** ♀ Fundus uteri Myometrium Perimetrium Uterine cornu **B Endometrium** ♀ **C Cervix** ♀ **F Cul-de-sac** ♀	**Ø Open** **3 Percutaneous** **4 Percutaneous Endoscopic** **7 Via Natural or Artificial Opening** **8 Via Natural or Artificial Opening Endoscopic**	**Z No Device**	**Z No Qualifier**
G Vagina ♀ **K Hymen** ♀	**Ø Open** **3 Percutaneous** **4 Percutaneous Endoscopic** **7 Via Natural or Artificial Opening** **8 Via Natural or Artificial Opening Endoscopic** **X External**	**Z No Device**	**Z No Qualifier**
J Clitoris ♀ **L Vestibular Gland** ♀ Bartholin's (greater vestibular) gland Greater vestibular (Bartholin's) gland Paraurethral (Skene's) gland Skene's (paraurethral) gland **M Vulva** ♀ Labia majora Labia minora	**Ø Open** **X External**	**Z No Device**	**Z No Qualifier**

NC ØU57[Ø,3,4,7,8]ZZ with principal or secondary diagnosis of Z3Ø.2 ♀ All body part, approach, device, and qualifier values

Ø Medical and Surgical
U Female Reproductive System
7 Dilation Definition: Expanding an orifice or the lumen of a tubular body part

Explanation: The orifice can be a natural orifice or an artificially created orifice. Accomplished by stretching a tubular body part using intraluminal pressure or by cutting part of the orifice or wall of the tubular body part.

Body Part Character 4	Approach Character 5	Device Character 6	Qualifier Character 7
5 Fallopian Tube, Right ♀ Oviduct Salpinx Uterine tube **6 Fallopian Tube, Left** ♀ *See 5 Fallopian Tube, Right* **7 Fallopian Tubes, Bilateral** ♀ **9 Uterus** ♀ Fundus uteri Myometrium Perimetrium Uterine cornu **C Cervix** ♀ **G Vagina** ♀	**Ø Open** **3 Percutaneous** **4 Percutaneous Endoscopic** **7 Via Natural or Artificial Opening** **8 Via Natural or Artificial Opening Endoscopic**	**D Intraluminal Device** **Z No Device**	**Z No Qualifier**
K Hymen ♀	**Ø Open** **3 Percutaneous** **4 Percutaneous Endoscopic** **7 Via Natural or Artificial Opening** **8 Via Natural or Artificial Opening Endoscopic** **X External**	**D Intraluminal Device** **Z No Device**	**Z No Qualifier**

Non-OR ØU7C[Ø,3,4,7,8][D,Z]Z
Non-OR ØU7G[7,8][D,Z]Z

♀ All body part, approach, device, and qualifier values

Ø Medical and Surgical
U Female Reproductive System
8 Division Definition: Cutting into a body part, without draining fluids and/or gases from the body part, in order to separate or transect a body part

Explanation: All or a portion of the body part is separated into two or more portions

Body Part Character 4	Approach Character 5	Device Character 6	Qualifier Character 7
Ø Ovary, Right ♀ **1 Ovary, Left** ♀ **2 Ovaries, Bilateral** ♀ **4 Uterine Supporting Structure** ♀ Broad ligament Infundibulopelvic ligament Ovarian ligament Round ligament of uterus	**Ø Open** **3 Percutaneous** **4 Percutaneous Endoscopic**	**Z No Device**	**Z No Qualifier**
K Hymen ♀	**7 Via Natural or Artificial Opening** **8 Via Natural or Artificial Opening Endoscopic** **X External**	**Z No Device**	**Z No Qualifier**

Non-OR ØU8K[7,8,X]ZZ

♀ All body part, approach, device, and qualifier values

Ø Medical and Surgical
U Female Reproductive System
9 Drainage Definition: Taking or letting out fluids and/or gases from a body part
Explanation: The qualifier DIAGNOSTIC is used to identify drainage procedures that are biopsies

Body Part Character 4	Approach Character 5	Device Character 6	Qualifier Character 7
Ø Ovary, Right ♀ **1** Ovary, Left ♀ **2** Ovaries, Bilateral ♀	**Ø** Open **3** Percutaneous **4** Percutaneous Endoscopic **8** Via Natural or Artificial Opening Endoscopic	**Ø** Drainage Device	**Z** No Qualifier
Ø Ovary, Right ♀ **1** Ovary, Left ♀ **2** Ovaries, Bilateral ♀	**Ø** Open **3** Percutaneous **4** Percutaneous Endoscopic **8** Via Natural or Artificial Opening Endoscopic	**Z** No Device	**X** Diagnostic **Z** No Qualifier
Ø Ovary, Right ♀ **1** Ovary, Left ♀ **2** Ovaries, Bilateral ♀	**X** External	**Z** No Device	**Z** No Qualifier
4 Uterine Supporting Structure ♀ Broad ligament Infundibulopelvic ligament Ovarian ligament Round ligament of uterus	**Ø** Open **3** Percutaneous **4** Percutaneous Endoscopic **8** Via Natural or Artificial Opening Endoscopic	**Ø** Drainage Device	**Z** No Qualifier
4 Uterine Supporting Structure ♀ Broad ligament Infundibulopelvic ligament Ovarian ligament Round ligament of uterus	**Ø** Open **3** Percutaneous **4** Percutaneous Endoscopic **8** Via Natural or Artificial Opening Endoscopic	**Z** No Device	**X** Diagnostic **Z** No Qualifier
5 Fallopian Tube, Right ♀ Oviduct Salpinx Uterine tube **6** Fallopian Tube, Left ♀ *See 5 Fallopian Tube, Right* **7** Fallopian Tubes, Bilateral ♀ **9** Uterus ♀ Fundus uteri Myometrium Perimetrium Uterine cornu **C** Cervix ♀ **F** Cul-de-sac ♀	**Ø** Open **3** Percutaneous **4** Percutaneous Endoscopic **7** Via Natural or Artificial Opening **8** Via Natural or Artificial Opening Endoscopic	**Ø** Drainage Device	**Z** No Qualifier
5 Fallopian Tube, Right ♀ Oviduct Salpinx Uterine tube **6** Fallopian Tube, Left ♀ *See 5 Fallopian Tube, Right* **7** Fallopian Tubes, Bilateral ♀ **9** Uterus ♀ Fundus uteri Myometrium Perimetrium Uterine cornu **C** Cervix ♀ **F** Cul-de-sac ♀	**Ø** Open **3** Percutaneous **4** Percutaneous Endoscopic **7** Via Natural or Artificial Opening **8** Via Natural or Artificial Opening Endoscopic	**Z** No Device	**X** Diagnostic **Z** No Qualifier

Non-OR ØU9[Ø,1,2][3,8]ØZ
Non-OR ØU9[Ø,1,2][3,8]ZZ
Non-OR ØU9[Ø,1,2]8ZX
Non-OR ØU94[3,8]ØZ
Non-OR ØU94[3,8]ZZ
Non-OR ØU948ZX
Non-OR ØU9[5,6,7,9,C]3ØZ
Non-OR ØU9F[3,4]ØZ
Non-OR ØU9[5,6,7][3,4,7,8]ZZ
Non-OR ØU9[9,C]3ZZ
Non-OR ØU9F[3,4]ZZ
♀ All body part, approach, device, and qualifier values

ØU9 Continued on next page

Ø Medical and Surgical
U Female Reproductive System
9 Drainage Definition: Taking or letting out fluids and/or gases from a body part
Explanation: The qualifier DIAGNOSTIC is used to identify drainage procedures that are biopsies

ØU9 Continued

Body Part Character 4	Approach Character 5	Device Character 6	Qualifier Character 7
G Vagina ♀ **K** Hymen ♀	**Ø** Open **3** Percutaneous **4** Percutaneous Endoscopic **7** Via Natural or Artificial Opening **8** Via Natural or Artificial Opening Endoscopic **X** External	**Ø** Drainage Device	**Z** No Qualifier
G Vagina ♀ **K** Hymen ♀	**Ø** Open **3** Percutaneous **4** Percutaneous Endoscopic **7** Via Natural or Artificial Opening **8** Via Natural or Artificial Opening Endoscopic **X** External	**Z** No Device	**X** Diagnostic **Z** No Qualifier
J Clitoris ♀ **L** Vestibular Gland ♀ Bartholin's (greater vestibular) gland Greater vestibular (Bartholin's) gland Paraurethral (Skene's) gland Skene's (paraurethral) gland **M** Vulva ♀ Labia majora Labia minora	**Ø** Open **X** External	**Ø** Drainage Device	**Z** No Qualifier
J Clitoris ♀ **L** Vestibular Gland ♀ Bartholin's (greater vestibular) gland Greater vestibular (Bartholin's) gland Paraurethral (Skene's) gland Skene's (paraurethral) gland **M** Vulva ♀ Labia majora Labia minora	**Ø** Open **X** External	**Z** No Device	**X** Diagnostic **Z** No Qualifier

Non-OR ØU9G3ØZ
Non-OR ØU9K[Ø,3,4,7,8,X]ØZ
Non-OR ØU9G3ZZ
Non-OR ØU9K[Ø,3,4,7,8,X]ZZ
Non-OR ØU9L[Ø,X]ØZ
Non-OR ØU9L[Ø,X]Z[X,Z]
♀ All body part, approach, device, and qualifier values

Ø Medical and Surgical
U Female Reproductive System
B Excision Definition: Cutting out or off, without replacement, a portion of a body part
Explanation: The qualifier DIAGNOSTIC is used to identify excision procedures that are biopsies

Body Part Character 4	Approach Character 5	Device Character 6	Qualifier Character 7
Ø Ovary, Right ♀ **1 Ovary, Left** ♀ **2 Ovaries, Bilateral** ♀ **4 Uterine Supporting Structure** ♀ Broad ligament Infundibulopelvic ligament Ovarian ligament Round ligament of uterus **5 Fallopian Tube, Right** ♀ Oviduct Salpinx Uterine tube **6 Fallopian Tube, Left** ♀ *See 5 Fallopian Tube, Right* **7 Fallopian Tubes, Bilateral** ♀ **9 Uterus** ♀ Fundus uteri Myometrium Perimetrium Uterine cornu **C Cervix** ♀ **F Cul-de-sac** ♀	**Ø Open** **3 Percutaneous** **4 Percutaneous Endoscopic** **7 Via Natural or Artificial Opening** **8 Via Natural or Artificial Opening Endoscopic**	**Z No Device**	**X Diagnostic** **Z No Qualifier**
G Vagina ♀ **K Hymen** ♀	**Ø Open** **3 Percutaneous** **4 Percutaneous Endoscopic** **7 Via Natural or Artificial Opening** **8 Via Natural or Artificial Opening Endoscopic** **X External**	**Z No Device**	**X Diagnostic** **Z No Qualifier**
J Clitoris ♀ **L Vestibular Gland** ♀ Bartholin's (greater vestibular) gland Greater vestibular (Bartholin's) gland Paraurethral (Skene's) gland Skene's (paraurethral) gland **M Vulva** ♀ Labia majora Labia minora	**Ø Open** **X External**	**Z No Device**	**X Diagnostic** **Z No Qualifier**

♀ All body part, approach, device, and qualifier values

Ø Medical and Surgical
U Female Reproductive System
C Extirpation Definition: Taking or cutting out solid matter from a body part

Explanation: The solid matter may be an abnormal byproduct of a biological function or a foreign body; it may be imbedded in a body part or in the lumen of a tubular body part. The solid matter may or may not have been previously broken into pieces.

Body Part Character 4	Approach Character 5	Device Character 6	Qualifier Character 7
Ø Ovary, Right ♀ **1 Ovary, Left** ♀ **2 Ovaries, Bilateral** ♀ **4 Uterine Supporting Structure** ♀ Broad ligament Infundibulopelvic ligament Ovarian ligament Round ligament of uterus	**Ø Open** **3 Percutaneous** **4 Percutaneous Endoscopic** **8 Via Natural or Artificial Opening Endoscopic**	**Z No Device**	**Z No Qualifier**
5 Fallopian Tube, Right ♀ Oviduct Salpinx Uterine tube **6 Fallopian Tube, Left** ♀ *See 5 Fallopian Tube, Right* **7 Fallopian Tubes, Bilateral** ♀ **9 Uterus** ♀ Fundus uteri Myometrium Perimetrium Uterine cornu **B Endometrium** ♀ **C Cervix** ♀ **F Cul-de-sac** ♀	**Ø Open** **3 Percutaneous** **4 Percutaneous Endoscopic** **7 Via Natural or Artificial Opening** **8 Via Natural or Artificial Opening Endoscopic**	**Z No Device**	**Z No Qualifier**
G Vagina ♀ **K Hymen** ♀	**Ø Open** **3 Percutaneous** **4 Percutaneous Endoscopic** **7 Via Natural or Artificial Opening** **8 Via Natural or Artificial Opening Endoscopic** **X External**	**Z No Device**	**Z No Qualifier**
J Clitoris ♀ **L Vestibular Gland** ♀ Bartholin's (greater vestibular) gland Greater vestibular (Bartholin's) gland Paraurethral (Skene's) gland Skene's (paraurethral) gland **M Vulva** ♀ Labia majora Labia minora	**Ø Open** **X External**	**Z No Device**	**Z No Qualifier**

Non-OR ØUC9[7,8]ZZ
Non-OR ØUCG[7,8,X]ZZ
Non-OR ØUCK[Ø,3,4,7,8,X]ZZ
Non-OR ØUCMXZZ
♀ All body part, approach, device, and qualifier values

Ø Medical and Surgical
U Female Reproductive System
D Extraction Definition: Pulling or stripping out or off all or a portion of a body part by the use of force

Explanation: The qualifier DIAGNOSTIC is used to identify extraction procedures that are biopsies

Body Part Character 4	Approach Character 5	Device Character 6	Qualifier Character 7
B Endometrium ♀	**7 Via Natural or Artificial Opening** **8 Via Natural or Artificial Opening Endoscopic**	**Z No Device**	**X Diagnostic** **Z No Qualifier**
N Ova ♀	**Ø Open** **3 Percutaneous** **4 Percutaneous Endoscopic**	**Z No Device**	**Z No Qualifier**

♀ All body part, approach, device, and qualifier values

Ø Medical and Surgical
U Female Reproductive System
F Fragmentation Definition: Breaking solid matter in a body part into pieces

Explanation: Physical force (e.g., manual, ultrasonic) applied directly or indirectly is used to break the solid matter into pieces. The solid matter may be an abnormal byproduct of a biological function or a foreign body. The pieces of solid matter are not taken out.

Body Part Character 4	Approach Character 5	Device Character 6	Qualifier Character 7
5 Fallopian Tube, Right NC ♀ Oviduct Salpinx Uterine tube **6 Fallopian Tube, Left** NC ♀ *See 5 Fallopian Tube, Right* **7 Fallopian Tubes, Bilateral** NC ♀ **9 Uterus** NC ♀ Fundus uteri Myometrium Perimetrium Uterine cornu	**Ø Open** **3 Percutaneous** **4 Percutaneous Endoscopic** **7 Via Natural or Artificial Opening** **8 Via Natural or Artificial Opening Endoscopic** **X External**	**Z No Device**	**Z No Qualifier**

Non-OR ØUF[5,6,7,9]XZZ
NC ØUF[5,6,7,9]XZZ
♀ All body part, approach, device, and qualifier values

Ø Medical and Surgical
U Female Reproductive System
H Insertion Definition: Putting in a nonbiological appliance that monitors, assists, performs, or prevents a physiological function but does not physically take the place of a body part

Explanation: None

Body Part Character 4	Approach Character 5	Device Character 6	Qualifier Character 7
3 Ovary ♀	**Ø Open** **3 Percutaneous** **4 Percutaneous Endoscopic**	**1 Radioactive Element** **3 Infusion Device** **Y Other Device**	**Z No Qualifier**
3 Ovary ♀	**7 Via Natural or Artificial Opening** **8 Via Natural or Artificial Opening Endoscopic**	**1 Radioactive Element** **Y Other Device**	**Z No Qualifier**
8 Fallopian Tube ♀ **D Uterus and Cervix** ♀ **H Vagina and Cul-de-sac** ♀	**Ø Open** **3 Percutaneous** **4 Percutaneous Endoscopic** **7 Via Natural or Artificial Opening** **8 Via Natural or Artificial Opening Endoscopic**	**3 Infusion Device** **Y Other Device**	**Z No Qualifier**
9 Uterus ♀ Fundus uteri Myometrium Perimetrium Uterine cornu	**Ø Open** **7 Via Natural or Artificial Opening** **8 Via Natural or Artificial Opening Endoscopic**	**1 Radioactive Element** **H Contraceptive Device**	**Z No Qualifier**
C Cervix ♀	**Ø Open** **3 Percutaneous** **4 Percutaneous Endoscopic**	**1 Radioactive Element**	**Z No Qualifier**
C Cervix ♀	**7 Via Natural or Artificial Opening** **8 Via Natural or Artificial Opening Endoscopic**	**1 Radioactive Element** **H Contraceptive Device**	**Z No Qualifier**
F Cul-de-sac ♀	**7 Via Natural or Artificial Opening** **8 Via Natural or Artificial Opening Endoscopic**	**G Intraluminal Device, Pessary**	**Z No Qualifier**
G Vagina ♀	**Ø Open** **3 Percutaneous** **4 Percutaneous Endoscopic** **X External**	**1 Radioactive Element**	**Z No Qualifier**
G Vagina ♀	**7 Via Natural or Artificial Opening** **8 Via Natural or Artificial Opening Endoscopic**	**1 Radioactive Element** **G Intraluminal Device, Pessary**	**Z No Qualifier**

Non-OR ØUH3[Ø,4][3,Y]Z
Non-OR ØUH33[1,3,Y]Z
Non-OR ØUH3[7,8][1,Y]Z
Non-OR ØUH[8,D][Ø,3,4,7,8][3,Y]Z
Non-OR ØUHH[3,4]YZ
Non-OR ØUHH[7,8][3,Y]Z
Non-OR ØUH9[Ø,7,8][1,H]Z
Non-OR ØUHC[7,8]HZ
Non-OR ØUHF[7,8]HZ
Non-OR ØUHG[7,8]HZ
♀ All body part, approach, device, and qualifier values

Ø Medical and Surgical
U Female Reproductive System
J Inspection Definition: Visually and/or manually exploring a body part

Explanation: Visual exploration may be performed with or without optical instrumentation. Manual exploration may be performed directly or through intervening body layers.

Body Part Character 4	Approach Character 5	Device Character 6	Qualifier Character 7
3 Ovary ♀	Ø Open 3 Percutaneous 4 Percutaneous Endoscopic 8 Via Natural or Artificial Opening Endoscopic X External	Z No Device	Z No Qualifier
8 Fallopian Tube ♀ D Uterus and Cervix ♀ H Vagina and Cul-de-sac ♀	Ø Open 3 Percutaneous 4 Percutaneous Endoscopic 7 Via Natural or Artificial Opening 8 Via Natural or Artificial Opening Endoscopic X External	Z No Device	Z No Qualifier
M Vulva ♀ Labia majora Labia minora	Ø Open X External	Z No Device	Z No Qualifier

Non-OR ØUJ3[3,8,X]ZZ
Non-OR ØUJ[8,D,H][3,7,8,X]ZZ
Non-OR ØUJMXZZ
♀ All body part, approach, device, and qualifier values

Ø Medical and Surgical
U Female Reproductive System
L Occlusion Definition: Completely closing an orifice or the lumen of a tubular body part

Explanation: The orifice can be a natural orifice or an artificially created orifice

Body Part Character 4	Approach Character 5	Device Character 6	Qualifier Character 7
5 Fallopian Tube, Right ♀ Oviduct Salpinx Uterine tube 6 Fallopian Tube, Left ♀ *See 5 Fallopian Tube, Right* 7 Fallopian Tubes, Bilateral NC ♀	Ø Open 3 Percutaneous 4 Percutaneous Endoscopic	C Extraluminal Device D Intraluminal Device Z No Device	Z No Qualifier
5 Fallopian Tube, Right ♀ Oviduct Salpinx Uterine tube 6 Fallopian Tube, Left ♀ *See 5 Fallopian Tube, Right* 7 Fallopian Tubes, Bilateral NC ♀	7 Via Natural or Artificial Opening 8 Via Natural or Artificial Opening Endoscopic	D Intraluminal Device Z No Device	Z No Qualifier
F Cul-de-sac ♀ G Vagina ♀	7 Via Natural or Artificial Opening 8 Via Natural or Artificial Opening Endoscopic	D Intraluminal Device Z No Device	Z No Qualifier

NC ØUL7[Ø,3,4][C,D,Z]Z with principal or secondary diagnosis of Z3Ø.2
NC ØUL7[7,8][D,Z]Z with principal or secondary diagnosis of Z3Ø.2
♀ All body part, approach, device, and qualifier values

Ø Medical and Surgical
U Female Reproductive System
M Reattachment Definition: Putting back in or on all or a portion of a separated body part to its normal location or other suitable location

Explanation: Vascular circulation and nervous pathways may or may not be reestablished

Body Part Character 4	Approach Character 5	Device Character 6	Qualifier Character 7
Ø Ovary, Right ♀ **1 Ovary, Left** ♀ **2 Ovaries, Bilateral** ♀ **4 Uterine Supporting Structure** ♀ Broad ligament Infundibulopelvic ligament Ovarian ligament Round ligament of uterus **5 Fallopian Tube, Right** ♀ Oviduct Salpinx Uterine tube **6 Fallopian Tube, Left** ♀ *See 5 Fallopian Tube, Right* **7 Fallopian Tubes, Bilateral** ♀ **9 Uterus** ♀ Fundus uteri Myometrium Perimetrium Uterine cornu **C Cervix** ♀ **F Cul-de-sac** ♀ **G Vagina** ♀	**Ø Open** **4 Percutaneous Endoscopic**	**Z No Device**	**Z No Qualifier**
J Clitoris ♀ **M Vulva** ♀ Labia majora Labia minora	**X External**	**Z No Device**	**Z No Qualifier**
K Hymen ♀	**Ø Open** **4 Percutaneous Endoscopic** **X External**	**Z No Device**	**Z No Qualifier**

♀ All body part, approach, device, and qualifier values

Ø Medical and Surgical
U Female Reproductive System
N Release Definition: Freeing a body part from an abnormal physical constraint by cutting or by the use of force
Explanation: Some of the restraining tissue may be taken out but none of the body part is taken out

Body Part Character 4	Approach Character 5	Device Character 6	Qualifier Character 7
Ø Ovary, Right ♀ **1 Ovary, Left** ♀ **2 Ovaries, Bilateral** ♀ **4 Uterine Supporting Structure** ♀ Broad ligament Infundibulopelvic ligament Ovarian ligament Round ligament of uterus	**Ø Open** **3 Percutaneous** **4 Percutaneous Endoscopic** **8 Via Natural or Artificial Opening Endoscopic**	**Z No Device**	**Z No Qualifier**
5 Fallopian Tube, Right ♀ Oviduct Salpinx Uterine tube **6 Fallopian Tube, Left** ♀ *See 5 Fallopian Tube, Right* **7 Fallopian Tubes, Bilateral** ♀ **9 Uterus** ♀ Fundus uteri Myometrium Perimetrium Uterine cornu **C Cervix** ♀ **F Cul-de-sac** ♀	**Ø Open** **3 Percutaneous** **4 Percutaneous Endoscopic** **7 Via Natural or Artificial Opening** **8 Via Natural or Artificial Opening Endoscopic**	**Z No Device**	**Z No Qualifier**
G Vagina ♀ **K Hymen** ♀	**Ø Open** **3 Percutaneous** **4 Percutaneous Endoscopic** **7 Via Natural or Artificial Opening** **8 Via Natural or Artificial Opening Endoscopic** **X External**	**Z No Device**	**Z No Qualifier**
J Clitoris ♀ **L Vestibular Gland** ♀ Bartholin's (greater vestibular) gland Greater vestibular (Bartholin's) gland Paraurethral (Skene's) gland Skene's (paraurethral) gland **M Vulva** ♀ Labia majora Labia minora	**Ø Open** **X External**	**Z No Device**	**Z No Qualifier**

♀ All body part, approach, device, and qualifier values

Ø Medical and Surgical
U Female Reproductive System
P Removal Definition: Taking out or off a device from a body part

Explanation: If a device is taken out and a similar device put in without cutting or puncturing the skin or mucous membrane, the procedure is coded to the root operation CHANGE. Otherwise, the procedure for taking out the device is coded to the root operation REMOVAL.

Body Part Character 4	Approach Character 5	Device Character 6	Qualifier Character 7
3 Ovary ♀	**Ø** Open **3** Percutaneous **4** Percutaneous Endoscopic	**Ø** Drainage Device **3** Infusion Device **Y** Other Device	**Z** No Qualifier
3 Ovary ♀	**7** Via Natural or Artificial Opening **8** Via Natural or Artificial Opening Endoscopic	**Y** Other Device	**Z** No Qualifier
3 Ovary ♀	**X** External	**Ø** Drainage Device **3** Infusion Device	**Z** No Qualifier
8 Fallopian Tube ♀	**Ø** Open **3** Percutaneous **4** Percutaneous Endoscopic **7** Via Natural or Artificial Opening **8** Via Natural or Artificial Opening Endoscopic	**Ø** Drainage Device **3** Infusion Device **7** Autologous Tissue Substitute **C** Extraluminal Device **D** Intraluminal Device **J** Synthetic Substitute **K** Nonautologous Tissue Substitute **Y** Other Device	**Z** No Qualifier
8 Fallopian Tube ♀	**X** External	**Ø** Drainage Device **3** Infusion Device **D** Intraluminal Device	**Z** No Qualifier
D Uterus and Cervix ♀	**Ø** Open **3** Percutaneous **4** Percutaneous Endoscopic **7** Via Natural or Artificial Opening **8** Via Natural or Artificial Opening Endoscopic	**Ø** Drainage Device **1** Radioactive Element **3** Infusion Device **7** Autologous Tissue Substitute **C** Extraluminal Device **D** Intraluminal Device **H** Contraceptive Device **J** Synthetic Substitute **K** Nonautologous Tissue Substitute **Y** Other Device	**Z** No Qualifier
D Uterus and Cervix ♀	**X** External	**Ø** Drainage Device **3** Infusion Device **D** Intraluminal Device **H** Contraceptive Device	**Z** No Qualifier
H Vagina and Cul-de-sac ♀	**Ø** Open **3** Percutaneous **4** Percutaneous Endoscopic **7** Via Natural or Artificial Opening **8** Via Natural or Artificial Opening Endoscopic	**Ø** Drainage Device **1** Radioactive Element **3** Infusion Device **7** Autologous Tissue Substitute **D** Intraluminal Device **J** Synthetic Substitute **K** Nonautologous Tissue Substitute **Y** Other Device	**Z** No Qualifier
H Vagina and Cul-de-sac ♀	**X** External	**Ø** Drainage Device **1** Radioactive Element **3** Infusion Device **D** Intraluminal Device	**Z** No Qualifier
M Vulva ♀ Labia majora Labia minora	**Ø** Open	**Ø** Drainage Device **7** Autologous Tissue Substitute **J** Synthetic Substitute **K** Nonautologous Tissue Substitute	**Z** No Qualifier
M Vulva ♀ Labia majora Labia minora	**X** External	**Ø** Drainage Device	**Z** No Qualifier

Non-OR ØUP3[3,4]YZ
Non-OR ØUP3[7,8]YZ
Non-OR ØUP3X[Ø,3]Z
Non-OR ØUP8[3,4]YZ
Non-OR ØUP8[7,8][Ø,3,D,Y]Z
Non-OR ØUP8X[Ø,3,D]Z
Non-OR ØUPD[3,4][C,Y]Z
Non-OR ØUPD[7,8][Ø,3,C,D,H,Y]Z
Non-OR ØUPDX[Ø,3,D,H]Z
Non-OR ØUPH[3,4]YZ
Non-OR ØUPH[7,8][Ø,3,D,Y]Z
Non-OR ØUPHX[Ø,1,3,D]Z
Non-OR ØUPMXØZ
♀ All body part, approach, device, and qualifier values

Ø Medical and Surgical
U Female Reproductive System
Q Repair Definition: Restoring, to the extent possible, a body part to its normal anatomic structure and function

Explanation: Used only when the method to accomplish the repair is not one of the other root operations

Body Part Character 4	Approach Character 5	Device Character 6	Qualifier Character 7
Ø Ovary, Right ♀ **1 Ovary, Left** ♀ **2 Ovaries, Bilateral** ♀ **4 Uterine Supporting Structure** ♀ Broad ligament Infundibulopelvic ligament Ovarian ligament Round ligament of uterus	**Ø Open** **3 Percutaneous** **4 Percutaneous Endoscopic** **8 Via Natural or Artificial Opening Endoscopic**	**Z No Device**	**Z No Qualifier**
5 Fallopian Tube, Right ♀ Oviduct Salpinx Uterine tube **6 Fallopian Tube, Left** ♀ *See 5 Fallopian Tube, Right* **7 Fallopian Tubes, Bilateral** ♀ **9 Uterus** ♀ Fundus uteri Myometrium Perimetrium Uterine cornu **C Cervix** ♀ **F Cul-de-sac** ♀	**Ø Open** **3 Percutaneous** **4 Percutaneous Endoscopic** **7 Via Natural or Artificial Opening** **8 Via Natural or Artificial Opening Endoscopic**	**Z No Device**	**Z No Qualifier**
G Vagina ♀ **K Hymen** ♀	**Ø Open** **3 Percutaneous** **4 Percutaneous Endoscopic** **7 Via Natural or Artificial Opening** **8 Via Natural or Artificial Opening Endoscopic** **X External**	**Z No Device**	**Z No Qualifier**
J Clitoris ♀ **L Vestibular Gland** ♀ Bartholin's (greater vestibular) gland Greater vestibular (Bartholin's) gland Paraurethral (Skene's) gland Skene's (paraurethral) gland **M Vulva** ♀ Labia majora Labia minora	**Ø Open** **X External**	**Z No Device**	**Z No Qualifier**

Non-OR ØUQG[7,X]ZZ
Non-OR ØUQKXZZ
Non-OR ØUQMXZZ
♀ All body part, approach, device, and qualifier values

Ø Medical and Surgical
U Female Reproductive System
S Reposition Definition: Moving to its normal location, or other suitable location, all or a portion of a body part

Explanation: The body part is moved to a new location from an abnormal location, or from a normal location where it is not functioning correctly. The body part may or may not be cut out or off to be moved to the new location.

Body Part Character 4	Approach Character 5	Device Character 6	Qualifier Character 7
Ø Ovary, Right ♀ **1 Ovary, Left** ♀ **2 Ovaries, Bilateral** ♀ **4 Uterine Supporting Structure** ♀ Broad ligament Infundibulopelvic ligament Ovarian ligament Round ligament of uterus **5 Fallopian Tube, Right** ♀ Oviduct Salpinx Uterine tube **6 Fallopian Tube, Left** ♀ *See 5 Fallopian Tube, Right* **7 Fallopian Tubes, Bilateral** ♀ **C Cervix** ♀ **F Cul-de-sac** ♀	**Ø Open** **4 Percutaneous Endoscopic** **8 Via Natural or Artificial Opening Endoscopic**	**Z No Device**	**Z No Qualifier**
9 Uterus ♀ Fundus uteri Myometrium Perimetrium Uterine cornu **G Vagina** ♀	**Ø Open** **4 Percutaneous Endoscopic** **7 Via Natural or Artificial Opening** **8 Via Natural or Artificial Opening Endoscopic** **X External**	**Z No Device**	**Z No Qualifier**

Non-OR ØUS9XZZ
♀ All body part, approach, device, and qualifier values

NC Noncovered Procedure LC Limited Coverage QA Questionable OB Admit NT New Tech Add-on Combination Member ♂ Male ♀ Female

Ø Medical and Surgical
U Female Reproductive System
T Resection Definition: Cutting out or off, without replacement, all of a body part
Explanation: None

Body Part Character 4	Approach Character 5	Device Character 6	Qualifier Character 7
Ø Ovary, Right ♀ **1 Ovary, Left** ♀ **2 Ovaries, Bilateral** ⊞♀ **5 Fallopian Tube, Right** ♀ Oviduct Salpinx Uterine tube **6 Fallopian Tube, Left** ♀ *See 5 Fallopian Tube, Right* **7 Fallopian Tubes, Bilateral** ⊞♀	**Ø Open** **4 Percutaneous Endoscopic** **7 Via Natural or Artificial Opening** **8 Via Natural or Artificial Opening Endoscopic** **F Via Natural or Artificial Opening With Percutaneous Endoscopic Assistance**	**Z No Device**	**Z No Qualifier**
4 Uterine Supporting Structure ⊞♀ Broad ligament Infundibulopelvic ligament Ovarian ligament Round ligament of uterus **C Cervix** ⊞♀ **F Cul-de-sac** ♀ **G Vagina** ⊞♀	**Ø Open** **4 Percutaneous Endoscopic** **7 Via Natural or Artificial Opening** **8 Via Natural or Artificial Opening Endoscopic**	**Z No Device**	**Z No Qualifier**
9 Uterus ⊞♀ Fundus uteri Myometrium Perimetrium Uterine cornu	**Ø Open** **4 Percutaneous Endoscopic** **7 Via Natural or Artificial Opening** **8 Via Natural or Artificial Opening Endoscopic** **F Via Natural or Artificial Opening With Percutaneous Endoscopic Assistance**	**Z No Device**	**L Supracervical** **Z No Qualifier**
J Clitoris ♀ **L Vestibular Gland** ♀ Bartholin's (greater vestibular) gland Greater vestibular (Bartholin's) gland Paraurethral (Skene's) gland Skene's (paraurethral) gland **M Vulva** ⊞♀ Labia majora Labia minora	**Ø Open** **X External**	**Z No Device**	**Z No Qualifier**
K Hymen ♀	**Ø Open** **4 Percutaneous Endoscopic** **7 Via Natural or Artificial Opening** **8 Via Natural or Artificial Opening Endoscopic** **X External**	**Z No Device**	**Z No Device**

♀ All body part, approach, device, and qualifier values

See Appendix L for Procedure Combinations
⊞ ØUT[2,7]ØZZ
⊞ ØUT[4,C][Ø,4,7,8]ZZ
⊞ ØUTGØZZ
⊞ ØUT9[Ø,4,7,8,F]ZZ
⊞ ØUTM[Ø,X]ZZ

Ø Medical and Surgical
U Female Reproductive System
U Supplement Definition: Putting in or on biological or synthetic material that physically reinforces and/or augments the function of a portion of a body part

Explanation: The biological material is non-living, or is living and from the same individual. The body part may have been previously replaced, and the SUPPLEMENT procedure is performed to physically reinforce and/or augment the function of the replaced body part.

Body Part Character 4	Approach Character 5	Device Character 6	Qualifier Character 7
4 Uterine Supporting Structure ♀ Broad ligament Infundibulopelvic ligament Ovarian ligament Round ligament of uterus	**Ø Open** **4 Percutaneous Endoscopic**	**7 Autologous Tissue Substitute** **J Synthetic Substitute** **K Nonautologous Tissue Substitute**	**Z No Qualifier**
5 Fallopian Tube, Right ♀ Oviduct Salpinx Uterine tube **6 Fallopian Tube, Left** ♀ *See 5 Fallopian Tube, Right* **7 Fallopian Tubes, Bilateral** ♀ **F Cul-de-sac** ♀	**Ø Open** **4 Percutaneous Endoscopic** **7 Via Natural or Artificial Opening** **8 Via Natural or Artificial Opening Endoscopic**	**7 Autologous Tissue Substitute** **J Synthetic Substitute** **K Nonautologous Tissue Substitute**	**Z No Qualifier**
G Vagina ♀ **K Hymen** ♀	**Ø Open** **4 Percutaneous Endoscopic** **7 Via Natural or Artificial Opening** **8 Via Natural or Artificial Opening Endoscopic** **X External**	**7 Autologous Tissue Substitute** **J Synthetic Substitute** **K Nonautologous Tissue Substitute**	**Z No Qualifier**
J Clitoris ♀ **M Vulva** ♀ Labia majora Labia minora	**Ø Open** **X External**	**7 Autologous Tissue Substitute** **J Synthetic Substitute** **K Nonautologous Tissue Substitute**	**Z No Qualifier**

♀ All body part, approach, device, and qualifier values

Ø Medical and Surgical
U Female Reproductive System
V Restriction Definition: Partially closing an orifice or the lumen of a tubular body part

Explanation: The orifice can be a natural orifice or an artificially created orifice

Body Part Character 4	Approach Character 5	Device Character 6	Qualifier Character 7
C Cervix ♀	**Ø Open** **3 Percutaneous** **4 Percutaneous Endoscopic**	**C Extraluminal Device** **D Intraluminal Device** **Z No Device**	**Z No Qualifier**
C Cervix ♀	**7 Via Natural or Artificial Opening** **8 Via Natural or Artificial Opening Endoscopic**	**D Intraluminal Device** **Z No Device**	**Z No Qualifier**

♀ All body part, approach, device, and qualifier values

Ø Medical and Surgical
U Female Reproductive System
W Revision Definition: Correcting, to the extent possible, a portion of a malfunctioning device or the position of a displaced device

Explanation: Revision can include correcting a malfunctioning or displaced device by taking out or putting in components of the device such as a screw or pin

Body Part Character 4	Approach Character 5	Device Character 6	Qualifier Character 7
3 Ovary ♀	Ø Open 3 Percutaneous 4 Percutaneous Endoscopic	Ø Drainage Device 3 Infusion Device Y Other Device	Z No Qualifier
3 Ovary ♀	7 Via Natural or Artificial Opening 8 Via Natural or Artificial Opening Endoscopic	Y Other Device	Z No Qualifier
3 Ovary ♀	X External	Ø Drainage Device 3 Infusion Device	Z No Qualifier
8 Fallopian Tube ♀	Ø Open 3 Percutaneous 4 Percutaneous Endoscopic 7 Via Natural or Artificial Opening 8 Via Natural or Artificial Opening Endoscopic	Ø Drainage Device 3 Infusion Device 7 Autologous Tissue Substitute C Extraluminal Device D Intraluminal Device J Synthetic Substitute K Nonautologous Tissue Substitute Y Other Device	Z No Qualifier
8 Fallopian Tube ♀	X External	Ø Drainage Device 3 Infusion Device 7 Autologous Tissue Substitute C Extraluminal Device D Intraluminal Device J Synthetic Substitute K Nonautologous Tissue Substitute	Z No Qualifier
D Uterus and Cervix ♀	Ø Open 3 Percutaneous 4 Percutaneous Endoscopic 7 Via Natural or Artificial Opening 8 Via Natural or Artificial Opening Endoscopic	Ø Drainage Device 1 Radioactive Element 3 Infusion Device 7 Autologous Tissue Substitute C Extraluminal Device D Intraluminal Device H Contraceptive Device J Synthetic Substitute K Nonautologous Tissue Substitute Y Other Device	Z No Qualifier
D Uterus and Cervix ♀	X External	Ø Drainage Device 3 Infusion Device 7 Autologous Tissue Substitute C Extraluminal Device D Intraluminal Device H Contraceptive Device J Synthetic Substitute K Nonautologous Tissue Substitute	Z No Qualifier
H Vagina and Cul-de-sac ♀	Ø Open 3 Percutaneous 4 Percutaneous Endoscopic 7 Via Natural or Artificial Opening 8 Via Natural or Artificial Opening Endoscopic	Ø Drainage Device 1 Radioactive Element 3 Infusion Device 7 Autologous Tissue Substitute D Intraluminal Device J Synthetic Substitute K Nonautologous Tissue Substitute Y Other Device	Z No Qualifier
H Vagina and Cul-de-sac ♀	X External	Ø Drainage Device 3 Infusion Device 7 Autologous Tissue Substitute D Intraluminal Device J Synthetic Substitute K Nonautologous Tissue Substitute	Z No Qualifier
M Vulva ♀ Labia majora Labia minora	Ø Open X External	Ø Drainage Device 7 Autologous Tissue Substitute J Synthetic Substitute K Nonautologous Tissue Substitute	Z No Qualifier

Non-OR ØUW3[3,4]YZ
Non-OR ØUW3[7,8]YZ
Non-OR ØUW3X[Ø,3]Z
Non-OR ØUW8[3,4,7,8]YZ
Non-OR ØUW8X[Ø,3,7,C,D,J,K]Z
Non-OR ØUWD[3,4,7,8]YZ
Non-OR ØUWDX[Ø,3,7,C,D,H,J,K]Z
Non-OR ØUWH[3,4,7,8]YZ
Non-OR ØUWHX[Ø,3,7,D,J,K]Z
Non-OR ØUWMX[Ø,7,J,K]Z
♀ All body part, approach, device, and qualifier values

Ø Medical and Surgical
U Female Reproductive System
Y Transplantation Definition: Putting in or on all or a portion of a living body part taken from another individual or animal to physically take the place and/or function of all or a portion of a similar body part

Explanation: The native body part may or may not be taken out, and the transplanted body part may take over all or a portion of its function

Body Part Character 4	Approach Character 5	Device Character 6	Qualifier Character 7
Ø Ovary, Right ♀ **1** Ovary, Left ♀ **9** Uterus ♀	**Ø** Open	**Z** No Device	**Ø** Allogeneic **1** Syngeneic **2** Zooplastic

♀ All body part, approach, device, and qualifier values

Male Reproductive System ØV1–ØVY

Character Meanings

This Character Meaning table is provided as a guide to assist the user in the identification of character members that may be found in this section of code tables. It **SHOULD NOT** be used to build a PCS code.

Operation–Character 3		Body Part–Character 4		Approach–Character 5		Device–Character 6		Qualifier–Character 7	
1	Bypass	Ø	Prostate	Ø	Open	Ø	Drainage Device	Ø	Allogeneic
2	Change	1	Seminal Vesicle, Right	3	Percutaneous	1	Radioactive Element	1	Syngeneic
5	Destruction	2	Seminal Vesicle, Left	4	Percutaneous Endoscopic	3	Infusion Device	2	Zooplastic
7	Dilation	3	Seminal Vesicles, Bilateral	7	Via Natural or Artificial Opening	7	Autologous Tissue Substitute	3	Laser Interstitial Thermal Therapy
9	Drainage	4	Prostate and Seminal Vesicles	8	Via Natural or Artificial Opening Endoscopic	C	Extraluminal Device	D	Urethra
B	Excision	5	Scrotum	X	External	D	Intraluminal Device	J	Epididymis, Right
C	Extirpation	6	Tunica Vaginalis, Right			J	Synthetic Substitute	K	Epididymis, Left
H	Insertion	7	Tunica Vaginalis, Left			K	Nonautologous Tissue Substitute	N	Vas Deferens, Right
J	Inspection	8	Scrotum and Tunica Vaginalis			Y	Other Device	P	Vas Deferens, Left
L	Occlusion	9	Testis, Right			Z	No Device	S	Penis
M	Reattachment	B	Testis, Left					X	Diagnostic
N	Release	C	Testes, Bilateral					Z	No Qualifier
P	Removal	D	Testis						
Q	Repair	F	Spermatic Cord, Right						
R	Replacement	G	Spermatic Cord, Left						
S	Reposition	H	Spermatic Cords, Bilateral						
T	Resection	J	Epididymis, Right						
U	Supplement	K	Epididymis, Left						
W	Revision	L	Epididymis, Bilateral						
X	Transfer	M	Epididymis and Spermatic Cord						
Y	Transplantation	N	Vas Deferens, Right						
		P	Vas Deferens, Left						
		Q	Vas Deferens, Bilateral						
		R	Vas Deferens						
		S	Penis						
		T	Prepuce						

AHA Coding Clinic for table ØV1
2018, 3Q, 12 Al-Ghorab distal penile shunt surgery

AHA Coding Clinic for table ØV5
2022, 4Q, 53-54 Laser interstitial thermal therapy

AHA Coding Clinic for table ØV9
2018, 3Q, 12 Al-Ghorab distal penile shunt surgery

AHA Coding Clinic for table ØVB
2020, 1Q, 31 Repair of buried penis
2019, 3Q, 18 Radical prostatectomy and lymph node dissection with biopsy of neurovascular bundle
2016, 1Q, 23 Transurethral resection of ejaculatory ducts
2014, 4Q, 33 Radical prostatectomy

AHA Coding Clinic for table ØVH
2020, 4Q, 43-44 Insertion of radioactive element

AHA Coding Clinic for table ØVP
2016, 2Q, 28 Removal of multi-component inflatable penile prosthesis with placement of new malleable device

AHA Coding Clinic for table ØVQ
2018, 3Q, 12 Al-Ghorab distal penile shunt surgery

AHA Coding Clinic for table ØVT
2020, 4Q, 99 Robotic-assisted prostatectomy with extension of incision for specimen removal
2019, 3Q, 18 Radical prostatectomy and lymph node dissection with biopsy of neurovascular bundle
2014, 4Q, 33 Radical prostatectomy

AHA Coding Clinic for table ØVU
2020, 1Q, 31 Repair of buried penis
2016, 2Q, 28 Removal of multi-component inflatable penile prosthesis with placement of new malleable device
2015, 3Q, 25 Placement of inflatable penile prosthesis

AHA Coding Clinic for table ØVX
2018, 4Q, 40 Transfer of prepuce

AHA Coding Clinic for table ØVY
2023, 2Q, 32 Preparation of donor organ before transplantation
2020, 4Q, 58 Male reproductive organ transplant

Male Reproductive System

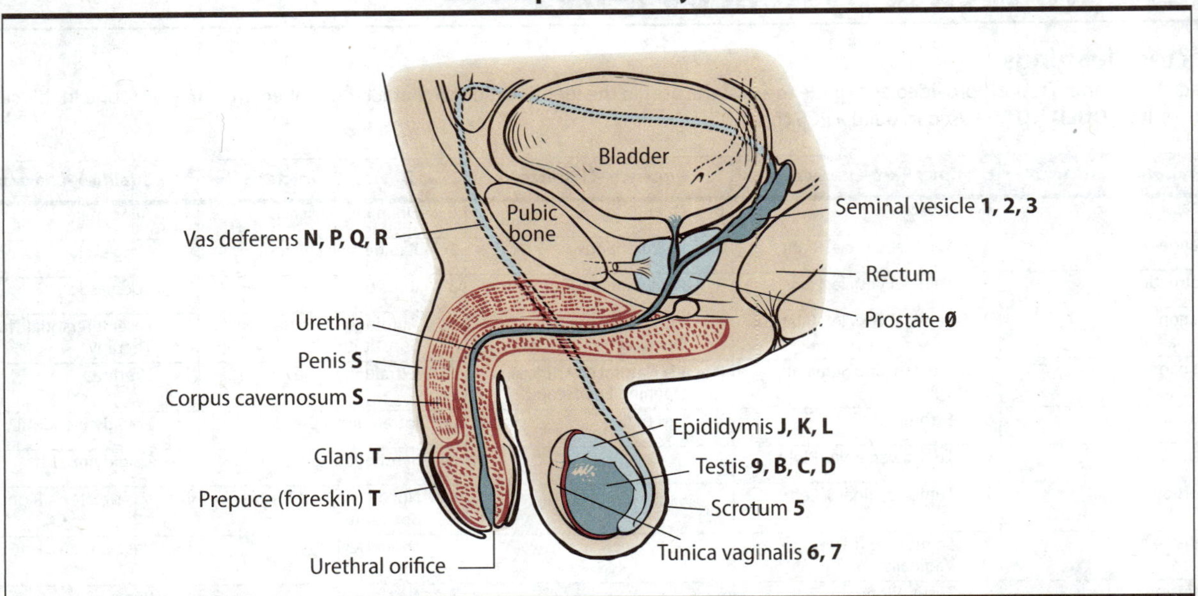

Penis

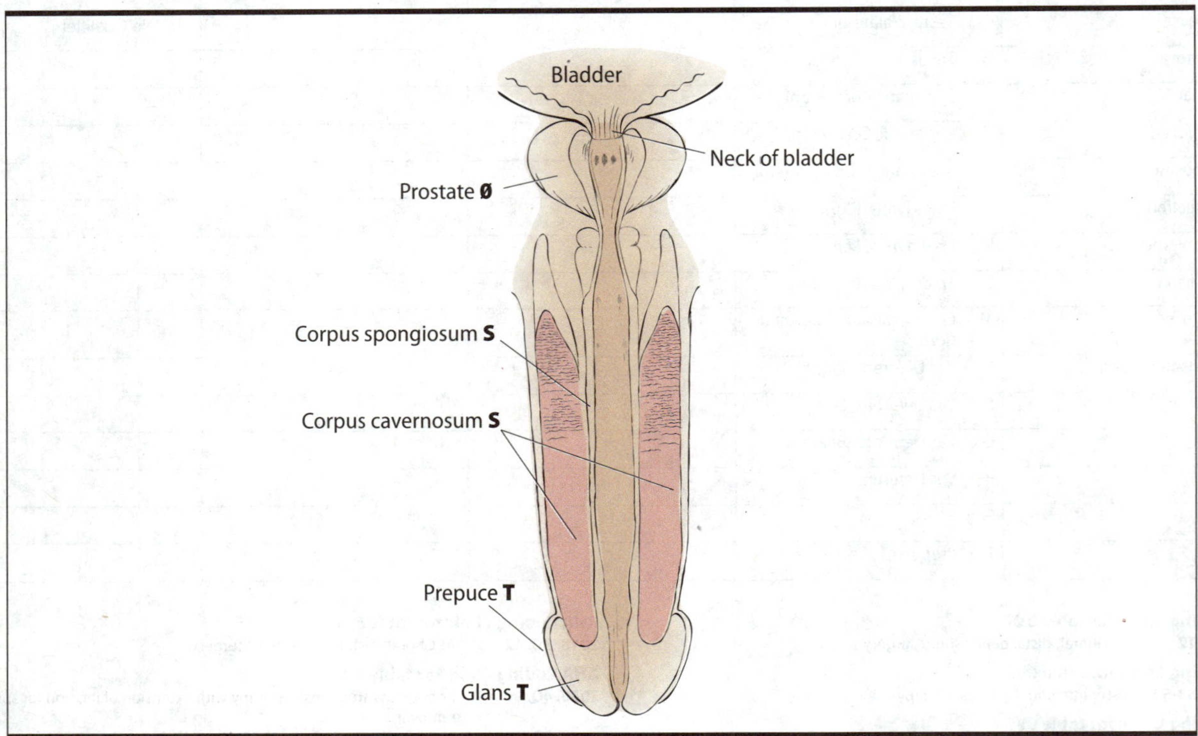

Ø Medical and Surgical
V Male Reproductive System
1 Bypass Definition: Altering the route of passage of the contents of a tubular body part

Explanation: Rerouting contents of a body part to a downstream area of the normal route, to a similar route and body part, or to an abnormal route and dissimilar body part. Includes one or more anastomoses, with or without the use of a device.

Body Part Character 4	Approach Character 5	Device Character 6	Qualifier Character 7
N Vas Deferens, Right ♂ Ductus deferens Ejaculatory duct P Vas Deferens, Left ♂ *See N Vas Deferens, Right* Q Vas Deferens, Bilateral ♂ *See N Vas Deferens, Right*	Ø Open 4 Percutaneous Endoscopic	7 Autologous Tissue Substitute J Synthetic Substitute K Nonautologous Tissue Substitute Z No Device	J Epididymis, Right K Epididymis, Left N Vas Deferens, Right P Vas Deferens, Left

♂ All body part, approach, device, and qualifier values

Ø Medical and Surgical
V Male Reproductive System
2 Change Definition: Taking out or off a device from a body part and putting back an identical or similar device in or on the same body part without cutting or puncturing the skin or a mucous membrane

Explanation: All CHANGE procedures are coded using the approach EXTERNAL

Body Part Character 4	Approach Character 5	Device Character 6	Qualifier Character 7
4 Prostate and Seminal Vesicles ♂ 8 Scrotum and Tunica Vaginalis ♂ D Testis ♂ M Epididymis and Spermatic Cord ♂ R Vas Deferens ♂ Ductus deferens Ejaculatory duct S Penis ♂ Corpus cavernosum Corpus spongiosum	X External	Ø Drainage Device Y Other Device	Z No Qualifier

Non-OR All body part, approach, device, and qualifier values
♂ All body part, approach, device, and qualifier values

Ø Medical and Surgical
V Male Reproductive System
5 Destruction Definition: Physical eradication of all or a portion of a body part by the direct use of energy, force, or a destructive agent

Explanation: None of the body part is physically taken out

Body Part Character 4	Approach Character 5	Device Character 6	Qualifier Character 7
Ø Prostate ♂	Ø Open 3 Percutaneous 4 Percutaneous Endoscopic	Z No Device	3 Laser Interstitial Thermal Therapy Z No Qualifier
Ø Prostate ♂	7 Via Natural or Artificial Opening 8 Via Natural or Artificial Opening Endoscopic	Z No Device	Z No Qualifier
1 Seminal Vesicle, Right ♂ 2 Seminal Vesicle, Left ♂ 3 Seminal Vesicles, Bilateral ♂ 6 Tunica Vaginalis, Right ♂ 7 Tunica Vaginalis, Left ♂ 9 Testis, Right ♂ B Testis, Left ♂ C Testes, Bilateral ♂	Ø Open 3 Percutaneous 4 Percutaneous Endoscopic	Z No Device	Z No Qualifier
5 Scrotum ♂ S Penis ♂ Corpus cavernosum Corpus spongiosum T Prepuce ♂ Foreskin Glans penis	Ø Open 3 Percutaneous 4 Percutaneous Endoscopic X External	Z No Device	Z No Qualifier
F Spermatic Cord, Right ♂ G Spermatic Cord, Left ♂ H Spermatic Cords, Bilateral ♂ J Epididymis, Right ♂ K Epididymis, Left ♂ L Epididymis, Bilateral ♂ N Vas Deferens, Right NC ♂ Ductus deferens Ejaculatory duct P Vas Deferens, Left NC ♂ *See N Vas Deferens, Right* Q Vas Deferens, Bilateral NC ♂ *See N Vas Deferens, Right*	Ø Open 3 Percutaneous 4 Percutaneous Endoscopic 8 Via Natural or Artificial Opening Endoscopic	Z No Device	Z No Qualifier

Non-OR ØV55[Ø,3,4,X]ZZ
Non-OR ØV5[N,P,Q][Ø,3,4,8]ZZ
NC ØV5[N,P,Q][Ø,3,4]ZZ with principal or secondary diagnosis of Z3Ø.2
♂ All body part, approach, device, and qualifier values

NC Noncovered Procedure | LC Limited Coverage | QA Questionable OB Admit | NT New Tech Add-on | Combination Member | ♂ Male | ♀ Female

Ø Medical and Surgical
V Male Reproductive System
7 Dilation

Definition: Expanding an orifice or the lumen of a tubular body part

Explanation: The orifice can be a natural orifice or an artificially created orifice. Accomplished by stretching a tubular body part using intraluminal pressure or by cutting part of the orifice or wall of the tubular body part.

Body Part Character 4	Approach Character 5	Device Character 6	Qualifier Character 7
N Vas Deferens, Right ♂ Ductus deferens Ejaculatory duct P Vas Deferens, Left ♂ *See N Vas Deferens, Right* Q Vas Deferens, Bilateral ♂ *See N Vas Deferens, Right*	Ø Open 3 Percutaneous 4 Percutaneous Endoscopic	D Intraluminal Device Z No Device	Z No Qualifier

♂ All body part, approach, device, and qualifier values

Ø Medical and Surgical
V Male Reproductive System
9 Drainage

Definition: Taking or letting out fluids and/or gases from a body part

Explanation: The qualifier DIAGNOSTIC is used to identify drainage procedures that are biopsies

Body Part Character 4	Approach Character 5	Device Character 6	Qualifier Character 7
Ø Prostate ♂	Ø Open 3 Percutaneous 4 Percutaneous Endoscopic 7 Via Natural or Artificial Opening 8 Via Natural or Artificial Opening Endoscopic	Ø Drainage Device	Z No Qualifier
Ø Prostate ♂	Ø Open 3 Percutaneous 4 Percutaneous Endoscopic 7 Via Natural or Artificial Opening 8 Via Natural or Artificial Opening Endoscopic	Z No Device	X Diagnostic Z No Qualifier
1 Seminal Vesicle, Right ♂ 2 Seminal Vesicle, Left ♂ 3 Seminal Vesicles, Bilateral ♂ 6 Tunica Vaginalis, Right ♂ 7 Tunica Vaginalis, Left ♂ 9 Testis, Right ♂ B Testis, Left ♂ C Testes, Bilateral ♂ F Spermatic Cord, Right ♂ G Spermatic Cord, Left ♂ H Spermatic Cords, Bilateral ♂ J Epididymis, Right ♂ K Epididymis, Left ♂ L Epididymis, Bilateral ♂ N Vas Deferens, Right ♂ Ductus deferens Ejaculatory duct P Vas Deferens, Left ♂ *See N Vas Deferens, Right* Q Vas Deferens, Bilateral ♂ *See N Vas Deferens, Right*	Ø Open 3 Percutaneous 4 Percutaneous Endoscopic	Ø Drainage Device	Z No Qualifier

Non-OR ØV9Ø[3,4]ØZ
Non-OR ØV9Ø[3,4]Z[X,Z]
Non-OR ØV9Ø[7,8]ZX
Non-OR ØV9[1,2,3,9,B,C][3,4]ØZ
Non-OR ØV9[6,7,F,G,H,N,P,Q][Ø,3,4]ØZ
Non-OR ØV9[J,K,L]3ØZ
♂ All body part, approach, device, and qualifier values

ØV9 Continued on next page

Ø Medical and Surgical
V Male Reproductive System
9 Drainage Definition: Taking or letting out fluids and/or gases from a body part
Explanation: The qualifier DIAGNOSTIC is used to identify drainage procedures that are biopsies

ØV9 Continued

Body Part Character 4	Approach Character 5	Device Character 6	Qualifier Character 7
1 Seminal Vesicle, Right ♂ **2 Seminal Vesicle, Left** ♂ **3 Seminal Vesicles, Bilateral** ♂ **6 Tunica Vaginalis, Right** ♂ **7 Tunica Vaginalis, Left** ♂ **9 Testis, Right** ♂ **B Testis, Left** ♂ **C Testes, Bilateral** ♂ **F Spermatic Cord, Right** ♂ **G Spermatic Cord, Left** ♂ **H Spermatic Cords, Bilateral** ♂ **J Epididymis, Right** ♂ **K Epididymis, Left** ♂ **L Epididymis, Bilateral** ♂ **N Vas Deferens, Right** ♂ Ductus deferens Ejaculatory duct **P Vas Deferens, Left** ♂ *See* *N Vas Deferens, Right* **Q Vas Deferens, Bilateral** ♂ *See* *N Vas Deferens, Right*	**Ø Open** **3 Percutaneous** **4 Percutaneous Endoscopic**	**Z No Device**	**X Diagnostic** **Z No Qualifier**
5 Scrotum ♂ **S Penis** ♂ Corpus cavernosum Corpus spongiosum **T Prepuce** ♂ Foreskin Glans penis	**Ø Open** **3 Percutaneous** **4 Percutaneous Endoscopic** **X External**	**Ø Drainage Device**	**Z No Qualifier**
5 Scrotum ♂ **S Penis** ♂ Corpus cavernosum Corpus spongiosum **T Prepuce** ♂ Foreskin Glans penis	**Ø Open** **3 Percutaneous** **4 Percutaneous Endoscopic** **X External**	**Z No Device**	**X Diagnostic** **Z No Qualifier**

Non-OR ØV9[1,2,3,9,B,C][3,4]Z[X,Z]
Non-OR ØV9[6,7,F,G,H,J,K,L,N,P,Q][Ø,3,4]ZX
Non-OR ØV9[6,7,F,G,H,N,P,Q][Ø,3,4]ZZ
Non-OR ØV9[J,K,L]3ZZ
Non-OR ØV95[Ø,3,4,X]ØZ
Non-OR ØV9[S,T]3ØZ
Non-OR ØV95ØZX
Non-OR ØV95[3,4,X]Z[X,Z]
Non-OR ØV9[S,T]3ZZ
♂ All body part, approach, device, and qualifier values

Ø Medical and Surgical
V Male Reproductive System
B Excision Definition: Cutting out or off, without replacement, a portion of a body part
Explanation: The qualifier DIAGNOSTIC is used to identify excision procedures that are biopsies

Body Part Character 4	Approach Character 5	Device Character 6	Qualifier Character 7
Ø Prostate ♂	**Ø Open** **3 Percutaneous** **4 Percutaneous Endoscopic** **7 Via Natural or Artificial Opening** **8 Via Natural or Artificial Opening Endoscopic**	**Z No Device**	**X Diagnostic** **Z No Qualifier**
1 Seminal Vesicle, Right ♂ **2 Seminal Vesicle, Left** ♂ **3 Seminal Vesicles, Bilateral** ♂ **6 Tunica Vaginalis, Right** ♂ **7 Tunica Vaginalis, Left** ♂ **9 Testis, Right** ♂ **B Testis, Left** ♂ **C Testes, Bilateral** ♂	**Ø Open** **3 Percutaneous** **4 Percutaneous Endoscopic**	**Z No Device**	**X Diagnostic** **Z No Qualifier**
5 Scrotum ♂ **S Penis** ♂ Corpus cavernosum Corpus spongiosum **T Prepuce** ♂ Foreskin Glans penis	**Ø Open** **3 Percutaneous** **4 Percutaneous Endoscopic** **X External**	**Z No Device**	**X Diagnostic** **Z No Qualifier**
F Spermatic Cord, Right ♂ **G Spermatic Cord, Left** ♂ **H Spermatic Cords, Bilateral** ♂ **J Epididymis, Right** ♂ **K Epididymis, Left** ♂ **L Epididymis, Bilateral** ♂ **N Vas Deferens, Right** NC ♂ Ductus deferens Ejaculatory duct **P Vas Deferens, Left** NC ♂ *See N Vas Deferens, Right* **Q Vas Deferens, Bilateral** NC ♂ *See N Vas Deferens, Right*	**Ø Open** **3 Percutaneous** **4 Percutaneous Endoscopic** **8 Via Natural or Artificial Opening Endoscopic**	**Z No Device**	**X Diagnostic** **Z No Qualifier**

Non-OR ØVBØ[3,4,7,8]ZX
Non-OR ØVB[1,2,3,9,B,C][3,4]ZX
Non-OR ØVB[6,7][Ø,3,4]ZX
Non-OR ØVB5ØZX
Non-OR ØVB5[3,4,X]Z[X,Z]
Non-OR ØVB[F,G,H,J,K,L][Ø,3,4,8]ZX
Non-OR ØVB[N,P,Q][Ø,3,4,8]Z[X,Z]
NC ØVB[N,P,Q][Ø,3,4]ZZ with principal or secondary diagnosis of Z3Ø.2
♂ All body part, approach, device, and qualifier values

Ø Medical and Surgical
V Male Reproductive System
C Extirpation Definition: Taking or cutting out solid matter from a body part

Explanation: The solid matter may be an abnormal byproduct of a biological function or a foreign body; it may be imbedded in a body part or in the lumen of a tubular body part. The solid matter may or may not have been previously broken into pieces.

Body Part Character 4	Approach Character 5	Device Character 6	Qualifier Character 7
Ø Prostate ♂	**Ø** Open **3** Percutaneous **4** Percutaneous Endoscopic **7** Via Natural or Artificial Opening **8** Via Natural or Artificial Opening Endoscopic	**Z** No Device	**Z** No Qualifier
1 Seminal Vesicle, Right ♂ **2** Seminal Vesicle, Left ♂ **3** Seminal Vesicles, Bilateral ♂ **6** Tunica Vaginalis, Right ♂ **7** Tunica Vaginalis, Left ♂ **9** Testis, Right ♂ **B** Testis, Left ♂ **C** Testes, Bilateral ♂ **F** Spermatic Cord, Right ♂ **G** Spermatic Cord, Left ♂ **H** Spermatic Cords, Bilateral ♂ **J** Epididymis, Right ♂ **K** Epididymis, Left ♂ **L** Epididymis, Bilateral ♂ **N** Vas Deferens, Right ♂ Ductus deferens Ejaculatory duct **P** Vas Deferens, Left ♂ *See N Vas Deferens, Right* **Q** Vas Deferens, Bilateral ♂ *See N Vas Deferens, Right*	**Ø** Open **3** Percutaneous **4** Percutaneous Endoscopic	**Z** No Device	**Z** No Qualifier
5 Scrotum ♂ **S** Penis ♂ Corpus cavernosum Corpus spongiosum **T** Prepuce ♂ Foreskin Glans penis	**Ø** Open **3** Percutaneous **4** Percutaneous Endoscopic **X** External	**Z** No Device	**Z** No Qualifier

Non-OR ØVC[6,7,N,P,Q][Ø,3,4]ZZ
Non-OR ØVC5[3,4,X]ZZ
Non-OR ØVCSXZZ
♂ All body part, approach, device, and qualifier values

Ø Medical and Surgical
V Male Reproductive System
H Insertion Definition: Putting in a nonbiological appliance that monitors, assists, performs, or prevents a physiological function but does not physically take the place of a body part

Explanation: None

Body Part Character 4	Approach Character 5	Device Character 6	Qualifier Character 7
Ø Prostate ♂	Ø Open 3 Percutaneous 4 Percutaneous Endoscopic 7 Via Natural or Artificial Opening 8 Via Natural or Artificial Opening Endoscopic	1 Radioactive Element	Z No Qualifier
4 Prostate and Seminal Vesicles ♂ 8 Scrotum and Tunica Vaginalis ♂ M Epididymis and Spermatic Cord ♂ R Vas Deferens ♂ Ductus deferens Ejaculatory duct	Ø Open 3 Percutaneous 4 Percutaneous Endoscopic 7 Via Natural or Artificial Opening 8 Via Natural or Artificial Opening Endoscopic	3 Infusion Device Y Other Device	Z No Qualifier
D Testis ♂	Ø Open 3 Percutaneous 4 Percutaneous Endoscopic 7 Via Natural or Artificial Opening 8 Via Natural or Artificial Opening Endoscopic	1 Radioactive Element 3 Infusion Device Y Other Device	Z No Qualifier
S Penis ♂ Corpus cavernosum Corpus spongiosum	Ø Open 3 Percutaneous 4 Percutaneous Endoscopic	3 Infusion Device Y Other Device	Z No Qualifier
S Penis ♂ Corpus cavernosum Corpus spongiosum	7 Via Natural or Artificial Opening 8 Via Natural or Artificial Opening Endoscopic	Y Other Device	Z No Qualifier
S Penis ♂ Corpus cavernosum Corpus spongiosum	X External	3 Infusion Device	Z No Qualifier

Non-OR ØVH[4,8,M,R][Ø,3,4,7,8][3,Y]Z
Non-OR ØVHD[Ø,3,4,7,8][1,3,Y]Z
Non-OR ØVHS[Ø,3,4][3,Y]Z
Non-OR ØVHS[7,8]YZ
Non-OR ØVHSX3Z
♂ All body part, approach, device, and qualifier values

Ø Medical and Surgical
V Male Reproductive System
J Inspection Definition: Visually and/or manually exploring a body part

Explanation: Visual exploration may be performed with or without optical instrumentation. Manual exploration may be performed directly or through intervening body layers.

Body Part Character 4	Approach Character 5	Device Character 6	Qualifier Character 7
4 Prostate and Seminal Vesicles ♂ 8 Scrotum and Tunica Vaginalis ♂ D Testis ♂ M Epididymis and Spermatic Cord ♂ R Vas Deferens ♂ Ductus deferens Ejaculatory duct S Penis ♂ Corpus cavernosum Corpus spongiosum	Ø Open 3 Percutaneous 4 Percutaneous Endoscopic X External	Z No Device	Z No Qualifier

Non-OR ØVJ[4,D,M,R][3,X]ZZ
Non-OR ØVJ8[Ø,3,4,X]ZZ
Non-OR ØVJS[3,4,X]ZZ
♂ All body part, approach, device, and qualifier values

Ø Medical and Surgical
V Male Reproductive System
L Occlusion Definition: Completely closing an orifice or the lumen of a tubular body part
Explanation: The orifice can be a natural orifice or an artificially created orifice

Body Part Character 4	Approach Character 5	Device Character 6	Qualifier Character 7
F Spermatic Cord, Right NC ♂ G Spermatic Cord, Left NC ♂ H Spermatic Cords, Bilateral NC ♂ N Vas Deferens, Right NC ♂ Ductus deferens Ejaculatory duct P Vas Deferens, Left NC ♂ *See N Vas Deferens, Right* Q Vas Deferens, Bilateral NC ♂ *See N Vas Deferens, Right*	Ø Open 3 Percutaneous 4 Percutaneous Endoscopic 8 Via Natural or Artificial Opening Endoscopic	C Extraluminal Device D Intraluminal Device Z No Device	Z No Qualifier

Non-OR ØVL[F,G,H][Ø,3,4,8][C,D,Z]Z
Non-OR ØVL[N,P,Q][Ø,3,4,8][C,Z]Z

NC ØVL[F,G,H][Ø,3,4][C,D,Z]Z with principal or secondary diagnosis of Z3Ø.2
NC ØVL[N,P,Q][Ø,3,4][C,Z]Z with principal or secondary diagnosis of Z3Ø.2
♂ All body part, approach, device, and qualifier values

Ø Medical and Surgical
V Male Reproductive System
M Reattachment Definition: Putting back in or on all or a portion of a separated body part to its normal location or other suitable location
Explanation: Vascular circulation and nervous pathways may or may not be reestablished

Body Part Character 4	Approach Character 5	Device Character 6	Qualifier Character 7
5 Scrotum ♂ S Penis ♂ Corpus cavernosum Corpus spongiosum	X External	Z No Device	Z No Qualifier
6 Tunica Vaginalis, Right ♂ 7 Tunica Vaginalis, Left ♂ 9 Testis, Right ♂ B Testis, Left ♂ C Testes, Bilateral ♂ F Spermatic Cord, Right ♂ G Spermatic Cord, Left ♂ H Spermatic Cords, Bilateral ♂	Ø Open 4 Percutaneous Endoscopic	Z No Device	Z No Qualifier

♂ All body part, approach, device, and qualifier values

Ø Medical and Surgical
V Male Reproductive System
N Release Definition: Freeing a body part from an abnormal physical constraint by cutting or by the use of force

Explanation: Some of the restraining tissue may be taken out but none of the body part is taken out

Body Part Character 4	Approach Character 5	Device Character 6	Qualifier Character 7
Ø Prostate ♂	**Ø Open** **3 Percutaneous** **4 Percutaneous Endoscopic** **7 Via Natural or Artificial Opening** **8 Via Natural or Artificial Opening Endoscopic**	**Z No Device**	**Z No Qualifier**
1 Seminal Vesicle, Right ♂ **2 Seminal Vesicle, Left** ♂ **3 Seminal Vesicles, Bilateral** ♂ **6 Tunica Vaginalis, Right** ♂ **7 Tunica Vaginalis, Left** ♂ **9 Testis, Right** ♂ **B Testis, Left** ♂ **C Testes, Bilateral** ♂	**Ø Open** **3 Percutaneous** **4 Percutaneous Endoscopic**	**Z No Device**	**Z No Qualifier**
5 Scrotum ♂ **S Penis** ♂ Corpus cavernosum Corpus spongiosum **T Prepuce** ♂ Foreskin Glans penis	**Ø Open** **3 Percutaneous** **4 Percutaneous Endoscopic** **X External**	**Z No Device**	**Z No Qualifier**
F Spermatic Cord, Right ♂ **G Spermatic Cord, Left** ♂ **H Spermatic Cords, Bilateral** ♂ **J Epididymis, Right** ♂ **K Epididymis, Left** ♂ **L Epididymis, Bilateral** ♂ **N Vas Deferens, Right** ♂ Ductus deferens Ejaculatory duct **P Vas Deferens, Left** ♂ *See N Vas Deferens, Right* **Q Vas Deferens, Bilateral** ♂ *See N Vas Deferens, Right*	**Ø Open** **3 Percutaneous** **4 Percutaneous Endoscopic** **8 Via Natural or Artificial Opening Endoscopic**	**Z No Device**	**Z No Qualifier**

Non-OR ØVN[9,B,C][Ø,3,4]ZZ
Non-OR ØVNT[Ø,3,4,X]ZZ

♂ All body part, approach, device, and qualifier values

Ø Medical and Surgical
V Male Reproductive System
P Removal Definition: Taking out or off a device from a body part

Explanation: If a device is taken out and a similar device put in without cutting or puncturing the skin or mucous membrane, the procedure is coded to the root operation CHANGE. Otherwise, the procedure for taking out the device is coded to the root operation REMOVAL.

Body Part Character 4	Approach Character 5	Device Character 6	Qualifier Character 7
4 Prostate and Seminal Vesicles ♂	Ø Open 3 Percutaneous 4 Percutaneous Endoscopic 7 Via Natural or Artificial Opening 8 Via Natural or Artificial Opening Endoscopic	Ø Drainage Device 1 Radioactive Element 3 Infusion Device 7 Autologous Tissue Substitute J Synthetic Substitute K Nonautologous Tissue Substitute Y Other Device	Z No Qualifier
4 Prostate and Seminal Vesicles ♂	X External	Ø Drainage Device 1 Radioactive Element 3 Infusion Device	Z No Qualifier
8 Scrotum and Tunica Vaginalis ♂ D Testis ♂ S Penis ♂ Corpus cavernosum Corpus spongiosum	Ø Open 3 Percutaneous 4 Percutaneous Endoscopic 7 Via Natural or Artificial Opening 8 Via Natural or Artificial Opening Endoscopic	Ø Drainage Device 3 Infusion Device 7 Autologous Tissue Substitute J Synthetic Substitute K Nonautologous Tissue Substitute Y Other Device	Z No Qualifier
8 Scrotum and Tunica Vaginalis ♂ D Testis ♂ S Penis ♂ Corpus cavernosum Corpus spongiosum	X External	Ø Drainage Device 3 Infusion Device	Z No Qualifier
M Epididymis and Spermatic Cord ♂	Ø Open 3 Percutaneous 4 Percutaneous Endoscopic 7 Via Natural or Artificial Opening 8 Via Natural or Artificial Opening Endoscopic	Ø Drainage Device 3 Infusion Device 7 Autologous Tissue Substitute C Extraluminal Device J Synthetic Substitute K Nonautologous Tissue Substitute Y Other Device	Z No Qualifier
M Epididymis and Spermatic Cord ♂	X External	Ø Drainage Device 3 Infusion Device	Z No Qualifier
R Vas Deferens ♂ Ductus deferens Ejaculatory duct	Ø Open 3 Percutaneous 4 Percutaneous Endoscopic 7 Via Natural or Artificial Opening 8 Via Natural or Artificial Opening Endoscopic	Ø Drainage Device 3 Infusion Device 7 Autologous Tissue Substitute C Extraluminal Device D Intraluminal Device J Synthetic Substitute K Nonautologous Tissue Substitute Y Other Device	Z No Qualifier
R Vas Deferens ♂ Ductus deferens Ejaculatory duct	X External	Ø Drainage Device 3 Infusion Device D Intraluminal Device	Z No Qualifier

Non-OR ØVP4[3,4]YZ
Non-OR ØVP4[7,8][Ø,3,Y]Z
Non-OR ØVP4X[Ø,1,3]Z
Non-OR ØVP8[Ø,3,4,7,8][Ø,3,7,J,K,Y]Z
Non-OR ØVP[D,S][3,4]YZ
Non-OR ØVP[D,S][7,8][Ø,3,Y]Z
Non-OR ØVP[8,D,S]X[Ø,3]Z
Non-OR ØVPM[3,4]YZ
Non-OR ØVPM[7,8][Ø,3,Y]Z
Non-OR ØVPMX[Ø,3]Z
Non-OR ØVPR[Ø,3,4][Ø,3,7,C,J,K,Y]Z
Non-OR ØVPR[7,8][Ø,3,7,C,D,J,K,Y]Z
Non-OR ØVPRX[Ø,3,D]Z
♂ All body part, approach, device, and qualifier values

Ø Medical and Surgical
V Male Reproductive System
Q Repair Definition: Restoring, to the extent possible, a body part to its normal anatomic structure and function

Explanation: Used only when the method to accomplish the repair is not one of the other root operations

Body Part Character 4	Approach Character 5	Device Character 6	Qualifier Character 7
Ø Prostate ♂	Ø Open 3 Percutaneous 4 Percutaneous Endoscopic 7 Via Natural or Artificial Opening 8 Via Natural or Artificial Opening Endoscopic	Z No Device	Z No Qualifier
1 Seminal Vesicle, Right ♂ 2 Seminal Vesicle, Left ♂ 3 Seminal Vesicles, Bilateral ♂ 6 Tunica Vaginalis, Right ♂ 7 Tunica Vaginalis, Left ♂ 9 Testis, Right ♂ B Testis, Left ♂ C Testes, Bilateral ♂	Ø Open 3 Percutaneous 4 Percutaneous Endoscopic	Z No Device	Z No Qualifier
5 Scrotum ♂ S Penis ♂ Corpus cavernosum Corpus spongiosum T Prepuce ♂ Foreskin Glans penis	Ø Open 3 Percutaneous 4 Percutaneous Endoscopic X External	Z No Device	Z No Qualifier
F Spermatic Cord, Right ♂ G Spermatic Cord, Left ♂ H Spermatic Cords, Bilateral ♂ J Epididymis, Right ♂ K Epididymis, Left ♂ L Epididymis, Bilateral ♂ N Vas Deferens, Right ♂ Ductus deferens Ejaculatory duct P Vas Deferens, Left ♂ *See* N Vas Deferens, Right Q Vas Deferens, Bilateral ♂ *See* N Vas Deferens, Right	Ø Open 3 Percutaneous 4 Percutaneous Endoscopic 8 Via Natural or Artificial Opening Endoscopic	Z No Device	Z No Qualifier

Non-OR ØVQ[6,7][Ø,3,4]ZZ
Non-OR ØVQ5[Ø,3,4,X]ZZ

♂ All body part, approach, device, and qualifier values

Ø Medical and Surgical
V Male Reproductive System
R Replacement Definition: Putting in or on biological or synthetic material that physically takes the place and/or function of all or a portion of a body part

Explanation: The body part may have been taken out or replaced, or may be taken out, physically eradicated, or rendered nonfunctional during the REPLACEMENT procedure. A REMOVAL procedure is coded for taking out the device used in a previous replacement procedure.

Body Part Character 4	Approach Character 5	Device Character 6	Qualifier Character 7
9 Testis, Right ♂ B Testis, Left ♂ C Testes, Bilateral ♂	Ø Open	J Synthetic Substitute	Z No Qualifier

♂ All body part, approach, device, and qualifier values

Ø Medical and Surgical
V Male Reproductive System
S Reposition Definition: Moving to its normal location, or other suitable location, all or a portion of a body part

Explanation: The body part is moved to a new location from an abnormal location, or from a normal location where it is not functioning correctly. The body part may or may not be cut out or off to be moved to the new location.

Body Part Character 4	Approach Character 5	Device Character 6	Qualifier Character 7
9 Testis, Right ♂ B Testis, Left ♂ C Testes, Bilateral ♂ F Spermatic Cord, Right ♂ G Spermatic Cord, Left ♂ H Spermatic Cords, Bilateral ♂	Ø Open 3 Percutaneous 4 Percutaneous Endoscopic 8 Via Natural or Artificial Opening Endoscopic	Z No Device	Z No Qualifier

♂ All body part, approach, device, and qualifier values

Ø Medical and Surgical
V Male Reproductive System
T Resection Definition: Cutting out or off, without replacement, all of a body part
Explanation: None

Body Part Character 4	Approach Character 5	Device Character 6	Qualifier Character 7
Ø Prostate ♂	Ø Open 4 Percutaneous Endoscopic 7 Via Natural or Artificial Opening 8 Via Natural or Artificial Opening Endoscopic	Z No Device	Z No Qualifier
1 Seminal Vesicle, Right ♂ 2 Seminal Vesicle, Left ♂ 3 Seminal Vesicles, Bilateral ♂ 6 Tunica Vaginalis, Right ♂ 7 Tunica Vaginalis, Left ♂ 9 Testis, Right ♂ B Testis, Left ♂ C Testes, Bilateral ♂ F Spermatic Cord, Right ♂ G Spermatic Cord, Left ♂ H Spermatic Cords, Bilateral ♂ J Epididymis, Right ♂ K Epididymis, Left ♂ L Epididymis, Bilateral ♂ N Vas Deferens, Right NC ♂ Ductus deferens Ejaculatory duct P Vas Deferens, Left NC ♂ *See* *N Vas Deferens, Right* Q Vas Deferens, Bilateral NC ♂ *See* *N Vas Deferens, Right*	Ø Open 4 Percutaneous Endoscopic	Z No Device	Z No Qualifier
5 Scrotum ♂ S Penis ♂ Corpus cavernosum Corpus spongiosum T Prepuce ♂ Foreskin Glans penis	Ø Open 4 Percutaneous Endoscopic X External	Z No Device	Z No Qualifier

Non-OR ØVT[N,P,Q][Ø,4]ZZ
Non-OR ØVT[5,T][Ø,4,X]ZZ
NC ØVT[N,P,Q][Ø,4]ZZ with principal or secondary diagnosis of Z3Ø.2
♂ All body part, approach, device, and qualifier values

See Appendix L for Procedure Combinations
ØVTØ[Ø,4,7,8]ZZ
ØVT3[Ø,4]ZZ

Ø Medical and Surgical
V Male Reproductive System
U Supplement Definition: Putting in or on biological or synthetic material that physically reinforces and/or augments the function of a portion of a body part

Explanation: The biological material is non-living, or is living and from the same individual. The body part may have been previously replaced, and the SUPPLEMENT procedure is performed to physically reinforce and/or augment the function of the replaced body part.

Body Part Character 4	Approach Character 5	Device Character 6	Qualifier Character 7
1 Seminal Vesicle, Right ♂ **2 Seminal Vesicle, Left** ♂ **3 Seminal Vesicles, Bilateral** ♂ **6 Tunica Vaginalis, Right** ♂ **7 Tunica Vaginalis, Left** ♂ **F Spermatic Cord, Right** ♂ **G Spermatic Cord, Left** ♂ **H Spermatic Cords, Bilateral** ♂ **J Epididymis, Right** ♂ **K Epididymis, Left** ♂ **L Epididymis, Bilateral** ♂ **N Vas Deferens, Right** ♂ Ductus deferens Ejaculatory duct **P Vas Deferens, Left** ♂ *See N Vas Deferens, Right* **Q Vas Deferens, Bilateral** ♂ *See N Vas Deferens, Right*	**Ø Open** **4 Percutaneous Endoscopic** **8 Via Natural or Artificial Opening Endoscopic**	**7 Autologous Tissue Substitute** **J Synthetic Substitute** **K Nonautologous Tissue Substitute**	**Z No Qualifier**
5 Scrotum ♂ **S Penis** ♂ Corpus cavernosum Corpus spongiosum **T Prepuce** ♂ Foreskin Glans penis	**Ø Open** **4 Percutaneous Endoscopic** **X External**	**7 Autologous Tissue Substitute** **J Synthetic Substitute** **K Nonautologous Tissue Substitute**	**Z No Qualifier**
9 Testis, Right ♂ **B Testis, Left** ♂ **C Testes, Bilateral** ♂	**Ø Open**	**7 Autologous Tissue Substitute** **J Synthetic Substitute** **K Nonautologous Tissue Substitute**	**Z No Qualifier**

Non-OR ØVUSX[7,J,K]Z

♂ All body part, approach, device, and qualifier values

Ø Medical and Surgical
V Male Reproductive System
W Revision

Definition: Correcting, to the extent possible, a portion of a malfunctioning device or the position of a displaced device

Explanation: Revision can include correcting a malfunctioning or displaced device by taking out or putting in components of the device such as a screw or pin

Body Part Character 4	Approach Character 5	Device Character 6	Qualifier Character 7
4 Prostate and Seminal Vesicles ♂ **8** Scrotum and Tunica Vaginalis ♂ **D** Testis ♂ **S** Penis ♂ Corpus cavernosum Corpus spongiosum	**Ø** Open **3** Percutaneous **4** Percutaneous Endoscopic **7** Via Natural or Artificial Opening **8** Via Natural or Artificial Opening Endoscopic	**Ø** Drainage Device **3** Infusion Device **7** Autologous Tissue Substitute **J** Synthetic Substitute **K** Nonautologous Tissue Substitute **Y** Other Device	**Z** No Qualifier
4 Prostate and Seminal Vesicles ♂ **8** Scrotum and Tunica Vaginalis ♂ **D** Testis ♂ **S** Penis ♂ Corpus cavernosum Corpus spongiosum	**X** External	**Ø** Drainage Device **3** Infusion Device **7** Autologous Tissue Substitute **J** Synthetic Substitute **K** Nonautologous Tissue Substitute	**Z** No Qualifier
M Epididymis and Spermatic Cord ♂	**Ø** Open **3** Percutaneous **4** Percutaneous Endoscopic **7** Via Natural or Artificial Opening **8** Via Natural or Artificial Opening Endoscopic	**Ø** Drainage Device **3** Infusion Device **7** Autologous Tissue Substitute **C** Extraluminal Device **J** Synthetic Substitute **K** Nonautologous Tissue Substitute **Y** Other Device	**Z** No Qualifier
M Epididymis and Spermatic Cord ♂	**X** External	**Ø** Drainage Device **3** Infusion Device **7** Autologous Tissue Substitute **C** Extraluminal Device **J** Synthetic Substitute **K** Nonautologous Tissue Substitute	**Z** No Qualifier
R Vas Deferens ♂ Ductus deferens Ejaculatory duct	**Ø** Open **3** Percutaneous **4** Percutaneous Endoscopic **7** Via Natural or Artificial Opening **8** Via Natural or Artificial Opening Endoscopic	**Ø** Drainage Device **3** Infusion Device **7** Autologous Tissue Substitute **C** Extraluminal Device **D** Intraluminal Device **J** Synthetic Substitute **K** Nonautologous Tissue Substitute **Y** Other Device	**Z** No Qualifier
R Vas Deferens ♂ Ductus deferens Ejaculatory duct	**X** External	**Ø** Drainage Device **3** Infusion Device **7** Autologous Tissue Substitute **C** Extraluminal Device **D** Intraluminal Device **J** Synthetic Substitute **K** Nonautologous Tissue Substitute	**Z** No Qualifier

Non-OR ØVW[4,D,S][3,4,7,8]YZ
Non-OR ØVW8[Ø,3,4,7,8][Ø,3,7,J,K,Y]Z
Non-OR ØVW[4,8,D,S]X[Ø,3,7,J,K]Z
Non-OR ØVWM[3,4,7,8]YZ
Non-OR ØVWMX[Ø,3,7,C,J,K]Z
Non-OR ØVWR[Ø,3,4,7,8][Ø,3,7,C,D,J,K,Y]Z
Non-OR ØVWRX[Ø,3,7,C,D,J,K]Z
♂ All body part, approach, device, and qualifier values

Ø Medical and Surgical
V Male Reproductive System
X Transfer Definition: Moving, without taking out, all or a portion of a body part to another location to take over the function of all or a portion of a body part

Explanation: The body part transferred remains connected to its vascular and nervous supply

Body Part Character 4	Approach Character 5	Device Character 6	Qualifier Character 7
T Prepuce Foreskin Glans penis	**Ø Open** **X External**	**Z No Device**	**D Urethra** **S Penis**

Ø Medical and Surgical
V Male Reproductive System
Y Transplantation Definition: Putting in or on all or a portion of a living body part taken from another individual or animal to physically take the place and/or function of all or a portion of a similar body part

Explanation: The native body part may or may not be taken out, and the transplanted body part may take over all or a portion of its function

Body Part Character 4	Approach Character 5	Device Character 6	Qualifier Character 7
5 Scrotum ♂ **S Penis** ♂ Corpus cavernosum Corpus spongiosum	**Ø Open**	**Z No Device**	**Ø Allogeneic** **1 Syngeneic** **2 Zooplastic**

♂ All body part, approach, device, and qualifier values

Anatomical Regions, General ØWØ–ØWY

Character Meanings

This Character Meaning table is provided as a guide to assist the user in the identification of character members that may be found in this section of code tables. It **SHOULD NOT** be used to build a PCS code.

Operation–Character 3	Body Region–Character 4	Approach–Character 5	Device–Character 6	Qualifier–Character 7
Ø Alteration	Ø Head	Ø Open	Ø Drainage Device	Ø Vagina OR Allogeneic
1 Bypass	1 Cranial Cavity	3 Percutaneous	1 Radioactive Element	1 Penis OR Syngeneic
2 Change	2 Face	4 Percutaneous Endoscopic	3 Infusion Device	2 Stoma
3 Control	3 Oral Cavity and Throat	7 Via Natural or Artificial Opening	7 Autologous Tissue Substitute	4 Cutaneous
4 Creation	4 Upper Jaw	8 Via Natural or Artificial Opening Endoscopic	G Defibrillator Lead	6 Bladder
8 Division	5 Lower Jaw	X External	J Synthetic Substitute	9 Pleural Cavity, Right
9 Drainage	6 Neck		K Nonautologous Tissue Substitute	B Pleural Cavity, Left
B Excision	8 Chest Wall		Y Other Device	G Peritoneal Cavity
C Extirpation	9 Pleural Cavity, Right		Z No Device	J Pelvic Cavity
F Fragmentation	B Pleural Cavity, Left			W Upper Vein
H Insertion	C Mediastinum			X Diagnostic
J Inspection	D Pericardial Cavity			Y Lower Vein
M Reattachment	F Abdominal Wall			Z No Qualifier
P Removal	G Peritoneal Cavity			
Q Repair	H Retroperitoneum			
U Supplement	J Pelvic Cavity			
W Revision	K Upper Back			
Y Transplantation	L Lower Back			
	M Perineum, Male			
	N Perineum, Female			
	P Gastrointestinal Tract			
	Q Respiratory Tract			
	R Genitourinary Tract			

AHA Coding Clinic for table ØWØ
2015, 1Q, 31 Bilateral browpexy

AHA Coding Clinic for table ØW1
2020, 4Q, 55 Insertion of subcutaneous pump system for ascites drainage
2018, 4Q, 41-42 Anatomical regions bypass qualifiers
2015, 2Q, 36 Insertion of infusion device into peritoneal cavity
2013, 4Q, 126-127 Creation of percutaneous cutaneoperitoneal fistula

AHA Coding Clinic for table ØW3
2023, 2Q, 26 Control of bleeding with Hemospray®
2021, 3Q, 26 Cavoatrial junction tear with repair and relief of cardiac tamponade
2019, 3Q, 4 Evacuation of subdural hematoma and control of bleeding artery
2018, 4Q, 38 Control of epistaxis
2018, 1Q, 19 Argon plasma coagulation of duodenal arteriovenous malformation
2018, 1Q, 19 Control of epistaxis via silver nitrate cauterization
2017, 4Q, 57-58 Added approach values - Transorifice esophageal vein banding
2017, 4Q, 105 Control of gastrointestinal bleeding
2017, 4Q, 106 Control of bleeding of external naris using suture
2017, 4Q, 106 Nasal packing for epistaxis
2016, 4Q, 99-100 Root operation Control
2014, 4Q, 44 Bakri balloon for control of postpartum hemorrhage
2013, 3Q, 23 Control of intraoperative bleeding

AHA Coding Clinic for table ØW4
2019, 4Q, 30 Transfer large intestine to vagina
2016, 4Q, 101 Root operation Creation

AHA Coding Clinic for table ØW9
2022, 4Q, 59-60 Drainage of the parapharyngeal space and retropharyngeal space
2021, 3Q, 17 Incision and drainage of retropharyngeal space abscess
2021, 3Q, 21 Drainage of midline neck abscess
2021, 3Q, 26 Cavoatrial junction tear with repair and relief of cardiac tamponade
2020, 4Q, 56 Transvaginal drainage of pelvis
2017, 3Q, 12 Therapeutic and diagnostic paracentesis
2017, 2Q, 16 Incision and drainage of floor of mouth

AHA Coding Clinic for table ØWB
2021, 3Q, 21 Excision of thyroglossal duct cyst
2019, 1Q, 27 Excision of pelvic sidewall mass
2017, 2Q, 16 Excision of floor of mouth
2016, 1Q, 21 Excision of urachal mass
2013, 4Q, 119 Excision of inclusion cyst of perineum

AHA Coding Clinic for table ØWC
2022, 1Q, 42 Removal of fat necrosis from retroperitoneum and space of Retzius
2019, 4Q, 35 Extirpation of jaw
2017, 2Q, 16 Excision of floor of mouth

AHA Coding Clinic for table ØWH
2021, 2Q, 14 Peritoneal dialysis catheter placement
2019, 4Q, 43 Unidirectional source brachytherapy
2018, 1Q, 25 Intrauterine brachytherapy & placement of tandems & ovoids
2017, 4Q, 104 Intrauterine brachytherapy & placement of tandems & ovoids
2016, 2Q, 14 Insertion of peritoneal totally implantable venous access device
2015, 2Q, 36 Insertion of infusion device into peritoneal cavity

AHA Coding Clinic for table ØWJ
2022, 3Q, 19 Aortic cross-clamping and exploratory thoracotomy
2021, 2Q, 19 Electromagnetic stealth guided ventriculoperitoneal shunt insertion with endoscopy
2019, 1Q, 3-8 Whipple procedure
2019, 1Q, 25 Laparoscopic appendectomy converted to open procedure
2018, 3Q, 29 Decommissioning of left ventricular assist device with exploration of mediastinum
2016, 4Q, 58 Longitudinal vaginal septum
2013, 2Q, 36 Insertion of ventriculoperitoneal shunt with laparoscopic assistance

AHA Coding Clinic for table ØWP
2021, 2Q, 14 Removal of peritoneal dialysis catheter

AHA Coding Clinic for table ØWQ
2017, 4Q, 106 Control of bleeding of external naris using suture
2017, 3Q, 8 Removal of silo and closure of gastroschisis
2016, 3Q, 3-7 Stoma creation & takedown procedures
2014, 4Q, 38 Abdominoplasty and abdominal wall plication for hernia repair
2014, 3Q, 28 Ileostomy takedown and parastomal hernia repair

AHA Coding Clinic for table ØWU
2017, 3Q, 8 First stage of gastroschisis repair with silo placement
2016, 3Q, 40 Omentoplasty
2015, 2Q, 29 Placement of Ioban™ antimicrobial drape over surgical wound
2014, 4Q, 39 Abdominal component release with placement of mesh for hernia repair
2012, 4Q, 101 Rib resection with reconstruction of anterior chest wall

AHA Coding Clinic for table ØWW
2015, 2Q, 9 Revision of ventriculoperitoneal (VP) shunt

AHA Coding Clinic for table ØWY
2016, 4Q, 112-113 Transplantation

Ø Medical and Surgical
W Anatomical Regions, General
Ø Alteration Definition: Modifying the anatomic structure of a body part without affecting the function of the body part

Explanation: Principal purpose is to improve appearance

Body Part Character 4	Approach Character 5	Device Character 6	Qualifier Character 7
Ø Head 2 Face 4 Upper Jaw 5 Lower Jaw 6 Neck Parapharyngeal space Retropharyngeal space 8 Chest Wall F Abdominal Wall K Upper Back L Lower Back M Perineum, Male ♂ N Perineum, Female ♀	Ø Open 3 Percutaneous 4 Percutaneous Endoscopic	7 Autologous Tissue Substitute J Synthetic Substitute K Nonautologous Tissue Substitute Z No Device	Z No Qualifier

♂ ØWØM[Ø,3,4][7,J,K,Z]Z
♀ ØWØN[Ø,3,4][7,J,K,Z]Z

Ø Medical and Surgical
W Anatomical Regions, General
1 Bypass Definition: Altering the route of passage of the contents of a tubular body part

Explanation: Rerouting contents of a body part to a downstream area of the normal route, to a similar route and body part, or to an abnormal route and dissimilar body part. Includes one or more anastomoses, with or without the use of a device.

Body Part Character 4	Approach Character 5	Device Character 6	Qualifier Character 7
1 Cranial Cavity	Ø Open	J Synthetic Substitute	9 Pleural Cavity, Right B Pleural Cavity, Left G Peritoneal Cavity J Pelvic Cavity
9 Pleural Cavity, Right B Pleural Cavity, Left J Pelvic Cavity Retropubic space Space of Retzius	Ø Open 3 Percutaneous 4 Percutaneous Endoscopic	J Synthetic Substitute	4 Cutaneous 9 Pleural Cavity, Right B Pleural Cavity, Left G Peritoneal Cavity J Pelvic Cavity W Upper Vein Y Lower Vein
G Peritoneal Cavity Abdominal cavity	Ø Open 3 Percutaneous 4 Percutaneous Endoscopic	J Synthetic Substitute	4 Cutaneous 6 Bladder 9 Pleural Cavity, Right B Pleural Cavity, Left G Peritoneal Cavity J Pelvic Cavity W Upper Vein Y Lower Vein

Non-OR ØW1[9,B][Ø,3,4]J[4,G,W,Y]
Non-OR ØW1J[Ø,3,4]J[4,W,Y]
Non-OR ØW1G[Ø,3,4]J[9,B,G,J]

Ø Medical and Surgical
W Anatomical Regions, General
2 Change Definition: Taking out or off a device from a body part and putting back an identical or similar device in or on the same body part without cutting or puncturing the skin or a mucous membrane

Explanation: All CHANGE procedures are coded using the approach EXTERNAL

Body Part Character 4	Approach Character 5	Device Character 6	Qualifier Character 7
Ø Head **1** Cranial Cavity **2** Face **4** Upper Jaw **5** Lower Jaw **6** Neck Parapharyngeal space Retropharyngeal space **8** Chest Wall **9** Pleural Cavity, Right **B** Pleural Cavity, Left **C** Mediastinum Mediastinal cavity Mediastinal space **D** Pericardial Cavity **F** Abdominal Wall **G** Peritoneal Cavity Abdominal cavity **H** Retroperitoneum Retroperitoneal cavity Retroperitoneal space **J** Pelvic Cavity Retropubic space Space of Retzius **K** Upper Back **L** Lower Back **M** Perineum, Male ♂ **N** Perineum, Female ♀	**X** External	**Ø** Drainage Device **Y** Other Device	**Z** No Qualifier

Non-OR All body part, approach, device, and qualifier values

♂ ØW2MX[Ø,Y]Z
♀ ØW2NX[Ø,Y]Z

Ø Medical and Surgical
W Anatomical Regions, General
3 Control Definition: Stopping, or attempting to stop, postprocedural or other acute bleeding
Explanation: None

Body Part Character 4	Approach Character 5	Device Character 6	Qualifier Character 7
Ø Head 1 Cranial Cavity 2 Face 4 Upper Jaw 5 Lower Jaw 6 Neck Parapharyngeal space Retropharyngeal space 8 Chest Wall 9 Pleural Cavity, Right B Pleural Cavity, Left C Mediastinum Mediastinal cavity Mediastinal space D Pericardial Cavity F Abdominal Wall G Peritoneal Cavity Abdominal cavity H Retroperitoneum Retroperitoneal cavity Retroperitoneal space J Pelvic Cavity Retropubic space Space of Retzius K Upper Back L Lower Back M Perineum, Male ♂ N Perineum, Female ♀	Ø Open 3 Percutaneous 4 Percutaneous Endoscopic	Z No Device	Z No Qualifier
3 Oral Cavity and Throat	Ø Open 3 Percutaneous 4 Percutaneous Endoscopic 7 Via Natural or Artificial Opening 8 Via Natural or Artificial Opening Endoscopic X External	Z No Device	Z No Qualifier
P Gastrointestinal Tract Q Respiratory Tract R Genitourinary Tract	Ø Open 3 Percutaneous 4 Percutaneous Endoscopic 7 Via Natural or Artificial Opening 8 Via Natural or Artificial Opening Endoscopic	Z No Device	Z No Qualifier

Non-OR ØW3P8ZZ
♂ ØW3M[Ø,3,4]ZZ
♀ ØW3N[Ø,3,4]ZZ

Ø Medical and Surgical
W Anatomical Regions, General
4 Creation Definition: Putting in or on biological or synthetic material to form a new body part that to the extent possible replicates the anatomic structure or function of an absent body part
Explanation: Used for gender reassignment surgery and corrective procedures in individuals with congenital anomalies

Body Part Character 4	Approach Character 5	Device Character 6	Qualifier Character 7
M Perineum, Male ♂	Ø Open	7 Autologous Tissue Substitute J Synthetic Substitute K Nonautologous Tissue Substitute	Ø Vagina
N Perineum, Female ♀	Ø Open	7 Autologous Tissue Substitute J Synthetic Substitute K Nonautologous Tissue Substitute	1 Penis

♂ ØW4MØ[7,J,K]Ø
♀ ØW4NØ[7,J,K]1

Ø Medical and Surgical
W Anatomical Regions, General
8 Division Definition: Cutting into a body part, without draining fluids and/or gases from the body part, in order to separate or transect a body part
Explanation: All or a portion of the body part is separated into two or more portions

Body Part Character 4	Approach Character 5	Device Character 6	Qualifier Character 7
N Perineum, Female ♀	X External	Z No Device	Z No Qualifier

Non-OR ØW8NXZZ
♀ ØW8NXZZ

Ø Medical and Surgical
W Anatomical Regions, General
9 Drainage Definition: Taking or letting out fluids and/or gases from a body part
Explanation: The qualifier DIAGNOSTIC is used to identify drainage procedures that are biopsies

Body Part Character 4	Approach Character 5	Device Character 6	Qualifier Character 7
Ø Head **1** Cranial Cavity **2** Face **3** Oral Cavity and Throat **4** Upper Jaw **5** Lower Jaw **8** Chest Wall **9** Pleural Cavity, Right **B** Pleural Cavity, Left **C** Mediastinum Mediastinal cavity Mediastinal space **D** Pericardial Cavity **F** Abdominal Wall **G** Peritoneal Cavity Abdominal cavity **H** Retroperitoneum Retroperitoneal cavity Retroperitoneal space **K** Upper Back **L** Lower Back **M** Perineum, Male ♂ **N** Perineum, Female ♀	**Ø** Open **3** Percutaneous **4** Percutaneous Endoscopic	**Ø** Drainage Device	**Z** No Qualifier
Ø Head **1** Cranial Cavity **2** Face **3** Oral Cavity and Throat **4** Upper Jaw **5** Lower Jaw **8** Chest Wall **9** Pleural Cavity, Right **B** Pleural Cavity, Left **C** Mediastinum Mediastinal cavity Mediastinal space **D** Pericardial Cavity **F** Abdominal Wall **G** Peritoneal Cavity Abdominal cavity **H** Retroperitoneum Retroperitoneal cavity Retroperitoneal space **K** Upper Back **L** Lower Back **M** Perineum, Male ♂ **N** Perineum, Female ♀	**Ø** Open **3** Percutaneous **4** Percutaneous Endoscopic	**Z** No Device	**X** Diagnostic **Z** No Qualifier
6 Neck Parapharyngeal space Retropharyngeal space **J** Pelvic Cavity Retropubic space Space of Retzius	**Ø** Open **3** Percutaneous **4** Percutaneous Endoscopic **7** Via Natural or Artificial Opening **8** Via Natural or Artificial Opening Endoscopic	**Ø** Drainage Device	**Z** No Qualifier
6 Neck Parapharyngeal space Retropharyngeal space **J** Pelvic Cavity Retropubic space Space of Retzius	**Ø** Open **3** Percutaneous **4** Percutaneous Endoscopic **7** Via Natural or Artificial Opening **8** Via Natural or Artificial Opening Endoscopic	**Z** No Device	**X** Diagnostic **Z** No Qualifier

Non-OR ØW9[Ø,8,9,B,K,L,M]ØØZ
Non-OR ØW9[Ø,1,2,3,4,5,8,9,B,C,D,F,G,H,K,L,M,N]3ØZ
Non-OR ØW9[Ø,1,8,F,K,L,M]4ØZ
Non-OR ØW9[Ø,2,3,4,5,8,9,B,K,L,M,N]ØZX
Non-OR ØW9[Ø,1,2,3,4,5,8,9,B,C,D,G,K,L,M,N]3ZX
Non-OR ØW9[Ø,1,2,3,4,5,8,C,K,L,M,N]4ZX
Non-OR ØW9[Ø,8,9,B,K,L,M]ØZZ
Non-OR ØW9[Ø,1,2,3,4,5,8,9,B,C,D,F,G,H,K,L,M,N]3ZZ
Non-OR ØW9[Ø,1,8,F,K,L,M]4ZZ
Non-OR ØW9[6,J][3,7,8]ØZ
Non-OR ØW96[Ø,4]ZX
Non-OR ØW9[6,J][3,7,8]Z[X,Z]

♂ ØW9M[Ø,3,4]ØZ
♂ ØW9M[Ø,3,4]Z[X,Z]
♀ ØW9N[Ø,3,4]ØZ
♀ ØW9N[Ø,3]Z[X,Z]
♀ ØW9N4ZZ

Ø Medical and Surgical
W Anatomical Regions, General
B Excision Definition: Cutting out or off, without replacement, a portion of a body part
Explanation: The qualifier DIAGNOSTIC is used to identify excision procedures that are biopsies

Body Part Character 4	Approach Character 5	Device Character 6	Qualifier Character 7
Ø Head 2 Face 3 Oral Cavity and Throat 4 Upper Jaw 5 Lower Jaw 8 Chest Wall K Upper Back L Lower Back M Perineum, Male ♂ N Perineum, Female ♀	Ø Open 3 Percutaneous 4 Percutaneous Endoscopic X External	Z No Device	X Diagnostic Z No Qualifier
6 Neck Parapharyngeal space Retropharyngeal space F Abdominal Wall	Ø Open 3 Percutaneous 4 Percutaneous Endoscopic	Z No Device	X Diagnostic Z No Qualifier
6 Neck Parapharyngeal space Retropharyngeal space F Abdominal Wall	X External	Z No Device	2 Stoma X Diagnostic Z No Qualifier
C Mediastinum Mediastinal cavity Mediastinal space H Retroperitoneum Retroperitoneal cavity Retroperitoneal space	Ø Open 3 Percutaneous 4 Percutaneous Endoscopic	Z No Device	X Diagnostic Z No Qualifier

Non-OR ØWB[Ø,2,4,5,8,K,L,M][Ø,3,4,X]ZX
Non-OR ØWB6[Ø,3,4]ZX
Non-OR ØWB6XZX
Non-OR ØWBH[3,4]ZX
♂ ØWEM[Ø,3,4,X]Z[X,Z]
♀ ØWEN[Ø,3,4,X]Z[X,Z]

Ø Medical and Surgical
W Anatomical Regions, General
C Extirpation Definition: Taking or cutting out solid matter from a body part
Explanation: The solid matter may be an abnormal byproduct of a biological function or a foreign body; it may be imbedded in a body part or in the lumen of a tubular body part. The solid matter may or may not have been previously broken into pieces.

Body Part Character 4	Approach Character 5	Device Character 6	Qualifier Character 7
1 Cranial Cavity 3 Oral Cavity and Throat 9 Pleural Cavity, Right B Pleural Cavity, Left C Mediastinum Mediastinal cavity Mediastinal space D Pericardial Cavity G Peritoneal Cavity Abdominal cavity H Retroperitoneum Retroperitoneal cavity Retroperitoneal space J Pelvic Cavity Retropubic space Space of Retzius	Ø Open 3 Percutaneous 4 Percutaneous Endoscopic X External	Z No Device	Z No Qualifier
4 Upper Jaw 5 Lower Jaw	Ø Open 3 Percutaneous 4 Percutaneous Endoscopic	Z No Device	Z No Qualifier
P Gastrointestinal Tract Q Respiratory Tract R Genitourinary Tract	Ø Open 3 Percutaneous 4 Percutaneous Endoscopic 7 Via Natural or Artificial Opening 8 Via Natural or Artificial Opening Endoscopic X External	Z No Device	Z No Qualifier

Non-OR ØWC[1,3]XZZ
Non-OR ØWC[9,B][Ø,3,4,X]ZZ
Non-OR ØWC[C,D,G,H,J]XZZ
Non-OR ØWC[4,5]3ZZ
Non-OR ØWC[P,R][7,8,X]ZZ
Non-OR ØWCQ[Ø,3,4,X]ZZ

Ø Medical and Surgical
W Anatomical Regions, General
F Fragmentation Definition: Breaking solid matter in a body part into pieces

Explanation: Physical force (e.g., manual, ultrasonic) applied directly or indirectly is used to break the solid matter into pieces. The solid matter may be an abnormal byproduct of a biological function or a foreign body. The pieces of solid matter are not taken out.

Body Part Character 4	Approach Character 5	Device Character 6	Qualifier Character 7
1 Cranial Cavity NC 3 Oral Cavity and Throat NC 9 Pleural Cavity, Right NC B Pleural Cavity, Left NC C Mediastinum NC Mediastinal cavity Mediastinal space D Pericardial Cavity G Peritoneal Cavity NC Abdominal cavity J Pelvic Cavity NC Retropubic space Space of Retzius	Ø Open 3 Percutaneous 4 Percutaneous Endoscopic X External	Z No Device	Z No Qualifier
P Gastrointestinal Tract NC Q Respiratory Tract NC R Genitourinary Tract	Ø Open 3 Percutaneous 4 Percutaneous Endoscopic 7 Via Natural or Artificial Opening 8 Via Natural or Artificial Opening Endoscopic X External	Z No Device	Z No Qualifier

Non-OR ØWF[1,3,9,B,C,G]XZZ
Non-OR ØWFJ[Ø,3,4,X]ZZ
Non-OR ØWFP[Ø,3,4,7,8,X]ZZ
Non-OR ØWFQXZZ
Non-OR ØWFR[Ø,3,4,7,8,X]ZZ
NC ØWF[1,3,9,B,C,G,J]XZZ
NC ØWF[P,Q]XZZ

Ø Medical and Surgical
W Anatomical Regions, General
H Insertion Definition: Putting in a nonbiological appliance that monitors, assists, performs, or prevents a physiological function but does not physically take the place of a body part

Explanation: None

Body Part Character 4	Approach Character 5	Device Character 6	Qualifier Character 7
Ø Head 1 Cranial Cavity 2 Face 3 Oral Cavity and Throat 4 Upper Jaw 5 Lower Jaw 6 Neck Parapharyngeal space Retropharyngeal space 8 Chest Wall 9 Pleural Cavity, Right B Pleural Cavity, Left D Pericardial Cavity F Abdominal Wall G Peritoneal Cavity Abdominal cavity H Retroperitoneum Retroperitoneal cavity Retroperitoneal space J Pelvic Cavity Retropubic space Space of Retzius K Upper Back L Lower Back M Perineum, Male N Perineum, Female ♀	Ø Open 3 Percutaneous 4 Percutaneous Endoscopic	1 Radioactive Element 3 Infusion Device Y Other Device	Z No Qualifier
C Mediastinum Mediastinal cavity Mediastinal space	Ø Open 3 Percutaneous 4 Percutaneous Endoscopic	1 Radioactive Element 3 Infusion Device G Defibrillator Lead Y Other Device	Z No Qualifier
P Gastrointestinal Tract Q Respiratory Tract R Genitourinary Tract	Ø Open 3 Percutaneous 4 Percutaneous Endoscopic 7 Via Natural or Artificial Opening 8 Via Natural or Artificial Opening Endoscopic	1 Radioactive Element 3 Infusion Device Y Other Device	Z No Qualifier

DRG Non-OR ØWH[Ø,2,4,5,6,K,L,M][Ø,3,4][3,Y]Z
Non-OR ØWH1[Ø,3,4]3Z
Non-OR ØWH[8,9,B][Ø,3,4][3,Y]Z
Non-OR ØWHPØYZ
Non-OR ØWHP[3,4,7,8][3,Y]Z
Non-OR ØWHQ[Ø,7,8][3,Y]Z
Non-OR ØWHR[Ø,3,4,7,8][3,Y]Z
♀ ØWHN[Ø,3,4][3,Y]Z

Ø Medical and Surgical
W Anatomical Regions, General
J Inspection Definition: Visually and/or manually exploring a body part

Explanation: Visual exploration may be performed with or without optical instrumentation. Manual exploration may be performed directly or through intervening body layers.

Body Part Character 4	Approach Character 5	Device Character 6	Qualifier Character 7
Ø Head 2 Face 3 Oral Cavity and Throat 4 Upper Jaw 5 Lower Jaw 6 Neck Parapharyngeal space Retropharyngeal space 8 Chest Wall F Abdominal Wall K Upper Back L Lower Back M Perineum, Male ♂ N Perineum, Female ♀	Ø Open 3 Percutaneous 4 Percutaneous Endoscopic X External	Z No Device	Z No Qualifier
1 Cranial Cavity 9 Pleural Cavity, Right B Pleural Cavity, Left C Mediastinum Mediastinal cavity Mediastinal space D Pericardial Cavity G Peritoneal Cavity Abdominal cavity H Retroperitoneum Retroperitoneal cavity Retroperitoneal space J Pelvic Cavity Retropubic space Space of Retzius	Ø Open 3 Percutaneous 4 Percutaneous Endoscopic	Z No Device	Z No Qualifier
P Gastrointestinal Tract Q Respiratory Tract R Genitourinary Tract	Ø Open 3 Percutaneous 4 Percutaneous Endoscopic 7 Via Natural or Artificial Opening 8 Via Natural or Artificial Opening Endoscopic	Z No Device	Z No Qualifier

DRG Non-OR ØWJ[Ø,2,4,5,K,L]ØZZ
DRG Non-OR ØWJM[Ø,4]ZZ
Non-OR ØWJ3ØZZ
Non-OR ØWJ[Ø,2,3,4,5,6,8,F,K,L,M,N][3,X]ZZ
Non-OR ØWJ[Ø,2,3,4,5,K,L]4ZZ
Non-OR ØWJDØZZ
Non-OR ØWJ[1,9,B,C,D,G,H,J]3ZZ
Non-OR ØWJ[P,Q,R][3,7,8]ZZ

♂ ØWJM[Ø,3,4,X]ZZ
♀ ØWJN[Ø,3,4,X]ZZ

Ø Medical and Surgical
W Anatomical Regions, General
M Reattachment Definition: Putting back in or on all or a portion of a separated body part to its normal location or other suitable location

Explanation: Vascular circulation and nervous pathways may or may not be reestablished

Body Part Character 4	Approach Character 5	Device Character 6	Qualifier Character 7
2 Face 4 Upper Jaw 5 Lower Jaw 6 Neck Parapharyngeal space Retropharyngeal space 8 Chest Wall F Abdominal Wall K Upper Back L Lower Back M Perineum, Male ♂ N Perineum, Female ♀	Ø Open	Z No Device	Z No Qualifier

♂ ØWMMØZZ
♀ ØWMNØZZ

Ø Medical and Surgical
W Anatomical Regions, General
P Removal Definition: Taking out or off a device from a body part

Explanation: If a device is taken out and a similar device put in without cutting or puncturing the skin or mucous membrane, the procedure is coded to the root operation CHANGE. Otherwise, the procedure for taking out the device is coded to the root operation REMOVAL.

Body Part Character 4	Approach Character 5	Device Character 6	Qualifier Character 7
Ø Head **2 Face** **4 Upper Jaw** **5 Lower Jaw** **6 Neck** Parapharyngeal space Retropharyngeal space **8 Chest Wall** **F Abdominal Wall** **K Upper Back** **L Lower Back** **M Perineum, Male** ♂ **N Perineum, Female** ♀	**Ø Open** **3 Percutaneous** **4 Percutaneous Endoscopic** **X External**	**Ø Drainage Device** **1 Radioactive Element** **3 Infusion Device** **7 Autologous Tissue Substitute** **J Synthetic Substitute** **K Nonautologous Tissue Substitute** **Y Other Device**	**Z No Qualifier**
1 Cranial Cavity **9 Pleural Cavity, Right** **B Pleural Cavity, Left** **G Peritoneal Cavity** Abdominal cavity **J Pelvic Cavity** Retropubic space Space of Retzius	**Ø Open** **3 Percutaneous** **4 Percutaneous Endoscopic**	**Ø Drainage Device** **1 Radioactive Element** **3 Infusion Device** **J Synthetic Substitute** **Y Other Device**	**Z No Qualifier**
1 Cranial Cavity **9 Pleural Cavity, Right** **B Pleural Cavity, Left** **G Peritoneal Cavity** Abdominal cavity **J Pelvic Cavity** Retropubic space Space of Retzius	**X External**	**Ø Drainage Device** **1 Radioactive Element** **3 Infusion Device**	**Z No Qualifier**
C Mediastinum Mediastinal cavity Mediastinal space	**Ø Open** **3 Percutaneous** **4 Percutaneous Endoscopic** **X External**	**Ø Drainage Device** **1 Radioactive Element** **3 Infusion Device** **7 Autologous Tissue Substitute** **G Defibrillator Lead** **J Synthetic Substitute** **K Nonautologous Tissue Substitute** **Y Other Device**	**Z No Qualifier**
D Pericardial Cavity **H Retroperitoneum** Retroperitoneal cavity Retroperitoneal space	**Ø Open** **3 Percutaneous** **4 Percutaneous Endoscopic**	**Ø Drainage Device** **1 Radioactive Element** **3 Infusion Device** **Y Other Device**	**Z No Qualifier**
D Pericardial Cavity **H Retroperitoneum** Retroperitoneal cavity Retroperitoneal space	**X External**	**Ø Drainage Device** **1 Radioactive Element** **3 Infusion Device**	**Z No Qualifier**
P Gastrointestinal Tract **Q Respiratory Tract** **R Genitourinary Tract**	**Ø Open** **3 Percutaneous** **4 Percutaneous Endoscopic** **7 Via Natural or Artificial Opening** **8 Via Natural or Artificial Opening Endoscopic** **X External**	**1 Radioactive Element** **3 Infusion Device** **Y Other Device**	**Z No Qualifier**

Non-OR ØWP[Ø,2,4,5,6,8][Ø,3,4,X][Ø,1,3,7,J,K,Y]Z
Non-OR ØWPFX[Ø,1,3,7,J,K,Y]Z
Non-OR ØWP[K,L][Ø,3,4,X][Ø,1,3,7,J,K,Y]Z
Non-OR ØWPM[Ø,3,4][Ø,1,3,J,Y]Z
Non-OR ØWPMX[Ø,1,3,Y]Z
Non-OR ØWPNX[Ø,1,3,7,J,K,Y]Z
Non-OR ØWP1[Ø,3,4]3Z
Non-OR ØWP[9,B,J][Ø,3,4][Ø,1,3,J,Y]Z
Non-OR ØWP[1,9,B,G,J]X[Ø,1,3]Z
Non-OR ØWPCX[Ø,1,3,7,J,K,Y]Z
Non-OR ØWP[D,H]X[Ø,1,3]Z
Non-OR ØWPP[3,4,7,8,X][1,3,Y]Z
Non-OR ØWPQ73Z
Non-OR ØWPQ8[3,Y]Z
Non-OR ØWPQ[Ø,X][1,3,Y]Z
Non-OR ØWPR[Ø,3,4,7,8,X][1,3,Y]Z

♂ ØWPM[Ø,3,4,X][Ø,1,3,7,J,K,Y]Z
♀ ØWPN[Ø,3,4,X][Ø,1,3,7,J,K,Y]Z

Ø Medical and Surgical
W Anatomical Regions, General
Q Repair

Definition: Restoring, to the extent possible, a body part to its normal anatomic structure and function

Explanation: Used only when the method to accomplish the repair is not one of the other root operations

Body Part Character 4	Approach Character 5	Device Character 6	Qualifier Character 7
Ø Head **2** Face **3** Oral Cavity and Throat **4** Upper Jaw **5** Lower Jaw **8** Chest Wall **K** Upper Back **L** Lower Back **M** Perineum, Male ♂ **N** Perineum, Female ♀	**Ø** Open **3** Percutaneous **4** Percutaneous Endoscopic **X** External	**Z** No Device	**Z** No Qualifier
6 Neck Parapharyngeal space Retropharyngeal space **F** Abdominal Wall	**Ø** Open **3** Percutaneous **4** Percutaneous Endoscopic	**Z** No Device	**Z** No Qualifier
6 Neck Parapharyngeal space Retropharyngeal space **F** Abdominal Wall ⊞	**X** External	**Z** No Device	**2** Stoma **Z** No Qualifier
C Mediastinum Mediastinal cavity Mediastinal space	**Ø** Open **3** Percutaneous **4** Percutaneous Endoscopic	**Z** No Device	**Z** No Qualifier

Non-OR ØWQNXZZ
♂ ØWQM[Ø,3,4,X]ZZ
♀ ØWQN[Ø,3,4,X]ZZ

See Appendix L for Procedure Combinations
⊞ ØWQFXZ[2,Z]

Ø Medical and Surgical
W Anatomical Regions, General
U Supplement

Definition: Putting in or on biological or synthetic material that physically reinforces and/or augments the function of a portion of a body part

Explanation: The biological material is non-living, or is living and from the same individual. The body part may have been previously replaced, and the SUPPLEMENT procedure is performed to physically reinforce and/or augment the function of the replaced body part.

Body Part Character 4	Approach Character 5	Device Character 6	Qualifier Character 7
Ø Head **2** Face **4** Upper Jaw **5** Lower Jaw **6** Neck Parapharyngeal space Retropharyngeal space **8** Chest Wall **C** Mediastinum Mediastinal cavity Mediastinal space **F** Abdominal Wall **K** Upper Back **L** Lower Back **M** Perineum, Male ♂ **N** Perineum, Female ♀	**Ø** Open **4** Percutaneous Endoscopic	**7** Autologous Tissue Substitute **J** Synthetic Substitute **K** Nonautologous Tissue Substitute	**Z** No Qualifier

♂ ØWUM[Ø,4][7,J,K]Z
♀ ØWUN[Ø,4][7,J,K]Z

Ø Medical and Surgical
W Anatomical Regions, General
W Revision Definition: Correcting, to the extent possible, a portion of a malfunctioning device or the position of a displaced device

Explanation: Revision can include correcting a malfunctioning or displaced device by taking out or putting in components of the device such as a screw or pin

Body Part Character 4	Approach Character 5	Device Character 6	Qualifier Character 7
Ø Head **2** Face **4** Upper Jaw **5** Lower Jaw **6** Neck Parapharyngeal space Retropharyngeal space **8** Chest Wall **F** Abdominal Wall **K** Upper Back **L** Lower Back **M** Perineum, Male ♂ **N** Perineum, Female ♀	**Ø** Open **3** Percutaneous **4** Percutaneous Endoscopic **X** External	**Ø** Drainage Device **1** Radioactive Element **3** Infusion Device **7** Autologous Tissue Substitute **J** Synthetic Substitute **K** Nonautologous Tissue Substitute **Y** Other Device	**Z** No Qualifier
1 Cranial Cavity **9** Pleural Cavity, Right **B** Pleural Cavity, Left **G** Peritoneal Cavity Abdominal cavity **J** Pelvic Cavity Retropubic space Space of Retzius	**Ø** Open **3** Percutaneous **4** Percutaneous Endoscopic **X** External	**Ø** Drainage Device **1** Radioactive Element **3** Infusion Device **J** Synthetic Substitute **Y** Other Device	**Z** No Qualifier
C Mediastinum Mediastinal cavity Mediastinal space	**Ø** Open **3** Percutaneous **4** Percutaneous Endoscopic **X** External	**Ø** Drainage Device **1** Radioactive Element **3** Infusion Device **7** Autologous Tissue Substitute **G** Defibrillator Lead **J** Synthetic Substitute **K** Nonautologous Tissue Substitute **Y** Other Device	**Z** No Qualifier
D Pericardial Cavity **H** Retroperitoneum Retroperitoneal cavity Retroperitoneal space	**Ø** Open **3** Percutaneous **4** Percutaneous Endoscopic **X** External	**Ø** Drainage Device **1** Radioactive Element **3** Infusion Device **Y** Other Device	**Z** No Qualifier
P Gastrointestinal Tract **Q** Respiratory Tract **R** Genitourinary Tract	**Ø** Open **3** Percutaneous **4** Percutaneous Endoscopic **7** Via Natural or Artificial Opening **8** Via Natural or Artificial Opening Endoscopic **X** External	**1** Radioactive Element **3** Infusion Device **Y** Other Device	**Z** No Qualifier

DRG Non-OR ØWW[Ø,2,4,5,6,K,L][Ø,3,4][Ø,1,3,7,J,K,Y]Z
DRG Non-OR ØWWM[Ø,3,4][Ø,1,3,J,Y]Z
Non-OR ØWW[Ø,2,4,5,6,F,K,L,M,N]X[Ø,1,3,7,J,K,Y]Z
Non-OR ØWW8[Ø,3,4,X][Ø,1,3,7,J,K,Y]Z
Non-OR ØWW[1,G,J]X[Ø,1,3,J,Y]Z
Non-OR ØWW[9,B][Ø,3,4,X][Ø,1,3,J,Y]Z
Non-OR ØWWCX[Ø,1,3,7,J,K,Y]Z
Non-OR ØWW[D,H]X[Ø,1,3,Y]Z
Non-OR ØWWP[3,4,7,8,X][1,3,Y]Z
Non-OR ØWWQ[Ø,X][1,3,Y]Z
Non-OR ØWWR[Ø,3,4,7,8,X][1,3,Y]Z

♂ ØWWM[Ø,3,4,X][Ø,1,3,7,K,Y]Z
♀ ØWWN[Ø,3,4,X][Ø,1,3,7,K,Y]Z

Ø Medical and Surgical
W Anatomical Regions, General
Y Transplantation Definition: Putting in or on all or a portion of a living body part taken from another individual or animal to physically take the place and/or function of all or a portion of a similar body part

Explanation: The native body part may or may not be taken out, and the transplanted body part may take over all or a portion of its function

Body Part Character 4	Approach Character 5	Device Character 6	Qualifier Character 7
2 Face	**Ø** Open	**Z** No Device	**Ø** Allogeneic **1** Syngeneic

Anatomical Regions, Upper Extremities ØXØ–ØXY

Character Meanings

This Character Meaning table is provided as a guide to assist the user in the identification of character members that may be found in this section of code tables. It **SHOULD NOT** be used to build a PCS code.

Operation–Character 3	Body Part–Character 4	Approach–Character 5	Device–Character 6	Qualifier–Character 7
Ø Alteration	Ø Forequarter, Right	Ø Open	Ø Drainage Device	Ø Allogeneic OR Complete
2 Change	1 Forequarter, Left	3 Percutaneous	1 Radioactive Element	1 High OR Syngeneic
3 Control	2 Shoulder Region, Right	4 Percutaneous Endoscopic	3 Infusion Device	2 Mid
6 Detachment	3 Shoulder Region, Left	X External	7 Autologous Tissue Substitute	3 Low
9 Drainage	4 Axilla, Right		J Synthetic Substitute	4 Complete 1st Ray
B Excision	5 Axilla, Left		K Nonautologous Tissue Substitute	5 Complete 2nd Ray
H Insertion	6 Upper Extremity, Right		Y Other Device	6 Complete 3rd Ray
J Inspection	7 Upper Extremity, Left		Z No Device	7 Complete 4th Ray
M Reattachment	8 Upper Arm, Right			8 Complete 5th Ray
P Removal	9 Upper Arm, Left			9 Partial 1st Ray
Q Repair	B Elbow Region, Right			B Partial 2nd Ray
R Replacement	C Elbow Region, Left			C Partial 3rd Ray
U Supplement	D Lower Arm, Right			D Partial 4th Ray
W Revision	F Lower Arm, Left			F Partial 5th Ray
X Transfer	G Wrist Region, Right			L Thumb, Right
Y Transplantation	H Wrist Region, Left			M Thumb, Left
	J Hand, Right			N Toe, Right
	K Hand, Left			P Toe, Left
	L Thumb, Right			X Diagnostic
	M Thumb, Left			Z No Qualifier
	N Index Finger, Right			
	P Index Finger, Left			
	Q Middle Finger, Right			
	R Middle Finger, Left			
	S Ring Finger, Right			
	T Ring Finger, Left			
	V Little Finger, Right			
	W Little Finger, Left			

AHA Coding Clinic for table ØX3
2016, 4Q, 99 Root operation Control
2015, 1Q, 35 Evacuation of hematoma for control of postprocedural bleeding
2013, 3Q, 23 Control of intraoperative bleeding

AHA Coding Clinic for table ØX6
2017, 2Q, 3-4 Qualifiers for the root operation detachment
2017, 2Q, 18 Removal of polydactyl digits
2017, 1Q, 52 Further distal phalangeal amputation
2016, 3Q, 33 Traumatic amputation of fingers with further revision amputation

AHA Coding Clinic for table ØXH
2017, 2Q, 20 Exchange of intramedullary antibiotic impregnated spacer

AHA Coding Clinic for table ØXP
2017, 2Q, 20 Exchange of intramedullary antibiotic impregnated spacer

AHA Coding Clinic for table ØXY
2016, 4Q, 112-113 Transplantation

Detachment Qualifier Descriptions

Qualifier Definition	Upper Arm	Lower Arm
1 **High:** Amputation at the proximal portion of the shaft of the:	Humerus	Radius/Ulna
2 **Mid:** Amputation at the middle portion of the shaft of the:	Humerus	Radius/Ulna
3 **Low:** Amputation at the distal portion of the shaft of the:	Humerus	Radius/Ulna

Qualifier Definition	Hand
0 Complete 1st through 5th Rays Ray: digit of hand or foot with corresponding metacarpus or metatarsus	Through carpo-metacarpal joint, **Wrist**
4 Complete 1st Ray	Through carpo-metacarpal joint, **Thumb**
5 Complete 2nd Ray	Through carpo-metacarpal joint, **Index Finger**
6 Complete 3rd Ray	Through carpo-metacarpal joint, **Middle Finger**
7 Complete 4th Ray	Through carpo-metacarpal joint, **Ring Finger**
8 Complete 5th Ray	Through carpo-metacarpal joint, **Little Finger**
9 Partial 1st Ray	Anywhere along shaft or head of metacarpal bone, **Thumb**
B Partial 2nd Ray	Anywhere along shaft or head of metacarpal bone, **Index Finger**
C Partial 3rd Ray	Anywhere along shaft or head of metacarpal bone, **Middle Finger**
D Partial 4th Ray	Anywhere along shaft or head of metacarpal bone, **Ring Finger**
F Partial 5th Ray	Anywhere along shaft or head of metacarpal bone, **Little Finger**

Qualifier Definition	Thumb/Finger
0 Complete	At the metacarpophalangeal joint
1 High	Anywhere along the proximal phalanx
2 Mid	Through the proximal interphalangeal joint or anywhere along the middle phalanx
3 Low	Through the distal interphalangeal joint or anywhere along the distal phalanx

Ø Medical and Surgical
X Anatomical Regions, Upper Extremities
Ø Alteration

Definition: Modifying the anatomic structure of a body part without affecting the function of the body part

Explanation: Principal purpose is to improve appearance

Body Part Character 4	Approach Character 5	Device Character 6	Qualifier Character 7
2 Shoulder Region, Right 3 Shoulder Region, Left 4 Axilla, Right 5 Axilla, Left 6 Upper Extremity, Right 7 Upper Extremity, Left 8 Upper Arm, Right 9 Upper Arm, Left B Elbow Region, Right C Elbow Region, Left D Lower Arm, Right F Lower Arm, Left G Wrist Region, Right H Wrist Region, Left	Ø Open 3 Percutaneous 4 Percutaneous Endoscopic	7 Autologous Tissue Substitute J Synthetic Substitute K Nonautologous Tissue Substitute Z No Device	Z No Qualifier

Ø Medical and Surgical
X Anatomical Regions, Upper Extremities
2 Change

Definition: Taking out or off a device from a body part and putting back an identical or similar device in or on the same body part without cutting or puncturing the skin or a mucous membrane

Explanation: All CHANGE procedures are coded using the approach EXTERNAL

Body Part Character 4	Approach Character 5	Device Character 6	Qualifier Character 7
6 Upper Extremity, Right 7 Upper Extremity, Left	X External	Ø Drainage Device Y Other Device	Z No Qualifier

Non-OR All body part, approach, device, and qualifier values

Ø Medical and Surgical
X Anatomical Regions, Upper Extremities
3 Control

Definition: Stopping, or attempting to stop, postprocedural or other acute bleeding

Explanation: None

Body Part Character 4	Approach Character 5	Device Character 6	Qualifier Character 7
2 Shoulder Region, Right 3 Shoulder Region, Left 4 Axilla, Right 5 Axilla, Left 6 Upper Extremity, Right 7 Upper Extremity, Left 8 Upper Arm, Right 9 Upper Arm, Left B Elbow Region, Right C Elbow Region, Left D Lower Arm, Right F Lower Arm, Left G Wrist Region, Right H Wrist Region, Left J Hand, Right K Hand, Left	Ø Open 3 Percutaneous 4 Percutaneous Endoscopic	Z No Device	Z No Qualifier

Ø Medical and Surgical
X Anatomical Regions, Upper Extremities
6 Detachment Definition: Cutting off all or a portion of the upper or lower extremities

Explanation: The body part value is the site of the detachment, with a qualifier if applicable to further specify the level where the extremity was detached

Body Part Character 4	Approach Character 5	Device Character 6	Qualifier Character 7
Ø Forequarter, Right 1 Forequarter, Left 2 Shoulder Region, Right 3 Shoulder Region, Left B Elbow Region, Right C Elbow Region, Left	Ø Open	Z No Device	Z No Qualifier
8 Upper Arm, Right 9 Upper Arm, Left D Lower Arm, Right F Lower Arm, Left	Ø Open	Z No Device	1 High 2 Mid 3 Low
J Hand, Right K Hand, Left	Ø Open	Z No Device	Ø Complete 4 Complete 1st Ray 5 Complete 2nd Ray 6 Complete 3rd Ray 7 Complete 4th Ray 8 Complete 5th Ray 9 Partial 1st Ray B Partial 2nd Ray C Partial 3rd Ray D Partial 4th Ray F Partial 5th Ray
L Thumb, Right M Thumb, Left N Index Finger, Right P Index Finger, Left Q Middle Finger, Right R Middle Finger, Left S Ring Finger, Right T Ring Finger, Left V Little Finger, Right W Little Finger, Left	Ø Open	Z No Device	Ø Complete 1 High 2 Mid 3 Low

Ø Medical and Surgical
X Anatomical Regions, Upper Extremities
9 Drainage
Definition: Taking or letting out fluids and/or gases from a body part
Explanation: The qualifier DIAGNOSTIC is used to identify drainage procedures that are biopsies

Body Part Character 4	Approach Character 5	Device Character 6	Qualifier Character 7
2 Shoulder Region, Right 3 Shoulder Region, Left 4 Axilla, Right 5 Axilla, Left 6 Upper Extremity, Right 7 Upper Extremity, Left 8 Upper Arm, Right 9 Upper Arm, Left B Elbow Region, Right C Elbow Region, Left D Lower Arm, Right F Lower Arm, Left G Wrist Region, Right H Wrist Region, Left J Hand, Right K Hand, Left	Ø Open 3 Percutaneous 4 Percutaneous Endoscopic	Ø Drainage Device	Z No Qualifier
2 Shoulder Region, Right 3 Shoulder Region, Left 4 Axilla, Right 5 Axilla, Left 6 Upper Extremity, Right 7 Upper Extremity, Left 8 Upper Arm, Right 9 Upper Arm, Left B Elbow Region, Right C Elbow Region, Left D Lower Arm, Right F Lower Arm, Left G Wrist Region, Right H Wrist Region, Left J Hand, Right K Hand, Left	Ø Open 3 Percutaneous 4 Percutaneous Endoscopic	Z No Device	X Diagnostic Z No Qualifier

Non-OR All body part, approach, device, and qualifier values

Ø Medical and Surgical
X Anatomical Regions, Upper Extremities
B Excision
Definition: Cutting out or off, without replacement, a portion of a body part
Explanation: The qualifier DIAGNOSTIC is used to identify excision procedures that are biopsies

Body Part Character 4	Approach Character 5	Device Character 6	Qualifier Character 7
2 Shoulder Region, Right 3 Shoulder Region, Left 4 Axilla, Right 5 Axilla, Left 6 Upper Extremity, Right 7 Upper Extremity, Left 8 Upper Arm, Right 9 Upper Arm, Left B Elbow Region, Right C Elbow Region, Left D Lower Arm, Right F Lower Arm, Left G Wrist Region, Right H Wrist Region, Left J Hand, Right K Hand, Left	Ø Open 3 Percutaneous 4 Percutaneous Endoscopic	Z No Device	X Diagnostic Z No Qualifier

Non-OR ØXB[2,3,4,5,6,7,8,9,B,C,D,F,G,H,J,K][Ø,3,4]ZX

Ø Medical and Surgical
X Anatomical Regions, Upper Extremities
H Insertion Definition: Putting in a nonbiological appliance that monitors, assists, performs, or prevents a physiological function but does not physically take the place of a body part

Explanation: None

Body Part Character 4	Approach Character 5	Device Character 6	Qualifier Character 7
2 Shoulder Region, Right 3 Shoulder Region, Left 4 Axilla, Right 5 Axilla, Left 6 Upper Extremity, Right 7 Upper Extremity, Left 8 Upper Arm, Right 9 Upper Arm, Left B Elbow Region, Right C Elbow Region, Left D Lower Arm, Right F Lower Arm, Left G Wrist Region, Right H Wrist Region, Left J Hand, Right K Hand, Left	Ø Open 3 Percutaneous 4 Percutaneous Endoscopic	1 Radioactive Element 3 Infusion Device Y Other Device	Z No Qualifier

DRG Non-OR ØXH[2,3,4,5,6,7,8,9,B,C,D,F,G,H,J,K][Ø,3,4][3,Y]Z

Ø Medical and Surgical
X Anatomical Regions, Upper Extremities
J Inspection Definition: Visually and/or manually exploring a body part

Explanation: Visual exploration may be performed with or without optical instrumentation. Manual exploration may be performed directly or through intervening body layers.

Body Part Character 4	Approach Character 5	Device Character 6	Qualifier Character 7
2 Shoulder Region, Right 3 Shoulder Region, Left 4 Axilla, Right 5 Axilla, Left 6 Upper Extremity, Right 7 Upper Extremity, Left 8 Upper Arm, Right 9 Upper Arm, Left B Elbow Region, Right C Elbow Region, Left D Lower Arm, Right F Lower Arm, Left G Wrist Region, Right H Wrist Region, Left J Hand, Right K Hand, Left	Ø Open 3 Percutaneous 4 Percutaneous Endoscopic X External	Z No Device	Z No Qualifier

DRG Non-OR ØXJ[2,3,4,5,6,7,8,9,B,C,D,F,G,H,J,K]ØZZ
Non-OR ØXJ[2,3,4,5,6,7,8,9,B,C,D,F,G,H][3,4,X]ZZ
Non-OR ØXJ[J,K][3,X]ZZ

Ø Medical and Surgical
X Anatomical Regions, Upper Extremities
M Reattachment Definition: Putting back in or on all or a portion of a separated body part to its normal location or other suitable location

Explanation: Vascular circulation and nervous pathways may or may not be reestablished

Body Part Character 4	Approach Character 5	Device Character 6	Qualifier Character 7
Ø Forequarter, Right 1 Forequarter, Left 2 Shoulder Region, Right 3 Shoulder Region, Left 4 Axilla, Right 5 Axilla, Left 6 Upper Extremity, Right 7 Upper Extremity, Left 8 Upper Arm, Right 9 Upper Arm, Left B Elbow Region, Right C Elbow Region, Left D Lower Arm, Right F Lower Arm, Left G Wrist Region, Right H Wrist Region, Left J Hand, Right K Hand, Left L Thumb, Right M Thumb, Left N Index Finger, Right P Index Finger, Left Q Middle Finger, Right R Middle Finger, Left S Ring Finger, Right T Ring Finger, Left V Little Finger, Right W Little Finger, Left	Ø Open	Z No Device	Z No Qualifier

Ø Medical and Surgical
X Anatomical Regions, Upper Extremities
P Removal Definition: Taking out or off a device from a body part

Explanation: If a device is taken out and a similar device put in without cutting or puncturing the skin or mucous membrane, the procedure is coded to the root operation CHANGE. Otherwise, the procedure for taking out the device is coded to the root operation REMOVAL.

Body Part Character 4	Approach Character 5	Device Character 6	Qualifier Character 7
6 Upper Extremity, Right 7 Upper Extremity, Left	Ø Open 3 Percutaneous 4 Percutaneous Endoscopic X External	Ø Drainage Device 1 Radioactive Element 3 Infusion Device 7 Autologous Tissue Substitute J Synthetic Substitute K Nonautologous Tissue Substitute Y Other Device	Z No Qualifier

Non-OR All body part, approach, device, and qualifier values

Ø Medical and Surgical
X Anatomical Regions, Upper Extremities
Q Repair Definition: Restoring, to the extent possible, a body part to its normal anatomic structure and function
Explanation: Used only when the method to accomplish the repair is not one of the other root operations

Body Part Character 4	Approach Character 5	Device Character 6	Qualifier Character 7
2 Shoulder Region, Right **3** Shoulder Region, Left **4** Axilla, Right **5** Axilla, Left **6** Upper Extremity, Right **7** Upper Extremity, Left **8** Upper Arm, Right **9** Upper Arm, Left **B** Elbow Region, Right **C** Elbow Region, Left **D** Lower Arm, Right **F** Lower Arm, Left **G** Wrist Region, Right **H** Wrist Region, Left **J** Hand, Right **K** Hand, Left **L** Thumb, Right **M** Thumb, Left **N** Index Finger, Right **P** Index Finger, Left **Q** Middle Finger, Right **R** Middle Finger, Left **S** Ring Finger, Right **T** Ring Finger, Left **V** Little Finger, Right **W** Little Finger, Left	**Ø** Open **3** Percutaneous **4** Percutaneous Endoscopic **X** External	**Z** No Device	**Z** No Qualifier

Ø Medical and Surgical
X Anatomical Regions, Upper Extremities
R Replacement Definition: Putting in or on biological or synthetic material that physically takes the place and/or function of all or a portion of a body part
Explanation: The body part may have been taken out or replaced, or may be taken out, physically eradicated, or rendered nonfunctional during the REPLACEMENT procedure. A REMOVAL procedure is coded for taking out the device used in a previous replacement procedure.

Body Part Character 4	Approach Character 5	Device Character 6	Qualifier Character 7
L Thumb, Right **M** Thumb, Left	**Ø** Open **4** Percutaneous Endoscopic	**7** Autologous Tissue Substitute	**N** Toe, Right **P** Toe, Left

Ø Medical and Surgical
X Anatomical Regions, Upper Extremities
U Supplement Definition: Putting in or on biological or synthetic material that physically reinforces and/or augments the function of a portion of a body part

Explanation: The biological material is non-living, or is living and from the same individual. The body part may have been previously replaced, and the SUPPLEMENT procedure is performed to physically reinforce and/or augment the function of the replaced body part.

Body Part Character 4	Approach Character 5	Device Character 6	Qualifier Character 7
2 Shoulder Region, Right 3 Shoulder Region, Left 4 Axilla, Right 5 Axilla, Left 6 Upper Extremity, Right 7 Upper Extremity, Left 8 Upper Arm, Right 9 Upper Arm, Left B Elbow Region, Right C Elbow Region, Left D Lower Arm, Right F Lower Arm, Left G Wrist Region, Right H Wrist Region, Left J Hand, Right K Hand, Left L Thumb, Right M Thumb, Left N Index Finger, Right P Index Finger, Left Q Middle Finger, Right R Middle Finger, Left S Ring Finger, Right T Ring Finger, Left V Little Finger, Right W Little Finger, Left	Ø Open 4 Percutaneous Endoscopic	7 Autologous Tissue Substitute J Synthetic Substitute K Nonautologous Tissue Substitute	Z No Qualifier

Ø Medical and Surgical
X Anatomical Regions, Upper Extremities
W Revision Definition: Correcting, to the extent possible, a portion of a malfunctioning device or the position of a displaced device

Explanation: Revision can include correcting a malfunctioning or displaced device by taking out or putting in components of the device such as a screw or pin

Body Part Character 4	Approach Character 5	Device Character 6	Qualifier Character 7
6 Upper Extremity, Right 7 Upper Extremity, Left	Ø Open 3 Percutaneous 4 Percutaneous Endoscopic X External	Ø Drainage Device 3 Infusion Device 7 Autologous Tissue Substitute J Synthetic Substitute K Nonautologous Tissue Substitute Y Other Device	Z No Qualifier

DRG Non-OR ØXW[6,7][Ø,3,4][Ø,3,7,J,K,Y]Z
Non-OR ØXW[6,7]X[Ø,3,7,J,K,Y]Z

Ø Medical and Surgical
X Anatomical Regions, Upper Extremities
X Transfer Definition: Moving, without taking out, all or a portion of a body part to another location to take over the function of all or a portion of a body part

Explanation: The body part transferred remains connected to its vascular and nervous supply

Body Part Character 4	Approach Character 5	Device Character 6	Qualifier Character 7
N Index Finger, Right	Ø Open	Z No Device	L Thumb, Right
P Index Finger, Left	Ø Open	Z No Device	M Thumb, Left

Ø Medical and Surgical
X Anatomical Regions, Upper Extremities
Y Transplantation Definition: Putting in or on all or a portion of a living body part taken from another individual or animal to physically take the place and/or function of all or a portion of a similar body part

Explanation: The native body part may or may not be taken out, and the transplanted body part may take over all or a portion of its function

Body Part Character 4	Approach Character 5	Device Character 6	Qualifier Character 7
J Hand, Right K Hand, Left	Ø Open	Z No Device	Ø Allogeneic 1 Syngeneic

Anatomical Regions, Lower Extremities ØYØ–ØYW

Character Meanings

This Character Meaning table is provided as a guide to assist the user in the identification of character members that may be found in this section of code tables. It **SHOULD NOT** be used to build a PCS code.

Operation–Character 3		Body Part–Character 4		Approach–Character 5		Device–Character 6		Qualifier–Character 7	
Ø	Alteration	Ø	Buttock, Right	Ø	Open	Ø	Drainage Device	Ø	Complete
2	Change	1	Buttock, Left	3	Percutaneous	1	Radioactive Element	1	High
3	Control	2	Hindquarter, Right	4	Percutaneous Endoscopic	3	Infusion Device	2	Mid
6	Detachment	3	Hindquarter, Left	X	External	7	Autologous Tissue Substitute	3	Low
9	Drainage	4	Hindquarter, Bilateral			J	Synthetic Substitute	4	Complete 1st Ray
B	Excision	5	Inguinal Region, Right			K	Nonautologous Tissue Substitute	5	Complete 2nd Ray
H	Insertion	6	Inguinal Region, Left			Y	Other Device	6	Complete 3rd Ray
J	Inspection	7	Femoral Region, Right			Z	No Device	7	Complete 4th Ray
M	Reattachment	8	Femoral Region, Left					8	Complete 5th Ray
P	Removal	9	Lower Extremity, Right					9	Partial 1st Ray
Q	Repair	A	Inguinal Region, Bilateral					B	Partial 2nd Ray
U	Supplement	B	Lower Extremity, Left					C	Partial 3rd Ray
W	Revision	C	Upper Leg, Right					D	Partial 4th Ray
		D	Upper Leg, Left					F	Partial 5th Ray
		E	Femoral Region, Bilateral					X	Diagnostic
		F	Knee Region, Right					Z	No Qualifier
		G	Knee Region, Left						
		H	Lower Leg, Right						
		J	Lower Leg, Left						
		K	Ankle Region, Right						
		L	Ankle Region, Left						
		M	Foot, Right						
		N	Foot, Left						
		P	1st Toe, Right						
		Q	1st Toe, Left						
		R	2nd Toe, Right						
		S	2nd Toe, Left						
		T	3rd Toe, Right						
		U	3rd Toe, Left						
		V	4th Toe, Right						
		W	4th Toe, Left						
		X	5th Toe, Right						
		Y	5th Toe, Left						

AHA Coding Clinic for table ØY3
2016, 4Q, 99 Root operation Control
2013, 3Q, 23 Control of intraoperative bleeding

AHA Coding Clinic for table ØY6
2019, 2Q, 17 Cryoamputation of lower leg
2017, 2Q, 3-4 Qualifiers for the root operation detachment
2017, 1Q, 22 Chopart amputation of foot
2015, 2Q, 28 Partial amputation of hallux at interphalangeal Joint
2015, 1Q, 28 Mid-foot amputation

AHA Coding Clinic for table ØY9
2015, 1Q, 22 Incision and drainage of abscess of femoropopliteal bypass site
2015, 1Q, 22 Incision and drainage of groin abscess

AHA Coding Clinic for table ØYH
2023, 1Q, 27 Bilateral traumatic amputation with Stage 1 placement of OPRA device
2023, 1Q, 29 Stage 2 placement of OPRA device

AHA Coding Clinic for table ØYW
2023, 1Q, 29 Stage 2 placement of OPRA device

Detachment Qualifier Descriptions

Qualifier Definition	Upper Leg	Lower Leg
1 **High:** Amputation at the proximal portion of the shaft of the:	Femur	Tibia/Fibula
2 **Mid:** Amputation at the middle portion of the shaft of the:	Femur	Tibia/Fibula
3 **Low:** Amputation at the distal portion of the shaft of the:	Femur	Tibia/Fibula

Qualifier Definition	Foot
0 Complete 1st through 5th Rays Ray: digit of hand or foot with corresponding metacarpus or metatarsus	Through tarso-metatarsal Joint, **Ankle**
4 Complete 1st Ray	Through tarso-metatarsal joint, **Great Toe**
5 Complete 2nd Ray	Through tarso-metatarsal joint, **2nd Toe**
6 Complete 3rd Ray	Through tarso-metatarsal joint, **3rd Toe**
7 Complete 4th Ray	Through tarso-metatarsal joint, **4th Toe**
8 Complete 5th Ray	Through tarso-metatarsal joint, **Little Toe**
9 Partial 1st Ray	Anywhere along shaft or head of metatarsal bone, **Great Toe**
B Partial 2nd Ray	Anywhere along shaft or head of metatarsal bone, **2nd Toe**
C Partial 3rd Ray	Anywhere along shaft or head of metatarsal bone, **3rd Toe**
D Partial 4th Ray	Anywhere along shaft or head of metatarsal bone, **4th Toe**
F Partial 5th Ray	Anywhere along shaft or head of metatarsal bone, **Little Toe**

Qualifier Definition	Toe
0 Complete	At the metatarsal-phalangeal joint
1 High	Anywhere along the proximal phalanx
2 Mid	Through the proximal interphalangeal joint or anywhere along the middle phalanx
3 Low	Through the distal interphalangeal joint or anywhere along the distal phalanx

Ø Medical and Surgical
Y Anatomical Regions, Lower Extremities
Ø Alteration Definition: Modifying the anatomic structure of a body part without affecting the function of the body part
Explanation: Principal purpose is to improve appearance

Body Part Character 4	Approach Character 5	Device Character 6	Qualifier Character 7
Ø Buttock, Right 1 Buttock, Left 9 Lower Extremity, Right B Lower Extremity, Left C Upper Leg, Right D Upper Leg, Left F Knee Region, Right G Knee Region, Left H Lower Leg, Right J Lower Leg, Left K Ankle Region, Right L Ankle Region, Left	Ø Open 3 Percutaneous 4 Percutaneous Endoscopic	7 Autologous Tissue Substitute J Synthetic Substitute K Nonautologous Tissue Substitute Z No Device	Z No Qualifier

Ø Medical and Surgical
Y Anatomical Regions, Lower Extremities
2 Change Definition: Taking out or off a device from a body part and putting back an identical or similar device in or on the same body part without cutting or puncturing the skin or a mucous membrane
Explanation: All CHANGE procedures are coded using the approach EXTERNAL

Body Part Character 4	Approach Character 5	Device Character 6	Qualifier Character 7
9 Lower Extremity, Right B Lower Extremity, Left	X External	Ø Drainage Device Y Other Device	Z No Qualifier

Non-OR All body part, approach, device, and qualifier values

Ø Medical and Surgical
Y Anatomical Regions, Lower Extremities
3 Control Definition: Stopping, or attempting to stop, postprocedural or other acute bleeding
Explanation: None

Body Part Character 4	Approach Character 5	Device Character 6	Qualifier Character 7
Ø Buttock, Right 1 Buttock, Left 5 Inguinal Region, Right Inguinal canal Inguinal triangle 6 Inguinal Region, Left *See 5 Inguinal Region, Right* 7 Femoral Region, Right 8 Femoral Region, Left 9 Lower Extremity, Right B Lower Extremity, Left C Upper Leg, Right D Upper Leg, Left F Knee Region, Right G Knee Region, Left H Lower Leg, Right J Lower Leg, Left K Ankle Region, Right L Ankle Region, Left M Foot, Right N Foot, Left	Ø Open 3 Percutaneous 4 Percutaneous Endoscopic	Z No Device	Z No Qualifier

Ø Medical and Surgical
Y Anatomical Regions, Lower Extremities
6 Detachment Definition: Cutting off all or a portion of the upper or lower extremities

Explanation: The body part value is the site of the detachment, with a qualifier if applicable to further specify the level where the extremity was detached

Body Part Character 4	Approach Character 5	Device Character 6	Qualifier Character 7
2 Hindquarter, Right **3** Hindquarter, Left **4** Hindquarter, Bilateral **7** Femoral Region, Right **8** Femoral Region, Left **F** Knee Region, Right **G** Knee Region, Left	**Ø** Open	**Z** No Device	**Z** No Qualifier
C Upper Leg, Right **D** Upper Leg, Left **H** Lower Leg, Right **J** Lower Leg, Left	**Ø** Open	**Z** No Device	**1** High **2** Mid **3** Low
M Foot, Right **N** Foot, Left	**Ø** Open	**Z** No Device	**Ø** Complete **4** Complete 1st Ray **5** Complete 2nd Ray **6** Complete 3rd Ray **7** Complete 4th Ray **8** Complete 5th Ray **9** Partial 1st Ray **B** Partial 2nd Ray **C** Partial 3rd Ray **D** Partial 4th Ray **F** Partial 5th Ray
P 1st Toe, Right Hallux **Q** 1st Toe, Left *See 1st Toe, Right* **R** 2nd Toe, Right **S** 2nd Toe, Left **T** 3rd Toe, Right **U** 3rd Toe, Left **V** 4th Toe, Right **W** 4th Toe, Left **X** 5th Toe, Right **Y** 5th Toe, Left	**Ø** Open	**Z** No Device	**Ø** Complete **1** High **2** Mid **3** Low

Ø Medical and Surgical
Y Anatomical Regions, Lower Extremities
9 Drainage Definition: Taking or letting out fluids and/or gases from a body part
Explanation: The qualifier DIAGNOSTIC is used to identify drainage procedures that are biopsies

Body Part Character 4	Approach Character 5	Device Character 6	Qualifier Character 7
Ø Buttock, Right **1** Buttock, Left **5** Inguinal Region, Right Inguinal canal Inguinal triangle **6** Inguinal Region, Left *See 5 Inguinal Region, Right* **7** Femoral Region, Right **8** Femoral Region, Left **9** Lower Extremity, Right **B** Lower Extremity, Left **C** Upper Leg, Right **D** Upper Leg, Left **F** Knee Region, Right **G** Knee Region, Left **H** Lower Leg, Right **J** Lower Leg, Left **K** Ankle Region, Right **L** Ankle Region, Left **M** Foot, Right **N** Foot, Left	**Ø** Open **3** Percutaneous **4** Percutaneous Endoscopic	**Ø** Drainage Device	**Z** No Qualifier
Ø Buttock, Right **1** Buttock, Left **5** Inguinal Region, Right Inguinal canal Inguinal triangle **6** Inguinal Region, Left *See 5 Inguinal Region, Right* **7** Femoral Region, Right **8** Femoral Region, Left **9** Lower Extremity, Right **B** Lower Extremity, Left **C** Upper Leg, Right **D** Upper Leg, Left **F** Knee Region, Right **G** Knee Region, Left **H** Lower Leg, Right **J** Lower Leg, Left **K** Ankle Region, Right **L** Ankle Region, Left **M** Foot, Right **N** Foot, Left	**Ø** Open **3** Percutaneous **4** Percutaneous Endoscopic	**Z** No Device	**X** Diagnostic **Z** No Qualifier

Non-OR ØY9[Ø,1,7,8,9,B,C,D,F,G,H,J,K,L,M,N][Ø,3,4]ØZ
Non-OR ØY9[5,6]3ØZ
Non-OR ØY9[Ø,1,7,8,9,B,C,D,F,G,H,J,K,L,M,N][Ø,3,4]Z[X,Z]
Non-OR ØY9[5,6]3ZZ

Ø Medical and Surgical
Y Anatomical Regions, Lower Extremities
B Excision Definition: Cutting out or off, without replacement, a portion of a body part
Explanation: The qualifier DIAGNOSTIC is used to identify excision procedures that are biopsies

Body Part Character 4	Approach Character 5	Device Character 6	Qualifier Character 7
Ø Buttock, Right 1 Buttock, Left 5 Inguinal Region, Right Inguinal canal Inguinal triangle 6 Inguinal Region, Left *See 5 Inguinal Region, Right* 7 Femoral Region, Right 8 Femoral Region, Left 9 Lower Extremity, Right B Lower Extremity, Left C Upper Leg, Right D Upper Leg, Left F Knee Region, Right G Knee Region, Left H Lower Leg, Right J Lower Leg, Left K Ankle Region, Right L Ankle Region, Left M Foot, Right N Foot, Left	Ø Open 3 Percutaneous 4 Percutaneous Endoscopic	Z No Device	X Diagnostic Z No Qualifier

Non-OR ØYB[Ø,1,9,B,C,D,F,G,H,J,K,L,M,N][Ø,3,4]ZX

Ø Medical and Surgical
Y Anatomical Regions, Lower Extremities
H Insertion Definition: Putting in a nonbiological appliance that monitors, assists, performs, or prevents a physiological function but does not physically take the place of a body part
Explanation: None

Body Part Character 4	Approach Character 5	Device Character 6	Qualifier Character 7
Ø Buttock, Right 1 Buttock, Left 5 Inguinal Region, Right Inguinal canal Inguinal triangle 6 Inguinal Region, Left *See 5 Inguinal Region, Right* 7 Femoral Region, Right 8 Femoral Region, Left 9 Lower Extremity, Right B Lower Extremity, Left C Upper Leg, Right D Upper Leg, Left F Knee Region, Right G Knee Region, Left H Lower Leg, Right J Lower Leg, Left K Ankle Region, Right L Ankle Region, Left M Foot, Right N Foot, Left	Ø Open 3 Percutaneous 4 Percutaneous Endoscopic	1 Radioactive Element 3 Infusion Device Y Other Device	Z No Qualifier

DRG Non-OR ØYH[Ø,1,5,6,7,8,9,B,C,D,F,G,H,J,K,L,M,N][Ø,3,4][3,Y]Z

Ø Medical and Surgical
Y Anatomical Regions, Lower Extremities
J Inspection Definition: Visually and/or manually exploring a body part

Explanation: Visual exploration may be performed with or without optical instrumentation. Manual exploration may be performed directly or through intervening body layers.

Body Part Character 4	Approach Character 5	Device Character 6	Qualifier Character 7
Ø Buttock, Right **1** Buttock, Left **5** Inguinal Region, Right Inguinal canal Inguinal triangle **6** Inguinal Region, Left *See* *5 Inguinal Region, Right* **7** Femoral Region, Right **8** Femoral Region, Left **9** Lower Extremity, Right **A** Inguinal Region, Bilateral *See* *5 Inguinal Region, Right* **B** Lower Extremity, Left **C** Upper Leg, Right **D** Upper Leg, Left **E** Femoral Region, Bilateral **F** Knee Region, Right **G** Knee Region, Left **H** Lower Leg, Right **J** Lower Leg, Left **K** Ankle Region, Right **L** Ankle Region, Left **M** Foot, Right **N** Foot, Left	**Ø** Open **3** Percutaneous **4** Percutaneous Endoscopic **X** External	**Z** No Device	**Z** No Qualifier

DRG Non-OR ØYJ[Ø,1,8,9,B,C,D,E,F,G,H,J,K,L,M,N]ØZZ
Non-OR ØYJ[Ø,1,9,B,C,D,F,G,H,J,K,L,M,N][3,4,X]ZZ
Non-OR ØYJ[5,6,7,8,A,E][3,X]ZZ

Ø Medical and Surgical
Y Anatomical Regions, Lower Extremities
M Reattachment Definition: Putting back in or on all or a portion of a separated body part to its normal location or other suitable location

Explanation: Vascular circulation and nervous pathways may or may not be reestablished

Body Part Character 4	Approach Character 5	Device Character 6	Qualifier Character 7
Ø Buttock, Right **1 Buttock, Left** **2 Hindquarter, Right** **3 Hindquarter, Left** **4 Hindquarter, Bilateral** **5 Inguinal Region, Right** Inguinal canal Inguinal triangle **6 Inguinal Region, Left** *See 5 Inguinal Region, Right* **7 Femoral Region, Right** **8 Femoral Region, Left** **9 Lower Extremity, Right** **B Lower Extremity, Left** **C Upper Leg, Right** **D Upper Leg, Left** **F Knee Region, Right** **G Knee Region, Left** **H Lower Leg, Right** **J Lower Leg, Left** **K Ankle Region, Right** **L Ankle Region, Left** **M Foot, Right** **N Foot, Left** **P 1st Toe, Right** Hallux **Q 1st Toe, Left** *See 1st Toe, Right* **R 2nd Toe, Right** **S 2nd Toe, Left** **T 3rd Toe, Right** **U 3rd Toe, Left** **V 4th Toe, Right** **W 4th Toe, Left** **X 5th Toe, Right** **Y 5th Toe, Left**	**Ø Open**	**Z No Device**	**Z No Qualifier**

Ø Medical and Surgical
Y Anatomical Regions, Lower Extremities
P Removal Definition: Taking out or off a device from a body part

Explanation: If a device is taken out and a similar device put in without cutting or puncturing the skin or mucous membrane, the procedure is coded to the root operation CHANGE. Otherwise, the procedure for taking out the device is coded to the root operation REMOVAL.

Body Part Character 4	Approach Character 5	Device Character 6	Qualifier Character 7
9 Lower Extremity, Right **B Lower Extremity, Left**	**Ø Open** **3 Percutaneous** **4 Percutaneous Endoscopic** **X External**	**Ø Drainage Device** **1 Radioactive Element** **3 Infusion Device** **7 Autologous Tissue Substitute** **J Synthetic Substitute** **K Nonautologous Tissue Substitute** **Y Other Device**	**Z No Qualifier**

Non-OR All body part, approach, device, and qualifier values

Ø Medical and Surgical
Y Anatomical Regions, Lower Extremities
Q Repair Definition: Restoring, to the extent possible, a body part to its normal anatomic structure and function
Explanation: Used only when the method to accomplish the repair is not one of the other root operations

Body Part Character 4	Approach Character 5	Device Character 6	Qualifier Character 7
Ø Buttock, Right **1** Buttock, Left **5** Inguinal Region, Right Inguinal canal Inguinal triangle **6** Inguinal Region, Left *See 5 Inguinal Region, Right* **7** Femoral Region, Right **8** Femoral Region, Left **9** Lower Extremity, Right **A** Inguinal Region, Bilateral *See 5 Inguinal Region, Right* **B** Lower Extremity, Left **C** Upper Leg, Right **D** Upper Leg, Left **E** Femoral Region, Bilateral **F** Knee Region, Right **G** Knee Region, Left **H** Lower Leg, Right **J** Lower Leg, Left **K** Ankle Region, Right **L** Ankle Region, Left **M** Foot, Right **N** Foot, Left **P** 1st Toe, Right Hallux **Q** 1st Toe, Left *See 1st Toe, Right* **R** 2nd Toe, Right **S** 2nd Toe, Left **T** 3rd Toe, Right **U** 3rd Toe, Left **V** 4th Toe, Right **W** 4th Toe, Left **X** 5th Toe, Right **Y** 5th Toe, Left	**Ø** Open **3** Percutaneous **4** Percutaneous Endoscopic **X** External	**Z** No Device	**Z** No Qualifier

Non-OR ØYQ[5,6,7,8,A,E]XZZ

Ø Medical and Surgical
Y Anatomical Regions, Lower Extremities
U Supplement Definition: Putting in or on biological or synthetic material that physically reinforces and/or augments the function of a portion of a body part

Explanation: The biological material is non-living, or is living and from the same individual. The body part may have been previously replaced, and the SUPPLEMENT procedure is performed to physically reinforce and/or augment the function of the replaced body part.

Body Part Character 4	Approach Character 5	Device Character 6	Qualifier Character 7
Ø Buttock, Right 1 Buttock, Left 5 Inguinal Region, Right Inguinal canal Inguinal triangle 6 Inguinal Region, Left *See 5 Inguinal Region, Right* 7 Femoral Region, Right 8 Femoral Region, Left 9 Lower Extremity, Right A Inguinal Region, Bilateral *See 5 Inguinal Region, Right* B Lower Extremity, Left C Upper Leg, Right D Upper Leg, Left E Femoral Region, Bilateral F Knee Region, Right G Knee Region, Left H Lower Leg, Right J Lower Leg, Left K Ankle Region, Right L Ankle Region, Left M Foot, Right N Foot, Left P 1st Toe, Right Hallux Q 1st Toe, Left *See 1st Toe, Right* R 2nd Toe, Right S 2nd Toe, Left T 3rd Toe, Right U 3rd Toe, Left V 4th Toe, Right W 4th Toe, Left X 5th Toe, Right Y 5th Toe, Left	Ø Open 4 Percutaneous Endoscopic	7 Autologous Tissue Substitute J Synthetic Substitute K Nonautologous Tissue Substitute	Z No Qualifier

Ø Medical and Surgical
Y Anatomical Regions, Lower Extremities
W Revision Definition: Correcting, to the extent possible, a portion of a malfunctioning device or the position of a displaced device

Explanation: Revision can include correcting a malfunctioning or displaced device by taking out or putting in components of the device such as a screw or pin

Body Part Character 4	Approach Character 5	Device Character 6	Qualifier Character 7
9 Lower Extremity, Right B Lower Extremity, Left	Ø Open 3 Percutaneous 4 Percutaneous Endoscopic X External	Ø Drainage Device 3 Infusion Device 7 Autologous Tissue Substitute J Synthetic Substitute K Nonautologous Tissue Substitute Y Other Device	Z No Qualifier

DRG Non-OR ØYW[9,B][Ø,3,4][Ø,3,7,J,K,Y]Z
Non-OR ØYW[9,B]X[Ø,3,7,J,K,Y]Z

Obstetrics 1Ø2–1ØY

Character Meanings

This Character Meaning table is provided as a guide to assist the user in the identification of character members that may be found in this section of code tables. It **SHOULD NOT** be used to build a PCS code.

Ø: Pregnancy

Operation–Character 3	Body Part–Character 4	Approach–Character 5	Device–Character 6	Qualifier–Character 7
2 Change	Ø Products of Conception	Ø Open	3 Monitoring Electrode	Ø High
9 Drainage	1 Products of Conception, Retained	3 Percutaneous	Y Other Device	1 Low
A Abortion	2 Products of Conception, Ectopic	4 Percutaneous Endoscopic	Z No Device	2 Extraperitoneal
D Extraction		7 Via Natural or Artificial Opening		3 Low Forceps
E Delivery		8 Via Natural or Artificial Opening Endoscopic		4 Mid Forceps
H Insertion		X External		5 High Forceps
J Inspection				6 Vacuum
P Removal				7 Internal Version
Q Repair				8 Other
S Reposition				9 Fetal Blood OR Manual
T Resection				A Fetal Cerebrospinal Fluid
Y Transplantation				B Fetal Fluid, Other
				C Amniotic Fluid, Therapeutic
				D Fluid, Other
				E Nervous System
				F Cardiovascular System
				G Lymphatics & Hemic
				H Eye
				J Ear, Nose & Sinus
				K Respiratory System
				L Mouth & Throat
				M Gastrointestinal System
				N Hepatobiliary & Pancreas
				P Endocrine System
				Q Skin
				R Musculoskeletal System
				S Urinary System
				T Female Reproductive System
				U Amniotic Fluid, Diagnostic
				V Male Reproductive System
				W Laminaria
				X Abortifacient
				Y Other Body System
				Z No Qualifier

AHA Coding Clinic for table 1Ø9
2014, 3Q, 12 Fetoscopic laser photocoagulation and laser microseptostomy for twin-twin transfusion syndrome
2014, 2Q, 9 Pitocin administration to augment labor

AHA Coding Clinic for table 1ØA
2022, 1Q, 21 Gravid hysterectomy due to placenta increta
2022, 1Q, 41 Intrauterine Cook balloon placement for ectopic pregnancy

AHA Coding Clinic for table 1ØD
2022, 1Q, 19 Spontaneous abortion with retained placenta of Twin B
2021, 1Q, 52 Removal of ectopic pregnancy via laparotomy
2020, 4Q, 59-60 Extraction of ectopic products of conception
2018, 4Q, 49-51 Revised qualifier values for root operation "extraction" (cesarean delivery)
2018, 2Q, 17 High transverse cesarean section
2016, 1Q, 9 Vaginal delivery assisted by vacuum and low forceps extraction
2014, 4Q, 43 Cesarean delivery assisted by vacuum extraction
2014, 4Q, 43 Vacuum dilation and curettage for blighted ovum

AHA Coding Clinic for table 1ØE
2017, 3Q, 5 Delivery of placenta
2016, 2Q, 34 Assisted vaginal delivery
2014, 4Q, 17 RH (D) alloimmunization (sensitization)
2014, 2Q, 9 Pitocin administration to augment labor

AHA Coding Clinic for table 1ØH
2013, 2Q, 36 Intrauterine pressure monitor

AHA Coding Clinic for table 1ØQ
2021, 2Q, 21 Ex Utero intrapartum treatment procedure
2014, 3Q, 12 Fetoscopic laser photocoagulation and laser microseptostomy for twin-twin transfusion syndrome

AHA Coding Clinic for table 1ØT
2020, 3Q, 47 Removal of ectopic cornual pregnancy
2015, 3Q, 31 Laparoscopic partial salpingectomy for ectopic pregnancy

1 Obstetrics
Ø Pregnancy
2 Change

Definition: Taking out or off a device from a body part and putting back an identical or similar device in or on the same body part without cutting or puncturing the skin or a mucous membrane

Explanation: None

Body Part Character 4	Approach Character 5	Device Character 6	Qualifier Character 7
Ø Products of Conception ♀	7 Via Natural or Artificial Opening	3 Monitoring Electrode Y Other Device	Z No Qualifier

Non-OR All body part, approach, device, and qualifier values
♀ All body part, approach, device, and qualifier values

1 Obstetrics
Ø Pregnancy
9 Drainage

Definition: Taking or letting out fluids and/or gases from a body part

Explanation: None

Body Part Character 4	Approach Character 5	Device Character 6	Qualifier Character 7
Ø Products of Conception ♀	Ø Open 3 Percutaneous 4 Percutaneous Endoscopic 7 Via Natural or Artificial Opening 8 Via Natural or Artificial Opening Endoscopic	Z No Device	9 Fetal Blood A Fetal Cerebrospinal Fluid B Fetal Fluid, Other C Amniotic Fluid, Therapeutic D Fluid, Other U Amniotic Fluid, Diagnostic

Non-OR All body part, approach, device, and qualifier values
♀ All body part, approach, device, and qualifier values

1 Obstetrics
Ø Pregnancy
A Abortion

Definition: Artificially terminating a pregnancy

Explanation: None

Body Part Character 4	Approach Character 5	Device Character 6	Qualifier Character 7
Ø Products of Conception ♀	Ø Open 3 Percutaneous 4 Percutaneous Endoscopic 8 Via Natural or Artificial Opening Endoscopic	Z No Device	Z No Qualifier
Ø Products of Conception ♀	7 Via Natural or Artificial Opening	Z No Device	6 Vacuum W Laminaria X Abortifacient Z No Qualifier

Non-OR 1ØAØ7Z[6,W,X]
♀ All body part, approach, device, and qualifier values

1 Obstetrics
Ø Pregnancy
D Extraction

Definition: Pulling or stripping out or off all or a portion of a body part by the use of force

Explanation: None

Body Part Character 4	Approach Character 5	Device Character 6	Qualifier Character 7
Ø Products of Conception QA ♀	Ø Open	Z No Device	Ø High 1 Low 2 Extraperitoneal
Ø Products of Conception QA ♀	7 Via Natural or Artificial Opening	Z No Device	3 Low Forceps 4 Mid Forceps 5 High Forceps 6 Vacuum 7 Internal Version 8 Other
1 Products of Conception, Retained ♀	7 Via Natural or Artificial Opening 8 Via Natural or Artificial Opening Endoscopic	Z No Device	9 Manual Z No Qualifier
2 Products of Conception, Ectopic ♀	Ø Open 4 Percutaneous Endoscopic 7 Via Natural or Artificial Opening 8 Via Natural or Artificial Opening Endoscopic	Z No Device	Z No Qualifier

DRG Non-OR 1ØDØ7Z[3,4,5,6,7,8]
QA 1ØDØØZ[Ø,1,2] except when a corresponding SDX of Z37.Ø-Z37.9 is also reported
QA 1ØDØ7Z[3,4,5,7] except when a corresponding SDX of Z37.Ø-Z37.9 is also reported
♀ All body part, approach, device, and qualifier values

1 Obstetrics
Ø Pregnancy
E Delivery

Definition: Assisting the passage of the products of conception from the genital canal

Explanation: None

Body Part Character 4	Approach Character 5	Device Character 6	Qualifier Character 7
Ø Products of Conception QA ♀	X External	Z No Device	Z No Qualifier

DRG Non-OR 1ØEØXZZ
QA 1ØEØXZZ except when a corresponding SDX of Z37.Ø-Z37.9 is also reported
♀ All body part, approach, device, and qualifier values

1 Obstetrics
Ø Pregnancy
H Insertion

Definition: Putting in a nonbiological appliance that monitors, assists, performs, or prevents a physiological function but does not physically take the place of a body part

Explanation: None

Body Part Character 4	Approach Character 5	Device Character 6	Qualifier Character 7
Ø Products of Conception ♀	Ø Open 7 Via Natural or Artificial Opening	3 Monitoring Electrode Y Other Device	Z No Qualifier

Non-OR All body part, approach, device, and qualifier values
♀ All body part, approach, device, and qualifier values

1 Obstetrics
Ø Pregnancy
J Inspection

Definition: Visually and/or manually exploring a body part

Explanation: Visual exploration may be performed with or without optical instrumentation. Manual exploration may be performed directly or through intervening body layers.

Body Part Character 4	Approach Character 5	Device Character 6	Qualifier Character 7
Ø Products of Conception ♀ 1 Products of Conception, Retained ♀ 2 Products of Conception, Ectopic ♀	Ø Open 3 Percutaneous 4 Percutaneous Endoscopic 7 Via Natural or Artificial Opening 8 Via Natural or Artificial Opening Endoscopic X External	Z No Device	Z No Qualifier

Non-OR All body part, approach, device, and qualifier values
♀ All body part, approach, device, and qualifier values

1 Obstetrics
Ø Pregnancy
P Removal

Definition: Taking out or off a device from a body part, region or orifice

Explanation: If a device is taken out and a similar device put in without cutting or puncturing the skin or mucous membrane, the procedure is coded to the root operation CHANGE. Otherwise, the procedure for taking out a device is coded to the root operation REMOVAL.

Body Part Character 4	Approach Character 5	Device Character 6	Qualifier Character 7
Ø Products of Conception ♀	Ø Open 7 Via Natural or Artificial Opening	3 Monitoring Electrode Y Other Device	Z No Qualifier

Non-OR All body part, approach, device, and qualifier values
♀ All body part, approach, device, and qualifier values

1 Obstetrics
Ø Pregnancy
Q Repair

Definition: Restoring, to the extent possible, a body part to its normal anatomic structure and function

Explanation: Used only when the method to accomplish the repair is not one of the other root operations

Body Part Character 4	Approach Character 5	Device Character 6	Qualifier Character 7
Ø Products of Conception ♀	Ø Open 3 Percutaneous 4 Percutaneous Endoscopic 7 Via Natural or Artificial Opening 8 Via Natural or Artificial Opening Endoscopic	Y Other Device Z No Device	E Nervous System F Cardiovascular System G Lymphatics and Hemic H Eye J Ear, Nose and Sinus K Respiratory System L Mouth and Throat M Gastrointestinal System N Hepatobiliary and Pancreas P Endocrine System Q Skin R Musculoskeletal System S Urinary System T Female Reproductive System V Male Reproductive System Y Other Body System

Non-OR All body part, approach, device, and qualifier values
♀ All body part, approach, device, and qualifier values

1 Obstetrics
Ø Pregnancy
S Reposition

Definition: Moving to its normal location, or other suitable location, all or a portion of a body part

Explanation: The body part is moved to a new location from an abnormal location, or from a normal location where it is not functioning correctly. The body part may or may not be cut out or off to be moved to the new location.

Body Part Character 4	Approach Character 5	Device Character 6	Qualifier Character 7
Ø Products of Conception ♀	7 Via Natural or Artificial Opening X External	Z No Device	Z No Qualifier
2 Products of Conception, Ectopic ♀	Ø Open 3 Percutaneous 4 Percutaneous Endoscopic 7 Via Natural or Artificial Opening 8 Via Natural or Artificial Opening Endoscopic	Z No Device	Z No Qualifier

Non-OR 1ØSØ[7,X]ZZ
♀ All body part, approach, device, and qualifier values

1 Obstetrics
Ø Pregnancy
T Resection

Definition: Cutting out or off, without replacement, all of a body part

Explanation: None

Body Part Character 4	Approach Character 5	Device Character 6	Qualifier Character 7
2 Products of Conception, Ectopic ♀	Ø Open 3 Percutaneous 4 Percutaneous Endoscopic 7 Via Natural or Artificial Opening 8 Via Natural or Artificial Opening Endoscopic	Z No Device	Z No Qualifier

♀ All body part, approach, device, and qualifier values

1 Obstetrics
Ø Pregnancy
Y Transplantation

Definition: Putting in or on all or a portion of a living body part taken from another individual or animal to physically take the place and/or function of all or a portion of a similar body part

Explanation: The native body part may or may not be taken out, and the transplanted body part may take over all or a portion of its function

Body Part Character 4	Approach Character 5	Device Character 6	Qualifier Character 7
Ø Products of Conception ♀	3 Percutaneous 4 Percutaneous Endoscopic 7 Via Natural or Artificial Opening	Z No Device	E Nervous System F Cardiovascular System G Lymphatics and Hemic H Eye J Ear, Nose and Sinus K Respiratory System L Mouth and Throat M Gastrointestinal System N Hepatobiliary and Pancreas P Endocrine System Q Skin R Musculoskeletal System S Urinary System T Female Reproductive System V Male Reproductive System Y Other Body System

Non-OR All body part, approach, device, and qualifier values
♀ All body part, approach, device, and qualifier values

Placement 2WØ–2Y5

AHA Coding Clinic for table 2W6
2015, 2Q, 35 Application of tongs to reduce and stabilize cervical fracture
2013, 2Q, 39 Application of cervical tongs for reduction of cervical fracture

AHA Coding Clinic for table 2Y4
2018, 4Q, 38 Control of epistaxis
2017, 4Q, 106 Nasal packing for epistaxis

2 Placement
W Anatomical Regions
Ø Change Definition: Taking out or off a device from a body part and putting back an identical or similar device in or on the same body part without cutting or puncturing the skin or a mucous membrane

Body Region Character 4	Approach Character 5	Device Character 6	Qualifier Character 7
Ø Head 2 Neck 3 Abdominal Wall 4 Chest Wall 5 Back 6 Inguinal Region, Right 7 Inguinal Region, Left 8 Upper Extremity, Right 9 Upper Extremity, Left A Upper Arm, Right B Upper Arm, Left C Lower Arm, Right D Lower Arm, Left E Hand, Right F Hand, Left G Thumb, Right H Thumb, Left J Finger, Right K Finger, Left L Lower Extremity, Right M Lower Extremity, Left N Upper Leg, Right P Upper Leg, Left Q Lower Leg, Right R Lower Leg, Left S Foot, Right T Foot, Left U Toe, Right V Toe, Left	X External	Ø Traction Apparatus 1 Splint 2 Cast 3 Brace 4 Bandage 5 Packing Material 6 Pressure Dressing 7 Intermittent Pressure Device Y Other Device	Z No Qualifier
1 Face	X External	Ø Traction Apparatus 1 Splint 2 Cast 3 Brace 4 Bandage 5 Packing Material 6 Pressure Dressing 7 Intermittent Pressure Device 9 Wire Y Other Device	Z No Qualifier

2 Placement
W Anatomical Regions
1 Compression Definition: Putting pressure on a body region

Body Region Character 4	Approach Character 5	Device Character 6	Qualifier Character 7
Ø Head 1 Face 2 Neck 3 Abdominal Wall 4 Chest Wall 5 Back 6 Inguinal Region, Right 7 Inguinal Region, Left 8 Upper Extremity, Right 9 Upper Extremity, Left A Upper Arm, Right B Upper Arm, Left C Lower Arm, Right D Lower Arm, Left E Hand, Right F Hand, Left G Thumb, Right H Thumb, Left J Finger, Right K Finger, Left L Lower Extremity, Right M Lower Extremity, Left N Upper Leg, Right P Upper Leg, Left Q Lower Leg, Right R Lower Leg, Left S Foot, Right T Foot, Left U Toe, Right V Toe, Left	X External	6 Pressure Dressing 7 Intermittent Pressure Device	Z No Qualifier

2 Placement
W Anatomical Regions
2 Dressing Definition: Putting material on a body region for protection

Body Region Character 4	Approach Character 5	Device Character 6	Qualifier Character 7
Ø Head 1 Face 2 Neck 3 Abdominal Wall 4 Chest Wall 5 Back 6 Inguinal Region, Right 7 Inguinal Region, Left 8 Upper Extremity, Right 9 Upper Extremity, Left A Upper Arm, Right B Upper Arm, Left C Lower Arm, Right D Lower Arm, Left E Hand, Right F Hand, Left G Thumb, Right H Thumb, Left J Finger, Right K Finger, Left L Lower Extremity, Right M Lower Extremity, Left N Upper Leg, Right P Upper Leg, Left Q Lower Leg, Right R Lower Leg, Left S Foot, Right T Foot, Left U Toe, Right V Toe, Left	X External	4 Bandage	Z No Qualifier

2 Placement
W Anatomical Regions
3 Immobilization Definition: Limiting or preventing motion of a body region

Body Region Character 4	Approach Character 5	Device Character 6	Qualifier Character 7
Ø Head **2** Neck **3** Abdominal Wall **4** Chest Wall **5** Back **6** Inguinal Region, Right **7** Inguinal Region, Left **8** Upper Extremity, Right **9** Upper Extremity, Left **A** Upper Arm, Right **B** Upper Arm, Left **C** Lower Arm, Right **D** Lower Arm, Left **E** Hand, Right **F** Hand, Left **G** Thumb, Right **H** Thumb, Left **J** Finger, Right **K** Finger, Left **L** Lower Extremity, Right **M** Lower Extremity, Left **N** Upper Leg, Right **P** Upper Leg, Left **Q** Lower Leg, Right **R** Lower Leg, Left **S** Foot, Right **T** Foot, Left **U** Toe, Right **V** Toe, Left	**X** External	**1** Splint **2** Cast **3** Brace **Y** Other Device	**Z** No Qualifier
1 Face	**X** External	**1** Splint **2** Cast **3** Brace **9** Wire **Y** Other Device	**Z** No Qualifier

2 Placement
W Anatomical Regions
4 Packing Definition: Putting material in a body region or orifice

Body Region Character 4	Approach Character 5	Device Character 6	Qualifier Character 7
Ø Head **1** Face **2** Neck **3** Abdominal Wall **4** Chest Wall **5** Back **6** Inguinal Region, Right **7** Inguinal Region, Left **8** Upper Extremity, Right **9** Upper Extremity, Left **A** Upper Arm, Right **B** Upper Arm, Left **C** Lower Arm, Right **D** Lower Arm, Left **E** Hand, Right **F** Hand, Left **G** Thumb, Right **H** Thumb, Left **J** Finger, Right **K** Finger, Left **L** Lower Extremity, Right **M** Lower Extremity, Left **N** Upper Leg, Right **P** Upper Leg, Left **Q** Lower Leg, Right **R** Lower Leg, Left **S** Foot, Right **T** Foot, Left **U** Toe, Right **V** Toe, Left	**X** External	**5** Packing Material	**Z** No Qualifier

2 Placement
W Anatomical Regions
5 Removal Definition: Taking out or off a device from a body part

Body Region Character 4	Approach Character 5	Device Character 6	Qualifier Character 7
Ø Head 2 Neck 3 Abdominal Wall 4 Chest Wall 5 Back 6 Inguinal Region, Right 7 Inguinal Region, Left 8 Upper Extremity, Right 9 Upper Extremity, Left A Upper Arm, Right B Upper Arm, Left C Lower Arm, Right D Lower Arm, Left E Hand, Right F Hand, Left G Thumb, Right H Thumb, Left J Finger, Right K Finger, Left L Lower Extremity, Right M Lower Extremity, Left N Upper Leg, Right P Upper Leg, Left Q Lower Leg, Right R Lower Leg, Left S Foot, Right T Foot, Left U Toe, Right V Toe, Left	X External	Ø Traction Apparatus 1 Splint 2 Cast 3 Brace 4 Bandage 5 Packing Material 6 Pressure Dressing 7 Intermittent Pressure Device Y Other Device	Z No Qualifier
1 Face	X External	Ø Traction Apparatus 1 Splint 2 Cast 3 Brace 4 Bandage 5 Packing Material 6 Pressure Dressing 7 Intermittent Pressure Device 9 Wire Y Other Device	Z No Qualifier

2 Placement
W Anatomical Regions
6 Traction Definition: Exerting a pulling force on a body region in a distal direction

Body Region Character 4	Approach Character 5	Device Character 6	Qualifier Character 7
Ø Head 1 Face 2 Neck 3 Abdominal Wall 4 Chest Wall 5 Back 6 Inguinal Region, Right 7 Inguinal Region, Left 8 Upper Extremity, Right 9 Upper Extremity, Left A Upper Arm, Right B Upper Arm, Left C Lower Arm, Right D Lower Arm, Left E Hand, Right F Hand, Left G Thumb, Right H Thumb, Left J Finger, Right K Finger, Left L Lower Extremity, Right M Lower Extremity, Left N Upper Leg, Right P Upper Leg, Left Q Lower Leg, Right R Lower Leg, Left S Foot, Right T Foot, Left U Toe, Right V Toe, Left	X External	Ø Traction Apparatus Z No Device	Z No Qualifier

2 Placement
Y Anatomical Orifices
Ø Change Definition: Taking out or off a device from a body part and putting back an identical or similar device in or on the same body part without cutting or puncturing the skin or a mucous membrane

Body Region Character 4	Approach Character 5	Device Character 6	Qualifier Character 7
Ø Mouth and Pharynx 1 Nasal 2 Ear 3 Anorectal 4 Female Genital Tract ♀ 5 Urethra	X External	5 Packing Material	Z No Qualifier

♀ 2YØ4X5Z

2 Placement
Y Anatomical Orifices
4 Packing Definition: Putting material in a body region or orifice

Body Region Character 4	Approach Character 5	Device Character 6	Qualifier Character 7
Ø Mouth and Pharynx 1 Nasal 2 Ear 3 Anorectal 4 Female Genital Tract ♀ 5 Urethra	X External	5 Packing Material	Z No Qualifier

♀ 2Y44X5Z

2 Placement
Y Anatomical Orifices
5 Removal Definition: Taking out or off a device from a body part

Body Region Character 4	Approach Character 5	Device Character 6	Qualifier Character 7
Ø Mouth and Pharynx 1 Nasal 2 Ear 3 Anorectal 4 Female Genital Tract ♀ 5 Urethra	X External	5 Packing Material	Z No Qualifier

♀ 2Y54X5Z

Administration 3Ø2–3E1

AHA Coding Clinic for table 3Ø2

2023, 1Q, 10-11 Intraosseous administration of blood products
2021, 4Q, 54 Nonautologous pathogen reduced cryoprecipitated fibrinogen complex
2020, 4Q, 60-61 Transfusion stem cell progenitor cells
2019, 4Q, 35 Transfusion of blood products
2019, 4Q, 36 T-cell depleted hematopoietic stem cells for transplantation
2016, 4Q, 113 Bone marrow and stem cell transfusion (Transplantation)

AHA Coding Clinic for table 3EØ

2023, 2Q, 33 Testing of premature rupture of membranes via indigo carmine injection
2022, 4Q, 60-61 Introduction of other therapeutic monoclonal antibody
2022, 4Q, 61 Introduction of bone-substitute material
2022, 3Q, 26 Tumor-infiltrating lymphocyte therapy
2022, 1Q, 8 Other monoclonal antibody
2021, 4Q, 54-55 Antineoplastic monoclonal antibody
2021, 4Q, 110 New/revised frequently asked questions regarding ICD-10-CM/PCS coding for COVID-19
2021, 1Q, 49 Frequently asked questions regarding ICD-10-CM and ICD-10-PCS coding for COVID-19
2020, 4Q, 49-50 Intravascular ultrasound assisted thrombolysis
2020, 4Q, 95 Frequently asked questions regarding ICD-10-PCS coding for COVID-19
2020, 3Q, 17-21 New procedure codes for introduction or infusion of therapeutics
2019, 4Q, 36-37 Hyperthermic antineoplastic chemotherapy
2018, 3Q, 7 Coronary brachytherapy with angioplasty
2018, 1Q, 8 Placement of bone morphogenetic protein & spinal fusion surgery
2017, 2Q, 14 Infusion of tPA into pleural cavity
2017, 1Q, 37 Injection of glue into enteric fistula tract
2016, 4Q, 113-114 Substances applied to cranial cavity and brain
2016, 3Q, 29 Closure of bilateral alveolar clefts
2016, 1Q, 20 Metatarsophalangeal joint resection arthroplasty

AHA Coding Clinic for table 3EØ (Continued)

2015, 3Q, 24 Esophagogastroduodenoscopy with epinephrine injection for control of bleeding
2015, 3Q, 29 Placement of adhesion barrier
2015, 2Q, 29 Insertion of nasogastric tube for drainage and feeding
2015, 2Q, 31 Thoracoscopic talc pleurodesis
2015, 1Q, 31 Intrathecal chemotherapy
2015, 1Q, 38 Chemoembolization of the hepatic artery
2014, 4Q, 16 Administration of RH (D) immunoglobulin
2014, 4Q, 17 RH (D) alloimmunization (sensitization)
2014, 4Q, 19 Ultrasound accelerated thrombolysis
2014, 4Q, 34 Resection of brain malignancy with implantation of chemotherapeutic wafer
2014, 4Q, 38 Placement of saline and Seprafilm solution into abdominal cavity
2014, 3Q, 26 Coil embolization of gastroduodenal artery with chemoembolization of hepatic artery
2014, 2Q, 8 Medical induction of labor with Cervidil tampon insertion
2014, 2Q, 10 Prophylactic Neulasta injection for infection prevention
2013, 4Q, 124 Administration of tPA for stroke treatment prior to transfer
2013, 1Q, 27 Injection of sclerosing agent into an esophageal varix

AHA Coding Clinic for table 3E1

2021, 4Q, 55 Laparoscopic irrigation of peritoneal cavity
2019, 4Q, 38 Irrigation of joint using irrigating substance
2017, 3Q, 14 Bronchoscopy with suctioning and washings for removal of mucus plug

3 Administration
Ø Circulatory
2 Transfusion Definition: Putting in blood or blood products

Body System/Region Character 4	Approach Character 5	Substance Character 6	Qualifier Character 7
3 Peripheral Vein NC 4 Central Vein NC	3 Percutaneous	A Stem Cells, Embryonic	Z No Qualifier
3 Peripheral Vein 4 Central Vein	3 Percutaneous	C Hematopoietic Stem/Progenitor Cells, Genetically Modified	Ø Autologous
3 Peripheral Vein 4 Central Vein	3 Percutaneous	D Pathogen Reduced Cryoprecipitated Fibrinogen Complex NT	1 Nonautologous
3 Peripheral Vein NC 4 Central Vein NC	3 Percutaneous	G Bone Marrow X Stem Cells, Cord Blood Y Stem Cells, Hematopoietic	Ø Autologous 2 Allogeneic, Related 3 Allogeneic, Unrelated 4 Allogeneic, Unspecified
3 Peripheral Vein 4 Central Vein	3 Percutaneous	H Whole Blood J Serum Albumin K Frozen Plasma L Fresh Plasma M Plasma Cryoprecipitate N Red Blood Cells P Frozen Red Cells Q White Cells R Platelets S Globulin T Fibrinogen V Antihemophilic Factors W Factor IX	Ø Autologous 1 Nonautologous
3 Peripheral Vein 4 Central Vein	3 Percutaneous	U Stem Cells, T-cell Depleted Hematopoietic	2 Allogeneic, Related 3 Allogeneic, Unrelated 4 Allogeneic, Unspecified
7 Products of Conception, Circulatory ♀	3 Percutaneous 7 Via Natural or Artificial Opening	H Whole Blood J Serum Albumin K Frozen Plasma L Fresh Plasma M Plasma Cryoprecipitate N Red Blood Cells P Frozen Red Cells Q White Cells R Platelets S Globulin T Fibrinogen V Antihemophilic Factors W Factor IX	1 Nonautologous
8 Vein	3 Percutaneous	B 4-Factor Prothrombin Complex Concentrate	1 Nonautologous
A Bone Marrow	3 Percutaneous	H Whole Blood J Serum Albumin K Frozen Plasma L Fresh Plasma N Red Blood Cells P Frozen Red Cells R Platelets	Ø Autologous 1 Nonautologous

DRG Non-OR 3Ø2[3,4]3AZ
DRG Non-OR 3Ø2[3,4]3CØ
DRG Non-OR 3Ø2[3,4]3[G,X,Y][Ø,2,3,4]
DRG Non-OR 3Ø2[3,4]3U[2,3,4]

NC 3Ø2[3,4]3AZ Only when reported with PDx or SDx of C91.ØØ, C92.ØØ, C92.1Ø, C92.11, C92.4Ø, C92.5Ø, C92.6Ø, C92.AØ, C93.ØØ, C94.ØØ, C95.ØØ
NC 3Ø2[3,4]3[G,Y]Ø Only when reported with PDx or SDx of C91.ØØ, C92.ØØ, C92.1Ø, C92.11, C92.4Ø, C92.5Ø, C92.6Ø, C92.AØ, C93.ØØ, C94.ØØ, C95.ØØ
NT 3Ø2[3,4]3D1 for Intercept® (PRCFC) in combination with dx code D62, D65, D68.2, D68.4, or D68.9
♀ 3Ø27[3,7][H,J,K,L,M,N,P,Q,R,S,T,V,W]1

3 Administration
C Indwelling Device
1 Irrigation Definition: Putting in or on a cleansing substance

Body System/Region Character 4	Approach Character 5	Substance Character 6	Qualifier Character 7
Z None	X External	8 Irrigating Substance	Z No Qualifier

3 Administration
E Physiological Systems and Anatomical Regions
Ø Introduction Definition: Putting in or on a therapeutic, diagnostic, nutritional, physiological, or prophylactic substance except blood or blood products

Body System/Region Character 4	Approach Character 5	Substance Character 6	Qualifier Character 7
Ø Skin and Mucous Membranes	X External	Ø Antineoplastic	5 Other Antineoplastic M Monoclonal Antibody
Ø Skin and Mucous Membranes	X External	2 Anti-infective	8 Oxazolidinones 9 Other Anti-infective
Ø Skin and Mucous Membranes	X External	3 Anti-inflammatory 4 Serum, Toxoid and Vaccine B Anesthetic Agent K Other Diagnostic Substance M Pigment N Analgesics, Hypnotics, Sedatives T Destructive Agent	Z No Qualifier
Ø Skin and Mucous Membranes	X External	G Other Therapeutic Substance	C Other Substance
1 Subcutaneous Tissue	Ø Open	2 Anti-infective	A Anti-Infective Envelope
1 Subcutaneous Tissue	3 Percutaneous	Ø Antineoplastic	5 Other Antineoplastic M Monoclonal Antibody
1 Subcutaneous Tissue	3 Percutaneous	2 Anti-infective	8 Oxazolidinones 9 Other Anti-infective A Anti-Infective Envelope
1 Subcutaneous Tissue	3 Percutaneous	3 Anti-inflammatory 6 Nutritional Substance 7 Electrolytic and Water Balance Substance B Anesthetic Agent H Radioactive Substance K Other Diagnostic Substance N Analgesics, Hypnotics, Sedatives T Destructive Agent	Z No Qualifier
1 Subcutaneous Tissue	3 Percutaneous	4 Serum, Toxoid and Vaccine	Ø Influenza Vaccine Z No Qualifier
1 Subcutaneous Tissue	3 Percutaneous	G Other Therapeutic Substance	C Other Substance
1 Subcutaneous Tissue	3 Percutaneous	V Hormone	G Insulin J Other Hormone
2 Muscle	3 Percutaneous	Ø Antineoplastic	5 Other Antineoplastic M Monoclonal Antibody
2 Muscle	3 Percutaneous	2 Anti-infective	8 Oxazolidinones 9 Other Anti-infective
2 Muscle	3 Percutaneous	3 Anti-inflammatory 6 Nutritional Substance 7 Electrolytic and Water Balance Substance B Anesthetic Agent H Radioactive Substance K Other Diagnostic Substance N Analgesics, Hypnotics, Sedatives T Destructive Agent	Z No Qualifier
2 Muscle	3 Percutaneous	4 Serum, Toxoid and Vaccine	Ø Influenza Vaccine Z No Qualifier
2 Muscle	3 Percutaneous	G Other Therapeutic Substance	C Other Substance
3 Peripheral Vein	Ø Open	Ø Antineoplastic	2 High-dose Interleukin-2 3 Low-dose Interleukin-2 5 Other Antineoplastic M Monoclonal Antibody P Clofarabine
3 Peripheral Vein	Ø Open	1 Thrombolytic	6 Recombinant Human- activated Protein C 7 Other Thrombolytic
3 Peripheral Vein	Ø Open	2 Anti-infective	8 Oxazolidinones 9 Other Anti-infective

DRG Non-OR 3EØ3ØØ2
DRG Non-OR 3EØ3Ø17

3EØ Continued on next page

3EØ Continued

3 Administration
E Physiological Systems and Anatomical Regions
Ø Introduction Definition: Putting in or on a therapeutic, diagnostic, nutritional, physiological, or prophylactic substance except blood or blood products

Body System/Region Character 4	Approach Character 5	Substance Character 6	Qualifier Character 7
3 Peripheral Vein	Ø Open	3 Anti-inflammatory 4 Serum, Toxoid and Vaccine 6 Nutritional Substance 7 Electrolytic and Water Balance Substance F Intracirculatory Anesthetic H Radioactive Substance K Other Diagnostic Substance N Analgesics, Hypnotics, Sedatives P Platelet Inhibitor R Antiarrhythmic T Destructive Agent X Vasopressor	Z No Qualifier
3 Peripheral Vein	Ø Open	G Other Therapeutic Substance	C Other Substance N Blood Brain Barrier Disruption
3 Peripheral Vein	Ø Open	U Pancreatic Islet Cells	Ø Autologous 1 Nonautologous
3 Peripheral Vein	Ø Open	V Hormone	G Insulin H Human B-type Natriuretic Peptide J Other Hormone
3 Peripheral Vein	Ø Open	W Immunotherapeutic	K Immunostimulator L Immunosuppressive
3 Peripheral Vein	3 Percutaneous	Ø Antineoplastic	2 High-dose Interleukin-2 3 Low-dose Interleukin-2 5 Other Antineoplastic M Monoclonal Antibody P Clofarabine
3 Peripheral Vein	3 Percutaneous	1 Thrombolytic	6 Recombinant Human- activated Protein C 7 Other Thrombolytic
3 Peripheral Vein	3 Percutaneous	2 Anti-infective	8 Oxazolidinones 9 Other Anti-infective
3 Peripheral Vein	3 Percutaneous	3 Anti-inflammatory 4 Serum, Toxoid and Vaccine 6 Nutritional Substance 7 Electrolytic and Water Balance Substance F Intracirculatory Anesthetic H Radioactive Substance K Other Diagnostic Substance N Analgesics, Hypnotics, Sedatives P Platelet Inhibitor R Antiarrhythmic T Destructive Agent X Vasopressor	Z No Qualifier
3 Peripheral Vein	3 Percutaneous	G Other Therapeutic Substance	C Other Substance N Blood Brain Barrier Disruption Q Glucarpidase R Other Therapeutic Monoclonal Antibody
3 Peripheral Vein	3 Percutaneous	U Pancreatic Islet Cells	Ø Autologous 1 Nonautologous
3 Peripheral Vein	3 Percutaneous	V Hormone	G Insulin H Human B-type Natriuretic Peptide J Other Hormone
3 Peripheral Vein	3 Percutaneous	W Immunotherapeutic	K Immunostimulator L Immunosuppressive
4 Central Vein	Ø Open	Ø Antineoplastic	2 High-dose Interleukin-2 3 Low-dose Interleukin-2 5 Other Antineoplastic M Monoclonal Antibody P Clofarabine
4 Central Vein	Ø Open	1 Thrombolytic	6 Recombinant Human- activated Protein C 7 Other Thrombolytic

Valid OR 3EØ3ØTZ
DRG Non-OR 3EØ3ØU[Ø,1]
DRG Non-OR 3EØ33Ø2
DRG Non-OR 3EØ3317
DRG Non-OR 3EØ33U[Ø,1]
DRG Non-OR 3EØ4ØØ2
DRG Non-OR 3EØ4Ø17

3EØ Continued on next page

3 Administration
E Physiological Systems and Anatomical Regions
Ø Introduction Definition: Putting in or on a therapeutic, diagnostic, nutritional, physiological, or prophylactic substance except blood or blood products

3EØ Continued

Body System/Region Character 4	Approach Character 5	Substance Character 6	Qualifier Character 7
4 Central Vein	Ø Open	2 Anti-infective	8 Oxazolidinones 9 Other Anti-infective
4 Central Vein	Ø Open	3 Anti-inflammatory 4 Serum, Toxoid and Vaccine 6 Nutritional Substance 7 Electrolytic and Water Balance Substance F Intracirculatory Anesthetic H Radioactive Substance K Other Diagnostic Substance N Analgesics, Hypnotics, Sedatives P Platelet Inhibitor R Antiarrhythmic T Destructive Agent X Vasopressor	Z No Qualifier
4 Central Vein	Ø Open	G Other Therapeutic Substance	C Other Substance N Blood Brain Barrier Disruption
4 Central Vein	Ø Open	V Hormone	G Insulin H Human B-type Natriuretic Peptide J Other Hormone
4 Central Vein	Ø Open	W Immunotherapeutic	K Immunostimulator L Immunosuppressive
4 Central Vein	3 Percutaneous	Ø Antineoplastic	2 High-dose Interleukin-2 3 Low-dose Interleukin-2 5 Other Antineoplastic M Monoclonal Antibody P Clofarabine
4 Central Vein	3 Percutaneous	1 Thrombolytic	6 Recombinant Human- activated Protein C 7 Other Thrombolytic
4 Central Vein	3 Percutaneous	2 Anti-infective	8 Oxazolidinones 9 Other Anti-infective
4 Central Vein	3 Percutaneous	3 Anti-inflammatory 4 Serum, Toxoid and Vaccine 6 Nutritional Substance 7 Electrolytic and Water Balance Substance F Intracirculatory Anesthetic H Radioactive Substance K Other Diagnostic Substance N Analgesics, Hypnotics, Sedatives P Platelet Inhibitor R Antiarrhythmic T Destructive Agent X Vasopressor	Z No Qualifier
4 Central Vein	3 Percutaneous	G Other Therapeutic Substance	C Other Substance N Blood Brain Barrier Disruption Q Glucarpidase R Other Therapeutic Monoclonal Antibody
4 Central Vein	3 Percutaneous	V Hormone	G Insulin H Human B-type Natriuretic Peptide J Other Hormone
4 Central Vein	3 Percutaneous	W Immunotherapeutic	K Immunostimulator L Immunosuppressive
5 Peripheral Artery 6 Central Artery	Ø Open 3 Percutaneous	Ø Antineoplastic	2 High-dose Interleukin-2 3 Low-dose Interleukin-2 5 Other Antineoplastic M Monoclonal Antibody P Clofarabine
5 Peripheral Artery 6 Central Artery	Ø Open 3 Percutaneous	1 Thrombolytic	6 Recombinant Human- activated Protein C 7 Other Thrombolytic
5 Peripheral Artery 6 Central Artery	Ø Open 3 Percutaneous	2 Anti-infective	8 Oxazolidinones 9 Other Anti-infective

Valid OR 3EØ4ØTZ
DRG Non-OR 3EØ43Ø2
DRG Non-OR 3EØ4317
DRG Non-OR 3EØ[5,6][Ø,3]Ø2
DRG Non-OR 3EØ[5,6][Ø,3]17

3EØ Continued on next page

3EØ Continued

3 Administration
E Physiological Systems and Anatomical Regions
Ø Introduction Definition: Putting in or on a therapeutic, diagnostic, nutritional, physiological, or prophylactic substance except blood or blood products

Body System/Region Character 4	Approach Character 5	Substance Character 6	Qualifier Character 7
5 Peripheral Artery 6 Central Artery	Ø Open 3 Percutaneous	3 Anti-inflammatory 4 Serum, Toxoid and Vaccine 6 Nutritional Substance 7 Electrolytic and Water Balance Substance F Intracirculatory Anesthetic H Radioactive Substance K Other Diagnostic Substance N Analgesics, Hypnotics, Sedatives P Platelet Inhibitor R Antiarrhythmic T Destructive Agent X Vasopressor	Z No Qualifier
5 Peripheral Artery 6 Central Artery	Ø Open 3 Percutaneous	G Other Therapeutic Substance	C Other Substance N Blood Brain Barrier Disruption
5 Peripheral Artery 6 Central Artery	Ø Open 3 Percutaneous	V Hormone	G Insulin H Human B-type Natriuretic Peptide J Other Hormone
5 Peripheral Artery 6 Central Artery	Ø Open 3 Percutaneous	W Immunotherapeutic	K Immunostimulator L Immunosuppressive
7 Coronary Artery 8 Heart	Ø Open 3 Percutaneous	1 Thrombolytic	6 Recombinant Human- activated Protein C 7 Other Thrombolytic
7 Coronary Artery 8 Heart	Ø Open 3 Percutaneous	G Other Therapeutic Substance	C Other Substance
7 Coronary Artery 8 Heart	Ø Open 3 Percutaneous	K Other Diagnostic Substance P Platelet Inhibitor	Z No Qualifier
7 Coronary Artery 8 Heart	4 Percutaneous Endoscopic	G Other Therapeutic Substance	C Other Substance
9 Nose	3 Percutaneous 7 Via Natural or Artificial Opening X External	Ø Antineoplastic	5 Other Antineoplastic M Monoclonal Antibody
9 Nose	3 Percutaneous 7 Via Natural or Artificial Opening X External	2 Anti-infective	8 Oxazolidinones 9 Other Anti-infective
9 Nose	3 Percutaneous 7 Via Natural or Artificial Opening X External	3 Anti-inflammatory 4 Serum, Toxoid and Vaccine B Anesthetic Agent H Radioactive Substance K Other Diagnostic Substance N Analgesics, Hypnotics, Sedatives T Destructive Agent	Z No Qualifier
9 Nose	3 Percutaneous 7 Via Natural or Artificial Opening X External	G Other Therapeutic Substance	C Other Substance
A Bone Marrow	3 Percutaneous	Ø Antineoplastic	5 Other Antineoplastic M Monoclonal Antibody
A Bone Marrow	3 Percutaneous	G Other Therapeutic Substance	C Other Substance
B Ear	3 Percutaneous 7 Via Natural or Artificial Opening X External	Ø Antineoplastic	4 Liquid Brachytherapy Radioisotope 5 Other Antineoplastic M Monoclonal Antibody
B Ear	3 Percutaneous 7 Via Natural or Artificial Opening X External	2 Anti-infective	8 Oxazolidinones 9 Other Anti-infective
B Ear	3 Percutaneous 7 Via Natural or Artificial Opening X External	3 Anti-inflammatory B Anesthetic Agent H Radioactive Substance K Other Diagnostic Substance N Analgesics, Hypnotics, Sedatives T Destructive Agent	Z No Qualifier
B Ear	3 Percutaneous 7 Via Natural or Artificial Opening X External	G Other Therapeutic Substance	C Other Substance

DRG Non-OR 3EØ8[Ø,3]17

3EØ Continued on next page

3 Administration
E Physiological Systems and Anatomical Regions
Ø Introduction Definition: Putting in or on a therapeutic, diagnostic, nutritional, physiological, or prophylactic substance except blood or blood products

3EØ Continued

Body System/Region Character 4	Approach Character 5	Substance Character 6	Qualifier Character 7
C Eye	**3** Percutaneous **7** Via Natural or Artificial Opening **X** External	**Ø** Antineoplastic	**4** Liquid Brachytherapy Radioisotope **5** Other Antineoplastic **M** Monoclonal Antibody
C Eye	**3** Percutaneous **7** Via Natural or Artificial Opening **X** External	**2** Anti-infective	**8** Oxazolidinones **9** Other Anti-infective
C Eye	**3** Percutaneous **7** Via Natural or Artificial Opening **X** External	**3** Anti-inflammatory **B** Anesthetic Agent **H** Radioactive Substance **K** Other Diagnostic Substance **M** Pigment **N** Analgesics, Hypnotics, Sedatives **T** Destructive Agent	**Z** No Qualifier
C Eye	**3** Percutaneous **7** Via Natural or Artificial Opening **X** External	**G** Other Therapeutic Substance	**C** Other Substance
C Eye	**3** Percutaneous **7** Via Natural or Artificial Opening **X** External	**S** Gas	**F** Other Gas
D Mouth and Pharynx	**3** Percutaneous **7** Via Natural or Artificial Opening **X** External	**Ø** Antineoplastic	**4** Liquid Brachytherapy Radioisotope **5** Other Antineoplastic **M** Monoclonal Antibody
D Mouth and Pharynx	**3** Percutaneous **7** Via Natural or Artificial Opening **X** External	**2** Anti-infective	**8** Oxazolidinones **9** Other Anti-infective
D Mouth and Pharynx	**3** Percutaneous **7** Via Natural or Artificial Opening **X** External	**3** Anti-inflammatory **4** Serum, Toxoid and Vaccine **6** Nutritional Substance **7** Electrolytic and Water Balance Substance **B** Anesthetic Agent **H** Radioactive Substance **K** Other Diagnostic Substance **N** Analgesics, Hypnotics, Sedatives **R** Antiarrhythmic **T** Destructive Agent	**Z** No Qualifier
D Mouth and Pharynx	**3** Percutaneous **7** Via Natural or Artificial Opening **X** External	**G** Other Therapeutic Substance	**C** Other Substance
E Products of Conception ♀ **G** Upper GI **H** Lower GI **K** Genitourinary Tract **N** Male Reproductive ♂	**3** Percutaneous **7** Via Natural or Artificial Opening **8** Via Natural or Artificial Opening Endoscopic	**Ø** Antineoplastic	**4** Liquid Brachytherapy Radioisotope **5** Other Antineoplastic **M** Monoclonal Antibody
E Products of Conception ♀ **G** Upper GI **H** Lower GI **K** Genitourinary Tract **N** Male Reproductive ♂	**3** Percutaneous **7** Via Natural or Artificial Opening **8** Via Natural or Artificial Opening Endoscopic	**2** Anti-infective	**8** Oxazolidinones **9** Other Anti-infective
E Products of Conception ♀ **G** Upper GI **H** Lower GI **K** Genitourinary Tract **N** Male Reproductive ♂	**3** Percutaneous **7** Via Natural or Artificial Opening **8** Via Natural or Artificial Opening Endoscopic	**3** Anti-inflammatory **6** Nutritional Substance **7** Electrolytic and Water Balance Substance **B** Anesthetic Agent **H** Radioactive Substance **K** Other Diagnostic Substance **N** Analgesics, Hypnotics, Sedatives **T** Destructive Agent	**Z** No Qualifier
E Products of Conception ♀ **G** Upper GI **H** Lower GI **K** Genitourinary Tract **N** Male Reproductive ♂	**3** Percutaneous **7** Via Natural or Artificial Opening **8** Via Natural or Artificial Opening Endoscopic	**G** Other Therapeutic Substance	**C** Other Substance

♂ All approach, substance, and qualifier values for body system/region (character 4) with this icon
♀ All approach, substance, and qualifier values for body system/region (character 4) with this icon

3EØ Continued on next page

3EØ Continued

3 **Administration**
E **Physiological Systems and Anatomical Regions**
Ø **Introduction** Definition: Putting in or on a therapeutic, diagnostic, nutritional, physiological, or prophylactic substance except blood or blood products

Body System/Region Character 4	Approach Character 5	Substance Character 6	Qualifier Character 7
E Products of Conception ♀ G Upper GI H Lower GI K Genitourinary Tract N Male Reproductive ♂	3 Percutaneous 7 Via Natural or Artificial Opening 8 Via Natural or Artificial Opening Endoscopic	S Gas	F Other Gas
E Products of Conception ♀ G Upper GI H Lower GI K Genitourinary Tract N Male Reproductive ♂	4 Percutaneous Endoscopic	G Other Therapeutic Substance	C Other Substance
F Respiratory Tract	3 Percutaneous 7 Via Natural or Artificial Opening 8 Via Natural or Artificial Opening Endoscopic	Ø Antineoplastic	4 Liquid Brachytherapy Radioisotope 5 Other Antineoplastic M Monoclonal Antibody
F Respiratory Tract	3 Percutaneous 7 Via Natural or Artificial Opening 8 Via Natural or Artificial Opening Endoscopic	2 Anti-infective	8 Oxazolidinones 9 Other Anti-infective
F Respiratory Tract	3 Percutaneous 7 Via Natural or Artificial Opening 8 Via Natural or Artificial Opening Endoscopic	3 Anti-inflammatory 6 Nutritional Substance 7 Electrolytic and Water Balance Substance B Anesthetic Agent H Radioactive Substance K Other Diagnostic Substance N Analgesics, Hypnotics, Sedatives T Destructive Agent	Z No Qualifier
F Respiratory Tract	3 Percutaneous 7 Via Natural or Artificial Opening 8 Via Natural or Artificial Opening Endoscopic	G Other Therapeutic Substance	C Other Substance
F Respiratory Tract	3 Percutaneous 7 Via Natural or Artificial Opening 8 Via Natural or Artificial Opening Endoscopic	S Gas	D Nitric Oxide F Other Gas
F Respiratory Tract	4 Percutaneous Endoscopic	G Other Therapeutic Substance	C Other Substance
J Biliary and Pancreatic Tract	3 Percutaneous 7 Via Natural or Artificial Opening 8 Via Natural or Artificial Opening Endoscopic	Ø Antineoplastic	4 Liquid Brachytherapy Radioisotope 5 Other Antineoplastic M Monoclonal Antibody
J Biliary and Pancreatic Tract	3 Percutaneous 7 Via Natural or Artificial Opening 8 Via Natural or Artificial Opening Endoscopic	2 Anti-infective	8 Oxazolidinones 9 Other Anti-infective
J Biliary and Pancreatic Tract	3 Percutaneous 7 Via Natural or Artificial Opening 8 Via Natural or Artificial Opening Endoscopic	3 Anti-inflammatory 6 Nutritional Substance 7 Electrolytic and Water Balance Substance B Anesthetic Agent H Radioactive Substance K Other Diagnostic Substance N Analgesics, Hypnotics, Sedatives T Destructive Agent	Z No Qualifier
J Biliary and Pancreatic Tract	3 Percutaneous 7 Via Natural or Artificial Opening 8 Via Natural or Artificial Opening Endoscopic	G Other Therapeutic Substance	C Other Substance
J Biliary and Pancreatic Tract	3 Percutaneous 7 Via Natural or Artificial Opening 8 Via Natural or Artificial Opening Endoscopic	S Gas	F Other Gas

♂ All approach, substance, and qualifier values for body system/region (character 4) with this icon
♀ All approach, substance, and qualifier values for body system/region (character 4) with this icon

3EØ Continued on next page

3EØ Continued

3 **Administration**
E **Physiological Systems and Anatomical Regions**
Ø **Introduction** Definition: Putting in or on a therapeutic, diagnostic, nutritional, physiological, or prophylactic substance except blood or blood products

Body System/Region Character 4	Approach Character 5	Substance Character 6	Qualifier Character 7
J Biliary and Pancreatic Tract	3 Percutaneous 7 Via Natural or Artificial Opening 8 Via Natural or Artificial Opening Endoscopic	U Pancreatic Islet Cells	Ø Autologous 1 Nonautologous
J Biliary and Pancreatic Tract	4 Percutaneous Endoscopic	G Other Therapeutic Substance	C Other Substance
L Pleural Cavity	Ø Open	5 Adhesion Barrier	Z No Qualifier
L Pleural Cavity	3 Percutaneous	Ø Antineoplastic	4 Liquid Brachytherapy Radioisotope 5 Other Antineoplastic M Monoclonal Antibody
L Pleural Cavity	3 Percutaneous	2 Anti-infective	8 Oxazolidinones 9 Other Anti-infective
L Pleural Cavity	3 Percutaneous	3 Anti-inflammatory 5 Adhesion Barrier 6 Nutritional Substance 7 Electrolytic and Water Balance Substance B Anesthetic Agent H Radioactive Substance K Other Diagnostic Substance N Analgesics, Hypnotics, Sedatives T Destructive Agent	Z No Qualifier
L Pleural Cavity	3 Percutaneous	G Other Therapeutic Substance	C Other Substance
L Pleural Cavity	3 Percutaneous	S Gas	F Other Gas
L Pleural Cavity	4 Percutaneous Endoscopic	5 Adhesion Barrier	Z No Qualifier
L Pleural Cavity	4 Percutaneous Endoscopic	G Other Therapeutic Substance	C Other Substance
L Pleural Cavity	7 Via Natural or Artificial Opening	Ø Antineoplastic	4 Liquid Brachytherapy Radioisotope 5 Other Antineoplastic M Monoclonal Antibody
L Pleural Cavity	7 Via Natural or Artificial Opening	S Gas	F Other Gas
M Peritoneal Cavity	Ø Open	5 Adhesion Barrier	Z No Qualifier
M Peritoneal Cavity	3 Percutaneous	Ø Antineoplastic	4 Liquid Brachytherapy Radioisotope 5 Other Antineoplastic M Monoclonal Antibody Y Hyperthermic
M Peritoneal Cavity	3 Percutaneous	2 Anti-infective	8 Oxazolidinones 9 Other Anti-infective
M Peritoneal Cavity	3 Percutaneous	3 Anti-inflammatory 5 Adhesion Barrier 6 Nutritional Substance 7 Electrolytic and Water Balance Substance B Anesthetic Agent H Radioactive Substance K Other Diagnostic Substance N Analgesics, Hypnotics, Sedatives T Destructive Agent	Z No Qualifier
M Peritoneal Cavity	3 Percutaneous	G Other Therapeutic Substance	C Other Substance
M Peritoneal Cavity	3 Percutaneous	S Gas	F Other Gas
M Peritoneal Cavity	4 Percutaneous Endoscopic	5 Adhesion Barrier	Z No Qualifier
M Peritoneal Cavity	4 Percutaneous Endoscopic	G Other Therapeutic Substance	C Other Substance
M Peritoneal Cavity	7 Via Natural or Artificial Opening	Ø Antineoplastic	4 Liquid Brachytherapy Radioisotope 5 Other Antineoplastic M Monoclonal Antibody
M Peritoneal Cavity	7 Via Natural or Artificial Opening	S Gas	F Other Gas
P Female Reproductive ♀	Ø Open	5 Adhesion Barrier	Z No Qualifier
P Female Reproductive ♀	3 Percutaneous	Ø Antineoplastic	4 Liquid Brachytherapy Radioisotope 5 Other Antineoplastic M Monoclonal Antibody
P Female Reproductive ♀	3 Percutaneous	2 Anti-infective	8 Oxazolidinones 9 Other Anti-infective

Valid OR 3EØL4GC
DRG Non-OR 3EØJ[3,7,8]U[Ø,1]
♀ All approach, substance, and qualifier values for body system/region (character 4) with this icon

3EØ Continued on next page

3EØ Continued

3 Administration
E Physiological Systems and Anatomical Regions
Ø Introduction Definition: Putting in or on a therapeutic, diagnostic, nutritional, physiological, or prophylactic substance except blood or blood products

Body System/Region Character 4	Approach Character 5	Substance Character 6	Qualifier Character 7
P Female Reproductive ♀	3 Percutaneous	3 Anti-inflammatory 5 Adhesion Barrier 6 Nutritional Substance 7 Electrolytic and Water Balance Substance B Anesthetic Agent H Radioactive Substance K Other Diagnostic Substance L Sperm N Analgesics, Hypnotics, Sedatives T Destructive Agent V Hormone	Z No Qualifier
P Female Reproductive ♀	3 Percutaneous	G Other Therapeutic Substance	C Other Substance
P Female Reproductive ♀	3 Percutaneous	Q Fertilized Ovum	Ø Autologous 1 Nonautologous
P Female Reproductive ♀	3 Percutaneous	S Gas	F Other Gas
P Female Reproductive ♀	4 Percutaneous Endoscopic	5 Adhesion Barrier	Z No Qualifier
P Female Reproductive ♀	4 Percutaneous Endoscopic	G Other Therapeutic Substance	C Other Substance
P Female Reproductive ♀	7 Via Natural or Artificial Opening	Ø Antineoplastic	4 Liquid Brachytherapy Radioisotope 5 Other Antineoplastic M Monoclonal Antibody
P Female Reproductive ♀	7 Via Natural or Artificial Opening	2 Anti-infective	8 Oxazolidinones 9 Other Anti-infective
P Female Reproductive ♀	7 Via Natural or Artificial Opening	3 Anti-inflammatory 6 Nutritional Substance 7 Electrolytic and Water Balance Substance B Anesthetic Agent H Radioactive Substance K Other Diagnostic Substance L Sperm N Analgesics, Hypnotics, Sedatives T Destructive Agent V Hormone	Z No Qualifier
P Female Reproductive ♀	7 Via Natural or Artificial Opening	G Other Therapeutic Substance	C Other Substance
P Female Reproductive ♀	7 Via Natural or Artificial Opening	Q Fertilized Ovum	Ø Autologous 1 Nonautologous
P Female Reproductive ♀	7 Via Natural or Artificial Opening	S Gas	F Other Gas
P Female Reproductive ♀	8 Via Natural or Artificial Opening Endoscopic	Ø Antineoplastic	4 Liquid Brachytherapy Radioisotope 5 Other Antineoplastic M Monoclonal Antibody
P Female Reproductive ♀	8 Via Natural or Artificial Opening Endoscopic	2 Anti-infective	8 Oxazolidinones 9 Other Anit-infective
P Female Reproductive ♀	8 Via Natural or Artificial Opening Endoscopic	3 Anti-inflammatory 6 Nutritional Substance 7 Electrolytic and Water Balance Substance B Anesthetic Agent H Radioactive Substance K Other Diagnostic Substance N Analgesics, Hypnotics, Sedatives T Destructive Agent	Z No Qualifier
P Female Reproductive ♀	8 Via Natural or Artificial Opening Endoscopic	G Other Therapeutic Substance	C Other Substance
P Female Reproductive ♀	8 Via Natural or Artificial Opening Endoscopic	S Gas	F Other Gas
Q Cranial Cavity and Brain	Ø Open 3 Percutaneous	Ø Antineoplastic	4 Liquid Brachytherapy Radioisotope 5 Other Antineoplastic M Monoclonal Antibody
Q Cranial Cavity and Brain	Ø Open 3 Percutaneous	2 Anti-infective	8 Oxazolidinones 9 Other Anti-infective

Valid OR 3EØP3Q[Ø,1]
Valid OR 3EØP7Q[Ø,1]
DRG Non-OR 3EØQ[Ø,3]Ø5
♀ All approach, substance, and qualifier values for body system/region (character 4) with this icon

3EØ Continued on next page

3 Administration
E Physiological Systems and Anatomical Regions
Ø Introduction Definition: Putting in or on a therapeutic, diagnostic, nutritional, physiological, or prophylactic substance except blood or blood products

3EØ Continued

Body System/Region Character 4	Approach Character 5	Substance Character 6	Qualifier Character 7
Q Cranial Cavity and Brain	Ø Open 3 Percutaneous	3 Anti-inflammatory 6 Nutritional Substance 7 Electrolytic and Water Balance Substance A Stem Cells, Embryonic B Anesthetic Agent H Radioactive Substance K Other Diagnostic Substance N Analgesics, Hypnotics, Sedatives T Destructive Agent	Z No Qualifier
Q Cranial Cavity and Brain	Ø Open 3 Percutaneous	E Stem Cells, Somatic	Ø Autologous 1 Nonautologous
Q Cranial Cavity and Brain	Ø Open 3 Percutaneous	G Other Therapeutic Substance	C Other Substance
Q Cranial Cavity and Brain	Ø Open 3 Percutaneous	S Gas	F Other Gas
Q Cranial Cavity and Brain	7 Via Natural or Artificial Opening	Ø Antineoplastic	4 Liquid Brachytherapy Radioisotope 5 Other Antineoplastic M Monoclonal Antibody
Q Cranial Cavity and Brain	7 Via Natural or Artificial Opening	S Gas	F Other Gas
R Spinal Canal	Ø Open	A Stem Cells, Embryonic	Z No Qualifier
R Spinal Canal	Ø Open	E Stem Cells, Somatic	Ø Autologous 1 Nonautologous
R Spinal Canal	3 Percutaneous	Ø Antineoplastic	2 High-dose Interleukin-2 3 Low-dose Interleukin-2 4 Liquid Brachytherapy Radioisotope 5 Other Antineoplastic M Monoclonal Antibody
R Spinal Canal	3 Percutaneous	2 Anti-infective	8 Oxazolidinones 9 Other Anti-infective
R Spinal Canal	3 Percutaneous	3 Anti-inflammatory 6 Nutritional Substance 7 Electrolytic and Water Balance Substance A Stem Cells, Embryonic B Anesthetic Agent H Radioactive Substance K Other Diagnostic Substance N Analgesics, Hypnotics, Sedatives T Destructive Agent	Z No Qualifier
R Spinal Canal	3 Percutaneous	E Stem Cells, Somatic	Ø Autologous 1 Nonautologous
R Spinal Canal	3 Percutaneous	G Other Therapeutic Substance	C Other Substance
R Spinal Canal	3 Percutaneous	S Gas	F Other Gas
R Spinal Canal	7 Via Natural or Artificial Opening	S Gas	F Other Gas
S Epidural Space	3 Percutaneous	Ø Antineoplastic	2 High-dose Interleukin-2 3 Low-dose Interleukin-2 4 Liquid Brachytherapy Radioisotope 5 Other Antineoplastic M Monoclonal Antibody
S Epidural Space	3 Percutaneous	2 Anti-infective	8 Oxazolidinones 9 Other Anti-infective
S Epidural Space	3 Percutaneous	3 Anti-inflammatory 6 Nutritional Substance 7 Electrolytic and Water Balance Substance B Anesthetic Agent H Radioactive Substance K Other Diagnostic Substance N Analgesics, Hypnotics, Sedatives T Destructive Agent	Z No Qualifier

DRG Non-OR 3EØQ7Ø5
DRG Non-OR 3EØR3Ø2
DRG Non-OR 3EØS3Ø2

3EØ Continued on next page

3EØ Continued

3 Administration
E Physiological Systems and Anatomical Regions
Ø Introduction Definition: Putting in or on a therapeutic, diagnostic, nutritional, physiological, or prophylactic substance except blood or blood products

Body System/Region Character 4	Approach Character 5	Substance Character 6	Qualifier Character 7
S Epidural Space	**3** Percutaneous	**G** Other Therapeutic Substance	**C** Other Substance
S Epidural Space	**3** Percutaneous	**S** Gas	**F** Other Gas
S Epidural Space	**7** Via Natural or Artificial Opening	**S** Gas	**F** Other Gas
T Peripheral Nerves and Plexi **X** Cranial Nerves	**3** Percutaneous	**3** Anti-inflammatory **B** Anesthetic Agent **T** Destructive Agent	**Z** No Qualifier
T Peripheral Nerves and Plexi **X** Cranial Nerves	**3** Percutaneous	**G** Other Therapeutic Substance	**C** Other Substance
U Joints	**Ø** Open	**2** Anti-infective	**8** Oxazolidinones **9** Other Anti-infective
U Joints	**Ø** Open	**G** Other Therapeutic Substance	**B** Recombinant Bone Morphogenetic Protein
U Joints	**3** Percutaneous	**Ø** Antineoplastic	**4** Liquid Brachytherapy Radioisotope **5** Other Antineoplastic **M** Monoclonal Antibody
U Joints	**3** Percutaneous	**2** Anti-infective	**8** Oxazolidinones **9** Other Anti-infective
U Joints	**3** Percutaneous	**3** Anti-inflammatory **6** Nutritional Substance **7** Electrolytic and Water Balance Substance **B** Anesthetic Agent **H** Radioactive Substance **K** Other Diagnostic Substance **N** Analgesics, Hypnotics, Sedatives **T** Destructive Agent	**Z** No Qualifier
U Joints	**3** Percutaneous	**G** Other Therapeutic Substance	**B** Recombinant Bone Morphogenetic Protein **C** Other Substance
U Joints	**3** Percutaneous	**S** Gas	**F** Other Gas
U Joints	**4** Percutaneous Endoscopic	**G** Other Therapeutic Substance	**C** Other Substance
V Bones	**Ø** Open	**G** Other Therapeutic Substance	**B** Recombinant Bone Morphogenetic Protein **C** Other Substance
V Bones	**3** Percutaneous	**Ø** Antineoplastic	**5** Other Antineoplastic **M** Monoclonal Antibody
V Bones	**3** Percutaneous	**2** Anti-infective	**8** Oxazolidinones **9** Other Anti-infective
V Bones	**3** Percutaneous	**3** Anti-inflammatory **6** Nutritional Substance **7** Electrolytic and Water Balance Substance **B** Anesthetic Agent **H** Radioactive Substance **K** Other Diagnostic Substance **N** Analgesics, Hypnotics, Sedatives **T** Destructive Agent	**Z** No Qualifier
V Bones	**3** Percutaneous	**G** Other Therapeutic Substance	**B** Recombinant Bone Morphogenetic Protein **C** Other Substance
V Bones	**4** Percutaneous Endoscopic	**G** Other Therapeutic Substance	**C** Other Substance
W Lymphatics	**3** Percutaneous	**Ø** Antineoplastic	**5** Other Antineoplastic **M** Monoclonal Antibody
W Lymphatics	**3** Percutaneous	**2** Anti-infective	**8** Oxazolidinones **9** Other Anti-infective
W Lymphatics	**3** Percutaneous	**3** Anti-inflammatory **6** Nutritional Substance **7** Electrolytic and Water Balance Substance **B** Anesthetic Agent **H** Radioactive Substance **K** Other Diagnostic Substance **N** Analgesics, Hypnotics, Sedatives **T** Destructive Agent	**Z** No Qualifier
W Lymphatics	**3** Percutaneous	**G** Other Therapeutic Substance	**C** Other Substance

3EØ Continued on next page

3 Administration
E Physiological Systems and Anatomical Regions
Ø Introduction Definition: Putting in or on a therapeutic, diagnostic, nutritional, physiological, or prophylactic substance except blood or blood products

3EØ Continued

Body System/Region Character 4	Approach Character 5	Substance Character 6	Qualifier Character 7
Y Pericardial Cavity	3 Percutaneous	Ø Antineoplastic	4 Liquid Brachytherapy Radioisotope 5 Other Antineoplastic M Monoclonal Antibody
Y Pericardial Cavity	3 Percutaneous	2 Anti-infective	8 Oxazolidinones 9 Other Anti-infective
Y Pericardial Cavity	3 Percutaneous	3 Anti-inflammatory 6 Nutritional Substance 7 Electrolytic and Water Balance Substance B Anesthetic Agent H Radioactive Substance K Other Diagnostic Substance N Analgesics, Hypnotics, Sedatives T Destructive Agent	Z No Qualifier
Y Pericardial Cavity	3 Percutaneous	G Other Therapeutic Substance	C Other Substance
Y Pericardial Cavity	3 Percutaneous	S Gas	F Other Gas
Y Pericardial Cavity	4 Percutaneous Endoscopic	G Other Therapeutic Substance	C Other Substance
Y Pericardial Cavity	7 Via Natural or Artificial Opening	Ø Antineoplastic	4 Liquid Brachytherapy Radioisotope 5 Other Antineoplastic M Monoclonal Antibody
Y Pericardial Cavity	7 Via Natural or Artificial Opening	S Gas	F Other Gas

3 Administration
E Physiological Systems and Anatomical Regions
1 Irrigation Definition: Putting in or on a cleansing substance

Body System/Region Character 4	Approach Character 5	Substance Character 6	Qualifier Character 7
Ø Skin and Mucous Membranes C Eye	3 Percutaneous X External	8 Irrigating Substance	X Diagnostic Z No Qualifier
9 Nose B Ear F Respiratory Tract G Upper GI H Lower GI J Biliary and Pancreatic Tract K Genitourinary Tract N Male Reproductive ♂ P Female Reproductive ♀	3 Percutaneous 7 Via Natural or Artificial Opening 8 Via Natural or Artificial Opening Endoscopic	8 Irrigating Substance	X Diagnostic Z No Qualifier
L Pleural Cavity Q Cranial Cavity and Brain R Spinal Canal S Epidural Space Y Pericardial Cavity	3 Percutaneous	8 Irrigating Substance	X Diagnostic Z No Qualifier
M Peritoneal Cavity	3 Percutaneous	8 Irrigating Substance	X Diagnostic Z No Qualifier
M Peritoneal Cavity	3 Percutaneous	9 Dialysate	Z No Qualifier
M Peritoneal Cavity	4 Percutaneous Endoscopic	8 Irrigating Substance	X Diagnostic Z No Qualifier
U Joints	3 Percutaneous 4 Percutaneous Endoscopic	8 Irrigating Substance	X Diagnostic Z No Qualifier

♂ 3E1N[3,7,8]8[X,Z]
♀ 3E1P[3,7,8]8[X,Z]

Measurement and Monitoring 4AØ–4BØ

AHA Coding Clinic for table 4AØ

2022, 1Q, 46 Internal cardioversion
2020, 4Q, 62 Measurement of intracranial arterial flow
2020, 4Q, 62 Percutaneous endoscopic measurement of portal venous pressure
2020, 4Q, 63 Intercompartmental pressure measurement
2019, 3Q, 32 Endomyocardial biopsy and right heart catheterization
2018, 1Q, 12 Percutaneous balloon valvuloplasty & cardiac catheterization with ventriculogram
2016, 3Q, 37 Fractional flow reserve
2015, 3Q, 29 Approach value for esophageal electrophysiology study

AHA Coding Clinic for table 4BØ

2021, 4Q, 55-56 Measurement of flow in a cerebral fluid shunt

AHA Coding Clinic for table 4A1

2019, 4Q, 38-39 Intraoperative fluorescence lymphatic mapping using Indocyanine green dye
2016, 4Q, 114 Fluorescence vascular angiography
2016, 2Q, 29 Decompressive craniectomy with cryopreservation and storage of bone flap
2016, 2Q, 33 Monitoring of arterial pressure & pulse
2015, 3Q, 35 Swan Ganz catheterization
2015, 2Q, 14 Intraoperative EMG monitoring via endotracheal tube
2015, 1Q, 26 Intraoperative monitoring using Sentio MMG®
2014, 4Q, 28 Removal and replacement of displaced growing rods

4 Measurement and Monitoring
A Physiological Systems
Ø Measurement Definition: Determining the level of a physiological or physical function at a point in time

Body System Character 4	Approach Character 5	Function/Device Character 6	Qualifier Character 7
Ø Central Nervous	Ø Open	2 Conductivity 4 Electrical Activity B Pressure	Z No Qualifier
Ø Central Nervous	3 Percutaneous 7 Via Natural or Artificial Opening 8 Via Natural or Artificial Opening Endoscopic	4 Electrical Activity	Z No Qualifier
Ø Central Nervous	3 Percutaneous 7 Via Natural or Artificial Opening 8 Via Natural or Artificial Opening Endoscopic	B Pressure K Temperature R Saturation	D Intracranial
Ø Central Nervous	X External	2 Conductivity 4 Electrical Activity	Z No Qualifier
1 Peripheral Nervous	Ø Open 3 Percutaneous 7 Via Natural or Artificial Opening 8 Via Natural or Artificial Opening Endoscopic X External	2 Conductivity	9 Sensory B Motor
1 Peripheral Nervous	Ø Open 3 Percutaneous 7 Via Natural or Artificial Opening 8 Via Natural or Artificial Opening Endoscopic X External	4 Electrical Activity	Z No Qualifier
2 Cardiac	Ø Open 3 Percutaneous 7 Via Natural or Artificial Opening 8 Via Natural or Artificial Opening Endoscopic	4 Electrical Activity 9 Output C Rate F Rhythm H Sound P Action Currents	Z No Qualifier
2 Cardiac	Ø Open 3 Percutaneous 7 Via Natural or Artificial Opening 8 Via Natural or Artificial Opening Endoscopic	N Sampling and Pressure	6 Right Heart 7 Left Heart 8 Bilateral
2 Cardiac	X External	4 Electrical Activity	A Guidance Z No Qualifier
2 Cardiac	X External	9 Output C Rate F Rhythm H Sound P Action Currents	Z No Qualifier
2 Cardiac	X External	M Total Activity	4 Stress
3 Arterial	Ø Open 3 Percutaneous	5 Flow J Pulse	1 Peripheral 3 Pulmonary C Coronary
3 Arterial	Ø Open 3 Percutaneous	B Pressure	1 Peripheral 3 Pulmonary C Coronary F Other Thoracic

DRG Non-OR 4AØ2[3,7,8]FZ
DRG Non-OR 4AØ2[Ø,3,7,8]N[6,7,8]

4AØ Continued on next page

4AØ Continued

4 Measurement and Monitoring
A Physiological Systems
Ø Measurement Definition: Determining the level of a physiological or physical function at a point in time

Body System Character 4	Approach Character 5	Function/Device Character 6	Qualifier Character 7
3 Arterial	Ø Open 3 Percutaneous	H Sound R Saturation	1 Peripheral
3 Arterial	X External	5 Flow	1 Peripheral D Intracranial
3 Arterial	X External	B Pressure H Sound J Pulse R Saturation	1 Peripheral
4 Venous	Ø Open 3 Percutaneous	5 Flow B Pressure J Pulse	Ø Central 1 Peripheral 2 Portal 3 Pulmonary
4 Venous	Ø Open 3 Percutaneous	R Saturation	1 Peripheral
4 Venous	4 Percutaneous Endoscopic	B Pressure	2 Portal
4 Venous	X External	5 Flow B Pressure J Pulse R Saturation	1 Peripheral
5 Circulatory	X External	L Volume	Z No Qualifier
6 Lymphatic	Ø Open 3 Percutaneous 7 Via Natural or Artificial Opening 8 Via Natural or Artificial Opening Endoscopic	5 Flow B Pressure	Z No Qualifier
7 Visual	X External	Ø Acuity 7 Mobility B Pressure	Z No Qualifier
8 Olfactory	X External	Ø Acuity	Z No Qualifier
9 Respiratory	7 Via Natural or Artificial Opening 8 Via Natural or Artificial Opening Endoscopic X External	1 Capacity 5 Flow C Rate D Resistance L Volume M Total Activity	Z No Qualifier
B Gastrointestinal	7 Via Natural or Artificial Opening 8 Via Natural or Artificial Opening Endoscopic	8 Motility B Pressure G Secretion	Z No Qualifier
C Biliary	3 Percutaneous 4 Percutaneous Endoscopic 7 Via Natural or Artificial Opening 8 Via Natural or Artificial Opening Endoscopic	5 Flow B Pressure	Z No Qualifier
D Urinary	7 Via Natural or Artificial Opening 8 Via Natural or Artificial Opening Endoscopic	3 Contractility 5 Flow B Pressure D Resistance L Volume	Z No Qualifier
F Musculoskeletal	3 Percutaneous	3 Contractility	Z No Qualifier
F Musculoskeletal	3 Percutaneous	B Pressure	E Compartment
F Musculoskeletal	X External	3 Contractility	Z No Qualifier
H Products of Conception, Cardiac ♀	7 Via Natural or Artificial Opening 8 Via Natural or Artificial Opening Endoscopic X External	4 Electrical Activity C Rate F Rhythm H Sound	Z No Qualifier
J Products of Conception, Nervous ♀	7 Via Natural or Artificial Opening 8 Via Natural or Artificial Opening Endoscopic X External	2 Conductivity 4 Electrical Activity B Pressure	Z No Qualifier
Z None	7 Via Natural or Artificial Opening	6 Metabolism K Temperature	Z No Qualifier
Z None	X External	6 Metabolism K Temperature Q Sleep	Z No Qualifier

Valid OR 4A06Ø[5,B]Z
Valid OR 4AØC4[5,B]Z
♀ 4AØH[7,8,X][4,C,F,H]Z
♀ 4AØJ[7,8,X][2,4,B]Z

4 Measurement and Monitoring
A Physiological Systems
1 Monitoring Definition: Determining the level of a physiological or physical function repetitively over a period of time

Body System Character 4	Approach Character 5	Function/Device Character 6	Qualifier Character 7
Ø Central Nervous	Ø Open	2 Conductivity B Pressure	Z No Qualifier
Ø Central Nervous	Ø Open	4 Electrical Activity	G Intraoperative Z No Qualifier
Ø Central Nervous	3 Percutaneous 7 Via Natural or Artificial Opening 8 Via Natural or Artificial Opening Endoscopic	4 Electrical Activity	G Intraoperative Z No Qualifier
Ø Central Nervous	3 Percutaneous 7 Via Natural or Artificial Opening 8 Via Natural or Artificial Opening Endoscopic	B Pressure K Temperature R Saturation	D Intracranial
Ø Central Nervous	X External	2 Conductivity	Z No Qualifier
Ø Central Nervous	X External	4 Electrical Activity	G Intraoperative Z No Qualifier
1 Peripheral Nervous	Ø Open 3 Percutaneous 7 Via Natural or Artificial Opening 8 Via Natural or Artificial Opening Endoscopic X External	2 Conductivity	9 Sensory B Motor
1 Peripheral Nervous	Ø Open 3 Percutaneous 7 Via Natural or Artificial Opening 8 Via Natural or Artificial Opening Endoscopic X External	4 Electrical Activity	G Intraoperative Z No Qualifier
2 Cardiac	Ø Open 3 Percutaneous 7 Via Natural or Artificial Opening 8 Via Natural or Artificial Opening Endoscopic	4 Electrical Activity 9 Output C Rate F Rhythm H Sound	Z No Qualifier
2 Cardiac	X External	4 Electrical Activity	5 Ambulatory Z No Qualifier
2 Cardiac	X External	9 Output C Rate F Rhythm H Sound	Z No Qualifier
2 Cardiac	X External	M Total Activity	4 Stress
2 Cardiac	X External	S Vascular Perfusion	H Indocyanine Green Dye
3 Arterial	Ø Open 3 Percutaneous	5 Flow B Pressure J Pulse	1 Peripheral 3 Pulmonary C Coronary
3 Arterial	Ø Open 3 Percutaneous	H Sound R Saturation	1 Peripheral
3 Arterial	X External	5 Flow B Pressure H Sound J Pulse R Saturation	1 Peripheral
4 Venous	Ø Open 3 Percutaneous	5 Flow B Pressure J Pulse	Ø Central 1 Peripheral 2 Portal 3 Pulmonary
4 Venous	Ø Open 3 Percutaneous	R Saturation	Ø Central 2 Portal 3 Pulmonary
4 Venous	X External	5 Flow B Pressure J Pulse	1 Peripheral
6 Lymphatic	Ø Open 3 Percutaneous 7 Via Natural or Artificial Opening 8 Via Natural or Artificial Opening Endoscopic	5 Flow	H Indocyanine Green Dye Z No Qualifier

Valid OR 4A16Ø5Z

4A1 Continued on next page

4A1 Continued

4 Measurement and Monitoring
A Physiological Systems
1 Monitoring Definition: Determining the level of a physiological or physical function repetitively over a period of time

Body System Character 4	Approach Character 5	Function/Device Character 6	Qualifier Character 7
6 Lymphatic	Ø Open 3 Percutaneous 7 Via Natural or Artificial Opening 8 Via Natural or Artificial Opening Endoscopic	B Pressure	Z No Qualifier
9 Respiratory	7 Via Natural or Artificial Opening X External	1 Capacity 5 Flow C Rate D Resistance L Volume	Z No Qualifier
B Gastrointestinal	7 Via Natural or Artificial Opening 8 Via Natural or Artificial Opening Endoscopic	8 Motility B Pressure G Secretion	Z No Qualifier
B Gastrointestinal	X External	S Vascular Perfusion	H Indocyanine Green Dye
D Urinary	7 Via Natural or Artificial Opening 8 Via Natural or Artificial Opening Endoscopic	3 Contractility 5 Flow B Pressure D Resistance L Volume	Z No Qualifier
G Skin and Breast	X External	S Vascular Perfusion	H Indocyanine Green Dye
H Products of Conception, Cardiac ♀	7 Via Natural or Artificial Opening 8 Via Natural or Artificial Opening Endoscopic X External	4 Electrical Activity C Rate F Rhythm H Sound	Z No Qualifier
J Products of Conception, Nervous ♀	7 Via Natural or Artificial Opening 8 Via Natural or Artificial Opening Endoscopic X External	2 Conductivity 4 Electrical Activity B Pressure	Z No Qualifier
Z None	7 Via Natural or Artificial Opening	K Temperature	Z No Qualifier
Z None	X External	K Temperature Q Sleep	Z No Qualifier

Valid OR 4A16ØBZ
♀ 4A1H[7,8,X][4,C,F,H]Z
♀ 4A1J[7,8,X][2,4,B]Z

4 Measurement and Monitoring
B Physiological Devices
Ø Measurement Definition: Determining the level of a physiological or physical function at a point in time

Body System Character 4	Approach Character 5	Function/Device Character 6	Qualifier Character 7
Ø Central Nervous	X External	V Stimulator	Z No Qualifier
Ø Central Nervous	X External	W Cerebrospinal Fluid Shunt	Ø Wireless Sensor
1 Peripheral Nervous F Musculoskeletal	X External	V Stimulator	Z No Qualifier
2 Cardiac	X External	S Pacemaker T Defibrillator	Z No Qualifier
9 Respiratory	X External	S Pacemaker	Z No Qualifier

Extracorporeal or Systemic Assistance and Performance 5AØ–5A2

AHA Coding Clinic for table 5AØ
2022, 4Q, 61-62 Cardiac perfusion with intra-arterial supersaturated oxygen
2022, 3Q, 23 Placement of preCARDIA device
2021, 2Q, 12 Repositioning of displaced intra-aortic balloon pump
2020, 4Q, 64-65 Ventilatory assistance by high flow or high velocity nasal cannula devices
2020, 1Q, 10 Intermittent use of continuous positive airway pressure
2018, 2Q, 3-5 Intra-aortic balloon pump
2017, 4Q, 43-44 Insertion of external heart assist devices
2017, 3Q, 18 Intra-aortic balloon pump removal
2017, 1Q, 10-11 External heart assist device
2017, 1Q, 29 Newborn resuscitation using positive pressure ventilation
2017, 1Q, 29 Newborn noninvasive ventilation
2016, 4Q, 137-139 Heart assist device systems
2014, 4Q, 9 Mechanical ventilation
2014, 3Q, 19 Ablation of ventricular tachycardia with Impella® support
2013, 3Q, 18 Heart transplant surgery

AHA Coding Clinic for table 5A1
2022, 2Q, 25 Temporary-permanent pacemaker placement
2021, 4Q, 56 Automated chest compression
2019, 4Q, 39-41 Intraoperative extracorporeal membrane oxygenation
2019, 3Q, 19 Insertion of left ventricular catheter
2019, 3Q, 20 Removal and revision of ECMO component
2019, 3Q, 21 Exchange of extracorporeal membrane oxygenation component (oxygenator)

AHA Coding Clinic for table 5A1 (Continued)
2019, 2Q, 36 Veno-arterial extracorporeal membrane oxygenation via sternotomy
2019, 3Q, 22 Extracorporeal membrane oxygenation and Centrimag™ pump
2019, 3Q, 22 Extracorporeal membrane oxygenation transfers
2018, 4Q, 52-54 Percutaneous extracorporeal membrane oxygenation
2018, 1Q, 13 Mechanical ventilation using patient's equipment
2017, 4Q, 71-73 Hemodialysis and renal replacement therapy
2017, 3Q, 7 Senning procedure (arterial switch)
2017, 1Q, 19 Norwood Sano procedure
2016, 1Q, 27 Aortocoronary bypass graft utilizing Y-graft
2016, 1Q, 28 Extracorporeal liver assist device
2016, 1Q, 29 Duration of hemodialysis
2015, 4Q, 22-24 Congenital heart corrective procedures
2014, 4Q, 3-10 Mechanical ventilation
2014, 4Q, 11-15 Sequencing of mechanical ventilation with other procedures
2014, 3Q, 16 Repair of Tetralogy of Fallot
2014, 3Q, 20 MAZE procedure performed with coronary artery bypass graft
2014, 1Q, 10 Repair of thoracic aortic aneurysm & coronary artery bypass graft
2013, 3Q, 18 Heart transplant surgery

AHA Coding Clinic for table 5A2
2022, 1Q, 46 Internal cardioversion

5 Extracorporeal or Systemic Assistance and Performance
A Physiological Systems
Ø Assistance Definition: Taking over a portion of a physiological function by extracorporeal means

Body System Character 4	Duration Character 5	Function Character 6	Qualifier Character 7
2 Cardiac	1 Intermittent	1 Output	Ø Balloon Pump 5 Pulsatile Compression 6 Other Pump D Impeller Pump
2 Cardiac	2 Continuous	1 Output	Ø Balloon Pump 5 Pulsatile Compression 6 Other Pump D Impeller Pump
2 Cardiac	2 Continuous	2 Oxygenation	C Supersaturated
5 Circulatory	1 Intermittent 2 Continuous	2 Oxygenation	1 Hyperbaric
9 Respiratory	2 Continuous	Ø Filtration NT	Z No Qualifier
9 Respiratory	3 Less than 24 Consecutive Hours 4 24-96 Consecutive Hours 5 Greater than 96 Consecutive Hours	5 Ventilation	7 Continuous Positive Airway Pressure 8 Intermittent Positive Airway Pressure 9 Continuous Negative Airway Pressure A High Nasal Flow/Velocity B Intermittent Negative Airway Pressure Z No Qualifier
9 Respiratory	B Less than 8 Consecutive Hours C 8-24 Consecutive Hours D Greater than 24 Consecutive Hours	5 Ventilation	K Intubated Prone Positioning

Valid OR 5AØ211[Ø,6,D]
Valid OR 5AØ221[Ø,6,D]
NT 5AØ92ØZ for Hemolung Respiratory Assist System (RAS)

5 Extracorporeal or Systemic Assistance and Performance
A Physiological Systems
1 Performance Definition: Completely taking over a physiological function by extracorporeal means

Body System Character 4	Duration Character 5	Function Character 6	Qualifier Character 7
2 Cardiac	Ø Single	1 Output	2 Manual
2 Cardiac	1 Intermittent	3 Pacing	Z No Qualifier
2 Cardiac	2 Continuous	1 Output	J Automated Z No Qualifier
2 Cardiac	2 Continuous	3 Pacing	Z No Qualifier
5 Circulatory	2 Continuous A Intraoperative	2 Oxygenation	F Membrane, Central G Membrane, Peripheral Veno-arterial H Membrane, Peripheral Veno-venous
9 Respiratory	Ø Single	5 Ventilation	4 Nonmechanical
9 Respiratory	3 Less than 24 Consecutive Hours 4 24-96 Consecutive Hours 5 Greater than 96 Consecutive Hours	5 Ventilation	Z No Qualifier
C Biliary	Ø Single 6 Multiple	Ø Filtration	Z No Qualifier
D Urinary	7 Intermittent, Less than 6 Hours per day 8 Prolonged Intermittent, 6-18 Hours per day 9 Continuous, Greater than 18 Hours per day	Ø Filtration	Z No Qualifier

Valid OR 5A1522F
DRG Non-OR 5A1522[G,H]
DRG Non-OR 5A19[3,4]5Z
DRG Non-OR 5A1955Z Length of stay must be > 4 consecutive days.
DRG Non-OR 5A1D[7,8,9]ØZ

5 Extracorporeal or Systemic Assistance and Performance
A Physiological Systems
2 Restoration Definition: Returning, or attempting to return, a physiological function to its original state by extracorporeal means.

Body System Character 4	Duration Character 5	Function Character 6	Qualifier Character 7
2 Cardiac	Ø Single	4 Rhythm	Z No Qualifier

Extracorporeal or Systemic Therapies 6AØ–6AB

AHA Coding Clinic for table 6A4
2019, 2Q, 17 Cryoamputation of lower leg

AHA Coding Clinic for table 6A5
2022, 1Q, 48 Umbilical cord blood sampling

AHA Coding Clinic for table 6A7
2014, 4Q, 19 Ultrasound accelerated thrombolysis

AHA Coding Clinic for table 6AB
2023, 2Q, 32 Preparation of donor organ before transplantation
2016, 4Q, 115 Donor organ perfusion

6 Extracorporeal or Systemic Therapies
A Physiological Systems
Ø Atmospheric Control Definition: Extracorporeal control of atmospheric pressure and composition

Body System Character 4	Duration Character 5	Qualifier Character 6	Qualifier Character 7
Z None	Ø Single 1 Multiple	Z No Qualifier	Z No Qualifier

6 Extracorporeal or Systemic Therapies
A Physiological Systems
1 Decompression Definition: Extracorporeal elimination of undissolved gas from body fluids

Body System Character 4	Duration Character 5	Qualifier Character 6	Qualifier Character 7
5 Circulatory	Ø Single 1 Multiple	Z No Qualifier	Z No Qualifier

6 Extracorporeal or Systemic Therapies
A Physiological Systems
2 Electromagnetic Therapy Definition: Extracorporeal treatment by electromagnetic rays

Body System Character 4	Duration Character 5	Qualifier Character 6	Qualifier Character 7
1 Urinary 2 Central Nervous	Ø Single 1 Multiple	Z No Qualifier	Z No Qualifier

6 Extracorporeal or Systemic Therapies
A Physiological Systems
3 Hyperthermia Definition: Extracorporeal raising of body temperature

Body System Character 4	Duration Character 5	Qualifier Character 6	Qualifier Character 7
Z None	Ø Single 1 Multiple	Z No Qualifier	Z No Qualifier

6 Extracorporeal or Systemic Therapies
A Physiological Systems
4 Hypothermia Definition: Extracorporeal lowering of body temperature

Body System Character 4	Duration Character 5	Qualifier Character 6	Qualifier Character 7
Z None	Ø Single 1 Multiple	Z No Qualifier	Z No Qualifier

6 Extracorporeal or Systemic Therapies
A Physiological Systems
5 Pheresis Definition: Extracorporeal separation of blood products

Body System Character 4	Duration Character 5	Qualifier Character 6	Qualifier Character 7
5 Circulatory	Ø Single 1 Multiple	Z No Qualifier	Ø Erythrocytes 1 Leukocytes 2 Platelets 3 Plasma T Stem Cells, Cord Blood V Stem Cells, Hematopoietic

6 Extracorporeal or Systemic Therapies
A Physiological Systems
6 Phototherapy Definition: Extracorporeal treatment by light rays

Body System Character 4	Duration Character 5	Qualifier Character 6	Qualifier Character 7
Ø Skin 5 Circulatory	Ø Single 1 Multiple	Z No Qualifier	Z No Qualifier

6 Extracorporeal or Systemic Therapies
A Physiological Systems
7 Ultrasound Therapy Definition: Extracorporeal treatment by ultrasound

Body System Character 4	Duration Character 5	Qualifier Character 6	Qualifier Character 7
5 Circulatory	Ø Single 1 Multiple	Z No Qualifier	4 Head and Neck Vessels 5 Heart 6 Peripheral Vessels 7 Other Vessels Z No Qualifier

6 Extracorporeal or Systemic Therapies
A Physiological Systems
8 Ultraviolet Light Therapy Definition: Extracorporeal treatment by ultraviolet light

Body System Character 4	Duration Character 5	Qualifier Character 6	Qualifier Character 7
Ø Skin	Ø Single 1 Multiple	Z No Qualifier	Z No Qualifier

6 Extracorporeal or Systemic Therapies
A Physiological Systems
9 Shock Wave Therapy Definition: Extracorporeal treatment by shock waves

Body System Character 4	Duration Character 5	Qualifier Character 6	Qualifier Character 7
3 Musculoskeletal	Ø Single 1 Multiple	Z No Qualifier	Z No Qualifier

6 Extracorporeal or Systemic Therapies
A Physiological Systems
B Perfusion Definition: Extracorporeal treatment by diffusion of therapeutic fluid

Body System Character 4	Duration Character 5	Qualifier Character 6	Qualifier Character 7
5 Circulatory B Respiratory System F Hepatobiliary System and Pancreas T Urinary System	Ø Single	B Donor Organ	Z No Qualifier

Osteopathic 7WØ

7 Osteopathic
W Anatomical Regions
Ø Treatment Definition: Manual treatment to eliminate or alleviate somatic dysfunction and related disorders

Body Region Character 4	Approach Character 5	Method Character 6	Qualifier Character 7
Ø Head **1** Cervical **2** Thoracic **3** Lumbar **4** Sacrum **5** Pelvis **6** Lower Extremities **7** Upper Extremities **8** Rib Cage **9** Abdomen	**X** External	**Ø** Articulatory-Raising **1** Fascial Release **2** General Mobilization **3** High Velocity-Low Amplitude **4** Indirect **5** Low Velocity-High Amplitude **6** Lymphatic Pump **7** Muscle Energy-Isometric **8** Muscle Energy-Isotonic **9** Other Method	**Z** None

Other Procedures 8CØ–8EØ

AHA Coding Clinic for table 8EØ

2021, 4Q, 49 Division of liver for staged hepatectomy
2021, 2Q, 19 Electromagnetic stealth guided ventriculoperitoneal shunt insertion with endoscopy
2020, 4Q, 53 Bypass pancreatic duct to stomach
2020, 4Q, 65-66 Near infrared spectroscopy for tissue viability assessment
2020, 4Q, 99 Robotic-assisted prostatectomy with extension of incision for specimen removal
2020, 4Q, 100 Robotic-assisted sigmoid colectomy with extension of incision for specimen removal
2019, 4Q, 41-42 Intraoperative fluorescence guidance
2019, 1Q, 30 Laparoscopic-assisted rectopexy with manual reduction of prolapse
2015, 1Q, 33 Robotic-assisted laparoscopic hysterectomy converted to open procedure
2014, 4Q, 33 Radical prostatectomy

8 Other Procedures
C Indwelling Device
Ø Other Procedures Definition: Methodologies which attempt to remediate or cure a disorder or disease

Body Region Character 4	Approach Character 5	Method Character 6	Qualifier Character 7
1 Nervous System	X External	6 Collection	J Cerebrospinal Fluid L Other Fluid
2 Circulatory System	X External	6 Collection	K Blood L Other Fluid

8 Other Procedures
E Physiological Systems and Anatomical Regions
Ø Other Procedures Definition: Methodologies which attempt to remediate or cure a disorder or disease

Body Region Character 4	Approach Character 5	Method Character 6	Qualifier Character 7
1 Nervous System	X External	Y Other Method	7 Examination
2 Circulatory System	3 Percutaneous X External	D Near Infrared Spectroscopy	Z No Qualifier
9 Head and Neck Region	Ø Open	C Robotic Assisted Procedure	Z No Qualifier
9 Head and Neck Region	Ø Open	E Fluorescence Guided Procedure	M Aminolevulinic Acid Z No Qualifier
9 Head and Neck Region	3 Percutaneous 4 Percutaneous Endoscopic 7 Via Natural or Artificial Opening 8 Via Natural or Artificial Opening Endoscopic	C Robotic Assisted Procedure E Fluorescence Guided Procedure	Z No Qualifier
9 Head and Neck Region	X External	B Computer Assisted Procedure	F With Fluoroscopy G With Computerized Tomography H With Magnetic Resonance Imaging Z No Qualifier
9 Head and Neck Region	X External	C Robotic Assisted Procedure	Z No Qualifier
9 Head and Neck Region	X External	Y Other Method	8 Suture Removal
H Integumentary System and Breast	3 Percutaneous	Ø Acupuncture	Ø Anesthesia Z No Qualifier
H Integumentary System and Breast ♀	X External	6 Collection	2 Breast Milk
H Integumentary System and Breast	X External	Y Other Method	9 Piercing
K Musculoskeletal System	X External	1 Therapeutic Massage	Z No Qualifier
K Musculoskeletal System	X External	Y Other Method	7 Examination
U Female Reproductive System ♀	Ø Open 3 Percutaneous 4 Percutaneous Endoscopic 7 Via Natural or Artificial Opening 8 Via Natural or Artificial Opening Endoscopic	E Fluorescence Guided Procedure	N Pafolacianine
U Female Reproductive System ♀	X External	Y Other Method	7 Examination
V Male Reproductive System ♂	X External	1 Therapeutic Massage	C Prostate D Rectum
V Male Reproductive System ♂	X External	6 Collection	3 Sperm
W Trunk Region	Ø Open 3 Percutaneous 4 Percutaneous Endoscopic 7 Via Natural or Artificial Opening 8 Via Natural or Artificial Opening Endoscopic	C Robotic Assisted Procedure	Z No Qualifier
W Trunk Region	Ø Open 3 Percutaneous 4 Percutaneous Endoscopic 7 Via Natural or Artificial Opening 8 Via Natural or Artificial Opening Endoscopic	E Fluorescence Guided Procedure	N Pafolacianine Z No Qualifier
W Trunk Region	X External	B Computer Assisted Procedure	F With Fluoroscopy G With Computerized Tomography H With Magnetic Resonance Imaging Z No Qualifier
W Trunk Region	X External	C Robotic Assisted Procedure	Z No Qualifier
W Trunk Region	X External	Y Other Method	8 Suture Removal
X Upper Extremity Y Lower Extremity	Ø Open 3 Percutaneous 4 Percutaneous Endoscopic	C Robotic Assisted Procedure E Fluorescence Guided Procedure	Z No Qualifier
X Upper Extremity Y Lower Extremity	X External	B Computer Assisted Procedure	F With Fluoroscopy G With Computerized Tomography H With Magnetic Resonance Imaging Z No Qualifier
X Upper Extremity Y Lower Extremity	X External	C Robotic Assisted Procedure	Z No Qualifier
X Upper Extremity Y Lower Extremity	X External	Y Other Method	8 Suture Removal
Z None	X External	Y Other Method	1 In Vitro Fertilization 4 Yoga Therapy 5 Meditation 6 Isolation

♂ 8EØVX1C ♀ 8EØUXY7
♂ 8EØVX63 ♀ 8EØHX62

Chiropractic 9WB

9 Chiropractic
W Anatomical Regions
B Manipulation Definition: Manual procedure that involves a directed thrust to move a joint past the physiological range of motion, without exceeding the anatomical limit

Body Region Character 4	Approach Character 5	Method Character 6	Qualifier Character 7
Ø Head **1** Cervical **2** Thoracic **3** Lumbar **4** Sacrum **5** Pelvis **6** Lower Extremities **7** Upper Extremities **8** Rib Cage **9** Abdomen	**X** External	**B** Non-Manual **C** Indirect Visceral **D** Extra-Articular **F** Direct Visceral **G** Long Lever Specific Contact **H** Short Lever Specific Contact **J** Long and Short Lever Specific Contact **K** Mechanically Assisted **L** Other Method	**Z** None

Imaging BØØ–BY4

AHA Coding Clinic for table B21
2018, 1Q, 12 Percutaneous balloon valvuloplasty & cardiac catheterization with ventriculogram
2016, 3Q, 36 Type of contrast medium for angiography (high osmolar, low osmolar, and other)

AHA Coding Clinic for table B41
2015, 3Q, 9 Aborted endovascular stenting of superficial femoral artery

AHA Coding Clinic for table B51
2015, 4Q, 30 Vascular access devices

AHA Coding Clinic for table BB3
2022, 4Q, 62 Hyperpolarized Xenon-129 gas for imaging of lung function

AHA Coding Clinic for table BF1
2021, 4Q, 57 Fluoroscopic guidance of hepatobiliary sites

AHA Coding Clinic for table BF4
2014, 3Q, 15 Drainage of pancreatic pseudocyst
2020, 4Q, 66 Other imaging type

AHA Coding Clinic for table BF5
2020, 4Q, 66 Other imaging type
2020, 4Q, 66-67 Fluorescence imaging of hepatobiliary system

AHA Coding Clinic for table BW5
2020, 4Q, 66 Other imaging type
2020, 4Q, 68 Bacterial autofluorescence detection

Contrast Agents

High Osmolar (Ø)	Low Osmolar (1)	Other Contrast (Y)
cholografin meglumine	hexabrix	iodixanol
conray	iohexol	iotrolan
cysto-conray II	iomeprol	isovist
cystografin	iomeron	visipaque
cystografin-dilute	iopamidol	
diatrizoate	iopromide	
gastrografin	ioversol	
hypaque	ioxaglate	
iothalamate	ioxilan	
isopaque	isovue	
md-76r	omnipaque	
metrizoate	optiray	
reno-dip	oxilan	
sinografin	ultravist	

B Imaging
Ø Central Nervous System
Ø Plain Radiography Definition: Planar display of an image developed from the capture of external ionizing radiation on photographic or photoconductive plate

Body Part Character 4	Contrast Character 5	Qualifier Character 6	Qualifier Character 7
B Spinal Cord	Ø High Osmolar 1 Low Osmolar Y Other Contrast Z None	Z None	Z None

B Imaging
Ø Central Nervous System
1 Fluoroscopy Definition: Single plane or bi-plane real time display of an image developed from the capture of external ionizing radiation on a fluorescent screen. The image may also be stored by either digital or analog means.

Body Part Character 4	Contrast Character 5	Qualifier Character 6	Qualifier Character 7
B Spinal Cord	Ø High Osmolar 1 Low Osmolar Y Other Contrast Z None	Z None	Z None

B Imaging
Ø Central Nervous System
2 Computerized Tomography (CT Scan) Definition: Computer reformatted digital display of multiplanar images developed from the capture of multiple exposures of external ionizing radiation

Body Part Character 4	Contrast Character 5	Qualifier Character 6	Qualifier Character 7
Ø Brain 7 Cisterna 8 Cerebral Ventricle(s) 9 Sella Turcica/Pituitary Gland B Spinal Cord	Ø High Osmolar 1 Low Osmolar Y Other Contrast	Ø Unenhanced and Enhanced Z None	Z None
Ø Brain 7 Cisterna 8 Cerebral Ventricle(s) 9 Sella Turcica/Pituitary Gland B Spinal Cord	Z None	Z None	Z None

B Imaging
Ø Central Nervous System
3 Magnetic Resonance Imaging (MRI) Definition: Computer reformatted digital display of multiplanar images developed from the capture of radio-frequency signals emitted by nuclei in a body site excited within a magnetic field

Body Part Character 4	Contrast Character 5	Qualifier Character 6	Qualifier Character 7
Ø Brain 9 Sella Turcica/Pituitary Gland B Spinal Cord C Acoustic Nerves	Y Other Contrast	Ø Unenhanced and Enhanced Z None	Z None
Ø Brain 9 Sella Turcica/Pituitary Gland B Spinal Cord C Acoustic Nerves	Z None	Z None	Z None

B Imaging
Ø Central Nervous System
4 Ultrasonography Definition: Real time display of images of anatomy or flow information developed from the capture of reflected and attenuated high frequency sound waves

Body Part Character 4	Contrast Character 5	Qualifier Character 6	Qualifier Character 7
Ø Brain B Spinal Cord	Z None	Z None	Z None

B Imaging
2 Heart
Ø Plain Radiography Definition: Planar display of an image developed from the capture of external ionizing radiation on photographic or photoconductive plate

Body Part Character 4	Contrast Character 5	Qualifier Character 6	Qualifier Character 7
Ø Coronary Artery, Single 1 Coronary Arteries, Multiple 2 Coronary Artery Bypass Graft, Single 3 Coronary Artery Bypass Grafts, Multiple 4 Heart, Right 5 Heart, Left 6 Heart, Right and Left 7 Internal Mammary Bypass Graft, Right 8 Internal Mammary Bypass Graft, Left F Bypass Graft, Other	Ø High Osmolar 1 Low Osmolar Y Other Contrast	Z None	Z None

DRG Non-OR All body part, contrast, and qualifier values

B Imaging
2 Heart
1 Fluoroscopy Definition: Single plane or bi-plane real time display of an image developed from the capture of external ionizing radiation on a fluorescent screen. The image may also be stored by either digital or analog means.

Body Part Character 4	Contrast Character 5	Qualifier Character 6	Qualifier Character 7
Ø Coronary Artery, Single 1 Coronary Arteries, Multiple 2 Coronary Artery Bypass Graft, Single 3 Coronary Artery Bypass Grafts, Multiple	Ø High Osmolar 1 Low Osmolar Y Other Contrast	1 Laser	Ø Intraoperative
Ø Coronary Artery, Single 1 Coronary Arteries, Multiple 2 Coronary Artery Bypass Graft, Single 3 Coronary Artery Bypass Grafts, Multiple	Ø High Osmolar 1 Low Osmolar Y Other Contrast	Z None	Z None
4 Heart, Right 5 Heart, Left 6 Heart, Right and Left 7 Internal Mammary Bypass Graft, Right 8 Internal Mammary Bypass Graft, Left F Bypass Graft, Other	Ø High Osmolar 1 Low Osmolar Y Other Contrast	Z None	Z None

DRG Non-OR B21[Ø,1,2,3][Ø,1,Y]ZZ
DRG Non-OR B21[4,5,6,7,8,F][Ø,1,Y]ZZ

B Imaging
2 Heart
2 Computerized Tomography (CT Scan) Definition: Computer reformatted digital display of multiplanar images developed from the capture of multiple exposures of external ionizing radiation

Body Part Character 4	Contrast Character 5	Qualifier Character 6	Qualifier Character 7
1 Coronary Arteries, Multiple 3 Coronary Artery Bypass Grafts, Multiple 6 Heart, Right and Left	Ø High Osmolar 1 Low Osmolar Y Other Contrast	Ø Unenhanced and Enhanced Z None	Z None
1 Coronary Arteries, Multiple 3 Coronary Artery Bypass Grafts, Multiple 6 Heart, Right and Left	Z None	2 Intravascular Optical Coherence Z None	Z None

B Imaging
2 Heart
3 Magnetic Resonance Imaging (MRI) Definition: Computer reformatted digital display of multiplanar images developed from the capture of radio-frequency signals emitted by nuclei in a body site excited within a magnetic field

Body Part Character 4	Contrast Character 5	Qualifier Character 6	Qualifier Character 7
1 Coronary Arteries, Multiple 3 Coronary Artery Bypass Grafts, Multiple 6 Heart, Right and Left	Y Other Contrast	Ø Unenhanced and Enhanced Z None	Z None
1 Coronary Arteries, Multiple 3 Coronary Artery Bypass Grafts, Multiple 6 Heart, Right and Left	Z None	Z None	Z None

B Imaging
2 Heart
4 Ultrasonography Definition: Real time display of images of anatomy or flow information developed from the capture of reflected and attenuated high frequency sound waves

Body Part Character 4	Contrast Character 5	Qualifier Character 6	Qualifier Character 7
Ø Coronary Artery, Single **1** Coronary Arteries, Multiple **4** Heart, Right **5** Heart, Left **6** Heart, Right and Left **B** Heart with Aorta **C** Pericardium **D** Pediatric Heart	**Y** Other Contrast	**Z** None	**Z** None
Ø Coronary Artery, Single **1** Coronary Arteries, Multiple **4** Heart, Right **5** Heart, Left **6** Heart, Right and Left **B** Heart with Aorta **C** Pericardium **D** Pediatric Heart	**Z** None	**Z** None	**3** Intravascular **4** Transesophageal **Z** None

B Imaging
3 Upper Arteries
Ø Plain Radiography Definition: Planar display of an image developed from the capture of external ionizing radiation on photographic or photoconductive plate

Body Part Character 4	Contrast Character 5	Qualifier Character 6	Qualifier Character 7
Ø Thoracic Aorta **1** Brachiocephalic-Subclavian Artery, Right **2** Subclavian Artery, Left **3** Common Carotid Artery, Right **4** Common Carotid Artery, Left **5** Common Carotid Arteries, Bilateral **6** Internal Carotid Artery, Right **7** Internal Carotid Artery, Left **8** Internal Carotid Arteries, Bilateral **9** External Carotid Artery, Right **B** External Carotid Artery, Left **C** External Carotid Arteries, Bilateral **D** Vertebral Artery, Right **F** Vertebral Artery, Left **G** Vertebral Arteries, Bilateral **H** Upper Extremity Arteries, Right **J** Upper Extremity Arteries, Left **K** Upper Extremity Arteries, Bilateral **L** Intercostal and Bronchial Arteries **M** Spinal Arteries **N** Upper Arteries, Other **P** Thoraco-Abdominal Aorta **Q** Cervico-Cerebral Arch **R** Intracranial Arteries **S** Pulmonary Artery, Right **T** Pulmonary Artery, Left	**Ø** High Osmolar **1** Low Osmolar **Y** Other Contrast **Z** None	**Z** None	**Z** None

B Imaging
3 Upper Arteries
1 Fluoroscopy Definition: Single plane or bi-plane real time display of an image developed from the capture of external ionizing radiation on a fluorescent screen. The image may also be stored by either digital or analog means.

Body Part Character 4	Contrast Character 5	Qualifier Character 6	Qualifier Character 7
Ø Thoracic Aorta 1 Brachiocephalic-Subclavian Artery, Right 2 Subclavian Artery, Left 3 Common Carotid Artery, Right 4 Common Carotid Artery, Left 5 Common Carotid Arteries, Bilateral 6 Internal Carotid Artery, Right 7 Internal Carotid Artery, Left 8 Internal Carotid Arteries, Bilateral 9 External Carotid Artery, Right B External Carotid Artery, Left C External Carotid Arteries, Bilateral D Vertebral Artery, Right F Vertebral Artery, Left G Vertebral Arteries, Bilateral H Upper Extremity Arteries, Right J Upper Extremity Arteries, Left K Upper Extremity Arteries, Bilateral L Intercostal and Bronchial Arteries M Spinal Arteries N Upper Arteries, Other P Thoraco-Abdominal Aorta Q Cervico-Cerebral Arch R Intracranial Arteries S Pulmonary Artery, Right T Pulmonary Artery, Left U Pulmonary Trunk	Ø High Osmolar 1 Low Osmolar Y Other Contrast	1 Laser	Ø Intraoperative
Ø Thoracic Aorta 1 Brachiocephalic-Subclavian Artery, Right 2 Subclavian Artery, Left 3 Common Carotid Artery, Right 4 Common Carotid Artery, Left 5 Common Carotid Arteries, Bilateral 6 Internal Carotid Artery, Right 7 Internal Carotid Artery, Left 8 Internal Carotid Arteries, Bilateral 9 External Carotid Artery, Right B External Carotid Artery, Left C External Carotid Arteries, Bilateral D Vertebral Artery, Right F Vertebral Artery, Left G Vertebral Arteries, Bilateral H Upper Extremity Arteries, Right J Upper Extremity Arteries, Left K Upper Extremity Arteries, Bilateral L Intercostal and Bronchial Arteries M Spinal Arteries N Upper Arteries, Other P Thoraco-Abdominal Aorta Q Cervico-Cerebral Arch R Intracranial Arteries S Pulmonary Artery, Right T Pulmonary Artery, Left U Pulmonary Trunk	Ø High Osmolar 1 Low Osmolar Y Other Contrast	Z None	Z None

B31 Continued on next page

B31 Continued

B Imaging
3 Upper Arteries
1 Fluoroscopy Definition: Single plane or bi-plane real time display of an image developed from the capture of external ionizing radiation on a fluorescent screen. The image may also be stored by either digital or analog means.

Body Part Character 4	Contrast Character 5	Qualifier Character 6	Qualifier Character 7
Ø Thoracic Aorta 1 Brachiocephalic-Subclavian Artery, Right 2 Subclavian Artery, Left 3 Common Carotid Artery, Right 4 Common Carotid Artery, Left 5 Common Carotid Arteries, Bilateral 6 Internal Carotid Artery, Right 7 Internal Carotid Artery, Left 8 Internal Carotid Arteries, Bilateral 9 External Carotid Artery, Right B External Carotid Artery, Left C External Carotid Arteries, Bilateral D Vertebral Artery, Right F Vertebral Artery, Left G Vertebral Arteries, Bilateral H Upper Extremity Arteries, Right J Upper Extremity Arteries, Left K Upper Extremity Arteries, Bilateral L Intercostal and Bronchial Arteries M Spinal Arteries N Upper Arteries, Other P Thoraco-Abdominal Aorta Q Cervico-Cerebral Arch R Intracranial Arteries S Pulmonary Artery, Right T Pulmonary Artery, Left U Pulmonary Trunk	Z None	Z None	Z None

B Imaging
3 Upper Arteries
2 Computerized Tomography (CT Scan) Definition: Computer reformatted digital display of multiplanar images developed from the capture of multiple exposures of external ionizing radiation

Body Part Character 4	Contrast Character 5	Qualifier Character 6	Qualifier Character 7
Ø Thoracic Aorta 5 Common Carotid Arteries, Bilateral 8 Internal Carotid Arteries, Bilateral G Vertebral Arteries, Bilateral R Intracranial Arteries S Pulmonary Artery, Right T Pulmonary Artery, Left	Ø High Osmolar 1 Low Osmolar Y Other Contrast	Z None	Z None
Ø Thoracic Aorta 5 Common Carotid Arteries, Bilateral 8 Internal Carotid Arteries, Bilateral G Vertebral Arteries, Bilateral R Intracranial Arteries S Pulmonary Artery, Right T Pulmonary Artery, Left	Z None	2 Intravascular Optical Coherence Z None	Z None

B Imaging
3 Upper Arteries
3 Magnetic Resonance Imaging (MRI) Definition: Computer reformatted digital display of multiplanar images developed from the capture of radio-frequency signals emitted by nuclei in a body site excited within a magnetic field

Body Part Character 4	Contrast Character 5	Qualifier Character 6	Qualifier Character 7
Ø Thoracic Aorta 5 Common Carotid Arteries, Bilateral 8 Internal Carotid Arteries, Bilateral G Vertebral Arteries, Bilateral H Upper Extremity Arteries, Right J Upper Extremity Arteries, Left K Upper Extremity Arteries, Bilateral M Spinal Arteries Q Cervico-Cerebral Arch R Intracranial Arteries	Y Other Contrast	Ø Unenhanced and Enhanced Z None	Z None
Ø Thoracic Aorta 5 Common Carotid Arteries, Bilateral 8 Internal Carotid Arteries, Bilateral G Vertebral Arteries, Bilateral H Upper Extremity Arteries, Right J Upper Extremity Arteries, Left K Upper Extremity Arteries, Bilateral M Spinal Arteries Q Cervico-Cerebral Arch R Intracranial Arteries	Z None	Z None	Z None

B Imaging
3 Upper Arteries
4 Ultrasonography Definition: Real time display of images of anatomy or flow information developed from the capture of reflected and attenuated high frequency sound waves

Body Part Character 4	Contrast Character 5	Qualifier Character 6	Qualifier Character 7
Ø Thoracic Aorta 1 Brachiocephalic-Subclavian Artery, Right 2 Subclavian Artery, Left 3 Common Carotid Artery, Right 4 Common Carotid Artery, Left 5 Common Carotid Arteries, Bilateral 6 Internal Carotid Artery, Right 7 Internal Carotid Artery, Left 8 Internal Carotid Arteries, Bilateral H Upper Extremity Arteries, Right J Upper Extremity Arteries, Left K Upper Extremity Arteries, Bilateral R Intracranial Arteries S Pulmonary Artery, Right T Pulmonary Artery, Left V Ophthalmic Arteries	Z None	Z None	3 Intravascular Z None

B Imaging
4 Lower Arteries
Ø Plain Radiography Definition: Planar display of an image developed from the capture of external ionizing radiation on photographic or photoconductive plate

Body Part Character 4	Contrast Character 5	Qualifier Character 6	Qualifier Character 7
Ø Abdominal Aorta 2 Hepatic Artery 3 Splenic Arteries 4 Superior Mesenteric Artery 5 Inferior Mesenteric Artery 6 Renal Artery, Right 7 Renal Artery, Left 8 Renal Arteries, Bilateral 9 Lumbar Arteries B Intra-Abdominal Arteries, Other C Pelvic Arteries D Aorta and Bilateral Lower Extremity Arteries F Lower Extremity Arteries, Right G Lower Extremity Arteries, Left J Lower Arteries, Other M Renal Artery Transplant	Ø High Osmolar 1 Low Osmolar Y Other Contrast	Z None	Z None

B Imaging
4 Lower Arteries
1 Fluoroscopy Definition: Single plane or bi-plane real time display of an image developed from the capture of external ionizing radiation on a fluorescent screen. The image may also be stored by either digital or analog means.

Body Part Character 4	Contrast Character 5	Qualifier Character 6	Qualifier Character 7
Ø Abdominal Aorta 2 Hepatic Artery 3 Splenic Arteries 4 Superior Mesenteric Artery 5 Inferior Mesenteric Artery 6 Renal Artery, Right 7 Renal Artery, Left 8 Renal Arteries, Bilateral 9 Lumbar Arteries B Intra-Abdominal Arteries, Other C Pelvic Arteries D Aorta and Bilateral Lower Extremity Arteries F Lower Extremity Arteries, Right G Lower Extremity Arteries, Left J Lower Arteries, Other	Ø High Osmolar 1 Low Osmolar Y Other Contrast	1 Laser	Ø Intraoperative
Ø Abdominal Aorta 2 Hepatic Artery 3 Splenic Arteries 4 Superior Mesenteric Artery 5 Inferior Mesenteric Artery 6 Renal Artery, Right 7 Renal Artery, Left 8 Renal Arteries, Bilateral 9 Lumbar Arteries B Intra-Abdominal Arteries, Other C Pelvic Arteries D Aorta and Bilateral Lower Extremity Arteries F Lower Extremity Arteries, Right G Lower Extremity Arteries, Left J Lower Arteries, Other	Ø High Osmolar 1 Low Osmolar Y Other Contrast	Z None	Z None
Ø Abdominal Aorta 2 Hepatic Artery 3 Splenic Arteries 4 Superior Mesenteric Artery 5 Inferior Mesenteric Artery 6 Renal Artery, Right 7 Renal Artery, Left 8 Renal Arteries, Bilateral 9 Lumbar Arteries B Intra-Abdominal Arteries, Other C Pelvic Arteries D Aorta and Bilateral Lower Extremity Arteries F Lower Extremity Arteries, Right G Lower Extremity Arteries, Left J Lower Arteries, Other	Z None	Z None	Z None

B Imaging
4 Lower Arteries
2 Computerized Tomography (CT Scan) Definition: Computer reformatted digital display of multiplanar images developed from the capture of multiple exposures of external ionizing radiation

Body Part Character 4	Contrast Character 5	Qualifier Character 6	Qualifier Character 7
Ø Abdominal Aorta **1** Celiac Artery **4** Superior Mesenteric Artery **8** Renal Arteries, Bilateral **C** Pelvic Arteries **F** Lower Extremity Arteries, Right **G** Lower Extremity Arteries, Left **H** Lower Extremity Arteries, Bilateral **M** Renal Artery Transplant	**Ø** High Osmolar **1** Low Osmolar **Y** Other Contrast	**Z** None	**Z** None
Ø Abdominal Aorta **1** Celiac Artery **4** Superior Mesenteric Artery **8** Renal Arteries, Bilateral **C** Pelvic Arteries **F** Lower Extremity Arteries, Right **G** Lower Extremity Arteries, Left **H** Lower Extremity Arteries, Bilateral **M** Renal Artery Transplant	**Z** None	**2** Intravascular Optical Coherence **Z** None	**Z** None

B Imaging
4 Lower Arteries
3 Magnetic Resonance Imaging (MRI) Definition: Computer reformatted digital display of multiplanar images developed from the capture of radio-frequency signals emitted by nuclei in a body site excited within a magnetic field

Body Part Character 4	Contrast Character 5	Qualifier Character 6	Qualifier Character 7
Ø Abdominal Aorta **1** Celiac Artery **4** Superior Mesenteric Artery **8** Renal Arteries, Bilateral **C** Pelvic Arteries **F** Lower Extremity Arteries, Right **G** Lower Extremity Arteries, Left **H** Lower Extremity Arteries, Bilateral	**Y** Other Contrast	**Ø** Unenhanced and Enhanced **Z** None	**Z** None
Ø Abdominal Aorta **1** Celiac Artery **4** Superior Mesenteric Artery **8** Renal Arteries, Bilateral **C** Pelvic Arteries **F** Lower Extremity Arteries, Right **G** Lower Extremity Arteries, Left **H** Lower Extremity Arteries, Bilateral	**Z** None	**Z** None	**Z** None

B Imaging
4 Lower Arteries
4 Ultrasonography Definition: Real time display of images of anatomy or flow information developed from the capture of reflected and attenuated high frequency sound waves

Body Part Character 4	Contrast Character 5	Qualifier Character 6	Qualifier Character 7
Ø Abdominal Aorta **4** Superior Mesenteric Artery **5** Inferior Mesenteric Artery **6** Renal Artery, Right **7** Renal Artery, Left **8** Renal Arteries, Bilateral **B** Intra-Abdominal Arteries, Other **F** Lower Extremity Arteries, Right **G** Lower Extremity Arteries, Left **H** Lower Extremity Arteries, Bilateral **K** Celiac and Mesenteric Arteries **L** Femoral Artery **N** Penile Arteries	**Z** None	**Z** None	**3** Intravascular **Z** None

B Imaging
5 Veins
Ø Plain Radiography Definition: Planar display of an image developed from the capture of external ionizing radiation on photographic or photoconductive plate

Body Part Character 4	Contrast Character 5	Qualifier Character 6	Qualifier Character 7
Ø Epidural Veins 1 Cerebral and Cerebellar Veins 2 Intracranial Sinuses 3 Jugular Veins, Right 4 Jugular Veins, Left 5 Jugular Veins, Bilateral 6 Subclavian Vein, Right 7 Subclavian Vein, Left 8 Superior Vena Cava 9 Inferior Vena Cava B Lower Extremity Veins, Right C Lower Extremity Veins, Left D Lower Extremity Veins, Bilateral F Pelvic (Iliac) Veins, Right G Pelvic (Iliac) Veins, Left H Pelvic (Iliac) Veins, Bilateral J Renal Vein, Right K Renal Vein, Left L Renal Veins, Bilateral M Upper Extremity Veins, Right N Upper Extremity Veins, Left P Upper Extremity Veins, Bilateral Q Pulmonary Vein, Right R Pulmonary Vein, Left S Pulmonary Veins, Bilateral T Portal and Splanchnic Veins V Veins, Other W Dialysis Shunt/Fistula	Ø High Osmolar 1 Low Osmolar Y Other Contrast	Z None	Z None

B Imaging
5 Veins
1 Fluoroscopy Definition: Single plane or bi-plane real time display of an image developed from the capture of external ionizing radiation on a fluorescent screen. The image may also be stored by either digital or analog means.

Body Part Character 4	Contrast Character 5	Qualifier Character 6	Qualifier Character 7
Ø Epidural Veins 1 Cerebral and Cerebellar Veins 2 Intracranial Sinuses 3 Jugular Veins, Right 4 Jugular Veins, Left 5 Jugular Veins, Bilateral 6 Subclavian Vein, Right 7 Subclavian Vein, Left 8 Superior Vena Cava 9 Inferior Vena Cava B Lower Extremity Veins, Right C Lower Extremity Veins, Left D Lower Extremity Veins, Bilateral F Pelvic (Iliac) Veins, Right G Pelvic (Iliac) Veins, Left H Pelvic (Iliac) Veins, Bilateral J Renal Vein, Right K Renal Vein, Left L Renal Veins, Bilateral M Upper Extremity Veins, Right N Upper Extremity Veins, Left P Upper Extremity Veins, Bilateral Q Pulmonary Vein, Right R Pulmonary Vein, Left S Pulmonary Veins, Bilateral T Portal and Splanchnic Veins V Veins, Other W Dialysis Shunt/Fistula	Ø High Osmolar 1 Low Osmolar Y Other Contrast Z None	Z None	A Guidance Z None

B Imaging
5 Veins
2 Computerized Tomography (CT Scan) Definition: Computer reformatted digital display of multiplanar images developed from the capture of multiple exposures of external ionizing radiation

Body Part Character 4	Contrast Character 5	Qualifier Character 6	Qualifier Character 7
2 Intracranial Sinuses 8 Superior Vena Cava 9 Inferior Vena Cava F Pelvic (Iliac) Veins, Right G Pelvic (Iliac) Veins, Left H Pelvic (Iliac) Veins, Bilateral J Renal Vein, Right K Renal Vein, Left L Renal Veins, Bilateral Q Pulmonary Vein, Right R Pulmonary Vein, Left S Pulmonary Veins, Bilateral T Portal and Splanchnic Veins	Ø High Osmolar 1 Low Osmolar Y Other Contrast	Ø Unenhanced and Enhanced Z None	Z None
2 Intracranial Sinuses 8 Superior Vena Cava 9 Inferior Vena Cava F Pelvic (Iliac) Veins, Right G Pelvic (Iliac) Veins, Left H Pelvic (Iliac) Veins, Bilateral J Renal Vein, Right K Renal Vein, Left L Renal Veins, Bilateral Q Pulmonary Vein, Right R Pulmonary Vein, Left S Pulmonary Veins, Bilateral T Portal and Splanchnic Veins	Z None	2 Intravascular Optical Coherence Z None	Z None

B Imaging
5 Veins
3 Magnetic Resonance Imaging (MRI) Definition: Computer reformatted digital display of multiplanar images developed from the capture of radio-frequency signals emitted by nuclei in a body site excited within a magnetic field

Body Part Character 4	Contrast Character 5	Qualifier Character 6	Qualifier Character 7
1 Cerebral and Cerebellar Veins 2 Intracranial Sinuses 5 Jugular Veins, Bilateral 8 Superior Vena Cava 9 Inferior Vena Cava B Lower Extremity Veins, Right C Lower Extremity Veins, Left D Lower Extremity Veins, Bilateral H Pelvic (Iliac) Veins, Bilateral L Renal Veins, Bilateral M Upper Extremity Veins, Right N Upper Extremity Veins, Left P Upper Extremity Veins, Bilateral S Pulmonary Veins, Bilateral T Portal and Splanchnic Veins V Veins, Other	Y Other Contrast	Ø Unenhanced and Enhanced Z None	Z None
1 Cerebral and Cerebellar Veins 2 Intracranial Sinuses 5 Jugular Veins, Bilateral 8 Superior Vena Cava 9 Inferior Vena Cava B Lower Extremity Veins, Right C Lower Extremity Veins, Left D Lower Extremity Veins, Bilateral H Pelvic (Iliac) Veins, Bilateral L Renal Veins, Bilateral M Upper Extremity Veins, Right N Upper Extremity Veins, Left P Upper Extremity Veins, Bilateral S Pulmonary Veins, Bilateral T Portal and Splanchnic Veins V Veins, Other	Z None	Z None	Z None

B Imaging
5 Veins
4 Ultrasonography Definition: Real time display of images of anatomy or flow information developed from the capture of reflected and attenuated high frequency sound waves

Body Part Character 4	Contrast Character 5	Qualifier Character 6	Qualifier Character 7
3 Jugular Veins, Right 4 Jugular Veins, Left 6 Subclavian Vein, Right 7 Subclavian Vein, Left 8 Superior Vena Cava 9 Inferior Vena Cava B Lower Extremity Veins, Right C Lower Extremity Veins, Left D Lower Extremity Veins, Bilateral J Renal Vein, Right K Renal Vein, Left L Renal Veins, Bilateral M Upper Extremity Veins, Right N Upper Extremity Veins, Left P Upper Extremity Veins, Bilateral T Portal and Splanchnic Veins	Z None	Z None	3 Intravascular A Guidance Z None

B Imaging
7 Lymphatic System
Ø Plain Radiography Definition: Planar display of an image developed from the capture of external ionizing radiation on photographic or photoconductive plate

Body Part Character 4	Contrast Character 5	Qualifier Character 6	Qualifier Character 7
Ø Abdominal/Retroperitoneal Lymphatics, Unilateral 1 Abdominal/Retroperitoneal Lymphatics, Bilateral 4 Lymphatics, Head and Neck 5 Upper Extremity Lymphatics, Right 6 Upper Extremity Lymphatics, Left 7 Upper Extremity Lymphatics, Bilateral 8 Lower Extremity Lymphatics, Right 9 Lower Extremity Lymphatics, Left B Lower Extremity Lymphatics, Bilateral C Lymphatics, Pelvic	Ø High Osmolar 1 Low Osmolar Y Other Contrast	Z None	Z None

B Imaging
8 Eye
Ø Plain Radiography Definition: Planar display of an image developed from the capture of external ionizing radiation on photographic or photoconductive plate

Body Part Character 4	Contrast Character 5	Qualifier Character 6	Qualifier Character 7
Ø Lacrimal Duct, Right 1 Lacrimal Duct, Left 2 Lacrimal Ducts, Bilateral	Ø High Osmolar 1 Low Osmolar Y Other Contrast	Z None	Z None
3 Optic Foramina, Right 4 Optic Foramina, Left 5 Eye, Right 6 Eye, Left 7 Eyes, Bilateral	Z None	Z None	Z None

B Imaging
8 Eye
2 Computerized Tomography (CT Scan) Definition: Computer reformatted digital display of multiplanar images developed from the capture of multiple exposures of external ionizing radiation

Body Part Character 4	Contrast Character 5	Qualifier Character 6	Qualifier Character 7
5 Eye, Right 6 Eye, Left 7 Eyes, Bilateral	Ø High Osmolar 1 Low Osmolar Y Other Contrast	Ø Unenhanced and Enhanced Z None	Z None
5 Eye, Right 6 Eye, Left 7 Eyes, Bilateral	Z None	Z None	Z None

B Imaging
8 Eye
3 Magnetic Resonance Imaging (MRI) Definition: Computer reformatted digital display of multiplanar images developed from the capture of radio-frequency signals emitted by nuclei in a body site excited within a magnetic field

Body Part Character 4	Contrast Character 5	Qualifier Character 6	Qualifier Character 7
5 Eye, Right 6 Eye, Left 7 Eyes, Bilateral	Y Other Contrast	Ø Unenhanced and Enhanced Z None	Z None
5 Eye, Right 6 Eye, Left 7 Eyes, Bilateral	Z None	Z None	Z None

B Imaging
8 Eye
4 Ultrasonography Definition: Real time display of images of anatomy or flow information developed from the capture of reflected and attenuated high frequency sound waves

Body Part Character 4	Contrast Character 5	Qualifier Character 6	Qualifier Character 7
5 Eye, Right 6 Eye, Left 7 Eyes, Bilateral	Z None	Z None	Z None

B Imaging
9 Ear, Nose, Mouth and Throat
Ø Plain Radiography Definition: Planar display of an image developed from the capture of external ionizing radiation on photographic or photoconductive plate

Body Part Character 4	Contrast Character 5	Qualifier Character 6	Qualifier Character 7
2 Paranasal Sinuses F Nasopharynx/Oropharynx H Mastoids	Z None	Z None	Z None
4 Parotid Gland, Right 5 Parotid Gland, Left 6 Parotid Glands, Bilateral 7 Submandibular Gland, Right 8 Submandibular Gland, Left 9 Submandibular Glands, Bilateral B Salivary Gland, Right C Salivary Gland, Left D Salivary Glands, Bilateral	Ø High Osmolar 1 Low Osmolar Y Other Contrast	Z None	Z None

B Imaging
9 Ear, Nose, Mouth and Throat
1 Fluoroscopy Definition: Single plane or bi-plane real time display of an image developed from the capture of external ionizing radiation on a fluorescent screen. The image may also be stored by either digital or analog means.

Body Part Character 4	Contrast Character 5	Qualifier Character 6	Qualifier Character 7
G Pharynx and Epiglottis J Larynx	Y Other Contrast Z None	Z None	Z None

B Imaging
9 Ear, Nose, Mouth and Throat
2 Computerized Tomography (CT Scan) Definition: Computer reformatted digital display of multiplanar images developed from the capture of multiple exposures of external ionizing radiation

Body Part Character 4	Contrast Character 5	Qualifier Character 6	Qualifier Character 7
Ø Ear 2 Paranasal Sinuses 6 Parotid Glands, Bilateral 9 Submandibular Glands, Bilateral D Salivary Glands, Bilateral F Nasopharynx/Oropharynx J Larynx	Ø High Osmolar 1 Low Osmolar Y Other Contrast	Ø Unenhanced and Enhanced Z None	Z None
Ø Ear 2 Paranasal Sinuses 6 Parotid Glands, Bilateral 9 Submandibular Glands, Bilateral D Salivary Glands, Bilateral F Nasopharynx/Oropharynx J Larynx	Z None	Z None	Z None

B Imaging
9 Ear, Nose, Mouth and Throat
3 Magnetic Resonance Imaging (MRI) Definition: Computer reformatted digital display of multiplanar images developed from the capture of radio-frequency signals emitted by nuclei in a body site excited within a magnetic field

Body Part Character 4	Contrast Character 5	Qualifier Character 6	Qualifier Character 7
Ø Ear 2 Paranasal Sinuses 6 Parotid Glands, Bilateral 9 Submandibular Glands, Bilateral D Salivary Glands, Bilateral F Nasopharynx/Oropharynx J Larynx	Y Other Contrast	Ø Unenhanced and Enhanced Z None	Z None
Ø Ear 2 Paranasal Sinuses 6 Parotid Glands, Bilateral 9 Submandibular Glands, Bilateral D Salivary Glands, Bilateral F Nasopharynx/Oropharynx J Larynx	Z None	Z None	Z None

B Imaging
B Respiratory System
Ø Plain Radiography Definition: Planar display of an image developed from the capture of external ionizing radiation on photographic or photoconductive plate

Body Part Character 4	Contrast Character 5	Qualifier Character 6	Qualifier Character 7
7 Tracheobronchial Tree, Right 8 Tracheobronchial Tree, Left 9 Tracheobronchial Trees, Bilateral	Y Other Contrast	Z None	Z None
D Upper Airways	Z None	Z None	Z None

B Imaging
B Respiratory System
1 Fluoroscopy Definition: Single plane or bi-plane real time display of an image developed from the capture of external ionizing radiation on a fluorescent screen. The image may also be stored by either digital or analog means.

Body Part Character 4	Contrast Character 5	Qualifier Character 6	Qualifier Character 7
2 Lung, Right 3 Lung, Left 4 Lungs, Bilateral 6 Diaphragm C Mediastinum D Upper Airways	Z None	Z None	Z None
7 Tracheobronchial Tree, Right 8 Tracheobronchial Tree, Left 9 Tracheobronchial Trees, Bilateral	Y Other Contrast	Z None	Z None

B Imaging
B Respiratory System
2 Computerized Tomography (CT Scan) Definition: Computer reformatted digital display of multiplanar images developed from the capture of multiple exposures of external ionizing radiation

Body Part Character 4	Contrast Character 5	Qualifier Character 6	Qualifier Character 7
4 Lungs, Bilateral 7 Tracheobronchial Tree, Right 8 Tracheobronchial Tree, Left 9 Tracheobronchial Trees, Bilateral F Trachea/Airways	Ø High Osmolar 1 Low Osmolar Y Other Contrast	Ø Unenhanced and Enhanced Z None	Z None
4 Lungs, Bilateral 7 Tracheobronchial Tree, Right 8 Tracheobronchial Tree, Left 9 Tracheobronchial Trees, Bilateral F Trachea/Airways	Z None	Z None	Z None

B Imaging
B Respiratory System
3 Magnetic Resonance Imaging (MRI) Definition: Computer reformatted digital display of multiplanar images developed from the capture of radio-frequency signals emitted by nuclei in a body site excited within a magnetic field

Body Part Character 4	Contrast Character 5	Qualifier Character 6	Qualifier Character 7
4 Lungs, Bilateral	Z None	3 Hyperpolarized Xenon 129 (Xe-129)	Z None
G Lung Apices	Y Other Contrast	Ø Unenhanced and Enhanced Z None	Z None
G Lung Apices	Z None	Z None	Z None

B Imaging
B Respiratory System
4 Ultrasonography Definition: Real time display of images of anatomy or flow information developed from the capture of reflected and attenuated high frequency sound waves

Body Part Character 4	Contrast Character 5	Qualifier Character 6	Qualifier Character 7
B Pleura C Mediastinum	Z None	Z None	Z None

B Imaging
D Gastrointestinal System
1 Fluoroscopy Definition: Single plane or bi-plane real time display of an image developed from the capture of external ionizing radiation on a fluorescent screen. The image may also be stored by either digital or analog means.

Body Part Character 4	Contrast Character 5	Qualifier Character 6	Qualifier Character 7
1 Esophagus 2 Stomach 3 Small Bowel 4 Colon 5 Upper GI 6 Upper GI and Small Bowel 9 Duodenum B Mouth/Oropharynx	Y Other Contrast Z None	Z None	Z None

B Imaging
D Gastrointestinal System
2 Computerized Tomography (CT Scan) Definition: Computer reformatted digital display of multiplanar images developed from the capture of multiple exposures of external ionizing radiation

Body Part Character 4	Contrast Character 5	Qualifier Character 6	Qualifier Character 7
4 Colon	Ø High Osmolar 1 Low Osmolar Y Other Contrast	Ø Unenhanced and Enhanced Z None	Z None
4 Colon	Z None	Z None	Z None

B Imaging
D Gastrointestinal System
4 Ultrasonography Definition: Real time display of images of anatomy or flow information developed from the capture of reflected and attenuated high frequency sound waves

Body Part Character 4	Contrast Character 5	Qualifier Character 6	Qualifier Character 7
1 Esophagus 2 Stomach 7 Gastrointestinal Tract 8 Appendix 9 Duodenum C Rectum	Z None	Z None	Z None

B Imaging
F Hepatobiliary System and Pancreas
Ø Plain Radiography Definition: Planar display of an image developed from the capture of external ionizing radiation on photographic or photoconductive plate

Body Part Character 4	Contrast Character 5	Qualifier Character 6	Qualifier Character 7
Ø Bile Ducts 3 Gallbladder and Bile Ducts C Hepatobiliary System, All	Ø High Osmolar 1 Low Osmolar Y Other Contrast	Z None	Z None

B Imaging
F Hepatobiliary System and Pancreas
1 Fluoroscopy Definition: Single plane or bi-plane real time display of an image developed from the capture of external ionizing radiation on a fluorescent screen. The image may also be stored by either digital or analog means.

Body Part Character 4	Contrast Character 5	Qualifier Character 6	Qualifier Character 7
Ø Bile Ducts 1 Biliary and Pancreatic Ducts 2 Gallbladder 3 Gallbladder and Bile Ducts 4 Gallbladder, Bile Ducts and Pancreatic Ducts 8 Pancreatic Ducts	Ø High Osmolar 1 Low Osmolar Y Other Contrast	Z None	Z None
5 Liver	Ø High Osmolar 1 Low Osmolar Y Other Contrast	Z None	Z None
5 Liver	Z None	Z None	A Guidance

B Imaging
F Hepatobiliary System and Pancreas
2 Computerized Tomography (CT Scan) Definition: Computer reformatted digital display of multiplanar images developed from the capture of multiple exposures of external ionizing radiation

Body Part Character 4	Contrast Character 5	Qualifier Character 6	Qualifier Character 7
5 Liver 6 Liver and Spleen 7 Pancreas C Hepatobiliary System, All	Ø High Osmolar 1 Low Osmolar Y Other Contrast	Ø Unenhanced and Enhanced Z None	Z None
5 Liver 6 Liver and Spleen 7 Pancreas C Hepatobiliary System, All	Z None	Z None	Z None

B Imaging
F Hepatobiliary System and Pancreas
3 Magnetic Resonance Imaging (MRI) Definition: Computer reformatted digital display of multiplanar images developed from the capture of radio-frequency signals emitted by nuclei in a body site excited within a magnetic field

Body Part Character 4	Contrast Character 5	Qualifier Character 6	Qualifier Character 7
5 Liver 6 Liver and Spleen 7 Pancreas	Y Other Contrast	Ø Unenhanced and Enhanced Z None	Z None
5 Liver 6 Liver and Spleen 7 Pancreas	Z None	Z None	Z None

B Imaging
F Hepatobiliary System and Pancreas
4 Ultrasonography Definition: Real time display of images of anatomy or flow information developed from the capture of reflected and attenuated high frequency sound waves

Body Part Character 4	Contrast Character 5	Qualifier Character 6	Qualifier Character 7
Ø Bile Ducts 2 Gallbladder 3 Gallbladder and Bile Ducts 5 Liver 6 Liver and Spleen 7 Pancreas C Hepatobiliary System, All	Z None	Z None	Z None

B Imaging
F Hepatobiliary System and Pancreas
5 Other Imaging Definition: Other specified modality for visualizing a body part

Body Part Character 4	Contrast Character 5	Qualifier Character 6	Qualifier Character 7
Ø Bile Ducts 2 Gallbladder 3 Gallbladder and Bile Ducts 5 Liver 6 Liver and Spleen 7 Pancreas C Hepatobiliary System, All	2 Fluorescing Agent	Ø Indocyanine Green Dye Z None	Ø Intraoperative Z None

B Imaging
G Endocrine System
2 Computerized Tomography (CT Scan) Definition: Computer reformatted digital display of multiplanar images developed from the capture of multiple exposures of external ionizing radiation

Body Part Character 4	Contrast Character 5	Qualifier Character 6	Qualifier Character 7
2 Adrenal Glands, Bilateral 3 Parathyroid Glands 4 Thyroid Gland	Ø High Osmolar 1 Low Osmolar Y Other Contrast	Ø Unenhanced and Enhanced Z None	Z None
2 Adrenal Glands, Bilateral 3 Parathyroid Glands 4 Thyroid Gland	Z None	Z None	Z None

B Imaging
G Endocrine System
3 Magnetic Resonance Imaging (MRI) Definition: Computer reformatted digital display of multiplanar images developed from the capture of radio-frequency signals emitted by nuclei in a body site excited within a magnetic field

Body Part Character 4	Contrast Character 5	Qualifier Character 6	Qualifier Character 7
2 Adrenal Glands, Bilateral 3 Parathyroid Glands 4 Thyroid Gland	Y Other Contrast	Ø Unenhanced and Enhanced Z None	Z None
2 Adrenal Glands, Bilateral 3 Parathyroid Glands 4 Thyroid Gland	Z None	Z None	Z None

B Imaging
G Endocrine System
4 Ultrasonography Definition: Real time display of images of anatomy or flow information developed from the capture of reflected and attenuated high frequency sound waves

Body Part Character 4	Contrast Character 5	Qualifier Character 6	Qualifier Character 7
Ø Adrenal Gland, Right 1 Adrenal Gland, Left 2 Adrenal Glands, Bilateral 3 Parathyroid Glands 4 Thyroid Gland	Z None	Z None	Z None

B Imaging
H Skin, Subcutaneous Tissue and Breast
Ø Plain Radiography Definition: Planar display of an image developed from the capture of external ionizing radiation on photographic or photoconductive plate

Body Part Character 4	Contrast Character 5	Qualifier Character 6	Qualifier Character 7
Ø Breast, Right 1 Breast, Left 2 Breasts, Bilateral	Z None	Z None	Z None
3 Single Mammary Duct, Right 4 Single Mammary Duct, Left 5 Multiple Mammary Ducts, Right 6 Multiple Mammary Ducts, Left	Ø High Osmolar 1 Low Osmolar Y Other Contrast Z None	Z None	Z None

B Imaging
H Skin, Subcutaneous Tissue and Breast
3 Magnetic Resonance Imaging (MRI) Definition: Computer reformatted digital display of multiplanar images developed from the capture of radio-frequency signals emitted by nuclei in a body site excited within a magnetic field

Body Part Character 4	Contrast Character 5	Qualifier Character 6	Qualifier Character 7
Ø Breast, Right 1 Breast, Left 2 Breasts, Bilateral D Subcutaneous Tissue, Head/Neck F Subcutaneous Tissue, Upper Extremity G Subcutaneous Tissue, Thorax H Subcutaneous Tissue, Abdomen and Pelvis J Subcutaneous Tissue, Lower Extremity	Y Other Contrast	Ø Unenhanced and Enhanced Z None	Z None
Ø Breast, Right 1 Breast, Left 2 Breasts, Bilateral D Subcutaneous Tissue, Head/Neck F Subcutaneous Tissue, Upper Extremity G Subcutaneous Tissue, Thorax H Subcutaneous Tissue, Abdomen and Pelvis J Subcutaneous Tissue, Lower Extremity	Z None	Z None	Z None

B Imaging
H Skin, Subcutaneous Tissue and Breast
4 Ultrasonography Definition: Real time display of images of anatomy or flow information developed from the capture of reflected and attenuated high frequency sound waves

Body Part Character 4	Contrast Character 5	Qualifier Character 6	Qualifier Character 7
Ø Breast, Right 1 Breast, Left 2 Breasts, Bilateral 7 Extremity, Upper 8 Extremity, Lower 9 Abdominal Wall B Chest Wall C Head and Neck	Z None	Z None	Z None

B Imaging
L Connective Tissue
3 Magnetic Resonance Imaging (MRI) Definition: Computer reformatted digital display of multiplanar images developed from the capture of radio-frequency signals emitted by nuclei in a body site excited within a magnetic field

Body Part Character 4	Contrast Character 5	Qualifier Character 6	Qualifier Character 7
Ø Connective Tissue, Upper Extremity 1 Connective Tissue, Lower Extremity 2 Tendons, Upper Extremity 3 Tendons, Lower Extremity	Y Other Contrast	Ø Unenhanced and Enhanced Z None	Z None
Ø Connective Tissue, Upper Extremity 1 Connective Tissue, Lower Extremity 2 Tendons, Upper Extremity 3 Tendons, Lower Extremity	Z None	Z None	Z None

B Imaging
L Connective Tissue
4 Ultrasonography Definition: Real time display of images of anatomy or flow information developed from the capture of reflected and attenuated high frequency sound waves

Body Part Character 4	Contrast Character 5	Qualifier Character 6	Qualifier Character 7
Ø Connective Tissue, Upper Extremity 1 Connective Tissue, Lower Extremity 2 Tendons, Upper Extremity 3 Tendons, Lower Extremity	Z None	Z None	Z None

B Imaging
N Skull and Facial Bones
Ø Plain Radiography Definition: Planar display of an image developed from the capture of external ionizing radiation on photographic or photoconductive plate

Body Part Character 4	Contrast Character 5	Qualifier Character 6	Qualifier Character 7
Ø Skull 1 Orbit, Right 2 Orbit, Left 3 Orbits, Bilateral 4 Nasal Bones 5 Facial Bones 6 Mandible B Zygomatic Arch, Right C Zygomatic Arch, Left D Zygomatic Arches, Bilateral G Tooth, Single H Teeth, Multiple J Teeth, All	Z None	Z None	Z None
7 Temporomandibular Joint, Right 8 Temporomandibular Joint, Left 9 Temporomandibular Joints, Bilateral	Ø High Osmolar 1 Low Osmolar Y Other Contrast Z None	Z None	Z None

B Imaging
N Skull and Facial Bones
1 Fluoroscopy Definition: Single plane or bi-plane real time display of an image developed from the capture of external ionizing radiation on a fluorescent screen. The image may also be stored by either digital or analog means.

Body Part Character 4	Contrast Character 5	Qualifier Character 6	Qualifier Character 7
7 Temporomandibular Joint, Right 8 Temporomandibular Joint, Left 9 Temporomandibular Joints, Bilateral	Ø High Osmolar 1 Low Osmolar Y Other Contrast Z None	Z None	Z None

B Imaging
N Skull and Facial Bones
2 Computerized Tomography (CT Scan) Definition: Computer reformatted digital display of multiplanar images developed from the capture of multiple exposures of external ionizing radiation

Body Part Character 4	Contrast Character 5	Qualifier Character 6	Qualifier Character 7
Ø Skull 3 Orbits, Bilateral 5 Facial Bones 6 Mandible 9 Temporomandibular Joints, Bilateral F Temporal Bones	Ø High Osmolar 1 Low Osmolar Y Other Contrast Z None	Z None	Z None

B Imaging
N Skull and Facial Bones
3 Magnetic Resonance Imaging (MRI) Definition: Computer reformatted digital display of multiplanar images developed from the capture of radio-frequency signals emitted by nuclei in a body site excited within a magnetic field

Body Part Character 4	Contrast Character 5	Qualifier Character 6	Qualifier Character 7
9 Temporomandibular Joints, Bilateral	Y Other Contrast Z None	Z None	Z None

B Imaging
P Non-Axial Upper Bones
Ø Plain Radiography Definition: Planar display of an image developed from the capture of external ionizing radiation on photographic or photoconductive plate

Body Part Character 4	Contrast Character 5	Qualifier Character 6	Qualifier Character 7
Ø Sternoclavicular Joint, Right 1 Sternoclavicular Joint, Left 2 Sternoclavicular Joints, Bilateral 3 Acromioclavicular Joints, Bilateral 4 Clavicle, Right 5 Clavicle, Left 6 Scapula, Right 7 Scapula, Left A Humerus, Right B Humerus, Left E Upper Arm, Right F Upper Arm, Left J Forearm, Right K Forearm, Left N Hand, Right P Hand, Left R Finger(s), Right S Finger(s), Left X Ribs, Right Y Ribs, Left	Z None	Z None	Z None
8 Shoulder, Right 9 Shoulder, Left C Hand/Finger Joint, Right D Hand/Finger Joint, Left G Elbow, Right H Elbow, Left L Wrist, Right M Wrist, Left	Ø High Osmolar 1 Low Osmolar Y Other Contrast Z None	Z None	Z None

B Imaging
P Non-Axial Upper Bones
1 Fluoroscopy Definition: Single plane or bi-plane real time display of an image developed from the capture of external ionizing radiation on a fluorescent screen. The image may also be stored by either digital or analog means.

Body Part Character 4	Contrast Character 5	Qualifier Character 6	Qualifier Character 7
Ø Sternoclavicular Joint, Right 1 Sternoclavicular Joint, Left 2 Sternoclavicular Joints, Bilateral 3 Acromioclavicular Joints, Bilateral 4 Clavicle, Right 5 Clavicle, Left 6 Scapula, Right 7 Scapula, Left A Humerus, Right B Humerus, Left E Upper Arm, Right F Upper Arm, Left J Forearm, Right K Forearm, Left N Hand, Right P Hand, Left R Finger(s), Right S Finger(s), Left X Ribs, Right Y Ribs, Left	Z None	Z None	Z None
8 Shoulder, Right 9 Shoulder, Left L Wrist, Right M Wrist, Left	Ø High Osmolar 1 Low Osmolar Y Other Contrast Z None	Z None	Z None
C Hand/Finger Joint, Right D Hand/Finger Joint, Left G Elbow, Right H Elbow, Left	Ø High Osmolar 1 Low Osmolar Y Other Contrast	Z None	Z None

B Imaging
P Non-Axial Upper Bones
2 Computerized Tomography (CT Scan) Definition: Computer reformatted digital display of multiplanar images developed from the capture of multiple exposures of external ionizing radiation

Body Part Character 4	Contrast Character 5	Qualifier Character 6	Qualifier Character 7
Ø Sternoclavicular Joint, Right 1 Sternoclavicular Joint, Left W Thorax	Ø High Osmolar 1 Low Osmolar Y Other Contrast	Z None	Z None
2 Sternoclavicular Joints, Bilateral 3 Acromioclavicular Joints, Bilateral 4 Clavicle, Right 5 Clavicle, Left 6 Scapula, Right 7 Scapula, Left 8 Shoulder, Right 9 Shoulder, Left A Humerus, Right B Humerus, Left E Upper Arm, Right F Upper Arm, Left G Elbow, Right H Elbow, Left J Forearm, Right K Forearm, Left L Wrist, Right M Wrist, Left N Hand, Right P Hand, Left Q Hands and Wrists, Bilateral R Finger(s), Right S Finger(s), Left T Upper Extremity, Right U Upper Extremity, Left V Upper Extremities, Bilateral X Ribs, Right Y Ribs, Left	Ø High Osmolar 1 Low Osmolar Y Other Contrast Z None	Z None	Z None
C Hand/Finger Joint, Right D Hand/Finger Joint, Left	Z None	Z None	Z None

B Imaging
P Non-Axial Upper Bones
3 Magnetic Resonance Imaging (MRI) Definition: Computer reformatted digital display of multiplanar images developed from the capture of radio-frequency signals emitted by nuclei in a body site excited within a magnetic field

Body Part Character 4	Contrast Character 5	Qualifier Character 6	Qualifier Character 7
8 Shoulder, Right 9 Shoulder, Left C Hand/Finger Joint, Right D Hand/Finger Joint, Left E Upper Arm, Right F Upper Arm, Left G Elbow, Right H Elbow, Left J Forearm, Right K Forearm, Left L Wrist, Right M Wrist, Left	Y Other Contrast	Ø Unenhanced and Enhanced Z None	Z None
8 Shoulder, Right 9 Shoulder, Left C Hand/Finger Joint, Right D Hand/Finger Joint, Left E Upper Arm, Right F Upper Arm, Left G Elbow, Right H Elbow, Left J Forearm, Right K Forearm, Left L Wrist, Right M Wrist, Left	Z None	Z None	Z None

B Imaging
P Non-Axial Upper Bones
4 Ultrasonography Definition: Real time display of images of anatomy or flow information developed from the capture of reflected and attenuated high frequency sound waves

Body Part Character 4	Contrast Character 5	Qualifier Character 6	Qualifier Character 7
8 Shoulder, Right 9 Shoulder, Left G Elbow, Right H Elbow, Left L Wrist, Right M Wrist, Left N Hand, Right P Hand, Left	Z None	Z None	1 Densitometry Z None

B Imaging
Q Non-Axial Lower Bones
Ø Plain Radiography Definition: Planar display of an image developed from the capture of external ionizing radiation on photographic or photoconductive plate

Body Part Character 4	Contrast Character 5	Qualifier Character 6	Qualifier Character 7
Ø Hip, Right 1 Hip, Left	Ø High Osmolar 1 Low Osmolar Y Other Contrast	Z None	Z None
Ø Hip, Right 1 Hip, Left	Z None	Z None	1 Densitometry Z None
3 Femur, Right 4 Femur, Left	Z None	Z None	1 Densitometry Z None
7 Knee, Right 8 Knee, Left G Ankle, Right H Ankle, Left	Ø High Osmolar 1 Low Osmolar Y Other Contrast Z None	Z None	Z None
D Lower Leg, Right F Lower Leg, Left J Calcaneus, Right K Calcaneus, Left L Foot, Right M Foot, Left P Toe(s), Right Q Toe(s), Left V Patella, Right W Patella, Left	Z None	Z None	Z None
X Foot/Toe Joint, Right Y Foot/Toe Joint, Left	Ø High Osmolar 1 Low Osmolar Y Other Contrast	Z None	Z None

B Imaging
Q Non-Axial Lower Bones
1 Fluoroscopy Definition: Single plane or bi-plane real time display of an image developed from the capture of external ionizing radiation on a fluorescent screen. The image may also be stored by either digital or analog means.

Body Part Character 4	Contrast Character 5	Qualifier Character 6	Qualifier Character 7
Ø Hip, Right 1 Hip, Left 7 Knee, Right 8 Knee, Left G Ankle, Right H Ankle, Left X Foot/Toe Joint, Right Y Foot/Toe Joint, Left	Ø High Osmolar 1 Low Osmolar Y Other Contrast Z None	Z None	Z None
3 Femur, Right 4 Femur, Left D Lower Leg, Right F Lower Leg, Left J Calcaneus, Right K Calcaneus, Left L Foot, Right M Foot, Left P Toe(s), Right Q Toe(s), Left V Patella, Right W Patella, Left	Z None	Z None	Z None

B Imaging
Q Non-Axial Lower Bones
2 Computerized Tomography (CT Scan) Definition: Computer reformatted digital display of multiplanar images developed from the capture of multiple exposures of external ionizing radiation

Body Part Character 4	Contrast Character 5	Qualifier Character 6	Qualifier Character 7
Ø Hip, Right 1 Hip, Left 3 Femur, Right 4 Femur, Left 7 Knee, Right 8 Knee, Left D Lower Leg, Right F Lower Leg, Left G Ankle, Right H Ankle, Left J Calcaneus, Right K Calcaneus, Left L Foot, Right M Foot, Left P Toe(s), Right Q Toe(s), Left R Lower Extremity, Right S Lower Extremity, Left V Patella, Right W Patella, Left X Foot/Toe Joint, Right Y Foot/Toe Joint, Left	Ø High Osmolar 1 Low Osmolar Y Other Contrast Z None	Z None	Z None
B Tibia/Fibula, Right C Tibia/Fibula, Left	Ø High Osmolar 1 Low Osmolar Y Other Contrast	Z None	Z None

B Imaging
Q Non-Axial Lower Bones
3 Magnetic Resonance Imaging (MRI) Definition: Computer reformatted digital display of multiplanar images developed from the capture of radio-frequency signals emitted by nuclei in a body site excited within a magnetic field

Body Part Character 4	Contrast Character 5	Qualifier Character 6	Qualifier Character 7
Ø Hip, Right 1 Hip, Left 3 Femur, Right 4 Femur, Left 7 Knee, Right 8 Knee, Left D Lower Leg, Right F Lower Leg, Left G Ankle, Right H Ankle, Left J Calcaneus, Right K Calcaneus, Left L Foot, Right M Foot, Left P Toe(s), Right Q Toe(s), Left V Patella, Right W Patella, Left	Y Other Contrast	Ø Unenhanced and Enhanced Z None	Z None
Ø Hip, Right 1 Hip, Left 3 Femur, Right 4 Femur, Left 7 Knee, Right 8 Knee, Left D Lower Leg, Right F Lower Leg, Left G Ankle, Right H Ankle, Left J Calcaneus, Right K Calcaneus, Left L Foot, Right M Foot, Left P Toe(s), Right Q Toe(s), Left V Patella, Right W Patella, Left	Z None	Z None	Z None

B Imaging
Q Non-Axial Lower Bones
4 Ultrasonography Definition: Real time display of images of anatomy or flow information developed from the capture of reflected and attenuated high frequency sound waves

Body Part Character 4	Contrast Character 5	Qualifier Character 6	Qualifier Character 7
Ø Hip, Right 1 Hip, Left 2 Hips, Bilateral 7 Knee, Right 8 Knee, Left 9 Knees, Bilateral	Z None	Z None	Z None

B Imaging
R Axial Skeleton, Except Skull and Facial Bones
Ø Plain Radiography Definition: Planar display of an image developed from the capture of external ionizing radiation on photographic or photoconductive plate

Body Part Character 4	Contrast Character 5	Qualifier Character 6	Qualifier Character 7
Ø Cervical Spine 7 Thoracic Spine 9 Lumbar Spine G Whole Spine	Z None	Z None	1 Densitometry Z None
1 Cervical Disc(s) 2 Thoracic Disc(s) 3 Lumbar Disc(s) 4 Cervical Facet Joint(s) 5 Thoracic Facet Joint(s) 6 Lumbar Facet Joint(s) D Sacroiliac Joints	Ø High Osmolar 1 Low Osmolar Y Other Contrast Z None	Z None	Z None
8 Thoracolumbar Joint B Lumbosacral Joint C Pelvis F Sacrum and Coccyx H Sternum	Z None	Z None	Z None

B Imaging
R Axial Skeleton, Except Skull and Facial Bones
1 Fluoroscopy Definition: Single plane or bi-plane real time display of an image developed from the capture of external ionizing radiation on a fluorescent screen. The image may also be stored by either digital or analog means.

Body Part Character 4	Contrast Character 5	Qualifier Character 6	Qualifier Character 7
Ø Cervical Spine 1 Cervical Disc(s) 2 Thoracic Disc(s) 3 Lumbar Disc(s) 4 Cervical Facet Joint(s) 5 Thoracic Facet Joint(s) 6 Lumbar Facet Joint(s) 7 Thoracic Spine 8 Thoracolumbar Joint 9 Lumbar Spine B Lumbosacral Joint C Pelvis D Sacroiliac Joints F Sacrum and Coccyx G Whole Spine H Sternum	Ø High Osmolar 1 Low Osmolar Y Other Contrast Z None	Z None	Z None

B Imaging
R Axial Skeleton, Except Skull and Facial Bones
2 Computerized Tomography (CT Scan) Definition: Computer reformatted digital display of multiplanar images developed from the capture of multiple exposures of external ionizing radiation

Body Part Character 4	Contrast Character 5	Qualifier Character 6	Qualifier Character 7
Ø Cervical Spine 7 Thoracic Spine 9 Lumbar Spine C Pelvis D Sacroiliac Joints F Sacrum and Coccyx	Ø High Osmolar 1 Low Osmolar Y Other Contrast Z None	Z None	Z None

B Imaging
R Axial Skeleton, Except Skull and Facial Bones
3 Magnetic Resonance Imaging (MRI) Definition: Computer reformatted digital display of multiplanar images developed from the capture of radio-frequency signals emitted by nuclei in a body site excited within a magnetic field

Body Part Character 4	Contrast Character 5	Qualifier Character 6	Qualifier Character 7
Ø Cervical Spine 1 Cervical Disc(s) 2 Thoracic Disc(s) 3 Lumbar Disc(s) 7 Thoracic Spine 9 Lumbar Spine C Pelvis F Sacrum and Coccyx	Y Other Contrast	Ø Unenhanced and Enhanced Z None	Z None
Ø Cervical Spine 1 Cervical Disc(s) 2 Thoracic Disc(s) 3 Lumbar Disc(s) 7 Thoracic Spine 9 Lumbar Spine C Pelvis F Sacrum and Coccyx	Z None	Z None	Z None

B Imaging
R Axial Skeleton, Except Skull and Facial Bones
4 Ultrasonography Definition: Real time display of images of anatomy or flow information developed from the capture of reflected and attenuated high frequency sound waves

Body Part Character 4	Contrast Character 5	Qualifier Character 6	Qualifier Character 7
Ø Cervical Spine 7 Thoracic Spine 9 Lumbar Spine F Sacrum and Coccyx	Z None	Z None	Z None

B Imaging
T Urinary System
Ø Plain Radiography Definition: Planar display of an image developed from the capture of external ionizing radiation on photographic or photoconductive plate

Body Part Character 4	Contrast Character 5	Qualifier Character 6	Qualifier Character 7
Ø Bladder 1 Kidney, Right 2 Kidney, Left 3 Kidneys, Bilateral 4 Kidneys, Ureters and Bladder 5 Urethra 6 Ureter, Right 7 Ureter, Left 8 Ureters, Bilateral B Bladder and Urethra C Ileal Diversion Loop	Ø High Osmolar 1 Low Osmolar Y Other Contrast Z None	Z None	Z None

B Imaging
T Urinary System
1 Fluoroscopy Definition: Single plane or bi-plane real time display of an image developed from the capture of external ionizing radiation on a fluorescent screen. The image may also be stored by either digital or analog means.

Body Part Character 4	Contrast Character 5	Qualifier Character 6	Qualifier Character 7
Ø Bladder 1 Kidney, Right 2 Kidney, Left 3 Kidneys, Bilateral 4 Kidneys, Ureters and Bladder 5 Urethra 6 Ureter, Right 7 Ureter, Left B Bladder and Urethra C Ileal Diversion Loop D Kidney, Ureter and Bladder, Right F Kidney, Ureter and Bladder, Left G Ileal Loop, Ureters and Kidneys	Ø High Osmolar 1 Low Osmolar Y Other Contrast Z None	Z None	Z None

B Imaging
T Urinary System
2 Computerized Tomography (CT Scan) Definition: Computer reformatted digital display of multiplanar images developed from the capture of multiple exposures of external ionizing radiation

Body Part Character 4	Contrast Character 5	Qualifier Character 6	Qualifier Character 7
Ø Bladder 1 Kidney, Right 2 Kidney, Left 3 Kidneys, Bilateral 9 Kidney Transplant	Ø High Osmolar 1 Low Osmolar Y Other Contrast	Ø Unenhanced and Enhanced Z None	Z None
Ø Bladder 1 Kidney, Right 2 Kidney, Left 3 Kidneys, Bilateral 9 Kidney Transplant	Z None	Z None	Z None

B Imaging
T Urinary System
3 Magnetic Resonance Imaging (MRI) Definition: Computer reformatted digital display of multiplanar images developed from the capture of radio-frequency signals emitted by nuclei in a body site excited within a magnetic field

Body Part Character 4	Contrast Character 5	Qualifier Character 6	Qualifier Character 7
Ø Bladder 1 Kidney, Right 2 Kidney, Left 3 Kidneys, Bilateral 9 Kidney Transplant	Y Other Contrast	Ø Unenhanced and Enhanced Z None	Z None
Ø Bladder 1 Kidney, Right 2 Kidney, Left 3 Kidneys, Bilateral 9 Kidney Transplant	Z None	Z None	Z None

B Imaging
T Urinary System
4 Ultrasonography Definition: Real time display of images of anatomy or flow information developed from the capture of reflected and attenuated high frequency sound waves

Body Part Character 4	Contrast Character 5	Qualifier Character 6	Qualifier Character 7
Ø Bladder 1 Kidney, Right 2 Kidney, Left 3 Kidneys, Bilateral 5 Urethra 6 Ureter, Right 7 Ureter, Left 8 Ureters, Bilateral 9 Kidney Transplant J Kidneys and Bladder	Z None	Z None	Z None

B Imaging
U Female Reproductive System
Ø Plain Radiography Definition: Planar display of an image developed from the capture of external ionizing radiation on photographic or photoconductive plate

Body Part Character 4	Contrast Character 5	Qualifier Character 6	Qualifier Character 7
Ø Fallopian Tube, Right ♀ 1 Fallopian Tube, Left ♀ 2 Fallopian Tubes, Bilateral ♀ 6 Uterus ♀ 8 Uterus and Fallopian Tubes ♀ 9 Vagina ♀	Ø High Osmolar 1 Low Osmolar Y Other Contrast	Z None	Z None

♀ All body part, contrast, and qualifier values

B Imaging
U Female Reproductive System
1 Fluoroscopy Definition: Single plane or bi-plane real time display of an image developed from the capture of external ionizing radiation on a fluorescent screen. The image may also be stored by either digital or analog means.

Body Part Character 4	Contrast Character 5	Qualifier Character 6	Qualifier Character 7
Ø Fallopian Tube, Right ♀ 1 Fallopian Tube, Left ♀ 2 Fallopian Tubes, Bilateral ♀ 6 Uterus ♀ 8 Uterus and Fallopian Tubes ♀ 9 Vagina ♀	Ø High Osmolar 1 Low Osmolar Y Other Contrast Z None	Z None	Z None

♀ All body part, contrast, and qualifier values

B Imaging
U Female Reproductive System
3 Magnetic Resonance Imaging (MRI) Definition: Computer reformatted digital display of multiplanar images developed from the capture of radio-frequency signals emitted by nuclei in a body site excited within a magnetic field

Body Part Character 4	Contrast Character 5	Qualifier Character 6	Qualifier Character 7
3 Ovary, Right ♀ 4 Ovary, Left ♀ 5 Ovaries, Bilateral ♀ 6 Uterus ♀ 9 Vagina ♀ B Pregnant Uterus ♀ C Uterus and Ovaries ♀	Y Other Contrast	Ø Unenhanced and Enhanced Z None	Z None
3 Ovary, Right ♀ 4 Ovary, Left ♀ 5 Ovaries, Bilateral ♀ 6 Uterus ♀ 9 Vagina ♀ B Pregnant Uterus ♀ C Uterus and Ovaries ♀	Z None	Z None	Z None

♀ All body part, contrast, and qualifier values

B Imaging
U Female Reproductive System
4 Ultrasonography Definition: Real time display of images of anatomy or flow information developed from the capture of reflected and attenuated high frequency sound waves

Body Part Character 4	Contrast Character 5	Qualifier Character 6	Qualifier Character 7
Ø Fallopian Tube, Right ♀ 1 Fallopian Tube, Left ♀ 2 Fallopian Tubes, Bilateral ♀ 3 Ovary, Right ♀ 4 Ovary, Left ♀ 5 Ovaries, Bilateral ♀ 6 Uterus ♀ C Uterus and Ovaries ♀	Y Other Contrast Z None	Z None	Z None

♀ All body part, contrast, and qualifier values

B Imaging
V Male Reproductive System
Ø Plain Radiography Definition: Planar display of an image developed from the capture of external ionizing radiation on photographic or photoconductive plate

Body Part Character 4	Contrast Character 5	Qualifier Character 6	Qualifier Character 7
Ø Corpora Cavernosa ♂ 1 Epididymis, Right ♂ 2 Epididymis, Left ♂ 3 Prostate ♂ 5 Testicle, Right ♂ 6 Testicle, Left ♂ 8 Vasa Vasorum ♂	Ø High Osmolar 1 Low Osmolar Y Other Contrast	Z None	Z None

♂ All body part, contrast, and qualifier values

B Imaging
V Male Reproductive System
1 Fluoroscopy Definition: Single plane or bi-plane real time display of an image developed from the capture of external ionizing radiation on a fluorescent screen. The image may also be stored by either digital or analog means.

Body Part Character 4	Contrast Character 5	Qualifier Character 6	Qualifier Character 7
Ø Corpora Cavernosa ♂ 8 Vasa Vasorum ♂	Ø High Osmolar 1 Low Osmolar Y Other Contrast Z None	Z None	Z None

♂ All body part, contrast, and qualifier values

B Imaging
V Male Reproductive System
2 Computerized Tomography (CT Scan) Definition: Computer reformatted digital display of multiplanar images developed from the capture of multiple exposures of external ionizing radiation

Body Part Character 4	Contrast Character 5	Qualifier Character 6	Qualifier Character 7
3 Prostate ♂	Ø High Osmolar 1 Low Osmolar Y Other Contrast	Ø Unenhanced and Enhanced Z None	Z None
3 Prostate ♂	Z None	Z None	Z None

♂ BV23[Ø,Y][Ø,Z]Z
♂ BV231ØZ
♂ BV23ZZZ

B Imaging
V Male Reproductive System
3 Magnetic Resonance Imaging (MRI) Definition: Computer reformatted digital display of multiplanar images developed from the capture of radio-frequency signals emitted by nuclei in a body site excited within a magnetic field

Body Part Character 4	Contrast Character 5	Qualifier Character 6	Qualifier Character 7
Ø Corpora Cavernosa ♂ 3 Prostate ♂ 4 Scrotum ♂ 5 Testicle, Right ♂ 6 Testicle, Left ♂ 7 Testicles, Bilateral ♂	Y Other Contrast	Ø Unenhanced and Enhanced Z None	Z None
Ø Corpora Cavernosa ♂ 3 Prostate ♂ 4 Scrotum ♂ 5 Testicle, Right ♂ 6 Testicle, Left ♂ 7 Testicles, Bilateral ♂	Z None	Z None	Z None

♂ All body part, contrast, and qualifier values

B Imaging
V Male Reproductive System
4 Ultrasonography Definition: Real time display of images of anatomy or flow information developed from the capture of reflected and attenuated high frequency sound waves

Body Part Character 4	Contrast Character 5	Qualifier Character 6	Qualifier Character 7
4 Scrotum ♂ 9 Prostate and Seminal Vesicles ♂ B Penis ♂	Z None	Z None	Z None

♂ All body part, contrast, and qualifier values

B Imaging
W Anatomical Regions
Ø Plain Radiography Definition: Planar display of an image developed from the capture of external ionizing radiation on photographic or photoconductive plate

Body Part Character 4	Contrast Character 5	Qualifier Character 6	Qualifier Character 7
Ø Abdomen 1 Abdomen and Pelvis 3 Chest B Long Bones, All C Lower Extremity J Upper Extremity K Whole Body L Whole Skeleton M Whole Body, Infant	Z None	Z None	Z None

B Imaging
W Anatomical Regions
1 Fluoroscopy Definition: Single plane or bi-plane real time display of an image developed from the capture of external ionizing radiation on a fluorescent screen. The image may also be stored by either digital or analog means.

Body Part Character 4	Contrast Character 5	Qualifier Character 6	Qualifier Character 7
1 Abdomen and Pelvis 9 Head and Neck C Lower Extremity J Upper Extremity	Ø High Osmolar 1 Low Osmolar Y Other Contrast Z None	Z None	Z None

B Imaging
W Anatomical Regions
2 Computerized Tomography (CT Scan) Definition: Computer reformatted digital display of multiplanar images developed from the capture of multiple exposures of external ionizing radiation

Body Part Character 4	Contrast Character 5	Qualifier Character 6	Qualifier Character 7
Ø Abdomen 1 Abdomen and Pelvis 4 Chest and Abdomen 5 Chest, Abdomen and Pelvis 8 Head 9 Head and Neck F Neck G Pelvic Region	Ø High Osmolar 1 Low Osmolar Y Other Contrast	Ø Unenhanced and Enhanced Z None	Z None
Ø Abdomen 1 Abdomen and Pelvis 4 Chest and Abdomen 5 Chest, Abdomen and Pelvis 8 Head 9 Head and Neck F Neck G Pelvic Region	Z None	Z None	Z None

B Imaging
W Anatomical Regions
3 Magnetic Resonance Imaging (MRI) Definition: Computer reformatted digital display of multiplanar images developed from the capture of radio-frequency signals emitted by nuclei in a body site excited within a magnetic field

Body Part Character 4	Contrast Character 5	Qualifier Character 6	Qualifier Character 7
Ø Abdomen 8 Head F Neck G Pelvic Region H Retroperitoneum P Brachial Plexus	Y Other Contrast	Ø Unenhanced and Enhanced Z None	Z None
Ø Abdomen 8 Head F Neck G Pelvic Region H Retroperitoneum P Brachial Plexus	Z None	Z None	Z None
3 Chest	Y Other Contrast	Ø Unenhanced and Enhanced Z None	Z None

B Imaging
W Anatomical Regions
4 Ultrasonography Definition: Real time display of images of anatomy or flow information developed from the capture of reflected and attenuated high frequency sound waves

Body Part Character 4	Contrast Character 5	Qualifier Character 6	Qualifier Character 7
Ø Abdomen 1 Abdomen and Pelvis F Neck G Pelvic Region	Z None	Z None	Z None

B Imaging
W Anatomical Regions
5 Other Imaging Definition: Other specified modality for visualizing a body part

Body Part Character 4	Contrast Character 5	Qualifier Character 6	Qualifier Character 7
2 Trunk 9 Head and Neck C Lower Extremity J Upper Extremity	Z None	1 Bacterial Autofluorescence	Z None

B Imaging
Y Fetus and Obstetrical
3 Magnetic Resonance Imaging (MRI) Definition: Computer reformatted digital display of multiplanar images developed from the capture of radio-frequency signals emitted by nuclei in a body site excited within a magnetic field

Body Part Character 4	Contrast Character 5	Qualifier Character 6	Qualifier Character 7
Ø Fetal Head ♀ 1 Fetal Heart ♀ 2 Fetal Thorax ♀ 3 Fetal Abdomen ♀ 4 Fetal Spine ♀ 5 Fetal Extremities ♀ 6 Whole Fetus ♀	Y Other Contrast	Ø Unenhanced and Enhanced Z None	Z None
Ø Fetal Head ♀ 1 Fetal Heart ♀ 2 Fetal Thorax ♀ 3 Fetal Abdomen ♀ 4 Fetal Spine ♀ 5 Fetal Extremities ♀ 6 Whole Fetus ♀	Z None	Z None	Z None

♀ BY3[Ø,1,2,3,5,6]Y[Ø,Z]Z
♀ BY34YZZ
♀ BY3[Ø,1,2,3,4,5,6]ZZZ

B Imaging
Y Fetus and Obstetrical
4 Ultrasonography Definition: Real time display of images of anatomy or flow information developed from the capture of reflected and attenuated high frequency sound waves

Body Part Character 4	Contrast Character 5	Qualifier Character 6	Qualifier Character 7
7 Fetal Umbilical Cord ♀ 8 Placenta ♀ 9 First Trimester, Single Fetus ♀ B First Trimester, Multiple Gestation ♀ C Second Trimester, Single Fetus ♀ D Second Trimester, Multiple Gestation ♀ F Third Trimester, Single Fetus ♀ G Third Trimester, Multiple Gestation ♀	Z None	Z None	Z None

♀ All body part, contrast, and qualifier values

Nuclear Medicine CØ1–CW7

C Nuclear Medicine
Ø Central Nervous System
1 Planar Nuclear Medicine Imaging

Definition: Introduction of radioactive materials into the body for single plane display of images developed from the capture of radioactive emissions

Body Part Character 4	Radionuclide Character 5	Qualifier Character 6	Qualifier Character 7
Ø Brain	1 Technetium 99m (Tc-99m) Y Other Radionuclide	Z None	Z None
5 Cerebrospinal Fluid	D Indium 111 (In-111) Y Other Radionuclide	Z None	Z None
Y Central Nervous System	Y Other Radionuclide	Z None	Z None

C Nuclear Medicine
Ø Central Nervous System
2 Tomographic (Tomo) Nuclear Medicine Imaging

Definition: Introduction of radioactive materials into the body for three dimensional display of images developed from the capture of radioactive emissions

Body Part Character 4	Radionuclide Character 5	Qualifier Character 6	Qualifier Character 7
Ø Brain	1 Technetium 99m (Tc-99m) F Iodine 123 (I-123) S Thallium 201 (Tl-201) Y Other Radionuclide	Z None	Z None
5 Cerebrospinal Fluid	D Indium 111 (In-111) Y Other Radionuclide	Z None	Z None
Y Central Nervous System	Y Other Radionuclide	Z None	Z None

C Nuclear Medicine
Ø Central Nervous System
3 Positron Emission Tomographic (PET) Imaging

Definition: Introduction of radioactive materials into the body for three dimensional display of images developed from the simultaneous capture, 180 degrees apart, of radioactive emissions

Body Part Character 4	Radionuclide Character 5	Qualifier Character 6	Qualifier Character 7
Ø Brain	B Carbon 11 (C-11) K Fluorine 18 (F-18) M Oxygen 15 (O-15) Y Other Radionuclide	Z None	Z None
Y Central Nervous System	Y Other Radionuclide	Z None	Z None

C Nuclear Medicine
Ø Central Nervous System
5 Nonimaging Nuclear Medicine Probe

Definition: Introduction of radioactive materials into the body for the study of distribution and fate of certain substances by the detection of radioactive emissions; or, alternatively, measurement of absorption of radioactive emissions from an external source

Body Part Character 4	Radionuclide Character 5	Qualifier Character 6	Qualifier Character 7
Ø Brain	V Xenon 133 (Xe-133) Y Other Radionuclide	Z None	Z None
Y Central Nervous System	Y Other Radionuclide	Z None	Z None

C Nuclear Medicine
2 Heart
1 Planar Nuclear Medicine Imaging

Definition: Introduction of radioactive materials into the body for single plane display of images developed from the capture of radioactive emissions

Body Part Character 4	Radionuclide Character 5	Qualifier Character 6	Qualifier Character 7
6 Heart, Right and Left	1 Technetium 99m (Tc-99m) Y Other Radionuclide	Z None	Z None
G Myocardium	1 Technetium 99m (Tc-99m) D Indium 111 (In-111) S Thallium 201 (Tl-201) Y Other Radionuclide Z None	Z None	Z None
Y Heart	Y Other Radionuclide	Z None	Z None

C Nuclear Medicine
2 Heart
2 Tomographic (Tomo) Nuclear Medicine Imaging Definition: Introduction of radioactive materials into the body for three dimensional display of images developed from the capture of radioactive emissions

Body Part Character 4	Radionuclide Character 5	Qualifier Character 6	Qualifier Character 7
6 Heart, Right and Left	1 Technetium 99m (Tc-99m) Y Other Radionuclide	Z None	Z None
G Myocardium	1 Technetium 99m (Tc-99m) D Indium 111 (In-111) K Fluorine 18 (F-18) S Thallium 201 (Tl-201) Y Other Radionuclide Z None	Z None	Z None
Y Heart	Y Other Radionuclide	Z None	Z None

C Nuclear Medicine
2 Heart
3 Positron Emission Tomographic (PET) Imaging Definition: Introduction of radioactive materials into the body for three dimensional display of images developed from the simultaneous capture, 180 degrees apart, of radioactive emissions

Body Part Character 4	Radionuclide Character 5	Qualifier Character 6	Qualifier Character 7
G Myocardium	K Fluorine 18 (F-18) M Oxygen 15 (O-15) Q Rubidium 82 (Rb-82) R Nitrogen 13 (N-13) Y Other Radionuclide	Z None	Z None
Y Heart	Y Other Radionuclide	Z None	Z None

C Nuclear Medicine
2 Heart
5 Nonimaging Nuclear Medicine Probe Definition: Introduction of radioactive materials into the body for the study of distribution and fate of certain substances by the detection of radioactive emissions; or, alternatively, measurement of absorption of radioactive emissions from an external source

Body Part Character 4	Radionuclide Character 5	Qualifier Character 6	Qualifier Character 7
6 Heart, Right and Left	1 Technetium 99m (Tc-99m) Y Other Radionuclide	Z None	Z None
Y Heart	Y Other Radionuclide	Z None	Z None

C Nuclear Medicine
5 Veins
1 Planar Nuclear Medicine Imaging Definition: Introduction of radioactive materials into the body for single plane display of images developed from the capture of radioactive emissions

Body Part Character 4	Radionuclide Character 5	Qualifier Character 6	Qualifier Character 7
B Lower Extremity Veins, Right C Lower Extremity Veins, Left D Lower Extremity Veins, Bilateral N Upper Extremity Veins, Right P Upper Extremity Veins, Left Q Upper Extremity Veins, Bilateral R Central Veins	1 Technetium 99m (Tc-99m) Y Other Radionuclide	Z None	Z None
Y Veins	Y Other Radionuclide	Z None	Z None

C Nuclear Medicine
7 Lymphatic and Hematologic System
1 Planar Nuclear Medicine Imaging

Definition: Introduction of radioactive materials into the body for single plane display of images developed from the capture of radioactive emissions

Body Part Character 4	Radionuclide Character 5	Qualifier Character 6	Qualifier Character 7
Ø Bone Marrow	**1** Technetium 99m (Tc-99m) **D** Indium 111 (In-111) **Y** Other Radionuclide	**Z** None	**Z** None
2 Spleen **5** Lymphatics, Head and Neck **D** Lymphatics, Pelvic **J** Lymphatics, Head **K** Lymphatics, Neck **L** Lymphatics, Upper Chest **M** Lymphatics, Trunk **N** Lymphatics, Upper Extremity **P** Lymphatics, Lower Extremity	**1** Technetium 99m (Tc-99m) **Y** Other Radionuclide	**Z** None	**Z** None
3 Blood	**D** Indium 111 (In-111) **Y** Other Radionuclide	**Z** None	**Z** None
Y Lymphatic and Hematologic System	**Y** Other Radionuclide	**Z** None	**Z** None

C Nuclear Medicine
7 Lymphatic and Hematologic System
2 Tomographic (Tomo) Nuclear Medicine Imaging

Definition: Introduction of radioactive materials into the body for three dimensional display of images developed from the capture of radioactive emissions

Body Part Character 4	Radionuclide Character 5	Qualifier Character 6	Qualifier Character 7
2 Spleen	**1** Technetium 99m (Tc-99m) **Y** Other Radionuclide	**Z** None	**Z** None
Y Lymphatic and Hematologic System	**Y** Other Radionuclide	**Z** None	**Z** None

C Nuclear Medicine
7 Lymphatic and Hematologic System
5 Nonimaging Nuclear Medicine Probe

Definition: Introduction of radioactive materials into the body for the study of distribution and fate of certain substances by the detection of radioactive emissions; or, alternatively, measurement of absorption of radioactive emissions from an external source

Body Part Character 4	Radionuclide Character 5	Qualifier Character 6	Qualifier Character 7
5 Lymphatics, Head and Neck **D** Lymphatics, Pelvic **J** Lymphatics, Head **K** Lymphatics, Neck **L** Lymphatics, Upper Chest **M** Lymphatics, Trunk **N** Lymphatics, Upper Extremity **P** Lymphatics, Lower Extremity	**1** Technetium 99m (Tc-99m) **Y** Other Radionuclide	**Z** None	**Z** None
Y Lymphatic and Hematologic System	**Y** Other Radionuclide	**Z** None	**Z** None

C Nuclear Medicine
7 Lymphatic and Hematologic System
6 Nonimaging Nuclear Medicine Assay

Definition: Introduction of radioactive materials into the body for the study of body fluids and blood elements, by the detection of radioactive emissions

Body Part Character 4	Radionuclide Character 5	Qualifier Character 6	Qualifier Character 7
3 Blood	**1** Technetium 99m (Tc-99m) **7** Cobalt 58 (Co-58) **C** Cobalt 57 (Co-57) **D** Indium 111 (In-111) **H** Iodine 125 (I-125) **W** Chromium (Cr-51) **Y** Other Radionuclide	**Z** None	**Z** None
Y Lymphatic and Hematologic System	**Y** Other Radionuclide	**Z** None	**Z** None

C Nuclear Medicine
8 Eye
1 Planar Nuclear Medicine Imaging

Definition: Introduction of radioactive materials into the body for single plane display of images developed from the capture of radioactive emissions

Body Part Character 4	Radionuclide Character 5	Qualifier Character 6	Qualifier Character 7
9 Lacrimal Ducts, Bilateral	1 Technetium 99m (Tc-99m) Y Other Radionuclide	Z None	Z None
Y Eye	Y Other Radionuclide	Z None	Z None

C Nuclear Medicine
9 Ear, Nose, Mouth and Throat
1 Planar Nuclear Medicine Imaging

Definition: Introduction of radioactive materials into the body for single plane display of images developed from the capture of radioactive emissions

Body Part Character 4	Radionuclide Character 5	Qualifier Character 6	Qualifier Character 7
B Salivary Glands, Bilateral	1 Technetium 99m (Tc-99m) Y Other Radionuclide	Z None	Z None
Y Ear, Nose, Mouth and Throat	Y Other Radionuclide	Z None	Z None

C Nuclear Medicine
B Respiratory System
1 Planar Nuclear Medicine Imaging

Definition: Introduction of radioactive materials into the body for single plane display of images developed from the capture of radioactive emissions

Body Part Character 4	Radionuclide Character 5	Qualifier Character 6	Qualifier Character 7
2 Lungs and Bronchi	1 Technetium 99m (Tc-99m) 9 Krypton (Kr-81m) T Xenon 127 (Xe-127) V Xenon 133 (Xe-133) Y Other Radionuclide	Z None	Z None
Y Respiratory System	Y Other Radionuclide	Z None	Z None

C Nuclear Medicine
B Respiratory System
2 Tomographic (Tomo) Nuclear Medicine Imaging

Definition: Introduction of radioactive materials into the body for three dimensional display of images developed from the capture of radioactive emissions

Body Part Character 4	Radionuclide Character 5	Qualifier Character 6	Qualifier Character 7
2 Lungs and Bronchi	1 Technetium 99m (Tc-99m) 9 Krypton (Kr-81m) Y Other Radionuclide	Z None	Z None
Y Respiratory System	Y Other Radionuclide	Z None	Z None

C Nuclear Medicine
B Respiratory System
3 Positron Emission Tomographic (PET) Imaging

Definition: Introduction of radioactive materials into the body for three dimensional display of images developed from the simultaneous capture, 180 degrees apart, of radioactive emissions

Body Part Character 4	Radionuclide Character 5	Qualifier Character 6	Qualifier Character 7
2 Lungs and Bronchi	K Fluorine 18 (F-18) Y Other Radionuclide	Z None	Z None
Y Respiratory System	Y Other Radionuclide	Z None	Z None

C Nuclear Medicine
D Gastrointestinal System
1 Planar Nuclear Medicine Imaging

Definition: Introduction of radioactive materials into the body for single plane display of images developed from the capture of radioactive emissions

Body Part Character 4	Radionuclide Character 5	Qualifier Character 6	Qualifier Character 7
5 Upper Gastrointestinal Tract 7 Gastrointestinal Tract	1 Technetium 99m (Tc-99m) D Indium 111 (In-111) Y Other Radionuclide	Z None	Z None
Y Digestive System	Y Other Radionuclide	Z None	Z None

C Nuclear Medicine
D Gastrointestinal System
2 Tomographic (Tomo) Nuclear Medicine Imaging Definition: Introduction of radioactive materials into the body for three dimensional display of images developed from the capture of radioactive emissions

Body Part Character 4	Radionuclide Character 5	Qualifier Character 6	Qualifier Character 7
7 Gastrointestinal Tract	1 Technetium 99m (Tc-99m) D Indium 111 (In-111) Y Other Radionuclide	Z None	Z None
Y Digestive System	Y Other Radionuclide	Z None	Z None

C Nuclear Medicine
F Hepatobiliary System and Pancreas
1 Planar Nuclear Medicine Imaging Definition: Introduction of radioactive materials into the body for single plane display of images developed from the capture of radioactive emissions

Body Part Character 4	Radionuclide Character 5	Qualifier Character 6	Qualifier Character 7
4 Gallbladder 5 Liver 6 Liver and Spleen C Hepatobiliary System, All	1 Technetium 99m (Tc-99m) Y Other Radionuclide	Z None	Z None
Y Hepatobiliary System and Pancreas	Y Other Radionuclide	Z None	Z None

C Nuclear Medicine
F Hepatobiliary System and Pancreas
2 Tomographic (Tomo) Nuclear Medicine Imaging Definition: Introduction of radioactive materials into the body for three dimensional display of images developed from the capture of radioactive emissions

Body Part Character 4	Radionuclide Character 5	Qualifier Character 6	Qualifier Character 7
4 Gallbladder 5 Liver 6 Liver and Spleen	1 Technetium 99m (Tc-99m) Y Other Radionuclide	Z None	Z None
Y Hepatobiliary System and Pancreas	Y Other Radionuclide	Z None	Z None

C Nuclear Medicine
G Endocrine System
1 Planar Nuclear Medicine Imaging Definition: Introduction of radioactive materials into the body for single plane display of images developed from the capture of radioactive emissions

Body Part Character 4	Radionuclide Character 5	Qualifier Character 6	Qualifier Character 7
1 Parathyroid Glands	1 Technetium 99m (Tc-99m) S Thallium 201 (Tl-201) Y Other Radionuclide	Z None	Z None
2 Thyroid Gland	1 Technetium 99m (Tc-99m) F Iodine 123 (I-123) G Iodine 131 (I-131) Y Other Radionuclide	Z None	Z None
4 Adrenal Glands, Bilateral	G Iodine 131 (I-131) Y Other Radionuclide	Z None	Z None
Y Endocrine System	Y Other Radionuclide	Z None	Z None

C Nuclear Medicine
G Endocrine System
2 Tomographic (Tomo) Nuclear Medicine Imaging Definition: Introduction of radioactive materials into the body for three dimensional display of images developed from the capture of radioactive emissions

Body Part Character 4	Radionuclide Character 5	Qualifier Character 6	Qualifier Character 7
1 Parathyroid Glands	1 Technetium 99m (Tc-99m) S Thallium 201 (Tl-201) Y Other Radionuclide	Z None	Z None
Y Endocrine System	Y Other Radionuclide	Z None	Z None

C Nuclear Medicine
G Endocrine System
4 Nonimaging Nuclear Medicine Uptake

Definition: Introduction of radioactive materials into the body for measurements of organ function, from the detection of radioactive emissions

Body Part Character 4	Radionuclide Character 5	Qualifier Character 6	Qualifier Character 7
2 Thyroid Gland	1 Technetium 99m (Tc-99m) F Iodine 123 (I-123) G Iodine 131 (I-131) Y Other Radionuclide	Z None	Z None
Y Endocrine System	Y Other Radionuclide	Z None	Z None

C Nuclear Medicine
H Skin, Subcutaneous Tissue and Breast
1 Planar Nuclear Medicine Imaging

Definition: Introduction of radioactive materials into the body for single plane display of images developed from the capture of radioactive emissions

Body Part Character 4	Radionuclide Character 5	Qualifier Character 6	Qualifier Character 7
Ø Breast, Right 1 Breast, Left 2 Breasts, Bilateral	1 Technetium 99m (Tc-99m) S Thallium 201 (Tl-201) Y Other Radionuclide	Z None	Z None
Y Skin, Subcutaneous Tissue and Breast	Y Other Radionuclide	Z None	Z None

C Nuclear Medicine
H Skin, Subcutaneous Tissue and Breast
2 Tomographic (Tomo) Nuclear Medicine Imaging

Definition: Introduction of radioactive materials into the body for three dimensional display of images developed from the capture of radioactive emissions

Body Part Character 4	Radionuclide Character 5	Qualifier Character 6	Qualifier Character 7
Ø Breast, Right 1 Breast, Left 2 Breasts, Bilateral	1 Technetium 99m (Tc-99m) S Thallium 201 (Tl-201) Y Other Radionuclide	Z None	Z None
Y Skin, Subcutaneous Tissue and Breast	Y Other Radionuclide	Z None	Z None

C Nuclear Medicine
P Musculoskeletal System
1 Planar Nuclear Medicine Imaging

Definition: Introduction of radioactive materials into the body for single plane display of images developed from the capture of radioactive emissions

Body Part Character 4	Radionuclide Character 5	Qualifier Character 6	Qualifier Character 7
1 Skull 4 Thorax 5 Spine 6 Pelvis 7 Spine and Pelvis 8 Upper Extremity, Right 9 Upper Extremity, Left B Upper Extremities, Bilateral C Lower Extremity, Right D Lower Extremity, Left F Lower Extremities, Bilateral Z Musculoskeletal System, All	1 Technetium 99m (Tc-99m) Y Other Radionuclide	Z None	Z None
Y Musculoskeletal System, Other	Y Other Radionuclide	Z None	Z None

C Nuclear Medicine
P Musculoskeletal System
2 Tomographic (Tomo) Nuclear Medicine Imaging Definition: Introduction of radioactive materials into the body for three dimensional display of images developed from the capture of radioactive emissions

Body Part Character 4	Radionuclide Character 5	Qualifier Character 6	Qualifier Character 7
1 Skull 2 Cervical Spine 3 Skull and Cervical Spine 4 Thorax 6 Pelvis 7 Spine and Pelvis 8 Upper Extremity, Right 9 Upper Extremity, Left B Upper Extremities, Bilateral C Lower Extremity, Right D Lower Extremity, Left F Lower Extremities, Bilateral G Thoracic Spine H Lumbar Spine J Thoracolumbar Spine	1 Technetium 99m (Tc-99m) Y Other Radionuclide	Z None	Z None
Y Musculoskeletal System, Other	Y Other Radionuclide	Z None	Z None

C Nuclear Medicine
P Musculoskeletal System
5 Nonimaging Nuclear Medicine Probe Definition: Introduction of radioactive materials into the body for the study of distribution and fate of certain substances by the detection of radioactive emissions; or, alternatively, measurement of absorption of radioactive emissions from an external source

Body Part Character 4	Radionuclide Character 5	Qualifier Character 6	Qualifier Character 7
5 Spine N Upper Extremities P Lower Extremities	Z None	Z None	Z None
Y Musculoskeletal System, Other	Y Other Radionuclide	Z None	Z None

C Nuclear Medicine
T Urinary System
1 Planar Nuclear Medicine Imaging Definition: Introduction of radioactive materials into the body for single plane display of images developed from the capture of radioactive emissions

Body Part Character 4	Radionuclide Character 5	Qualifier Character 6	Qualifier Character 7
3 Kidneys, Ureters and Bladder	1 Technetium 99m (Tc-99m) F Iodine 123 (I-123) G Iodine 131 (I-131) Y Other Radionuclide	Z None	Z None
H Bladder and Ureters	1 Technetium 99m (Tc-99m) Y Other Radionuclide	Z None	Z None
Y Urinary System	Y Other Radionuclide	Z None	Z None

C Nuclear Medicine
T Urinary System
2 Tomographic (Tomo) Nuclear Medicine Imaging Definition: Introduction of radioactive materials into the body for three dimensional display of images developed from the capture of radioactive emissions

Body Part Character 4	Radionuclide Character 5	Qualifier Character 6	Qualifier Character 7
3 Kidneys, Ureters and Bladder	1 Technetium 99m (Tc-99m) Y Other Radionuclide	Z None	Z None
Y Urinary System	Y Other Radionuclide	Z None	Z None

C Nuclear Medicine
T Urinary System
6 Nonimaging Nuclear Medicine Assay Definition: Introduction of radioactive materials into the body for the study of body fluids and blood elements, by the detection of radioactive emissions

Body Part Character 4	Radionuclide Character 5	Qualifier Character 6	Qualifier Character 7
3 Kidneys, Ureters and Bladder	1 Technetium 99m (Tc-99m) F Iodine 123 (I-123) G Iodine 131 (I-131) H Iodine 125 (I-125) Y Other Radionuclide	Z None	Z None
Y Urinary System	Y Other Radionuclide	Z None	Z None

C Nuclear Medicine
V Male Reproductive System
1 Planar Nuclear Medicine Imaging

Definition: Introduction of radioactive materials into the body for single plane display of images developed from the capture of radioactive emissions

Body Part Character 4	Radionuclide Character 5	Qualifier Character 6	Qualifier Character 7
9 Testicles, Bilateral ♂	1 Technetium 99m (Tc-99m) Y Other Radionuclide	Z None	Z None
Y Male Reproductive System ♂	Y Other Radionuclide	Z None	Z None

♂ All body part, radionuclide, and qualifier values

C Nuclear Medicine
W Anatomical Regions
1 Planar Nuclear Medicine Imaging

Definition: Introduction of radioactive materials into the body for single plane display of images developed from the capture of radioactive emissions

Body Part Character 4	Radionuclide Character 5	Qualifier Character 6	Qualifier Character 7
Ø Abdomen 1 Abdomen and Pelvis 4 Chest and Abdomen 6 Chest and Neck B Head and Neck D Lower Extremity J Pelvic Region M Upper Extremity N Whole Body	1 Technetium 99m (Tc-99m) D Indium 111 (In-111) F Iodine 123 (I-123) G Iodine 131 (I-131) L Gallium 67 (Ga-67) S Thallium 201 (Tl-201) Y Other Radionuclide	Z None	Z None
3 Chest	1 Technetium 99m (Tc-99m) D Indium 111 (In-111) F Iodine 123 (I-123) G Iodine 131 (I-131) K Fluorine 18 (F-18) L Gallium 67 (Ga-67) S Thallium 201 (Tl-201) Y Other Radionuclide	Z None	Z None
Y Anatomical Regions, Multiple	Y Other Radionuclide	Z None	Z None
Z Anatomical Region, Other	Z None	Z None	Z None

C Nuclear Medicine
W Anatomical Regions
2 Tomographic (Tomo) Nuclear Medicine Imaging

Definition: Introduction of radioactive materials into the body for three dimensional display of images developed from the capture of radioactive emissions

Body Part Character 4	Radionuclide Character 5	Qualifier Character 6	Qualifier Character 7
Ø Abdomen 1 Abdomen and Pelvis 3 Chest 4 Chest and Abdomen 6 Chest and Neck B Head and Neck D Lower Extremity J Pelvic Region M Upper Extremity	1 Technetium 99m (Tc-99m) D Indium 111 (In-111) F Iodine 123 (I-123) G Iodine 131 (I-131) K Fluorine 18 (F-18) L Gallium 67 (Ga-67) S Thallium 201 (Tl-201) Y Other Radionuclide	Z None	Z None
Y Anatomical Regions, Multiple	Y Other Radionuclide	Z None	Z None

C Nuclear Medicine
W Anatomical Regions
3 Positron Emission Tomographic (PET) Imaging

Definition: Introduction of radioactive materials into the body for three dimensional display of images developed from the simultaneous capture, 180 degrees apart, of radioactive emissions

Body Part Character 4	Radionuclide Character 5	Qualifier Character 6	Qualifier Character 7
N Whole Body	Y Other Radionuclide	Z None	Z None

C Nuclear Medicine
W Anatomical Regions
5 Nonimaging Nuclear Medicine Probe Definition: Introduction of radioactive materials into the body for the study of distribution and fate of certain substances by the detection of radioactive emissions; or, alternatively, measurement of absorption of radioactive emissions from an external source

Body Part Character 4	Radionuclide Character 5	Qualifier Character 6	Qualifier Character 7
Ø Abdomen 1 Abdomen and Pelvis 3 Chest 4 Chest and Abdomen 6 Chest and Neck B Head and Neck D Lower Extremity J Pelvic Region M Upper Extremity	1 Technetium 99m (Tc-99m) D Indium 111 (In-111) Y Other Radionuclide	Z None	Z None

C Nuclear Medicine
W Anatomical Regions
7 Systemic Nuclear Medicine Therapy Definition: Introduction of unsealed radioactive materials into the body for treatment

Body Part Character 4	Radionuclide Character 5	Qualifier Character 6	Qualifier Character 7
Ø Abdomen 3 Chest	N Phosphorus 32 (P-32) Y Other Radionuclide	Z None	Z None
G Thyroid	G Iodine 131 (I-131) Y Other Radionuclide	Z None	Z None
N Whole Body	8 Samarium 153 (Sm-153) G Iodine 131 (I-131) N Phosphorus 32 (P-32) P Strontium 89 (Sr-89) Y Other Radionuclide	Z None	Z None
Y Anatomical Regions, Multiple	Y Other Radionuclide	Z None	Z None

Radiation Therapy DØØ–DWY

AHA Coding Clinic for table DØ1
2020, 4Q, 43-44 Insertion of radioactive element
2020, 4Q, 69-70 Cesium 131 brachytherapy
2019, 4Q, 42-44 Unidirectional source brachytherapy

AHA Coding Clinic for table DØY
2022, 4Q, 62 Deletion of qualifier value for laser interstitial thermal therapy
2020, 4Q, 70 Intraoperative radiation therapy

AHA Coding Clinic for table D71
2020, 4Q, 43-44 Insertion of radioactive element
2020, 4Q, 69-70 Cesium 131 brachytherapy
2019, 4Q, 42-44 Unidirectional source brachytherapy

AHA Coding Clinic for table D81
2020, 4Q, 43-44 Insertion of radioactive element
2020, 4Q, 69-70 Cesium 131 brachytherapy
2019, 4Q, 42-44 Unidirectional source brachytherapy

AHA Coding Clinic for table D91
2020, 4Q, 43-44 Insertion of radioactive element
2020, 4Q, 69-70 Cesium 131 brachytherapy
2019, 4Q, 42-44 Unidirectional source brachytherapy

AHA Coding Clinic for table DB1
2020, 4Q, 43-44 Insertion of radioactive element
2020, 4Q, 69-70 Cesium 131 brachytherapy
2019, 4Q, 42-44 Unidirectional source brachytherapy

AHA Coding Clinic for table DBY
2022, 4Q, 62 Deletion of qualifier value for laser interstitial thermal therapy

AHA Coding Clinic for table DD1
2020, 4Q, 43-44 Insertion of radioactive element
2020, 4Q, 69-70 Cesium 131 brachytherapy
2019, 4Q, 42-44 Unidirectional source brachytherapy

AHA Coding Clinic for table DDY
2022, 4Q, 62 Deletion of qualifier value for laser interstitial thermal therapy

AHA Coding Clinic for table DF1
2022, 2Q, 26 Radioembolization of right hepatic lobe
2020, 4Q, 43-44 Insertion of radioactive element
2020, 4Q, 69-70 Cesium 131 brachytherapy
2019, 4Q, 42-44 Unidirectional source brachytherapy

AHA Coding Clinic for table DFY
2022, 4Q, 62 Deletion of qualifier value for laser interstitial thermal therapy

AHA Coding Clinic for table DG1
2020, 4Q, 43-44 Insertion of radioactive element
2020, 4Q, 69-70 Cesium 131 brachytherapy
2019, 4Q, 42-44 Unidirectional source brachytherapy

AHA Coding Clinic for table DGY
2022, 4Q, 62 Deletion of qualifier value for laser interstitial thermal therapy

AHA Coding Clinic for table DM1
2020, 4Q, 43-44 Insertion of radioactive element
2020, 4Q, 69-70 Cesium 131 brachytherapy
2019, 4Q, 42-44 Unidirectional source brachytherapy

AHA Coding Clinic for table DMY
2022, 4Q, 62 Deletion of qualifier value for laser interstitial thermal therapy

AHA Coding Clinic for table DT1
2020, 4Q, 43-44 Insertion of radioactive element
2020, 4Q, 69-70 Cesium 131 brachytherapy
2019, 4Q, 42-44 Unidirectional source brachytherapy

AHA Coding Clinic for table DU1
2020, 4Q, 43-44 Insertion of radioactive element
2020, 4Q, 69-70 Cesium 131 brachytherapy
2019, 4Q, 42-44 Unidirectional source brachytherapy
2017, 4Q, 104 Intrauterine brachytherapy & placement of tandems & ovoids

AHA Coding Clinic for table DV1
2020, 4Q, 43-44 Insertion of radioactive element
2020, 4Q, 69-70 Cesium 131 brachytherapy
2019, 4Q, 42-44 Unidirectional source brachytherapy

AHA Coding Clinic for table DVY
2022, 4Q, 62 Deletion of qualifier value for laser interstitial thermal therapy

AHA Coding Clinic for table DW1
2020, 4Q, 43-44 Insertion of radioactive element
2020, 4Q, 69-70 Cesium 131 brachytherapy
2019, 4Q, 42-44 Unidirectional source brachytherapy

AHA Coding Clinic for table DWY
2019, 4Q, 37 Hyperthermic antineoplastic chemotherapy

D Radiation Therapy
Ø Central and Peripheral Nervous System
Ø Beam Radiation

Treatment Site Character 4	Modality Qualifier Character 5	Isotope Character 6	Qualifier Character 7
Ø Brain 1 Brain Stem 6 Spinal Cord 7 Peripheral Nerve	Ø Photons <1 MeV 1 Photons 1- 10 MeV 2 Photons >10 MeV 4 Heavy Particles (Protons, Ions) 5 Neutrons 6 Neutron Capture	Z None	Z None
Ø Brain 1 Brain Stem 6 Spinal Cord 7 Peripheral Nerve	3 Electrons	Z None	Ø Intraoperative Z None

D Radiation Therapy
Ø Central and Peripheral Nervous System
1 Brachytherapy

Treatment Site Character 4	Modality Qualifier Character 5	Isotope Character 6	Qualifier Character 7
Ø Brain 1 Brain Stem 6 Spinal Cord 7 Peripheral Nerve	9 High Dose Rate (HDR)	7 Cesium 137 (Cs-137) 8 Iridium 192 (Ir-192) 9 Iodine 125 (I-125) B Palladium 103 (Pd-103) C Californium 252 (Cf-252) Y Other Isotope	Z None
Ø Brain 1 Brain Stem 6 Spinal Cord 7 Peripheral Nerve	B Low Dose Rate (LDR)	6 Cesium 131 (Cs-131) 7 Cesium 137 (Cs-137) 8 Iridium 192 (Ir-192) 9 Iodine 125 (I-125) C Californium 252 (Cf-252) Y Other Isotope	Z None
Ø Brain 1 Brain Stem 6 Spinal Cord 7 Peripheral Nerve	B Low Dose Rate (LDR)	B Palladium 103 (Pd-103)	1 Unidirectional Source Z None

D Radiation Therapy
Ø Central and Peripheral Nervous System
2 Stereotactic Radiosurgery

Treatment Site Character 4	Modality Qualifier Character 5	Isotope Character 6	Qualifier Character 7
Ø Brain 1 Brain Stem 6 Spinal Cord 7 Peripheral Nerve	D Stereotactic Other Photon Radiosurgery H Stereotactic Particulate Radiosurgery J Stereotactic Gamma Beam Radiosurgery	Z None	Z None

DRG Non-OR All treatment site, modality, isotope, and qualifier values

D Radiation Therapy
Ø Central and Peripheral Nervous System
Y Other Radiation

Treatment Site Character 4	Modality Qualifier Character 5	Isotope Character 6	Qualifier Character 7
Ø Brain 1 Brain Stem 6 Spinal Cord 7 Peripheral Nerve	7 Contact Radiation 8 Hyperthermia C Intraoperative Radiation Therapy (IORT) F Plaque Radiation	Z None	Z None

D Radiation Therapy
7 Lymphatic and Hematologic System
Ø Beam Radiation

Treatment Site Character 4	Modality Qualifier Character 5	Isotope Character 6	Qualifier Character 7
Ø Bone Marrow 1 Thymus 2 Spleen 3 Lymphatics, Neck 4 Lymphatics, Axillary 5 Lymphatics, Thorax 6 Lymphatics, Abdomen 7 Lymphatics, Pelvis 8 Lymphatics, Inguinal	Ø Photons <1 MeV 1 Photons 1- 10 MeV 2 Photons >10 MeV 4 Heavy Particles (Protons, Ions) 5 Neutrons 6 Neutron Capture	Z None	Z None
Ø Bone Marrow 1 Thymus 2 Spleen 3 Lymphatics, Neck 4 Lymphatics, Axillary 5 Lymphatics, Thorax 6 Lymphatics, Abdomen 7 Lymphatics, Pelvis 8 Lymphatics, Inguinal	3 Electrons	Z None	Ø Intraoperative Z None

D Radiation Therapy
7 Lymphatic and Hematologic System
1 Brachytherapy

Treatment Site Character 4	Modality Qualifier Character 5	Isotope Character 6	Qualifier Character 7
Ø Bone Marrow **1** Thymus **2** Spleen **3** Lymphatics, Neck **4** Lymphatics, Axillary **5** Lymphatics, Thorax **6** Lymphatics, Abdomen **7** Lymphatics, Pelvis **8** Lymphatics, Inguinal	**9** High Dose Rate (HDR)	**7** Cesium 137 (Cs-137) **8** Iridium 192 (Ir-192) **9** Iodine 125 (I-125) **B** Palladium 103 (Pd-103) **C** Californium 252 (Cf-252) **Y** Other Isotope	**Z** None
Ø Bone Marrow **1** Thymus **2** Spleen **3** Lymphatics, Neck **4** Lymphatics, Axillary **5** Lymphatics, Thorax **6** Lymphatics, Abdomen **7** Lymphatics, Pelvis **8** Lymphatics, Inguinal	**B** Low Dose Rate (LDR)	**6** Cesium 131 (Cs-131) **7** Cesium 137 (Cs-137) **8** Iridium 192 (Ir-192) **9** Iodine 125 (I-125) **C** Californium 252 (Cf-252) **Y** Other Isotope	**Z** None
Ø Bone Marrow **1** Thymus **2** Spleen **3** Lymphatics, Neck **4** Lymphatics, Axillary **5** Lymphatics, Thorax **6** Lymphatics, Abdomen **7** Lymphatics, Pelvis **8** Lymphatics, Inguinal	**B** Low Dose Rate (LDR)	**B** Palladium 103 (Pd-103)	**1** Unidirectional Source **Z** None

D Radiation Therapy
7 Lymphatic and Hematologic System
2 Stereotactic Radiosurgery

Treatment Site Character 4	Modality Qualifier Character 5	Isotope Character 6	Qualifier Character 7
Ø Bone Marrow **1** Thymus **2** Spleen **3** Lymphatics, Neck **4** Lymphatics, Axillary **5** Lymphatics, Thorax **6** Lymphatics, Abdomen **7** Lymphatics, Pelvis **8** Lymphatics, Inguinal	**D** Stereotactic Other Photon Radiosurgery **H** Stereotactic Particulate Radiosurgery **J** Stereotactic Gamma Beam Radiosurgery	**Z** None	**Z** None

DRG Non-OR All treatment site, modality, isotope, and qualifier values

D Radiation Therapy
7 Lymphatic and Hematologic System
Y Other Radiation

Treatment Site Character 4	Modality Qualifier Character 5	Isotope Character 6	Qualifier Character 7
Ø Bone Marrow **1** Thymus **2** Spleen **3** Lymphatics, Neck **4** Lymphatics, Axillary **5** Lymphatics, Thorax **6** Lymphatics, Abdomen **7** Lymphatics, Pelvis **8** Lymphatics, Inguinal	**8** Hyperthermia **F** Plaque Radiation	**Z** None	**Z** None

D Radiation Therapy
8 Eye
Ø Beam Radiation

Treatment Site Character 4	Modality Qualifier Character 5	Isotope Character 6	Qualifier Character 7
Ø Eye	Ø Photons <1 MeV 1 Photons 1- 10 MeV 2 Photons >10 MeV 4 Heavy Particles (Protons, Ions) 5 Neutrons 6 Neutron Capture	Z None	Z None
Ø Eye	3 Electrons	Z None	Ø Intraoperative Z None

D Radiation Therapy
8 Eye
1 Brachytherapy

Treatment Site Character 4	Modality Qualifier Character 5	Isotope Character 6	Qualifier Character 7
Ø Eye	9 High Dose Rate (HDR)	7 Cesium 137 (Cs-137) 8 Iridium 192 (Ir-192) 9 Iodine 125 (I-125) B Palladium 103 (Pd-103) C Californium 252 (Cf-252) Y Other Isotope	Z None
Ø Eye	B Low Dose Rate (LDR)	6 Cesium 131 (Cs-131) 7 Cesium 137 (Cs-137) 8 Iridium 192 (Ir-192) 9 Iodine 125 (I-125) C Californium 252 (Cf-252) Y Other Isotope	Z None
Ø Eye	B Low Dose Rate (LDR)	B Palladium 103 (Pd-103)	1 Unidirectional Source Z None

D Radiation Therapy
8 Eye
2 Stereotactic Radiosurgery

Treatment Site Character 4	Modality Qualifier Character 5	Isotope Character 6	Qualifier Character 7
Ø Eye	D Stereotactic Other Photon Radiosurgery H Stereotactic Particulate Radiosurgery J Stereotactic Gamma Beam Radiosurgery	Z None	Z None

DRG Non-OR All treatment site, modality, isotope, and qualifier values

D Radiation Therapy
8 Eye
Y Other Radiation

Treatment Site Character 4	Modality Qualifier Character 5	Isotope Character 6	Qualifier Character 7
Ø Eye	7 Contact Radiation 8 Hyperthermia F Plaque Radiation	Z None	Z None

D Radiation Therapy
9 Ear, Nose, Mouth and Throat
Ø Beam Radiation

Treatment Site Character 4	Modality Qualifier Character 5	Isotope Character 6	Qualifier Character 7
Ø Ear 1 Nose 3 Hypopharynx 4 Mouth 5 Tongue 6 Salivary Glands 7 Sinuses 8 Hard Palate 9 Soft Palate B Larynx D Nasopharynx F Oropharynx	Ø Photons <1 MeV 1 Photons 1- 10 MeV 2 Photons >10 MeV 4 Heavy Particles (Protons, Ions) 5 Neutrons 6 Neutron Capture	Z None	Z None
Ø Ear 1 Nose 3 Hypopharynx 4 Mouth 5 Tongue 6 Salivary Glands 7 Sinuses 8 Hard Palate 9 Soft Palate B Larynx D Nasopharynx F Oropharynx	3 Electrons	Z None	Ø Intraoperative Z None

D Radiation Therapy
9 Ear, Nose, Mouth and Throat
1 Brachytherapy

Treatment Site Character 4	Modality Qualifier Character 5	Isotope Character 6	Qualifier Character 7
Ø Ear 1 Nose 3 Hypopharynx 4 Mouth 5 Tongue 6 Salivary Glands 7 Sinuses 8 Hard Palate 9 Soft Palate B Larynx D Nasopharynx F Oropharynx	9 High Dose Rate (HDR)	7 Cesium 137 (Cs-137) 8 Iridium 192 (Ir-192) 9 Iodine 125 (I-125) B Palladium 103 (Pd-103) C Californium 252 (Cf-252) Y Other Isotope	Z None
Ø Ear 1 Nose 3 Hypopharynx 4 Mouth 5 Tongue 6 Salivary Glands 7 Sinuses 8 Hard Palate 9 Soft Palate B Larynx D Nasopharynx F Oropharynx	B Low Dose Rate (LDR)	6 Cesium 131 (Cs-131) 7 Cesium 137 (Cs-137) 8 Iridium 192 (Ir-192) 9 Iodine 125 (I-125) C Californium 252 (Cf-252) Y Other Isotope	Z None
Ø Ear 1 Nose 3 Hypopharynx 4 Mouth 5 Tongue 6 Salivary Glands 7 Sinuses 8 Hard Palate 9 Soft Palate B Larynx D Nasopharynx F Oropharynx	B Low Dose Rate (LDR)	B Palladium 103 (Pd-103)	1 Unidirectional Source Z None

D Radiation Therapy
9 Ear, Nose, Mouth and Throat
2 Stereotactic Radiosurgery

Treatment Site Character 4	Modality Qualifier Character 5	Isotope Character 6	Qualifier Character 7
Ø Ear 1 Nose 4 Mouth 5 Tongue 6 Salivary Glands 7 Sinuses 8 Hard Palate 9 Soft Palate B Larynx C Pharynx D Nasopharynx	D Stereotactic Other Photon Radiosurgery H Stereotactic Particulate Radiosurgery J Stereotactic Gamma Beam Radiosurgery	Z None	Z None

DRG Non-OR All treatment site, modality, isotope, and qualifier values

D Radiation Therapy
9 Ear, Nose, Mouth and Throat
Y Other Radiation

Treatment Site Character 4	Modality Qualifier Character 5	Isotope Character 6	Qualifier Character 7
Ø Ear 1 Nose 5 Tongue 6 Salivary Glands 7 Sinuses 8 Hard Palate 9 Soft Palate	7 Contact Radiation 8 Hyperthermia F Plaque Radiation	Z None	Z None
3 Hypopharynx F Oropharynx	7 Contact Radiation 8 Hyperthermia	Z None	Z None
4 Mouth B Larynx D Nasopharynx	7 Contact Radiation 8 Hyperthermia C Intraoperative Radiation Therapy (IORT) F Plaque Radiation	Z None	Z None
C Pharynx	C Intraoperative Radiation Therapy (IORT) F Plaque Radiation	Z None	Z None

D Radiation Therapy
B Respiratory System
Ø Beam Radiation

Treatment Site Character 4	Modality Qualifier Character 5	Isotope Character 6	Qualifier Character 7
Ø Trachea 1 Bronchus 2 Lung 5 Pleura 6 Mediastinum 7 Chest Wall 8 Diaphragm	Ø Photons <1 MeV 1 Photons 1- 10 MeV 2 Photons >10 MeV 4 Heavy Particles (Protons, Ions) 5 Neutrons 6 Neutron Capture	Z None	Z None
Ø Trachea 1 Bronchus 2 Lung 5 Pleura 6 Mediastinum 7 Chest Wall 8 Diaphragm	3 Electrons	Z None	Ø Intraoperative Z None

D Radiation Therapy
B Respiratory System
1 Brachytherapy

Treatment Site Character 4	Modality Qualifier Character 5	Isotope Character 6	Qualifier Character 7
Ø Trachea **1** Bronchus **2** Lung **5** Pleura **6** Mediastinum **7** Chest Wall **8** Diaphragm	**9** High Dose Rate (HDR)	**7** Cesium 137 (Cs-137) **8** Iridium 192 (Ir-192) **9** Iodine 125 (I-125) **B** Palladium 103 (Pd-103) **C** Californium 252 (Cf-252) **Y** Other Isotope	**Z** None
Ø Trachea **1** Bronchus **2** Lung **5** Pleura **6** Mediastinum **7** Chest Wall **8** Diaphragm	**B** Low Dose Rate (LDR)	**6** Cesium 131 (Cs-131) **7** Cesium 137 (Cs-137) **8** Iridium 192 (Ir-192) **9** Iodine 125 (I-125) **C** Californium 252 (Cf-252) **Y** Other Isotope	**Z** None
Ø Trachea **1** Bronchus **2** Lung **5** Pleura **6** Mediastinum **7** Chest Wall **8** Diaphragm	**B** Low Dose Rate (LDR)	**B** Palladium 103 (Pd-103)	**1** Unidirectional Source **Z** None

D Radiation Therapy
B Respiratory System
2 Stereotactic Radiosurgery

Treatment Site Character 4	Modality Qualifier Character 5	Isotope Character 6	Qualifier Character 7
Ø Trachea **1** Bronchus **2** Lung **5** Pleura **6** Mediastinum **7** Chest Wall **8** Diaphragm	**D** Stereotactic Other Photon Radiosurgery **H** Stereotactic Particulate Radiosurgery **J** Stereotactic Gamma Beam Radiosurgery	**Z** None	**Z** None

DRG Non-OR All treatment site, modality, isotope, and qualifier values

D Radiation Therapy
B Respiratory System
Y Other Radiation

Treatment Site Character 4	Modality Qualifier Character 5	Isotope Character 6	Qualifier Character 7
Ø Trachea **1** Bronchus **2** Lung **5** Pleura **6** Mediastinum **7** Chest Wall **8** Diaphragm	**7** Contact Radiation **8** Hyperthermia **F** Plaque Radiation	**Z** None	**Z** None

D Radiation Therapy
D Gastrointestinal System
Ø Beam Radiation

Treatment Site Character 4	Modality Qualifier Character 5	Isotope Character 6	Qualifier Character 7
Ø Esophagus 1 Stomach 2 Duodenum 3 Jejunum 4 Ileum 5 Colon 7 Rectum	Ø Photons <1 MeV 1 Photons 1- 10 MeV 2 Photons >10 MeV 4 Heavy Particles (Protons, Ions) 5 Neutrons 6 Neutron Capture	Z None	Z None
Ø Esophagus 1 Stomach 2 Duodenum 3 Jejunum 4 Ileum 5 Colon 7 Rectum	3 Electrons	Z None	Ø Intraoperative Z None

D Radiation Therapy
D Gastrointestinal System
1 Brachytherapy

Treatment Site Character 4	Modality Qualifier Character 5	Isotope Character 6	Qualifier Character 7
Ø Esophagus 1 Stomach 2 Duodenum 3 Jejunum 4 Ileum 5 Colon 7 Rectum	9 High Dose Rate (HDR)	7 Cesium 137 (Cs-137) 8 Iridium 192 (Ir-192) 9 Iodine 125 (I-125) B Palladium 103 (Pd-103) C Californium 252 (Cf-252) Y Other Isotope	Z None
Ø Esophagus 1 Stomach 2 Duodenum 3 Jejunum 4 Ileum 5 Colon 7 Rectum	B Low Dose Rate (LDR)	6 Cesium 131 (Cs-131) 7 Cesium 137 (Cs-137) 8 Iridium 192 (Ir-192) 9 Iodine 125 (I-125) C Californium 252 (Cf-252) Y Other Isotope	Z None
Ø Esophagus 1 Stomach 2 Duodenum 3 Jejunum 4 Ileum 5 Colon 7 Rectum	B Low Dose Rate (LDR)	B Palladium 103 (Pd-103)	1 Unidirectional Source Z None

D Radiation Therapy
D Gastrointestinal System
2 Stereotactic Radiosurgery

Treatment Site Character 4	Modality Qualifier Character 5	Isotope Character 6	Qualifier Character 7
Ø Esophagus 1 Stomach 2 Duodenum 3 Jejunum 4 Ileum 5 Colon 7 Rectum	D Stereotactic Other Photon Radiosurgery H Stereotactic Particulate Radiosurgery J Stereotactic Gamma Beam Radiosurgery	Z None	Z None

DRG Non-OR All treatment site, modality, isotope, and qualifier values

D Radiation therapy
D Gastrointestinal System
Y Other Radiation

Treatment Site Character 4	Modality Qualifier Character 5	Isotope Character 6	Qualifier Character 7
Ø Esophagus	7 Contact Radiation 8 Hyperthermia F Plaque Radiation	Z None	Z None
1 Stomach 2 Duodenum 3 Jejunum 4 Ileum 5 Colon 7 Rectum	7 Contact Radiation 8 Hyperthermia C Intraoperative Radiation Therapy (IORT) F Plaque Radiation	Z None	Z None
8 Anus	C Intraoperative Radiation Therapy (IORT) F Plaque Radiation	Z None	Z None

D Radiation Therapy
F Hepatobiliary System and Pancreas
Ø Beam Radiation

Treatment Site Character 4	Modality Qualifier Character 5	Isotope Character 6	Qualifier Character 7
Ø Liver 1 Gallbladder 2 Bile Ducts 3 Pancreas	Ø Photons <1 MeV 1 Photons 1- 10 MeV 2 Photons >10 MeV 4 Heavy Particles (Protons, Ions) 5 Neutrons 6 Neutron Capture	Z None	Z None
Ø Liver 1 Gallbladder 2 Bile Ducts 3 Pancreas	3 Electrons	Z None	Ø Intraoperative Z None

D Radiation Therapy
F Hepatobiliary System and Pancreas
1 Brachytherapy

Treatment Site Character 4	Modality Qualifier Character 5	Isotope Character 6	Qualifier Character 7
Ø Liver 1 Gallbladder 2 Bile Ducts 3 Pancreas	9 High Dose Rate (HDR)	7 Cesium 137 (Cs-137) 8 Iridium 192 (Ir-192) 9 Iodine 125 (I-125) B Palladium 103 (Pd-103) C Californium 252 (Cf-252) Y Other Isotope	Z None
Ø Liver 1 Gallbladder 2 Bile Ducts 3 Pancreas	B Low Dose Rate (LDR)	6 Cesium 131 (Cs-131) 7 Cesium 137 (Cs-137) 8 Iridium 192 (Ir-192) 9 Iodine 125 (I-125) C Californium 252 (Cf-252) Y Other Isotope	Z None
Ø Liver 1 Gallbladder 2 Bile Ducts 3 Pancreas	B Low Dose Rate (LDR)	B Palladium 103 (Pd-103)	1 Unidirectional Source Z None

D Radiation Therapy
F Hepatobiliary System and Pancreas
2 Stereotactic Radiosurgery

Treatment Site Character 4	Modality Qualifier Character 5	Isotope Character 6	Qualifier Character 7
Ø Liver 1 Gallbladder 2 Bile Ducts 3 Pancreas	D Stereotactic Other Photon Radiosurgery H Stereotactic Particulate Radiosurgery J Stereotactic Gamma Beam Radiosurgery	Z None	Z None

DRG Non-OR All treatment site, modality, isotope, and qualifier values

D Radiation Therapy
F Hepatobiliary System and Pancreas
Y Other Radiation

Treatment Site Character 4	Modality Qualifier Character 5	Isotope Character 6	Qualifier Character 7
Ø Liver 1 Gallbladder 2 Bile Ducts 3 Pancreas	7 Contact Radiation 8 Hyperthermia C Intraoperative Radiation Therapy (IORT) F Plaque Radiation	Z None	Z None

D Radiation Therapy
G Endocrine System
Ø Beam Radiation

Treatment Site Character 4	Modality Qualifier Character 5	Isotope Character 6	Qualifier Character 7
Ø Pituitary Gland 1 Pineal Body 2 Adrenal Glands 4 Parathyroid Glands 5 Thyroid	Ø Photons <1 MeV 1 Photons 1- 10 MeV 2 Photons >10 MeV 5 Neutrons 6 Neutron Capture	Z None	Z None
Ø Pituitary Gland 1 Pineal Body 2 Adrenal Glands 4 Parathyroid Glands 5 Thyroid	3 Electrons	Z None	Ø Intraoperative Z None

D Radiation Therapy
G Endocrine System
1 Brachytherapy

Treatment Site Character 4	Modality Qualifier Character 5	Isotope Character 6	Qualifier Character 7
Ø Pituitary Gland 1 Pineal Body 2 Adrenal Glands 4 Parathyroid Glands 5 Thyroid	9 High Dose Rate (HDR)	7 Cesium 137 (Cs-137) 8 Iridium 192 (Ir-192) 9 Iodine 125 (I-125) B Palladium 103 (Pd-103) C Californium 252 (Cf-252) Y Other Isotope	Z None
Ø Pituitary Gland 1 Pineal Body 2 Adrenal Glands 4 Parathyroid Glands 5 Thyroid	B Low Dose Rate (LDR)	6 Cesium 131 (Cs-131) 7 Cesium 137 (Cs-137) 8 Iridium 192 (Ir-192) 9 Iodine 125 (I-125) C Californium 252 (Cf-252) Y Other Isotope	Z None
Ø Pituitary Gland 1 Pineal Body 2 Adrenal Glands 4 Parathyroid Glands 5 Thyroid	B Low Dose Rate (LDR)	B Palladium 103 (Pd-103)	1 Unidirectional Source Z None

D Radiation Therapy
G Endocrine System
2 Stereotactic Radiosurgery

Treatment Site Character 4	Modality Qualifier Character 5	Isotope Character 6	Qualifier Character 7
Ø Pituitary Gland 1 Pineal Body 2 Adrenal Glands 4 Parathyroid Glands 5 Thyroid	D Stereotactic Other Photon Radiosurgery H Stereotactic Particulate Radiosurgery J Stereotactic Gamma Beam Radiosurgery	Z None	Z None

DRG Non-OR All treatment site, modality, isotope, and qualifier values

D Radiation therapy
G Endocrine System
Y Other Radiation

Treatment Site Character 4	Modality Qualifier Character 5	Isotope Character 6	Qualifier Character 7
Ø Pituitary Gland 1 Pineal Body 2 Adrenal Glands 4 Parathyroid Glands 5 Thyroid	7 Contact Radiation 8 Hyperthermia F Plaque Radiation	Z None	Z None

D Radiation Therapy
H Skin
Ø Beam Radiation

Treatment Site Character 4	Modality Qualifier Character 5	Isotope Character 6	Qualifier Character 7
2 Skin, Face 3 Skin, Neck 4 Skin, Arm 6 Skin, Chest 7 Skin, Back 8 Skin, Abdomen 9 Skin, Buttock B Skin, Leg	Ø Photons <1 MeV 1 Photons 1- 10 MeV 2 Photons >10 MeV 4 Heavy Particles (Protons, Ions) 5 Neutrons 6 Neutron Capture	Z None	Z None
2 Skin, Face 3 Skin, Neck 4 Skin, Arm 6 Skin, Chest 7 Skin, Back 8 Skin, Abdomen 9 Skin, Buttock B Skin, Leg	3 Electrons	Z None	Ø Intraoperative Z None

D Radiation Therapy
H Skin
Y Other Radiation

Treatment Site Character 4	Modality Qualifier Character 5	Isotope Character 6	Qualifier Character 7
2 Skin, Face 3 Skin, Neck 4 Skin, Arm 6 Skin, Chest 7 Skin, Back 8 Skin, Abdomen 9 Skin, Buttock B Skin, Leg	7 Contact Radiation 8 Hyperthermia F Plaque Radiation	Z None	Z None
5 Skin, Hand C Skin, Foot	F Plaque Radiation	Z None	Z None

D Radiation Therapy
M Breast
Ø Beam Radiation

Treatment Site Character 4	Modality Qualifier Character 5	Isotope Character 6	Qualifier Character 7
Ø Breast, Left 1 Breast, Right	Ø Photons <1 MeV 1 Photons 1- 10 MeV 2 Photons >10 MeV 4 Heavy Particles (Protons, Ions) 5 Neutrons 6 Neutron Capture	Z None	Z None
Ø Breast, Left 1 Breast, Right	3 Electrons	Z None	Ø Intraoperative Z None

D Radiation Therapy
M Breast
1 Brachytherapy

Treatment Site Character 4	Modality Qualifier Character 5	Isotope Character 6	Qualifier Character 7
Ø Breast, Left 1 Breast, Right	9 High Dose Rate (HDR)	7 Cesium 137 (Cs-137) 8 Iridium 192 (Ir-192) 9 Iodine 125 (I-125) B Palladium 103 (Pd-103) C Californium 252 (Cf-252) Y Other Isotope	Z None
Ø Breast, Left 1 Breast, Right	B Low Dose Rate (LDR)	6 Cesium 131 (Cs-131) 7 Cesium 137 (Cs-137) 8 Iridium 192 (Ir-192) 9 Iodine 125 (I-125) C Californium 252 (Cf-252) Y Other Isotope	Z None
Ø Breast, Left 1 Breast, Right	B Low Dose Rate (LDR)	B Palladium 103 (Pd-103)	1 Unidirectional Source Z None

D Radiation Therapy
M Breast
2 Stereotactic Radiosurgery

Treatment Site Character 4	Modality Qualifier Character 5	Isotope Character 6	Qualifier Character 7
Ø Breast, Left 1 Breast, Right	D Stereotactic Other Photon Radiosurgery H Stereotactic Particulate Radiosurgery J Stereotactic Gamma Beam Radiosurgery	Z None	Z None

DRG Non-OR All treatment site, modality, isotope, and qualifier values

D Radiation Therapy
M Breast
Y Other Radiation

Treatment Site Character 4	Modality Qualifier Character 5	Isotope Character 6	Qualifier Character 7
Ø Breast, Left 1 Breast, Right	7 Contact Radiation 8 Hyperthermia F Plaque Radiation	Z None	Z None

D Radiation Therapy
P Musculoskeletal System
Ø Beam Radiation

Treatment Site Character 4	Modality Qualifier Character 5	Isotope Character 6	Qualifier Character 7
Ø Skull 2 Maxilla 3 Mandible 4 Sternum 5 Rib(s) 6 Humerus 7 Radius/Ulna 8 Pelvic Bones 9 Femur B Tibia/Fibula C Other Bone	Ø Photons <1 MeV 1 Photons 1- 10 MeV 2 Photons >10 MeV 4 Heavy Particles (Protons, Ions) 5 Neutrons 6 Neutron Capture	Z None	Z None
Ø Skull 2 Maxilla 3 Mandible 4 Sternum 5 Rib(s) 6 Humerus 7 Radius/Ulna 8 Pelvic Bones 9 Femur B Tibia/Fibula C Other Bone	3 Electrons	Z None	Ø Intraoperative Z None

D Radiation Therapy
P Musculoskeletal System
Y Other Radiation

Treatment Site Character 4	Modality Qualifier Character 5	Isotope Character 6	Qualifier Character 7
Ø Skull 2 Maxilla 3 Mandible 4 Sternum 5 Rib(s) 6 Humerus 7 Radius/Ulna 8 Pelvic Bones 9 Femur B Tibia/Fibula C Other Bone	7 Contact Radiation 8 Hyperthermia F Plaque Radiation	Z None	Z None

D Radiation Therapy
T Urinary System
Ø Beam Radiation

Treatment Site Character 4	Modality Qualifier Character 5	Isotope Character 6	Qualifier Character 7
Ø Kidney 1 Ureter 2 Bladder 3 Urethra	Ø Photons <1 MeV 1 Photons 1- 10 MeV 2 Photons >10 MeV 4 Heavy Particles (Protons, Ions) 5 Neutrons 6 Neutron Capture	Z None	Z None
Ø Kidney 1 Ureter 2 Bladder 3 Urethra	3 Electrons	Z None	Ø Intraoperative Z None

D Radiation Therapy
T Urinary System
1 Brachytherapy

Treatment Site Character 4	Modality Qualifier Character 5	Isotope Character 6	Qualifier Character 7
Ø Kidney 1 Ureter 2 Bladder 3 Urethra	9 High Dose Rate (HDR)	7 Cesium 137 (Cs-137) 8 Iridium 192 (Ir-192) 9 Iodine 125 (I-125) B Palladium 103 (Pd-103) C Californium 252 (Cf-252) Y Other Isotope	Z None
Ø Kidney 1 Ureter 2 Bladder 3 Urethra	B Low Dose Rate (LDR)	6 Cesium 131 (Cs-131) 7 Cesium 137 (Cs-137) 8 Iridium 192 (Ir-192) 9 Iodine 125 (I-125) C Californium 252 (Cf-252) Y Other Isotope	Z None
Ø Kidney 1 Ureter 2 Bladder 3 Urethra	B Low Dose Rate (LDR)	B Palladium 103 (Pd-103)	1 Unidirectional Source Z None

D Radiation Therapy
T Urinary System
2 Stereotactic Radiosurgery

Treatment Site Character 4	Modality Qualifier Character 5	Isotope Character 6	Qualifier Character 7
Ø Kidney 1 Ureter 2 Bladder 3 Urethra	D Stereotactic Other Photon Radiosurgery H Stereotactic Particulate Radiosurgery J Stereotactic Gamma Beam Radiosurgery	Z None	Z None

DRG Non-OR All treatment site, modality, isotope, and qualifier values

NC Noncovered Procedure LC Limited Coverage QA Questionable OB Admit NT New Tech Add-on Combination Member ♂ Male ♀ Female

D Radiation Therapy
T Urinary System
Y Other Radiation

Treatment Site Character 4	Modality Qualifier Character 5	Isotope Character 6	Qualifier Character 7
Ø Kidney 1 Ureter 2 Bladder 3 Urethra	7 Contact Radiation 8 Hyperthermia C Intraoperative Radiation Therapy (IORT) F Plaque Radiation	Z None	Z None

D Radiation Therapy
U Female Reproductive System
Ø Beam Radiation

Treatment Site Character 4	Modality Qualifier Character 5	Isotope Character 6	Qualifier Character 7
Ø Ovary ♀ 1 Cervix ♀ 2 Uterus ♀	Ø Photons <1 MeV 1 Photons 1- 10 MeV 2 Photons >10 MeV 4 Heavy Particles (Protons, Ions) 5 Neutrons 6 Neutron Capture	Z None	Z None
Ø Ovary ♀ 1 Cervix ♀ 2 Uterus ♀	3 Electrons	Z None	Ø Intraoperative Z None

♀ All treatment site, modality, isotope, and qualifier values

D Radiation Therapy
U Female Reproductive System
1 Brachytherapy

Treatment Site Character 4	Modality Qualifier Character 5	Isotope Character 6	Qualifier Character 7
Ø Ovary ♀ 1 Cervix ♀ 2 Uterus ♀	9 High Dose Rate (HDR)	7 Cesium 137 (Cs-137) 8 Iridium 192 (Ir-192) 9 Iodine 125 (I-125) B Palladium 103 (Pd-103) C Californium 252 (Cf-252) Y Other Isotope	Z None
Ø Ovary ♀ 1 Cervix ♀ 2 Uterus ♀	B Low Dose Rate (LDR)	6 Cesium 131 (Cs-131) 7 Cesium 137 (Cs-137) 8 Iridium 192 (Ir-192) 9 Iodine 125 (I-125) C Californium 252 (Cf-252) Y Other Isotope	Z None
Ø Ovary ♀ 1 Cervix ♀ 2 Uterus ♀	B Low Dose Rate (LDR)	B Palladium 103 (Pd-103)	1 Unidirectional Source Z None

♀ All treatment site, modality, isotope, and qualifier values

D Radiation Therapy
U Female Reproductive System
2 Stereotactic Radiosurgery

Treatment Site Character 4	Modality Qualifier Character 5	Isotope Character 6	Qualifier Character 7
Ø Ovary ♀ 1 Cervix ♀ 2 Uterus ♀	D Stereotactic Other Photon Radiosurgery H Stereotactic Particulate Radiosurgery J Stereotactic Gamma Beam Radiosurgery	Z None	Z None

DRG Non-OR All treatment site, modality, isotope, and qualifier values
♀ All treatment site, modality, isotope, and qualifier values

D Radiation Therapy
U Female Reproductive System
Y Other Radiation

Treatment Site Character 4	Modality Qualifier Character 5	Isotope Character 6	Qualifier Character 7
Ø Ovary ♀ 1 Cervix ♀ 2 Uterus ♀	7 Contact Radiation 8 Hyperthermia C Intraoperative Radiation Therapy (IORT) F Plaque Radiation	Z None	Z None

♀ All treatment site, modality, isotope, and qualifier values

D Radiation Therapy
V Male Reproductive System
Ø Beam Radiation

Treatment Site Character 4	Modality Qualifier Character 5	Isotope Character 6	Qualifier Character 7
Ø Prostate ♂ 1 Testis ♂	Ø Photons <1 MeV 1 Photons 1- 10 MeV 2 Photons >10 MeV 4 Heavy Particles (Protons, Ions) 5 Neutrons 6 Neutron Capture	Z None	Z None
Ø Prostate ♂ 1 Testis ♂	3 Electrons	Z None	Ø Intraoperative Z None

♂ All treatment site, modality, isotope, and qualifier values

D Radiation Therapy
V Male Reproductive System
1 Brachytherapy

Treatment Site Character 4	Modality Qualifier Character 5	Isotope Character 6	Qualifier Character 7
Ø Prostate ♂ 1 Testis ♂	9 High Dose Rate (HDR)	7 Cesium 137 (Cs-137) 8 Iridium 192 (Ir-192) 9 Iodine 125 (I-125) B Palladium 103 (Pd-103) C Californium 252 (Cf-252) Y Other Isotope	Z None
Ø Prostate ♂ 1 Testis ♂	B Low Dose Rate (LDR)	6 Cesium 131 (Cs-131) 7 Cesium 137 (Cs-137) 8 Iridium 192 (Ir-192) 9 Iodine 125 (I-125) C Californium 252 (Cf-252) Y Other Isotope	Z None
Ø Prostate ♂ 1 Testis ♂	B Low Dose Rate (LDR)	B Palladium 103 (Pd-103)	1 Unidirectional Source Z None

♂ All treatment site, modality, isotope, and qualifier values

D Radiation Therapy
V Male Reproductive System
2 Stereotactic Radiosurgery

Treatment Site Character 4	Modality Qualifier Character 5	Isotope Character 6	Qualifier Character 7
Ø Prostate ♂ 1 Testis ♂	D Stereotactic Other Photon Radiosurgery H Stereotactic Particulate Radiosurgery J Stereotactic Gamma Beam Radiosurgery	Z None	Z None

DRG Non-OR All treatment site, modality, isotope, and qualifier values
♂ All treatment site, modality, isotope, and qualifier values

D Radiation Therapy
V Male Reproductive System
Y Other Radiation

Treatment Site Character 4	Modality Qualifier Character 5	Isotope Character 6	Qualifier Character 7
Ø Prostate ♂	7 Contact Radiation 8 Hyperthermia C Intraoperative Radiation Therapy (IORT) F Plaque Radiation	Z None	Z None
1 Testis ♂	7 Contact Radiation 8 Hyperthermia F Plaque Radiation	Z None	Z None

♂ All treatment site, modality, isotope, and qualifier values

D Radiation Therapy
W Anatomical Regions
Ø Beam Radiation

Treatment Site Character 4	Modality Qualifier Character 5	Isotope Character 6	Qualifier Character 7
1 Head and Neck 2 Chest 3 Abdomen 4 Hemibody 5 Whole Body 6 Pelvic Region	Ø Photons <1 MeV 1 Photons 1- 10 MeV 2 Photons >10 MeV 4 Heavy Particles (Protons, Ions) 5 Neutrons 6 Neutron Capture	Z None	Z None
1 Head and Neck 2 Chest 3 Abdomen 4 Hemibody 5 Whole Body 6 Pelvic Region	3 Electrons	Z None	Ø Intraoperative Z None

D Radiation Therapy
W Anatomical Regions
1 Brachytherapy

Treatment Site Character 4	Modality Qualifier Character 5	Isotope Character 6	Qualifier Character 7
Ø Cranial Cavity K Upper Back L Lower Back P Gastrointestinal Tract Q Respiratory Tract R Genitourinary Tract X Upper Extremity Y Lower Extremity	B Low Dose Rate (LDR)	B Palladium 103 (Pd-103)	1 Unidirectional Source Z None
1 Head and Neck 2 Chest 3 Abdomen 6 Pelvic Region	9 High Dose Rate (HDR)	7 Cesium 137 (Cs-137) 8 Iridium 192 (Ir-192) 9 Iodine 125 (I-125) B Palladium 103 (Pd-103) C Californium 252 (Cf-252) Y Other Isotope	Z None
1 Head and Neck 2 Chest 3 Abdomen 6 Pelvic Region	B Low Dose Rate (LDR)	6 Cesium 131 (Cs-131) 7 Cesium 137 (Cs-137) 8 Iridium 192 (Ir-192) 9 Iodine 125 (I-125) C Californium 252 (Cf-252) Y Other Isotope	Z None
1 Head and Neck 2 Chest 3 Abdomen 6 Pelvic Region	B Low Dose Rate (LDR)	B Palladium 103 (Pd-103)	1 Unidirectional Source Z None

D Radiation Therapy
W Anatomical Regions
2 Stereotactic Radiosurgery

Treatment Site Character 4	Modality Qualifier Character 5	Isotope Character 6	Qualifier Character 7
1 Head and Neck 2 Chest 3 Abdomen 6 Pelvic Region	D Stereotactic Other Photon Radiosurgery H Stereotactic Particulate Radiosurgery J Stereotactic Gamma Beam Radiosurgery	Z None	Z None

DRG Non-OR All treatment site, modality, isotope, and qualifier values

D Radiation Therapy
W Anatomical Regions
Y Other Radiation

Treatment Site Character 4	Modality Qualifier Character 5	Isotope Character 6	Qualifier Character 7
1 Head and Neck 2 Chest 3 Abdomen 4 Hemibody 6 Pelvic Region	7 Contact Radiation 8 Hyperthermia F Plaque Radiation	Z None	Z None
5 Whole Body	7 Contact Radiation 8 Hyperthermia F Plaque Radiation	Z None	Z None
5 Whole Body	G Isotope Administration	D Iodine 131 (I-131) F Phosphorus 32 (P-32) G Strontium 89 (Sr-89) H Strontium 90 (Sr-90) Y Other Isotope	Z None

Physical Rehabilitation and Diagnostic Audiology FØØ–F15

F Physical Rehabilitation and Diagnostic Audiology
Ø Rehabilitation
Ø Speech Assessment Definition: Measurement of speech and related functions

Body System/Region Character 4	Type Qualifier Character 5	Equipment Character 6	Qualifier Character 7
3 Neurological System - Whole Body	G Communicative/Cognitive Integration Skills	K Audiovisual M Augmentative / Alternative Communication P Computer Y Other Equipment Z None	Z None
Z None	Ø Filtered Speech 3 Staggered Spondaic Word Q Performance Intensity Phonetically Balanced Speech Discrimination R Brief Tone Stimuli S Distorted Speech T Dichotic Stimuli V Temporal Ordering of Stimuli W Masking Patterns	1 Audiometer 2 Sound Field / Booth K Audiovisual Z None	Z None
Z None	1 Speech Threshold 2 Speech/Word Recognition	1 Audiometer 2 Sound Field / Booth 9 Cochlear Implant K Audiovisual Z None	Z None
Z None	4 Sensorineural Acuity Level	1 Audiometer 2 Sound Field / Booth Z None	Z None
Z None	5 Synthetic Sentence Identification	1 Audiometer 2 Sound Field / Booth 9 Cochlear Implant K Audiovisual	Z None
Z None	6 Speech and/or Language Screening 7 Nonspoken Language 8 Receptive/Expressive Language C Aphasia G Communicative/Cognitive Integration Skills L Augmentative/Alternative Communication System	K Audiovisual M Augmentative / Alternative Communication P Computer Y Other Equipment Z None	Z None
Z None	9 Articulation/Phonology	K Audiovisual P Computer Q Speech Analysis Y Other Equipment Z None	Z None
Z None	B Motor Speech	K Audiovisual N Biosensory Feedback P Computer Q Speech Analysis T Aerodynamic Function Y Other Equipment Z None	Z None
Z None	D Fluency	K Audiovisual N Biosensory Feedback P Computer Q Speech Analysis S Voice Analysis T Aerodynamic Function Y Other Equipment Z None	Z None
Z None	F Voice	K Audiovisual N Biosensory Feedback P Computer S Voice Analysis T Aerodynamic Function Y Other Equipment Z None	Z None

DRG Non-OR All body system/region, type qualifier, equipment, and qualifier values

FØØ Continued on next page

F00 Continued

F Physical Rehabilitation and Diagnostic Audiology
0 Rehabilitation
0 Speech Assessment Definition: Measurement of speech and related functions

Body System/Region Character 4	Type Qualifier Character 5	Equipment Character 6	Qualifier Character 7
Z None	H Bedside Swallowing and Oral Function P Oral Peripheral Mechanism	Y Other Equipment Z None	Z None
Z None	J Instrumental Swallowing and Oral Function	T Aerodynamic Function W Swallowing Y Other Equipment	Z None
Z None	K Orofacial Myofunctional	K Audiovisual P Computer Y Other Equipment Z None	Z None
Z None	M Voice Prosthetic	K Audiovisual P Computer S Voice Analysis V Speech Prosthesis Y Other Equipment Z None	Z None
Z None	N Non-invasive Instrumental Status	N Biosensory Feedback P Computer Q Speech Analysis S Voice Analysis T Aerodynamic Function Y Other Equipment	Z None
Z None	X Other Specified Central Auditory Processing	Z None	Z None

DRG Non-OR All body system/region, type qualifier, equipment, and qualifier values

F Physical Rehabilitation and Diagnostic Audiology
0 Rehabilitation
1 Motor and/or Nerve Function Assessment Definition: Measurement of motor, nerve, and related functions

Body System/Region Character 4	Type Qualifier Character 5	Equipment Character 6	Qualifier Character 7
0 Neurological System - Head and Neck 1 Neurological System - Upper Back/ Upper Extremity 2 Neurological System - Lower Back/ Lower Extremity 3 Neurological System - Whole Body	0 Muscle Performance	E Orthosis F Assistive, Adaptive, Supportive or Protective U Prosthesis Y Other Equipment Z None	Z None
0 Neurological System - Head and Neck 1 Neurological System - Upper Back/ Upper Extremity 2 Neurological System - Lower Back/ Lower Extremity 3 Neurological System - Whole Body	1 Integumentary Integrity 3 Coordination/Dexterity 4 Motor Function G Reflex Integrity	Z None	Z None
0 Neurological System - Head and Neck 1 Neurological System - Upper Back/ Upper Extremity 2 Neurological System - Lower Back/ Lower Extremity 3 Neurological System - Whole Body	5 Range of Motion and Joint Integrity 6 Sensory Awareness/Processing/ Integrity	Y Other Equipment Z None	Z None
D Integumentary System - Head and Neck F Integumentary System - Upper Back/ Upper Extremity G Integumentary System - Lower Back/ Lower Extremity H Integumentary System - Whole Body J Musculoskeletal System - Head and Neck K Musculoskeletal System - Upper Back/ Upper Extremity L Musculoskeletal System - Lower Back/ Lower Extremity M Musculoskeletal System - Whole Body	0 Muscle Performance	E Orthosis F Assistive, Adaptive, Supportive or Protective U Prosthesis Y Other Equipment Z None	Z None

DRG Non-OR All body system/region, type qualifier, equipment, and qualifier values

F01 Continued on next page

F Physical Rehabilitation and Diagnostic Audiology
Ø Rehabilitation
1 Motor and/or Nerve Function Assessment Definition: Measurement of motor, nerve, and related functions

FØ1 Continued

Body System/Region Character 4	Type Qualifier Character 5	Equipment Character 6	Qualifier Character 7
D Integumentary System - Head and Neck F Integumentary System - Upper Back/ Upper Extremity G Integumentary System - Lower Back/ Lower Extremity H Integumentary System - Whole Body J Musculoskeletal System - Head and Neck K Musculoskeletal System - Upper Back/ Upper Extremity L Musculoskeletal System - Lower Back/ Lower Extremity M Musculoskeletal System - Whole Body	1 Integumentary Integrity	Z None	Z None
D Integumentary System - Head and Neck F Integumentary System - Upper Back/ Upper Extremity G Integumentary System - Lower Back/ Lower Extremity H Integumentary System - Whole Body J Musculoskeletal System - Head and Neck K Musculoskeletal System - Upper Back/ Upper Extremity L Musculoskeletal System - Lower Back/ Lower Extremity M Musculoskeletal System - Whole Body	5 Range of Motion and Joint Integrity 6 Sensory Awareness/Processing/ Integrity	Y Other Equipment Z None	Z None
N Genitourinary System	Ø Muscle Performance	E Orthosis F Assistive, Adaptive, Supportive or Protective U Prosthesis Y Other Equipment Z None	Z None
Z None	2 Visual Motor Integration	K Audiovisual M Augmentative / Alternative Communication N Biosensory Feedback P Computer Q Speech Analysis S Voice Analysis Y Other Equipment Z None	Z None
Z None	7 Facial Nerve Function	7 Electrophysiologic	Z None
Z None	9 Somatosensory Evoked Potentials	J Somatosensory	Z None
Z None	B Bed Mobility C Transfer F Wheelchair Mobility	E Orthosis F Assistive, Adaptive, Supportive or Protective U Prosthesis Z None	Z None
Z None	D Gait and/or Balance	E Orthosis F Assistive, Adaptive, Supportive or Protective U Prosthesis Y Other Equipment Z None	Z None

DRG Non-OR All body system/region, type qualifier, equipment, and qualifier values

F Physical Rehabilitation and Diagnostic Audiology
Ø Rehabilitation
2 Activities of Daily Living Assessment Definition: Measurement of functional level for activities of daily living

Body System/Region Character 4	Type Qualifier Character 5	Equipment Character 6	Qualifier Character 7
Ø Neurological System - Head and Neck	9 Cranial Nerve Integrity D Neuromotor Development	Y Other Equipment Z None	Z None
1 Neurological System - Upper Back/ Upper Extremity 2 Neurological System - Lower Back/ Lower Extremity 3 Neurological System - Whole Body	D Neuromotor Development	Y Other Equipment Z None	Z None
4 Circulatory System - Head and Neck 5 Circulatory System - Upper Back/ Upper Extremity 6 Circulatory System - Lower Back/ Lower Extremity 8 Respiratory System - Head and Neck 9 Respiratory System - Upper Back/ Upper Extremity B Respiratory System - Lower Back/ Lower Extremity	G Ventilation, Respiration and Circulation	C Mechanical G Aerobic Endurance and Conditioning Y Other Equipment Z None	Z None
7 Circulatory System - Whole Body C Respiratory System - Whole Body	7 Aerobic Capacity and Endurance	E Orthosis G Aerobic Endurance and Conditioning U Prosthesis Y Other Equipment Z None	Z None
7 Circulatory System - Whole Body C Respiratory System - Whole Body	G Ventilation, Respiration and Circulation	C Mechanical G Aerobic Endurance and Conditioning Y Other Equipment Z None	Z None
Z None	Ø Bathing/Showering 1 Dressing 3 Grooming/Personal Hygiene 4 Home Management	E Orthosis F Assistive, Adaptive, Supportive or Protective U Prosthesis Z None	Z None
Z None	2 Feeding/Eating 8 Anthropometric Characteristics F Pain	Y Other Equipment Z None	Z None
Z None	5 Perceptual Processing	K Audiovisual M Augmentative / Alternative Communication N Biosensory Feedback P Computer Q Speech Analysis S Voice Analysis Y Other Equipment Z None	Z None
Z None	6 Psychosocial Skills	Z None	Z None
Z None	B Environmental, Home and Work Barriers C Ergonomics and Body Mechanics	E Orthosis F Assistive, Adaptive, Supportive or Protective U Prosthesis Y Other Equipment Z None	Z None
Z None	H Vocational Activities and Functional Community or Work Reintegration Skills	E Orthosis F Assistive, Adaptive, Supportive or Protective G Aerobic Endurance and Conditioning U Prosthesis Y Other Equipment Z None	Z None

DRG Non-OR All body system/region, type qualifier, equipment, and qualifier values

F Physical Rehabilitation and Diagnostic Audiology
Ø Rehabilitation
6 Speech Treatment Definition: Application of techniques to improve, augment, or compensate for speech and related functional impairment

Body System/Region Character 4	Type Qualifier Character 5	Equipment Character 6	Qualifier Character 7
3 Neurological System - Whole Body	6 Communicative/Cognitive Integration Skills	K Audiovisual M Augmentative / Alternative Communication P Computer Y Other Equipment Z None	Z None
Z None	Ø Nonspoken Language 3 Aphasia 6 Communicative/Cognitive Integration Skills	K Audiovisual M Augmentative / Alternative Communication P Computer Y Other Equipment Z None	Z None
Z None	1 Speech-Language Pathology and Related Disorders Counseling 2 Speech-Language Pathology and Related Disorders Prevention	K Audiovisual Z None	Z None
Z None	4 Articulation/Phonology	K Audiovisual P Computer Q Speech Analysis T Aerodynamic Function Y Other Equipment Z None	Z None
Z None	5 Aural Rehabilitation	K Audiovisual L Assistive Listening M Augmentative / Alternative Communication N Biosensory Feedback P Computer Q Speech Analysis S Voice Analysis Y Other Equipment Z None	Z None
Z None	7 Fluency	4 Electroacoustic Immitance / Acoustic Reflex K Audiovisual N Biosensory Feedback Q Speech Analysis S Voice Analysis T Aerodynamic Function Y Other Equipment Z None	Z None
Z None	8 Motor Speech	K Audiovisual N Biosensory Feedback P Computer Q Speech Analysis S Voice Analysis T Aerodynamic Function Y Other Equipment Z None	Z None
Z None	9 Orofacial Myofunctional	K Audiovisual P Computer Y Other Equipment Z None	Z None
Z None	B Receptive/Expressive Language	K Audiovisual L Assistive Listening M Augmentative / Alternative Communication P Computer Y Other Equipment Z None	Z None

DRG Non-OR All body system/region, type qualifier, equipment, and qualifier values

FØ6 Continued on next page

F06 Continued

F Physical Rehabilitation and Diagnostic Audiology
Ø Rehabilitation
6 Speech Treatment Definition: Application of techniques to improve, augment, or compensate for speech and related functional impairment

Body System/Region Character 4	Type Qualifier Character 5	Equipment Character 6	Qualifier Character 7
Z None	C Voice	K Audiovisual N Biosensory Feedback P Computer S Voice Analysis T Aerodynamic Function V Speech Prosthesis Y Other Equipment Z None	Z None
Z None	D Swallowing Dysfunction	M Augmentative / Alternative Communication T Aerodynamic Function V Speech Prosthesis Y Other Equipment Z None	Z None

DRG Non-OR All body system/region, type qualifier, equipment, and qualifier values

F Physical Rehabilitation and Diagnostic Audiology
Ø Rehabilitation
7 Motor Treatment Definition: Exercise or activities to increase or facilitate motor function

Body System/Region Character 4	Type Qualifier Character 5	Equipment Character 6	Qualifier Character 7
Ø Neurological System - Head and Neck 1 Neurological System - Upper Back/Upper Extremity 2 Neurological System - Lower Back/Lower Extremity 3 Neurological System - Whole Body D Integumentary System - Head and Neck F Integumentary System - Upper Back/ Upper Extremity G Integumentary System - Lower Back/ Lower Extremity H Integumentary System - Whole Body J Musculoskeletal System - Head and Neck K Musculoskeletal System - Upper Back/ Upper Extremity L Musculoskeletal System - Lower Back/ Lower Extremity M Musculoskeletal System - Whole Body	Ø Range of Motion and Joint Mobility 1 Muscle Performance 2 Coordination/Dexterity 3 Motor Function	E Orthosis F Assistive, Adaptive, Supportive or Protective U Prosthesis Y Other Equipment Z None	Z None
Ø Neurological System - Head and Neck 1 Neurological System - Upper Back/Upper Extremity 2 Neurological System - Lower Back/Lower Extremity 3 Neurological System - Whole Body D Integumentary System - Head and Neck F Integumentary System - Upper Back/ Upper Extremity G Integumentary System - Lower Back/ Lower Extremity H Integumentary System - Whole Body J Musculoskeletal System - Head and Neck K Musculoskeletal System - Upper Back/ Upper Extremity L Musculoskeletal System - Lower Back/ Lower Extremity M Musculoskeletal System - Whole Body	6 Therapeutic Exercise	B Physical Agents C Mechanical D Electrotherapeutic E Orthosis F Assistive, Adaptive, Supportive or Protective G Aerobic Endurance and Conditioning H Mechanical or Electromechanical U Prosthesis Y Other Equipment Z None	Z None

DRG Non-OR All body system/region, type qualifier, equipment, and qualifier values

F07 Continued on next page

F Physical Rehabilitation and Diagnostic Audiology
Ø Rehabilitation
7 Motor Treatment Definition: Exercise or activities to increase or facilitate motor function

FØ7 Continued

Body System/Region Character 4	Type Qualifier Character 5	Equipment Character 6	Qualifier Character 7
Ø Neurological System - Head and Neck 1 Neurological System - Upper Back/Upper Extremity 2 Neurological System - Lower Back/Lower Extremity 3 Neurological System - Whole Body D Integumentary System - Head and Neck F Integumentary System - Upper Back/ Upper Extremity G Integumentary System - Lower Back/ Lower Extremity H Integumentary System - Whole Body J Musculoskeletal System - Head and Neck K Musculoskeletal System - Upper Back/ Upper Extremity L Musculoskeletal System - Lower Back/ Lower Extremity M Musculoskeletal System - Whole Body	7 Manual Therapy Techniques	Z None	Z None
4 Circulatory System - Head and Neck 5 Circulatory System - Upper Back / Upper Extremity 6 Circulatory System - Lower Back / Lower Extremity 7 Circulatory System - Whole Body 8 Respiratory System - Head and Neck 9 Respiratory System - Upper Back / Upper Extremity B Respiratory System - Lower Back / Lower Extremity C Respiratory System - Whole Body	6 Therapeutic Exercise	B Physical Agents C Mechanical D Electrotherapeutic E Orthosis F Assistive, Adaptive, Supportive or Protective G Aerobic Endurance and Conditioning H Mechanical or Electromechanical U Prosthesis Y Other Equipment Z None	Z None
N Genitourinary System	1 Muscle Performance	E Orthosis F Assistive, Adaptive, Supportive or Protective U Prosthesis Y Other Equipment Z None	Z None
N Genitourinary System	6 Therapeutic Exercise	B Physical Agents C Mechanical D Electrotherapeutic E Orthosis F Assistive, Adaptive, Supportive or Protective G Aerobic Endurance and Conditioning H Mechanical or Electromechanical U Prosthesis Y Other Equipment Z None	Z None
Z None	4 Wheelchair Mobility	D Electrotherapeutic E Orthosis F Assistive, Adaptive, Supportive or Protective U Prosthesis Y Other Equipment Z None	Z None
Z None	5 Bed Mobility	C Mechanical E Orthosis F Assistive, Adaptive, Supportive or Protective U Prosthesis Y Other Equipment Z None	Z None
Z None	8 Transfer Training	C Mechanical D Electrotherapeutic E Orthosis F Assistive, Adaptive, Supportive or Protective U Prosthesis Y Other Equipment Z None	Z None

DRG Non-OR All body system/region, type qualifier, equipment, and qualifier values

FØ7 Continued on next page

FØ7 Continued

F Physical Rehabilitation and Diagnostic Audiology
Ø Rehabilitation
7 Motor Treatment Definition: Exercise or activities to increase or facilitate motor function

Body System/Region Character 4	Type Qualifier Character 5	Equipment Character 6	Qualifier Character 7
Z None	9 Gait Training/Functional Ambulation	C Mechanical D Electrotherapeutic E Orthosis F Assistive, Adaptive, Supportive or Protective G Aerobic Endurance and Conditioning U Prosthesis Y Other Equipment Z None	Z None

DRG Non-OR All body system/region, type qualifier, equipment, and qualifier values

F Physical Rehabilitation and Diagnostic Audiology
Ø Rehabilitation
8 Activities of Daily Living Treatment Definition: Exercise or activities to facilitate functional competence for activities of daily living

Body System/Region Character 4	Type Qualifier Character 5	Equipment Character 6	Qualifier Character 7
D Integumentary System - Head and Neck F Integumentary System - Upper Back/ Upper Extremity G Integumentary System - Lower Back/ Lower Extremity H Integumentary System - Whole Body J Musculoskeletal System - Head and Neck K Musculoskeletal System - Upper Back/ Upper Extremity L Musculoskeletal System - Lower Back/ Lower Extremity M Musculoskeletal System - Whole Body	5 Wound Management	B Physical Agents C Mechanical D Electrotherapeutic E Orthosis F Assistive, Adaptive, Supportive or Protective U Prosthesis Y Other Equipment Z None	Z None
Z None	Ø Bathing/Showering Techniques 1 Dressing Techniques 2 Grooming/Personal Hygiene	E Orthosis F Assistive, Adaptive, Supportive or Protective U Prosthesis Y Other Equipment Z None	Z None
Z None	3 Feeding/Eating	C Mechanical D Electrotherapeutic E Orthosis F Assistive, Adaptive, Supportive or Protective U Prosthesis Y Other Equipment Z None	Z None
Z None	4 Home Management	D Electrotherapeutic E Orthosis F Assistive, Adaptive, Supportive or Protective U Prosthesis Y Other Equipment Z None	Z None
Z None	6 Psychosocial Skills	Z None	Z None
Z None	7 Vocational Activities and Functional Community or Work Reintegration Skills	B Physical Agents C Mechanical D Electrotherapeutic E Orthosis F Assistive, Adaptive, Supportive or Protective G Aerobic Endurance and Conditioning U Prosthesis Y Other Equipment Z None	Z None

DRG Non-OR All body system/region, type qualifier, equipment, and qualifier values

Physical Rehabilitation and Diagnostic Audiology FØ7–FØ8

F Physical Rehabilitation and Diagnostic Audiology
Ø Rehabilitation
9 Hearing Treatment Definition: Application of techniques to improve, augment, or compensate for hearing and related functional impairment

Body System/Region Character 4	Type Qualifier Character 5	Equipment Character 6	Qualifier Character 7
Z None	Ø Hearing and Related Disorders Counseling 1 Hearing and Related Disorders Prevention	K Audiovisual Z None	Z None
Z None	2 Auditory Processing	K Audiovisual L Assistive Listening P Computer Y Other Equipment Z None	Z None
Z None	3 Cerumen Management	X Cerumen Management Z None	Z None

DRG Non-OR All body system/region, type qualifier, equipment, and qualifier values

F Physical Rehabilitation and Diagnostic Audiology
Ø Rehabilitation
B Cochlear Implant Treatment Definition: Application of techniques to improve the communication abilities of individuals with cochlear implant

Body System/Region Character 4	Type Qualifier Character 5	Equipment Character 6	Qualifier Character 7
Z None	Ø Cochlear Implant Rehabilitation	1 Audiometer 2 Sound Field / Booth 9 Cochlear Implant K Audiovisual P Computer Y Other Equipment	Z None

DRG Non-OR All body system/region, type qualifier, equipment, and qualifier values

F Physical Rehabilitation and Diagnostic Audiology
Ø Rehabilitation
C Vestibular Treatment Definition: Application of techniques to improve, augment, or compensate for vestibular and related functional impairment

Body System/Region Character 4	Type Qualifier Character 5	Equipment Character 6	Qualifier Character 7
3 Neurological System - Whole Body H Integumentary System - Whole Body M Musculoskeletal System - Whole Body	3 Postural Control	E Orthosis F Assistive, Adaptive, Supportive or Protective U Prosthesis Y Other Equipment Z None	Z None
Z None	Ø Vestibular	8 Vestibular / Balance Z None	Z None
Z None	1 Perceptual Processing 2 Visual Motor Integration	K Audiovisual L Assistive Listening N Biosensory Feedback P Computer Q Speech Analysis S Voice Analysis T Aerodynamic Function Y Other Equipment Z None	Z None

DRG Non-OR All body system/region, type qualifier, equipment, and qualifier values

F Physical Rehabilitation and Diagnostic Audiology
Ø Rehabilitation
D Device Fitting Definition: Fitting of a device designed to facilitate or support achievement of a higher level of function

Body System/Region Character 4	Type Qualifier Character 5	Equipment Character 6	Qualifier Character 7
Z None	Ø Tinnitus Masker	5 Hearing Aid Selection / Fitting / Test Z None	Z None
Z None	1 Monaural Hearing Aid 2 Binaural Hearing Aid 5 Assistive Listening Device	1 Audiometer 2 Sound Field / Booth 5 Hearing Aid Selection / Fitting / Test K Audiovisual L Assistive Listening Z None	Z None
Z None	3 Augmentative/Alternative Communication System	M Augmentative / Alternative Communication	Z None
Z None	4 Voice Prosthetic	S Voice Analysis V Speech Prosthesis	Z None
Z None	6 Dynamic Orthosis 7 Static Orthosis 8 Prosthesis 9 Assistive, Adaptive, Supportive or Protective Devices	E Orthosis F Assistive, Adaptive, Supportive or Protective U Prosthesis Z None	Z None

DRG Non-OR FØDZØ[5,Z]Z
DRG Non-OR FØDZ[1, 2,5][1,2,5, K,L,Z]Z
DRG Non-OR FØDZ3MZ
DRG Non-OR FØDZ4[S,V]Z
DRG Non-OR FØDZ[6,7][E,F,U,Z]Z
DRG Non-OR FØDZ8[E,F,U]Z

F Physical Rehabilitation and Diagnostic Audiology
Ø Rehabilitation
F Caregiver Training Definition: Training in activities to support patient's optimal level of function

Body System/Region Character 4	Type Qualifier Character 5	Equipment Character 6	Qualifier Character 7
Z None	Ø Bathing/Showering Technique 1 Dressing 2 Feeding and Eating 3 Grooming/Personal Hygiene 4 Bed Mobility 5 Transfer 6 Wheelchair Mobility 7 Therapeutic Exercise 8 Airway Clearance Techniques 9 Wound Management B Vocational Activities and Functional Community or Work Reintegration Skills C Gait Training/Functional Ambulation D Application, Proper Use and Care of Devices F Application, Proper Use and Care of Orthoses G Application, Proper Use and Care of Prosthesis H Home Management	E Orthosis F Assistive, Adaptive, Supportive or Protective U Prosthesis Z None	Z None
Z None	J Communication Skills	K Audiovisual L Assistive Listening M Augmentative / Alternative Communication P Computer Z None	Z None

DRG Non-OR All body system/region, type qualifier, equipment, and qualifier values

F Physical Rehabilitation and Diagnostic Audiology
1 Diagnostic Audiology
3 Hearing Assessment Definition: Measurement of hearing and related functions

Body System/Region Character 4	Type Qualifier Character 5	Equipment Character 6	Qualifier Character 7
Z None	Ø Hearing Screening	Ø Occupational Hearing 1 Audiometer 2 Sound Field / Booth 3 Tympanometer 8 Vestibular / Balance 9 Cochlear Implant Z None	Z None
Z None	1 Pure Tone Audiometry, Air 2 Pure Tone Audiometry, Air and Bone	Ø Occupational Hearing 1 Audiometer 2 Sound Field / Booth Z None	Z None
Z None	3 Bekesy Audiometry 6 Visual Reinforcement Audiometry 9 Short Increment Sensitivity Index B Stenger C Pure Tone Stenger	1 Audiometer 2 Sound Field / Booth Z None	Z None
Z None	4 Conditioned Play Audiometry 5 Select Picture Audiometry	1 Audiometer 2 Sound Field / Booth K Audiovisual Z None	Z None
Z None	7 Alternate Binaural or Monaural Loudness Balance	1 Audiometer K Audiovisual Z None	Z None
Z None	8 Tone Decay D Tympanometry F Eustachian Tube Function G Acoustic Reflex Patterns H Acoustic Reflex Threshold J Acoustic Reflex Decay	3 Tympanometer 4 Electroacoustic Immitance / Acoustic Reflex Z None	Z None
Z None	K Electrocochleography L Auditory Evoked Potentials	7 Electrophysiologic Z None	Z None
Z None	M Evoked Otoacoustic Emissions, Screening N Evoked Otoacoustic Emissions, Diagnostic	6 Otoacoustic Emission (OAE) Z None	Z None
Z None	P Aural Rehabilitation Status	1 Audiometer 2 Sound Field / Booth 4 Electroacoustic Immitance / Acoustic Reflex 9 Cochlear Implant K Audiovisual L Assistive Listening P Computer Z None	Z None
Z None	Q Auditory Processing	K Audiovisual P Computer Y Other Equipment Z None	Z None

F Physical Rehabilitation and Diagnostic Audiology
1 Diagnostic Audiology
4 Hearing Aid Assessment

Definition: Measurement of the appropriateness and/or effectiveness of a hearing device

Body System/Region Character 4	Type Qualifier Character 5	Equipment Character 6	Qualifier Character 7
Z None	Ø Cochlear Implant	1 Audiometer 2 Sound Field / Booth 3 Tympanometer 4 Electroacoustic Immitance / Acoustic Reflex 5 Hearing Aid Selection / Fitting / Test 7 Electrophysiologic 9 Cochlear Implant K Audiovisual L Assistive Listening P Computer Y Other Equipment Z None	Z None
Z None	1 Ear Canal Probe Microphone 6 Binaural Electroacoustic Hearing Aid Check 8 Monaural Electroacoustic Hearing Aid Check	5 Hearing Aid Selection / Fitting / Test Z None	Z None
Z None	2 Monaural Hearing Aid 3 Binaural Hearing Aid	1 Audiometer 2 Sound Field / Booth 3 Tympanometer 4 Electroacoustic Immitance / Acoustic Reflex 5 Hearing Aid Selection / Fitting / Test K Audiovisual L Assistive Listening P Computer Z None	Z None
Z None	4 Assistive Listening System/Device Selection	1 Audiometer 2 Sound Field / Booth 3 Tympanometer 4 Electroacoustic Immitance / Acoustic Reflex K Audiovisual L Assistive Listening Z None	Z None
Z None	5 Sensory Aids	1 Audiometer 2 Sound Field / Booth 3 Tympanometer 4 Electroacoustic Immitance / Acoustic Reflex 5 Hearing Aid Selection / Fitting / Test K Audiovisual L Assistive Listening Z None	Z None
Z None	7 Ear Protector Attentuation	Ø Occupational Hearing Z None	Z None

F Physical Rehabilitation and Diagnostic Audiology
1 Diagnostic Audiology
5 Vestibular Assessment

Definition: Measurement of the vestibular system and related functions

Body System/Region Character 4	Type Qualifier Character 5	Equipment Character 6	Qualifier Character 7
Z None	Ø Bithermal, Binaural Caloric Irrigation 1 Bithermal, Monaural Caloric Irrigation 2 Unithermal Binaural Screen 3 Oscillating Tracking 4 Sinusoidal Vertical Axis Rotational 5 Dix-Hallpike Dynamic 6 Computerized Dynamic Posturography	8 Vestibular / Balance Z None	Z None
Z None	7 Tinnitus Masker	5 Hearing Aid Selection / Fitting / Test Z None	Z None

Mental Health GZ1–GZJ

G Mental Health
Z None
1 Psychological Tests Definition: The administration and interpretation of standardized psychological tests and measurement instruments for the assessment of psychological function

Qualifier Character 4	Qualifier Character 5	Qualifier Character 6	Qualifier Character 7
Ø Developmental 1 Personality and Behavioral 2 Intellectual and Psychoeducational 3 Neuropsychological 4 Neurobehavioral and Cognitive Status	Z None	Z None	Z None

G Mental Health
Z None
2 Crisis Intervention Definition: Treatment of a traumatized, acutely disturbed or distressed individual for the purpose of short-term stabilization

Qualifier Character 4	Qualifier Character 5	Qualifier Character 6	Qualifier Character 7
Z None	Z None	Z None	Z None

G Mental Health
Z None
3 Medication Management Definition: Monitoring and adjusting the use of medications for the treatment of a mental health disorder

Qualifier Character 4	Qualifier Character 5	Qualifier Character 6	Qualifier Character 7
Z None	Z None	Z None	Z None

G Mental Health
Z None
5 Individual Psychotherapy Definition: Treatment of an individual with a mental health disorder by behavioral, cognitive, psychoanalytic, psychodynamic or psychophysiological means to improve functioning or well-being

Qualifier Character 4	Qualifier Character 5	Qualifier Character 6	Qualifier Character 7
Ø Interactive 1 Behavioral 2 Cognitive 3 Interpersonal 4 Psychoanalysis 5 Psychodynamic 6 Supportive 8 Cognitive-Behavioral 9 Psychophysiological	Z None	Z None	Z None

G Mental Health
Z None
6 Counseling Definition: The application of psychological methods to treat an individual with normal developmental issues and psychological problems in order to increase function, improve well-being, alleviate distress, maladjustment or resolve crises

Qualifier Character 4	Qualifier Character 5	Qualifier Character 6	Qualifier Character 7
Ø Educational 1 Vocational 3 Other Counseling	Z None	Z None	Z None

G Mental Health
Z None
7 Family Psychotherapy Definition: Treatment that includes one or more family members of an individual with a mental health disorder by behavioral, cognitive, psychoanalytic, psychodynamic or psychophysiological means to improve functioning or well-being

Explanation: Remediation of emotional or behavioral problems presented by one or more family members in cases where psychotherapy with more than one family member is indicated

Qualifier Character 4	Qualifier Character 5	Qualifier Character 6	Qualifier Character 7
2 Other Family Psychotherapy	Z None	Z None	Z None

G Mental Health
Z None
B Electroconvulsive Therapy Definition: The application of controlled electrical voltages to treat a mental health disorder

Qualifier Character 4	Qualifier Character 5	Qualifier Character 6	Qualifier Character 7
Ø Unilateral-Single Seizure 1 Unilateral-Multiple Seizure 2 Bilateral-Single Seizure 3 Bilateral-Multiple Seizure 4 Other Electroconvulsive Therapy	Z None	Z None	Z None

G Mental Health
Z None
C Biofeedback Definition: Provision of information from the monitoring and regulating of physiological processes in conjunction with cognitive-behavioral techniques to improve patient functioning or well-being

Qualifier Character 4	Qualifier Character 5	Qualifier Character 6	Qualifier Character 7
9 Other Biofeedback	Z None	Z None	Z None

G Mental Health
Z None
F Hypnosis Definition: Induction of a state of heightened suggestibility by auditory, visual and tactile techniques to elicit an emotional or behavioral response

Qualifier Character 4	Qualifier Character 5	Qualifier Character 6	Qualifier Character 7
Z None	Z None	Z None	Z None

G Mental Health
Z None
G Narcosynthesis Definition: Administration of intravenous barbiturates in order to release suppressed or repressed thoughts

Qualifier Character 4	Qualifier Character 5	Qualifier Character 6	Qualifier Character 7
Z None	Z None	Z None	Z None

G Mental Health
Z None
H Group Psychotherapy Definition: Treatment of two or more individuals with a mental health disorder by behavioral, cognitive, psychoanalytic, psychodynamic or psychophysiological means to improve functioning or well-being

Qualifier Character 4	Qualifier Character 5	Qualifier Character 6	Qualifier Character 7
Z None	Z None	Z None	Z None

G Mental Health
Z None
J Light Therapy Definition: Application of specialized light treatments to improve functioning or well-being

Qualifier Character 4	Qualifier Character 5	Qualifier Character 6	Qualifier Character 7
Z None	Z None	Z None	Z None

Substance Abuse Treatment HZ2–HZ9

AHA Coding Clinic for table HZ2
2020, 1Q, 21 Inpatient detoxification services

AHA Coding Clinic for table HZ9
2020, 1Q, 21 Inpatient detoxification services

H Substance Abuse Treatment
Z None
2 Detoxification Services

Definition: Detoxification from alcohol and/or drugs
Explanation: Not a treatment modality, but helps the patient stabilize physically and psychologically until the body becomes free of drugs and the effects of alcohol

Qualifier Character 4	Qualifier Character 5	Qualifier Character 6	Qualifier Character 7
Z None	Z None	Z None	Z None

H Substance Abuse Treatment
Z None
3 Individual Counseling

Definition: The application of psychological methods to treat an individual with addictive behavior
Explanation: Comprised of several different techniques, which apply various strategies to address drug addiction

Qualifier Character 4	Qualifier Character 5	Qualifier Character 6	Qualifier Character 7
Ø Cognitive 1 Behavioral 2 Cognitive-Behavioral 3 12-Step 4 Interpersonal 5 Vocational 6 Psychoeducation 7 Motivational Enhancement 8 Confrontational 9 Continuing Care B Spiritual C Pre/Post-Test Infectious Disease	Z None	Z None	Z None

DRG Non-OR HZ3[Ø,1,2,3,4,5,6,7,8,9,B]ZZZ

H Substance Abuse Treatment
Z None
4 Group Counseling

Definition: The application of psychological methods to treat two or more individuals with addictive behavior
Explanation: Provides structured group counseling sessions and healing power through the connection with others

Qualifier Character 4	Qualifier Character 5	Qualifier Character 6	Qualifier Character 7
Ø Cognitive 1 Behavioral 2 Cognitive-Behavioral 3 12-Step 4 Interpersonal 5 Vocational 6 Psychoeducation 7 Motivational Enhancement 8 Confrontational 9 Continuing Care B Spiritual C Pre/Post-Test Infectious Disease	Z None	Z None	Z None

DRG Non-OR HZ4[Ø,1,2,3,4,5,6,7,8,9,B]ZZZ

H Substance Abuse Treatment
Z None
5 Individual Psychotherapy

Definition: Treatment of an individual with addictive behavior by behavioral, cognitive, psychoanalytic, psychodynamic or psychophysiological means

Qualifier Character 4	Qualifier Character 5	Qualifier Character 6	Qualifier Character 7
Ø Cognitive 1 Behavioral 2 Cognitive-Behavioral 3 12-Step 4 Interpersonal 5 Interactive 6 Psychoeducation 7 Motivational Enhancement 8 Confrontational 9 Supportive B Psychoanalysis C Psychodynamic D Psychophysiological	Z None	Z None	Z None

DRG Non-OR For all qualifier values

H Substance Abuse Treatment
Z None
6 Family Counseling

Definition: The application of psychological methods that includes one or more family members to treat an individual with addictive behavior

Explanation: Provides support and education for family members of addicted individuals. Family member participation is seen as a critical area of substance abuse treatment

Qualifier Character 4	Qualifier Character 5	Qualifier Character 6	Qualifier Character 7
3 Other Family Counseling	Z None	Z None	Z None

H Substance Abuse Treatment
Z None
8 Medication Management

Definition: Monitoring or adjusting the use of replacement medications for the treatment of addiction

Qualifier Character 4	Qualifier Character 5	Qualifier Character 6	Qualifier Character 7
Ø Nicotine Replacement 1 Methadone Maintenance 2 Levo-alpha-acetyl-methadol (LAAM) 3 Antabuse 4 Naltrexone 5 Naloxone 6 Clonidine 7 Bupropion 8 Psychiatric Medication 9 Other Replacement Medication	Z None	Z None	Z None

H Substance Abuse Treatment
Z None
9 Pharmacotherapy

Definition: The use of replacement medications for the treatment of addiction

Qualifier Character 4	Qualifier Character 5	Qualifier Character 6	Qualifier Character 7
Ø Nicotine Replacement 1 Methadone Maintenance 2 Levo-alpha-acetyl-methadol (LAAM) 3 Antabuse 4 Naltrexone 5 Naloxone 6 Clonidine 7 Bupropion 8 Psychiatric Medication 9 Other Replacement Medication	Z None	Z None	Z None

New Technology XØ5–XYØ

AHA Coding Clinic for all tables in the New Technology Section
2015, 4Q, 8-11 New Section X codes - New Technology procedures

AHA Coding Clinic for table XØH
2022, 4Q, 63-64 Implantation of sphenopalatine ganglion stimulator for ischemic stroke
2022, 4Q, 64-65 Implantation of paired vagus nerve stimulator using an external controller

AHA Coding Clinic for table XØZ
2022, 4Q, 65-66 Computer-assisted transcranial magnetic stimulation of the prefrontal cortex

AHA Coding Clinic for table X27
2019, 4Q, 45-46 Sustained released drug-eluting stent

AHA Coding Clinic for table X2A
2022, 4Q, 66 Pressure-controlled intermittent coronary sinus occlusion
2021, 1Q, 16 Placement of Sentinel™ embolic protection device with deployment of single filter
2020, 4Q, 70-71 Cerebral embolic filtration extracorporeal flow reversal circuit
2019, 4Q, 46 Cerebral embolic filtration
2016, 4Q, 115-116 Cerebral embolic filtration

AHA Coding Clinic for table X2C
2021, 4Q, 58-59 Computer-aided mechanical aspiration thrombectomy
2016, 4Q, 82-83 Coronary artery, number of arteries
2015, 4Q, 8-14 New Section X codes—New Technology procedures

AHA Coding Clinic for table X2J
2021, 4Q, 59 Transthoracic echocardiography with computer-aided image acquisition

AHA Coding Clinic for table X2K
2021, 4Q, 60 Percutaneous creation of arteriovenous fistula using thermal resistance energy

AHA Coding Clinic for table X2R
2022, 4Q, 54-55 Rapid deployment technique for replacement of aortic valve using zooplastic tissue
2021, 4Q, 61-62 Replacement combined with restriction of descending thoracic aorta
2016, 4Q, 116 Aortic valve rapid deployment
2015, 4Q, 8-12 New Section X codes—New Technology procedures

AHA Coding Clinic for table X2V
2021, 4Q, 61-62 Replacement combined with restriction of descending thoracic aorta
2021, 4Q, 63 Restriction of coronary sinus

AHA Coding Clinic for table XD2
2021, 4Q, 63-64 Monitoring of tissue oxygen saturation in gastrointestinal tract

AHA Coding Clinic for table XDP
2021, 4Q, 64-65 Colonic irrigation for colonoscopy

AHA Coding Clinic for table XF5
2022, 4Q, 67 Extracorporeal histotripsy of targeted liver tissue using ultrasound-guided cavitation

AHA Coding Clinic for table XFJ
2021, 4Q, 65-66 Single-use duodenoscope during endoscopic retrograde cholangiopancreatography

AHA Coding Clinic for table XHR
2021, 4Q, 66 Application of bioengineered allogeneic construct
2016, 4Q, 116 Application of wound matrix

AHA Coding Clinic for table XKØ
2017, 4Q, 74 Intramuscular autologous bone marrow cell therapy

AHA Coding Clinic for table XKU
2022, 4Q, 67-68 Posterior vertebral body tethering

AHA Coding Clinic for table XNH
2022, 4Q, 69 Internal fixation device with Tulip connector

AHA Coding Clinic for table XNS
2021, 4Q, 67 Posterior dynamic distraction
2017, 4Q, 74-75 Magnetic growth rods
2016, 4Q, 117 Placement of magnetic growth rods

AHA Coding Clinic for table XNU
2020, 4Q, 72 Implantation of vertebral mechanically expandable device

AHA Coding Clinic for table XRG
2022, 4Q, 69 Internal fixation device with Tulip connector
2021, 4Q, 68 Customizable interbody fusion
2017, 4Q, 76 Radiolucent porous interbody fusion device

AHA Coding Clinic for table XRH
2022, 4Q, 70 Insertion of posterior spinal motion preservation device

AHA Coding Clinic for table XRR
2022, 4Q, 70-71 Replacement of synthetic substitute meniscus of knee

AHA Coding Clinic for table XT2
2019, 4Q, 46-47 Renal function monitoring

AHA Coding Clinic for table XV5
2018, 4Q, 55 Robotic waterjet ablation

AHA Coding Clinic for table XWØ
2023, 2Q, 26 Control of bleeding with Hemospray®
2023, 1Q, 12 REGN-COV2 monoclonal antibody
2023, 1Q, 12 Sabizabulin
2022, 4Q, 60-61 Introduction of other therapeutic monoclonal antibody
2022, 4Q, 71-72 Spesolimab monoclonal antibody
2022, 4Q, 72 Daratumumab and hyaluronidase-fihj
2022, 4Q, 72 Maribavir anti-infective
2022, 4Q, 72 Teclistamab antineoplastic
2022, 4Q, 72-73 Mosunetuzumab antineoplatic
2022, 4Q, 73 Afamitresgene autoleucel immunotherapy
2022, 4Q, 73 Tabelecleucel immunotherapy
2022, 4Q, 74 Treosulfan
2022, 4Q, 74 Inebilizumab-cdon
2022, 4Q, 74 Engineered allogeneic thymus tissue
2022, 4Q, 74 Broad consortium microbiota-based live biotherapeutic suspension
2022, 3Q, 26 Tumor-infiltrating lymphocyte therapy
2022, 1Q, 5-6 COVID-19 vaccine administration
2022, 1Q, 7 Fostamatinib
2022, 1Q, 7-8 Tixagevimab and cilgavimab
2022, 1Q, 8 Other monoclonal antibody
2021, 4Q, 69-71 Introduction of new therapeutic substances
2021, 4Q, 71-74 Chimeric antigen receptor T-cell immunotherapy
2021, 4Q, 74-75 Antibiotic-eluting bone void filler
2021, 4Q, 110 New/revised frequently asked questions regarding ICD-10-CM/PCS coding for COVID-19
2021, 1Q, 49 Frequently asked questions regarding ICD-10-CM and ICD-10-PCS coding for COVID-19
2020, 4Q, 72-76 Introduction of new therapeutic substances
2020, 4Q, 95 Frequently asked questions regarding ICD-10-PCS coding for COVID-19
2020, 3Q, 17-21 New procedure codes for introduction or infusion of therapeutics
2019, 4Q, 47-50 New therapeutic substances
2018, 4Q, 56 New therapeutic substances
2015, 4Q, 8-15 New Section X codes—New Technology procedures

AHA Coding Clinic for table XW1
2023, 1Q, 13 Exagamglogene autotemcel
2022, 4Q, 75 Betibeglogene autotemcel
2022, 4Q, 75 Omidubicel
2022, 4Q, 76 OTL-103
2022, 4Q, 76 OTL-200
2021, 4Q, 76 Transfusion of hyperimmune globulin and high-dose immune globulin
2020, 3Q, 17-21 New procedure codes for introduction or infusion of therapeutics

AHA Coding Clinic for table XWH
2021, 4Q, 76-77 Pharyngeal electrical stimulation

AHA Coding Clinic for table XXE
2022, 4Q, 76 Computer-aided analysis for the detection and classification of epileptic events
2022, 4Q, 77 Quantitative flow rate for noninvasive analysis of coronary angiography
2022, 4Q, 77 Simulation for assessment of coronary obstruction risk
2022, 4Q, 78 Gene expression assay
2021, 4Q, 77 Computer-aided assessment of intracranial vascular activity
2021, 4Q, 77-78 Computer-aided triage and notification of pulmonary artery flow
2021, 4Q, 78-79 Mechanical initial specimen diversion of whole blood using active negative pressure
2021, 4Q, 79-80 Concurrent measurement of mRNA, PCR test and detection of antibodies
2020, 4Q, 78-79 Measurement of infection
2020, 4Q, 78-79 Positive blood culture fluorescence hybridization
2020, 4Q, 79 Nucleic acid-base microbial detection
2019, 4Q, 50-51 Whole blood nucleic acid-base microbial detection

AHA Coding Clinic for table XYØ
2022, 4Q, 78 Extracorporeal antimicrobial administration during renal replacement therapy
2021, 4Q, 80 Regional anticoagulation for renal replacement therapy
2017, 4Q, 78 Intraoperative treatment of vascular grafts

X New Technology
Ø Nervous System
5 Destruction

Definition: Physical eradication of all or a portion of a body part by the direct use of energy, force, or a destructive agent
Explanation: None

Body Part Character 4	Approach Character 5	Device/Substance/Technology Character 6	Qualifier Character 7
1 Renal Sympathetic Nerve(s)	3 Percutaneous	2 Ultrasound Ablation	9 New Technology Group 9

X New Technology
Ø Nervous System
H Insertion

Definition: Putting in a nonbiological appliance that monitors, assists, performs, or prevents a physiological function but does not physically take the place of a body part
Explanation: None

Body Part Character 4	Approach Character 5	Device/Substance/Technology Character 6	Qualifier Character 7
K Sphenopalatine Ganglion	3 Percutaneous	Q Neurostimulator Lead	8 New Technology Group 8
Q Vagus Nerve	3 Percutaneous	R Neurostimulator Lead with Paired Stimulation System NT	8 New Technology Group 8

Valid OR All body part, approach, device/substance/technology, and qualifier values
NT XØHQ3R8 for ViviStim® Paired VNS System

See Appendix L for Procedure Combinations
XØHQ3R8

X New Technology
Ø Nervous System
Z Other Procedures

Definition: Methodologies which attempt to remediate or cure a disorder or disease
Explanation: None

Body Part Character 4	Approach Character 5	Device/Substance/Technology Character 6	Qualifier Character 7
Ø Prefrontal Cortex	X External	1 Computer-assisted Transcranial Magnetic Stimulation	8 New Technology Group 8

X New Technology
2 Cardiovascular System
7 Dilation

Definition: Expanding an orifice or the lumen of a tubular body part
Explanation: The orifice can be a natural orifice or an artificially created orifice. Accomplished by stretching a tubular body part using intraluminal pressure or by cutting part of the orifice or wall of the tubular body part.

Body Part Character 4	Approach Character 5	Device/Substance/Technology Character 6	Qualifier Character 7
H Femoral Artery, Right J Femoral Artery, Left K Popliteal Artery, Proximal Right L Popliteal Artery, Proximal Left M Popliteal Artery, Distal Right N Popliteal Artery, Distal Left P Anterior Tibial Artery, Right Q Anterior Tibial Artery, Left R Posterior Tibial Artery, Right S Posterior Tibial Artery, Left T Peroneal Artery, Right U Peroneal Artery, Left	3 Percutaneous	8 Intraluminal Device, Sustained Release Drug-eluting 9 Intraluminal Device, Sustained Release Drug-eluting, Two B Intraluminal Device, Sustained Release Drug-eluting, Three C Intraluminal Device, Sustained Release Drug-eluting, Four or More	5 New Technology Group 5

Valid OR All body part, approach, device/substance/technology, and qualifier values

X New Technology
2 Cardiovascular System
A Assistance

Definition: Taking over a portion of a physiological function by extracorporeal means
Explanation: None

Body Part Character 4	Approach Character 5	Device/Substance/Technology Character 6	Qualifier Character 7
5 Innominate Artery and Left Common Carotid Artery	3 Percutaneous	1 Cerebral Embolic Filtration, Dual Filter	2 New Technology Group 2
6 Aortic Arch	3 Percutaneous	2 Cerebral Embolic Filtration, Single Deflection Filter	5 New Technology Group 5
7 Coronary Sinus	3 Percutaneous	5 Intermittent Coronary Sinus Occlusion	8 New Technology Group 8
H Common Carotid Artery, Right J Common Carotid Artery, Left	3 Percutaneous	3 Cerebral Embolic Filtration, Extracorporeal Flow Reversal Circuit	6 New Technology Group 6

DRG Non-OR X2A7358

X New Technology
2 Cardiovascular System
C Extirpation Definition: Taking or cutting out solid matter from a body part

Explanation: The solid matter may be an abnormal byproduct of a biological function or a foreign body; it may be imbedded in a body part or in the lumen of a tubular body part. The solid matter may or may not have been previously broken into pieces.

Body Part Character 4	Approach Character 5	Device/Substance/Technology Character 6	Qualifier Character 7
P Abdominal Aorta Q Upper Extremity Vein, Right R Upper Extremity Vein, Left S Lower Extremity Artery, Right T Lower Extremity Artery, Left U Lower Extremity Vein, Right V Lower Extremity Vein, Left Y Great Vessel	3 Percutaneous	T Computer-aided Mechanical Aspiration	7 New Technology Group 7

Valid OR All body part, approach, device/substance/technology, and qualifier values

X New Technology
2 Cardiovascular System
H Insertion Definition: Putting in a nonbiological appliance that monitors, assists, performs, or prevents a physiological function but does not physically take the place of a body part

Explanation: None

Body Part Character 4	Approach Character 5	Device/Substance/Technology Character 6	Qualifier Character 7
Ø Inferior Vena Cava 1 Superior Vena Cava	3 Percutaneous	R Intraluminal Device, Bioprosthetic Valve	9 New Technology Group 9
2 Femoral Vein, Right 3 Femoral Vein, Left	Ø Open	R Intraluminal Device, Bioprosthetic Valve	9 New Technology Group 9
6 Atrium, Right K Ventricle, Right	3 Percutaneous	V Intracardiac Pacemaker, Dual-Chamber	9 New Technology Group 9
L Axillary Artery, Right M Axillary Artery, Left X Thoracic Aorta, Ascending	Ø Open	F Conduit to Short-term External Heart Assist System	9 New Technology Group 9

Valid OR X2H13R9

X New Technology
2 Cardiovascular System
J Inspection Definition: Visually and/or manually exploring a body part

Explanation: None

Body Part Character 4	Approach Character 5	Device/Substance/Technology Character 6	Qualifier Character 7
A Heart	X External	4 Transthoracic Echocardiography, Computer-aided Guidance NT	7 New Technology Group 7

NT X2JAX47 for Caption Guidance™

X New Technology
2 Cardiovascular System
K Bypass Definition: Altering the route of passage of the contents of a tubular body part

Explanation: None

Body Part Character 4	Approach Character 5	Device/Substance/Technology Character 6	Qualifier Character 7
B Radial Artery, Right C Radial Artery, Left	3 Percutaneous	1 Thermal Resistance Energy	7 New Technology Group 7
H Femoral Artery, Right J Femoral Artery, Left	3 Percutaneous	D Conduit through Femoral Vein to Superficial Femoral Artery E Conduit through Femoral Vein to Popliteal Artery	9 New Technology Group 9

Valid OR All body part, approach, device/substance/technology, and qualifier values

X New Technology
2 Cardiovascular System
R Replacement Definition: Putting in or on biological or synthetic material that physically takes the place and/or function of all or a portion of a body part

Explanation: None

Body Part Character 4	Approach Character 5	Device/Substance/Technology Character 6	Qualifier Character 7
X Thoracic Aorta, Arch	Ø Open	N Branched Synthetic Substitute with Intraluminal Device NT	7 New Technology Group 7

Valid OR All body part, approach, device/substance/technology, and qualifier values

NT X2RXØN7 with X2VWØN7 for Thoraflex™ Hybrid System

X New Technology
2 Cardiovascular System
U Supplememt Definition: Putting in or on biological or synthetic material that physically reinforces and/or augments the function of a portion of a body part

Explanation: None

Body Part Character 4	Approach Character 5	Device/Substance/Technology Character 6	Qualifier Character 7
4 Coronary Artery/Arteries	Ø Open	7 Vein Graft Extraluminal Support Device(s)	9 New Technology Group 9
Q Upper Extremity Vein, Right R Upper Extremity Vein, Left	Ø Open	P Synthetic Substitute, Extraluminal Support Device	9 New Technology Group 9

Valid OR X2U[Q,R]ØP9

X New Technology
2 Cardiovascular System
V Restriction Definition: Partially closing an orifice or the lumen of a tubular body part

Explanation: None

Body Part Character 4	Approach Character 5	Device/Substance/Technology Character 6	Qualifier Character 7
7 Coronary Sinus	3 Percutaneous	Q Reduction Device	7 New Technology Group 7
W Thoracic Aorta, Descending	Ø Open	N Branched Synthetic Substitute NT with Intraluminal Device	7 New Technology Group 7

Valid OR All body part, approach, device/substance/technology, and qualifier values

NT X2VWØN7 with X2RXØN7 for Thoraflex™ Hybrid System

X New Technology
D Gastrointestinal System
2 Monitoring Definition: Determining the level of a physiological or physical function repetitively over a period of time

Explanation: None

Body Part Character 4	Approach Character 5	Device/Substance/Technology Character 6	Qualifier Character 7
G Upper GI H Lower GI	4 Percutaneous Endoscopic 8 Via Natural or Artificial Opening Endoscopic	V Oxygen Saturation	7 New Technology Group 7

X New Technology
D Gastrointestinal System
P Irrigation Definition: Putting in or on a cleansing substance

Explanation: None

Body Part Character 4	Approach Character 5	Device/Substance/Technology Character 6	Qualifier Character 7
H Lower GI	8 Via Natural or Artificial Opening Endoscopic	K Intraoperative Single-use Oversleeve	7 New Technology Group 7

X New Technology
F Hepatobiliary System and Pancreas
5 Destruction Definition: Physical eradication of all or a portion of a body part by the direct use of energy, force, or a destructive agent

Explanation: None of the body part is physically taken out

Body Part Character 4	Approach Character 5	Device/Substance/Technology Character 6	Qualifier Character 7
Ø Liver 1 Liver, Right Lobe 2 Liver, Left Lobe	X External	Ø Ultrasound-guided Cavitation	8 New Technology Group 8

DRG Non-OR All body part, approach, device/substance/technology, and qualifier values

X New Technology
F Hepatobiliary System and Pancreas
J Inspection Definition: Visually and/or manually exploring a body part

Explanation: None

Body Part Character 4	Approach Character 5	Device/Substance/Technology Character 6	Qualifier Character 7
B Hepatobiliary Duct D Pancreatic Duct	8 Via Natural or Artificial Opening Endoscopic	A Single-use Duodenoscope NT	7 New Technology Group 7

NT XFJ[B,D]8A7 for aScope® Duodeno

X New Technology
H Skin, Subcutaneous Tissue, Fascia and Breast
R Replacement Definition: Putting in or on biological or synthetic material that physically takes the place and/or function of all or a portion of a body part

Explanation: None

Body Part Character 4	Approach Character 5	Device/Substance/Technology Character 6	Qualifier Character 7
P Skin	X External	F Bioengineered Allogeneic NT Construct	7 New Technology Group 7

Valid OR XHRPXF7

NT XHRPXF7 for StrataGraft®

Non-OR Procedure DRG Non-OR Procedure Valid OR Procedure HAC Associated Procedure Combination Only New/Revised April New/Revised October

X New Technology
K Muscles, Tendons, Bursae and Ligaments
U Supplement Definition: Putting in or on biological or synthetic material that physically reinforces and/or augments the function of a portion of a body part
Explanation: None

Body Part Character 4	Approach Character 5	Device/Substance/Technology Character 6	Qualifier Character 7
C Upper Spine Bursa and Ligament D Lower Spine Bursa and Ligament	Ø Open	6 Posterior Vertebral Tether	8 New Technology Group 8

Valid OR All body part, approach, device/substance/technology, and qualifier values

X New Technology
N Bones
H Insertion Definition: Putting in a nonbiological appliance that monitors, assists, performs, or prevents a physiological function but does not physically take the place of a body part
Explanation: None

Body Part Character 4	Approach Character 5	Device/Substance/Technology Character 6	Qualifier Character 7
6 Pelvic Bone, Right 7 Pelvic Bone, Left	Ø Open 3 Percutaneous	5 Internal Fixation Device with Tulip Connector NT	8 New Technology Group 8
G Tibia, Right H Tibia, Left	Ø Open	F Tibial Extension with Motion Sensors	9 New Technology Group 9

Valid OR All body part, approach, device/substance/technology, and qualifier values
NT XNH[6,7][Ø,3]58 for iFuse Bedrock Granite Implant System

X New Technology
N Bones
R Replacement Definition: Putting in or on biological or synthetic material that physically takes the place and/or function of all or a portion of a body part
Explanation: None

Body Part Character 4	Approach Character 5	Device/Substance/Technology Character 6	Qualifier Character 7
8 Skull	Ø Open	D Synthetic Substitute, Ultrasound Penetrable	9 New Technology Group 9
L Tarsal, Right M Tarsal, Left	Ø Open	9 Synthetic Substitute, Talar Prosthesis	9 New Technology Group 9

Valid OR XNR8ØD9

X New Technology
N Bones
S Reposition Definition: Moving to its normal location, or other suitable location, all or a portion of a body part
Explanation: The body part is moved to a new location from an abnormal location, or from a normal location where it is not functioning correctly. The body part may or may not be cut out or off to be moved to the new location.

Body Part Character 4	Approach Character 5	Device/Substance/Technology Character 6	Qualifier Character 7
Ø Lumbar Vertebra	Ø Open	3 Magnetically Controlled Growth Rod(s)	2 New Technology Group 2
Ø Lumbar Vertebra	Ø Open	C Posterior (Dynamic) Distraction Device	7 New Technology Group 7
Ø Lumbar Vertebra	3 Percutaneous	3 Magnetically Controlled Growth Rod(s)	2 New Technology Group 2
Ø Lumbar Vertebra	3 Percutaneous	C Posterior (Dynamic) Distraction Device	7 New Technology Group 7
3 Cervical Vertebra	Ø Open 3 Percutaneous	3 Magnetically Controlled Growth Rod(s)	2 New Technology Group 2
4 Thoracic Vertebra	Ø Open	3 Magnetically Controlled Growth Rod(s)	2 New Technology Group 2
4 Thoracic Vertebra	Ø Open	C Posterior (Dynamic) Distraction Device	7 New Technology Group 7
4 Thoracic Vertebra	3 Percutaneous	3 Magnetically Controlled Growth Rod(s)	2 New Technology Group 2
4 Thoracic Vertebra	3 Percutaneous	C Posterior (Dynamic) Distraction Device	7 New Technology Group 7

Valid OR All body part, approach, device/substance/technology, and qualifier values

X New Technology
N Bones
U Supplement Definition: Putting in or on biological or synthetic material that physically reinforces and/or augments the function of a portion of a body part
Explanation: None

Body Part Character 4	Approach Character 5	Device/Substance/Technology Character 6	Qualifier Character 7
Ø Lumbar Vertebra 4 Thoracic Vertebra	3 Percutaneous	5 Synthetic Substitute, Mechanically Expandable (Paired)	6 New Technology Group 6

Valid OR XNU[Ø,4]356

X New Technology
R Joints
G Fusion

Definition: Joining together portions of an articular body part rendering the articular body part immobile

Explanation: None

Body Part Character 4	Approach Character 5	Device/Substance/Technology Character 6	Qualifier Character 7
A Thoracolumbar Vertebral Joint B Lumbar Vertebral Joint C Lumbar Vertebral Joints, 2 or more D Lumbosacral Joint	Ø Open 3 Percutaneous 4 Percutaneous Endoscopic	R Interbody Fusion Device, Custom-Made Anatomically Designed NT	7 New Technology Group 7
E Sacroiliac Joint, Right F Sacroiliac Joint, Left	Ø Open 3 Percutaneous	5 Internal Fixation Device with Tulip Connector NT	8 New Technology Group 8
J Ankle Joint, Right K Ankle Joint, Left L Tarsal Joint, Right M Tarsal Joint, Left	Ø Open	B Internal Fixation Device, Open-truss Design	9 New Technology Group 9

Valid OR All body part, approach, device/substance/technology, and qualifier values

HAC XRG[A,B,C,D][Ø,3,4]R7 when reported with SDx K68.11 or T81.4Ø-T81.49, T84.6Ø-T84.619, T84.63-T84.7 with 7th character A

HAC XRG[E,F][Ø,3]58 when reported with SDx K68.11 or T81.4Ø-T81.49,T84.6Ø-T84.619, T84.63-T84.7 with 7th character A

NT XRG[A,B,C,D][Ø,3,4]R7 for aprevo® Intervertebral Body Fusion Device

NT XRG[E,F][Ø,3]58 for iFuse Bedrock Granit Implant System

See Appendix L for Procedure Combinations

XRGC[Ø,3,4]R7

X New Technology
R Joints
H Insertion

Definition: Putting in a nonbiological appliance that monitors, assists, performs, or prevents a physiological function but does not physically take the place of a body part

Explanation: None

Body Part Character 4	Approach Character 5	Device/Substance/Technology Character 6	Qualifier Character 7
B Lumbar Vertebral Joint D Lumbosacral Joint	Ø Open	1 Posterior Spinal Motion Preservation Device	8 New Technology Group 8

Valid OR All body part, approach, device/substance/technology, and qualifier values

X New Technology
R Joints
R Replacement

Definition: Putting in or on biological or synthetic material that physically takes the place and/or function of all or a portion of a body part

Explanation: None

Body Part Character 4	Approach Character 5	Device/Substance/Technology Character 6	Qualifier Character 7
G Knee Joint, Right H Knee Joint, Left	Ø Open	L Synthetic Substitute, Lateral Meniscus M Synthetic Substitute, Medial Meniscus	8 New Technology Group 8

Valid OR All body part, approach, device/substance/technology, and qualifier values

HAC XRR[G,H]Ø[L,M]8 when reported with SDx of I26.Ø2-I26.Ø9, I26.92-I26.99, or I82.4Ø1-I82.4Z9

See Appendix L for Procedure Combinations

XRR[G,H]Ø[L,M]8

X New Technology
T Urinary System
2 Monitoring

Definition: Determining the level of a physiological or physical function repetitively over a period of time

Explanation: None

Body Part Character 4	Approach Character 5	Device/Substance/Technology Character 6	Qualifier Character 7
5 Kidney	X External	E Fluorescent Pyrazine	5 New Technology Group 5

X New Technology
W Anatomical Regions
Ø Introduction Definition: Putting in or on a therapeutic, diagnostic, nutritional, physiological, or prophylactic substance except blood or blood products
Explanation: None

Body Part Character 4	Approach Character 5	Device/Substance/Technology Character 6	Qualifier Character 7
Ø Skin	X External	2 Anacaulase-bcdb	7 New Technology Group 7
1 Subcutaneous Tissue	3 Percutaneous	1 Daratumumab and Hyaluronidase-fihj NT 4 Teclistamab Antineoplastic	8 New Technology Group 8
1 Subcutaneous Tissue	3 Percutaneous	9 Satralizumab-mwge	7 New Technology Group 7
1 Subcutaneous Tissue	3 Percutaneous	F Other New Technology Therapeutic Substance	5 New Technology Group 5
1 Subcutaneous Tissue	3 Percutaneous	G REGN-COV2 Monoclonal Antibody H Other New Technology Monoclonal Antibody K Leronlimab Monoclonal Antibody	6 New Technology Group 6
1 Subcutaneous Tissue	3 Percutaneous	L Elranatamab Antineoplastic	9 New Technology Group 9
1 Subcutaneous Tissue	3 Percutaneous	S COVID-19 Vaccine Dose 1	6 New Technology Group 6
1 Subcutaneous Tissue	3 Percutaneous	S Epcoritamab Monoclonal Antibody	9 New Technology Group 9
1 Subcutaneous Tissue	3 Percutaneous	T COVID-19 Vaccine Dose 2 U COVID-19 Vaccine	6 New Technology Group 6
1 Subcutaneous Tissue	3 Percutaneous	V COVID-19 Vaccine Dose 3	7 New Technology Group 7
1 Subcutaneous Tissue	3 Percutaneous	W Caplacizumab	5 New Technology Group 5
1 Subcutaneous Tissue	3 Percutaneous	W COVID-19 Vaccine Booster	7 New Technology Group 7
1 Subcutaneous Tissue	X External	2 Anacaulase-bcdb	7 New Technology Group 7
2 Muscle	Ø Open	D Engineered Allogeneic Thymus Tissue	8 New Technology Group 8
2 Muscle	3 Percutaneous	S COVID-19 Vaccine Dose 1 T COVID-19 Vaccine Dose 2 U COVID-19 Vaccine	6 New Technology Group 6
2 Muscle	3 Percutaneous	V COVID-19 Vaccine Dose 3 W COVID-19 Vaccine Booster X Tixagevimab and Cilgavimab Monoclonal Antibody Y Other New Technology Monoclonal Antibody	7 New Technology Group 7
3 Peripheral Vein	3 Percutaneous	Ø Brexanolone	6 New Technology Group 6
3 Peripheral Vein	3 Percutaneous	Ø Spesolimab Monoclonal Antibody	8 New Technology Group 8
3 Peripheral Vein	3 Percutaneous	2 Nerinitide 3 Durvalumab Antineoplastic	6 New Technology Group 6
3 Peripheral Vein	3 Percutaneous	5 Narsoplimab Monoclonal Antibody	7 New Technology Group 7
3 Peripheral Vein	3 Percutaneous	5 Mosunetuzumab Antineoplastic	8 New Technology Group 8
3 Peripheral Vein	3 Percutaneous	6 Lefamulin Anti-infective	6 New Technology Group 6
3 Peripheral Vein	3 Percutaneous	6 Terlipressin	7 New Technology Group 7
3 Peripheral Vein	3 Percutaneous	6 Afamitresgene Autoleucel Immunotherapy	8 New Technology Group 8
3 Peripheral Vein	3 Percutaneous	7 Coagulation Factor Xa, Inactivated	2 New Technology Group 2
3 Peripheral Vein	3 Percutaneous	7 Trilaciclib NT	7 New Technology Group 7
3 Peripheral Vein	3 Percutaneous	7 Tabelecleucel Immunotherapy	8 New Technology Group 8
3 Peripheral Vein	3 Percutaneous	8 Lurbinectedin NT	7 New Technology Group 7
3 Peripheral Vein	3 Percutaneous	8 Treosulfan	8 New Technology Group 8
3 Peripheral Vein	3 Percutaneous	9 Ceftolozane/Tazobactam Anti-infective	6 New Technology Group 6
3 Peripheral Vein	3 Percutaneous	9 Inebilizumab-cdon	8 New Technology Group 8
3 Peripheral Vein	3 Percutaneous	A Cefiderocol Anti-infective NT	6 New Technology Group 6
3 Peripheral Vein	3 Percutaneous	A Ciltacabtagene Autoleucel NT	7 New Technology Group 7
3 Peripheral Vein	3 Percutaneous	B Cytarabine and Daunorubicin Liposome Antineoplastic	3 New Technology Group 3
3 Peripheral Vein	3 Percutaneous	B Omadacycline Anti-infective	6 New Technology Group 6
3 Peripheral Vein	3 Percutaneous	B Amivantamab Monoclonal Antibody NT	7 New Technology Group 7
3 Peripheral Vein	3 Percutaneous	C Eculizumab	6 New Technology Group 6
3 Peripheral Vein	3 Percutaneous	C Engineered Chimeric Antigen Receptor T-cell Immunotherapy, Autologous	7 New Technology Group 7
3 Peripheral Vein	3 Percutaneous	D Atezolizumab Antineoplastic	6 New Technology Group 6
3 Peripheral Vein	3 Percutaneous	E Remdesivir Anti-infective	5 New Technology Group 5
3 Peripheral Vein	3 Percutaneous	E Etesevimab Monoclonal Antibody	6 New Technology Group 6
3 Peripheral Vein	3 Percutaneous	F Other New Technology Therapeutic Substance	3 New Technology Group 3

Valid OR XWØ2ØD8
DRG Non-OR XWØ3368
DRG Non-OR XWØ3378
DRG Non-OR XWØ33A7
DRG Non-OR XWØ33C7

NT XWØ1318 in combination with code E85.81
NT XWØ3377
NT XWØ3387
NT XWØ33A6 in combination with code Y95 and one of the following: J14, J15.Ø, J15.1, J15.5, J15.6, J15.8, OR code J95.851 and one of the following: B96.1, B96.2Ø, B96.21, B96.22, B96.23, B96.29, B96.3, B96.5, or B96.89
NT XWØ33A7
NT XWØ33B7
* For all codes with NT icon *see* Appendix I for registered or trade name of substance

XWØ Continued on next page

XWØ Continued

X New Technology
W Anatomical Regions
Ø Introduction Definition: Putting in or on a therapeutic, diagnostic, nutritional, physiological, or prophylactic substance except blood or blood products
Explanation: None

Body Part Character 4	Approach Character 5	Device/Substance/Technology Character 6	Qualifier Character 7
3 Peripheral Vein	3 Percutaneous	F Other New Technology Therapeutic Substance	5 New Technology Group 5
3 Peripheral Vein	3 Percutaneous	F Bamlanivimab Monoclonal Antibody	6 New Technology Group 6
3 Peripheral Vein	3 Percutaneous	G Sarilumab	5 New Technology Group 5
3 Peripheral Vein	3 Percutaneous	G REGN-COV2 Monoclonal Antibody	6 New Technology Group 6
3 Peripheral Vein	3 Percutaneous	G Engineered Chimeric Antigen Receptor T-cell Immunotherapy, Allogeneic	7 New Technology Group 7
3 Peripheral Vein	3 Percutaneous	H Tocilizumab	5 New Technology Group 5
3 Peripheral Vein	3 Percutaneous	H Other New Technology Monoclonal Antibody	6 New Technology Group 6
3 Peripheral Vein	3 Percutaneous	H Axicabtagene Ciloleucel Immunotherapy J Tisagenlecleucel Immunotherapy	7 New Technology Group 7
3 Peripheral Vein	3 Percutaneous	K Fosfomycin Anti-infective	5 New Technology Group 5
3 Peripheral Vein	3 Percutaneous	K Idecabtagene Vicleucel Immunotherapy NT	7 New Technology Group 7
3 Peripheral Vein	3 Percutaneous	K Sulbactam-Durlobactam	9 New Technology Group 9
3 Peripheral Vein	3 Percutaneous	L CD24Fc Immunomodulator	6 New Technology Group 6
3 Peripheral Vein	3 Percutaneous	L Lifileucel Immunotherapy M Brexucabtagene Autoleucel Immunotherapy NT	7 New Technology Group 7
3 Peripheral Vein	3 Percutaneous	N Meropenem-vaborbactam Anti-infective	5 New Technology Group 5
3 Peripheral Vein	3 Percutaneous	N Lisocabtagene Maraleucel Immunotherapy	7 New Technology Group 7
3 Peripheral Vein	3 Percutaneous	P Glofitamab Antineoplastic	9 New Technology Group 9
3 Peripheral Vein	3 Percutaneous	Q Tagraxofusp-erzs Antineoplastic	5 New Technology Group 5
3 Peripheral Vein	3 Percutaneous	Q Posoleucel R Rezafungin	9 New Technology Group 9
3 Peripheral Vein	3 Percutaneous	S Iobenguane I-131 Antineoplastic U Imipenem-cilastatin-relebactam Anti-infective NT W Caplacizumab	5 New Technology Group 5
4 Central Vein	3 Percutaneous	Ø Brexanolone	6 New Technology Group 6
4 Central Vein	3 Percutaneous	Ø Spesolimab Monoclonal Antibody	8 New Technology Group 8
4 Central Vein	3 Percutaneous	2 Nerinitide 3 Durvalumab Antineoplastic	6 New Technology Group 6
4 Central Vein	3 Percutaneous	5 Narsoplimab Monoclonal Antibody	7 New Technology Group 7
4 Central Vein	3 Percutaneous	5 Mosunetuzumab Antineoplastic	8 New Technology Group 8
4 Central Vein	3 Percutaneous	6 Lefamulin Anti-infective	6 New Technology Group 6
4 Central Vein	3 Percutaneous	6 Terlipressin	7 New Technology Group 7
4 Central Vein	3 Percutaneous	6 Afamitresgene Autoleucel Immunotherapy	8 New Technology Group 8
4 Central Vein	3 Percutaneous	7 Coagulation Factor Xa, Inactivated	2 New Technology Group 2
4 Central Vein	3 Percutaneous	7 Trilaciclib NT	7 New Technology Group 7
4 Central Vein	3 Percutaneous	7 Tabelecleucel Immunotherapy	8 New Technology Group 8
4 Central Vein	3 Percutaneous	8 Lurbinectedin NT	7 New Technology Group 7
4 Central Vein	3 Percutaneous	8 Treosulfan	8 New Technology Group 8
4 Central Vein	3 Percutaneous	9 Ceftolozane/Tazobactam Anti-infective	6 New Technology Group 6
4 Central Vein	3 Percutaneous	9 Inebilizumab-cdon	8 New Technology Group 8
4 Central Vein	3 Percutaneous	A Cefiderocol Anti-infective NT	6 New Technology Group 6
4 Central Vein	3 Percutaneous	A Ciltacabtagene Autoleucel NT	7 New Technology Group 7
4 Central Vein	3 Percutaneous	B Cytarabine and Daunorubicin Liposome Antineoplastic	3 New Technology Group 3
4 Central Vein	3 Percutaneous	B Omadacycline Anti-infective	6 New Technology Group 6
4 Central Vein	3 Percutaneous	B Amivantamab Monoclonal Antibody NT	7 New Technology Group 7
4 Central Vein	3 Percutaneous	C Eculizumab	6 New Technology Group 6
4 Central Vein	3 Percutaneous	C Engineered Chimeric Antigen Receptor T-cell Immunotherapy, Autologous	7 New Technology Group 7
4 Central Vein	3 Percutaneous	D Atezolizumab Antineoplastic	6 New Technology Group 6

DRG Non-OR XWØ33G7
DRG Non-OR XWØ33[H,J]7
DRG Non-OR XWØ33K7
DRG Non-OR XWØ33[L,M]7
DRG Non-OR XWØ33N7
DRG Non-OR XWØ4368
DRG Non-OR XWØ4378
DRG Non-OR XWØ43A7
DRG Non-OR XWØ43C7

NT XWØ33K7
NT XWØ33M7
NT XWØ33U5 in combination with code Y95 and one of the following: J14, J15.Ø, J15.1, J15.5, J15.6, J15.8, OR code J95.851 and one of the following: B96.1, B96.2Ø, B96.21, B96.22, B96.23, B96.29, B96.3, B96.5, or B96.89
NT XWØ4377
NT XWØ4387
NT XWØ43A6 in combination with code Y95 and one of the following: J14, J15.Ø, J15.1, J15.5, J15.6, J15.8 OR code J95.851 and one of the following: B96.1, B96.2Ø, B96.21, B96.22, B96.23, B96.29, B96.3, B96.5, or B96.89
NT XWØ43A7
NT XWØ43B7

* For all codes with NT icon *see* Appendix I for registered or trade name of substance

XWØ Continued on next page

X New Technology
W Anatomical Regions
Ø Introduction

XWØ Continued

Definition: Putting in or on a therapeutic, diagnostic, nutritional, physiological, or prophylactic substance except blood or blood products
Explanation: None

Body Part Character 4	Approach Character 5	Device/Substance/Technology Character 6	Qualifier Character 7
4 Central Vein	3 Percutaneous	E Remdesivir Anti-infective	5 New Technology Group 5
4 Central Vein	3 Percutaneous	E Etesevimab Monoclonal Antibody	6 New Technology Group 6
4 Central Vein	3 Percutaneous	F Other New Technology Therapeutic Substance	3 New Technology Group 3
4 Central Vein	3 Percutaneous	F Other New Technology Therapeutic Substance	5 New Technology Group 5
4 Central Vein	3 Percutaneous	F Bamlanivimab Monoclonal Antibody	6 New Technology Group 6
4 Central Vein	3 Percutaneous	G Sarilumab	5 New Technology Group 5
4 Central Vein	3 Percutaneous	G REGN-COV2 Monoclonal Antibody	6 New Technology Group 6
4 Central Vein	3 Percutaneous	G Engineered Chimeric Antigen Receptor T-cell Immunotherapy, Allogeneic	7 New Technology Group 7
4 Central Vein	3 Percutaneous	H Tocilizumab	5 New Technology Group 5
4 Central Vein	3 Percutaneous	H Other New Technology Monoclonal Antibody	6 New Technology Group 6
4 Central Vein	3 Percutaneous	H Axicabtagene Ciloleucel Immunotherapy J Tisagenlecleucel Immunotherapy	7 New Technology Group 7
4 Central Vein	3 Percutaneous	K Fosfomycin Anti-infective	5 New Technology Group 5
4 Central Vein	3 Percutaneous	K Idecabtagene Vicleucel Immunotherapy NT	7 New Technology Group 7
4 Central Vein	3 Percutaneous	K Sulbactam-Durlobactam	9 New Technology Group 9
4 Central Vein	3 Percutaneous	L CD24Fc Immunomodulator	6 New Technology Group 6
4 Central Vein	3 Percutaneous	L Lifileucel Immunotherapy M Brexucabtagene Autoleucel Immunotherapy NT	7 New Technology Group 7
4 Central Vein	3 Percutaneous	N Meropenem-vaborbactam Anti-infective	5 New Technology Group 5
4 Central Vein	3 Percutaneous	N Lisocabtagene Maraleucel Immunotherapy	7 New Technology Group 7
4 Central Vein	3 Percutaneous	P Glofitamab Antineoplastic	9 New Technology Group 9
4 Central Vein	3 Percutaneous	Q Tagraxofusp-erzs Antineoplastic	5 New Technology Group 5
4 Central Vein	3 Percutaneous	Q Posoleucel R Rezafungin	9 New Technology Group 9
4 Central Vein	3 Percutaneous	S Iobenguane I-131 Antineoplastic U Imipenem-cilastatin-relebactam Anti-infective NT W Caplacizumab	5 New Technology Group 5
5 Peripheral Artery	3 Percutaneous	T Melphalan Hydrochloride Antineoplastic	9 New Technology Group 9
9 Nose	7 Via Natural or Artificial Opening	M Esketamine Hydrochloride	5 New Technology Group 5
D Mouth and Pharynx	X External	3 Maribavir Anti-infective NT	8 New Technology Group 8
D Mouth and Pharynx	X External	6 Lefamulin Anti-infective	6 New Technology Group 6
D Mouth and Pharynx	X External	8 Uridine Triacetate	2 New Technology Group 2
D Mouth and Pharynx	X External	F Other New Technology Therapeutic Substance J Apalutamide Antineoplastic	5 New Technology Group 5
D Mouth and Pharynx	X External	J Quizartinib Antineoplastic	9 New Technology Group 9
D Mouth and Pharynx	X External	K Sabizabulin	8 New Technology Group 8
D Mouth and Pharynx	X External	L Erdafitinib Antineoplastic	5 New Technology Group 5
D Mouth and Pharynx	X External	M Baricitinib	6 New Technology Group 6
D Mouth and Pharynx	X External	N SER-109	9 New Technology Group 9
D Mouth and Pharynx	X External	R Venetoclax Antineoplastic	5 New Technology Group 5
D Mouth and Pharynx	X External	R Fostamatinib	7 New Technology Group 7
D Mouth and Pharynx	X External	T Ruxolitinib V Gilteritinib Antineoplastic	5 New Technology Group 5
G Upper GI	7 Via Natural or Artificial Opening	3 Maribavir Anti-infective NT K Sabizabulin	8 New Technology Group 8
G Upper GI	7 Via Natural or Artificial Opening	M Baricitinib	6 New Technology Group 6
G Upper GI	7 Via Natural or Artificial Opening	R Fostamatinib	7 New Technology Group 7
G Upper GI	8 Via Natural or Artificial Opening Endoscopic	8 Mineral-based Topical Hemostatic Agent	6 New Technology Group 6

DRG Non-OR XWØ43G7
DRG Non-OR XWØ43[H,J]7
DRG Non-OR XWØ43K7
DRG Non-OR XWØ43[L,M]7
DRG Non-OR XWØ43N7

NT XWØ43K7
NT XWØ43M7
NT XWØ43U5 in combination with code Y95 and one of the following: J14, J15.Ø, J15.1, J15.5, J15.6, J15.8, OR code J95.851 and one of the following: B96.1, B96.2Ø, B96.21, B96.22, B96.23, B96.29, B96.3, B96.5, or B96.89
NT XWØDX38
NT XWØG738

* For all codes with NT icon *see* Appendix I for registered or trade name of substance

XWØ Continued on next page

XWØ Continued

X New Technology
W Anatomical Regions
Ø Introduction Definition: Putting in or on a therapeutic, diagnostic, nutritional, physiological, or prophylactic substance except blood or blood products

Explanation: None

Body Part Character 4	Approach Character 5	Device/Substance/Technology Character 6	Qualifier Character 7
H Lower GI	7 Via Natural or Artificial Opening	3 Maribavir Anti-infective NT K Sabizabulin	8 New Technology Group 8
H Lower GI	7 Via Natural or Artificial Opening	M Baricitinib	6 New Technology Group 6
H Lower GI	7 Via Natural or Artificial Opening	R Fostamatinib	7 New Technology Group 7
H Lower GI	7 Via Natural or Artificial Opening	X Broad Consortium Microbiota-based Live Biotherapeutic Suspension	8 New Technology Group 8
H Lower GI	8 Via Natural or Artificial Opening Endoscopic	8 Mineral-based Topical HemostaticAgent	6 New Technology Group 6
Q Cranial Cavity and Brain	3 Percutaneous	1 Eladocagene exuparvovec	6 New Technology Group 6
V Bones	Ø Open	P Antibiotic-eluting Bone Void Filler NT	7 New Technology Group 7

Valid OR XWØQ316
NT XWØH738
NT XWØVØP7 for Cerament® G

X New Technology
W Anatomical Regions
1 Transfusion Definition: Putting in blood or blood products

Explanation: None

Body Part Character 4	Approach Character 5	Device/Substance/Technology Character 6	Qualifier Character 7
3 Peripheral Vein	3 Percutaneous	2 Plasma, Convalescent (Nonautologous)	5 New Technology Group 5
3 Peripheral Vein	3 Percutaneous	B Betibeglogene Autotemcel C Omidubicel	8 New Technology Group 8
3 Peripheral Vein	3 Percutaneous	D High-Dose Intravenous Immune Globulin E Hyperimmune Globulin	7 New Technology Group 7
3 Peripheral Vein	3 Percutaneous	F OTL-103 G OTL-200	8 New Technology Group 8
3 Peripheral Vein	3 Percutaneous	H Lovotibeglogene Autotemcel	9 New Technology Group 9
3 Peripheral Vein	3 Percutaneous	J Exagamglogene Autotemcel	8 New Technology Group 8
4 Central Vein	3 Percutaneous	2 Plasma, Convalescent (Nonautologous)	5 New Technology Group 5
4 Central Vein	3 Percutaneous	B Betibeglogene Autotemcel C Omidubicel	8 New Technology Group 8
4 Central Vein	3 Percutaneous	D High-Dose Intravenous Immune Globulin E Hyperimmune Globulin	7 New Technology Group 7
4 Central Vein	3 Percutaneous	F OTL-103 G OTL-200	8 New Technology Group 8
4 Central Vein	3 Percutaneous	H Lovotibeglogene Autotemcel	9 New Technology Group 9
4 Central Vein	3 Percutaneous	J Exagamglogene Autotemcel	8 New Technology Group 8

DRG Non-OR XW133[B,C]8
DRG Non-OR XW133[F,G]8
DRG Non-OR XW133H9
DRG Non-OR XW133J8
DRG Non-OR XW143[B,C]8
DRG Non-OR XW143[F,G]8
DRG Non-OR XW143H9
DRG Non-OR XW143J8

X New Technology
W Anatomical Regions
H Insertion Definition: Putting in a nonbiological appliance that monitors, assists, performs, or prevents a physiological function but does not physically take the place of a body part

Explanation: None

Body Part Character 4	Approach Character 5	Device/Substance/Technology Character 6	Qualifier Character 7
D Mouth and Pharynx	7 Via Natural or Artificial Opening	Q Neurostimulator Lead	7 New Technology Group 7

X New Technology
X Physiological Systems
2 Monitoring

Definition: Determining the level of a physiological or physical function repetitively over a period of time

Explanation: None

Body Part Character 4	Approach Character 5	Device/Substance/Technology Character 6	Qualifier Character 7
Ø Central Nervous	X External	8 Brain Electrical Activity, Computer-aided Detection and Notification	9 New Technology Group 9
F Musculoskeletal	3 Percutaneous	W Muscle Compartment Pressure, Micro-Electro-Mechanical System	9 New Technology Group 9

X New Technology
X Physiological Systems
E Measurement

Definition: Determining the level of a physiological or physical function at a point in time

Explanation: None

Body Part Character 4	Approach Character 5	Device/Substance/Technology Character 6	Qualifier Character 7
Ø Central Nervous	X External	Ø Intracranial Vascular Activity, Computer-aided Assessment	7 New Technology Group 7
Ø Central Nervous	X External	4 Brain Electrical Activity, Computer-aided Semiologic Analysis	8 New Technology Group 8
2 Cardiac	X External	1 Output, Computer-aided Assessment	9 New Technology Group 9
3 Arterial	X External	2 Pulmonary Artery Flow, Computer-aided Triage and Notification	7 New Technology Group 7
3 Arterial	X External	5 Coronary Artery Flow, Quantitative Flow Ratio Analysis 6 Coronary Artery Flow, Computer-aided Valve Modeling and Notification	8 New Technology Group 8
5 Circulatory	X External	3 Infection, Whole Blood Reverse Transcription and Quantitative Real-time Polymerase Chain Reaction	8 New Technology Group 8
5 Circulatory	X External	M Infection, Whole Blood Nucleic Acid-base Microbial Detection	5 New Technology Group 5
5 Circulatory	X External	N Infection, Positive Blood Culture Fluorescence Hybridization for Organism Identification, Concentration and Susceptibility	6 New Technology Group 6
5 Circulatory	X External	R Infection, Mechanical Initial Specimen Diversion Technique Using Active Negative Pressure T Intracranial Arterial Flow, Whole Blood mRNA V Infection, Serum/Plasma Nanoparticle Fluorescence SARS-CoV-2 Antibody Detection	7 New Technology Group 7
5 Circulatory	X External	Y Infection, Other Positive Blood/ Isolated Colonies Bimodal Phenotypic Susceptibility Technology	9 New Technology Group 9
9 Nose	7 Via Natural or Artificial Opening	U Infection, Nasopharyngeal Fluid SARS-CoV-2 Polymerase Chain Reaction	7 New Technology Group 7
B Respiratory	X External	Q Infection, Lower Respiratory Fluid Nucleic Acid-base Microbial Detection	6 New Technology Group 6

X New Technology
Y Extracorporeal
Ø Introduction

Definition: Putting in or on a therapeutic, diagnostic, nutritional, physiological, or prophylactic substance except blood or blood products

Explanation: None

Body Part Character 4	Approach Character 5	Device/Substance/Technology Character 6	Qualifier Character 7
V Vein Graft	X External	8 Endothelial Damage Inhibitor	3 New Technology Group 3
Y Extracorporeal	X External	2 Taurolidine Anti-infective and Heparin Anticoagulant NT	8 New Technology Group 8
Y Extracorporeal	X External	3 Nafamostat Anticoagulant	7 New Technology Group 7

NT XYØYX28 for DefenCath™

Appendixes

Appendix A: Components of the Medical and Surgical Approach Definitions

ICD-10-PCS Value	Definition	Access Location	Method	Type of Instrumentation	Example
Open (Ø)	Cutting through the skin or mucous membrane and any other body layers necessary to expose the site of the procedure	Skin or mucous membrane, any other body layers	Cutting	None	Abdominal hysterectomy
Percutaneous (3)	Entry, by puncture or minor incision, of instrumentation through the skin or mucous membrane and any other body layers necessary to reach the site of the procedure	Skin or mucous membrane, any other body layers	Puncture or minor incision	Without visualization	Needle biopsy of liver, Liposuction
Percutaneous endoscopic (4)	Entry, by puncture or minor incision, of instrumentation through the skin or mucous membrane and any other body layers necessary to reach and visualize the site of the procedure	Skin or mucous membrane, any other body layers	Puncture or minor incision	With visualization	Arthroscopy, Laparoscopic cholecystectomy
Via natural or artificial opening (7)	Entry of instrumentation through a natural or artificial external opening to reach the site of the procedure	Natural or artificial external opening	Direct entry	Without visualization	Endotracheal tube insertion, Foley catheter placement
Via natural or artificial opening endoscopic (8)	Entry of instrumentation through a natural or artificial external opening to reach and visualize the site of the procedure	Natural or artificial external opening	Direct entry	With visualization	Sigmoidoscopy, EGD, ERCP
Via natural or artificial opening with percutaneous endoscopic assistance (F)	Entry of instrumentation through a natural or artificial external opening and entry, by puncture or minor incision, of instrumentation through the skin or mucous membrane and any other body layers necessary to aid in the performance of the procedure	Skin or mucous membrane, any other body layers	Direct entry with puncture or minor incision for instrumentation only	With visualization	Laparoscopic-assisted vaginal hysterectomy
External (X)	Procedures performed directly on the skin or mucous membrane and procedures performed indirectly by the application of external force through the skin or mucous membrane	Skin or mucous membrane	Direct or indirect application	None	Closed fracture reduction, Resection of tonsils

The approach comprises three components: the access location, method, and type of instrumentation.

Access location: For procedures performed on an internal body part, the access location specifies the external site through which the site of the procedure is reached. There are two general types of access locations: skin or mucous membranes, and external orifices. Every approach value except external includes one of these two access locations. The skin or mucous membrane can be cut or punctured to reach the procedure site. All open and percutaneous approach values use this access location. The site of a procedure can also be reached through an external opening. External openings can be natural (e.g., mouth) or artificial (e.g., colostomy stoma).

Method: For procedures performed on an internal body part, the method specifies how the external access location is entered. An open method specifies cutting through the skin or mucous membrane and any other intervening body layers necessary to expose the site of the procedure. An instrumentation method specifies the entry of instrumentation through the access location to the internal procedure site. Instrumentation can be introduced by puncture or minor incision, or through an external opening. The puncture or minor incision does not constitute an open approach because it does not expose the site of the procedure. An approach can define multiple methods. For example, Via Natural or Artificial Opening with Percutaneous Endoscopic Assistance includes both the initial entry of instrumentation to reach the site of the procedure, and the placement of additional percutaneous instrumentation into the body part to visualize and assist in the performance of the procedure.

Type of instrumentation: For procedures performed on an internal body part, instrumentation means that specialized equipment is used to perform the procedure. Instrumentation is used in all internal approaches other than the basic open approach. Instrumentation may or may not include the capacity to visualize the procedure site. For example, the instrumentation used to perform a sigmoidoscopy permits the internal site of the procedure to be visualized, while the instrumentation used to perform a needle biopsy of the liver does not. The term "endoscopic" as used in approach values refers to instrumentation that permits a site to be visualized.

Procedures performed directly on the skin or mucous membrane are identified by the external approach (e.g., skin excision). Procedures performed indirectly by the application of external force are also identified by the external approach (e.g., closed reduction of fracture).

Open (Ø)

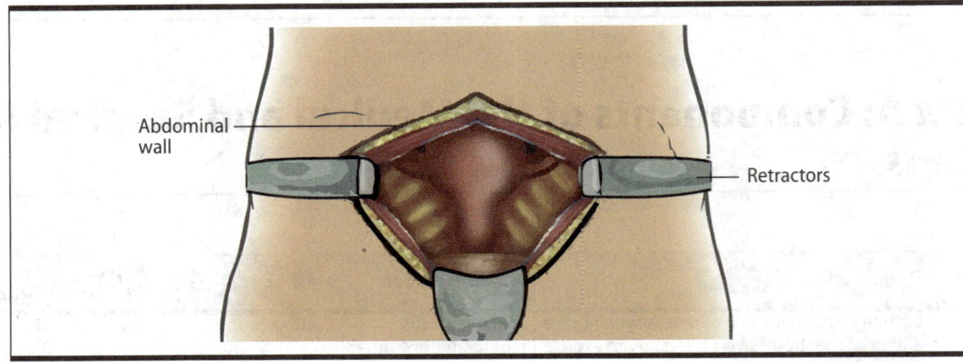

Percutaneous (3)

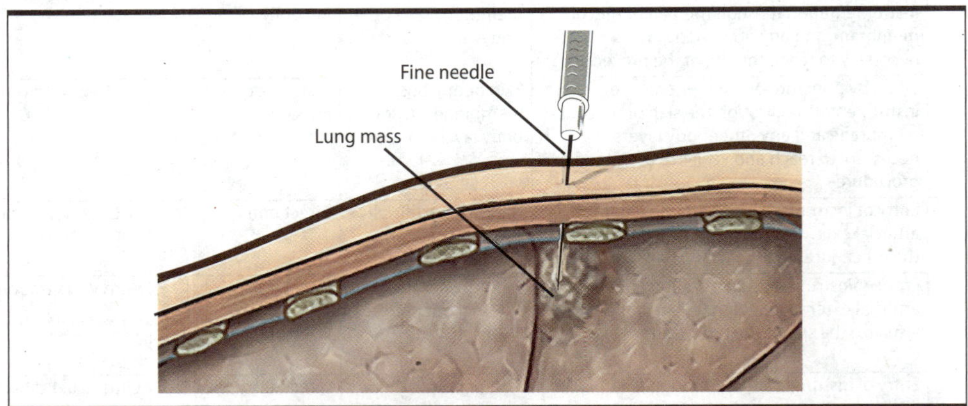

Percutaneous Endoscopic (4)

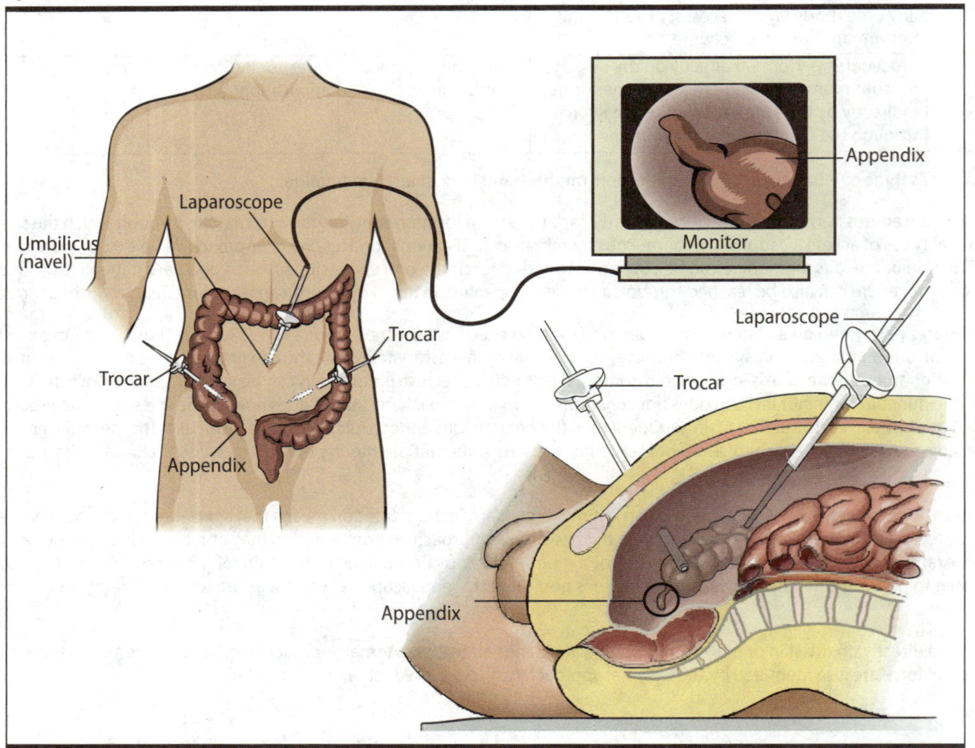

Via Natural or Artificial Opening (7)

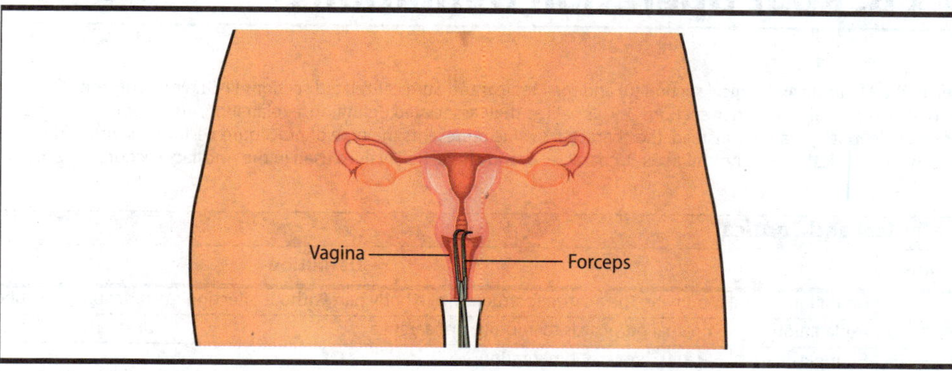

Via Natural or Artificial Opening, Endoscopic (8)

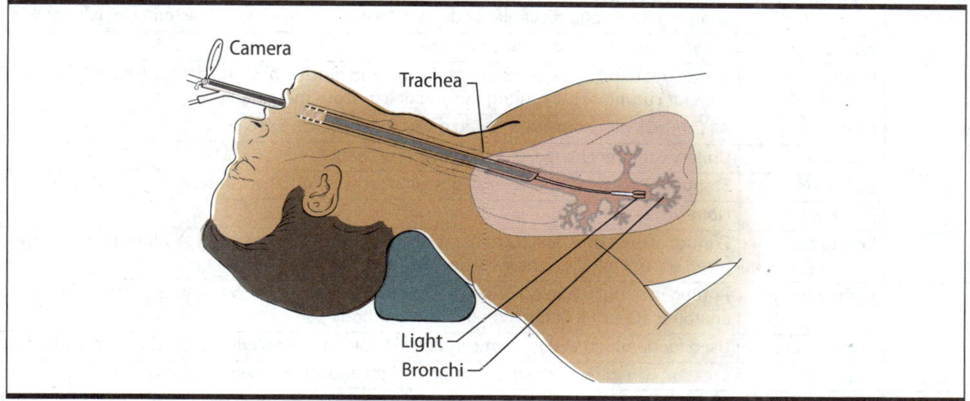

Via Natural or Artificial Opening with Percutaneous Endoscopic Assistance (F)

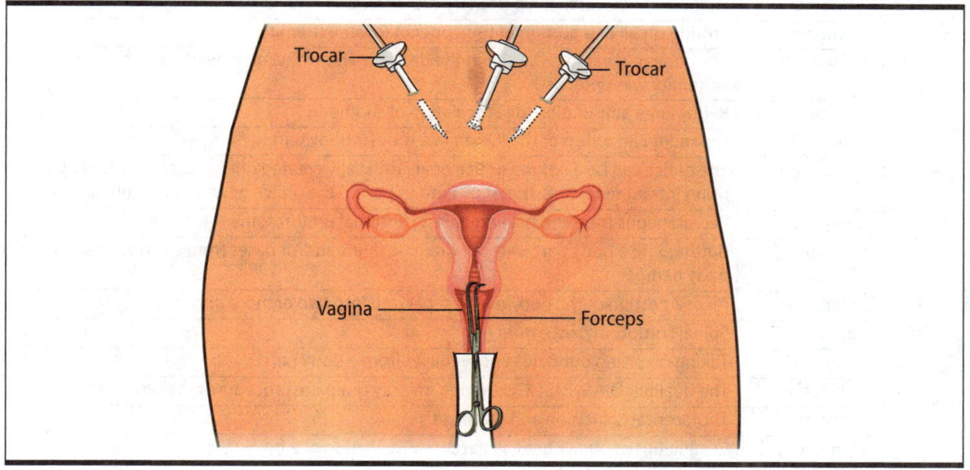

External (X)

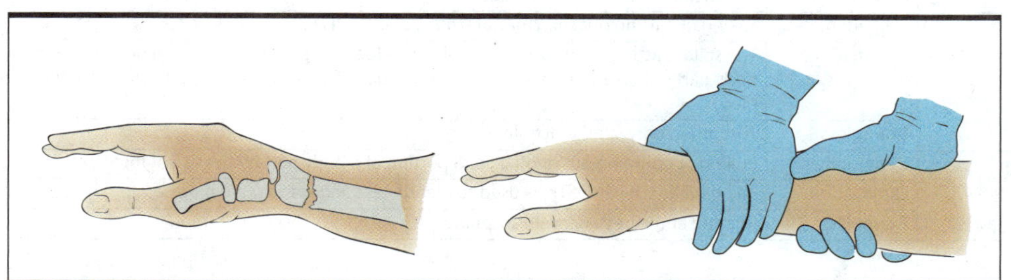

Appendix B: Root Operation Definitions

The character 3 value in the Medical and Surgical section (0) and the Medical and Surgical-related sections (1-9) represents the root operation. This resource provides each root operation (character 3) value, found in sections 0-9, as well as their associated definition, explanation, and examples, where applicable. The Ancillary sections (B-H) do not include root operations; instead, the character 3 value represents the type of procedure performed with additional detail provided by the character 4 or 5 value, when applicable. For the character 3, character 4, and character 5 values used in the Ancillary sections of B-H, along with their definitions, see appendix J.

Ø	Medical and Surgical		
ICD-10-PCS Value		Definition	
Ø	Alteration	Definition:	Modifying the anatomic structure of a body part without affecting the function of the body part
		Explanation:	Principal purpose is to improve appearance
		Examples:	Face lift, breast augmentation
1	Bypass	Definition:	Altering the route of passage of the contents of a tubular body part
		Explanation:	Rerouting contents of a body part to a downstream area of the normal route, to a similar route and body part, or to an abnormal route and dissimilar body part. Includes one or more anastomoses, with or without the use of a device.
		Examples:	Coronary artery bypass, colostomy formation
2	Change	Definition:	Taking out or off a device from a body part and putting back an identical or similar device in or on the same body part without cutting or puncturing the skin or a mucous membrane
		Explanation:	All CHANGE procedures are coded using the approach EXTERNAL
		Examples:	Urinary catheter change, gastrostomy tube change
3	Control	Definition:	Stopping, or attempting to stop, postprocedural or other acute bleeding
		Explanation:	None
		Examples:	Control of post-prostatectomy hemorrhage, control of intracranial subdural hemorrhage, control of bleeding duodenal ulcer, control of retroperitoneal hemorrhage
4	Creation	Definition:	Putting in or on biological or synthetic material to form a new body part that to the extent possible replicates the anatomic structure or function of an absent body part
		Explanation:	Used for gender reassignment surgery and corrective procedures in individuals with congenital anomalies
		Examples:	Creation of vagina in a male, creation of right and left atrioventricular valve from common atrioventricular valve
5	Destruction	Definition:	Physical eradication of all or a portion of a body part by the direct use of energy, force, or a destructive agent
		Explanation:	None of the body part is physically taken out
		Examples:	Fulguration of rectal polyp, cautery of skin lesion
6	Detachment	Definition:	Cutting off all or a portion of the upper or lower extremities
		Explanation:	The body part value is the site of the detachment, with a qualifier if applicable to further specify the level where the extremity was detached
		Examples:	Below knee amputation, disarticulation of shoulder
7	Dilation	Definition:	Expanding an orifice or the lumen of a tubular body part
		Explanation:	The orifice can be a natural orifice or an artificially created orifice. Accomplished by stretching a tubular body part using intraluminal pressure or by cutting part of the orifice or wall of the tubular body part.
		Examples:	Percutaneous transluminal angioplasty, internal urethrotomy
8	Division	Definition:	Cutting into a body part, without draining fluids and/or gases from the body part, in order to separate or transect a body part
		Explanation:	All or a portion of the body part is separated into two or more portions
		Examples:	Spinal cordotomy, osteotomy
9	Drainage	Definition:	Taking or letting out fluids and/or gases from a body part
		Explanation:	The qualifier DIAGNOSTIC is used to identify drainage procedures that are biopsies
		Examples:	Thoracentesis, incision and drainage
B	Excision	Definition:	Cutting out or off, without replacement, a portion of a body part
		Explanation:	The qualifier DIAGNOSTIC is used to identify excision procedures that are biopsies
		Examples:	Partial nephrectomy, liver biopsy
C	Extirpation	Definition:	Taking or cutting out solid matter from a body part
		Explanation:	The solid matter may be an abnormal byproduct of a biological function or a foreign body; it may be imbedded in a body part or in the lumen of a tubular body part. The solid matter may or may not have been previously broken into pieces.
		Examples:	Thrombectomy, choledocholithotomy
D	Extraction	Definition:	Pulling or stripping out or off all or a portion of a body part by the use of force
		Explanation:	The qualifier DIAGNOSTIC is used to identify extractions that are biopsies
		Examples:	Dilation and curettage, vein stripping

Continued on next page

Ø	Medical and Surgical		*Continued from previous page*
ICD-10-PCS Value		**Definition**	
F	Fragmentation	Definition:	Breaking solid matter in a body part into pieces
		Explanation:	Physical force (e.g., manual, ultrasonic) applied directly or indirectly is used to break the solid matter into pieces. The solid matter may be an abnormal byproduct of a biological function or a foreign body. The pieces of solid matter are not taken out.
		Examples:	Extracorporeal shockwave lithotripsy, transurethral lithotripsy
G	Fusion	Definition:	Joining together portions of an articular body part rendering the articular body part immobile
		Explanation:	The body part is joined together by fixation device, bone graft, or other means
		Examples:	Spinal fusion, ankle arthrodesis
H	Insertion	Definition:	Putting in a nonbiological appliance that monitors, assists, performs, or prevents a physiological function but does not physically take the place of a body part
		Explanation:	None
		Examples:	Insertion of radioactive implant, insertion of central venous catheter
J	Inspection	Definition:	Visually and/or manually exploring a body part
		Explanation:	Visual exploration may be performed with or without optical instrumentation. Manual exploration may be performed directly or through intervening body layers.
		Examples:	Diagnostic arthroscopy, exploratory laparotomy
K	Map	Definition:	Locating the route of passage of electrical impulses and/or locating functional areas in a body part
		Explanation:	Applicable only to the cardiac conduction mechanism and the central nervous system
		Examples:	Cardiac mapping, cortical mapping
L	Occlusion	Definition:	Completely closing an orifice or lumen of a tubular body part
		Explanation:	The orifice can be a natural orifice or an artificially created orifice
		Examples:	Fallopian tube ligation, ligation of inferior vena cava
M	Reattachment	Definition:	Putting back in or on all or a portion of a separated body part to its normal location or other suitable location
		Explanation:	Vascular circulation and nervous pathways may or may not be reestablished
		Examples:	Reattachment of hand, reattachment of avulsed kidney
N	Release	Definition:	Freeing a body part from an abnormal physical constraint by cutting or by use of force
		Explanation:	Some of the restraining tissue may be taken out but none of the body part is taken out
		Examples:	Adhesiolysis, carpal tunnel release
P	Removal	Definition:	Taking out or off a device from a body part
		Explanation:	If a device is taken out and a similar device put in without cutting or puncturing the skin or mucous membrane, the procedure is coded to the root operation CHANGE. Otherwise, the procedure for taking out a device is coded to the root operation REMOVAL.
		Examples:	Drainage tube removal, cardiac pacemaker removal
Q	Repair	Definition:	Restoring, to the extent possible, a body part to its normal anatomic structure and function
		Explanation:	Used only when the method to accomplish the repair is not one of the other root operations
		Examples:	Colostomy takedown, suture of laceration
R	Replacement	Definition:	Putting in or on biological or synthetic material that physically takes the place and/or function of all or a portion of a body part
		Explanation:	The body part may have been taken out or replaced, or may be taken out, physically eradicated, or rendered nonfunctional during the REPLACEMENT procedure. A REMOVAL procedure is coded for taking out the device used in a previous replacement procedure.
		Examples:	Total hip replacement, bone graft, free skin graft
S	Reposition	Definition:	Moving to its normal location, or other suitable location, all or a portion of a body part
		Explanation:	The body part is moved to a new location from an abnormal location, or from a normal location where it is not functioning correctly. The body part may or may not be cut out or off to be moved to the new location.
		Examples:	Reposition of undescended testicle, fracture reduction
T	Resection	Definition:	Cutting out or off, without replacement, all of a body part
		Explanation:	None
		Examples:	Total nephrectomy, total lobectomy of lung
V	Restriction	Definition:	Partially closing an orifice or the lumen of a tubular body part
		Explanation:	The orifice can be a natural orifice or an artificially created orifice
		Examples:	Esophagogastric fundoplication, cervical cerclage
W	Revision	Definition:	Correcting, to the extent possible, a portion of a malfunctioning device or the position of a displaced device
		Explanation:	Revision can include correcting a malfunctioning or displaced device by taking out or putting in components of the device such as a screw or pin
		Examples:	Adjustment of position of pacemaker lead, recementing of hip prosthesis

Continued on next page

Ø	Medical and Surgical		*Continued from previous page*
ICD-10-PCS Value		**Definition**	
U	Supplement	Definition:	Putting in or on biological or synthetic material that physically reinforces and/or augments the function of a portion of a body part
		Explanation:	The biological material is non-living, or is living and from the same individual. The body part may have been previously replaced, and the SUPPLEMENT procedure is performed to physically reinforce and/or augment the function of the replaced body part.
		Examples:	Herniorrhaphy using mesh, mitral valve ring annuloplasty, put a new acetabular liner in a previous hip replacement
X	Transfer	Definition:	Moving, without taking out, all or a portion of a body part to another location to take over the function of all or a portion of a body part
		Explanation:	The body part transferred remains connected to its vascular and nervous supply
		Examples:	Tendon transfer, skin pedicle flap transfer
Y	Transplantation	Definition:	Putting in or on all or a portion of a living body part taken from another individual or animal to physically take the place and/or function of all or a portion of a similar body part
		Explanation:	The native body part may or may not be taken out, and the transplanted body part may take over all or a portion of its function
		Examples:	Kidney transplant, heart transplant

Root Operation Definitions for Other Sections

1	Obstetrics		
ICD-10-PCS Value		**Definition**	
2	Change	Definition:	Taking out or off a device from a body part and putting back an identical or similar device in or on the same body part without cutting or puncturing the skin or a mucous membrane
		Explanation:	None
		Example:	Replacement of fetal scalp electrode
9	Drainage	Definition:	Taking or letting out fluids and/or gases from a body part
		Explanation:	None
		Example:	Biopsy of amniotic fluid
A	Abortion	Definition:	Artificially terminating a pregnancy
		Explanation:	None
		Example:	Transvaginal abortion using vacuum aspiration technique
D	Extraction	Definition:	Pulling or stripping out or off all or a portion of a body part by the use of force
		Explanation:	None
		Example:	Low-transverse C-section
E	Delivery	Definition:	Assisting the passage of the products of conception from the genital canal
		Explanation:	None
		Example:	Manually-assisted delivery
H	Insertion	Definition:	Putting in a nonbiological appliance that monitors, assists, performs, or prevents a physiological function but does not physically take the place of a body part
		Explanation:	None
		Example:	Placement of fetal scalp electrode
J	Inspection	Definition:	Visually and/or manually exploring a body part
		Explanation:	Visual exploration may be performed with or without optical instrumentation. Manual exploration may be performed directly or through intervening body layers.
		Example:	Bimanual pregnancy exam
P	Removal	Definition:	Taking out or off a device from a body part, region or orifice
		Explanation:	If a device is taken out and a similar device put in without cutting or puncturing the skin or mucous membrane, the procedure is coded to the root operation CHANGE. Otherwise, the procedure for taking out a device is coded to the root operation REMOVAL.
		Example:	Removal of fetal monitoring electrode
Q	Repair	Definition:	Restoring, to the extent possible, a body part to its normal anatomic structure and function
		Explanation:	Used only when the method to accomplish the repair is not one of the other root operations
		Example:	In utero repair of congenital diaphragmatic hernia
S	Reposition	Definition:	Moving to its normal location, or other suitable location, all or a portion of a body part
		Explanation:	The body part is moved to a new location from an abnormal location, or from a normal location where it is not functioning correctly. The body part may or may not be cut out or off to be moved to the new location.
		Example:	External version of fetus
T	Resection	Definition:	Cutting out or off, without replacement, all of a body part
		Explanation:	None
		Example:	Total excision of tubal pregnancy

Continued on next page

1 Obstetrics

Continued from previous page

ICD-10-PCS Value		Definition	
Y	Transplantation	Definition:	Putting in or on all or a portion of a living body part taken from another individual or animal to physically take the place and/or function of all or a portion of a similar body part
		Explanation:	The native body part may or may not be taken out, and the transplanted body part may take over all or a portion of its function
		Example:	In utero fetal kidney transplant

2 Placement

ICD-10-PCS Value		Definition	
Ø	Change	Definition:	Taking out or off a device from a body part and putting back an identical or similar device in or on the same body part without cutting or puncturing the skin or a mucous membrane
		Example:	Change of vaginal packing
1	Compression	Definition:	Putting pressure on a body region
		Example:	Placement of pressure dressing on abdominal wall
2	Dressing	Definition:	Putting material on a body region for protection
		Example:	Application of sterile dressing to head wound
3	Immobilization	Definition:	Limiting or preventing motion of a body region
		Example:	Placement of splint on left finger
4	Packing	Definition:	Putting material in a body region or orifice
		Example:	Placement of nasal packing
5	Removal	Definition:	Taking out or off a device from a body part
		Example:	Removal of stereotactic head frame
6	Traction	Definition:	Exerting a pulling force on a body region in a distal direction
		Example:	Lumbar traction using motorized split-traction table

3 Administration

ICD-10-PCS Value		Definition	
Ø	Introduction	Definition:	Putting in or on a therapeutic, diagnostic, nutritional, physiological, or prophylactic substance except blood or blood products
		Example:	Nerve block injection to median nerve
1	Irrigation	Definition:	Putting in or on a cleansing substance
		Example:	Flushing of eye
2	Transfusion	Definition:	Putting in blood or blood products
		Example:	Transfusion of cell saver red cells into central venous line

4 Measurement and Monitoring

ICD-10-PCS Value		Definition	
Ø	Measurement	Definition:	Determining the level of a physiological or physical function at a point in time
		Example:	External electrocardiogram(EKG), single reading
1	Monitoring	Definition:	Determining the level of a physiological or physical function repetitively over a period of time
		Example:	Urinary pressure monitoring

5 Extracorporeal or Systemic Assistance and Performance

ICD-10-PCS Value		Definition	
Ø	Assistance	Definition:	Taking over a portion of a physiological function by extracorporeal means
		Example:	Hyperbaric oxygenation of wound
1	Performance	Definition:	Completely taking over a physiological function by extracorporeal means
		Example:	Cardiopulmonary bypass in conjunction with CABG
2	Restoration	Definition:	Returning, or attempting to return, a physiological function to its original state by extracorporeal means
		Example:	Attempted cardiac defibrillation, unsuccessful

6	Extracorporeal or Systemic Therapies		
ICD-10-PCS Value		Definition	
Ø	Atmospheric Control	Definition:	Extracorporeal control of atmospheric pressure and composition
		Example:	Antigen-free air conditioning, series treatment
1	Decompression	Definition:	Extracorporeal elimination of undissolved gas from body fluids
		Example:	Hyperbaric decompression treatment, single
2	Electromagnetic Therapy	Definition:	Extracorporeal treatment by electromagnetic rays
		Example:	TMS (transcranial magnetic stimulation), series treatment
3	Hyperthermia	Definition:	Extracorporeal raising of body temperature
		Example:	None
4	Hypothermia	Definition:	Extracorporeal lowering of body temperature
		Example:	Whole body hypothermia treatment for temperature imbalances, series
5	Pheresis	Definition:	Extracorporeal separation of blood products
		Example:	Therapeutic leukopheresis, single treatment
6	Phototherapy	Definition:	Extracorporeal treatment by light rays
		Example:	Phototherapy of circulatory system, series treatment
7	Ultrasound Therapy	Definition:	Extracorporeal treatment by ultrasound
		Example:	Therapeutic ultrasound of peripheral vessels, single treatment
8	Ultraviolet Light Therapy	Definition:	Extracorporeal treatment by ultraviolet light
		Example:	Ultraviolet light phototherapy, series treatment
9	Shock Wave Therapy	Definition:	Extracorporeal treatment by shock waves
		Example:	Shockwave therapy of plantar fascia, single treatment
B	Perfusion	Definition:	Extracorporeal treatment by diffusion of therapeutic fluid
		Example:	Perfusion of donor liver while preparing transplant patient

7	Osteopathic		
ICD-10-PCS Value		Definition	
Ø	Treatment	Definition:	Manual treatment to eliminate or alleviate somatic dysfunction and related disorders
		Examples:	Fascial release of abdomen, osteopathic treatment

8	Other Procedures		
ICD-10-PCS Value		Definition	
Ø	Other Procedures	Definition:	Methodologies which attempt to remediate or cure a disorder or disease
		Examples:	Acupuncture, yoga therapy

9	Chiropractic		
ICD-10-PCS Value		Definition	
B	Manipulation	Definition:	Manual procedure that involves a directed thrust to move a joint past the physiological range of motion, without exceeding the anatomical limit
		Example:	Chiropractic treatment of cervical spine, short lever specific contact

Appendix C: Comparison of Medical and Surgical Root Operations

Note: The character associated with each operation appears in parentheses after its title.

Procedures That Take Out Some or All of a Body Part

Root Operation	Objective of Procedure	Site of Procedure	Example
Destruction (5)	Eradicating without taking out or replacement	Some/all of a body part	Fulguration of endometrium
Detachment (6)	Cutting out/off without replacement	Extremity only, any level	Amputation above elbow
Excision (B)	Cutting out/off without replacement	Some of a body part	Breast lumpectomy
Extraction (D)	Pulling out/off without replacement	Some/all of a body part	Suction D&C
Resection (T)	Cutting out/off without replacement	All of a body part	Total mastectomy

Procedures That Put In/Put Back or Move Some/All of a Body Part

Root Operation	Objective of Procedure	Site of Procedure	Example
Reattachment (M)	Putting back a detached body part	Some/all of a body part	Reattach finger
Reposition (S)	Moving a body part to normal or other suitable location	Some/all of a body part	Move undescended testicle
Transfer (X)	Moving a body part to function for a similar body part	Some/all of a body part	Skin pedicle transfer flap
Transplantation (Y)	Putting in a living body part from a person/animal	Some/all of a body part	Kidney transplant

Procedures That Take Out or Eliminate Solid Matter, Fluids, or Gases From a Body Part

Root Operation	Objective of Procedure	Site of Procedure	Example
Drainage (9)	Taking or letting out	Fluids and/or gases from a body part	Incision and drainage
Extirpation (C)	Taking or cutting out	Solid matter in a body part	Thrombectomy
Fragmentation (F)	Breaking into pieces	Solid matter within a body part	Lithotripsy

Procedures That Involve Only Examination of Body Parts and Regions

Root Operation	Objective of Procedure	Site of Procedure	Example
Inspection (J)	Visual/manual exploration	Some/all of a body part	Diagnostic cystoscopy Exploratory laparoscopy
Map (K)	Locating electrical impulse route/functional areas	Brain/cardiac conduction mechanism	Cardiac mapping

Procedures That Alter the Diameter/Route of a Tubular Body Part

Root Operation	Objective of Procedure	Site of Procedure	Example
Bypass (1)	Altering route of passage of contents	Tubular body part	Coronary artery bypass graft (CABG)
Dilation (7)	Expanding natural or artificially created orifice/lumen	Tubular body part	Percutaneous transluminal coronary angioplasty (PTCA)
Occlusion (L)	Completely closing natural or artificially created orifice/lumen	Tubular body part	Fallopian tube ligation
Restriction (V)	Partially closing natural or artificially created orifice/lumen	Tubular body part	Gastroesophageal fundoplication

Procedures That Always Involve Devices

Root Operation	Objective of Procedure	Site of Procedure	Example
Change (2) DVC	Exchanging device w/out cutting/puncturing	In/on a body part	Gastrostomy tube change
Insertion (H) DVC	Putting in nonbiological device	In/on a body part	Central line insertion
Removal (P) DVC	Taking out device	In/on a body part	Central line removal
Replacement (R) DVC	Putting in device that replaces a body part	Some/all of a body part	Total hip replacement
Revision (W) DVC	Correcting a malfunctioning/displaced device	In/on a body part	Revision of pacemaker
Supplement (U) DVC	Putting in device that reinforces or augments a body part	In/on a body part	Abdominal wall herniorrhaphy using mesh

DVC = Device involved in root operation

Procedures Involving Cutting or Separation Only

Root Operation	Objective of Procedure	Site of Procedure	Example
Division (8)	Cutting into/separating	A body part	Neurotomy
Release (N)	Freeing a body part from constraint	Around a body part	Adhesiolysis

Procedures That Define Other Repairs

Root Operation	Objective of Procedure	Site of Procedure	Example
Control (3)	Stopping/attempting to stop postprocedural or other acute bleeding	Anatomical region or nasal mucosa/soft tissue	Post-prostatectomy bleeding control, control subdural hemorrhage, bleeding ulcer, retroperitoneal hemorrhage
Repair (Q)	Restoring body part to its normal structure/function	Some/all of a body part	Suture laceration

Procedures That Define Other Objectives

Root Operation	Objective of Procedure	Site of Procedure	Example
Alteration (Ø)	Modifying body part for cosmetic purposes without affecting function	Some/all of a body part	Face lift
Creation (4)	Using biological or synthetic material to form a new body part that replicates the anatomic structure or function of a missing body part	Perineum, valve	Sex change/artificial vagina/penis, atrioventricular valve creation
Fusion (G)	Unification or immobilization	Joint or articular body part	Spinal fusion

Appendix C: Comparison of Medical and Surgical Root Operations

Appendix D: Body Part Key

Term	ICD-10-PCS Value
Abdominal aortic plexus	Abdominal Sympathetic Nerve
Abdominal cavity	Peritoneal Cavity
Abdominal esophagus	Esophagus, Lower
Abductor hallucis muscle	Foot Muscle, Right
	Foot Muscle, Left
Accessory cephalic vein	Cephalic Vein, Right
	Cephalic Vein, Left
Accessory obturator nerve	Lumbar Plexus
Accessory phrenic nerve	Phrenic nerve
Accessory spleen	Spleen
Acetabulofemoral joint	Hip Joint, Right
	Hip Joint, Left
Achilles tendon	Lower Leg Tendon, Right
	Lower Leg Tendon, Left
Acromioclavicular ligament	Shoulder Bursa and Ligament, Right
	Shoulder Bursa and Ligament, Left
Acromion (process)	Scapula, Right
	Scapula, Left
Adductor brevis muscle	Upper Leg Muscle, Right
	Upper Leg Muscle, Left
Adductor hallucis muscle	Foot Muscle, Right
	Foot Muscle, Left
Adductor longus muscle	Upper Leg Muscle, Right
	Upper Leg Muscle, Left
Adductor magnus muscle	Upper Leg Muscle, Right
	Upper Leg Muscle, Left
Adenohypophysis	Pituitary Gland
Alar ligament of axis	Head and Neck Bursa and Ligament
Alveolar process of mandible	Mandible, Right
	Mandible, Left
Alveolar process of maxilla	Maxilla
Anal orifice	Anus
Anatomical snuffbox	Lower Arm and Wrist Muscle, Right
	Lower Arm and Wrist Muscle, Left
Angular artery	Face Artery
Angular vein	Face Vein, Right
	Face Vein, Left
Annular ligament	Elbow Bursa and Ligament, Right
	Elbow Bursa and Ligament, Left
Anorectal junction	Rectum
Ansa cervicalis	Cervical Plexus
Antebrachial fascia	Subcutaneous Tissue and Fascia, Right Lower Arm
	Subcutaneous Tissue and Fascia, Left Lower Arm
Anterior (pectoral) lymph node	Lymphatic, Right Axillary
	Lymphatic, Left Axillary
Anterior cerebral artery	Intracranial Artery
Anterior cerebral vein	Intracranial Vein
Anterior choroidal artery	Intracranial Artery
Anterior circumflex humeral artery	Axillary Artery, Right
	Axillary Artery, Left
Anterior communicating artery	Intracranial Artery
Anterior cruciate ligament (ACL)	Knee Bursa and Ligament, Right
	Knee Bursa and Ligament, Left
Anterior crural nerve	Femoral Nerve

Term	ICD-10-PCS Value
Anterior facial vein	Face Vein, Right
	Face Vein, Left
Anterior intercostal artery	Internal Mammary Artery, Right
	Internal Mammary Artery, Left
Anterior interosseous nerve	Median Nerve
Anterior lateral malleolar artery	Anterior Tibial Artery, Right
	Anterior Tibial Artery, Left
Anterior lingual gland	Minor Salivary Gland
Anterior medial malleolar artery	Anterior Tibial Artery, Right
	Anterior Tibial Artery, Left
Anterior spinal artery	Vertebral Artery, Right
	Vertebral Artery, Left
Anterior tibial recurrent artery	Anterior Tibial Artery, Right
	Anterior Tibial Artery, Left
Anterior ulnar recurrent artery	Ulnar Artery, Right
	Ulnar Artery, Left
Anterior vagal trunk	Vagus Nerve
Anterior vertebral muscle	Neck Muscle, Right
	Neck Muscle, Left
Antihelix	External Ear, Right
	External Ear, Left
	External Ear, Bilateral
Antitragus	External Ear, Right
	External Ear, Left
	External Ear, Bilateral
Antrum of Highmore	Maxillary Sinus, Right
	Maxillary Sinus, Left
Aortic annulus	Aortic Valve
Aortic arch	Thoracic Aorta, Ascending/Arch
Aortic intercostal artery	Upper Artery
Apical (subclavicular) lymph node	Lymphatic, Right Axillary
	Lymphatic, Left Axillary
Apneustic center	Pons
Appendiceal orifice	Appendix
Aqueduct of Sylvius	Cerebral Ventricle
Aqueous humour	Anterior Chamber, Right
	Anterior Chamber, Left
Arachnoid mater, intracranial	Cerebral Meninges
Arachnoid mater, spinal	Spinal Meninges
Arcuate artery	Foot Artery, Right
	Foot Artery, Left
Areola	Nipple, Right
	Nipple, Left
Arterial canal (duct)	Pulmonary Artery, Left
Aryepiglottic fold	Larynx
Arytenoid cartilage	Larynx
Arytenoid muscle	Neck Muscle, Right
	Neck Muscle, Left
Ascending aorta	Thoracic Aorta, Ascending/Arch
Ascending palatine artery	Face Artery
Ascending pharyngeal artery	External Carotid Artery, Right
	External Carotid Artery, Left
Atlantoaxial joint	Cervical Vertebral Joint
Atrioventricular node	Conduction Mechanism
Atrium dextrum cordis	Atrium, Right
Atrium pulmonale	Atrium, Left

Term	ICD-10-PCS Value
Auditory tube	Eustachian Tube, Right
	Eustachian Tube, Left
Auerbach's (myenteric) plexus	Abdominal Sympathetic Nerve
Auricle	External Ear, Right
	External Ear, Left
	External Ear, Bilateral
Auricularis muscle	Head Muscle
Axillary fascia	Subcutaneous Tissue and Fascia, Right Upper Arm
	Subcutaneous Tissue and Fascia, Left Upper Arm
Axillary nerve	Brachial Plexus
Bartholin's (greater vestibular) gland	Vestibular Gland
Basal (internal) cerebral vein	Intracranial Vein
Basal nuclei	Basal Ganglia
Base of tongue	Pharynx
Basilar artery	Intracranial Artery
Basis pontis	Pons
Biceps brachii muscle	Upper Arm Muscle, Right
	Upper Arm Muscle, Left
Biceps femoris muscle	Upper Leg Muscle, Right
	Upper Leg Muscle, Left
Bicipital aponeurosis	Subcutaneous Tissue and Fascia, Right Lower Arm
	Subcutaneous Tissue and Fascia, Left Lower Arm
Bicuspid valve	Mitral Valve
Body of femur	Femoral Shaft, Right
	Femoral Shaft, Left
Body of fibula	Fibula, Right
	Fibula, Left
Bony labyrinth	Inner Ear, Right
	Inner Ear, Left
Bony orbit	Orbit, Right
	Orbit, Left
Bony vestibule	Inner Ear, Right
	Inner Ear, Left
Botallo's duct	Pulmonary Artery, Left
Brachial (lateral) lymph node	Lymphatic, Right Axillary
	Lymphatic, Left Axillary
Brachialis muscle	Upper Arm Muscle, Right
	Upper Arm Muscle, Left
Brachiocephalic artery	Innominate Artery
Brachiocephalic trunk	Innominate Artery
Brachiocephalic vein	Innominate Vein, Right
	Innominate Vein, Left
Brachioradialis muscle	Lower Arm and Wrist Muscle, Right
	Lower Arm and Wrist Muscle, Left
Breast procedures, skin only	Skin, Chest
Broad ligament	Uterine Supporting Structure
Bronchial artery	Upper Artery
Bronchus intermedius	Main Bronchus, Right
Buccal gland	Buccal Mucosa
Buccinator lymph node	Lymphatic, Head
Buccinator muscle	Facial Muscle
Bulbospongiosus muscle	Perineum Muscle
Bulbourethral (Cowper's) gland	Urethra
Bundle of His	Conduction Mechanism

Term	ICD-10-PCS Value
Bundle of Kent	Conduction Mechanism
Calcaneocuboid joint	Tarsal Joint, Right
	Tarsal Joint, Left
Calcaneocuboid ligament	Foot Bursa and Ligament, Right
	Foot Bursa and Ligament, Left
Calcaneofibular ligament	Ankle Bursa and Ligament, Right
	Ankle Bursa and Ligament, Left
Calcaneus	Tarsal, Right
	Tarsal, Left
Capitate bone	Carpal, Right
	Carpal, Left
Cardia	Esophagogastric Junction
Cardiac plexus	Thoracic Sympathetic Nerve
Cardioesophageal junction	Esophagogastric Junction
Caroticotympanic artery	Internal Carotid Artery, Right
	Internal Carotid Artery, Left
Carotid glomus	Carotid Body, Right
	Carotid Body, Left
	Carotid Bodies, Bilateral
Carotid sinus	Internal Carotid Artery, Right
	Internal Carotid Artery, Left
Carotid sinus nerve	Glossopharyngeal Nerve
Carpometacarpal ligament	Hand Bursa and Ligament, Right
	Hand Bursa and Ligament, Left
Cauda equina	Lumbar Spinal Cord
Cavernous plexus	Head and Neck Sympathetic Nerve
Cavoatrial junction	Superior Vena Cava
Celiac ganglion	Abdominal Sympathetic Nerve
Celiac (solar) plexus	Abdominal Sympathetic Nerve
Celiac lymph node	Lymphatic, Aortic
Celiac trunk	Celiac Artery
Central axillary lymph node	Lymphatic, Right Axillary
	Lymphatic, Left Axillary
Cerebral aqueduct (Sylvius)	Cerebral Ventricle
Cerebrum	Brain
Cervical esophagus	Esophagus, Upper
Cervical facet joint	Cervical Vertebral Joint
	Cervical Vertebral Joints, 2 or more
Cervical ganglion	Head and Neck Sympathetic Nerve
Cervical interspinous ligament	Head and Neck Bursa and Ligament
Cervical intertransverse ligament	Head and Neck Bursa and Ligament
Cervical ligamentum flavum	Head and Neck Bursa and Ligament
Cervical lymph node	Lymphatic, Right Neck
	Lymphatic, Left Neck
Cervicothoracic facet joint	Cervicothoracic Vertebral Joint
Chin	Subcutaneous Tissue and Fascia, Face
Choana	Nasopharynx
Chondroglossus muscle	Tongue, Palate, Pharynx Muscle
Chorda tympani	Facial Nerve
Choroid plexus	Cerebral Ventricle
Ciliary body	Eye, Right
	Eye, Left
Ciliary ganglion	Head and Neck Sympathetic Nerve
Circle of Willis	Intracranial Artery
Circumflex iliac artery	Femoral Artery, Right
	Femoral Artery, Left
Claustrum	Basal Ganglia
Coccygeal body	Coccygeal Glomus

Term	ICD-10-PCS Value
Coccygeus muscle	Trunk Muscle, Right
	Trunk Muscle, Left
Cochlea	Inner Ear, Right
	Inner Ear, Left
Cochlear nerve	Acoustic Nerve
Columella	Nasal Mucosa and Soft Tissue
Common digital vein	Foot Vein, Right
	Foot Vein, Left
Common facial vein	Face Vein, Right
	Face Vein, Left
Common fibular nerve	Peroneal Nerve
Common hepatic artery	Hepatic Artery
Common iliac (subaortic) lymph node	Lymphatic, Pelvis
Common interosseous artery	Ulnar Artery, Right
	Ulnar Artery, Left
Common peroneal nerve	Peroneal Nerve
Condyloid process	Mandible, Right
	Mandible, Left
Conus arteriosus	Ventricle, Right
Conus medullaris	Lumbar Spinal Cord
Coracoacromial ligament	Shoulder Bursa and Ligament, Right
	Shoulder Bursa and Ligament, Left
Coracobrachialis muscle	Upper Arm Muscle, Right
	Upper Arm Muscle, Left
Coracoclavicular ligament	Shoulder Bursa and Ligament, Right
	Shoulder Bursa and Ligament, Left
Coracohumeral ligament	Shoulder Bursa and Ligament, Right
	Shoulder Bursa and Ligament, Left
Coracoid process	Scapula, Right
	Scapula, Left
Corniculate cartilage	Larynx
Corpus callosum	Brain
Corpus cavernosum	Penis
Corpus spongiosum	Penis
Corpus striatum	Basal Ganglia
Corrugator supercilii muscle	Facial Muscle
Costocervical trunk	Subclavian Artery, Right
	Subclavian Artery, Left
Costoclavicular ligament	Shoulder Bursa and Ligament, Right
	Shoulder Bursa and Ligament, Left
Costotransverse joint	Thoracic Vertebral Joint
Costotransverse ligament	Rib(s) Bursa and Ligament
Costovertebral joint	Thoracic Vertebral Joint
Costoxiphoid ligament	Sternum Bursa and Ligament
Cowper's (bulbourethral) gland	Urethra
Cremaster muscle	Perineum Muscle
Cribriform plate	Ethmoid Bone, Right
	Ethmoid Bone, Left
Cricoid cartilage	Trachea
Cricothyroid artery	Thyroid Artery, Right
	Thyroid Artery, Left
Cricothyroid muscle	Neck Muscle, Right
	Neck Muscle, Left
Crural fascia	Subcutaneous Tissue and Fascia, Right Upper Leg
	Subcutaneous Tissue and Fascia, Left Upper Leg
Cubital lymph node	Lymphatic, Right Upper Extremity
	Lymphatic, Left Upper Extremity

Term	ICD-10-PCS Value
Cubital nerve	Ulnar Nerve
Cuboid bone	Tarsal, Right
	Tarsal, Left
Cuboideonavicular joint	Tarsal Joint, Right
	Tarsal Joint, Left
Culmen	Cerebellum
Cuneiform cartilage	Larynx
Cuneonavicular joint	Tarsal Joint, Right
	Tarsal Joint, Left
Cuneonavicular ligament	Foot Bursa and Ligament, Right
	Foot Bursa and Ligament, Left
Cutaneous (transverse) cervical nerve	Cervical Plexus
Deep cervical fascia	Subcutaneous Tissue and Fascia, Right Neck
	Subcutaneous Tissue and Fascia, Left Neck
Deep cervical vein	Vertebral Vein, Right
	Vertebral Vein, Left
Deep circumflex iliac artery	External Iliac Artery, Right
	External Iliac Artery, Left
Deep facial vein	Face Vein, Right
	Face Vein, Left
Deep femoral artery	Femoral Artery, Right
	Femoral Artery, Left
Deep femoral (profunda femoris) vein	Femoral Vein, Right
	Femoral Vein, Left
Deep palmar arch	Hand Artery, Right
	Hand Artery, Left
Deep transverse perineal muscle	Perineum Muscle
Deferential artery	Internal Iliac Artery, Right
	Internal Iliac Artery, Left
Deltoid fascia	Subcutaneous Tissue and Fascia, Right Upper Arm
	Subcutaneous Tissue and Fascia, Left Upper Arm
Deltoid ligament	Ankle Bursa and Ligament, Right
	Ankle Bursa and Ligament, Left
Deltoid muscle	Shoulder Muscle, Right
	Shoulder Muscle, Left
Deltopectoral (infraclavicular) lymph node	Lymphatic, Right Upper Extremity
	Lymphatic, Left Upper Extremity
Dens	Cervical Vertebra
Denticulate (dentate) ligament	Spinal Meninges
Depressor anguli oris muscle	Facial Muscle
Depressor labii inferioris muscle	Facial Muscle
Depressor septi nasi muscle	Facial Muscle
Depressor supercilii muscle	Facial Muscle
Dermis	Skin
Descending genicular artery	Femoral Artery, Right
	Femoral Artery, Left
Diaphragma sellae	Dura Mater
Distal humerus	Humeral Shaft, Right
	Humeral Shaft, Left
Distal humerus, involving joint	Elbow Joint, Right
	Elbow Joint, Left
Distal radioulnar joint	Wrist Joint, Right
	Wrist Joint, Left
Dorsal digital nerve	Radial Nerve

Term	ICD-10-PCS Value
Dorsal metacarpal vein	Hand Vein, Right
	Hand Vein, Left
Dorsal metatarsal artery	Foot Artery, Right
	Foot Artery, Left
Dorsal metatarsal vein	Foot Vein, Right
	Foot Vein, Left
Dorsal root ganglion	Cervical Spinal Cord
	Lumbar Spinal Cord
	Spinal Cord
	Thoracic Spinal Cord
Dorsal scapular artery	Subclavian Artery, Right
	Subclavian Artery, Left
Dorsal scapular nerve	Brachial Plexus
Dorsal venous arch	Foot Vein, Right
	Foot Vein, Left
Dorsalis pedis artery	Anterior Tibial Artery, Right
	Anterior Tibial Artery, Left
Duct of Santorini	Pancreatic Duct, Accessory
Duct of Wirsung	Pancreatic Duct
Ductus deferens	Vas Deferens, Right
	Vas Deferens, Left
	Vas Deferens, Bilateral
	Vas Deferens
Duodenal ampulla	Ampulla of Vater
Duodenojejunal flexure	Jejunum
Dura mater, intracranial	Dura Mater
Dura mater, spinal	Spinal Meninges
Dural venous sinus	Intracranial Vein
Earlobe	External Ear, Right
	External Ear, Left
	External Ear, Bilateral
Eighth cranial nerve	Acoustic Nerve
Ejaculatory duct	Vas Deferens, Right
	Vas Deferens, Left
	Vas Deferens, Bilateral
	Vas Deferens
Eleventh cranial nerve	Accessory Nerve
Encephalon	Brain
Ependyma	Cerebral Ventricle
Epidermis	Skin
Epidural space, spinal	Spinal Canal
Epiploic foramen	Peritoneum
Epithalamus	Thalamus
Epitrochlear lymph node	Lymphatic, Right Upper Extremity
	Lymphatic, Left Upper Extremity
Erector spinae muscle	Trunk Muscle, Right
	Trunk Muscle, Left
Esophageal artery	Upper Artery
Esophageal plexus	Thoracic Sympathetic Nerve
Ethmoidal air cell	Ethmoid Sinus, Right
	Ethmoid Sinus, Left
Extensor carpi radialis muscle	Lower Arm and Wrist Muscle, Right
	Lower Arm and Wrist Muscle, Left
Extensor carpi ulnaris muscle	Lower Arm and Wrist Muscle, Right
	Lower Arm and Wrist Muscle, Left
Extensor digitorum brevis muscle	Foot Muscle, Right
	Foot Muscle, Left
Extensor digitorum longus muscle	Lower Leg Muscle, Right
	Lower Leg Muscle, Left
Extensor hallucis brevis muscle	Foot Muscle, Right
	Foot Muscle, Left
Extensor hallucis longus muscle	Lower Leg Muscle, Right
	Lower Leg Muscle, Left
External anal sphincter	Anal Sphincter
External auditory meatus	External Auditory Canal, Right
	External Auditory Canal, Left
External maxillary artery	Face Artery
External naris	Nasal Mucosa and Soft Tissue
External oblique aponeurosis	Subcutaneous Tissue and Fascia, Trunk
External oblique muscle	Abdomen Muscle, Right
	Abdomen Muscle, Left
External popliteal nerve	Peroneal Nerve
External pudendal artery	Femoral Artery, Right
	Femoral Artery, Left
External pudendal vein	Saphenous Vein, Right
	Saphenous Vein, Left
External urethral sphincter	Urethra
Extradural space, intracranial	Epidural Space, Intracranial
Extradural space, spinal	Spinal Canal
Facial artery	Face Artery
False vocal cord	Larynx
Falx cerebri	Dura Mater
Fascia lata	Subcutaneous Tissue and Fascia, Right Upper Leg
	Subcutaneous Tissue and Fascia, Left Upper Leg
Femoral head	Upper Femur, Right
	Upper Femur, Left
Femoral lymph node	Lymphatic, Right Lower Extremity
	Lymphatic, Left Lower Extremity
Femoropatellar joint	Knee Joint, Right
	Knee Joint, Left
	Knee Joint, Femoral Surface, Right
	Knee Joint, Femoral Surface, Left
Femorotibial joint	Knee Joint, Right
	Knee Joint, Left
	Knee Joint, Tibial Surface, Right
	Knee Joint, Tibial Surface, Left
Fibular artery	Peroneal Artery, Right
	Peroneal Artery, Left
Fibular sesamoid	Metatarsal, Right
	Metatarsal, Left
Fibularis brevis muscle	Lower Leg Muscle, Right
	Lower Leg Muscle, Left
Fibularis longus muscle	Lower Leg Muscle, Right
	Lower Leg Muscle, Left
Fifth cranial nerve	Trigeminal Nerve
Filum terminale	Spinal Meninges
First cranial nerve	Olfactory Nerve
First intercostal nerve	Brachial Plexus
Flexor carpi radialis muscle	Lower Arm and Wrist Muscle, Right
	Lower Arm and Wrist Muscle, Left
Flexor carpi ulnaris muscle	Lower Arm and Wrist Muscle, Right
	Lower Arm and Wrist Muscle, Left
Flexor digitorum brevis muscle	Foot Muscle, Right
	Foot Muscle, Left
Flexor digitorum longus muscle	Lower Leg Muscle, Right
	Lower Leg Muscle, Left
Flexor hallucis brevis muscle	Foot Muscle, Right
	Foot Muscle, Left

Term	ICD-10-PCS Value
Flexor hallucis longus muscle	Lower Leg Muscle, Right
	Lower Leg Muscle, Left
Flexor pollicis longus muscle	Lower Arm and Wrist Muscle, Right
	Lower Arm and Wrist Muscle, Left
Foramen magnum	Occipital Bone
Foramen of Monro (intraventricular)	Cerebral Ventricle
Foreskin	Prepuce
Fossa of Rosenmuller	Nasopharynx
Fourth cranial nerve	Trochlear Nerve
Fourth ventricle	Cerebral Ventricle
Fovea	Retina, Right
	Retina, Left
Frenulum labii inferioris	Lower Lip
Frenulum labii superioris	Upper Lip
Frenulum linguae	Tongue
Frontal lobe	Cerebral Hemisphere
Frontal vein	Face Vein, Right
	Face Vein, Left
Fundus uteri	Uterus
Galea aponeurotica	Subcutaneous Tissue and Fascia, Scalp
Ganglion impar (ganglion of Walther)	Sacral Sympathetic Nerve
Gasserian ganglion	Trigeminal Nerve
Gastric lymph node	Lymphatic, Aortic
Gastric plexus	Abdominal Sympathetic Nerve
Gastrocnemius muscle	Lower Leg Muscle, Right
	Lower Leg Muscle, Left
Gastrocolic ligament	Omentum
Gastrocolic omentum	Omentum
Gastroduodenal artery	Hepatic Artery
Gastroesophageal (GE) junction	Esophagogastric Junction
Gastrohepatic omentum	Omentum
Gastrophrenic ligament	Omentum
Gastrosplenic ligament	Omentum
Gemellus muscle	Hip Muscle, Right
	Hip Muscle, Left
Geniculate ganglion	Facial Nerve
Geniculate nucleus	Thalamus
Genioglossus muscle	Tongue, Palate, Pharynx Muscle
Genitofemoral nerve	Lumbar Plexus
Glans penis	Prepuce
Glenohumeral joint	Shoulder Joint, Right
	Shoulder Joint, Left
Glenohumeral ligament	Shoulder Bursa and Ligament, Right
	Shoulder Bursa and Ligament, Left
Glenoid fossa (of scapula)	Glenoid Cavity, Right
	Glenoid Cavity, Left
Glenoid ligament (labrum)	Shoulder Joint, Right
	Shoulder Joint, Left
Globus pallidus	Basal Ganglia
Glossoepiglottic fold	Epiglottis
Glottis	Larynx
Gluteal lymph node	Lymphatic, Pelvis
Gluteal vein	Hypogastric Vein, Right
	Hypogastric Vein, Left
Gluteus maximus muscle	Hip Muscle, Right
	Hip Muscle, Left
Gluteus medius muscle	Hip Muscle, Right
	Hip Muscle, Left

Term	ICD-10-PCS Value
Gluteus minimus muscle	Hip Muscle, Right
	Hip Muscle, Left
Gracilis muscle	Upper Leg Muscle, Right
	Upper Leg Muscle, Left
Great auricular nerve	Cervical Plexus
Great cerebral vein	Intracranial Vein
Great(er) saphenous vein	Saphenous Vein, Right
	Saphenous Vein, Left
Greater alar cartilage	Nasal Mucosa and Soft Tissue
Greater occipital nerve	Cervical Nerve
Greater omentum	Omentum
Greater splanchnic nerve	Thoracic Sympathetic Nerve
Greater superficial petrosal nerve	Facial Nerve
Greater trochanter	Upper Femur, Right
	Upper Femur, Left
Greater tuberosity	Humeral Head, Right
	Humeral Head, Left
Greater vestibular (Bartholin's) gland	Vestibular Gland
Greater wing	Sphenoid Bone
Hallux	1st Toe, Right
	1st Toe, Left
Hamate bone	Carpal, Right
	Carpal, Left
Head of fibula	Fibula, Right
	Fibula, Left
Helix	External Ear, Right
	External Ear, Left
	External Ear, Bilateral
Hepatic artery proper	Hepatic Artery
Hepatic flexure	Transverse Colon
Hepatic lymph node	Lymphatic, Aortic
Hepatic plexus	Abdominal Sympathetic Nerve
Hepatic portal vein	Portal Vein
Hepatogastric ligament	Omentum
Hepatopancreatic ampulla	Ampulla of Vater
Humeroradial joint	Elbow Joint, Right
	Elbow Joint, Left
Humeroulnar joint	Elbow Joint, Right
	Elbow Joint, Left
Humerus, distal	Humeral Shaft, Right
	Humeral Shaft, Left
Hyoglossus muscle	Tongue, Palate, Pharynx Muscle
Hyoid artery	Thyroid Artery, Right
	Thyroid Artery, Left
Hypogastric artery	Internal Iliac Artery, Right
	Internal Iliac Artery, Left
Hypopharynx	Pharynx
Hypophysis	Pituitary Gland
Hypothenar muscle	Hand Muscle, Right
	Hand Muscle, Left
Ileal artery	Superior Mesenteric Artery
Ileocolic artery	Superior Mesenteric Artery
Ileocolic vein	Colic Vein
Iliac crest	Pelvic Bone, Right
	Pelvic Bone, Left
Iliac fascia	Subcutaneous Tissue and Fascia, Right Upper Leg
	Subcutaneous Tissue and Fascia, Left Upper Leg

Term	ICD-10-PCS Value
Iliac lymph node	Lymphatic, Pelvis
Iliacus muscle	Hip Muscle, Right
	Hip Muscle, Left
Iliofemoral ligament	Hip Bursa and Ligament, Right
	Hip Bursa and Ligament, Left
Iliohypogastric nerve	Lumbar Plexus
Ilioinguinal nerve	Lumbar Plexus
Iliolumbar artery	Internal Iliac Artery, Right
	Internal Iliac Artery, Left
Iliolumbar ligament	Lower Spine Bursa and Ligament
Iliotibial tract (band)	Subcutaneous Tissue and Fascia, Right Upper Leg
	Subcutaneous Tissue and Fascia, Left Upper Leg
Ilium	Pelvic Bone, Right
	Pelvic Bone, Left
Incus	Auditory Ossicle, Right
	Auditory Ossicle, Left
Inferior cardiac nerve	Thoracic Sympathetic Nerve
Inferior cerebellar vein	Intracranial Vein
Inferior cerebral vein	Intracranial Vein
Inferior epigastric artery	External Iliac Artery, Right
	External Iliac Artery, Left
Inferior epigastric lymph node	Lymphatic, Pelvis
Inferior genicular artery	Popliteal Artery, Right
	Popliteal Artery, Left
Inferior gluteal artery	Internal Iliac Artery, Right
	Internal Iliac Artery, Left
Inferior gluteal nerve	Sacral Plexus
Inferior hypogastric plexus	Abdominal Sympathetic Nerve
Inferior labial artery	Face Artery
Inferior longitudinal muscle	Tongue, Palate, Pharynx Muscle
Inferior mesenteric ganglion	Abdominal Sympathetic Nerve
Inferior mesenteric lymph node	Lymphatic, Mesenteric
Inferior mesenteric plexus	Abdominal Sympathetic Nerve
Inferior oblique muscle	Extraocular Muscle, Right
	Extraocular Muscle, Left
Inferior pancreaticoduo-denal artery	Superior Mesenteric Artery
Inferior phrenic artery	Abdominal Aorta
Inferior rectus muscle	Extraocular Muscle, Right
	Extraocular Muscle, Left
Inferior suprarenal artery	Renal Artery, Right
	Renal Artery, Left
Inferior tarsal plate	Lower Eyelid, Right
	Lower Eyelid, Left
Inferior thyroid vein	Innominate Vein, Right
	Innominate Vein, Left
Inferior tibiofibular joint	Ankle Joint, Right
	Ankle Joint, Left
Inferior turbinate	Nasal Turbinate
Inferior ulnar collateral artery	Brachial Artery, Right
	Brachial Artery, Left
Inferior vesical artery	Internal Iliac Artery, Right
	Internal Iliac Artery, Left
Infraauricular lymph node	Lymphatic, Head
Infraclavicular (deltopectoral) lymph node	Lymphatic, Right Upper Extremity
	Lymphatic, Left Upper Extremity

Term	ICD-10-PCS Value
Infrahyoid muscle	Neck Muscle, Right
	Neck Muscle, Left
Infraparotid lymph node	Lymphatic, Head
Infraspinatus fascia	Subcutaneous Tissue and Fascia, Right Upper Arm
	Subcutaneous Tissue and Fascia, Left Upper Arm
Infraspinatus muscle	Shoulder Muscle, Right
	Shoulder Muscle, Left
Infundibulopelvic ligament	Uterine Supporting Structure
Inguinal canal	Inguinal Region, Right
	Inguinal Region, Left
	Inguinal Region, Bilateral
Inguinal triangle	Inguinal Region, Right
	Inguinal Region, Left
	Inguinal Region, Bilateral
Interatrial septum	Atrial Septum
Intercarpal joint	Carpal Joint, Right
	Carpal Joint, Left
Intercarpal ligament	Hand Bursa and Ligament, Right
	Hand Bursa and Ligament, Left
Interclavicular ligament	Shoulder Bursa and Ligament, Right
	Shoulder Bursa and Ligament, Left
Intercostal lymph node	Lymphatic, Thorax
Intercostal muscle	Thorax Muscle, Right
	Thorax Muscle, Left
Intercostal nerve	Thoracic Nerve
Intercostobrachial nerve	Thoracic Nerve
Intercuneiform joint	Tarsal Joint, Right
	Tarsal Joint, Left
Intercuneiform ligament	Foot Bursa and Ligament, Right
	Foot Bursa and Ligament, Left
Intermediate bronchus	Main Bronchus, Right
Intermediate cuneiform bone	Tarsal, Right
	Tarsal, Left
Internal anal sphincter	Anal Sphincter
Internal (basal) cerebral vein	Intracranial Vein
Internal carotid artery, intracranial portion	Intracranial Artery
Internal carotid plexus	Head and Neck Sympathetic Nerve
Internal iliac vein	Hypogastric Vein, Right
	Hypogastric Vein, Left
Internal maxillary artery	External Carotid Artery, Right
	External Carotid Artery, Left
Internal naris	Nasal Mucosa and Soft Tissue
Internal oblique muscle	Abdomen Muscle, Right
	Abdomen Muscle, Left
Internal pudendal artery	Internal Iliac Artery, Right
	Internal Iliac Artery, Left
Internal pudendal vein	Hypogastric Vein, Right
	Hypogastric Vein, Left
Internal thoracic artery	Internal Mammary Artery, Right
	Internal Mammary Artery, Left
	Subclavian Artery, Right
	Subclavian Artery, Left
Internal urethral sphincter	Urethra
Interphalangeal (IP) joint	Finger Phalangeal Joint, Right
	Finger Phalangeal Joint, Left
	Toe Phalangeal Joint, Right
	Toe Phalangeal Joint, Left

Term	ICD-10-PCS Value
Interphalangeal ligament	Foot Bursa and Ligament, Right
	Foot Bursa and Ligament, Left
	Hand Bursa and Ligament, Right
	Hand Bursa and Ligament, Left
Interspinalis muscle	Trunk Muscle, Right
	Trunk Muscle, Left
Interspinous ligament, cervical	Head and Neck Bursa and Ligament
Interspinous ligament, lumbar	Lower Spine Bursa and Ligament
Interspinous ligament, thoracic	Upper Spine Bursa and Ligament
Intertransversarius muscle	Trunk Muscle, Right
	Trunk Muscle, Left
Intertransverse ligament, cervical	Head and Neck Bursa and Ligament
Intertransverse ligament, lumbar	Lower Spine Bursa and Ligament
Intertransverse ligament, thoracic	Upper Spine Bursa and Ligament
Interventricular foramen (Monro)	Cerebral Ventricle
Interventricular septum	Ventricular Septum
Intestinal lymphatic trunk	Cisterna Chyli
Ischiatic nerve	Sciatic Nerve
Ischiocavernosus muscle	Perineum Muscle
Ischiofemoral ligament	Hip Bursa and Ligament, Right
	Hip Bursa and Ligament, Left
Ischium	Pelvic Bone, Right
	Pelvic Bone, Left
Jejunal artery	Superior Mesenteric Artery
Jugular body	Glomus Jugulare
Jugular lymph node	Lymphatic, Right Neck
	Lymphatic, Left Neck
Labia majora	Vulva
Labia minora	Vulva
Labial gland	Upper Lip
	Lower Lip
Lacrimal canaliculus	Lacrimal Duct, Right
	Lacrimal Duct, Left
Lacrimal punctum	Lacrimal Duct, Right
	Lacrimal Duct, Left
Lacrimal sac	Lacrimal Duct, Right
	Lacrimal Duct, Left
Laryngopharynx	Pharynx
Lateral (brachial) lymph node	Lymphatic, Right Axillary
	Lymphatic, Left Axillary
Lateral canthus	Upper Eyelid, Right
	Upper Eyelid, Left
Lateral collateral ligament (LCL)	Knee Bursa and Ligament, Right
	Knee Bursa and Ligament, Left
Lateral condyle of femur	Lower Femur, Right
	Lower Femur, Left
Lateral condyle of tibia	Tibia, Right
	Tibia, Left
Lateral cuneiform bone	Tarsal, Right
	Tarsal, Left
Lateral epicondyle of femur	Lower Femur, Right
	Lower Femur, Left
Lateral epicondyle of humerus	Humeral Shaft, Right
	Humeral Shaft, Left

Term	ICD-10-PCS Value
Lateral femoral cutaneous nerve	Lumbar Plexus
Lateral malleolus	Fibula, Right
	Fibula, Left
Lateral meniscus	Knee Joint, Right
	Knee Joint, Left
Lateral nasal cartilage	Nasal Mucosa and Soft Tissue
Lateral plantar artery	Foot Artery, Right
	Foot Artery, Left
Lateral plantar nerve	Tibial Nerve
Lateral rectus muscle	Extraocular Muscle, Right
	Extraocular Muscle, Left
Lateral sacral artery	Internal Iliac Artery, Right
	Internal Iliac Artery, Left
Lateral sacral vein	Hypogastric Vein, Right
	Hypogastric Vein, Left
Lateral sural cutaneous nerve	Peroneal Nerve
Lateral tarsal artery	Foot Artery, Right
	Foot Artery, Left
Lateral temporo- mandibular ligament	Head and Neck Bursa and Ligament
Lateral thoracic artery	Axillary Artery, Right
	Axillary Artery, Left
Latissimus dorsi muscle	Trunk Muscle, Right
	Trunk Muscle, Left
Least splanchnic nerve	Thoracic Sympathetic Nerve
Left ascending lumbar vein	Hemiazygos Vein
Left atrioventricular valve	Mitral Valve
Left auricular appendix	Atrium, Left
Left colic vein	Colic Vein
Left coronary sulcus	Heart, Left
Left gastric artery	Gastric Artery
Left gastroepiploic artery	Splenic Artery
Left gastroepiploic vein	Splenic Vein
Left inferior phrenic vein	Renal Vein, Left
Left inferior pulmonary vein	Pulmonary Vein, Left
Left jugular trunk	Thoracic Duct
Left lateral ventricle	Cerebral Ventricle
Left ovarian vein	Renal Vein, Left
Left second lumbar vein	Renal Vein, Left
Left subclavian trunk	Thoracic Duct
Left subcostal vein	Hemiazygos Vein
Left superior pulmonary vein	Pulmonary Vein, Left
Left suprarenal vein	Renal Vein, Left
Left testicular vein	Renal Vein, Left
Leptomeninges, intracranial	Cerebral Meninges
Leptomeninges, spinal	Spinal Meninges
Lesser alar cartilage	Nasal Mucosa and Soft Tissue
Lesser occipital nerve	Cervical Plexus
Lesser omentum	Omentum
Lesser saphenous vein	Saphenous Vein, Right
	Saphenous Vein, Left
Lesser splanchnic nerve	Thoracic Sympathetic Nerve
Lesser trochanter	Upper Femur, Right
	Upper Femur, Left
Lesser tuberosity	Humeral Head, Right
	Humeral Head, Left
Lesser wing	Sphenoid Bone
Levator anguli oris muscle	Facial Muscle
Levator ani muscle	Perineum Muscle

Term	ICD-10-PCS Value
Levator labii superioris alaeque nasi muscle	Facial Muscle
Levator labii superioris muscle	Facial Muscle
Levator palpebrae superioris muscle	Upper Eyelid, Right
	Upper Eyelid, Left
Levator scapulae muscle	Neck Muscle, Right
	Neck Muscle, Left
Levator veli palatini muscle	Tongue, Palate, Pharynx Muscle
Levatores costarum muscle	Thorax Muscle, Right
	Thorax Muscle, Left
Ligament of head of fibula	Knee Bursa and Ligament, Right
	Knee Bursa and Ligament, Left
Ligament of the lateral malleolus	Ankle Bursa and Ligament, Right
	Ankle Bursa and Ligament, Left
Ligamentum flavum, cervical	Head and Neck Bursa and Ligament
Ligamentum flavum, lumbar	Lower Spine Bursa and Ligament
Ligamentum flavum, thoracic	Upper Spine Bursa and Ligament
Lingual artery	External Carotid Artery, Right
	External Carotid Artery, Left
Lingual tonsil	Pharynx
Locus ceruleus	Pons
Long thoracic nerve	Brachial Plexus
Lumbar artery	Abdominal Aorta
Lumbar facet joint	Lumbar Vertebral Joint
Lumbar ganglion	Lumbar Sympathetic Nerve
Lumbar lymph node	Lymphatic, Aortic
Lumbar lymphatic trunk	Cisterna Chyli
Lumbar splanchnic nerve	Lumbar Sympathetic Nerve
Lumbosacral facet joint	Lumbosacral Joint
Lumbosacral trunk	Lumbar Nerve
Lunate bone	Carpal, Right
	Carpal, Left
Lunotriquetral ligament	Hand Bursa and Ligament, Right
	Hand Bursa and Ligament, Left
Macula	Retina, Right
	Retina, Left
Malleus	Auditory Ossicle, Right
	Auditory Ossicle, Left
Mammary duct	Breast, Right
	Breast, Left
	Breast, Bilateral
Mammary gland	Breast, Right
	Breast, Left
	Breast, Bilateral
Mammillary body	Hypothalamus
Mandibular nerve	Trigeminal Nerve
Mandibular notch	Mandible, Right
	Mandible, Left
Manubrium	Sternum
Masseter muscle	Head Muscle
Masseteric fascia	Subcutaneous Tissue and Fascia, Face
Mastoid (postauricular) lymph node	Lymphatic, Right Neck
	Lymphatic, Left Neck
Mastoid air cells	Mastoid Sinus, Right
	Mastoid Sinus, Left
Mastoid process	Temporal Bone, Right
	Temporal Bone, Left
Maxillary artery	External Carotid Artery, Right
	External Carotid Artery, Left
Maxillary nerve	Trigeminal Nerve

Term	ICD-10-PCS Value
Medial canthus	Lower Eyelid, Right
	Lower Eyelid, Left
Medial collateral ligament (MCL)	Knee Bursa and Ligament, Right
	Knee Bursa and Ligament, Left
Medial condyle of femur	Lower Femur, Right
	Lower Femur, Left
Medial condyle of tibia	Tibia, Right
	Tibia, Left
Medial cuneiform bone	Tarsal, Right
	Tarsal, Left
Medial epicondyle of femur	Lower Femur, Right
	Lower Femur, Left
Medial epicondyle of humerus	Humeral Shaft, Right
	Humeral Shaft, Left
Medial malleolus	Tibia, Right
	Tibia, Left
Medial meniscus	Knee Joint, Right
	Knee Joint, Left
Medial plantar artery	Foot Artery, Right
	Foot Artery, Left
Medial plantar nerve	Tibial Nerve
Medial popliteal nerve	Tibial Nerve
Medial rectus muscle	Extraocular Muscle, Right
	Extraocular Muscle, Left
Medial sural cutaneous nerve	Tibial Nerve
Median antebrachial vein	Basilic Vein, Right
	Basilic Vein, Left
Median cubital vein	Basilic Vein, Right
	Basilic Vein, Left
Median sacral artery	Abdominal Aorta
Mediastinal cavity	Mediastinum
Mediastinal lymph node	Lymphatic, Thorax
Mediastinal space	Mediastinum
Meissner's (submucous) plexus	Abdominal Sympathetic Nerve
Membranous urethra	Urethra
Mental foramen	Mandible, Right
	Mandible, Left
Mentalis muscle	Facial Muscle
Mesoappendix	Mesentery
Mesocolon	Mesentery
Metacarpal ligament	Hand Bursa and Ligament, Right
	Hand Bursa and Ligament, Left
Metacarpophalangeal ligament	Hand Bursa and Ligament, Right
	Hand Bursa and Ligament, Left
Metatarsal ligament	Foot Bursa and Ligament, Right
	Foot Bursa and Ligament, Left
Metatarsophalangeal ligament	Foot Bursa and Ligament, Right
	Foot Bursa and Ligament, Left
Metatarsophalangeal (MTP) joint	Metatarsal-Phalangeal Joint, Right
	Metatarsal-Phalangeal Joint, Left
Metathalamus	Thalamus
Midcarpal joint	Carpal Joint, Right
	Carpal Joint, Left
Middle cardiac nerve	Thoracic Sympathetic Nerve
Middle cerebral artery	Intracranial Artery
Middle cerebral vein	Intracranial Vein
Middle colic vein	Colic Vein
Middle genicular artery	Popliteal Artery, Right
	Popliteal Artery, Left

Term	ICD-10-PCS Value
Middle hemorrhoidal vein	Hypogastric Vein, Right
	Hypogastric Vein, Left
Middle meningeal artery, intracranial portion	Intracranial Artery
Middle rectal artery	Internal Iliac Artery, Right
	Internal Iliac Artery, Left
Middle suprarenal artery	Abdominal Aorta
Middle temporal artery	Temporal Artery, Right
	Temporal Artery, Left
Middle turbinate	Nasal Turbinate
Mitral annulus	Mitral Valve
Molar gland	Buccal Mucosa
Musculocutaneous nerve	Brachial Plexus
Musculophrenic artery	Internal Mammary Artery, Right
	Internal Mammary Artery, Left
Musculospiral nerve	Radial Nerve
Myelencephalon	Medulla Oblongata
Myenteric (Auerbach's) plexus	Abdominal Sympathetic Nerve
Myometrium	Uterus
Nail bed	Finger Nail
	Toe Nail
Nail plate	Finger Nail
	Toe Nail
Nasal cavity	Nasal Mucosa and Soft Tissue
Nasal concha	Nasal Turbinate
Nasalis muscle	Facial Muscle
Nasolacrimal duct	Lacrimal Duct, Right
	Lacrimal Duct, Left
Navicular bone	Tarsal, Right
	Tarsal, Left
Neck of femur	Upper Femur, Right
	Upper Femur, Left
Neck of humerus (anatomical) (surgical)	Humeral Head, Right
	Humeral Head, Left
Nerve to the stapedius	Facial Nerve
Neurohypophysis	Pituitary Gland
Ninth cranial nerve	Glossopharyngeal Nerve
Nostril	Nasal Mucosa and Soft Tissue
Obturator artery	Internal Iliac Artery, Right
	Internal Iliac Artery, Left
Obturator lymph node	Lymphatic, Pelvis
Obturator muscle	Hip Muscle, Right
	Hip Muscle, Left
Obturator nerve	Lumbar Plexus
Obturator vein	Hypogastric Vein, Right
	Hypogastric Vein, Left
Obtuse margin	Heart, Left
Occipital artery	External Carotid Artery, Right
	External Carotid Artery, Left
Occipital lobe	Cerebral Hemisphere
Occipital lymph node	Lymphatic, Right Neck
	Lymphatic, Left Neck
Occipitofrontalis muscle	Facial Muscle
Odontoid process	Cervical Vertebra
Olecranon bursa	Elbow Bursa and Ligament, Right
	Elbow Bursa and Ligament, Left
Olecranon process	Ulna, Right
	Ulna, Left
Olfactory bulb	Olfactory Nerve

Term	ICD-10-PCS Value
Ophthalmic artery	Intracranial Artery
Ophthalmic nerve	Trigeminal Nerve
Ophthalmic vein	Intracranial Vein
Optic chiasma	Optic Nerve
Optic disc	Retina, Right
	Retina, Left
Optic foramen	Sphenoid Bone
Orbicularis oculi muscle	Upper Eyelid, Right
	Upper Eyelid, Left
Orbicularis oris muscle	Facial Muscle
Orbital fascia	Subcutaneous Tissue and Fascia, Face
Orbital portion of ethmoid bone	Orbit, Right
	Orbit, Left
Orbital portion of frontal bone	Orbit, Right
	Orbit, Left
Orbital portion of lacrimal bone	Orbit, Right
	Orbit, Left
Orbital portion of maxilla	Orbit, Right
	Orbit, Left
Orbital portion of palatine bone	Orbit, Right
	Orbit, Left
Orbital portion of sphenoid bone	Orbit, Right
	Orbit, Left
Orbital portion of zygomatic bone	Orbit, Right
	Orbit, Left
Oropharynx	Pharynx
Otic ganglion	Head and Neck Sympathetic Nerve
Oval window	Middle Ear, Right
	Middle Ear, Left
Ovarian artery	Abdominal Aorta
Ovarian ligament	Uterine Supporting Structure
Oviduct	Fallopian Tube, Right
	Fallopian Tube, Left
Palatine gland	Buccal Mucosa
Palatine tonsil	Tonsils
Palatine uvula	Uvula
Palatoglossal muscle	Tongue, Palate, Pharynx Muscle
Palatopharyngeal muscle	Tongue, Palate, Pharynx Muscle
Palmar (volar) digital vein	Hand Vein, Right
	Hand Vein, Left
Palmar (volar) metacarpal vein	Hand Vein, Right
	Hand Vein, Left
Palmar cutaneous nerve	Median Nerve
	Radial Nerve
Palmar fascia (aponeurosis)	Subcutaneous Tissue and Fascia, Right Hand
	Subcutaneous Tissue and Fascia, Left Hand
Palmar interosseous muscle	Hand Muscle, Right
	Hand Muscle, Left
Palmar ulnocarpal ligament	Wrist Bursa and Ligament, Right
	Wrist Bursa and Ligament, Left
Palmaris longus muscle	Lower Arm and Wrist Muscle, Right
	Lower Arm and Wrist Muscle, Left
Pancreatic artery	Splenic Artery
Pancreatic plexus	Abdominal Sympathetic Nerve
Pancreatic vein	Splenic Vein
Pancreaticosplenic lymph node	Lymphatic, Aortic
Paraaortic lymph node	Lymphatic, Aortic
Parapharyngeal space	Neck
Pararectal lymph node	Lymphatic, Mesenteric

Term	ICD-10-PCS Value
Parasternal lymph node	Lymphatic, Thorax
Paratracheal lymph node	Lymphatic, Thorax
Paraurethral (Skene's) gland	Vestibular Gland
Parietal lobe	Cerebral Hemisphere
Parotid lymph node	Lymphatic, Head
Parotid plexus	Facial Nerve
Pars flaccida	Tympanic Membrane, Right
	Tympanic Membrane, Left
Patellar ligament	Knee Bursa and Ligament, Right
	Knee Bursa and Ligament, Left
Patellar tendon	Knee Tendon, Right
	Knee Tendon, Left
Patellofemoral joint	Knee Joint, Right
	Knee Joint, Left
	Knee Joint, Femoral Surface, Right
	Knee Joint, Femoral Surface, Left
Pectineus muscle	Upper Leg Muscle, Right
	Upper Leg Muscle, Left
Pectoral (anterior) lymph node	Lymphatic, Right Axillary
	Lymphatic, Left Axillary
Pectoral fascia	Subcutaneous Tissue and Fascia, Chest
Pectoralis major muscle	Thorax Muscle, Right
	Thorax Muscle, Left
Pectoralis minor muscle	Thorax Muscle, Right
	Thorax Muscle, Left
Pelvic splanchnic nerve	Abdominal Sympathetic Nerve
	Sacral Sympathetic Nerve
Penile urethra	Urethra
Perianal skin	Skin, Perineum
Pericardiophrenic artery	Internal Mammary Artery, Right
	Internal Mammary Artery, Left
Perimetrium	Uterus
Peroneus brevis muscle	Lower Leg Muscle, Right
	Lower Leg Muscle, Left
Peroneus longus muscle	Lower Leg Muscle, Right
	Lower Leg Muscle, Left
Petrous part of temoporal bone	Temporal Bone, Right
	Temporal Bone, Left
Pharyngeal constrictor muscle	Tongue, Palate, Pharynx Muscle
Pharyngeal plexus	Vagus Nerve
Pharyngeal recess	Nasopharynx
Pharyngeal tonsil	Adenoids
Pharyngotympanic tube	Eustachian Tube, Right
	Eustachian Tube, Left
Pia mater, intracranial	Cerebral Meninges
Pia mater, spinal	Spinal Meninges
Pinna	External Ear, Right
	External Ear, Left
	External Ear, Bilateral
Piriform recess (sinus)	Pharynx
Piriformis muscle	Hip Muscle, Right
	Hip Muscle, Left
Pisiform bone	Carpal, Right
	Carpal, Left
Pisohamate ligament	Hand Bursa and Ligament, Right
	Hand Bursa and Ligament, Left
Pisometacarpal ligament	Hand Bursa and Ligament, Right
	Hand Bursa and Ligament, Left

Term	ICD-10-PCS Value
Plantar digital vein	Foot Vein, Right
	Foot Vein, Left
Plantar fascia (aponeurosis)	Subcutaneous Tissue and Fascia, Right Foot
	Subcutaneous Tissue and Fascia, Left Foot
Plantar metatarsal vein	Foot Vein, Right
	Foot Vein, Left
Plantar venous arch	Foot Vein, Right
	Foot Vein, Left
Platysma muscle	Neck Muscle, Right
	Neck Muscle, Left
Plica semilunaris	Conjunctiva, Right
	Conjunctiva, Left
Pneumogastric nerve	Vagus Nerve
Pneumotaxic center	Pons
Pontine tegmentum	Pons
Popliteal ligament	Knee Bursa and Ligament, Right
	Knee Bursa and Ligament, Left
Popliteal lymph node	Lymphatic, Left Lower Extremity
	Lymphatic, Right Lower Extremity
Popliteal vein	Femoral Vein, Right
	Femoral Vein, Left
Popliteus muscle	Lower Leg Muscle, Right
	Lower Leg Muscle, Left
Postauricular (mastoid) lymph node	Lymphatic, Right Neck
	Lymphatic, Left Neck
Postcava	Inferior Vena Cava
Posterior (subscapular) lymph node	Lymphatic, Right Axillary
	Lymphatic, Left Axillary
Posterior auricular artery	External Carotid Artery, Right
	External Carotid Artery, Left
Posterior auricular nerve	Facial Nerve
Posterior auricular vein	External Jugular Vein, Right
	External Jugular Vein, Left
Posterior cerebral artery	Intracranial Artery
Posterior chamber	Eye, Right
	Eye, Left
Posterior circumflex humeral artery	Axillary Artery, Right
	Axillary Artery, Left
Posterior communicating artery	Intracranial Artery
Posterior cruciate ligament (PCL)	Knee Bursa and Ligament, Right
	Knee Bursa and Ligament, Left
Posterior facial (retromandibular) vein	Face Vein, Right
	Face Vein, Left
Posterior femoral cutaneous nerve	Sacral Plexus
Posterior inferior cerebellar artery (PICA)	Intracranial Artery
Posterior interosseous nerve	Radial Nerve
Posterior labial nerve	Pudendal Nerve
Posterior scrotal nerve	Pudendal Nerve
Posterior spinal artery	Vertebral Artery, Right
	Vertebral Artery, Left
Posterior tibial recurrent artery	Anterior Tibial Artery, Right
	Anterior Tibial Artery, Left
Posterior ulnar recurrent artery	Ulnar Artery, Right
	Ulnar Artery, Left
Posterior vagal trunk	Vagus Nerve
Preauricular lymph node	Lymphatic, Head
Precava	Superior Vena Cava

Term	ICD-10-PCS Value
Prepatellar bursa	Knee Bursa and Ligament, Right
	Knee Bursa and Ligament, Left
Pretracheal fascia	Subcutaneous Tissue and Fascia, Right Neck
	Subcutaneous Tissue and Fascia, Left Neck
Prevertebral fascia	Subcutaneous Tissue and Fascia, Right Neck
	Subcutaneous Tissue and Fascia, Left Neck
Princeps pollicis artery	Hand Artery, Right
	Hand Artery, Left
Procerus muscle	Facial Muscle
Profunda brachii	Brachial Artery, Right
	Brachial Artery, Left
Profunda femoris (deep femoral) vein	Femoral Vein, Right
	Femoral Vein, Left
Pronator quadratus muscle	Lower Arm and Wrist Muscle, Right
	Lower Arm and Wrist Muscle, Left
Pronator teres muscle	Lower Arm and Wrist Muscle, Right
	Lower Arm and Wrist Muscle, Left
Prostatic artery	Internal Iliac Artery, Right
	Internal Iliac Artery, Left
Prostatic urethra	Urethra
Proximal radioulnar joint	Elbow Joint, Right
	Elbow Joint, Left
Psoas muscle	Hip Muscle, Right
	Hip Muscle, Left
Pterygoid muscle	Head Muscle
Pterygoid process	Sphenoid Bone
Pterygopalatine (sphenopalatine) ganglion	Head and Neck Sympathetic Nerve
Pubis	Pelvic Bone, Right
	Pelvic Bone, Left
Pubofemoral ligament	Hip Bursa and Ligament, Right
	Hip Bursa and Ligament, Left
Pudendal nerve	Sacral Plexus
Pulmoaortic canal	Pulmonary Artery, Left
Pulmonary annulus	Pulmonary Valve
Pulmonary plexus	Thoracic Sympathetic Nerve
	Vagus Nerve
Pulmonic valve	Pulmonary Valve
Pulvinar	Thalamus
Pyloric antrum	Stomach, Pylorus
Pyloric canal	Stomach, Pylorus
Pyloric sphincter	Stomach, Pylorus
Pyramidalis muscle	Abdomen Muscle, Right
	Abdomen Muscle, Left
Quadrangular cartilage	Nasal Septum
Quadrate lobe	Liver
Quadratus femoris muscle	Hip Muscle, Right
	Hip Muscle, Left
Quadratus lumborum muscle	Trunk Muscle, Right
	Trunk Muscle, Left
Quadratus plantae muscle	Foot Muscle, Right
	Foot Muscle, Left
Quadriceps (femoris)	Upper Leg Muscle, Right
	Upper Leg Muscle, Left
Radial collateral carpal ligament	Wrist Bursa and Ligament, Right
	Wrist Bursa and Ligament, Left
Radial collateral ligament	Elbow Bursa and Ligament, Right
	Elbow Bursa and Ligament, Left
Radial notch	Ulna, Right
	Ulna, Left

Term	ICD-10-PCS Value
Radial recurrent artery	Radial Artery, Right
	Radial Artery, Left
Radial vein	Brachial Vein, Right
	Brachial Vein, Left
Radialis indicis	Hand Artery, Right
	Hand Artery, Left
Radiocarpal joint	Wrist Joint, Right
	Wrist Joint, Left
Radiocarpal ligament	Wrist Bursa and Ligament, Right
	Wrist Bursa and Ligament, Left
Radioulnar ligament	Wrist Bursa and Ligament, Right
	Wrist Bursa and Ligament, Left
Rectosigmoid junction	Sigmoid Colon
Rectus abdominis muscle	Abdomen Muscle, Right
	Abdomen Muscle, Left
Rectus femoris muscle	Upper Leg Muscle, Right
	Upper Leg Muscle, Left
Recurrent laryngeal nerve	Vagus Nerve
Renal calyx	Kidney, Right
	Kidney, Left
	Kidneys, Bilateral
	Kidney
Renal capsule	Kidney, Right
	Kidney, Left
	Kidneys, Bilateral
	Kidney
Renal cortex	Kidney, Right
	Kidney, Left
	Kidneys, Bilateral
	Kidney
Renal nerve	Abdominal sympathetic Nerve
Renal plexus	Abdominal Sympathetic Nerve
Renal segment	Kidney, Right
	Kidney, Left
	Kidneys, Bilateral
	Kidney
Renal segmental artery	Renal Artery, Right
	Renal Artery, Left
Retroperitoneal cavity	Retroperitoneum
Retroperitoneal lymph node	Lymphatic, Aortic
Retroperitoneal space	Retroperitoneum
Retropharyngeal lymph node	Lymphatic, Right Neck
	Lymphatic, Left Neck
Retropharyngeal space	Neck
Retropubic space	Pelvic Cavity
Rhinopharynx	Nasopharynx
Rhomboid major muscle	Trunk Muscle, Right
	Trunk Muscle, Left
Rhomboid minor muscle	Trunk Muscle, Right
	Trunk Muscle, Left
Right ascending lumbar vein	Azygos Vein
Right atrioventricular valve	Tricuspid Valve
Right auricular appendix	Atrium, Right
Right colic vein	Colic Vein
Right coronary sulcus	Heart, Right
Right gastric artery	Gastric Artery
Right gastroepiploic vein	Superior Mesenteric Vein
Right inferior phrenic vein	Inferior Vena Cava
Right inferior pulmonary vein	Pulmonary Vein, Right
Right jugular trunk	Lymphatic, Right Neck

Term	ICD-10-PCS Value
Right lateral ventricle	Cerebral Ventricle
Right lymphatic duct	Lymphatic, Right Neck
Right ovarian vein	Inferior Vena Cava
Right second lumbar vein	Inferior Vena Cava
Right subclavian trunk	Lymphatic, Right Neck
Right subcostal vein	Azygos Vein
Right superior pulmonary vein	Pulmonary Vein, Right
Right suprarenal vein	Inferior Vena Cava
Right testicular vein	Inferior Vena Cava
Rima glottidis	Larynx
Risorius muscle	Facial Muscle
Round ligament of uterus	Uterine Supporting Structure
Round window	Inner Ear, Right
	Inner Ear, Left
Sacral ganglion	Sacral Sympathetic Nerve
Sacral lymph node	Lymphatic, Pelvis
Sacral splanchnic nerve	Sacral Sympathetic Nerve
Sacrococcygeal ligament	Lower Spine Bursa and Ligament
Sacrococcygeal symphysis	Sacrococcygeal Joint
Sacroiliac ligament	Lower Spine Bursa and Ligament
Sacrospinous ligament	Lower Spine Bursa and Ligament
Sacrotuberous ligament	Lower Spine Bursa and Ligament
Salpingopharyngeus muscle	Tongue, Palate, Pharynx Muscle
Salpinx	Fallopian Tube, Right
	Fallopian Tube, Left
Saphenous nerve	Femoral Nerve
Sartorius muscle	Upper Leg Muscle, Right
	Upper Leg Muscle, Left
Scalene muscle	Neck Muscle, Right
	Neck Muscle, Left
Scaphoid bone	Carpal, Right
	Carpal, Left
Scapholunate ligament	Wrist Bursa and Ligament, Right
	Wrist Bursa and Ligament, Left
Scaphotrapezium ligament	Hand Bursa and Ligament, Right
	Hand Bursa and Ligament, Left
Scarpa's (vestibular) ganglion	Acoustic Nerve
Sebaceous gland	Skin
Second cranial nerve	Optic Nerve
Sella turcica	Sphenoid Bone
Semicircular canal	Inner Ear, Right
	Inner Ear, Left
Semimembranosus muscle	Upper Leg Muscle, Right
	Upper Leg Muscle, Left
Semitendinosus muscle	Upper Leg Muscle, Right
	Upper Leg Muscle, Left
Septal cartilage	Nasal Septum
Serratus anterior muscle	Thorax Muscle, Right
	Thorax Muscle, Left
Serratus posterior muscle	Trunk Muscle, Right
	Trunk Muscle, Left
Seventh cranial nerve	Facial Nerve
Short gastric artery	Splenic Artery
Sigmoid artery	Inferior Mesenteric Artery
Sigmoid flexure	Sigmoid Colon
Sigmoid vein	Inferior Mesenteric Vein
Sinoatrial node	Conduction Mechanism
Sinus venosus	Atrium, Right
Sixth cranial nerve	Abducens Nerve

Term	ICD-10-PCS Value
Skene's (paraurethral) gland	Vestibular Gland
Small saphenous vein	Saphenous Vein, Right
	Saphenous Vein, Left
Solar (celiac) plexus	Abdominal Sympathetic Nerve
Soleus muscle	Lower Leg Muscle, Right
	Lower Leg Muscle, Left
Space of Retzius	Pelvic Cavity
Sphenomandibular ligament	Head and Neck Bursa and Ligament
Sphenopalatine (pterygopalatine) ganglion	Head and Neck Sympathetic Nerve
Spinal nerve, cervical	Cervical Nerve
Spinal nerve, lumbar	Lumbar Nerve
Spinal nerve, sacral	Sacral Nerve
Spinal nerve, thoracic	Thoracic Nerve
Spinous process	Cervical Vertebra
	Lumbar Vertebra
	Thoracic Vertebra
Spiral ganglion	Acoustic Nerve
Splenic flexure	Transverse Colon
Splenic plexus	Abdominal Sympathetic Nerve
Splenius capitis muscle	Head Muscle
Splenius cervicis muscle	Neck Muscle, Right
	Neck Muscle, Left
Stapes	Auditory Ossicle, Right
	Auditory Ossicle, Left
Stellate ganglion	Head and Neck Sympathetic Nerve
Stensen's duct	Parotid Duct, Right
	Parotid Duct, Left
Sternoclavicular ligament	Shoulder Bursa and Ligament, Right
	Shoulder Bursa and Ligament, Left
Sternocleidomastoid artery	Thyroid Artery, Right
	Thyroid Artery, Left
Sternocleidomastoid muscle	Neck Muscle, Right
	Neck Muscle, Left
Sternocostal ligament	Sternum Bursa and Ligament
Styloglossus muscle	Tongue, Palate, Pharynx Muscle
Stylomandibular ligament	Head and Neck Bursa and Ligament
Stylopharyngeus muscle	Tongue, Palate, Pharynx Muscle
Subacromial bursa	Shoulder Bursa and Ligament, Right
	Shoulder Bursa and Ligament, Left
Subaortic (common iliac) lymph node	Lymphatic, Pelvis
Subarachnoid space, spinal	Spinal Canal
Subclavicular (apical) lymph node	Lymphatic, Right Axillary
	Lymphatic, Left Axillary
Subclavius muscle	Thorax Muscle, Right
	Thorax Muscle, Left
Subclavius nerve	Brachial Plexus
Subcostal artery	Upper Artery
Subcostal muscle	Thorax Muscle, Right
	Thorax Muscle, Left
Subcostal nerve	Thoracic Nerve
Subdural space, spinal	Spinal Canal
Submandibular ganglion	Facial Nerve
	Head and Neck Sympathetic Nerve
Submandibular gland	Submaxillary Gland, Right
	Submaxillary Gland, Left
Submandibular lymph node	Lymphatic, Head
Submandibular space	Subcutaneous Tissue and Fascia, Face
Submaxillary ganglion	Head and Neck Sympathetic Nerve
Submaxillary lymph node	Lymphatic, Head

Term	ICD-10-PCS Value
Submental artery	Face Artery
Submental lymph node	Lymphatic, Head
Submucous (Meissner's) plexus	Abdominal Sympathetic Nerve
Suboccipital nerve	Cervical Nerve
Suboccipital venous plexus	Vertebral Vein, Right
	Vertebral Vein, Left
Subparotid lymph node	Lymphatic, Head
Subscapular aponeurosis	Subcutaneous Tissue and Fascia, Right Upper Arm
	Subcutaneous Tissue and Fascia, Left Upper Arm
Subscapular artery	Axillary Artery, Right
	Axillary Artery, Left
Subscapular (posterior) lymph node	Lymphatic, Right Axillary
	Lymphatic, Left Axillary
Subscapularis muscle	Shoulder Muscle, Right
	Shoulder Muscle, Left
Substantia nigra	Basal Ganglia
Subtalar (talocalcaneal) joint	Tarsal Joint, Right
	Tarsal Joint, Left
Subtalar ligament	Foot Bursa and Ligament, Right
	Foot Bursa and Ligament, Left
Subthalamic nucleus	Basal Ganglia
Superficial circumflex iliac vein	Saphenous Vein, Right
	Saphenous Vein, Left
Superficial epigastric artery	Femoral Artery, Right
	Femoral Artery, Left
Superficial epigastric vein	Saphenous Vein, Right
	Saphenous Vein, Left
Superficial palmar arch	Hand Artery, Right
	Hand Artery, Left
Superficial palmar venous arch	Hand Vein, Right
	Hand Vein, Left
Superficial temporal artery	Temporal Artery, Right
	Temporal Artery, Left
Superficial transverse perineal muscle	Perineum Muscle
Superior cardiac nerve	Thoracic Sympathetic Nerve
Superior cerebellar vein	Intracranial Vein
Superior cerebral vein	Intracranial Vein
Superior clunic (cluneal) nerve	Lumbar Nerve
Superior epigastric artery	Internal Mammary Artery, Right
	Internal Mammary Artery, Left
Superior genicular artery	Popliteal Artery, Right
	Popliteal Artery, Left
Superior gluteal artery	Internal Iliac Artery, Right
	Internal Iliac Artery, Left
Superior gluteal nerve	Lumbar Plexus
Superior hypogastric plexus	Abdominal Sympathetic Nerve
Superior labial artery	Face Artery
Superior laryngeal artery	Thyroid Artery, Right
	Thyroid Artery, Left
Superior laryngeal nerve	Vagus Nerve
Superior longitudinal muscle	Tongue, Palate, Pharynx Muscle
Superior mesenteric ganglion	Abdominal Sympathetic Nerve
Superior mesenteric lymph node	Lymphatic, Mesenteric
Superior mesenteric plexus	Abdominal Sympathetic Nerve

Term	ICD-10-PCS Value
Superior oblique muscle	Extraocular Muscle, Right
	Extraocular Muscle, Left
Superior olivary nucleus	Pons
Superior rectal artery	Inferior Mesenteric Artery
Superior rectal vein	Inferior Mesenteric Vein
Superior rectus muscle	Extraocular Muscle, Right
	Extraocular Muscle, Left
Superior tarsal plate	Upper Eyelid, Right
	Upper Eyelid, Left
Superior thoracic artery	Axillary Artery, Right
	Axillary Artery, Left
Superior thyroid artery	External Carotid Artery, Right
	External Carotid Artery, Left
	Thyroid Artery, Right
	Thyroid Artery, Left
Superior turbinate	Nasal Turbinate
Superior ulnar collateral artery	Brachial Artery, Right
	Brachial Artery, Left
Superior vesical artery	Internal Iliac Artery, Right
	Internal Iliac Artery, Left
Supraclavicular nerve	Cervical Plexus
Supraclavicular (Virchow's) lymph node	Lymphatic, Right Neck
	Lymphatic, Left Neck
Suprahyoid lymph node	Lymphatic, Head
Suprahyoid muscle	Neck Muscle, Right
	Neck Muscle, Left
Suprainguinal lymph node	Lymphatic, Pelvis
Supraorbital vein	Face Vein, Right
	Face Vein, Left
Suprarenal gland	Adrenal Gland, Right
	Adrenal Gland, Left
	Adrenal Glands, Bilateral
	Adrenal Gland
Suprarenal plexus	Abdominal Sympathetic Nerve
Suprascapular nerve	Brachial Plexus
Supraspinatus fascia	Subcutaneous Tissue and Fascia, Right Upper Arm
	Subcutaneous Tissue and Fascia, Left Upper Arm
Supraspinatus muscle	Shoulder Muscle, Right
	Shoulder Muscle, Left
Supraspinous ligament	Upper Spine Bursa and Ligament
	Lower Spine Bursa and Ligament
Suprasternal notch	Sternum
Supratrochlear lymph node	Lymphatic, Right Upper Extremity
	Lymphatic, Left Upper Extremity
Sural artery	Popliteal Artery, Right
	Popliteal Artery, Left
Sweat gland	Skin
Talocalcaneal ligament	Foot Bursa and Ligament, Right
	Foot Bursa and Ligament, Left
Talocalcaneal (subtalar) joint	Tarsal Joint, Right
	Tarsal Joint, Left
Talocalcaneonavicular joint	Tarsal Joint, Right
	Tarsal Joint, Left
Talocalcaneonavicular ligament	Foot Bursa and Ligament, Right
	Foot Bursa and Ligament, Left
Talocrural joint	Ankle Joint, Right
	Ankle Joint, Left
Talofibular ligament	Ankle Bursa and Ligament, Right
	Ankle Bursa and Ligament, Left

Term	ICD-10-PCS Value
Talus bone	Tarsal, Right
	Tarsal, Left
Tarsometatarsal ligament	Foot Bursa and Ligament, Right
	Foot Bursa and Ligament, Left
Temporal lobe	Cerebral Hemisphere
Temporalis muscle	Head Muscle
Temporoparietalis muscle	Head Muscle
Tensor fasciae latae muscle	Hip Muscle, Right
	Hip Muscle, Left
Tensor veli palatini muscle	Tongue, Palate, Pharynx Muscle
Tenth cranial nerve	Vagus Nerve
Tentorium cerebelli	Dura Mater
Teres major muscle	Shoulder Muscle, Right
	Shoulder Muscle, Left
Teres minor muscle	Shoulder Muscle, Right
	Shoulder Muscle, Left
Testicular artery	Abdominal Aorta
Thenar muscle	Hand Muscle, Right
	Hand Muscle, Left
Third cranial nerve	Oculomotor Nerve
Third occipital nerve	Cervical Nerve
Third ventricle	Cerebral Ventricle
Thoracic aortic plexus	Thoracic Sympathetic Nerve
Thoracic esophagus	Esophagus, Middle
Thoracic facet joint	Thoracic Vertebral Joint
Thoracic ganglion	Thoracic Sympathetic Nerve
Thoracoacromial artery	Axillary Artery, Right
	Axillary Artery, Left
Thoracolumbar facet joint	Thoracolumbar Vertebral Joint
Thymus gland	Thymus
Thyroarytenoid muscle	Neck Muscle, Right
	Neck Muscle, Left
Thyrocervical trunk	Thyroid Artery, Right
	Thyroid Artery, Left
Thyroid cartilage	Larynx
Tibial sesamoid	Metatarsal, Right
	Metatarsal, Left
Tibialis anterior muscle	Lower Leg Muscle, Right
	Lower Leg Muscle, Left
Tibialis posterior muscle	Lower Leg Muscle, Right
	Lower Leg Muscle, Left
Tibiofemoral joint	Knee Joint, Right
	Knee Joint, Left
	Knee Joint, Tibial Surface, Right
	Knee Joint, Tibial Surface, Left
Tibioperoneal trunk	Popliteal Artery, Right
	Popliteal Artery, Left
Tongue, base of	Pharynx
Tracheobronchial lymph node	Lymphatic, Thorax
Tragus	External Ear, Right
	External Ear, Left
	External Ear, Bilateral
Transversalis fascia	Subcutaneous Tissue and Fascia, Trunk
Transverse acetabular ligament	Hip Bursa and Ligament, Right
	Hip Bursa and Ligament, Left
Transverse (cutaneous) cervical nerve	Cervical Plexus
Transverse facial artery	Temporal Artery, Right
	Temporal Artery, Left
Transverse foramen	Cervical Vertebra
Transverse humeral ligament	Shoulder Bursa and Ligament, Right
	Shoulder Bursa and Ligament, Left
Transverse ligament of atlas	Head and Neck Bursa and Ligament
Transverse process	Cervical Vertebra
	Thoracic Vertebra
	Lumbar Vertebra
Transverse scapular ligament	Shoulder Bursa and Ligament, Right
	Shoulder Bursa and Ligament, Left
Transverse thoracis muscle	Thorax Muscle, Right
	Thorax Muscle, Left
Transversospinalis muscle	Trunk Muscle, Right
	Trunk Muscle, Left
Transversus abdominis muscle	Abdomen Muscle, Right
	Abdomen Muscle, Left
Trapezium bone	Carpal, Right
	Carpal, Left
Trapezius muscle	Trunk Muscle, Right
	Trunk Muscle, Left
Trapezoid bone	Carpal, Right
	Carpal, Left
Triceps brachii muscle	Upper Arm Muscle, Right
	Upper Arm Muscle, Left
Tricuspid annulus	Tricuspid Valve
Trifacial nerve	Trigeminal Nerve
Trigone of bladder	Bladder
Triquetral bone	Carpal, Right
	Carpal, Left
Trochanteric bursa	Hip Bursa and Ligament, Right
	Hip Bursa and Ligament, Left
Twelfth cranial nerve	Hypoglossal Nerve
Tympanic cavity	Middle Ear, Right
	Middle Ear, Left
Tympanic nerve	Glossopharyngeal Nerve
Tympanic part of temoporal bone	Temporal Bone, Right
	Temporal Bone, Left
Ulnar collateral carpal ligament	Wrist Bursa and Ligament, Right
	Wrist Bursa and Ligament, Left
Ulnar collateral ligament	Elbow Bursa and Ligament, Right
	Elbow Bursa and Ligament, Left
Ulnar notch	Radius, Right
	Radius, Left
Ulnar vein	Brachial Vein, Right
	Brachial Vein, Left
Umbilical artery	Internal Iliac Artery, Right
	Internal Iliac Artery, Left
	Lower Artery
Ureteral orifice	Ureter, Right
	Ureter, Left
	Ureters, Bilateral
	Ureter
Ureteropelvic junction (UPJ)	Kidney Pelvis, Right
	Kidney Pelvis, Left
Ureterovesical orifice	Ureter, Right
	Ureter, Left
	Ureters, Bilateral
	Ureter
Uterine artery	Internal Iliac Artery, Right
	Internal Iliac Artery, Left
Uterine cornu	Uterus

Term	ICD-10-PCS Value
Uterine tube	Fallopian Tube, Right
	Fallopian Tube, Left
Uterine vein	Hypogastric Vein, Right
	Hypogastric Vein, Left
Vaginal artery	Internal Iliac Artery, Right
	Internal Iliac Artery, Left
Vaginal vein	Hypogastric Vein, Right
	Hypogastric Vein, Left
Vastus intermedius muscle	Upper Leg Muscle, Right
	Upper Leg Muscle, Left
Vastus lateralis muscle	Upper Leg Muscle, Right
	Upper Leg Muscle, Left
Vastus medialis muscle	Upper Leg Muscle, Right
	Upper Leg Muscle, Left
Ventricular fold	Larynx
Vermiform appendix	Appendix
Vermilion border	Upper Lip
	Lower Lip
Vertebral arch	Cervical Vertebra
	Lumbar Vertebra
	Thoracic Vertebra
Vertebral artery, intracranial portion	Intracranial Artery
Vertebral body	Cervical Vertebra
	Lumbar Vertebra
	Thoracic Vertebra
Vertebral canal	Spinal Canal
Vertebral foramen	Cervical Vertebra
	Lumbar Vertebra
	Thoracic Vertebra
Vertebral lamina	Cervical Vertebra
	Lumbar Vertebra
	Thoracic Vertebra
Vertebral pedicle	Cervical Vertebra
	Lumbar Vertebra
	Thoracic Vertebra

Term	ICD-10-PCS Value
Vesical vein	Hypogastric Vein, Right
	Hypogastric Vein, Left
Vestibular (Scarpa's) ganglion	Acoustic Nerve
Vestibular nerve	Acoustic Nerve
Vestibulocochlear nerve	Acoustic Nerve
Virchow's (supraclavicular) lymph node	Lymphatic, Right Neck
	Lymphatic, Left Neck
Vitreous body	Vitreous, Right
	Vitreous, Left
Vocal fold	Vocal Cord, Right
	Vocal Cord, Left
Volar (palmar) digital vein	Hand Vein, Right
	Hand Vein, Left
Volar (palmar) metacarpal vein	Hand Vein, Right
	Hand Vein, Left
Vomer bone	Nasal Septum
Vomer of nasal septum	Nasal Bone
Xiphoid process	Sternum
Zonule of Zinn	Lens, Right
	Lens, Left
Zygomatic process of frontal bone	Frontal Bone
Zygomatic process of temporal bone	Temporal Bone, Right
	Temporal Bone, Left
Zygomaticus muscle	Facial Muscle

Appendix E: Body Part Definitions

ICD-10-PCS Value	Definition
1st Toe, Left 1st Toe, Right	Hallux
Abdomen Muscle, Left Abdomen Muscle, Right	External oblique muscle Internal oblique muscle Pyramidalis muscle Rectus abdominis muscle Transversus abdominis muscle
Abdominal Aorta	Inferior phrenic artery Lumbar artery Median sacral artery Middle suprarenal artery Ovarian artery Testicular artery
Abdominal Sympathetic Nerve	Abdominal aortic plexus Auerbach's (myenteric) plexus Celiac (solar) plexus Celiac ganglion Gastric plexus Hepatic plexus Inferior hypogastric plexus Inferior mesenteric ganglion Inferior mesenteric plexus Meissner's (submucous) plexus Myenteric (Auerbach's) plexus Pancreatic plexus Pelvic splanchnic nerve Renal nerve Renal plexus Solar (celiac) plexus Splenic plexus Submucous (Meissner's) plexus Superior hypogastric plexus Superior mesenteric ganglion Superior mesenteric plexus Suprarenal plexus
Abducens Nerve	Sixth cranial nerve
Accessory Nerve	Eleventh cranial nerve
Acoustic Nerve	Cochlear nerve Eighth cranial nerve Scarpa's (vestibular) ganglion Spiral ganglion Vestibular (Scarpa's) ganglion Vestibular nerve Vestibulocochlear nerve
Adenoids	Pharyngeal tonsil
Adrenal Gland Adrenal Gland, Left Adrenal Gland, Right Adrenal Glands, Bilateral	Suprarenal gland
Ampulla of Vater	Duodenal ampulla Hepatopancreatic ampulla
Anal Sphincter	External anal sphincter Internal anal sphincter
Ankle Bursa and Ligament, Left Ankle Bursa and Ligament, Right	Calcaneofibular ligament Deltoid ligament Ligament of the lateral malleolus Talofibular ligament
Ankle Joint, Left Ankle Joint, Right	Inferior tibiofibular joint Talocrural joint
Anterior Chamber, Left Anterior Chamber, Right	Aqueous humour
Anterior Tibial Artery, Left Anterior Tibial Artery, Right	Anterior lateral malleolar artery Anterior medial malleolar artery Anterior tibial recurrent artery Dorsalis pedis artery Posterior tibial recurrent artery

ICD-10-PCS Value	Definition
Anus	Anal orifice
Aortic Valve	Aortic annulus
Appendix	Appendiceal orifice Vermiform appendix
Atrial Septum	Interatrial septum
Atrium, Left	Atrium pulmonale Left auricular appendix
Atrium, Right	Atrium dextrum cordis Right auricular appendix Sinus venosus
Auditory Ossicle, Left Auditory Ossicle, Right	Incus Malleus Stapes
Axillary Artery, Left Axillary Artery, Right	Anterior circumflex humeral artery Lateral thoracic artery Posterior circumflex humeral artery Subscapular artery Superior thoracic artery Thoracoacromial artery
Azygos Vein	Right ascending lumbar vein Right subcostal vein
Basal Ganglia	Basal nuclei Claustrum Corpus striatum Globus pallidus Substantia nigra Subthalamic nucleus
Basilic Vein, Left Basilic Vein, Right	Median antebrachial vein Median cubital vein
Bladder	Trigone of bladder
Brachial Artery, Left Brachial Artery, Right	Inferior ulnar collateral artery Profunda brachii Superior ulnar collateral artery
Brachial Plexus	Axillary nerve Dorsal scapular nerve First intercostal nerve Long thoracic nerve Musculocutaneous nerve Subclavius nerve Suprascapular nerve
Brachial Vein, Left Brachial Vein, Right	Radial vein Ulnar vein
Brain	Cerebrum Corpus callosum Encephalon
Breast, Bilateral Breast, Left Breast, Right	Mammary duct Mammary gland
Buccal Mucosa	Buccal gland Molar gland Palatine gland
Carotid Bodies, Bilateral Carotid Body, Left Carotid Body, Right	Carotid glomus
Carpal Joint, Left Carpal Joint, Right	Intercarpal joint Midcarpal joint
Carpal, Left Carpal, Right	Capitate bone Hamate bone Lunate bone Pisiform bone Scaphoid bone Trapezium bone Trapezoid bone Triquetral bone
Celiac Artery	Celiac trunk

ICD-10-PCS Value	Definition
Cephalic Vein, Left **Cephalic Vein, Right**	Accessory cephalic vein
Cerebellum	Culmen
Cerebral Hemisphere	Frontal lobe Occipital lobe Parietal lobe Temporal lobe
Cerebral Meninges	Arachnoid mater, intracranial Leptomeninges, intracranial Pia mater, intracranial
Cerebral Ventricle	Aqueduct of Sylvius Cerebral aqueduct (Sylvius) Choroid plexus Ependyma Foramen of Monro (intraventricular) Fourth ventricle Interventricular foramen (Monro) Left lateral ventricle Right lateral ventricle Third ventricle
Cervical Nerve	Greater occipital nerve Spinal nerve, cervical Suboccipital nerve Third occipital nerve
Cervical Plexus	Ansa cervicalis Cutaneous (transverse) cervical nerve Great auricular nerve Lesser occipital nerve Supraclavicular nerve Transverse (cutaneous) cervical nerve
Cervical Spinal Cord	Dorsal root ganglion
Cervical Vertebra	Dens Odontoid process Spinous process Transverse foramen Transverse process Vertebral arch Vertebral body Vertebral foramen Vertebral lamina Vertebral pedicle
Cervical Vertebral Joint	Atlantoaxial joint Cervical facet joint
Cervical Vertebral Joints, 2 or more	Cervical facet joint
Cervicothoracic Vertebral Joint	Cervicothoracic facet joint
Cisterna Chyli	Intestinal lymphatic trunk Lumbar lymphatic trunk
Coccygeal Glomus	Coccygeal body
Colic Vein	Ileocolic vein Left colic vein Middle colic vein Right colic vein
Conduction Mechanism	Atrioventricular node Bundle of His Bundle of Kent Sinoatrial node
Conjunctiva, Left **Conjunctiva, Right**	Plica semilunaris
Dura Mater	Diaphragma sellae Dura mater, intracranial Falx cerebri Tentorium cerebelli
Elbow Bursa and Ligament, Left **Elbow Bursa and Ligament, Right**	Annular ligament Olecranon bursa Radial collateral ligament Ulnar collateral ligament

ICD-10-PCS Value	Definition
Elbow Joint, Left **Elbow Joint, Right**	Distal humerus, involving joint Humeroradial joint Humeroulnar joint Proximal radioulnar joint
Epidural Space, Intracranial	Extradural space, intracranial
Epiglottis	Glossoepiglottic fold
Esophagogastric Junction	Cardia Cardioesophageal junction Gastroesophageal (GE) junction
Esophagus, Lower	Abdominal esophagus
Esophagus, Middle	Thoracic esophagus
Esophagus, Upper	Cervical esophagus
Ethmoid Bone, Left **Ethmoid Bone, Right**	Cribriform plate
Ethmoid Sinus, Left **Ethmoid Sinus, Right**	Ethmoidal air cell
Eustachian Tube, Left **Eustachian Tube, Right**	Auditory tube Pharyngotympanic tube
External Auditory Canal, Left **External Auditory Canal, Right**	External auditory meatus
External Carotid Artery, Left **External Carotid Artery, Right**	Ascending pharyngeal artery Internal maxillary artery Lingual artery Maxillary artery Occipital artery Posterior auricular artery Superior thyroid artery
External Ear, Bilateral **External Ear, Left** **External Ear, Right**	Antihelix Antitragus Auricle Earlobe Helix Pinna Tragus
External Iliac Artery, Left **External Iliac Artery, Right**	Deep circumflex iliac artery Inferior epigastric artery
External Jugular Vein, Left **External Jugular Vein, Right**	Posterior auricular vein
Extraocular Muscle, Left **Extraocular Muscle, Right**	Inferior oblique muscle Inferior rectus muscle Lateral rectus muscle Medial rectus muscle Superior oblique muscle Superior rectus muscle
Eye, Left **Eye, Right**	Ciliary body Posterior chamber
Face Artery	Angular artery Ascending palatine artery External maxillary artery Facial artery Inferior labial artery Submental artery Superior labial artery
Face Vein, Left **Face Vein, Right**	Angular vein Anterior facial vein Common facial vein Deep facial vein Frontal vein Posterior facial (retromandibular) vein Supraorbital vein

ICD-10-PCS Value	Definition
Facial Muscle	Buccinator muscle Corrugator supercilii muscle Depressor anguli oris muscle Depressor labii inferioris muscle Depressor septi nasi muscle Depressor supercilii muscle Levator anguli oris muscle Levator labii superioris alaeque nasi muscle Levator labii superioris muscle Mentalis muscle Nasalis muscle Occipitofrontalis muscle Orbicularis oris muscle Procerus muscle Risorius muscle Zygomaticus muscle
Facial Nerve	Chorda tympani Geniculate ganglion Greater superficial petrosal nerve Nerve to the stapedius Parotid plexus Posterior auricular nerve Seventh cranial nerve Submandibular ganglion
Fallopian Tube, Left **Fallopian Tube, Right**	Oviduct Salpinx Uterine tube
Femoral Artery, Left **Femoral Artery, Right**	Circumflex iliac artery Deep femoral artery Descending genicular artery External pudendal artery Superficial epigastric artery
Femoral Nerve	Anterior crural nerve Saphenous nerve
Femoral Shaft, Left **Femoral Shaft, Right**	Body of femur
Femoral Vein, Left **Femoral Vein, Right**	Deep femoral (profunda femoris) vein Popliteal vein Profunda femoris (deep femoral) vein
Fibula, Left **Fibula, Right**	Body of fibula Head of fibula Lateral malleolus
Finger Nail	Nail bed Nail plate
Finger Phalangeal Joint, Left **Finger Phalangeal Joint, Right**	Interphalangeal (IP) joint
Foot Artery, Left **Foot Artery, Right**	Arcuate artery Dorsal metatarsal artery Lateral plantar artery Lateral tarsal artery Medial plantar artery
Foot Bursa and Ligament, Left **Foot Bursa and Ligament, Right**	Calcaneocuboid ligament Cuneonavicular ligament Intercuneiform ligament Interphalangeal ligament Metatarsal ligament Metatarsophalangeal ligament Subtalar ligament Talocalcaneal ligament Talocalcaneonavicular ligament Tarsometatarsal ligament
Foot Muscle, Left **Foot Muscle, Right**	Abductor hallucis muscle Adductor hallucis muscle Extensor digitorum brevis muscle Extensor hallucis brevis muscle Flexor digitorum brevis muscle Flexor hallucis brevis muscle Quadratus plantae muscle

ICD-10-PCS Value	Definition
Foot Vein, Left **Foot Vein, Right**	Common digital vein Dorsal metatarsal vein Dorsal venous arch Plantar digital vein Plantar metatarsal vein Plantar venous arch
Frontal Bone	Zygomatic process of frontal bone
Gastric Artery	Left gastric artery Right gastric artery
Glenoid Cavity, Left **Glenoid Cavity, Right**	Glenoid fossa (of scapula)
Glomus Jugulare	Jugular body
Glossopharyngeal Nerve	Carotid sinus nerve Ninth cranial nerve Tympanic nerve
Hand Artery, Left **Hand Artery, Right**	Deep palmar arch Princeps pollicis artery Radialis indicis Superficial palmar arch
Hand Bursa and Ligament, Left **Hand Bursa and Ligament, Right**	Carpometacarpal ligament Intercarpal ligament Interphalangeal ligament Lunotriquetral ligament Metacarpal ligament Metacarpophalangeal ligament Pisohamate ligament Pisometacarpal ligament Scaphotrapezium ligament
Hand Muscle, Left **Hand Muscle, Right**	Hypothenar muscle Palmar interosseous muscle Thenar muscle
Hand Vein, Left **Hand Vein, Right**	Dorsal metacarpal vein Palmar (volar) digital vein Palmar (volar) metacarpal vein Superficial palmar venous arch Volar (palmar) digital vein Volar (palmar) metacarpal vein
Head and Neck Bursa and Ligament	Alar ligament of axis Cervical interspinous ligament Cervical intertransverse ligament Cervical ligamentum flavum Interspinous ligament, cervical Intertransverse ligament, cervical Lateral temporomandibular ligament Ligamentum flavum, cervical Sphenomandibular ligament Stylomandibular ligament Transverse ligament of atlas
Head and Neck Sympathetic Nerve	Cavernous plexus Cervical ganglion Ciliary ganglion Internal carotid plexus Otic ganglion Pterygopalatine (sphenopalatine) ganglion Sphenopalatine (pterygopalatine) ganglion Stellate ganglion Submandibular ganglion Submaxillary ganglion
Head Muscle	Auricularis muscle Masseter muscle Pterygoid muscle Splenius capitis muscle Temporalis muscle Temporoparietalis muscle
Heart, Left	Left coronary sulcus Obtuse margin
Heart, Right	Right coronary sulcus
Hemiazygos Vein	Left ascending lumbar vein Left subcostal vein

ICD-10-PCS Value	Definition
Hepatic Artery	Common hepatic artery Gastroduodenal artery Hepatic artery proper
Hip Bursa and Ligament, Left **Hip Bursa and Ligament, Right**	Iliofemoral ligament Ischiofemoral ligament Pubofemoral ligament Transverse acetabular ligament Trochanteric bursa
Hip Joint, Left **Hip Joint, Right**	Acetabulofemoral joint
Hip Muscle, Left **Hip Muscle, Right**	Gemellus muscle Gluteus maximus muscle Gluteus medius muscle Gluteus minimus muscle Iliacus muscle Obturator muscle Piriformis muscle Psoas muscle Quadratus femoris muscle Tensor fasciae latae muscle
Humeral Head, Left **Humeral Head, Right**	Greater tuberosity Lesser tuberosity Neck of humerus (anatomical)(surgical)
Humeral Shaft, Left **Humeral Shaft, Right**	Distal humerus Humerus, distal Lateral epicondyle of humerus Medial epicondyle of humerus
Hypogastric Vein, Left **Hypogastric Vein, Right**	Gluteal vein Internal iliac vein Internal pudendal vein Lateral sacral vein Middle hemorrhoidal vein Obturator vein Uterine vein Vaginal vein Vesical vein
Hypoglossal Nerve	Twelfth cranial nerve
Hypothalamus	Mammillary body
Inferior Mesenteric Artery	Sigmoid artery Superior rectal artery
Inferior Mesenteric Vein	Sigmoid vein Superior rectal vein
Inferior Vena Cava	Postcava Right inferior phrenic vein Right ovarian vein Right second lumbar vein Right suprarenal vein Right testicular vein
Inguinal Region, Bilateral **Inguinal Region, Left** **Inguinal Region, Right**	Inguinal canal Inguinal triangle
Inner Ear, Left **Inner Ear, Right**	Bony labyrinth Bony vestibule Cochlea Round window Semicircular canal
Innominate Artery	Brachiocephalic artery Brachiocephalic trunk
Innominate Vein, Left **Innominate Vein, Right**	Brachiocephalic vein Inferior thyroid vein
Internal Carotid Artery, Left **Internal Carotid Artery, Right**	Caroticotympanic artery Carotid sinus
Internal Iliac Artery, Left **Internal Iliac Artery, Right**	Deferential artery Hypogastric artery Iliolumbar artery Inferior gluteal artery Inferior vesical artery Internal pudendal artery Lateral sacral artery Middle rectal artery Obturator artery Prostatic artery Superior gluteal artery Superior vesical artery Umbilical artery Uterine artery Vaginal artery
Internal Mammary Artery, Left **Internal Mammary Artery, Right**	Anterior intercostal artery Internal thoracic artery Musculophrenic artery Pericardiophrenic artery Superior epigastric artery
Intracranial Artery	Anterior cerebral artery Anterior choroidal artery Anterior communicating artery Basilar artery Circle of Willis Internal carotid artery, intracranial portion Middle cerebral artery Middle meningeal artery, intracranial portion Ophthalmic artery Posterior cerebral artery Posterior communicating artery Posterior inferior cerebellar artery (PICA) Vertebral artery, intracranial portion
Intracranial Vein	Anterior cerebral vein Basal (internal) cerebral vein Dural venous sinus Great cerebral vein Inferior cerebellar vein Inferior cerebral vein Internal (basal) cerebral vein Middle cerebral vein Ophthalmic vein Superior cerebellar vein Superior cerebral vein
Jejunum	Duodenojejunal flexure
Kidney	Renal calyx Renal capsule Renal cortex Renal segment
Kidney Pelvis, Left **Kidney Pelvis, Right**	Ureteropelvic junction (UPJ)
Kidney, Left **Kidney, Right** **Kidneys, Bilateral**	Renal calyx Renal capsule Renal cortex Renal segment
Knee Bursa and Ligament, Left **Knee Bursa and Ligament, Right**	Anterior cruciate ligament (ACL) Lateral collateral ligament (LCL) Ligament of head of fibula Medial collateral ligament (MCL) Patellar ligament Popliteal ligament Posterior cruciate ligament (PCL) Prepatellar bursa
Knee Joint, Femoral Surface, Left **Knee Joint, Femoral Surface, Right**	Femoropatellar joint Patellofemoral joint

ICD-10-PCS Value	Definition
Knee Joint, Left **Knee Joint, Right**	Femoropatellar joint Femorotibial joint Lateral meniscus Medial meniscus Patellofemoral joint Tibiofemoral joint
Knee Joint, Tibial Surface, Left **Knee Joint, Tibial Surface, Right**	Femorotibial joint Tibiofemoral joint
Knee Tendon, Left **Knee Tendon, Right**	Patellar tendon
Lacrimal Duct, Left **Lacrimal Duct, Right**	Lacrimal canaliculus Lacrimal punctum Lacrimal sac Nasolacrimal duct
Larynx	Aryepiglottic fold Arytenoid cartilage Corniculate cartilage Cuneiform cartilage False vocal cord Glottis Rima glottidis Thyroid cartilage Ventricular fold
Lens, Left **Lens, Right**	Zonule of Zinn
Liver	Quadrate lobe
Lower Arm and Wrist Muscle, Left **Lower Arm and Wrist Muscle, Right**	Anatomical snuffbox Brachioradialis muscle Extensor carpi radialis muscle Extensor carpi ulnaris muscle Flexor carpi radialis muscle Flexor carpi ulnaris muscle Flexor pollicis longus muscle Palmaris longus muscle Pronator quadratus muscle Pronator teres muscle
Lower Artery	Umbilical artery
Lower Eyelid, Left **Lower Eyelid, Right**	Inferior tarsal plate Medial canthus
Lower Femur, Left **Lower Femur, Right**	Lateral condyle of femur Lateral epicondyle of femur Medial condyle of femur Medial epicondyle of femur
Lower Leg Muscle, Left **Lower Leg Muscle, Right**	Extensor digitorum longus muscle Extensor hallucis longus muscle Fibularis brevis muscle Fibularis longus muscle Flexor digitorum longus muscle Flexor hallucis longus muscle Gastrocnemius muscle Peroneus brevis muscle Peroneus longus muscle Popliteus muscle Soleus muscle Tibialis anterior muscle Tibialis posterior muscle
Lower Leg Tendon, Left **Lower Leg Tendon, Right**	Achilles tendon
Lower Lip	Frenulum labii inferioris Labial gland Vermilion border
Lower Spine Bursa and Ligament	Iliolumbar ligament Interspinous ligament, lumbar Intertransverse ligament, lumbar Ligamentum flavum, lumbar Sacrococcygeal ligament Sacroiliac ligament Sacrospinous ligament Sacrotuberous ligament Supraspinous ligament
Lumbar Nerve	Lumbosacral trunk Spinal nerve, lumbar Superior clunic (cluneal) nerve
Lumbar Plexus	Accessory obturator nerve Genitofemoral nerve Iliohypogastric nerve Ilioinguinal nerve Lateral femoral cutaneous nerve Obturator nerve Superior gluteal nerve
Lumbar Spinal Cord	Cauda equina Conus medullaris Dorsal root ganglion
Lumbar Sympathetic Nerve	Lumbar ganglion Lumbar splanchnic nerve
Lumbar Vertebra	Spinous process Transverse process Vertebral arch Vertebral body Vertebral foramen Vertebral lamina Vertebral pedicle
Lumbar Vertebral Joint	Lumbar facet joint
Lumbosacral Joint	Lumbosacral facet joint
Lymphatic, Aortic	Celiac lymph node Gastric lymph node Hepatic lymph node Lumbar lymph node Pancreaticosplenic lymph node Paraaortic lymph node Retroperitoneal lymph node
Lymphatic, Head	Buccinator lymph node Infraauricular lymph node Infraparotid lymph node Parotid lymph node Preauricular lymph node Submandibular lymph node Submaxillary lymph node Submental lymph node Subparotid lymph node Suprahyoid lymph node
Lymphatic, Left Axillary	Anterior (pectoral) lymph node Apical (subclavicular) lymph node Brachial (lateral) lymph node Central axillary lymph node Lateral (brachial) lymph node Pectoral (anterior) lymph node Posterior (subscapular) lymph node Subclavicular (apical) lymph node Subscapular (posterior) lymph node
Lymphatic, Left Lower Extremity	Femoral lymph node Popliteal lymph node
Lymphatic, Left Neck	Cervical lymph node Jugular lymph node Mastoid (postauricular) lymph node Occipital lymph node Postauricular (mastoid) lymph node Retropharyngeal lymph node Supraclavicular (Virchow's) lymph node Virchow's (supraclavicular) lymph node
Lymphatic, Left Upper Extremity	Cubital lymph node Deltopectoral (infraclavicular) lymph node Epitrochlear lymph node Infraclavicular (deltopectoral) lymph node Supratrochlear lymph node
Lymphatic, Mesenteric	Inferior mesenteric lymph node Pararectal lymph node Superior mesenteric lymph node

ICD-10-PCS Value	Definition
Lymphatic, Pelvis	Common iliac (subaortic) lymph node Gluteal lymph node Iliac lymph node Inferior epigastric lymph node Obturator lymph node Sacral lymph node Subaortic (common iliac) lymph node Suprainguinal lymph node
Lymphatic, Right Axillary	Anterior (pectoral) lymph node Apical (subclavicular) lymph node Brachial (lateral) lymph node Central axillary lymph node Lateral (brachial) lymph node Pectoral (anterior) lymph node Posterior (subscapular) lymph node Subclavicular (apical) lymph node Subscapular (posterior) lymph node
Lymphatic, Right Lower Extremity	Femoral lymph node Popliteal lymph node
Lymphatic, Right Neck	Cervical lymph node Jugular lymph node Mastoid (postauricular) lymph node Occipital lymph node Postauricular (mastoid) lymph node Retropharyngeal lymph node Right jugular trunk Right lymphatic duct Right subclavian trunk Supraclavicular (Virchow's) lymph node Virchow's (supraclavicular) lymph node
Lymphatic, Right Upper Extremity	Cubital lymph node Deltopectoral (infraclavicular) lymph node Epitrochlear lymph node Infraclavicular (deltopectoral) lymph node Supratrochlear lymph node
Lymphatic, Thorax	Intercostal lymph node Mediastinal lymph node Parasternal lymph node Paratracheal lymph node Tracheobronchial lymph node
Main Bronchus, Right	Bronchus intermedius Intermediate bronchus
Mandible, Left **Mandible, Right**	Alveolar process of mandible Condyloid process Mandibular notch Mental foramen
Mastoid Sinus, Left **Mastoid Sinus, Right**	Mastoid air cells
Metatarsal, Left **Metatarsal, Right**	Fibular sesamoid Tibial sesamoid
Maxilla	Alveolar process of maxilla
Maxillary Sinus, Left **Maxillary Sinus, Right**	Antrum of Highmore
Median Nerve	Anterior interosseous nerve Palmar cutaneous nerve
Mediastinum	Mediastinal cavity Mediastinal space
Medulla Oblongata	Myelencephalon
Mesentery	Mesoappendix Mesocolon
Metatarsal, Right **Metatarsal, Left**	Fibular sesamoid Tibial sesamoid
Metatarsal-Phalangeal Joint, Left **Metatarsal-Phalangeal Joint, Right**	Metatarsophalangeal (MTP) joint
Middle Ear, Left **Middle Ear, Right**	Oval window Tympanic cavity
Minor Salivary Gland	Anterior lingual gland
Mitral Valve	Bicuspid valve Left atrioventricular valve Mitral annulus
Nasal Bone	Vomer of nasal septum
Nasal Mucosa and Soft Tissue	Columella External naris Greater alar cartilage Internal naris Lateral nasal cartilage Lesser alar cartilage Nasal cavity Nostril
Nasal Septum	Quadrangular cartilage Septal cartilage Vomer bone
Nasal Turbinate	Inferior turbinate Middle turbinate Nasal concha Superior turbinate
Nasopharynx	Choana Fossa of Rosenmuller Pharyngeal recess Rhinopharynx
Neck	Parapharyngeal space Retropharyngeal space
Neck Muscle, Left **Neck Muscle, Right**	Anterior vertebral muscle Arytenoid muscle Cricothyroid muscle Infrahyoid muscle Levator scapulae muscle Platysma muscle Scalene muscle Splenius cervicis muscle Sternocleidomastoid muscle Suprahyoid muscle Thyroarytenoid muscle
Nipple, Left **Nipple, Right**	Areola
Occipital Bone	Foramen magnum
Oculomotor Nerve	Third cranial nerve
Olfactory Nerve	First cranial nerve Olfactory bulb
Omentum	Gastrocolic ligament Gastrocolic omentum Gastrohepatic omentum Gastrophrenic ligament Gastrosplenic ligament Greater Omentum Hepatogastric ligament Lesser Omentum
Optic Nerve	Optic chiasma Second cranial nerve
Orbit, Left **Orbit, Right**	Bony orbit Orbital portion of ethmoid bone Orbital portion of frontal bone Orbital portion of lacrimal bone Orbital portion of maxilla Orbital portion of palatine bone Orbital portion of sphenoid bone Orbital portion of zygomatic bone
Pancreatic Duct	Duct of Wirsung
Pancreatic Duct, Accessory	Duct of Santorini
Parotid Duct, Left **Parotid Duct, Right**	Stensen's duct
Pelvic Bone, Left **Pelvic Bone, Right**	Iliac crest Ilium Ischium Pubis
Pelvic Cavity	Retropubic space Space of Retzius

ICD-10-PCS Value	Definition
Penis	Corpus cavernosum Corpus spongiosum
Perineum Muscle	Bulbospongiosus muscle Cremaster muscle Deep transverse perineal muscle Ischiocavernosus muscle Levator ani muscle Superficial transverse perineal muscle
Peritoneal Cavity	Abdominal cavity
Peritoneum	Epiploic foramen
Peroneal Artery, Left **Peroneal Artery, Right**	Fibular artery
Peroneal Nerve	Common fibular nerve Common peroneal nerve External popliteal nerve Lateral sural cutaneous nerve
Pharynx	Base of Tongue Hypopharynx Laryngopharynx Lingual tonsil Oropharynx Piriform recess (sinus) Tongue, base of
Phrenic Nerve	Accessory phrenic nerve
Pituitary Gland	Adenohypophysis Hypophysis Neurohypophysis
Pons	Apneustic center Basis pontis Locus ceruleus Pneumotaxic center Pontine tegmentum Superior olivary nucleus
Popliteal Artery, Left **Popliteal Artery, Right**	Inferior genicular artery Middle genicular artery Superior genicular artery Sural artery Tibioperoneal trunk
Portal Vein	Hepatic portal vein
Prepuce	Foreskin Glans penis
Pudendal Nerve	Posterior labial nerve Posterior scrotal nerve
Pulmonary Artery, Left	Arterial canal (duct) Botallo's duct Pulmoaortic canal
Pulmonary Valve	Pulmonary annulus Pulmonic valve
Pulmonary Vein, Left	Left inferior pulmonary vein Left superior pulmonary vein
Pulmonary Vein, Right	Right inferior pulmonary vein Right superior pulmonary vein
Radial Artery, Left **Radial Artery, Right**	Radial recurrent artery
Radial Nerve	Dorsal digital nerve Musculospiral nerve Palmar cutaneous nerve Posterior interosseous nerve
Radius, Left **Radius, Right**	Ulnar notch
Rectum	Anorectal junction
Renal Artery, Left **Renal Artery, Right**	Inferior suprarenal artery Renal segmental artery
Renal Vein, Left	Left inferior phrenic vein Left ovarian vein Left second lumbar vein Left suprarenal vein Left testicular vein

ICD-10-PCS Value	Definition
Retina, Left **Retina, Right**	Fovea Macula Optic disc
Retroperitoneum	Retroperitoneal cavity Retroperitoneal space
Rib(s) Bursa and Ligament	Costotransverse ligament
Sacral Nerve	Spinal nerve, sacral
Sacral Plexus	Inferior gluteal nerve Posterior femoral cutaneous nerve Pudendal nerve
Sacral Sympathetic Nerve	Ganglion impar (ganglion of Walther) Pelvic splanchnic nerve Sacral ganglion Sacral splanchnic nerve
Sacrococcygeal Joint	Sacrococcygeal symphysis
Saphenous Vein, Left **Saphenous Vein, Right**	External pudendal vein Great(er) saphenous vein Lesser saphenous vein Small saphenous vein Superficial circumflex iliac vein Superficial epigastric vein
Scapula, Left **Scapula, Right**	Acromion (process) Coracoid process
Sciatic Nerve	Ischiatic nerve
Shoulder Bursa and Ligament, Left **Shoulder Bursa and Ligament, Right**	Acromioclavicular ligament Coracoacromial ligament Coracoclavicular ligament Coracohumeral ligament Costoclavicular ligament Glenohumeral ligament Interclavicular ligament Sternoclavicular ligament Subacromial bursa Transverse humeral ligament Transverse scapular ligament
Shoulder Joint, Left **Shoulder Joint, Right**	Glenohumeral joint Glenoid ligament (labrum)
Shoulder Muscle, Left **Shoulder Muscle, Right**	Deltoid muscle Infraspinatus muscle Subscapularis muscle Supraspinatus muscle Teres major muscle Teres minor muscle
Sigmoid Colon	Rectosigmoid junction Sigmoid flexure
Skin	Dermis Epidermis Sebaceous gland Sweat gland
Skin, Chest	Breast procedures, skin only
Skin, Perineum	Perianal skin
Sphenoid Bone	Greater wing Lesser wing Optic foramen Pterygoid process Sella turcica
Spinal Canal	Epidural space, spinal Extradural space, spinal Subarachnoid space, spinal Subdural space, spinal Vertebral canal
Spinal Cord	Dorsal root ganglion
Spinal Meninges	Arachnoid mater, spinal Denticulate (dentate) ligament Dura mater, spinal Filum terminale Leptomeninges, spinal Pia mater, spinal

ICD-10-PCS Value	Definition
Spleen	Accessory spleen
Splenic Artery	Left gastroepiploic artery Pancreatic artery Short gastric artery
Splenic Vein	Left gastroepiploic vein Pancreatic vein
Sternum	Manubrium Suprasternal notch Xiphoid process
Sternum Bursa and Ligament	Costoxiphoid ligament Sternocostal ligament
Stomach, Pylorus	Pyloric antrum Pyloric canal Pyloric sphincter
Subclavian Artery, Left Subclavian Artery, Right	Costocervical trunk Dorsal scapular artery Internal thoracic artery
Subcutaneous Tissue and Fascia, Chest	Pectoral fascia
Subcutaneous Tissue and Fascia, Face	Chin Masseteric fascia Orbital fascia Submandibular space
Subcutaneous Tissue and Fascia, Left Foot	Plantar fascia (aponeurosis)
Subcutaneous Tissue and Fascia, Left Hand	Palmar fascia (aponeurosis)
Subcutaneous Tissue and Fascia, Left Lower Arm	Antebrachial fascia Bicipital aponeurosis
Subcutaneous Tissue and Fascia, Left Neck	Deep cervical fascia Pretracheal fascia Prevertebral fascia
Subcutaneous Tissue and Fascia, Left Upper Arm	Axillary fascia Deltoid fascia Infraspinatus fascia Subscapular aponeurosis Supraspinatus fascia
Subcutaneous Tissue and Fascia, Left Upper Leg	Crural fascia Fascia lata Iliac fascia Iliotibial tract (band)
Subcutaneous Tissue and Fascia, Right Foot	Plantar fascia (aponeurosis)
Subcutaneous Tissue and Fascia, Right Hand	Palmar fascia (aponeurosis)
Subcutaneous Tissue and Fascia, Right Lower Arm	Antebrachial fascia Bicipital aponeurosis
Subcutaneous Tissue and Fascia, Right Neck	Deep cervical fascia Pretracheal fascia Prevertebral fascia
Subcutaneous Tissue and Fascia, Right Upper Arm	Axillary fascia Deltoid fascia Infraspinatus fascia Subscapular aponeurosis Supraspinatus fascia
Subcutaneous Tissue and Fascia, Right Upper Leg	Crural fascia Fascia lata Iliac fascia Iliotibial tract (band)
Subcutaneous Tissue and Fascia, Scalp	Galea aponeurotica
Subcutaneous Tissue and Fascia, Trunk	External oblique aponeurosis Transversalis fascia
Submaxillary Gland, Left Submaxillary Gland, Right	Submandibular gland

ICD-10-PCS Value	Definition
Superior Mesenteric Artery	Ileal artery Ileocolic artery Inferior pancreaticoduodenal artery Jejunal artery
Superior Mesenteric Vein	Right gastroepiploic vein
Superior Vena Cava	Cavoatrial junction Precava
Tarsal Joint, Left Tarsal Joint, Right	Calcaneocuboid joint Cuboideonavicular joint Cuneonavicular joint Intercuneiform joint Subtalar (talocalcaneal) joint Talocalcaneal (subtalar) joint Talocalcaneonavicular joint
Tarsal, Left Tarsal, Right	Calcaneus Cuboid bone Intermediate cuneiform bone Lateral cuneiform bone Medial cuneiform bone Navicular bone Talus bone
Temporal Artery, Left Temporal Artery, Right	Middle temporal artery Superficial temporal artery Transverse facial artery
Temporal Bone, Left Temporal Bone, Right	Mastoid process Petrous part of temoporal bone Tympanic part of temoporal bone Zygomatic process of temporal bone
Thalamus	Epithalamus Geniculate nucleus Metathalamus Pulvinar
Thoracic Aorta, Ascending/Arch	Aortic arch Ascending aorta
Thoracic Duct	Left jugular trunk Left subclavian trunk
Thoracic Nerve	Intercostal nerve Intercostobrachial nerve Spinal nerve, thoracic Subcostal nerve
Thoracic Spinal Cord	Dorsal root ganglion
Thoracic Sympathetic Nerve	Cardiac plexus Esophageal plexus Greater splanchnic nerve Inferior cardiac nerve Least splanchnic nerve Lesser splanchnic nerve Middle cardiac nerve Pulmonary plexus Superior cardiac nerve Thoracic aortic plexus Thoracic ganglion
Thoracic Vertebra	Spinous process Transverse process Vertebral arch Vertebral body Vertebral foramen Vertebral lamina Vertebral pedicle
Thoracic Vertebral Joint	Costotransverse joint Costovertebral joint Thoracic facet joint
Thoracolumbar Vertebral Joint	Thoracolumbar facet joint

ICD-10-PCS Value	Definition
Thorax Muscle, Left **Thorax Muscle, Right**	Intercostal muscle Levatores costarum muscle Pectoralis major muscle Pectoralis minor muscle Serratus anterior muscle Subclavius muscle Subcostal muscle Transverse thoracis muscle
Thymus	Thymus gland
Thyroid Artery, Left **Thyroid Artery, Right**	Cricothyroid artery Hyoid artery Sternocleidomastoid artery Superior laryngeal artery Superior thyroid artery Thyrocervical trunk
Tibia, Left **Tibia, Right**	Lateral condyle of tibia Medial condyle of tibia Medial malleolus
Tibial Nerve	Lateral plantar nerve Medial plantar nerve Medial popliteal nerve Medial sural cutaneous nerve
Toe Nail	Nail bed Nail plate
Toe Phalangeal Joint, Left **Toe Phalangeal Joint, Right**	Interphalangeal (IP) joint
Tongue	Frenulum linguae
Tongue, Palate, Pharynx Muscle	Chondroglossus muscle Genioglossus muscle Hyoglossus muscle Inferior longitudinal muscle Levator veli palatini muscle Palatoglossal muscle Palatopharyngeal muscle Pharyngeal constrictor muscle Salpingopharyngeus muscle Styloglossus muscle Stylopharyngeus muscle Superior longitudinal muscle Tensor veli palatini muscle
Tonsils	Palatine tonsil
Trachea	Cricoid cartilage
Transverse Colon	Hepatic flexure Splenic flexure
Tricuspid Valve	Right atrioventricular valve Tricuspid annulus
Trigeminal Nerve	Fifth cranial nerve Gasserian ganglion Mandibular nerve Maxillary nerve Ophthalmic nerve Trifacial nerve
Trochlear Nerve	Fourth cranial nerve
Trunk Muscle, Left **Trunk Muscle, Right**	Coccygeus muscle Erector spinae muscle Interspinalis muscle Intertransversarius muscle Latissimus dorsi muscle Quadratus lumborum muscle Rhomboid major muscle Rhomboid minor muscle Serratus posterior muscle Transversospinalis muscle Trapezius muscle
Tympanic Membrane, Left **Tympanic Membrane, Right**	Pars flaccida
Ulna, Left **Ulna, Right**	Olecranon process Radial notch

ICD-10-PCS Value	Definition
Ulnar Artery, Left **Ulnar Artery, Right**	Anterior ulnar recurrent artery Common interosseous artery Posterior ulnar recurrent artery
Ulnar Nerve	Cubital nerve
Upper Arm Muscle, Left **Upper Arm Muscle, Right**	Biceps brachii muscle Brachialis muscle Coracobrachialis muscle Triceps brachii muscle
Upper Artery	Aortic intercostal artery Bronchial artery Esophageal artery Subcostal artery
Upper Eyelid, Left **Upper Eyelid, Right**	Lateral canthus Levator palpebrae superioris muscle Orbicularis oculi muscle Superior tarsal plate
Upper Femur, Left **Upper Femur, Right**	Femoral head Greater trochanter Lesser trochanter Neck of femur
Upper Leg Muscle, Left **Upper Leg Muscle, Right**	Adductor brevis muscle Adductor longus muscle Adductor magnus muscle Biceps femoris muscle Gracilis muscle Pectineus muscle Quadriceps (femoris) Rectus femoris muscle Sartorius muscle Semimembranosus muscle Semitendinosus muscle Vastus intermedius muscle Vastus lateralis muscle Vastus medialis muscle
Upper Lip	Frenulum labii superioris Labial gland Vermilion border
Upper Spine Bursa and Ligament	Interspinous ligament, thoracic Intertransverse ligament, thoracic Ligamentum flavum, thoracic Supraspinous ligament
Ureter **Ureter, Left** **Ureter, Right** **Ureters, Bilateral**	Ureteral orifice Ureterovesical orifice
Urethra	Bulbourethral (Cowper's) gland Cowper's (bulbourethral) gland External urethral sphincter Internal urethral sphincter Membranous urethra Penile urethra Prostatic urethra
Uterine Supporting Structure	Broad ligament Infundibulopelvic ligament Ovarian ligament Round ligament of uterus
Uterus	Fundus uteri Myometrium Perimetrium Uterine cornu
Uvula	Palatine uvula
Vagus Nerve	Anterior vagal trunk Pharyngeal plexus Pneumogastric nerve Posterior vagal trunk Pulmonary plexus Recurrent laryngeal nerve Superior laryngeal nerve Tenth cranial nerve

ICD-10-PCS Value	Definition
Vas Deferens **Vas Deferens, Bilateral** **Vas Deferens, Left** **Vas Deferens, Right**	Ductus deferens Ejaculatory duct
Ventricle, Right	Conus arteriosus
Ventricular Septum	Interventricular septum
Vertebral Artery, Left **Vertebral Artery, Right**	Anterior spinal artery Posterior spinal artery
Vertebral Vein, Left **Vertebral Vein, Right**	Deep cervical vein Suboccipital venous plexus
Vestibular Gland	Bartholin's (greater vestibular) gland Greater vestibular (Bartholin's) gland Paraurethral (Skene's) gland Skene's (paraurethral) gland
Vitreous, Left **Vitreous, Right**	Vitreous body

ICD-10-PCS Value	Definition
Vocal Cord, Left **Vocal Cord, Right**	Vocal fold
Vulva	Labia majora Labia minora
Wrist Bursa and Ligament, Left **Wrist Bursa and Ligament, Right**	Palmar ulnocarpal ligament Radial collateral carpal ligament Radiocarpal ligament Radioulnar ligament Scapholunate ligament Ulnar collateral carpal ligament
Wrist Joint, Left **Wrist Joint, Right**	Distal radioulnar joint Radiocarpal joint

Appendix F: Device Classification

In most PCS codes, the sixth character of the code classifies the device. The sixth character device value "defines the material or appliance used to accomplish the objective of the procedure that remains in or on the procedure site at the end of the procedure." If the device is the means by which the procedural objective is accomplished, then a specific device value is coded in the sixth character. If no device is used to accomplish the objective of the procedure, the device value *No Device* is coded in the sixth character. In limited root operations, the classification provides the qualifier values *Temporary* and *Intraoperative*, for specific procedures involving clinically significant devices whose purpose is brief use during the procedure or current inpatient stay.

Material that is classified as a PCS device is distinguished from material classified as a PCS substance by its having a specific location. A device is intended to maintain a fixed location at the procedure site where it was put, whereas a substance is intended to disperse or be absorbed in the body. There are circumstances in which a device does not stay where it was put and may need to be "revised" in a subsequent procedure to move the device back to its intended location.

Material classified as a PCS device is also distinguishable by the fact that it is removable. Although it may not be practical to remove some types of devices, once they become established at the site, it is physically possible to remove a device for some time after the procedure. A skin graft, for example, once it "takes," may be nearly indistinguishable from the surrounding skin and so is no longer clearly identifiable as a device. Nevertheless, procedures that involve material coded as a device can for the most part be "reversed" by removing the device from the procedure site.

General Device Types

Device Type	Definition	Examples
Grafts	Biological or synthetic material that **takes the place of all or a portion of a body part.**	Full- or partial-thickness skin grafts: • Autologous • Nonautologous • Synthetic • Zooplastic Other tissue grafts: • Bone • Tendon • Vascular
Prosthesis	Biological or synthetic material that **takes the place of all or a portion of a body part.**	Joint prosthesis: • Autologous • Nonautologous • Synthetic
Implants	**Therapeutic** material that is not absorbed by, eliminated by, or incorporated into a body part.	External fixation device Internal fixation device: • Orthopaedic pins • Intramedullary rods Radioactive element implant Mesh
Simple or mechanical appliances	Biological or synthetic material that **assists or prevents a physiological function.**	Drainage device Extraluminal device Endobrachial device Fusion device Intraluminal device (can be temporary) Tracheostomy device IUD
Electronic appliances	Electronic appliances used to **assist, monitor, take the pace of, or prevent a physiological function.**	Cardiac leads Diaphragmatic pacemaker External heart assist system Short-term external heart assist system (Intraoperative) Fetal monitoring Hearing device Monitoring device Neurostimulator
External appliances	Performed without making an incision or a puncture, external appliances are used for the purpose of **protection, immobilization, stretching, compression, or packing.**	Bandage Cast Packing material Pressure dressing Traction apparatus

Transplant/Grafting Tissue Type Terminology

Tissue Type	Terminology
Tissue or organ transferred into a new position in **the body of the same individual**	Autograft Autologous Autoplastic
Having to do with individuals or tissues that have **identical genes**, such as identical twins	Isograft Isologous Syngeneic Syngraft
Tissue or organ taken from **different individuals** of the same species	Allogeneic Allograft Homologous Homograft
Tissue or organ from a **cadaver**	Nonautologous
Tissue or organ from individuals of **different species**	Heterogeneic Heterologous Xenogeneic Xenograft Zooplastic

Appendix G: Device Key and Aggregation Table

This NT symbol next to a device in the Term column identifies that the device has been approved for NTAP (new technology add-on payment). CMS provides incremental payment, in addition to the DRG payment, for technologies that have received an NTAP designation.

Device Key

Terms	ICD-10-PCS Value
3f (Aortic) Bioprosthesis valve	Zooplastic Tissue in Heart and Great Vessels
AbioCor® Total Replacement Heart	Synthetic Substitute
Absolute Pro Vascular (OTW) Self-Expanding Stent System	Intraluminal Device
Acculink (RX) Carotid Stent System	Intraluminal Device
Acellular Hydrated Dermis	Nonautologous Tissue Substitute
Acetabular cup	Liner in Lower Joints
Activa PC neurostimulator	Stimulator Generator, Multiple Array for Insertion in Subcutaneous Tissue and Fascia
Activa RC neurostimulator	Stimulator Generator, Multiple Array Rechargeable for Insertion in Subcutaneous Tissue and Fascia
Activa SC neurostimulator	Stimulator Generator, Single Array for Insertion in Subcutaneous Tissue and Fascia
ACUITY™ Steerable Lead	Cardiac Lead, Pacemaker for Insertion in Heart and Great Vessels Cardiac Lead, Defibrillator for Insertion in Heart and Great Vessels
Advisa (MRI)	Pacemaker, Dual Chamber for Insertion in Subcutaneous Tissue and Fascia
AFX® Endovascular AAA System	Intraluminal Device
Alfapump® system	Other Device
AMPLATZER® Muscular VSD Occluder	Synthetic Substitute
AMS 800® Urinary Control System	Artificial Sphincter in Urinary System
AneuRx® AAA Advantage®	Intraluminal Device
Ankle Truss System™ (ATS)	Internal Fixation Device, Open-truss Design in New Technology
Annuloplasty ring	Synthetic Substitute
Aortix™ System	Short-term External Heart Assist System in Heart and Great Vessels
ApiFix® Minimally Invasive Deformity Correction (MID-C) System (C)	Posterior (Dynamic) Distraction Device in New Technology
aprevo™	Interbody Fusion Device, Custom-made Anatomically Designed in New Technology
Articulating Spacer (Antibiotic)	Articulating Spacer in Lower Joints
Artificial anal sphincter (AAS)	Artificial Sphincter in Gastrointestinal System
Artificial bowel sphincter (neosphincter)	Artificial Sphincter in Gastrointestinal System
Artificial urinary sphincter (AUS)	Artificial Sphincter in Urinary System
Ascenda Intrathecal Catheter	Infusion Device
Assurant (Cobalt) stent	Intraluminal Device
AtriClip LAA Exclusion System	Extraluminal Device
Attain Ability® Lead	Cardiac Lead, Pacemaker for Insertion in Heart and Great Vessels Cardiac Lead, Defibrillator for Insertion in Heart and Great Vessels
Attain StarFix® (OTW) Lead	Cardiac Lead, Pacemaker for Insertion in Heart and Great Vessels Cardiac Lead, Defibrillator for Insertion in Heart and Great Vessels
Autograft	Autologous Tissue Substitute
Autologous artery graft	Autologous Arterial Tissue in Heart and Great Vessels Autologous Arterial Tissue in Upper Arteries Autologous Arterial Tissue in Lower Arteries Autologous Arterial Tissue in Upper Veins Autologous Arterial Tissue in Lower Veins
Autologous vein graft	Autologous Venous Tissue in Heart and Great Vessels Autologous Venous Tissue in Upper Arteries Autologous Venous Tissue in Lower Arteries Autologous Venous Tissue in Upper Veins Autologous Venous Tissue in Lower Veins
Aveir™ AR, as dual chamber	Intracardiac Pacemaker, Dual-Chamber in New Technology
Aveir™ DR, dual chamber	Intracardiac Pacemaker, Dual-Chamber in New Technology
Aveir™ VR, as single chamber	Intracardiac Pacemaker in the Heart and Great Vessels
Axial Lumbar Interbody Fusion System	Interbody Fusion Device in Lower Joints
AxiaLIF® System	Interbody Fusion Device in Lower Joints
BAK/C® Interbody Cervical Fusion System	Interbody Fusion Device in Upper Joints
Bard® Composix® (E/X)(LP) mesh	Synthetic Substitute
Bard® Composix® Kugel® patch	Synthetic Substitute
Bard® Dulex™ mesh	Synthetic Substitute
Bard® Ventralex™ hernia patch	Synthetic Substitute
Baroreflex Activation Therapy® (BAT®)	Stimulator Lead in Upper Arteries Stimulator Generator in Subcutaneous Tissue and Fascia
Barricaid® Annular Closure Device (ACD)	Synthetic Substitute
Berlin Heart Ventricular Assist Device	Implantable Heart Assist System in Heart and Great Vessels
Bioactive embolization coil(s)	Intraluminal Device, Bioactive in Upper Arteries
Biventricular external heart assist system	Short-term External Heart Assist System in Heart and Great Vessels
Blood glucose monitoring system	Monitoring Device
Bone anchored hearing device	Hearing Device, Bone Conduction for Insertion in Ear, Nose, Sinus Hearing Device, in Head and Facial Bones
Bone bank bone graft	Nonautologous Tissue Substitute
Bone screw (interlocking)(lag)(pedicle)(recessed)	Internal Fixation Device in Head and Facial Bones Internal Fixation Device in Upper Bones Internal Fixation Device in Lower Bones
Bovine pericardial valve	Zooplastic Tissue in Heart and Great Vessels
Bovine pericardium graft	Zooplastic Tissue in Heart and Great Vessels
Brachytherapy seeds	Radioactive Element
BRYAN® Cervical Disc System	Synthetic Substitute
BVS 5000 Ventricular Assist Device	Short-term External Heart Assist System in Heart and Great Vessels

Terms	ICD-10-PCS Value
Canturio™ te (Tibial Extension)	Tibial Extension with Motion Sensors in New Technology
Cardiac contractility modulation lead	Cardiac Lead in Heart and Great Vessels
Cardiac event recorder	Monitoring Device
Cardiac resynchronization therapy (CRT) lead	Cardiac Lead, Pacemaker for Insertion in Heart and Great Vessels Cardiac Lead, Defibrillator for Insertion in Heart and Great Vessels
CardioMEMS® pressure sensor	Monitoring Device, Pressure Sensor for Insertion in Heart and Great Vessels
Carmat total artificial heart (TAH)	Biologic with Synthetic Substitute, Autoregulated Electrohydraulic for Replacement in Heart and Great Vessels
Carotid (artery) sinus (baroreceptor) lead	Stimulator Lead in Upper Arteries
Carotid WALLSTENT® Monorail® Endoprosthesis	Intraluminal Device
Centrimag® Blood Pump	Short-term External Heart Assist System in Heart and Great Vessels
Ceramic on ceramic bearing surface	Synthetic Substitute, Ceramic for Replacement in Lower Joints
Cesium-131 Collagen Implant	Radioactive Element, Cesium-131 Collagen Implant for Insertion in Central Nervous System and Cranial Nerves
CivaSheet®	Radioactive Element
Clamp and rod internal fixation system (CRIF)	Internal Fixation Device in Upper Bones Internal Fixation Device in Lower Bones
COALESCE® radiolucent interbody fusion device	Interbody Fusion Device in Upper Joints Interbody Fusion Device in Lower Joints
CoAxia NeuroFlo catheter	Intraluminal Device
Cobalt/chromium head and polyethylene socket	Synthetic Substitute, Metal on Polyethylene for Replacement in Lower Joints
Cobalt/chromium head and socket	Synthetic Substitute, Metal for Replacement in Lower Joints
Cochlear implant (CI), multiple channel (electrode)	Hearing Device, Multiple Channel Cochlear Prosthesis for Insertion in Ear, Nose, Sinus
Cochlear implant (CI), single channel (electrode)	Hearing Device, Single Channel Cochlear Prosthesis for Insertion in Ear, Nose, Sinus
COGNIS® CRT-D	Cardiac Resynchronization Defibrillator Pulse Generator for Insertion in Subcutaneous Tissue and Fascia
COHERE® radiolucent interbody fusion device	Interbody Fusion Device in Upper Joints Interbody Fusion Device in Lower Joints
Colonic Z-Stent®	Intraluminal Device
Complete (SE) stent	Intraluminal Device
Concerto II CRT-D	Cardiac Resynchronization Defibrillator Pulse Generator for Insertion in Subcutaneous Tissue and Fascia
CONSERVE® PLUS Total Resurfacing Hip System	Resurfacing Device in Lower Joints
Consulta CRT-D	Cardiac Resynchronization Defibrillator Pulse Generator for Insertion in Subcutaneous Tissue and Fascia
Consulta CRT-P	Cardiac Resynchronization Pacemaker Pulse Generator for Insertion in Subcutaneous Tissue and Fascia
CONTAK RENEWAL® 3 RF (HE) CRT-D	Cardiac Resynchronization Defibrillator Pulse Generator for Insertion in Subcutaneous Tissue and Fascia
Contegra Pulmonary Valved Conduit	Zooplastic Tissue in Heart and Great Vessels
Continuous Glucose Monitoring (CGM) device	Monitoring Device
Cook Biodesign® Fistula Plug(s)	Nonautologous Tissue Substitute
Cook Biodesign® Hernia Graft(s)	Nonautologous Tissue Substitute
Cook Biodesign® Layered Graft(s)	Nonautologous Tissue Substitute
Cook Zenapro™ Layered Graft(s)	Nonautologous Tissue Substitute
Cook Zenith AAA Endovascular Graft	Intraluminal Device
Cook Zenith® Fenestrated AAA Endovascular Graft	Intraluminal Device, Branched or Fenestrated, One or Two Arteries for Restriction in Lower Arteries Intraluminal Device, Branched or Fenestrated, Three or More Arteries for Restriction in Lower Arteries
CoreValve transcatheter aortic valve	Zooplastic Tissue in Heart and Great Vessels
Cormet Hip Resurfacing System	Resurfacing Device in Lower Joints
CoRoent® XL	Interbody Fusion Device in Lower Joints
Corox (OTW) Bipolar Lead	Cardiac Lead, Pacemaker for Insertion in Heart and Great Vessels Cardiac Lead, Defibrillator for Insertion in Heart and Great Vessels
Cortical strip neurostimulator lead	Neurostimulator Lead in Central Nervous System and Cranial Nerves
Corvia IASD®	Synthetic Substitute
Cultured epidermal cell autograft	Autologous Tissue Substitute
CYPHER® Stent	Intraluminal Device, Drug-eluting in Heart and Great Vessels
Cystostomy tube	Drainage Device
DBS lead	Neurostimulator Lead in Central Nervous System and Cranial Nerves
DeBakey Left Ventricular Assist Device	Implantable Heart Assist System in Heart and Great Vessels
Deep brain neurostimulator lead	Neurostimulator Lead in Central Nervous System and Cranial Nerves
Delta frame external fixator	External Fixation Device, Hybrid for Insertion in Upper Bones External Fixation Device, Hybrid for Reposition in Upper Bones External Fixation Device, Hybrid for Insertion in Lower Bones External Fixation Device, Hybrid for Reposition in Lower Bones
Delta III Reverse shoulder prosthesis	Synthetic Substitute, Reverse Ball and Socket for Replacement in Upper Joints
DETOUR® System	Conduit through Femoral Vein to Popliteal Artery in New Technology Conduit through Femoral Vein to Superficial Femoral Artery in New Technology
Diaphragmatic pacemaker generator	Stimulator Generator in Subcutaneous Tissue and Fascia
Direct Lateral Interbody Fusion (DLIF) device	Interbody Fusion Device in Lower Joints
Driver stent (RX) (OTW)	Intraluminal Device
DuraHeart Left Ventricular Assist System	Implantable Heart Assist System in Heart and Great Vessels
Durata® Defibrillation Lead	Cardiac Lead, Defibrillator for Insertion in Heart and Great Vessels
DynaClip® (Forte)	Internal Fixation Device, Sustained Compression for Fusion in Upper Joints Internal Fixation Device, Sustained Compression for Fusion in Lower Joints
DynaNail® (Helix) (Hybrid) (Mini)	Internal Fixation Device, Sustained Compression for Fusion in Upper Joints Internal Fixation Device, Sustained Compression for Fusion in Lower Joints

Terms	ICD-10-PCS Value
Dynesys® Dynamic Stabilization System	Spinal Stabilization Device, Pedicle-Based for Insertion in Upper Joints Spinal Stabilization Device, Pedicle-Based for Insertion in Lower Joints
E-Luminexx™ (Biliary) (Vascular) Stent	Intraluminal Device
Electrical bone growth stimulator (EBGS)	Bone Growth Stimulator in Head and Facial Bones Bone Growth Stimulator in Upper Bones Bone Growth Stimulator in Lower Bones
Electrical muscle stimulation (EMS) lead	Stimulator Lead in Muscles
Electronic muscle stimulator lead	Stimulator Lead in Muscles
Eluvia™ Drug-eluting Vascular Stent System	Intraluminal Device, Sustained Release Drug-eluting in New Technology Intraluminal Device, Sustained Release Drug-eluting, Two in New Technology Intraluminal Device, Sustained Release Drug-eluting, Three in New Technology Intraluminal Device, Sustained Release Drug-eluting, Four or More in New Technology
Embolization coil(s)	Intraluminal Device
Endeavor® (III) (IV) (Sprint) Zotarolimus-eluting Coronary Stent System	Intraluminal Device, Drug-eluting in Heart and Great Vessels
Endologix AFX® Endovascular AAA System	Intraluminal Device
EndoSure® sensor	Monitoring Device, Pressure Sensor for Insertion in Heart and Great Vessels
ENDOTAK RELIANCE® (G) Defibrillation Lead	Cardiac Lead, Defibrillator for Insertion in Heart and Great Vessels
Endotracheal tube (cuffed) (double-lumen)	Intraluminal Device, Endotracheal Airway in Respiratory System
Endurant® Endovascular Stent Graft	Intraluminal Device
Endurant® II AAA stent graft system	Intraluminal Device
EnRhythm	Pacemaker, Dual Chamber for Insertion in Subcutaneous Tissue and Fascia
Enterra gastric neurostimulator	Stimulator Generator, Multiple Array for Insertion in Subcutaneous Tissue and Fascia
Epic™ Stented Tissue Valve (aortic)	Zooplastic Tissue in Heart and Great Vessels
Epicel® cultured epidermal autograft	Autologous Tissue Substitute
Esophageal obturator airway (EOA)	Intraluminal Device, Airway in Gastrointestinal System
Esteem® implantable hearing system	Hearing Device in Ear, Nose, Sinus
EV ICD System (Extravascular implantable defibrillator lead)	Defibrillator Lead in Anatomical Regions, General
Evera (XT)(S)(DR/VR)	Defibrillator Generator for Insertion in Subcutaneous Tissue and Fascia
Everolimus-eluting coronary stent	Intraluminal Device, Drug-eluting in Heart and Great Vessels
Ex-PRESS™ mini glaucoma shunt	Synthetic Substitute
EXCLUDER® AAA Endoprosthesis	Intraluminal Device Intraluminal Device, Branched or Fenestrated, One or Two Arteries for Restriction in Lower Arteries Intraluminal Device, Branched or Fenestrated, Three or More Arteries for Restriction in Lower Arteries
EXCLUDER® IBE Endoprosthesis	Intraluminal Device, Branched or Fenestrated, One or Two Arteries for Restriction in Lower Arteries
Express® (LD) Premounted Stent System	Intraluminal Device
Express® Biliary SD Monorail® Premounted Stent System	Intraluminal Device
Express® SD Renal Monorail® Premounted Stent System	Intraluminal Device
External fixator	External Fixation Device in Head and Facial Bones External Fixation Device in Upper Bones External Fixation Device in Lower Bones External Fixation Device in Upper Joints External Fixation Device in Lower Joints
EXtreme Lateral Interbody Fusion (XLIF) device	Interbody Fusion Device in Lower Joints
Facet replacement spinal stabilization device	Spinal Stabilization Device, Facet Replacement for Insertion in Upper Joints Spinal Stabilization Device, Facet Replacement for Insertion in Lower Joints
FLAIR® Endovascular Stent Graft	Intraluminal Device
Flexible Composite Mesh	Synthetic Substitute
Flourish® Pediatric Esophageal Atresia Device	Magnetic Lengthening Device in Gastrointestinal System
Flow Diverter embolization device	Intraluminal Device, Flow Diverter for Restriction in Upper Arteries
Foley catheter	Drainage Device
Formula™ Balloon-Expandable Renal Stent System	Intraluminal Device
Freestyle (Stentless) Aortic Root Bioprosthesis	Zooplastic Tissue in Heart and Great Vessels
Fusion screw (compression)(lag)(locking)	Internal Fixation Device in Upper Joints Internal Fixation Device in Lower Joints
GammaTile™	Radioactive Element, Cesium-131 Collagen Implant for Insertion in Central Nervous System and Cranial Nerves
Gastric electrical stimulation (GES) lead	Stimulator Lead in Gastrointestinal System
Gastric pacemaker lead	Stimulator Lead in Gastrointestinal System
GORE EXCLUDER® AAA Endoprosthesis	Intraluminal Device Intraluminal Device, Branched or Fenestrated, One or Two Arteries for Restriction in Lower Arteries Intraluminal Device, Branched or Fenestrated, Three or More Arteries for Restriction in Lower Arteries
GORE EXCLUDER® IBE Endoprosthesis	Intraluminal Device, Branched or Fenestrated, One or Two Arteries for Restriction in Lower Arteries
GORE TAG® Thoracic Endoprosthesis NT	Intraluminal Device
GORE® DUALMESH®	Synthetic Substitute
Guedel airway	Intraluminal Device, Airway in Mouth and Throat
Hancock Bioprosthesis (aortic)(mitral) valve	Zooplastic Tissue in Heart and Great Vessels
Hancock Bioprosthetic Valved Conduit	Zooplastic Tissue in Heart and Great Vessels
HeartMate 3™ LVAS	Implantable Heart Assist System in Heart and Great Vessels
HeartMate II® Left Ventricular Assist Device (LVAD)	Implantable Heart Assist System in Heart and Great Vessels
HeartMate XVE® Left Ventricular Assist Device (LVAD)	Implantable Heart Assist System in Heart and Great Vessels

Terms	ICD-10-PCS Value
Herculink (RX) Elite Renal Stent System	Intraluminal Device
Hip (joint) liner	Liner in Lower Joints
Holter valve ventricular shunt	Synthetic Substitute
IASD® (InterAtrial Shunt Device), Corvia	Synthetic Substitute
iFuse Bedrock™ Granite Implant System NT	Internal Fixation Device with Tulip Connector in New Technology
Ilizarov external fixator	External Fixation Device, Ring for Insertion in Upper Bones External Fixation Device, Ring for Reposition in Upper Bones External Fixation Device, Ring for Insertion in Lower Bones External Fixation Device, Ring for Reposition in Lower Bones
Ilizarov-Vecklich device	External Fixation Device, Limb Lengthening for Insertion in Upper Bones External Fixation Device, Limb Lengthening for Insertion in Lower Bones
Impella® 5.5 with SmartAssist® System	Conduit To Short-term External Heart Assist System in New Technology
Impella® heart pump	Short-term External Heart Assist System in Heart and Great Vessels
Implantable cardioverter-defibrillator (ICD)	Defibrillator Generator for Insertion in Subcutaneous Tissue and Fascia
Implantable drug infusion pump (anti-spasmodic) (chemotherapy)(pain)	Infusion Device, Pump in Subcutaneous Tissue and Fascia
Implantable glucose monitoring device	Monitoring Device
Implantable hemodynamic monitor (IHM)	Monitoring Device, Hemodynamic for Insertion in Subcutaneous Tissue and Fascia
Implantable hemodynamic monitoring system (IHMS)	Monitoring Device, Hemodynamic for Insertion in Subcutaneous Tissue and Fascia
Implantable Miniature Telescope™ (IMT)	Synthetic Substitute, Intraocular Telescope for Replacement in Eye
Implanted (venous)(access) port	Vascular Access Device, Totally Implantable in Subcutaneous Tissue and Fascia
InDura, intrathecal catheter (1P) (spinal)	Infusion Device
Injection reservoir, port	Vascular Access Device, Totally Implantable in Subcutaneous Tissue and Fascia
Injection reservoir, pump	Infusion Device, Pump in Subcutaneous Tissue and Fascia
Intellis™ neurostimulator	Stimulator Generator, Multiple Array Rechargeable for Insertion in Subcutaneous Tissue and Fascia
InterAtrial Shunt Device IASD®, Corvia	Synthetic Substitute
Interbody fusion (spine) cage	Interbody Fusion Device in Upper Joints Interbody Fusion Device in Lower Joints
Interspinous process spinal stabilization device	Spinal Stabilization Device, Interspinous Process for Insertion in Upper Joints Spinal Stabilization Device, Interspinous Process for Insertion in Lower Joints
InterStim™ Micro Therapy neurostimulator	Stimulator Generator, Single Array Rechargeable for Insertion in Subcutaneous Tissue and Fascia
InterStim® Therapy lead	Neurostimulator Lead in Peripheral Nervous System
InterStim™ II Therapy neurostimulator	Stimulator Generator, Single Array for Insertion in Subcutaneous Tissue and Fascia
Intramedullary (IM) rod (nail)	Internal Fixation Device, Intramedullary in Upper Bones Internal Fixation Device, Intramedullary in Lower Bones
Intramedullary skeletal kinetic distractor (ISKD)	Internal Fixation Device, Intramedullary in Upper Bones Internal Fixation Device, Intramedullary in Lower Bones
Intrauterine Device (IUD)	Contraceptive Device in Female Reproductive System
Ischemic Stroke System (ISS500)	Neurostimulator Lead in New Technology
ISS500 (Ischemic Stroke System)	Neurostimulator Lead in New Technology
Itrel (3)(4) neurostimulator	Stimulator Generator, Single Array for Insertion in Subcutaneous Tissue and Fascia
Joint fixation plate	Internal Fixation Device in Upper Joints Internal Fixation Device in Lower Joints
Joint liner (insert)	Liner in Lower Joints
Joint spacer (antibiotic)	Spacer in Upper Joints Spacer in Lower Joints
Kappa	Pacemaker, Dual Chamber for Insertion in Subcutaneous Tissue and Fascia
Kirschner wire (K-wire)	Internal Fixation Device in Head and Facial Bones Internal Fixation Device in Upper Bones Internal Fixation Device in Lower Bones Internal Fixation Device in Upper Joints Internal Fixation Device in Lower Joints
Knee (implant) insert	Liner in Lower Joints
Kuntscher nail	Internal Fixation Device, Intramedullary in Upper Bones Internal Fixation Device, Intramedullary in Lower Bones
LAP-BAND® adjustable gastric banding system	Extraluminal Device
LifeStent® (Flexstar)(XL) Vascular Stent System	Intraluminal Device
LigaPASS 2.0™ PJK Prevention System	Posterior Vertebral Tether in New Technology
LIVIAN™ CRT-D	Cardiac Resynchronization Defibrillator Pulse Generator for Insertion in Subcutaneous Tissue and Fascia
Longeviti ClearFit® Cranial Implant	Synthetic Substitute, Ultrasound Penetrable in New Technology
Longeviti ClearFit® OTS Cranial Implant	Synthetic Substitute, Ultrasound Penetrable in New Technology
Loop recorder, implantable	Monitoring Device
MAGEC® Spinal Bracing and Distraction System	Magnetically Controlled Growth Rod(s) in New Technology
Mark IV Breathing Pacemaker System	Stimulator Generator in Subcutaneous Tissue and Fascia
Maximo II DR (VR)	Defibrillator Generator for Insertion in Subcutaneous Tissue and Fascia
Maximo II DR CRT-D	Cardiac Resynchronization Defibrillator Pulse Generator for Insertion in Subcutaneous Tissue and Fascia
Medtronic Endurant® II AAA stent graft system	Intraluminal Device
Melody® transcatheter pulmonary valve	Zooplastic Tissue in Heart and Great Vessels
Metal on metal bearing surface	Synthetic Substitute, Metal for Replacement in Lower Joints
Micro-Driver stent (RX) (OTW)	Intraluminal Device
MicroMed HeartAssist	Implantable Heart Assist System in Heart and Great Vessels

Terms	ICD-10-PCS Value
Micrus CERECYTE microcoil	Intraluminal Device, Bioactive in Upper Arteries
MIRODERM™ Biologic Wound Matrix	Nonautologous Tissue Substitute
MitraClip valve repair system	Synthetic Substitute
Mitroflow® Aortic Pericardial Heart Valve	Zooplastic Tissue in Heart and Great Vessels
Mosaic Bioprosthesis (aortic) (mitral) valve	Zooplastic Tissue in Heart and Great Vessels
MULTI-LINK (VISION)(MINI-VISION)(ULTRA) Coronary Stent System	Intraluminal Device
nanoLOCK™ interbody fusion device	Interbody Fusion Device in Upper Joints Interbody Fusion Device in Lower Joints
Nasopharyngeal airway (NPA)	Intraluminal Device, Airway in Ear, Nose, Sinus
Neovasc Reducer™	Reduction Device in New Technology
Neuromuscular electrical stimulation (NEMS) lead	Stimulator Lead in Muscles
Neurostimulator generator, multiple channel	Stimulator Generator, Multiple Array for Insertion in Subcutaneous Tissue and Fascia
Neurostimulator generator, multiple channel rechargeable	Stimulator Generator, Multiple Array Rechargeable for Insertion in Subcutaneous Tissue and Fascia
Neurostimulator generator, single channel	Stimulator Generator, Single Array for Insertion in Subcutaneous Tissue and Fascia
Neurostimulator generator, single channel rechargeable	Stimulator Generator, Single Array Rechargeable for Insertion in Subcutaneous Tissue and Fascia
Neutralization plate	Internal Fixation Device in Head and Facial Bones Internal Fixation Device in Upper Bones Internal Fixation Device in Lower Bones
Nitinol framed polymer mesh	Synthetic Substitute
Non-tunneled central venous catheter	Infusion Device
Novacor Left Ventricular Assist Device	Implantable Heart Assist System in Heart and Great Vessels
Novation® Ceramic AHS® (Articulation Hip System)	Synthetic Substitute, Ceramic for Replacement in Lower Joints
NUsurface® Meniscus Implant	Synthetic Substitute, Lateral Meniscus in New Technology Synthetic Substitute, Medial Meniscus in New Technology
Omnilink Elite Vascular Balloon Expandable Stent System	Intraluminal Device
Open Pivot Aortic Valve Graft (AVG)	Synthetic Substitute
Open Pivot (mechanical) Valve	Synthetic Substitute
Optimizer™ III implantable pulse generator	Contractility Modulation Device for Insertion in Subcutaneous Tissue and Fascia
Oropharyngeal airway (OPA)	Intraluminal Device, Airway in Mouth and Throat
Ovatio™ CRT-D	Cardiac Resynchronization Defibrillator Pulse Generator for Insertion in Subcutaneous Tissue and Fascia
OXINIUM	Synthetic Substitute, Oxidized Zirconium on Polyethylene for Replacement in Lower Joints
Paclitaxel-eluting coronary stent	Intraluminal Device, Drug-eluting in Heart and Great Vessels
Paclitaxel-eluting peripheral stent	Intraluminal Device, Drug-eluting in Upper Arteries Intraluminal Device, Drug-eluting in Lower Arteries
Partially absorbable mesh	Synthetic Substitute
Pedicle-based dynamic stabilization device	Spinal Stabilization Device, Pedicle-Based for Insertion in Upper Joints Spinal Stabilization Device, Pedicle-Based for Insertion in Lower Joints
PERCEPT™ PC neurostimulator	Stimulator Generator, Multiple Array for Insertion in Subcutaneous Tissue and Fascia
Percutaneous endoscopic gastrojejunostomy (PEG/J) tube	Feeding Device in Gastrointestinal System
Percutaneous endoscopic gastrostomy (PEG) tube	Feeding Device in Gastrointestinal System
Percutaneous nephrostomy catheter	Drainage Device
Peripherally inserted central catheter (PICC)	Infusion Device
Pessary ring	Intraluminal Device, Pessary in Female Reproductive System
Phrenic nerve stimulator generator	Stimulator Generator in Subcutaneous Tissue and Fascia
Phrenic nerve stimulator lead	Diaphragmatic Pacemaker Lead in Respiratory System
PHYSIOMESH™ Flexible Composite Mesh	Synthetic Substitute
Pipeline™ (Flex) embolization device	Intraluminal Device, Flow Diverter for Restriction in Upper Arteries
Polyethylene socket	Synthetic Substitute, Polyethylene for Replacement in Lower Joints
Polymethylmethacrylate (PMMA)	Synthetic Substitute
Polypropylene mesh	Synthetic Substitute
Porcine (bioprosthetic) valve	Zooplastic Tissue in Heart and Great Vessels
PRECICE intramedullary limb lengthening system	Internal Fixation Device, Intramedullary Limb Lengthening for Insertion in Upper Bones Internal Fixation Device, Intramedullary Limb Lengthening for Insertion in Lower Bones
PRESTIGE® Cervical Disc	Synthetic Substitute
PrimeAdvanced neurostimulator (SureScan)(MRI Safe)	Stimulator Generator, Multiple Array for Insertion in Subcutaneous Tissue and Fascia
PROCEED™ Ventral Patch	Synthetic Substitute
Prodisc-C	Synthetic Substitute
Prodisc-L	Synthetic Substitute
PROLENE Polypropylene Hernia System (PHS)	Synthetic Substitute
Protecta XT CRT-D	Cardiac Resynchronization Defibrillator Pulse Generator for Insertion in Subcutaneous Tissue and Fascia
Protecta XT DR (XT VR)	Defibrillator Generator for Insertion in Subcutaneous Tissue and Fascia
Protégé® RX Carotid Stent System	Intraluminal Device
Pump reservoir	Infusion Device, Pump in Subcutaneous Tissue and Fascia
REALIZE® Adjustable Gastric Band	Extraluminal Device
Rebound HRD® (Hernia Repair Device)	Synthetic Substitute
Reducer™ System	Reduction Device in New Technology
RestoreAdvanced neurostimulator (SureScan)(MRI Safe)	Stimulator Generator, Multiple Array Rechargeable for Insertion in Subcutaneous Tissue and Fascia
RestoreSensor neurostimulator (SureScan)(MRI Safe)	Stimulator Generator, Multiple Array Rechargeable for Insertion in Subcutaneous Tissue and Fascia

Terms	ICD-10-PCS Value
RestoreUltra neurostimulator (SureScan)(MRI Safe)	Stimulator Generator, Multiple Array Rechargeable for Insertion in Subcutaneous Tissue and Fascia
Reveal (LINQ)(DX)(XT)	Monitoring Device
Reverse® Shoulder Prosthesis	Synthetic Substitute, Reverse Ball and Socket for Replacement in Upper Joints
Revo MRI™ SureScan® pacemaker	Pacemaker, Dual Chamber for Insertion in Subcutaneous Tissue and Fascia
Rheos® System device	Stimulator Generator in Subcutaneous Tissue and Fascia
Rheos® System lead	Stimulator Lead in Upper Arteries
RNS System lead	Neurostimulator Lead in Central Nervous System and Cranial Nerves
RNS system neurostimulator generator	Neurostimulator Generator in Head and Facial Bones
S-ICD™ lead	Subcutaneous Defibrillator Lead in Subcutaneous Tissue and Fascia
Sacral nerve modulation (SNM) lead	Stimulator Lead in Urinary System
Sacral neuromodulation lead	Stimulator Lead in Urinary System
SAPIEN transcatheter aortic valve	Zooplastic Tissue in Heart and Great Vessels
SAVAL below-the-knee (BTK) drug-eluting stent system	Intraluminal Device, Sustained Release Drug-eluting in New Technology Intraluminal Device, Sustained Release Drug-eluting, Two in New Technology Intraluminal Device, Sustained Release Drug-eluting, Three in New Technology Intraluminal Device, Sustained Release Drug-eluting, Four or More in New Technology
Secura (DR) (VR)	Defibrillator Generator for Insertion in Subcutaneous Tissue and Fascia
Sheffield hybrid external fixator	External Fixation Device, Hybrid for Insertion in Upper Bones External Fixation Device, Hybrid for Reposition in Upper Bones External Fixation Device, Hybrid for Insertion in Lower Bones External Fixation Device, Hybrid for Reposition in Lower Bones
Sheffield ring external fixator	External Fixation Device, Ring for Insertion in Upper Bones External Fixation Device, Ring for Reposition in Upper Bones External Fixation Device, Ring for Insertion in Lower Bones External Fixation Device, Ring for Reposition in Lower Bones
Single lead pacemaker (atrium)(ventricle)	Pacemaker, Single Chamber for Insertion in Subcutaneous Tissue and Fascia
Single lead rate responsive pacemaker (atrium)(ventricle)	Pacemaker, Single Chamber Rate Responsive for Insertion in Subcutaneous Tissue and Fascia
Sirolimus-eluting coronary stent	Intraluminal Device, Drug-eluting in Heart and Great Vessels
SJM Biocor® Stented Valve System	Zooplastic Tissue in Heart and Great Vessels
Spacer, Articulating (Antibiotic)	Articulating Spacer in Lower Joints
Spacer, Static (Antibiotic)	Spacer in Lower Joints
Spinal cord neurostimulator lead	Neurostimulator Lead in Central Nervous System and Cranial Nerves
Spinal growth rods, magnetically controlled	Magnetically Controlled Growth Rod(s) in New Technology
SpineJack® system	Synthetic Substitute, Mechanically Expandable (Paired) in New Technology

Terms	ICD-10-PCS Value
Spiration IBV™ Valve System	Intraluminal Device, Endobronchial Valve in Respiratory System
Static Spacer (Antibiotic)	Spacer in Lower Joints
Stent, intraluminal (cardiovascular) (gastrointestinal) (hepatobiliary)(urinary)	Intraluminal Device
Stented tissue valve	Zooplastic Tissue in Heart and Great Vessels
Stratos LV	Cardiac Resynchronization Pacemaker Pulse Generator for Insertion in Subcutaneous Tissue and Fascia
Subcutaneous injection reservoir, port	Vascular Access Device, Totally Implantable in Subcutaneous Tissue and Fascia
Subcutaneous injection reservoir, pump	Infusion Device, Pump in Subcutaneous Tissue and Fascia
Subdermal progesterone implant	Contraceptive Device in Subcutaneous Tissue and Fascia
Surpass Streamline™ Flow Diverter	Intraluminal Device, Flow Diverter for Restriction in Upper Arteries
SynCardia (temporary) Total Artificial Heart (TAH)	Synthetic Substitute, Pneumatic for Replacement in Heart and Great Vessels
SynCardia Total Artificial Heart	Synthetic Substitute
Synchra CRT-P	Cardiac Resynchronization Pacemaker Pulse Generator for Insertion in Subcutaneous Tissue and Fascia
SynchroMed Pump	Infusion Device, Pump in Subcutaneous Tissue and Fascia
Talent® Converter	Intraluminal Device
Talent® Occluder	Intraluminal Device
Talent® Stent Graft (abdominal)(thoracic)	Intraluminal Device
TandemHeart® System	Short-term External Heart Assist System in Heart and Great Vessels
TAXUS® Liberté® Paclitaxel-eluting Coronary Stent System	Intraluminal Device, Drug-eluting in Heart and Great Vessels
Therapeutic occlusion coil(s)	Intraluminal Device
Thoracostomy tube	Drainage Device
Thoraflex™ Hybrid device NT	Branched Synthetic Substitute with Intraluminal Device in New Technology
Thoratec IVAD (Implantable Ventricular Assist Device)	Implantable Heart Assist System in Heart and Great Vessels
Thoratec Paracorporeal Ventricular Assist Device	Short-term External Heart Assist System in Heart and Great Vessels
Tibial insert	Liner in Lower Joints
Tissue bank graft	Nonautologous Tissue Substitute
Tissue expander (inflatable)(injectable)	Tissue Expander in Skin and Breast Tissue Expander in Subcutaneous Tissue and Fascia
Titan Endoskeleton™	Interbody Fusion Device in Upper Joints Interbody Fusion Device in Lower Joints
Titanium Sternal Fixation System (TSFS)	Internal Fixation Device, Rigid Plate for Insertion in Upper Bones Internal Fixation Device, Rigid Plate for Reposition in Upper Bones
TOPS™ System	Posterior Spinal Motion Preservation Device in New Technology
Total Ankle Talar Replacement™ (TATR)	Synthetic Substitute, Talar Prosthesis in New Technology
Total artificial (replacement) heart	Synthetic Substitute
Tracheostomy tube	Tracheostomy Device in Respiratory System
TricValve® Transcatheter Bicaval Valve System	Intraluminal Device, Bioprosthetic Valve in New Technology
Trifecta™ Valve (aortic)	Zooplastic Tissue in Heart and Great Vessels

Terms	ICD-10-PCS Value
Tunneled central venous catheter	Vascular Access Device, Tunneled in Subcutaneous Tissue and Fascia
Tunneled spinal (intrathecal) catheter	Infusion Device
Two lead pacemaker	Pacemaker, Dual Chamber for Insertion in Subcutaneous Tissue and Fascia
Ultraflex™ Precision Colonic Stent System	Intraluminal Device
ULTRAPRO Hernia System (UHS)	Synthetic Substitute
ULTRAPRO Partially Absorbable Lightweight Mesh	Synthetic Substitute
ULTRAPRO Plug	Synthetic Substitute
Ultrasonic osteogenic stimulator	Bone Growth Stimulator in Head and Facial Bones Bone Growth Stimulator in Upper Bones Bone Growth Stimulator in Lower Bones
Ultrasound bone healing system	Bone Growth Stimulator in Head and Facial Bones Bone Growth Stimulator in Upper Bones Bone Growth Stimulator in Lower Bones
Uniplanar external fixator	External Fixation Device, Monoplanar for Insertion in Upper Bones External Fixation Device, Monoplanar for Reposition in Upper Bones External Fixation Device, Monoplanar for Insertion in Lower Bones External Fixation Device, Monoplanar for Reposition in Lower Bones
Urinary incontinence stimulator lead	Stimulator Lead in Urinary System
V-Wave Interatrial Shunt System	Synthetic Substitute
Vaginal pessary	Intraluminal Device, Pessary in Female Reproductive System
Valiant Thoracic Stent Graft	Intraluminal Device
Vanta™ PC neurostimulator	Stimulator Generator, Multiple Array for Insertion in Subcutaneous Tissue and Fascia
VasQ™ External Support device	Synthetic Substitute, Extraluminal Support Device in New Technology
Vectra® Vascular Access Graft	Vascular Access Device, Tunneled in Subcutaneous Tissue and Fascia
VenoValve®	Intraluminal Device, Bioprosthetic Valve in New Technology
Ventrio™ Hernia Patch	Synthetic Substitute
Versa	Pacemaker, Dual Chamber for Insertion in Subcutaneous Tissue and Fascia
VEST™ Venous External Support device	Vein Graft Extraluminal Support Device(s) in New Technology
Virtuoso (II) (DR) (VR)	Defibrillator Generator for Insertion in Subcutaneous Tissue and Fascia
Viva(XT)(S)	Cardiac Resynchronization Defibrillator Pulse Generator for Insertion in Subcutaneous Tissue and Fascia
Vivistim® Paired VNS System Lead NT	Neurostimulator Lead with Paired Stimulation System in New Technology
WALLSTENT® Endoprosthesis	Intraluminal Device
X-Spine Axle Cage	Spinal Stabilization Device, Interspinous Process for Insertion in Upper Joints Spinal Stabilization Device, Interspinous Process for Insertion in Lower Joints
X-STOP® Spacer	Spinal Stabilization Device, Interspinous Process for Insertion in Upper Joints Spinal Stabilization Device, Interspinous Process for Insertion in Lower Joints
Xact Carotid Stent System	Intraluminal Device
Xenograft	Zooplastic Tissue in Heart and Great Vessels
XIENCE Everolimus Eluting Coronary Stent System	Intraluminal Device, Drug-eluting in Heart and Great Vessels
XLIF® System	Interbody Fusion Device in Lower Joints
Zenith AAA Endovascular Graft	Intraluminal Device
Zenith® Fenestrated AAA Endovascular Graft	Intraluminal Device, Branched or Fenestrated, One or Two Arteries for Restriction in Lower Arteries Intraluminal Device, Branched or Fenestrated, Three or More Arteries for Restriction in Lower Arteries
Zenith Flex® AAA Endovascular Graft	Intraluminal Device
Zenith® Renu™ AAA Ancillary Graft	Intraluminal Device
Zenith TX2® TAA Endovascular Graft	Intraluminal Device
Zilver® PTX® (paclitaxel) Drug-Eluting Peripheral Stent	Intraluminal Device, Drug-eluting in Upper Arteries Intraluminal Device, Drug-eluting in Lower Arteries
Zimmer® NexGen® LPS Mobile Bearing Knee	Synthetic Substitute
Zimmer® NexGen® LPS-Flex Mobile Knee	Synthetic Substitute
Zotarolimus-eluting coronary stent	Intraluminal Device, Drug-eluting in Heart and Great Vessels

Device Aggregation Table

This table crosswalks specific device character value definitions for specific root operations in a specific body system to the more general device character value to be used when the root operation covers a wide range of body parts and the device character represents an entire family of devices.

Specific Device	for Operation	in Body System	General Device
Autologous Arterial Tissue (A)	All applicable	Heart and Great Vessels Lower Arteries Lower Veins Upper Arteries Upper Veins	**7** Autologous Tissue Substitute
Autologous Venous Tissue (9)	All applicable	Heart and Great Vessels Lower Arteries Lower Veins Upper Arteries Upper Veins	**7** Autologous Tissue Substitute
Cardiac Lead, Defibrillator (K)	Insertion	Heart and Great Vessels	**M** Cardiac Lead
Cardiac Lead, Pacemaker (J)	Insertion	Heart and Great Vessels	**M** Cardiac Lead
Cardiac Resynchronization Defibrillator Pulse Generator (9)	Insertion	Subcutaneous Tissue and Fascia	**P** Cardiac Rhythm Related Device
Cardiac Resynchronization Pacemaker Pulse Generator (7)	Insertion	Subcutaneous Tissue and Fascia	**P** Cardiac Rhythm Related Device
Contractility Modulation Device (A)	Insertion	Subcutaneous Tissue and Fascia	**P** Cardiac Rhythm Related Device
Defibrillator Generator (8)	Insertion	Subcutaneous Tissue and Fascia	**P** Cardiac Rhythm Related Device
Epiretinal Visual Prosthesis (5)	All applicable	Eye	**J** Synthetic Substitute
External Fixation Device, Hybrid (D)	Insertion	Lower Bones Upper Bones	**5** External Fixation Device
External Fixation Device, Hybrid (D)	Reposition	Lower Bones Upper Bones	**5** External Fixation Device
External Fixation Device, Limb Lengthening (8)	Insertion	Lower Bones Upper Bones	**5** External Fixation Device
External Fixation Device, Monoplanar (B)	Insertion	Lower Bones Upper Bones	**5** External Fixation Device
External Fixation Device, Monoplanar (B)	Reposition	Lower Bones Upper Bones	**5** External Fixation Device
External Fixation Device, Ring (C)	Insertion	Lower Bones Upper Bones	**5** External Fixation Device
External Fixation Device, Ring (C)	Reposition	Lower Bones Upper Bones	**5** External Fixation Device
Hearing Device, Bone Conduction (4)	Insertion	Ear, Nose, Sinus	**S** Hearing Device
Hearing Device, Multiple Channel Cochlear Prosthesis (6)	Insertion	Ear, Nose, Sinus	**S** Hearing Device
Hearing Device, Single Channel Cochlear Prosthesis (5)	Insertion	Ear, Nose, Sinus	**S** Hearing Device
Internal Fixation Device, Intramedullary (6)	All applicable	Lower Bones Upper Bones	**4** Internal Fixation Device
Internal Fixation Device, Intramedullary Limb Lengthening (7)	Insertion	Lower Bones Upper Bones	**6** Internal Fixation Device, Intramedullary
Internal Fixation Device, Rigid Plate (Ø)	Insertion	Upper Bones	**4** Internal Fixation Device
Internal Fixation Device, Rigid Plate (Ø)	Reposition	Upper Bones	**4** Internal Fixation Device
Intraluminal Device, Airway (B)	All applicable	Ear, Nose, Sinus Gastrointestinal System Mouth and Throat	**D** Intraluminal Device
Intraluminal Device, Bioactive (B)	All applicable	Upper Arteries	**D** Intraluminal Device
Intraluminal Device, Branched or Fenestrated, One or Two Arteries (E)	Restriction	Heart and Great Vessels Lower Arteries	**D** Intraluminal Device
Intraluminal Device, Branched or Fenestrated, Three or More Arteries (F)	Restriction	Heart and Great Vessels Lower Arteries	**D** Intraluminal Device
Intraluminal Device, Drug-eluting (4)	All applicable	Heart and Great Vessels Lower Arteries Upper Arteries	**D** Intraluminal Device
Intraluminal Device, Drug-eluting, Four or More (7)	All applicable	Heart and Great Vessels Lower Arteries Upper Arteries	**D** Intraluminal Device
Intraluminal Device, Drug-eluting, Three (6)	All applicable	Heart and Great Vessels Lower Arteries Upper Arteries	**D** Intraluminal Device
Intraluminal Device, Drug-eluting, Two (5)	All applicable	Heart and Great Vessels Lower Arteries Upper Arteries	**D** Intraluminal Device
Intraluminal Device, Endobronchial Valve (G)	All applicable	Respiratory System	**D** Intraluminal Device
Intraluminal Device, Endotracheal Airway (E)	All applicable	Respiratory System	**D** Intraluminal Device

Specific Device	for Operation	in Body System	General Device
Intraluminal Device, Flow Diverter (H)	Restriction	Upper Arteries	**D** Intraluminal Device
Intraluminal Device, Four or More (G)	All applicable	Heart and Great Vessels Lower Arteries Upper Arteries	**D** Intraluminal Device
Intraluminal Device, Pessary (G)	All applicable	Female Reproductive System	**D** Intraluminal Device
Intraluminal Device, Radioactive (T)	All applicable	Heart and Great Vessels	**D** Intraluminal Device
Intraluminal Device, Three (F)	All applicable	Heart and Great Vessels Lower Arteries Upper Arteries	**D** Intraluminal Device
Intraluminal Device, Two (E)	All applicable	Heart and Great Vessels Lower Arteries Upper Arteries	**D** Intraluminal Device
Monitoring Device, Hemodynamic (Ø)	Insertion	Subcutaneous Tissue and Fascia	**2** Monitoring Device
Monitoring Device, Pressure Sensor (Ø)	Insertion	Heart and Great Vessels	**2** Monitoring Device
Pacemaker, Dual Chamber (6)	Insertion	Subcutaneous Tissue and Fascia	**P** Cardiac Rhythm Related Device
Pacemaker, Single Chamber (4)	Insertion	Subcutaneous Tissue and Fascia	**P** Cardiac Rhythm Related Device
Pacemaker, Single Chamber Rate Responsive (5)	Insertion	Subcutaneous Tissue and Fascia	**P** Cardiac Rhythm Related Device
Spinal Stabilization Device, Facet Replacement (D)	Insertion	Lower Joints Upper Joints	**4** Internal Fixation Device
Spinal Stabilization Device, Interspinous Process (B)	Insertion	Lower Joints Upper Joints	**4** Internal Fixation Device
Spinal Stabilization Device, Pedicle-Based (C)	Insertion	Lower Joints Upper Joints	**4** Internal Fixation Device
Spinal Stabilization Device, Vertebral Body Tether (3)	Reposition	Lower Bones Upper Bones	**4** Internal Fixation Device
Stimulator Generator, Multiple Array (D)	Insertion	Subcutaneous Tissue and Fascia	**M** Stimulator Generator
Stimulator Generator, Multiple Array Rechargeable (E)	Insertion	Subcutaneous Tissue and Fascia	**M** Stimulator Generator
Stimulator Generator, Single Array (B)	Insertion	Subcutaneous Tissue and Fascia	**M** Stimulator Generator
Stimulator Generator, Single Array Rechargeable (C)	Insertion	Subcutaneous Tissue and Fascia	**M** Stimulator Generator
Synthetic Substitute, Ceramic (3)	Replacement	Lower Joints	**J** Synthetic Substitute
Synthetic Substitute, Ceramic on Polyethylene (4)	Replacement	Lower Joints	**J** Synthetic Substitute
Synthetic Substitute, Intraocular Telescope (Ø)	Replacement	Eye	**J** Synthetic Substitute
Synthetic Substitute, Metal (1)	Replacement	Lower Joints	**J** Synthetic Substitute
Synthetic Substitute, Metal on Polyethylene (2)	Replacement	Lower Joints	**J** Synthetic Substitute
Synthetic Substitute, Oxidized Zirconium on Polyethylene (6)	Replacement	Lower Joints	**J** Synthetic Substitute
Synthetic Substitute, Polyethylene (Ø)	Replacement	Lower Joints	**J** Synthetic Substitute
Synthetic Substitute, Reverse Ball and Socket (Ø)	Replacement	Upper Joints	**J** Synthetic Substitute

Appendix H: Device Definitions

This NT symbol next to a device in the Definition column identifies that the device has been approved for NTAP (new technology add-on payment). CMS provides incremental payment, in addition to the DRG payment, for technologies that have received an NTAP designation.

ICD-10-PCS Value	Definition
Articulating Spacer in Lower Joints	Articulating Spacer (Antibiotic) Spacer, Articulating (Antibiotic)
Artificial Sphincter in Gastrointestinal System	Artificial anal sphincter (AAS) Artificial bowel sphincter (neosphincter)
Artificial Sphincter in Urinary System	AMS 800® Urinary Control System Artificial urinary sphincter (AUS)
Autologous Arterial Tissue in Heart and Great Vessels	Autologous artery graft
Autologous Arterial Tissue in Lower Arteries	Autologous artery graft
Autologous Arterial Tissue in Lower Veins	Autologous artery graft
Autologous Arterial Tissue in Upper Arteries	Autologous artery graft
Autologous Arterial Tissue in Upper Veins	Autologous artery graft
Autologous Tissue Substitute	Autograft Cultured epidermal cell autograft Epicel® cultured epidermal autograft
Autologous Venous Tissue in Heart and Great Vessels	Autologous vein graft
Autologous Venous Tissue in Lower Arteries	Autologous vein graft
Autologous Venous Tissue in Lower Veins	Autologous vein graft
Autologous Venous Tissue in Upper Arteries	Autologous vein graft
Autologous Venous Tissue in Upper Veins	Autologous vein graft
Biologic with Synthetic Substitute, Autoregulated Electrohydraulic for Replacement in Heart and Great Vessels	Carmat total artificial heart (TAH)
Bone Growth Stimulator in Head and Facial Bones	Electrical bone growth stimulator (EBGS) Ultrasonic osteogenic stimulator Ultrasound bone healing system
Bone Growth Stimulator in Lower Bones	Electrical bone growth stimulator (EBGS) Ultrasonic osteogenic stimulator Ultrasound bone healing system
Bone Growth Stimulator in Upper Bones	Electrical bone growth stimulator (EBGS) Ultrasonic osteogenic stimulator Ultrasound bone healing system
Branched Synthetic Substitute with Intraluminal Device in New Technology	Thoraflex™ Hybrid device NT
Cardiac Lead in Heart and Great Vessels	Cardiac contractility modulation lead
Cardiac Lead, Defibrillator for Insertion in Heart and Great Vessels	ACUITY™ Steerable Lead Attain Ability® lead Attain StarFix® (OTW) lead Cardiac resynchronization therapy (CRT) lead Corox (OTW) Bipolar Lead Durata® Defibrillation Lead ENDOTAK RELIANCE® (G) Defibrillation Lead
Cardiac Lead, Pacemaker for Insertion in Heart and Great Vessels	ACUITY™ Steerable Lead Attain Ability® lead Attain StarFix® (OTW) lead Cardiac resynchronization therapy (CRT) lead Corox (OTW) Bipolar Lead

ICD-10-PCS Value	Definition
Cardiac Resynchronization Defibrillator Pulse Generator for Insertion in Subcutaneous Tissue and Fascia	COGNIS® CRT-D Concerto II CRT-D Consulta CRT-D CONTAK RENEWA® 3 RF (HE) CRT-D LIVIAN™ CRT-D Maximo II DR CRT-D Ovatio™ CRT-D Protecta XT CRT-D Viva (XT)(S)
Cardiac Resynchronization Pacemaker Pulse Generator for Insertion in Subcutaneous Tissue and Fascia	Consulta CRT-P Stratos LV Synchra CRT-P
Conduit through Femoral Vein to Popliteal Artery in New Technology	DETOUR® System
Conduit through Femoral Vein to Superficial Femoral Artery in New Technology	DETOUR® System
Conduit to Short-term External Heart Assist System in New Technology	Impella® 5.5 with SmartAssist® System
Contraceptive Device in Female Reproductive System	Intrauterine device (IUD)
Contraceptive Device in Subcutaneous Tissue and Fascia	Subdermal progesterone implant
Contractility Modulation Device for Insertion in Subcutaneous Tissue and Fascia	Optimizer™ III implantable pulse generator
Defibrillator Generator for Insertion in Subcutaneous Tissue and Fascia	Evera (XT)(S)(DR/VR) Implantable cardioverter-defibrillator (ICD) Maximo II DR (VR) Protecta XT DR (XT VR) Secura (DR) (VR) Virtuoso (II) (DR) (VR)
Defibrillator Lead in Anatomical Regions, General	EV ICD System (Extravascular implantable defibrillator lead)
Diaphragmatic Pacemaker Lead in Respiratory System	Phrenic nerve stimulator lead
Drainage Device	Cystostomy tube Foley catheter Percutaneous nephrostomy catheter Thoracostomy tube
External Fixation Device in Head and Facial Bones	External fixator
External Fixation Device in Lower Bones	External fixator
External Fixation Device in Lower Joints	External fixator
External Fixation Device in Upper Bones	External fixator
External Fixation Device in Upper Joints	External fixator
External Fixation Device, Hybrid for Insertion in Lower Bones	Delta frame external fixator Sheffield hybrid external fixator
External Fixation Device, Hybrid for Insertion in Upper Bones	Delta frame external fixator Sheffield hybrid external fixator

ICD-10-PCS Value	Definition
External Fixation Device, Hybrid for Reposition in Lower Bones	Delta frame external fixator Sheffield hybrid external fixator
External Fixation Device, Hybrid for Reposition in Upper Bones	Delta frame external fixator Sheffield hybrid external fixator
External Fixation Device, Limb Lengthening for Insertion in Lower Bones	Ilizarov-Vecklich device
External Fixation Device, Limb Lengthening for Insertion in Upper Bones	Ilizarov-Vecklich device
External Fixation Device, Monoplanar for Insertion in Lower Bones	Uniplanar external fixator
External Fixation Device, Monoplanar for Insertion in Upper Bones	Uniplanar external fixator
External Fixation Device, Monoplanar for Reposition in Lower Bones	Uniplanar external fixator
External Fixation Device, Monoplanar for Reposition in Upper Bones	Uniplanar external fixator
External Fixation Device, Ring for Insertion in Lower Bones	Ilizarov external fixator Sheffield ring external fixator
External Fixation Device, Ring for Insertion in Upper Bones	Ilizarov external fixator Sheffield ring external fixator
External Fixation Device, Ring for Reposition in Lower Bones	Ilizarov external fixator Sheffield ring external fixator
External Fixation Device, Ring for Reposition in Upper Bones	Ilizarov external fixator Sheffield ring external fixator
Extraluminal Device	AtriClip LAA Exclusion System LAP-BAND® adjustable gastric banding system REALIZE® Adjustable Gastric Band
Feeding Device in Gastrointestinal System	Percutaneous endoscopic gastrojejunostomy (PEG/J) tube Percutaneous endoscopic gastrostomy (PEG) tube
Hearing Device in Ear, Nose, Sinus	Esteem® implantable hearing system
Hearing Device in Head and Facial Bones	Bone anchored hearing device
Hearing Device, Bone Conduction for Insertion in Ear, Nose, Sinus	Bone anchored hearing device
Hearing Device, Multiple Channel Cochlear Prosthesis for Insertion in Ear, Nose, Sinus	Cochlear implant (CI), multiple channel (electrode)
Hearing Device, Single Channel Cochlear Prosthesis for Insertion in Ear, Nose, Sinus	Cochlear implant (CI), single channel (electrode)

ICD-10-PCS Value	Definition
Implantable Heart Assist System in Heart and Great Vessels	Berlin Heart Ventricular Assist Device DeBakey Left Ventricular Assist Device DuraHeart Left Ventricular Assist System HeartMate 3™ LVAS HeartMate II® Left Ventricular Assist Device (LVAD) HeartMate XVE® Left Ventricular Assist Device (LVAD) MicroMed HeartAssist Novacor Left Ventricular Assist Device Thoratec IVAD (Implantable Ventricular Assist Device)
Infusion Device	Ascenda Intrathecal Catheter InDura, intrathecal catheter (1P) (spinal) Non-tunneled central venous catheter Peripherally inserted central catheter (PICC) Tunneled spinal (intrathecal) catheter
Infusion Device, Pump in Subcutaneous Tissue and Fascia	Implantable drug infusion pump (anti-spasmodic)(chemotherapy)(pain) Injection reservoir, pump Pump reservoir Subcutaneous injection reservoir, pump SynchroMed pump
Interbody Fusion Device, Custom-made Anatomically Designedin New Technology	aprevo™
Interbody Fusion Device in Lower Joints	Axial Lumbar Interbody Fusion System AxiaLIF® System COALESCE® radiolucent interbody fusion device COHERE® radiolucent interbody fusion device CoRoent® XL Direct Lateral Interbody Fusion (DLIF) device EXtreme Lateral Interbody Fusion (XLIF) device Interbody fusion (spine) cage nanoLOCK™ interbody fusion device Titan Endoskeleton™ XLIF® System
Interbody Fusion Device in Upper Joints	BAK/C® Interbody Cervical Fusion System COALESCE® radiolucent interbody fusion device COHERE® radiolucent interbody fusion device Interbody fusion (spine) cage nanoLOCK™ interbody fusion device Titan Endoskeleton™
Internal Fixation Device in Head and Facial Bones	Bone screw (interlocking)(lag)(pedicle) (recessed) Kirschner wire (K-wire) Neutralization plate
Internal Fixation Device in Lower Bones	Bone screw (interlocking)(lag)(pedicle) (recessed) Clamp and rod internal fixation system (CRIF) Kirschner wire (K-wire) Neutralization plate
Internal Fixation Device in Lower Joints	Fusion screw (compression)(lag)(locking) Joint fixation plate Kirschner wire (K-wire)
Internal Fixation Device in Upper Bones	Bone screw (interlocking)(lag)(pedicle) (recessed) Clamp and rod internal fixation system (CRIF) Kirschner wire (K-wire) Neutralization plate
Internal Fixation Device in Upper Joints	Fusion screw (compression)(lag)(locking) Joint fixation plate Kirschner wire (K-wire)
Internal Fixation Device, Intramedullary in Lower Bones	Intramedullary (IM) rod (nail) Intramedullary skeletal kinetic distractor (ISKD) Kuntscher nail

ICD-10-PCS Value	Definition
Internal Fixation Device, Intramedullary in Upper Bones	Intramedullary (IM) rod (nail) Intramedullary skeletal kinetic distractor (ISKD) Kuntscher nail
Internal Fixation Device Intramedullary Limb Lengthening for Insertion in Lower Bones	PRECICE intramedullary limb lengthening system
Internal Fixation Device Intramedullary Limb Lengthening for Insertion in Upper Bones	PRECICE intramedullary limb lengthening system
Internal Fixation Device, Open-truss Design in New Technology	Ankle Truss System™ (ATS)
Internal Fixation Device, Rigid Plate for Insertion in Upper Bones	Titanium Sternal Fixation System (TSFS)
Internal Fixation Device, Rigid Plate for Reposition in Upper Bones	Titanium Sternal Fixation System (TSFS)
Internal Fixation Device, Sustained Compression for Fusion in Lower Joints	DynaClip® (Forte) DynaNail® (Helix) (Hybrid) (Mini)
Internal Fixation Device, Sustained Compression for Fusion in Upper Joints	DynaClip® (Forte) DynaNail® (Helix) (Hybrid) (Mini)
Internal Fixation Device with Tulip Connector in New Technology	iFuse Bedrock™ Granite Implant System NT
Intracardiac Pacemaker, Dual-Chamber in New Technology	Aveir™ AR, as dual chamber Aveir™ DR, dual chamber
Intracardiac Pacemaker in Heart and Great Vessels	Aveir™ VR, as single chamber
Intraluminal Device	Absolute Pro Vascular (OTW) Self-Expanding Stent System Acculink (RX) Carotid Stent System AFX® Endovascular AAA System AneuRx® AAA Advantage® Assurant (Cobalt) stent Carotid WALLSTENT® Monorail® Endoprosthesis CoAxia NeuroFlo catheter Colonic Z-Stent® Complete (SE) stent Cook Zenith AAA Endovascular Graft Driver stent (RX) (OTW) E-Luminexx™ (Biliary)(Vascular) Stent Embolization coil(s) Endologix AFX® Endovascular AAA System Endurant® Endovascular Stent Graft Endurant® II AAA stent graft system EXCLUDER® AAA Endoprosthesis Express® (LD) Premounted Stent System Express® Biliary SD Monorail® Premounted Stent System Express® SD Renal Monorail® Premounted Stent System FLAIR® Endovascular Stent Graft Formula™ Balloon-Expandable Renal Stent System GORE EXCLUDER® AAA Endoprosthesis GORE TAG® Thoracic Endoprosthesis NT Herculink (RX) Elite Renal Stent System LifeStent® (Flexstar)(XL) Vascular Stent System Medtronic Endurant® II AAA stent graft system Micro-Driver stent (RX) (OTW) MULTI-LINK (VISION)(MINI-VISION)(ULTRA) Coronary Stent System Omnilink Elite Vascular Balloon Expandable Stent System Protege® RX Carotid Stent System Stent, intraluminal (cardiovascular) (gastrointestinal)(hepatobiliary) (urinary) Talent® Converter Talent® Occluder Talent® Stent Graft (abdominal)(thoracic) Therapeutic occlusion coil(s) Ultraflex™ Precision Colonic Stent System Valiant Thoracic Stent Graft WALLSTENT® Endoprosthesis Xact Carotid Stent System Zenith AAA Endovascular Graft Zenith Flex® AAA Endovascular Graft Zenith TX2® TAA Endovascular Graft Zenith® Renu™ AAA Ancillary Graft
Intraluminal Device, Airway in Ear, Nose, Sinus	Nasopharyngeal airway (NPA)
Intraluminal Device, Airway in Gastrointestinal System	Esophageal obturator airway (EOA)
Intraluminal Device, Airway in Mouth and Throat	Guedel airway Oropharyngeal airway (OPA)
Intraluminal Device, Bioactive in Upper Arteries	Bioactive embolization coil(s) Micrus CERECYTE microcoil
Intraluminal Device, Bioprosthetic Valve in New Technology	TricValve® Transcatheter Bicaval Valve System VenoValve®
Intraluminal Device, Branched or Fenestrated, One or Two Arteries for Restriction in Lower Arteries	Cook Zenith® Fenestrated AAA Endovascular Graft EXCLUDER® AAA Endoprosthesis EXCLUDER® IBE Endoprosthesis GORE EXCLUDER® AAA Endoprosthesis GORE EXCLUDER®IBE Endoprosthesis Zenith® Fenestrated AAA Endovascular Graft

ICD-10-PCS Value	Definition
Intraluminal Device, Branched or Fenestrated, Three or More Arteries for Restriction in Lower Arteries	Cook Zenith® Fenestrated AAA Endovascular Graft EXCLUDER® AAA Endoprosthesis GORE EXCLUDER® AAA Endoprosthesis Zenith® Fenestrated AAA Endovascular Graft
Intraluminal Device, Drug-eluting in Heart and Great Vessels	CYPHER® Stent Endeavor® (III)(IV) (Sprint) Zotarolimus-eluting Coronary Stent System Everolimus-eluting coronary stent Paclitaxel-eluting coronary stent Sirolimus-eluting coronary stent TAXUS® Liberte® Paclitaxel-eluting Coronary Stent System XIENCE Everolimus Eluting Coronary Stent System Zotarolimus-eluting coronary stent
Intraluminal Device, Drug-eluting in Lower Arteries	Paclitaxel-eluting peripheral stent Zilver® PTX® (paclitaxel) Drug-Eluting Peripheral Stent
Intraluminal Device, Drug-eluting in Upper Arteries	Paclitaxel-eluting peripheral stent Zilver® PTX® (paclitaxel) Drug-Eluting Peripheral Stent
Intraluminal Device, Endobronchial Valve in Respiratory System	Spiration IBV™ Valve System
Intraluminal Device, Endotracheal Airway in Respiratory System	Endotracheal tube (cuffed)(double-lumen)
Intraluminal Device, Flow Diverter for Restriction in Upper Arteries	Flow Diverter embolization device Pipeline™ (Flex) embolization device Surpass Streamline™ Flow Diverter
Intraluminal Device, Pessary in Female Reproductive System	Pessary ring Vaginal pessary
Intraluminal Device, Sustained Release Drug-eluting in New Technology	Eluvia™ Drug-eluting Vascular Stent System SAVAL below-the-knee (BTK) drug-eluting stent system
Intraluminal Device, Sustained Release Drug-eluting, Four or More in New Technology	Eluvia™ Drug-eluting Vascular Stent System SAVAL below-the-knee (BTK) drug-eluting stent system
Intraluminal Device, Sustained Release Drug-eluting, Three in New Technology	Eluvia™ Drug-eluting Vascular Stent System SAVAL below-the-knee (BTK) drug-eluting stent system
Intraluminal Device, Sustained Release Drug-eluting, Two in New Technology	Eluvia™ Drug-eluting Vascular Stent System SAVAL below-the-knee (BTK) drug-eluting stent system
Liner in Lower Joints	Acetabular cup Hip (joint) liner Joint liner (insert) Knee (implant) insert Tibial insert
Magnetically Controlled Growth Rod(s) in New Technology	MAGEC® Spinal Bracing and Distraction System Spinal growth rods, magnetically controlled
Magnetic Lengthening Device in Gastrointestinal System	Flourish® Pediatric Esophageal Atresia Device
Monitoring Device	Blood glucose monitoring system Cardiac event recorder Continuous Glucose Monitoring (CGM) device Implantable glucose monitoring device Loop recorder, implantable Reveal (LINQ)(DX)(XT)

ICD-10-PCS Value	Definition
Monitoring Device, Hemodynamic for Insertion in Subcutaneous Tissue and Fascia	Implantable hemodynamic monitor (IHM) Implantable hemodynamic monitoring system (IHMS)
Monitoring Device, Pressure Sensor for Insertion in Heart and Great Vessels	CardioMEMS® pressure sensor EndoSure® sensor
Neurostimulator Generator in Head and Facial Bones	RNS system neurostimulator generator
Neurostimulator Lead in Central Nervous System and Cranial Nerves	Cortical strip neurostimulator lead DBS lead Deep brain neurostimulator lead RNS System lead Spinal cord neurostimulator lead
Neurostimulator Lead in Peripheral Nervous System	InterStim® Therapy lead
Neurostimulator Lead in New Technology	Ischemic Stroke System (ISS500) ISS500 (Ischemic Stroke System)
Neurostimulator Lead with Paired Stimulation System in New Technology	Vivistim® Paired VNS System Lead NT
Nonautologous Tissue Substitute	Acellular Hydrated Dermis Bone bank bone graft Cook Biodesign® Fistula Plug(s) Cook Biodesign® Hernia Graft(s) Cook Biodesign® Layered Graft(s) Cook Zenapro™ Layered Graft(s) MIRODERM™ Biologic Wound Matrix Tissue bank graft
Other Device	Alfapump® system
Pacemaker, Dual Chamber for Insertion in Subcutaneous Tissue and Fascia	Advisa (MRI) EnRhythm Kappa Revo MRI™ SureScan® pacemaker Two lead pacemaker Versa
Pacemaker, Single Chamber for Insertion in Subcutaneous Tissue and Fascia	Single lead pacemaker (atrium)(ventricle)
Pacemaker, Single Chamber Rate Responsive for Insertion in Subcutaneous Tissue and Fascia	Single lead rate responsive pacemaker (atrium)(ventricle)
Posterior (Dynamic) Distraction Device in New Technology	ApiFix® Minimally Invasive Deformity Correction (MID-C) System
Posterior Spinal Motion Preservation Device in New Technology	TOPS™ System
Posterior Vertebral Tether in New Technology	LigaPASS 2.0™ PJK Prevention System
Radioactive Element	Brachytherapy seeds CivaSheet®
Radioactive Element, Cesium-131 Collagen Implant for Insertion in Central Nervous System and Cranial Nerves	Cesium-131 Collagen Implant GammaTile™
Reduction Device in New Technology	Neovasc Reducer™ Reducer™ System
Resurfacing Device in Lower Joints	CONSERVE® PLUS Total Resurfacing Hip System Cormet Hip Resurfacing System

ICD-10-PCS Value	Definition
Short-term External Heart Assist System in Heart and Great Vessels	Aortix™ System Biventricular external heart assist system BVS 5000 Ventricular Assist Device Centrimag® Blood Pump Impella® heart pump TandemHeart® System Thoratec Paracorporeal Ventricular Assist Device
Spacer in Lower Joints	Joint spacer (antibiotic) Spacer, Static (Antibiotic) Static Spacer (Antibiotic)
Spacer in Upper Joints	Joint spacer (antibiotic)
Spinal Stabilization Device, Facet Replacement for Insertion in Lower Joints	Facet replacement spinal stabilization device
Spinal Stabilization Device, Facet Replacement for Insertion in Upper Joints	Facet replacement spinal stabilization device
Spinal Stabilization Device, Interspinous Process for Insertion in Lower Joints	Interspinous process spinal stabilization device X-Spine Axle Cage X-STOP® Spacer
Spinal Stabilization Device, Interspinous Process for Insertion in Upper Joints	Interspinous process spinal stabilization device X-Spine Axle Cage X-STOP® Spacer
Spinal Stabilization Device, Pedicle- Based for Insertion in Lower Joints	Dynesys® Dynamic Stabilization System Pedicle-based dynamic stabilization device
Spinal Stabilization Device, Pedicle-Based for Insertion in Upper Joints	Dynesys® Dynamic Stabilization System Pedicle-based dynamic stabilization device
Stimulator Generator in Subcutaneous Tissue and Fascia	Baroreflex Activation Therapy® (BAT®) Diaphragmatic pacemaker generator Mark IV Breathing Pacemaker System Phrenic nerve stimulator generator Rheos® System device
Stimulator Generator, Multiple Array for Insertion in Subcutaneous Tissue and Fascia	Activa PC neurostimulator Enterra gastric neurostimulator Neurostimulator generator, multiple channel PERCEPT™ PC neurostimulator PrimeAdvanced neurostimulator (SureScan)(MRI Safe) Vanta™ PC neurostimulator
Stimulator Generator, Multiple Array Rechargeable for Insertion in Subcutaneous Tissue and Fascia	Activa RC neurostimulator Intellis™ neurostimulator Neurostimulator generator, multiple channel rechargeable RestoreAdvanced neurostimulator (SureScan)(MRI Safe) RestoreSensor neurostimulator (SureScan)(MRI Safe) RestoreUltra neurostimulator (SureScan)(MRI Safe)
Stimulator Generator, Single Array for Insertion in Subcutaneous Tissue and Fascia	Activa SC neurostimulator InterStim™ II Therapy neurostimulator Itrel (3)(4) neurostimulator Neurostimulator generator, single channel
Stimulator Generator, Single Array Rechargeable for Insertion in Subcutaneous Tissue and Fascia	InterStim™ Micro Therapy neurostimulator Neurostimulator generator, single channel rechargeable
Stimulator Lead in Gastrointestinal System	Gastric electrical stimulation (GES) lead Gastric pacemaker lead
Stimulator Lead in Muscles	Electrical muscle stimulation (EMS) lead Electronic muscle stimulator lead Neuromuscular electrical stimulation (NEMS) lead
Stimulator Lead in Upper Arteries	Baroreflex Activation Therapy® (BAT®) Carotid (artery) sinus (baroreceptor) lead Rheos® System lead
Stimulator Lead in Urinary System	Sacral nerve modulation (SNM) lead Sacral neuromodulation lead Urinary incontinence stimulator lead
Subcutaneous Defibrillator Lead in Subcutaneous Tissue and Fascia	S-ICD™ lead
Synthetic Substitute	AbioCor® Total Replacement Heart AMPLATZER® Muscular VSD Occluder Annuloplasty ring Bard® Composix® (E/X) (LP) mesh Bard® Composix® Kugel® patch Bard® Dulex™ mesh Bard® Ventralex™ hernia patch Barricaid® Annular Closure Device (ACD) BRYAN® Cervical Disc System Corvia IASD® Ex-PRESS™ mini glaucoma shunt Flexible Composite Mesh GORE® DUALMESH® Holter valve ventricular shunt IASD® (InterAtrial Shunt Device), Corvia InterAtrial Shunt Device IASD®, Corvia MitraClip valve repair system Nitinol framed polymer mesh Open Pivot (mechanical) valve Open Pivot Aortic Valve Graft (AVG) Partially absorbable mesh PHYSIOMESH™ Flexible Composite Mesh Polymethylmethacrylate (PMMA) Polypropylene mesh PRESTIGE® Cervical Disc PROCEED™ Ventral Patch Prodisc-C Prodisc-L PROLENE Polypropylene Hernia System (PHS) Rebound HRD® (Hernia Repair Device) SynCardia Total Artificial Heart Total artificial (replacement) heart ULTRAPRO Hernia System (UHS) ULTRAPRO Partially Absorbable Lightweight Mesh ULTRAPRO Plug V-Wave Interatrial Shunt System Ventrio™ Hernia Patch Zimmer® NexGen® LPS Mobile Bearing Knee Zimmer® NexGen® LPS-Flex Mobile Knee
Synthetic Substitute, Ceramic for Replacement in Lower Joints	Ceramic on ceramic bearing surface Novation® Ceramic AHS® (Articulation Hip System)
Synthetic Substitute, Extraluminal Support Device in New Technology	VasQ™ External Support device
Synthetic Substitute, Intraocular Telescope for Replacement in Eye	Implantable Miniature Telescope™ (IMT)
Synthetic Substitute, Lateral Meniscus in New Technology	NUsurface® Meniscus Implant
Synthetic Substitute, Mechanically Expandable (Paired) in New Technology	SpineJack® system
Synthetic Substitute, Medial Meniscus in New Technology	NUsurface® Meniscus Implant
Synthetic Substitute, Metal for Replacement in Lower Joints	Cobalt/chromium head and socket Metal on metal bearing surface
Synthetic Substitute, Metal on Polyethylene for Replacement in Lower Joints	Cobalt/chromium head and polyethylene socket

ICD-10-PCS Value	Definition
Synthetic Substitute, Oxidized Zirconium on Polyethylene for Replacement in Lower Joints	OXINIUM
Synthetic Substitute, Pneumatic for Replacement in Heart and Great Vessels	SynCardia (temporary) total artificial heart (TAH)
Synthetic Substitute, Polyethylene for Replacement in Lower Joints	Polyethylene socket
Synthetic Substitute, Reverse Ball and Socket for Replacement in Upper Joints	Delta III Reverse shoulder prosthesis Reverse® Shoulder Prosthesis
Synthetic Substitute, Talar Prosthesis in New Technology	Total Ankle Talar Replacement™ (TATR)
Synthetic Substitute, Ultrasound Penetrable in New Technology	Longeviti ClearFit® Cranial Implant Longeviti ClearFit® OTS Cranial Implant
Tibial Extension with Motion Sensors in New Technology	Canturio™ te (Tibial Extension)
Tissue Expander in Skin and Breast	Tissue expander (inflatable) (injectable)
Tissue Expander in Subcutaneous Tissue and Fascia	Tissue expander (inflatable) (injectable)
Tracheostomy Device in Respiratory System	Tracheostomy tube
Vascular Access Device, Totally Implantable in Subcutaneous Tissue and Fascia	Implanted (venous)(access) port Injection reservoir, port Subcutaneous injection reservoir, port
Vascular Access Device, Tunneled in Subcutaneous Tissue and Fascia	Tunneled central venous catheter Vectra® Vascular Access Graft
Vein Graft Extraluminal Support Device(s) in New Technology	VEST™ Venous External Support device
Zooplastic Tissue in Heart and Great Vessels	3f (Aortic) Bioprosthesis valve Bovine pericardial valve Bovine pericardium graft Contegra Pulmonary Valved Conduit CoreValve transcatheter aortic valve Epic™ Stented Tissue Valve (aortic) Freestyle (Stentless) Aortic Root Bioprosthesis Hancock Bioprosthesis (aortic) (mitral) valve Hancock Bioprosthetic Valved Conduit Melody® transcatheter pulmonary valve Mitroflow® Aortic Pericardial Heart Valve Mosaic Bioprosthesis (aortic) (mitral) valve Porcine (bioprosthetic) valve SAPIEN transcatheter aortic valve SJM Biocor® Stented Valve System Stented tissue valve Trifecta™ Valve (aortic) Xenograft

Appendix I: Substance Key/Substance Definitions

Substance Key

This table crosswalks a specific substance, listed by trade name or synonym, to the PCS value that would be used to represent that substance in either the Administration or New Technology section. The ICD-10-PCS value may be located in either the 6th-character Substance column or the 7th-character Qualifier column depending on the section/table to which it is classified. The most specific character is listed in the table.

This NT symbol next to a substance/technology in the Trade Name or Synonym column identifies that the substance/technology has been approved for NTAP (new technology add-on payment). CMS provides incremental payment, in addition to the DRG payment, for technologies that have received an NTAP designation.

Substances denoted by an asterisk (*) in the Trade Name or Synonym column, although not included in the official ICD-10-PCS classification, were added based on information provided in the FY 2024 IPPS proposed rule.

Trade Name or Synonym	ICD-10-PCS Value	PCS Section
ABECMA® NT	Idecabtagene Vicleucel Immunotherapy (K)	New Technology (X)
ACTEMRA®	Tocilizumab (H)	New Technology (X)
afami-cel	Afamitresgene Autoleucel Immunotherapy (6)	New Technology (X)
AIGISRx Antibacterial Envelope	Anti-Infective Envelope (A)	Administration (3)
Andexanet Alfa, Factor Xa Inhibitor Reversal Agent	Coagulation Factor Xa, Inactivated (7)	New Technology (X)
Andexxa	Coagulation Factor Xa, Inactivated (7)	New Technology (X)
Angiotensin II	Vasopressor (X)	Administration (3)
Antibacterial Envelope (TYRX) (AIGISRx)	Anti-Infective Envelope (A)	Administration (3)
Antimicrobial envelope	Anti-Infective Envelope (A)	Administration (3)
Anti-SARS-CoV-2 hyperimmune globulin	Hyperimmune Globulin (E)	New Technology (X)
AVYCAZ® (ceftazidime-avibactam)	Other Anti-infective (9)	Administration (3)
Axicabtagene Ciloleucel	Axicabtagene Ciloleucel Immunotherapy (H)	New Technology (X)
AZEDRA®	Iobenguane I-131 Antineoplastic (S)	New Technology (X)
***Balversa™**	Erdafitinib Antineoplastic (L)	New Technology (X)
beti-cel	Betibeglogene Autotemcel (B)	New Technology (X)
Blinatumomab	Other Antineoplastic (5)	Administration (3)
BLINCYTO® (blinatumomab)	Other Antineoplastic (5)	Administration (3)
Bone morphogenetic protein 2 (BMP 2)	Recombinant Bone Morphogenetic Protein (B)	Administration (3)
Brexucabtagene Autoleucel	Brexucabtagene Autoleucel Immunotherapy (4)	New Technology (X)
Breyanzi®	Lisocabtagene Maraleucel Immunotherapy (N)	New Technology (X)
Bromelain-enriched Proteolytic Enzyme	Anacaulase-bcdb (2)	New Technology (X)
***CABLIVI®**	Caplacizumab (W)	New Technology (X)
CARVYKTI™ NT	Ciltacabtagene Autoleucel (A)	New Technology (X)
Casirivimab (REGN10933) and Imdevimab (REGN10987)	REGN-COV2 Monoclonal Antibody (G)	New Technology (X)
CBMA (Concentrated Bone Marrow Aspirate)	Other Substance (C)	Administration (3)
Ceftazidime-avibactam	Other Anti-infective (9)	Administration (3)
CERAMENT® G NT	Antibiotic-eluting Bone Void Filler (P)	New Technology (X)
cilta-cel	Ciltacabtagene Autoleucel (A)	New Technology (X)
Clolar	Clofarabine (P)	Administration (3)
Coagulation Factor Xa, (Recombinant) Inactivated	Coagulation Factor Xa, Inactivated (7)	New Technology (X)
COMIRNATY®	COVID-19 Vaccine (U) COVID-19 Booster (W) COVID-19 Vaccine Dose 1 (S) COVID-19 Vaccine Dose 2 (T) COVID-19 Vaccine Dose 3 (V)	New Technology (X)
CONTEPO™	Fosfomycin Anti-infective (K)	New Technology (X)
COSELA™ NT	Trilaciclib (7)	New Technology (X)
CRESEMBA® (isavuconazonium sulfate)	Other Anti-infective (9)	Administration (3)
CTX001™	Exagamglogene Autotemcel (J)	New Technology (X)
Darzalex Faspro® NT	Daratumumab and Hyaluronidase-fihj (1)	New Technology (X)
DefenCath™ NT	Taurolidine Anti-infective and Heparin Anticoagulant (2)	New Technology (X)
Defitelio	Other Substance (C)	Administration (3)
DuraGraft® Endothelial Damage Inhibitor	Endothelial Damage Inhibitor (8)	New Technology (X)
ELZONRIS™	Tagraxofusp-erzs Antineoplastic (Q)	New Technology (X)
ENSPRYNG™	Satralizumab-mwge (9)	New Technology (X)
ERLEADA™	Apalutamide Antineoplastic (J)	New Technology (X)
EVUSHELD™	Tixagevimab and Cilgavimab Monoclonal Antibody (X)	New Technology (X)
Factor Xa Inhibitor Reversal Agent, Andexanet Alfa	Coagulation Factor Xa, Inactivated (7)	New Technology (X)
FETROJA® NT	Cefiderocol Anti-infective (A)	New Technology (X)

Trade Name or Synonym	ICD-10-PCS Value	PCS Section
Fosfomycin injection	Fosfomycin Anti-infective (K)	New Technology (X)
Gammaglobulin	Globulin (S)	Administration (3)
GAMUNEX-C, for COVID-19 treatment	High-Dose Intravenous Immune Globulin (D)	New Technology (X)
GIAPREZA™	Vasopressor (X)	Administration (3)
GS-5734	Remdesivir Anti-infective (E)	New Technology (X)
hdIVIG (high-dose intravenous immunoglobulin), for COVID-19 treatment	High-Dose Intravenous Immune Globulin (D)	New Technology (X)
Hemospray® Endoscopic Hemostat	Mineral-based Topical Hemostatic Agent (8)	New Technology (X)
HEPZATO™ KIT (melphalan hydrochloride Hepatic Delivery System)	Melphalan Hydrochloride Antineoplastic (T)	New Technology (X)
HIG (hyperimmune globulin), for COVID-19 treatment	Hyperimmune Globulin (E)	New Technology (X)
High-dose intravenous immunoglobulin (hdIVIG), for COVID-19 treatment	High-Dose Intravenous Immune Globulin (D)	New Technology (X)
hIVIG (hyperimmune intravenous immunoglobulin), for COVID-19 treatment	Hyperimmune Globulin (E)	New Technology (X)
Human angiotensin II, synthetic	Vasopressor (X)	Administration (3)
Hyperimmune globulin	Globulin (S)	Administration (3)
Hyperimmune intravenous immunoglobulin (hIVIG), for COVID-19 treatment	Hyperimmune Globulin (E)	New Technology (X)
Idarucizumab, Pradaxa® (dabigatran) reversal agent	Other Therapeutic Substance (G)	Administration (3)
Idecabtagene Vicleucel	Idecabtagene Vicleucel Immunotherapy (K)	New Technology (X)
Ide-cel	Idecabtagene Vicleucel Immunotherapy (K)	New Technology (X)
IGIV-C, for COVID-19 treatment	Hyperimmune Globulin (E)	New Technology (X)
Imdevimab (REGN10987) and Casirivimab (REGN10933)	REGN-COV2 Monoclonal Antibody (G)	New Technology (X)
IMFINZI®	Durvalumab Antineoplastic (3)	New Technology (X)
IMI/REL	Imipenem-cilastatin-relebactam Anti-infective (U)	New Technology (X)
Immunoglobulin	Globulin (S)	Administration (3)
INTERCEPT Blood System for Plasma Pathogen Reduced Cryoprecipitated Fibrinogen Complex	Pathogen Reduced Cryoprecipitated Fibrinogen Complex (D)	Administration (3)
INTERCEPT Fibrinogen Complex	Pathogen Reduced Cryoprecipitated Fibrinogen Complex (D)	Administration (3)
Iobenguane I-131, High Specific Activity (HSA)	Iobenguane I-131 Antineoplastic (S)	New Technology (X)
Isavuconazole (isavuconazonium sulfate)	Other Anti-infective (9)	Administration (3)
Jakafi®	Ruxolitinib (T)	New Technology (X)
Kcentra	4-Factor Prothrombin Complex Concentrate (B)	Administration (3)
KEVZARA®	Sarilumab (G)	New Technology (X)
KYMRIAH®	Tisagenlecleucel Immunotherapy (J)	New Technology (X)
Lifileucel	Lifileucel Immunotherapy (L)	New Technology (X)
Lisocabtagene Maraleucel	Lisocabtagene Maraleucel Immunotherapy (7)	New Technology (X)
LIVTENCITY™ NT	Maribavir Anti-infective (3)	New Technology (X)
LTX Regional Anticoagulant	Nafamostat Anticoagulant (3)	New Technology (X)
LUNSUMIO™	Mosunetuzumab Antineoplastic (5)	New Technology (X)
MarrowStim™ PAD Kit for CBMA (Concentrated Bone Marrow Aspirate)	Other Substance (C)	Administration (3)
NA-1 (Nerinitide)	Nerinitide (2)	New Technology (X)
Nesiritide	Human B-type Natriuretic Peptide (H)	Administration (3)
NexoBrid™	Anacaulase-bcdb (2)	New Technology (X)
Niyad™	Nafamostat Anticoagulant (3)	New Technology (X)
NUZYRA™	Omadacycline Anti-infective (B)	New Technology (X)
Octagam 10%, for COVID-19 treatment	High-Dose Intravenous Immune Globulin (D)	New Technology (X)
Olumiant®	Baricitinib (M)	New Technology (X)
OTL-101	Hematopoietic Stem/Progenitor Cells, Genetically Modified (C)	Administration (3)
Plazomicin	Other Anti-infective (9)	Administration (3)
Polyclonal hyperimmune globulin	Globulin (S)	Administration (3)
Praxbind® (idarucizumab), Pradaxa® (dabigatran) reversal agent	Other Therapeutic Substance (G)	Administration (3)
REBYOTA®	Broad Consortium Microbiota-based Live Biotherapeutic Suspension (X)	New Technology (X)
***RECARBRIO™** NT	Imipenem-cilastatin-relebactam Anti-infective (U)	New Technology (X)
RETHYMIC®	Engineered Allogeneic Thymus Tissue (D)	New Technology (X)
rhBMP-2	Recombinant Bone Morphogenetic Protein (B)	Administration (3)
RYBREVANT™ NT	Amivantamab Monoclonal Antibody (B)	New Technology (X)

Trade Name or Synonym	ICD-10-PCS Value	PCS Section
Seprafilm	Adhesion Barrier (5)	Administration (3)
Soliris®	Eculizumab (C)	New Technology (X)
SPIKEVAX™	COVID-19 Vaccine (U) COVID-19 Booster (W) COVID-19 Vaccine Dose 1 (S) COVID-19 Vaccine Dose 2 (T) COVID-19 Vaccine Dose 3 (V)	New Technology (X)
SPRAVATO™	Esketamine Hydrochloride (M)	New Technology (X)
STELARA®	Other New Technology Therapeutic Substance (F)	New Technology (X)
StrataGraft® NT	Bioengineered Allogeneic Construct (F)	New Technology (X)
SUL-DUR	Sulbactam-Durlobactam (K)	New Technology (X)
tab-cel®	Tabelecleucel Immunotherapy (7)	New Technology (X)
TECARTUS™ NT	Brexucabtagene Autoleucel Immunotherapy (M)	New Technology (X)
TECENTRIQ®	Atezolizumab Antineoplastic (D)	New Technology (X)
TERLIVAZ®	Terlipressin (6)	New Technology (X)
Tisagenlecleucel	Tisagenlecleucel Immunotherapy (J)	New Technology (X)
Tissue Plasminogen Activator (tPA)(r-tPA)	Other Thrombolytic (7)	Administration (3)
TYRX Antibacterial Envelope	Anti-Infective Envelope (A)	Administration (3)
UPLIZNA®	Inebilizumab-cdon (9)	New Technology (X)
Ustekinumab	Other New Technology Therapeutic Substance (F)	New Technology (X)
Vabomere™	Meropenem-vaborbactam Anti-infective (N)	New Technology (X)
Veklury	Remdesivir Anti-infective (E)	New Technology (X)
Venclexta®	Venetoclax Antineoplastic (R)	New Technology (X)
Vistogard®	Uridine Triacetate (8)	New Technology (X)
Voraxaze	Glucarpidase (Q)	Administration (3)
VYXEOS™	Cytarabine and Daunorubicin Liposome Antineoplastic (B)	New Technology (X)
XENLETA™	Lefamulin Anti-infective (6)	New Technology (X)
XOSPATA®	Gilteritinib Antineoplastic (V)	New Technology (X)
Yescarta®	Axicabtagene Ciloleucel Immunotherapy (H)	New Technology (X)
***ZEMDRI®**	Plazomicin Anti-infective (6)	New Technology (X)
ZEPZELCA™ NT	Lurbinectedin (8)	New Technology (X)
ZERBAXA®	Ceftolozane/Tazobactam Anti-infective (9)	New Technology (X)
ZULRESSO™	Brexanolone (Ø)	New Technology (X)
ZYNTEGLO®	Betibeglogene Autotemcel (B)	New Technology (X)
Zyvox	Oxazolidinones (8)	Administration (3)

Substance Definitions

This table crosswalks a PCS value, used in the Administration or New Technology section, to a specific substance. The specific substances are listed by trade name or synonym. The ICD-10-PCS value may be located in either the 6th-character Substance column or the 7th-character Qualifier column depending on the section/table to which it is classified.

This NT symbol next to a substance/technology in the Trade Name or Synonym column identifies that the substance/technology has been approved for NTAP (new technology add-on payment). CMS provides incremental payment, in addition to the DRG payment, for technologies that have received an NTAP designation.

Substances denoted by an asterisk (*) in the Trade Name or Synonym column, although not included in the official ICD-10-PCS classification, were added based on information provided in the FY 2024 IPPS proposed rule.

ICD-10-PCS Value	Trade Name or Synonym	PCS Section
4-Factor Prothrombin Complex Concentrate (B)	Kcentra	Administration (3)
Afamitresgene Autoleucel Immunotherapy (6)	afami-cel	New Technology (X)
Adhesion Barrier (5)	Seprafilm	Administration (3)
Amivantamab Monoclonal Antibody (B)	RYBREVANT™ NT	New Technology (X)
Anacaulase-bcdb (2)	Bromelain-enriched Proteolytic Enzyme NexoBrid™	New Technology (X)
Antibiotic-eluting Bone Void Filler (P)	CERAMENT® G NT	New Technology (X)
Anti-Infective Envelope (A)	AIGISRx Antibacterial Envelope Antibacterial Envelope (TYRX) (AIGISRx) Antimicrobial envelope TYRX Antibacterial Envelope	Administration (3)
Apalutamide Antineoplastic (J)	ERLEADA™	New Technology (X)
Atezolizumab Antineoplastic (D)	TECENTRIQ®	New Technology (X)
Axicabtagene Ciloleucel Immunotherapy (H)	Axicabtagene Ciloleucel Yescarta®	New Technology (X)
Baricitinib (M)	Olumiant®	New Technology (X)

ICD-10-PCS Value	Trade Name or Synonym	PCS Section
Betibeglogene Autotemcel (B)	beti-cel ZYNTEGLO®	New Technology (X)
Bioengineered Allogeneic Construct (F)	StrataGraft® NT	New Technology (X)
Brexanolone (Ø)	ZULRESSO™	New Technology (X)
Brexucabtagene Autoleucel Immunotherapy (M)	TECARTUS™ NT	New Technology (X)
Broad Consortium Microbiota-based Live Biotherapeutic Suspension (X)	REBYOTA®	New Technology (X)
Caplacizumab (W)	*CABLIVI®	New Technology (X)
Cefiderocol Anti-infective (A)	FETROJA® NT	New Technology (X)
Ceftolozane/Tazobactam Anti- infective (9)	ZERBAXA®	New Technology (X)
Ciltacabtagene Autoleucel (A)	CARVYKTI™ NT cilta-cel	New Technology (X)
Clofarabine (P)	Clolar	Administration (3)
Coagulation Factor Xa, Inactivated (7)	Andexanet Alfa, Factor Xa Inhibitor Reversal Agent Andexxa Coagulation Factor Xa, (Recombinant) Inactivated Factor Xa Inhibitor Reversal Agent, Andexanet Alfa	New Technology (X)
COVID-19 Vaccine (U)	COMIRNATY® SPIKEVAX™	New Technology (X)
COVID-19 Booster (W)	COMIRNATY® SPIKEVAX™	New Technology (X)
COVID-19 Vaccine Dose 1 (S)	COMIRNATY® SPIKEVAX™	New Technology (X)
COVID-19 Vaccine Dose 2 (T)	COMIRNATY® SPIKEVAX™	New Technology (X)
COVID-19 Vaccine Dose 3 (V)	COMIRNATY® SPIKEVAX™	New Technology (X)
Cytarabine and Daunorubicin Liposome Antineoplastic (B)	VYXEOS™	New Technology (X)
Daratumumab and Hyaluronidase-fihj (1)	Darzalex Faspro® NT	New Technology (X)
Durvalumab Antineoplastic (3)	IMFINZI®	New Technology (X)
Eculizumab (C)	Soliris®	New Technology (X)
Endothelial Damage Inhibitor (8)	DuraGraft® Endothelial Damage Inhibitor	New Technology (X)
Erdafitinib Antineoplastic (L)	*Balversa™	New Technology (X)
Engineered Allogeneic Thymus Tissue (D)	RETHYMIC®	New Technology (X)
Esketamine Hydrochloride (M)	SPRAVATO™	New Technology (X)
Exagamglogene Autotemcel (J)	CTX001™	New Technology (X)
Fosfomycin Anti-infective (K)	CONTEPO™ Fosfomycin injection	New Technology (X)
Gilteritinib Antineoplastic (V)	XOSPATA®	New Technology (X)
Globulin (S)	Gammaglobulin Hyperimmune globulin Immunoglobulin Polyclonal hyperimmune globulin	Administration (3)
Glucarpidase (Q)	Voraxaze	Administration (3)
Hematopoietic Stem/Progenitor Cells, Genetically Modified (C)	OTL-101	Administration (3)
High-Dose Intravenous Immune Globulin (D)	GAMUNEX-C, for COVID-19 treatment hdIVIG (high-dose intravenous immunoglobulin), for COVID-19 treatment High-dose intravenous immunoglobulin (hdIVIG), for COVID-19 treatment Octagam 10%, for COVID-19 treatment	New Technology (X)
Human B-type Natriuretic Peptide (H)	Nesiritide	Administration (3)
Hyperimmune Globulin (E)	Anti-SARS-CoV-2 hyperimmune globulin HIG (hyperimmune globulin), for COVID-19 treatment hIVIG (hyperimmune intravenous immunoglobulin), for COVID-19 treatment Hyperimmune intravenous immunoglobulin (hIVIG), for COVID-19 treatment IGIV-C, for COVID-19 treatment	New Technology (X)
Idecabtagene Vicleucel Immunotherapy (K)	ABECMA® NT Idecabtagene Vicleucel Ide-cel	New Technology (X)
Imipenem-cilastatin-relebactam Anti-infective (U)	IMI/REL *RECARBRIO™ NT	New Technology (X)
Inebilizumab-cdon (9)	UPLIZNA®	New Technology (X)

ICD-10-PCS Value	Trade Name or Synonym	PCS Section
Iobenguane I-131 Antineoplastic (S)	AZEDRA® Iobenguane I-131, High Specific Activity (HSA)	New Technology (X)
Lefamulin Anti-infective (6)	XENLETA™	New Technology (X)
Lifileucel Immunotherapy (L)	Lifileucel	New Technology (X)
Lisocabtagene Maraleucel Immunotherapy (7)	Breyanzi® Lisocabtagene Maraleucel	New Technology (X)
Lurbinectedin (8)	ZEPZELCA™ NT	New Technology (X)
Maribavir Anti-infective (3)	LIVTENCITY™ NT	New Technology (X)
Melphalan Hydrochloride Antineoplastic (T)	HEPZATO™ KIT (melphalan hydrochloride Hepatic Delivery System)	New Technology (X)
Meropenem-vaborbactam Anti-infective (N)	Vabomere™	New Technology (X)
Mineral-based Topical Hemostatic Agent (8)	Hemospray® Endoscopic Hemostat	New Technology (X)
Mosunetuzumab Antineoplastic (5)	LUNSUMIO™	New Technology (X)
Nafamostat Anticoagulant (3)	LTX Regional Anticoagulant Niyad™	New Technology (X)
Nerinitide (2)	NA-1 (Nerinitide)	New Technology (X)
Omadacycline Anti-infective (B)	NUZYRA™	New Technology (X)
Other Anti-infective (9)	AVYCAZ® (ceftazidime-avibactam) Ceftazidime-avibactam CRESEMBA® (isavuconazonium sulfate) Isavuconazole (isavuconazonium sulfate) Plazomicin *ZEMDRI	Administration (3)
Other Antineoplastic (5)	Blinatumomab BLINCYTO® (blinatumomab)	Administration (3)
Other New Technology Therapeutic Substance (F)	STELARA® Ustekinumab	New Technology (X)
Other Substance (C)	CBMA (Concentrated Bone Marrow Aspirate) Defitelio MarrowStim™ PAD Kit for CBMA (Concentrated Bone Marrow Aspirate)	Administration (3)
Other Therapeutic Substance (G)	Idarucizumab, Pradaxa® (dabigatran) reversal agent Praxbind® (idarucizumab), Pradaxa® (dabigatran) reversal agent	Administration (3)
Other Thrombolytic (7)	Tissue Plasminogen Activator (tPA)(r-tPA)	Administration (3)
Oxazolidinones (8)	Zyvox	Administration (3)
Pathogen Reduced Cryoprecipitated Fibrinogen Complex (D)	INTERCEPT Blood System for Plasma Pathogen Reduced Cryoprecipitated Fibrinogen Complex INTERCEPT Fibrinogen Complex	Administration (3)
Recombinant Bone Morphogenetic Protein (B)	Bone morphogenetic protein 2 (BMP 2) rhBMP-2	Administration (3)
REGN-COV2 Monoclonal Antibody (G)	Casirivimab (REGN10933) and Imdevimab (REGN10987) Imdevimab (REGN10987) and Casirivimab (REGN10933)	New Technology (X)
Remdesivir Anti-infective (E)	GS-5734 Veklury NT	New Technology (X)
Ruxolitinib (T)	Jakafi®	New Technology (X)
Sarilumab (G)	KEVZARA®	New Technology (X)
Satralizumab-mwge (9)	ENSPRYNG™	New Technology (X)
Sulbactam-Durlobactam (K)	SUL-DUR	New Technology (X)
Tabelecleucel Immunotherapy (7)	tab-cel®	New Technology (X)
Tagraxofusp-erzs Antineoplastic (Q)	ELZONRIS™	New Technology (X)
Taurolidine Anti-infective and Heparin Anticoagulant (2)	DefenCath™ NT	New Technology (X)
Terlipressin (6)	TERLIVAZ®	New Technology (X)
Tisagenlecleucel Immunotherapy (J)	KYMRIAH® Tisagenlecleucel	New Technology (X)
Tixagevimab and Cilgavimab Monoclonal Antibody (X)	EVUSHELD™	New Technology (X)
Tocilizumab (H)	ACTEMRA®	New Technology (X)
Trilaciclib (7)	COSELA™ NT	New Technology (X)
Uridine Triacetate (8)	Vistogard®	New Technology (X)
Vasopressor (X)	Angiotensin II GIAPREZA™ Human angiotensin II, synthetic	Administration (3)
Venetoclax Antineoplastic (R)	Venclexta®	New Technology (X)

Appendix J: Sections B–H Character Definitions

Sections B-H (Imaging through Substance Abuse Treatment) do not include root operations. Instead, the character 3 value represents the type of procedure performed with additional details about that procedure provided by the character 4 or 5 value, when appropriate. This resource provides the specific ICD-10-PCS value and its associated definition for the character 3, character 4, and character 5 values in the ancillary sections of B-H.

Section B–Imaging

ICD-10-PCS Value (Character 3)	Definition
Computerized Tomography (CT Scan) (2)	Computer reformatted digital display of multiplanar images developed from the capture of multiple exposures of external ionizing radiation
Fluoroscopy (1)	Single plane or bi-plane real time display of an image developed from the capture of external ionizing radiation on a fluorescent screen. The image may also be stored by either digital or analog means.
Magnetic Resonance Imaging (MRI) (3)	Computer reformatted digital display of multiplanar images developed from the capture of radiofrequency signals emitted by nuclei in a body site excited within a magnetic field
Other Imaging (5)	Other specified modality for visualizing a body part
Plain Radiography (Ø)	Planar display of an image developed from the capture of external ionizing radiation on photographic or photoconductive plate
Ultrasonography (4)	Real time display of images of anatomy or flow information developed from the capture of reflected and attenuated high frequency sound waves

Section C–Nuclear Medicine

ICD-10-PCS Value (Character 3)	Definition
Nonimaging Nuclear Medicine Assay (6)	Introduction of radioactive materials into the body for the study of body fluids and blood elements, by the detection of radioactive emissions
Nonimaging Nuclear Medicine Probe (5)	Introduction of radioactive materials into the body for the study of distribution and fate of certain substances by the detection of radioactive emissions; or, alternatively, measurement of absorption of radioactive emissions from an external source
Nonimaging Nuclear Medicine Uptake (4)	Introduction of radioactive materials into the body for measurements of organ function, from the detection of radioactive emissions
Planar Nuclear Medicine Imaging (1)	Introduction of radioactive materials into the body for single plane display of images developed from the capture of radioactive emissions
Positron Emission Tomographic (PET) Imaging (3)	Introduction of radioactive materials into the body for three dimensional display of images developed from the simultaneous capture, 18Ø degrees apart, of radioactive emissions
Systemic Nuclear Medicine Therapy (7)	Introduction of unsealed radioactive materials into the body for treatment
Tomographic (Tomo) Nuclear Medicine Imaging (2)	Introduction of radioactive materials into the body for three dimensional display of images developed from the capture of radioactive emissions

Section F–Physical Rehabilitation and Diagnostic Audiology

ICD-10-PCS Value (Character 3)	Definition
Activities of Daily Living Assessment (2)	Measurement of functional level for activities of daily living
Activities of Daily Living Treatment (8)	Exercise or activities to facilitate functional competence for activities of daily living
Caregiver Training (F)	Training in activities to support patient's optimal level of function
Cochlear Implant Treatment (B)	Application of techniques to improve the communication abilities of individuals with cochlear implant
Device Fitting (D)	Fitting of a device designed to facilitate or support achievement of a higher level of function
Hearing Aid Assessment (4)	Measurement of the appropriateness and/or effectiveness of a hearing device
Hearing Assessment (3)	Measurement of hearing and related functions
Hearing Treatment (9)	Application of techniques to improve, augment, or compensate for hearing and related functional impairment
Motor and/or Nerve Function Assessment (1)	Measurement of motor, nerve, and related functions
Motor Treatment (7)	Exercise or activities to increase or facilitate motor function
Speech Assessment (Ø)	Measurement of speech and related functions

Continued on next page

Section F–Physical Rehabilitation and Diagnostic Audiology

Continued from previous page

ICD-10-PCS Value (Character 3)	Definition
Speech Treatment (6)	Application of techniques to improve, augment, or compensate for speech and related functional impairment
Vestibular Assessment (5)	Measurement of the vestibular system and related functions
Vestibular Treatment (C)	Application of techniques to improve, augment, or compensate for vestibular and related functional impairment

Section F–Physical Rehabilitation and Diagnostic Audiology

ICD-10-PCS Value Qualifier (Character 5)	Definition
Acoustic Reflex Decay (J)	Measures reduction in size/strength of acoustic reflex over time Includes/Examples: Includes site of lesion test
Acoustic Reflex Patterns (G)	Defines site of lesion based upon presence/absence of acoustic reflexes with ipsilateral vs. contralateral stimulation
Acoustic Reflex Threshold (H)	Determines minimal intensity that acoustic reflex occurs with ipsilateral and/or contralateral stimulation
Aerobic Capacity and Endurance (7)	Measures autonomic responses to positional changes; perceived exertion, dyspnea or angina during activity; performance during exercise protocols; standard vital signs; and blood gas analysis or oxygen consumption
Alternate Binaural or Monaural Loudness Balance (7)	Determines auditory stimulus parameter that yields the same objective sensation Includes/Examples: Sound intensities that yield same loudness perception
Anthropometric Characteristics (B)	Measures edema, body fat composition, height, weight, length and girth
Aphasia (Assessment) (C)	Measures expressive and receptive speech and language function including reading and writing
Aphasia (Treatment) (3)	Applying techniques to improve, augment, or compensate for receptive/ expressive language impairments
Articulation/Phonology (Assessment) (9)	Measures speech production
Articulation/Phonology (Treatment) (4)	Applying techniques to correct, improve, or compensate for speech productive impairment
Assistive Listening Device (5)	Assists in use of effective and appropriate assistive listening device/system
Assistive Listening System/Device Selection (4)	Measures the effectiveness and appropriateness of assistive listening systems/devices
Assistive, Adaptive, Supportive or Protective Devices (9)	Explanation: Devices to facilitate or support achievement of a higher level of function in wheelchair mobility; bed mobility; transfer or ambulation ability; bath and showering ability; dressing; grooming; personal hygiene; play or leisure
Auditory Evoked Potentials (L)	Measures electric responses produced by the VIIIth cranial nerve and brainstem following auditory stimulation
Auditory Processing (Assessment) (Q)	Evaluates ability to receive and process auditory information and comprehension of spoken language
Auditory Processing (Treatment) (2)	Applying techniques to improve the receiving and processing of auditory information and comprehension of spoken language
Augmentative/Alternative Communication System (Assessment) (L)	Determines the appropriateness of aids, techniques, symbols, and/or strategies to augment or replace speech and enhance communication Includes/Examples: Includes the use of telephones, writing equipment, emergency equipment, and TDD
Augmentative/Alternative Communication System (Treatment) (3)	Includes/Examples: Includes augmentative communication devices and aids
Aural Rehabilitation (5)	Applying techniques to improve the communication abilities associated with hearing loss
Aural Rehabilitation Status (P)	Measures impact of a hearing loss including evaluation of receptive and expressive communication skills
Bathing/Showering (Ø)	Includes/Examples: Includes obtaining and using supplies; soaping, rinsing, and drying body parts; maintaining bathing position; and transferring to and from bathing positions
Bathing/Showering Techniques (Ø)	Activities to facilitate obtaining and using supplies, soaping, rinsing and drying body parts, maintaining bathing position, and transferring to and from bathing positions
Bed Mobility (Assessment) (B)	Transitional movement within bed
Bed Mobility (Treatment) (5)	Exercise or activities to facilitate transitional movements within bed
Bedside Swallowing and Oral Function (H)	Includes/Examples: Bedside swallowing includes assessment of sucking, masticating, coughing, and swallowing. Oral function includes assessment of musculature for controlled movements, structures, and functions to determine coordination and phonation.

Continued on next page

Section F–Physical Rehabilitation and Diagnostic Audiology

Continued from previous page

ICD-10-PCS Value Qualifier (Character 5)	Definition
Bekesy Audiometry (3)	Uses an instrument that provides a choice of discrete or continuously varying pure tones; choice of pulsed or continuous signal
Binaural Electroacoustic Hearing Aid Check (6)	Determines mechanical and electroacoustic function of bilateral hearing aids using hearing aid test box
Binaural Hearing Aid (Assessment) (3)	Measures the candidacy, effectiveness, and appropriateness of a hearing aid Explanation: Measures bilateral fit
Binaural Hearing Aid (Treatment) (2)	Explanation: Assists in achieving maximum understanding and performance
Bithermal, Binaural Caloric Irrigation (Ø)	Measures the rhythmic eye movements stimulated by changing the temperature of the vestibular system
Bithermal, Monaural Caloric Irrigation (1)	Measures the rhythmic eye movements stimulated by changing the temperature of the vestibular system in one ear
Brief Tone Stimuli (R)	Measures specific central auditory process
Cerumen Management (3)	Includes examination of external auditory canal and tympanic membrane and removal of cerumen from external ear canal
Cochlear Implant (Ø)	Measures candidacy for cochlear implant
Cochlear Implant Rehabilitation (Ø)	Applying techniques to improve the communication abilities of individuals with cochlear implant; includes programming the device, providing patients/families with information
Communicative/Cognitive Integration Skills (Assessment) (G)	Measures ability to use higher cortical functions Includes/Examples: Includes orientation, recognition, attention span, initiation and termination of activity, memory, sequencing, categorizing, concept formation, spatial operations, judgment, problem solving, generalization and pragmatic communication
Communicative/Cognitive Integration Skills (Treatment) (6)	Activities to facilitate the use of higher cortical functions Includes/Examples: Includes level of arousal, orientation, recognition, attention span, initiation and termination of activity, memory sequencing, judgment and problem solving, learning and generalization, and pragmatic communication
Computerized Dynamic Posturography (6)	Measures the status of the peripheral and central vestibular system and the sensory/motor component of balance; evaluates the efficacy of vestibular rehabilitation
Conditioned Play Audiometry (4)	Behavioral measures using nonspeech and speech stimuli to obtain frequency-specific and ear-specific information on auditory status from the patient Explanation: Obtains speech reception threshold by having patient point to pictures of spondaic words
Coordination/Dexterity (Assessment) (3)	Measures large and small muscle groups for controlled goal-directed movements Explanation: Dexterity includes object manipulation
Coordination/Dexterity (Treatment) (2)	Exercise or activities to facilitate gross coordination and fine coordination
Cranial Nerve Integrity (9)	Measures cranial nerve sensory and motor functions, including tastes, smell and facial expression
Dichotic Stimuli (T)	Measures specific central auditory process
Distorted Speech (S)	Measures specific central auditory process
Dix-Hallpike Dynamic (5)	Measures nystagmus following Dix-Hallpike maneuver
Dressing (1)	Includes/Examples: Includes selecting clothing and accessories, obtaining clothing from storage, dressing, fastening and adjusting clothing and shoes, and applying and removing personal devices, prosthesis or orthosis
Dressing Techniques (1)	Activities to facilitate selecting clothing and accessories, dressing and undressing, adjusting clothing and shoes, applying and removing devices, prostheses or orthoses
Dynamic Orthosis (6)	Includes/Examples: Includes customized and prefabricated splints, inhibitory casts, spinal and other braces, and protective devices; allows motion through transfer of movement from other body parts or by use of outside forces
Ear Canal Probe Microphone (1)	Real ear measures
Ear Protector Attentuation (7)	Measures ear protector fit and effectiveness
Electrocochleography (K)	Measures the VIIIth cranial nerve action potential
Environmental, Home, Work Barriers (B)	Measures current and potential barriers to optimal function, including safety hazards, access problems and home or office design
Ergonomics and Body Mechanics (C)	Ergonomic measurement of job tasks, work hardening or work conditioning needs; functional capacity; and body mechanics
Eustachian Tube Function (F)	Measures eustachian tube function and patency of eustachian tube

Continued on next page

Section F–Physical Rehabilitation and Diagnostic Audiology

Continued from previous page

ICD-10-PCS Value Qualifier (Character 5)	Definition
Evoked Otoacoustic Emissions, Diagnostic (N)	Measures auditory evoked potentials in a diagnostic format
Evoked Otoacoustic Emissions, Screening (M)	Measures auditory evoked potentials in a screening format
Facial Nerve Function (7)	Measures electrical activity of the VIIth cranial nerve (facial nerve)
Feeding/Eating (Assessment) (2)	Includes/Examples: Includes setting up food, selecting and using utensils and tableware, bringing food or drink to mouth, cleaning face, hands, and clothing, and management of alternative methods of nourishment
Feeding/Eating (Treatment) (3)	Exercise or activities to facilitate setting up food, selecting and using utensils and tableware, bringing food or drink to mouth, cleaning face, hands, and clothing, and management of alternative methods of nourishment
Filtered Speech (Ø)	Uses high or low pass filtered speech stimuli to assess central auditory processing disorders, site of lesion testing
Fluency (Assessment) (D)	Measures speech fluency or stuttering
Fluency (Treatment) (7)	Applying techniques to improve and augment fluent speech
Gait and/or Balance (D)	Measures biomechanical, arthrokinematic and other spatial and temporal characteristics of gait and balance
Gait Training/Functional Ambulation (9)	Exercise or activities to facilitate ambulation on a variety of surfaces and in a variety of environments
Grooming/Personal Hygiene (Assessment) (3)	Includes/Examples: Includes ability to obtain and use supplies in a sequential fashion, general grooming, oral hygiene, toilet hygiene, personal care devices, including care for artificial airways
Grooming/Personal Hygiene (Treatment) (2)	Activities to facilitate obtaining and using supplies in a sequential fashion: general grooming, oral hygiene, toilet hygiene, cleaning body, and personal care devices, including artificial airways
Hearing and Related Disorders Counseling (Ø)	Provides patients/families/caregivers with information, support, referrals to facilitate recovery from a communication disorder Includes/Examples: Includes strategies for psychosocial adjustment to hearing loss for clients and families/caregivers
Hearing and Related Disorders Prevention (1)	Provides patients/families/caregivers with information and support to prevent communication disorders
Hearing Screening (Ø)	Pass/refer measures designed to identify need for further audiologic assessment
Home Management (Assessment) (4)	Obtaining and maintaining personal and household possessions and environment Includes/Examples: Includes clothing care, cleaning, meal preparation and cleanup, shopping, money management, household maintenance, safety procedures, and childcare/parenting
Home Management (Treatment) (4)	Activities to facilitate obtaining and maintaining personal household possessions and environment Includes/Examples: Includes clothing care, cleaning, meal preparation and clean-up, shopping, money management, household maintenance, safety procedures, childcare/parenting
Instrumental Swallowing and Oral Function (J)	Measures swallowing function using instrumental diagnostic procedures Explanation: Methods include videofluoroscopy, ultrasound, manometry, endoscopy
Integumentary Integrity (1)	Includes/Examples: Includes burns, skin conditions, ecchymosis, bleeding, blisters, scar tissue, wounds and other traumas, tissue mobility, turgor and texture
Manual Therapy Techniques (7)	Techniques in which the therapist uses his/her hands to administer skilled movements Includes/Examples: Includes connective tissue massage, joint mobilization and manipulation, manual lymph drainage, manual traction, soft tissue mobilization and manipulation
Masking Patterns (W)	Measures central auditory processing status
Monaural Electroacoustic Hearing Aid Check (8)	Determines mechanical and electroacoustic function of one hearing aid using hearing aid test box
Monaural Hearing Aid (Assessment) (2)	Measures the candidacy, effectiveness, and appropriateness of a hearing aid Explanation: Measures unilateral fit
Monaural Hearing Aid (Treatment) (1)	Explanation: Assists in achieving maximum understanding and performance
Motor Function (Assessment) (4)	Measures the body's functional and versatile movement patterns Includes/Examples: Includes motor assessment scales, analysis of head, trunk and limb movement, and assessment of motor learning
Motor Function (Treatment) (3)	Exercise or activities to facilitate crossing midline, laterality, bilateral integration, praxis, neuromuscular relaxation, inhibition, facilitation, motor function and motor learning
Motor Speech (Assessment) (B)	Measures neurological motor aspects of speech production
Motor Speech (Treatment) (8)	Applying techniques to improve and augment the impaired neurological motor aspects of speech production

Continued on next page

Section F–Physical Rehabilitation and Diagnostic Audiology

Continued from previous page

ICD-10-PCS Value Qualifier (Character 5)	Definition
Muscle Performance (Assessment) (Ø)	Measures muscle strength, power and endurance using manual testing, dynamometry or computer-assisted electromechanical muscle test; functional muscle strength, power and endurance; muscle pain, tone, or soreness; or pelvic-floor musculature Explanation: Muscle endurance refers to the ability to contract a muscle repeatedly over time
Muscle Performance (Treatment) (1)	Exercise or activities to increase the capacity of a muscle to do work in terms of strength, power, and/or endurance Explanation: Muscle strength is the force exerted to overcome resistance in one maximal effort. Muscle power is work produced per unit of time, or the product of strength and speed. Muscle endurance is the ability to contract a muscle repeatedly over time.
Neuromotor Development (D)	Measures motor development, righting and equilibrium reactions, and reflex and equilibrium reactions
Non-invasive Instrumental Status (N)	Instrumental measures of oral, nasal, vocal, and velopharyngeal functions as they pertain to speech production
Nonspoken Language (Assessment) (7)	Measures nonspoken language (print, sign, symbols) for communication
Nonspoken Language (Treatment) (Ø)	Applying techniques that improve, augment, or compensate spoken communication
Oral Peripheral Mechanism (P)	Structural measures of face, jaw, lips, tongue, teeth, hard and soft palate, pharynx as related to speech production
Orofacial Myofunctional (Assessment) (K)	Measures orofacial myofunctional patterns for speech and related functions
Orofacial Myofunctional (Treatment) (9)	Applying techniques to improve, alter, or augment impaired orofacial myofunctional patterns and related speech production errors
Oscillating Tracking (3)	Measures ability to visually track
Pain (F)	Measures muscle soreness, pain and soreness with joint movement, and pain perception Includes/Examples: Includes questionnaires, graphs, symptom magnification scales or visual analog scales
Perceptual Processing (Assessment) (5)	Measures stereognosis, kinesthesia, body schema, right-left discrimination, form constancy, position in space, visual closure, figure-ground, depth perception, spatial relations and topographical orientation
Perceptual Processing (Treatment) (1)	Exercise and activities to facilitate perceptual processing Explanation: Includes stereognosis, kinesthesia, body schema, right-left discrimination, form constancy, position in space, visual closure, figure-ground, depth perception, spatial relations, and topographical orientation Includes/Examples: Includes stereognosis, kinesthesia, body schema, right-left discrimination, form constancy, position in space, visual closure, figure-ground, depth perception, spatial relations, and topographical orientation
Performance Intensity Phonetically Balanced Speech Discrimination (Q)	Measures word recognition over varying intensity levels
Postural Control (3)	Exercise or activities to increase postural alignment and control
Prosthesis (8)	Explanation: Artificial substitutes for missing body parts that augment performance or function Includes/Examples: Limb prosthesis, ocular prosthesis
Psychosocial Skills (Assessment) (6)	The ability to interact in society and to process emotions Includes/Examples: Includes psychological (values, interests, self-concept); social (role performance, social conduct, interpersonal skills, self expression); self-management (coping skills, time management, self-control)
Psychosocial Skills (Treatment) (6)	The ability to interact in society and to process emotions Includes/Examples: Includes psychological (values, interests, self-concept); social (role performance, social conduct, interpersonal skills, self expression); self-management (coping skills, time management, self-control)
Pure Tone Audiometry, Air (1)	Air-conduction pure tone threshold measures with appropriate masking
Pure Tone Audiometry, Air and Bone (2)	Air-conduction and bone-conduction pure tone threshold measures with appropriate masking
Pure Tone Stenger (C)	Measures unilateral nonorganic hearing loss based on simultaneous presentation of pure tones of differing volume
Range of Motion and Joint Integrity (5)	Measures quantity, quality, grade, and classification of joint movement and/or mobility Explanation: Range of Motion is the space, distance or angle through which movement occurs at a joint or series of joints. Joint integrity is the conformance of joints to expected anatomic, biomechanical and kinematic norms.
Range of Motion and Joint Mobility (Ø)	Exercise or activities to increase muscle length and joint mobility
Receptive/Expressive Language (Assessment) (8)	Measures receptive and expressive language
Receptive/Expressive Language (Treatment) (B)	Applying techniques to improve and augment receptive/expressive language
Reflex Integrity (G)	Measures the presence, absence, or exaggeration of developmentally appropriate, pathologic or normal reflexes

Continued on next page

Section F–Physical Rehabilitation and Diagnostic Audiology

Continued from previous page

ICD-10-PCS Value Qualifier (Character 5)	Definition
Select Picture Audiometry (5)	Establishes hearing threshold levels for speech using pictures
Sensorineural Acuity Level (4)	Measures sensorineural acuity masking presented via bone conduction
Sensory Aids (5)	Determines the appropriateness of a sensory prosthetic device, other than a hearing aid or assistive listening system/device
Sensory Awareness/ Processing/ Integrity (6)	Includes/Examples: Includes light touch, pressure, temperature, pain, sharp/dull, proprioception, vestibular, visual, auditory, gustatory, and olfactory
Short Increment Sensitivity Index (9)	Measures the ear's ability to detect small intensity changes; site of lesion test requiring a behavioral response
Sinusoidal Vertical Axis Rotational (4)	Measures nystagmus following rotation
Somatosensory Evoked Potentials (9)	Measures neural activity from sites throughout the body
Speech/Language Screening (6)	Identifies need for further speech and/or language evaluation
Speech Threshold (1)	Measures minimal intensity needed to repeat spondaic words
Speech-Language Pathology and Related Disorders Counseling (1)	Provides patients/families with information, support, referrals to facilitate recovery from a communication disorder
Speech-Language Pathology and Related Disorders Prevention (2)	Applying techniques to avoid or minimize onset and/or development of a communication disorder
Speech/Word Recognition (2)	Measures ability to repeat/identify single syllable words; scores given as a percentage; includes word recognition/speech discrimination
Staggered Spondaic Word (3)	Measures central auditory processing site of lesion based upon dichotic presentation of spondaic words
Static Orthosis (7)	Includes/Examples: Includes customized and prefabricated splints, inhibitory casts, spinal and other braces, and protective devices; has no moving parts, maintains joint(s) in desired position
Stenger (B)	Measures unilateral nonorganic hearing loss based on simultaneous presentation of signals of differing volume
Swallowing Dysfunction (D)	Activities to improve swallowing function in coordination with respiratory function Includes/Examples: Includes function and coordination of sucking, mastication, coughing, swallowing
Synthetic Sentence Identification (5)	Measures central auditory dysfunction using identification of third order approximations of sentences and competing messages
Temporal Ordering of Stimuli (V)	Measures specific central auditory process
Therapeutic Exercise (6)	Exercise or activities to facilitate sensory awareness, sensory processing, sensory integration, balance training, conditioning, reconditioning Includes/Examples: Includes developmental activities, breathing exercises, aerobic endurance activities, aquatic exercises, stretching and ventilatory muscle training
Tinnitus Masker (Assessment) (7)	Determines candidacy for tinnitus masker
Tinnitus Masker (Treatment) (Ø)	Explanation: Used to verify physical fit, acoustic appropriateness, and benefit; assists in achieving maximum benefit
Tone Decay (8)	Measures decrease in hearing sensitivity to a tone; site of lesion test requiring a behavioral response
Transfer (C)	Transitional movement from one surface to another
Transfer Training (8)	Exercise or activities to facilitate movement from one surface to another
Tympanometry (D)	Measures the integrity of the middle ear; measures ease at which sound flows through the tympanic membrane while air pressure against the membrane is varied
Unithermal Binaural Screen (2)	Measures the rhythmic eye movements stimulated by changing the temperature of the vestibular system in both ears using warm water, screening format
Ventilation/Respiration/Circulation (G)	Measures ventilatory muscle strength, power and endurance, pulmonary function and ventilatory mechanics Includes/Examples: Includes ability to clear airway, activities that aggravate or relieve edema, pain, dyspnea or other symptoms, chest wall mobility, cardiopulmonary response to performance of ADL and IAD, cough and sputum, standard vital signs
Vestibular (Ø)	Applying techniques to compensate for balance disorders; includes habituation, exercise therapy, and balance retraining
Visual Motor Integration (Assessment) (2)	Coordinating the interaction of information from the eyes with body movement during activity

Continued on next page

Section F–Physical Rehabilitation and Diagnostic Audiology

Continued from previous page

ICD-10-PCS Value Qualifier (Character 5)	Definition
Visual Motor Integration (Treatment) (2)	Exercise or activities to facilitate coordinating the interaction of information from eyes with body movement during activity
Visual Reinforcement Audiometry (6)	Behavioral measures using nonspeech and speech stimuli to obtain frequency/ear-specific information on auditory status Includes/Examples: Includes a conditioned response of looking toward a visual reinforcer (e.g., lights, animated toy) every time auditory stimuli are heard
Vocational Activities and Functional Community or Work Reintegration Skills (Assessment) (H)	Measures environmental, home, work (job/school/play) barriers that keep patients from functioning optimally in their environment Includes/Examples: Includes assessment of vocational skills and interests, environment of work (job/school/play), injury potential and injury prevention or reduction, ergonomic stressors, transportation skills, and ability to access and use community resources
Vocational Activities and Functional Community or Work Reintegration Skills (Treatment) (7)	Activities to facilitate vocational exploration, body mechanics training, job acquisition, and environmental or work (job/school/play) task adaptation Includes/Examples: Includes injury prevention and reduction, ergonomic stressor reduction, job coaching and simulation, work hardening and conditioning, driving training, transportation skills, and use of community resources
Voice (Assessment) (F)	Measures vocal structure, function and production
Voice (Treatment) (C)	Applying techniques to improve voice and vocal function
Voice Prosthetic (Assessment) (M)	Determines the appropriateness of voice prosthetic/adaptive device to enhance or facilitate communication
Voice Prosthetic (Treatment) (4)	Includes/Examples: Includes electrolarynx, and other assistive, adaptive, supportive devices
Wheelchair Mobility (Assessment) (F)	Measures fit and functional abilities within wheelchair in a variety of environments
Wheelchair Mobility (Treatment) (4)	Management, maintenance and controlled operation of a wheelchair, scooter or other device, in and on a variety of surfaces and environments
Wound Management (5)	Includes/Examples: Includes non-selective and selective debridement (enzymes, autolysis, sharp debridement), dressings (wound coverings, hydrogel, vacuum-assisted closure), topical agents, etc.

Section G–Mental Health

ICD-10-PCS Value (Character 3)	Definition
Biofeedback (C)	Provision of information from the monitoring and regulating of physiological processes in conjunction with cognitive-behavioral techniques to improve patient functioning or well-being Includes/Examples: Includes EEG, blood pressure, skin temperature or peripheral blood flow, ECG, electrooculogram, EMG, respirometry or capnometry, GSR/EDR, perineometry to monitor/regulate bowel/bladder activity, electrogastrogram to monitor/regulate gastric motility
Counseling (6)	The application of psychological methods to treat an individual with normal developmental issues and psychological problems in order to increase function, improve well-being, alleviate distress, maladjustment or resolve crises
Crisis Intervention (2)	Treatment of a traumatized, acutely disturbed or distressed individual for the purpose of short-term stabilization Includes/Examples: Includes defusing, debriefing, counseling, psychotherapy and/or coordination of care with other providers or agencies
Electroconvulsive Therapy (B)	The application of controlled electrical voltages to treat a mental health disorder Includes/Examples: Includes appropriate sedation and other preparation of the individual
Family Psychotherapy (7)	Treatment that includes one or more family members of an individual with a mental health disorder by behavioral, cognitive, psychoanalytic, psychodynamic or psychophysiological means to improve functioning or well-being Explanation: Remediation of emotional or behavioral problems presented by one or more family members in cases where psychotherapy with more than one family member is indicated
Group Psychotherapy (H)	Treatment of two or more individuals with a mental health disorder by behavioral, cognitive, psychoanalytic, psychodynamic or psychophysiological means to improve functioning or well-being
Hypnosis (F)	Induction of a state of heightened suggestibility by auditory, visual and tactile techniques to elicit an emotional or behavioral response
Individual Psychotherapy (5)	Treatment of an individual with a mental health disorder by behavioral, cognitive, psychoanalytic, psychodynamic or psychophysiological means to improve functioning or well-being
Light Therapy (J)	Application of specialized light treatments to improve functioning or well-being
Medication Management (3)	Monitoring and adjusting the use of medications for the treatment of a mental health disorder
Narcosynthesis (G)	Administration of intravenous barbiturates in order to release suppressed or repressed thoughts
Psychological Tests (1)	The administration and interpretation of standardized psychological tests and measurement instruments for the assessment of psychological function

Continued on next page

Section G–Mental Health

Continued from previous page

ICD-10-PCS Value (Character 3)	Definition
Behavioral (1)	Primarily to modify behavior Includes/Examples: Includes modeling and role playing, positive reinforcement of target behaviors, response cost, and training of self-management skills
Cognitive (2)	Primarily to correct cognitive distortions and errors
Cognitive-Behavioral (8)	Combining cognitive and behavioral treatment strategies to improve functioning Explanation: Maladaptive responses are examined to determine how cognitions relate to behavior patterns in response to an event. Uses learning principles and information-processing models.
Developmental (Ø)	Age-normed developmental status of cognitive, social and adaptive behavior skills
Intellectual and Psychoeducational (2)	Intellectual abilities, academic achievement and learning capabilities (including behaviors and emotional factors affecting learning)
Interactive (Ø)	Uses primarily physical aids and other forms of non-oral interaction with a patient who is physically, psychologically or developmentally unable to use ordinary language for communication Includes/Examples: Includes the use of toys in symbolic play
Interpersonal (3)	Helps an individual make changes in interpersonal behaviors to reduce psychological dysfunction Includes/Examples: Includes exploratory techniques, encouragement of affective expression, clarification of patient statements, analysis of communication patterns, use of therapy relationship and behavior change techniques
Neurobehavioral and Cognitive Status (4)	Includes neurobehavioral status exam, interview(s), and observation for the clinical assessment of thinking, reasoning and judgment, acquired knowledge, attention, memory, visual spatial abilities, language functions, and planning
Neuropsychological (3)	Thinking, reasoning and judgment, acquired knowledge, attention, memory, visual spatial abilities, language functions, planning
Personality and Behavioral (1)	Mood, emotion, behavior, social functioning, psychopathological conditions, personality traits and characteristics
Psychoanalysis (4)	Methods of obtaining a detailed account of past and present mental and emotional experiences to determine the source and eliminate or diminish the undesirable effects of unconscious conflicts Explanation: Accomplished by making the individual aware of their existence, origin, and inappropriate expression in emotions and behavior
Psychodynamic (5)	Exploration of past and present emotional experiences to understand motives and drives using insight-oriented techniques to reduce the undesirable effects of internal conflicts on emotions and behavior Explanation: Techniques include empathetic listening, clarifying self-defeating behavior patterns, and exploring adaptive alternatives
Psychophysiological (9)	Monitoring and alteration of physiological processes to help the individual associate physiological reactions combined with cognitive and behavioral strategies to gain improved control of these processes to help the individual cope more effectively
Supportive (6)	Formation of therapeutic relationship primarily for providing emotional support to prevent further deterioration in functioning during periods of particular stress Explanation: Often used in conjunction with other therapeutic approaches
Vocational (1)	Exploration of vocational interests, aptitudes and required adaptive behavior skills to develop and carry out a plan for achieving a successful vocational placement Includes/Examples: Includes enhancing work related adjustment and/or pursuing viable options in training education or preparation

Section H–Substance Abuse Treatment

ICD-10-PCS Value (Character 3)	Definition
Detoxification Services (2)	Detoxification from alcohol and/or drugs Explanation: Not a treatment modality, but helps the patient stabilize physically and psychologically until the body becomes free of drugs and the effects of alcohol
Family Counseling (6)	The application of psychological methods that includes one or more family members to treat an individual with addictive behavior Explanation: Provides support and education for family members of addicted individuals. Family member participation is seen as a critical area of substance abuse treatment.
Group Counseling (4)	The application of psychological methods to treat two or more individuals with addictive behavior Explanation: Provides structured group counseling sessions and healing power through the connection with others
Individual Counseling (3)	The application of psychological methods to treat an individual with addictive behavior Explanation: Comprised of several different techniques, which apply various strategies to address drug addiction
Individual Psychotherapy (5)	Treatment of an individual with addictive behavior by behavioral, cognitive, psychoanalytic, psychodynamic or psychophysiological means
Medication Management (8)	Monitoring and adjusting the use of replacement medications for the treatment of addiction
Pharmacotherapy (9)	The use of replacement medications for the treatment of addiction

Appendix K: Hospital Acquired Conditions

Hospital acquired conditions (HACs) are conditions considered reasonably preventable through the application of evidence-based guidelines. Although it is the ICD-10-CM diagnosis code that drives a HAC designation, in some cases a specific ICD-10-PCS procedure code must also be present before that diagnosis code can be considered a HAC. This resource provides only those HAC categories that require both an ICD-10-PCS code and an ICD-10-CM diagnosis code. The official descriptions for each code are also provided. To see all 14 HAC categories and their corresponding codes, refer to Optum's *ICD-10-CM Expert for Hospitals*.

Note: The resource used to compile this list is the proposed, version 40, MS-DRG Grouper software and Definitions Manual files published with the fiscal 2024 IPPS proposed rule. For the most current files, refer to the following: https://www.cms.gov/Medicare/Medicare-Fee-for-Service-Payment/AcuteInpatientPPS/MS-DRG-Classifications-and-Software.

HAC 08: Surgical Site Infection of Mediastinitis After Coronary Bypass Graft (CABG) Procedures

Secondary diagnosis not POA:

J98.51 Mediastinitis
J98.59 Other diseases of mediastinum, not elsewhere classified

AND

Any of the following procedures:

Ø21ØØ83 Bypass Coronary Artery, One Artery from Coronary Artery with Zooplastic Tissue, Open Approach
Ø21ØØ88 Bypass Coronary Artery, One Artery from Right Internal Mammary with Zooplastic Tissue, Open Approach
Ø21ØØ89 Bypass Coronary Artery, One Artery from Left Internal Mammary with Zooplastic Tissue, Open Approach
Ø21ØØ8C Bypass Coronary Artery, One Artery from Thoracic Artery with Zooplastic Tissue, Open Approach
Ø21ØØ8F Bypass Coronary Artery, One Artery from Abdominal Artery with Zooplastic Tissue, Open Approach
Ø21ØØ8W Bypass Coronary Artery, One Artery from Aorta with Zooplastic Tissue, Open Approach
Ø21ØØ93 Bypass Coronary Artery, One Artery from Coronary Artery with Autologous Venous Tissue, Open Approach
Ø21ØØ98 Bypass Coronary Artery, One Artery from Right Internal Mammary with Autologous Venous Tissue, Open Approach
Ø21ØØ99 Bypass Coronary Artery, One Artery from Left Internal Mammary with Autologous Venous Tissue, Open Approach
Ø21ØØ9C Bypass Coronary Artery, One Artery from Thoracic Artery with Autologous Venous Tissue, Open Approach
Ø21ØØ9F Bypass Coronary Artery, One Artery from Abdominal Artery with Autologous Venous Tissue, Open Approach
Ø21ØØ9W Bypass Coronary Artery, One Artery from Aorta with Autologous Venous Tissue, Open Approach
Ø21ØØA3 Bypass Coronary Artery, One Artery from Coronary Artery with Autologous Arterial Tissue, Open Approach
Ø21ØØA8 Bypass Coronary Artery, One Artery from Right Internal Mammary with Autologous Arterial Tissue, Open Approach
Ø21ØØA9 Bypass Coronary Artery, One Artery from Left Internal Mammary with Autologous Arterial Tissue, Open Approach
Ø21ØØAC Bypass Coronary Artery, One Artery from Thoracic Artery with Autologous Arterial Tissue, Open Approach
Ø21ØØAF Bypass Coronary Artery, One Artery from Abdominal Artery with Autologous Arterial Tissue, Open Approach
Ø21ØØAW Bypass Coronary Artery, One Artery from Aorta with Autologous Arterial Tissue, Open Approach
Ø21ØØJ3 Bypass Coronary Artery, One Artery from Coronary Artery with Synthetic Substitute, Open Approach
Ø21ØØJ8 Bypass Coronary Artery, One Artery from Right Internal Mammary with Synthetic Substitute, Open Approach
Ø21ØØJ9 Bypass Coronary Artery, One Artery from Left Internal Mammary with Synthetic Substitute, Open Approach
Ø21ØØJC Bypass Coronary Artery, One Artery from Thoracic Artery with Synthetic Substitute, Open Approach
Ø21ØØJF Bypass Coronary Artery, One Artery from Abdominal Artery with Synthetic Substitute, Open Approach
Ø21ØØJW Bypass Coronary Artery, One Artery from Aorta with Synthetic Substitute, Open Approach
Ø21ØØK3 Bypass Coronary Artery, One Artery from Coronary Artery with Nonautologous Tissue Substitute, Open Approach
Ø21ØØK8 Bypass Coronary Artery, One Artery from Right Internal Mammary with Nonautologous Tissue Substitute, Open Approach
Ø21ØØK9 Bypass Coronary Artery, One Artery from Left Internal Mammary with Nonautologous Tissue Substitute, Open Approach
Ø21ØØKC Bypass Coronary Artery, One Artery from Thoracic Artery with Nonautologous Tissue Substitute, Open Approach
Ø21ØØKF Bypass Coronary Artery, One Artery from Abdominal Artery with Nonautologous Tissue Substitute, Open Approach
Ø21ØØKW Bypass Coronary Artery, One Artery from Aorta with Nonautologous Tissue Substitute, Open Approach
Ø21ØØZ3 Bypass Coronary Artery, One Artery from Coronary Artery, Open Approach
Ø21ØØZ8 Bypass Coronary Artery, One Artery from Right Internal Mammary, Open Approach
Ø21ØØZ9 Bypass Coronary Artery, One Artery from Left Internal Mammary, Open Approach
Ø21ØØZC Bypass Coronary Artery, One Artery from Thoracic Artery, Open Approach
Ø21ØØZF Bypass Coronary Artery, One Artery from Abdominal Artery, Open Approach
Ø21Ø483 Bypass Coronary Artery, One Artery from Coronary Artery with Zooplastic Tissue, Percutaneous Endoscopic Approach
Ø21Ø488 Bypass Coronary Artery, One Artery from Right Internal Mammary with Zooplastic Tissue, Percutaneous Endoscopic Approach
Ø21Ø489 Bypass Coronary Artery, One Artery from Left Internal Mammary with Zooplastic Tissue, Percutaneous Endoscopic Approach
Ø21Ø48C Bypass Coronary Artery, One Artery from Thoracic Artery with Zooplastic Tissue, Percutaneous Endoscopic Approach
Ø21Ø48F Bypass Coronary Artery, One Artery from Abdominal Artery with Zooplastic Tissue, Percutaneous Endoscopic Approach
Ø21Ø48W Bypass Coronary Artery, One Artery from Aorta with Zooplastic Tissue, Percutaneous Endoscopic Approach
Ø21Ø493 Bypass Coronary Artery, One Artery from Coronary Artery with Autologous Venous Tissue, Percutaneous Endoscopic Approach
Ø21Ø498 Bypass Coronary Artery, One Artery from Right Internal Mammary with Autologous Venous Tissue, Percutaneous Endoscopic Approach
Ø21Ø499 Bypass Coronary Artery, One Artery from Left Internal Mammary with Autologous Venous Tissue, Percutaneous Endoscopic Approach
Ø21Ø49C Bypass Coronary Artery, One Artery from Thoracic Artery with Autologous Venous Tissue, Percutaneous Endoscopic Approach
Ø21Ø49F Bypass Coronary Artery, One Artery from Abdominal Artery with Autologous Venous Tissue, Percutaneous Endoscopic Approach
Ø21Ø49W Bypass Coronary Artery, One Artery from Aorta with Autologous Venous Tissue, Percutaneous Endoscopic Approach
Ø21Ø4A3 Bypass Coronary Artery, One Artery from Coronary Artery with Autologous Arterial Tissue, Percutaneous Endoscopic Approach
Ø21Ø4A8 Bypass Coronary Artery, One Artery from Right Internal Mammary with Autologous Arterial Tissue, Percutaneous Endoscopic Approach
Ø21Ø4A9 Bypass Coronary Artery, One Artery from Left Internal Mammary with Autologous Arterial Tissue, Percutaneous Endoscopic Approach
Ø21Ø4AC Bypass Coronary Artery, One Artery from Thoracic Artery with Autologous Arterial Tissue, Percutaneous Endoscopic Approach
Ø21Ø4AF Bypass Coronary Artery, One Artery from Abdominal Artery with Autologous Arterial Tissue, Percutaneous Endoscopic Approach
Ø21Ø4AW Bypass Coronary Artery, One Artery from Aorta with Autologous Arterial Tissue, Percutaneous Endoscopic Approach
Ø21Ø4J3 Bypass Coronary Artery, One Artery from Coronary Artery with Synthetic Substitute, Percutaneous Endoscopic Approach
Ø21Ø4J8 Bypass Coronary Artery, One Artery from Right Internal Mammary with Synthetic Substitute, Percutaneous Endoscopic Approach
Ø21Ø4J9 Bypass Coronary Artery, One Artery from Left Internal Mammary with Synthetic Substitute, Percutaneous Endoscopic Approach

HAC 08: Surgical Site Infection of Mediastinitis After Coronary Bypass Graft (CABG) Procedures (continued)

Ø2104JC Bypass Coronary Artery, One Artery from Thoracic Artery with Synthetic Substitute, Percutaneous Endoscopic Approach
Ø2104JF Bypass Coronary Artery, One Artery from Abdominal Artery with Synthetic Substitute, Percutaneous Endoscopic Approach
Ø2104JW Bypass Coronary Artery, One Artery from Aorta with Synthetic Substitute, Percutaneous Endoscopic Approach
Ø2104K3 Bypass Coronary Artery, One Artery from Coronary Artery with Nonautologous Tissue Substitute, Percutaneous Endoscopic Approach
Ø2104K8 Bypass Coronary Artery, One Artery from Right Internal Mammary with Nonautologous Tissue Substitute, Percutaneous Endoscopic Approach
Ø2104K9 Bypass Coronary Artery, One Artery from Left Internal Mammary with Nonautologous Tissue Substitute, Percutaneous Endoscopic Approach
Ø2104KC Bypass Coronary Artery, One Artery from Thoracic Artery with Nonautologous Tissue Substitute, Percutaneous Endoscopic Approach
Ø2104KF Bypass Coronary Artery, One Artery from Abdominal Artery with Nonautologous Tissue Substitute, Percutaneous Endoscopic Approach
Ø2104KW Bypass Coronary Artery, One Artery from Aorta with Nonautologous Tissue Substitute, Percutaneous Endoscopic Approach
Ø2104Z3 Bypass Coronary Artery, One Artery from Coronary Artery, Percutaneous Endoscopic Approach
Ø2104Z8 Bypass Coronary Artery, One Artery from Right Internal Mammary, Percutaneous Endoscopic Approach
Ø2104Z9 Bypass Coronary Artery, One Artery from Left Internal Mammary, Percutaneous Endoscopic Approach
Ø2104ZC Bypass Coronary Artery, One Artery from Thoracic Artery, Percutaneous Endoscopic Approach
Ø2104ZF Bypass Coronary Artery, One Artery from Abdominal Artery, Percutaneous Endoscopic Approach
Ø211Ø83 Bypass Coronary Artery, Two Arteries from Coronary Artery with Zooplastic Tissue, Open Approach
Ø211Ø88 Bypass Coronary Artery, Two Arteries from Right Internal Mammary with Zooplastic Tissue, Open Approach
Ø211Ø89 Bypass Coronary Artery, Two Arteries from Left Internal Mammary with Zooplastic Tissue, Open Approach
Ø211Ø8C Bypass Coronary Artery, Two Arteries from Thoracic Artery with Zooplastic Tissue, Open Approach
Ø211Ø8F Bypass Coronary Artery, Two Arteries from Abdominal Artery with Zooplastic Tissue, Open Approach
Ø211Ø8W Bypass Coronary Artery, Two Arteries from Aorta with Zooplastic Tissue, Open Approach
Ø211Ø93 Bypass Coronary Artery, Two Arteries from Coronary Artery with Autologous Venous Tissue, Open Approach
Ø211Ø98 Bypass Coronary Artery, Two Arteries from Right Internal Mammary with Autologous Venous Tissue, Open Approach
Ø211Ø99 Bypass Coronary Artery, Two Arteries from Left Internal Mammary with Autologous Venous Tissue, Open Approach
Ø211Ø9C Bypass Coronary Artery, Two Arteries from Thoracic Artery with Autologous Venous Tissue, Open Approach
Ø211Ø9F Bypass Coronary Artery, Two Arteries from Abdominal Artery with Autologous Venous Tissue, Open Approach
Ø211Ø9W Bypass Coronary Artery, Two Arteries from Aorta with Autologous Venous Tissue, Open Approach
Ø211ØA3 Bypass Coronary Artery, Two Arteries from Coronary Artery with Autologous Arterial Tissue, Open Approach
Ø211ØA8 Bypass Coronary Artery, Two Arteries from Right Internal Mammary with Autologous Arterial Tissue, Open Approach
Ø211ØA9 Bypass Coronary Artery, Two Arteries from Left Internal Mammary with Autologous Arterial Tissue, Open Approach
Ø211ØAC Bypass Coronary Artery, Two Arteries from Thoracic Artery with Autologous Arterial Tissue, Open Approach
Ø211ØAF Bypass Coronary Artery, Two Arteries from Abdominal Artery with Autologous Arterial Tissue, Open Approach
Ø211ØAW Bypass Coronary Artery, Two Arteries from Aorta with Autologous Arterial Tissue, Open Approach
Ø211ØJ3 Bypass Coronary Artery, Two Arteries from Coronary Artery with Synthetic Substitute, Open Approach
Ø211ØJ8 Bypass Coronary Artery, Two Arteries from Right Internal Mammary with Synthetic Substitute, Open Approach
Ø211ØJ9 Bypass Coronary Artery, Two Arteries from Left Internal Mammary with Synthetic Substitute, Open Approach
Ø211ØJC Bypass Coronary Artery, Two Arteries from Thoracic Artery with Synthetic Substitute, Open Approach
Ø211ØJF Bypass Coronary Artery, Two Arteries from Abdominal Artery with Synthetic Substitute, Open Approach
Ø211ØJW Bypass Coronary Artery, Two Arteries from Aorta with Synthetic Substitute, Open Approach
Ø211ØK3 Bypass Coronary Artery, Two Arteries from Coronary Artery with Nonautologous Tissue Substitute, Open Approach
Ø211ØK8 Bypass Coronary Artery, Two Arteries from Right Internal Mammary with Nonautologous Tissue Substitute, Open Approach
Ø211ØK9 Bypass Coronary Artery, Two Arteries from Left Internal Mammary with Nonautologous Tissue Substitute, Open Approach
Ø211ØKC Bypass Coronary Artery, Two Arteries from Thoracic Artery with Nonautologous Tissue Substitute, Open Approach
Ø211ØKF Bypass Coronary Artery, Two Arteries from Abdominal Artery with Nonautologous Tissue Substitute, Open Approach
Ø211ØKW Bypass Coronary Artery, Two Arteries from Aorta with Nonautologous Tissue Substitute, Open Approach
Ø211ØZ3 Bypass Coronary Artery, Two Arteries from Coronary Artery, Open Approach
Ø211ØZ8 Bypass Coronary Artery, Two Arteries from Right Internal Mammary, Open Approach
Ø211ØZ9 Bypass Coronary Artery, Two Arteries from Left Internal Mammary, Open Approach
Ø211ØZC Bypass Coronary Artery, Two Arteries from Thoracic Artery, Open Approach
Ø211ØZF Bypass Coronary Artery, Two Arteries from Abdominal Artery, Open Approach
Ø211483 Bypass Coronary Artery, Two Arteries from Coronary Artery with Zooplastic Tissue, Percutaneous Endoscopic Approach
Ø211488 Bypass Coronary Artery, Two Arteries from Right Internal Mammary with Zooplastic Tissue, Percutaneous Endoscopic Approach
Ø211489 Bypass Coronary Artery, Two Arteries from Left Internal Mammary with Zooplastic Tissue, Percutaneous Endoscopic Approach
Ø21148C Bypass Coronary Artery, Two Arteries from Thoracic Artery with Zooplastic Tissue, Percutaneous Endoscopic Approach
Ø21148F Bypass Coronary Artery, Two Arteries from Abdominal Artery with Zooplastic Tissue, Percutaneous Endoscopic Approach
Ø21148W Bypass Coronary Artery, Two Arteries from Aorta with Zooplastic Tissue, Percutaneous Endoscopic Approach
Ø211493 Bypass Coronary Artery, Two Arteries from Coronary Artery with Autologous Venous Tissue, Percutaneous Endoscopic Approach
Ø211498 Bypass Coronary Artery, Two Arteries from Right Internal Mammary with Autologous Venous Tissue, Percutaneous Endoscopic Approach
Ø211499 Bypass Coronary Artery, Two Arteries from Left Internal Mammary with Autologous Venous Tissue, Percutaneous Endoscopic Approach
Ø21149C Bypass Coronary Artery, Two Arteries from Thoracic Artery with Autologous Venous Tissue, Percutaneous Endoscopic Approach
Ø21149F Bypass Coronary Artery, Two Arteries from Abdominal Artery with Autologous Venous Tissue, Percutaneous Endoscopic Approach
Ø21149W Bypass Coronary Artery, Two Arteries from Aorta with Autologous Venous Tissue, Percutaneous Endoscopic Approach
Ø2114A3 Bypass Coronary Artery, Two Arteries from Coronary Artery with Autologous Arterial Tissue, Percutaneous Endoscopic Approach
Ø2114A8 Bypass Coronary Artery, Two Arteries from Right Internal Mammary with Autologous Arterial Tissue, Percutaneous Endoscopic Approach
Ø2114A9 Bypass Coronary Artery, Two Arteries from Left Internal Mammary with Autologous Arterial Tissue, Percutaneous Endoscopic Approach
Ø2114AC Bypass Coronary Artery, Two Arteries from Thoracic Artery with Autologous Arterial Tissue, Percutaneous Endoscopic Approach
Ø2114AF Bypass Coronary Artery, Two Arteries from Abdominal Artery with Autologous Arterial Tissue, Percutaneous Endoscopic Approach
Ø2114AW Bypass Coronary Artery, Two Arteries from Aorta with Autologous Arterial Tissue, Percutaneous Endoscopic Approach
Ø2114J3 Bypass Coronary Artery, Two Arteries from Coronary Artery with Synthetic Substitute, Percutaneous Endoscopic Approach
Ø2114J8 Bypass Coronary Artery, Two Arteries from Right Internal Mammary with Synthetic Substitute, Percutaneous Endoscopic Approach

HAC 08: Surgical Site Infection of Mediastinitis After Coronary Bypass Graft (CABG) Procedures (continued)

Ø2114J9 Bypass Coronary Artery, Two Arteries from Left Internal Mammary with Synthetic Substitute, Percutaneous Endoscopic Approach
Ø2114JC Bypass Coronary Artery, Two Arteries from Thoracic Artery with Synthetic Substitute, Percutaneous Endoscopic Approach
Ø2114JF Bypass Coronary Artery, Two Arteries from Abdominal Artery with Synthetic Substitute, Percutaneous Endoscopic Approach
Ø2114JW Bypass Coronary Artery, Two Arteries from Aorta with Synthetic Substitute, Percutaneous Endoscopic Approach
Ø2114K3 Bypass Coronary Artery, Two Arteries from Coronary Artery with Nonautologous Tissue Substitute, Percutaneous Endoscopic Approach
Ø2114K8 Bypass Coronary Artery, Two Arteries from Right Internal Mammary with Nonautologous Tissue Substitute, Percutaneous Endoscopic Approach
Ø2114K9 Bypass Coronary Artery, Two Arteries from Left Internal Mammary with Nonautologous Tissue Substitute, Percutaneous Endoscopic Approach
Ø2114KC Bypass Coronary Artery, Two Arteries from Thoracic Artery with Nonautologous Tissue Substitute, Percutaneous Endoscopic Approach
Ø2114KF Bypass Coronary Artery, Two Arteries from Abdominal Artery with Nonautologous Tissue Substitute, Percutaneous Endoscopic Approach
Ø2114KW Bypass Coronary Artery, Two Arteries from Aorta with Nonautologous Tissue Substitute, Percutaneous Endoscopic Approach
Ø2114Z3 Bypass Coronary Artery, Two Arteries from Coronary Artery, Percutaneous Endoscopic Approach
Ø2114Z8 Bypass Coronary Artery, Two Arteries from Right Internal Mammary, Percutaneous Endoscopic Approach
Ø2114Z9 Bypass Coronary Artery, Two Arteries from Left Internal Mammary, Percutaneous Endoscopic Approach
Ø2114ZC Bypass Coronary Artery, Two Arteries from Thoracic Artery, Percutaneous Endoscopic Approach
Ø2114ZF Bypass Coronary Artery, Two Arteries from Abdominal Artery, Percutaneous Endoscopic Approach
Ø212Ø83 Bypass Coronary Artery, Three Arteries from Coronary Artery with Zooplastic Tissue, Open Approach
Ø212Ø88 Bypass Coronary Artery, Three Arteries from Right Internal Mammary with Zooplastic Tissue, Open Approach
Ø212Ø89 Bypass Coronary Artery, Three Arteries from Left Internal Mammary with Zooplastic Tissue, Open Approach
Ø212Ø8C Bypass Coronary Artery, Three Arteries from Thoracic Artery with Zooplastic Tissue, Open Approach
Ø212Ø8F Bypass Coronary Artery, Three Arteries from Abdominal Artery with Zooplastic Tissue, Open Approach
Ø212Ø8W Bypass Coronary Artery, Three Arteries from Aorta with Zooplastic Tissue, Open Approach
Ø212Ø93 Bypass Coronary Artery, Three Arteries from Coronary Artery with Autologous Venous Tissue, Open Approach
Ø212Ø98 Bypass Coronary Artery, Three Arteries from Right Internal Mammary with Autologous Venous Tissue, Open Approach
Ø212Ø99 Bypass Coronary Artery, Three Arteries from Left Internal Mammary with Autologous Venous Tissue, Open Approach
Ø212Ø9C Bypass Coronary Artery, Three Arteries from Thoracic Artery with Autologous Venous Tissue, Open Approach
Ø212Ø9F Bypass Coronary Artery, Three Arteries from Abdominal Artery with Autologous Venous Tissue, Open Approach
Ø212Ø9W Bypass Coronary Artery, Three Arteries from Aorta with Autologous Venous Tissue, Open Approach
Ø212ØA3 Bypass Coronary Artery, Three Arteries from Coronary Artery with Autologous Arterial Tissue, Open Approach
Ø212ØA8 Bypass Coronary Artery, Three Arteries from Right Internal Mammary with Autologous Arterial Tissue, Open Approach
Ø212ØA9 Bypass Coronary Artery, Three Arteries from Left Internal Mammary with Autologous Arterial Tissue, Open Approach
Ø212ØAC Bypass Coronary Artery, Three Arteries from Thoracic Artery with Autologous Arterial Tissue, Open Approach
Ø212ØAF Bypass Coronary Artery, Three Arteries from Abdominal Artery with Autologous Arterial Tissue, Open Approach
Ø212ØAW Bypass Coronary Artery, Three Arteries from Aorta with Autologous Arterial Tissue, Open Approach
Ø212ØJ3 Bypass Coronary Artery, Three Arteries from Coronary Artery with Synthetic Substitute, Open Approach
Ø212ØJ8 Bypass Coronary Artery, Three Arteries from Right Internal Mammary with Synthetic Substitute, Open Approach
Ø212ØJ9 Bypass Coronary Artery, Three Arteries from Left Internal Mammary with Synthetic Substitute, Open Approach
Ø212ØJC Bypass Coronary Artery, Three Arteries from Thoracic Artery with Synthetic Substitute, Open Approach
Ø212ØJF Bypass Coronary Artery, Three Arteries from Abdominal Artery with Synthetic Substitute, Open Approach
Ø212ØJW Bypass Coronary Artery, Three Arteries from Aorta with Synthetic Substitute, Open Approach
Ø212ØK3 Bypass Coronary Artery, Three Arteries from Coronary Artery with Nonautologous Tissue Substitute, Open Approach
Ø212ØK8 Bypass Coronary Artery, Three Arteries from Right Internal Mammary with Nonautologous Tissue Substitute, Open Approach
Ø212ØK9 Bypass Coronary Artery, Three Arteries from Left Internal Mammary with Nonautologous Tissue Substitute, Open Approach
Ø212ØKC Bypass Coronary Artery, Three Arteries from Thoracic Artery with Nonautologous Tissue Substitute, Open Approach
Ø212ØKF Bypass Coronary Artery, Three Arteries from Abdominal Artery with Nonautologous Tissue Substitute, Open Approach
Ø212ØKW Bypass Coronary Artery, Three Arteries from Aorta with Nonautologous Tissue Substitute, Open Approach
Ø212ØZ3 Bypass Coronary Artery, Three Arteries from Coronary Artery, Open Approach
Ø212ØZ8 Bypass Coronary Artery, Three Arteries from Right Internal Mammary, Open Approach
Ø212ØZ9 Bypass Coronary Artery, Three Arteries from Left Internal Mammary, Open Approach
Ø212ØZC Bypass Coronary Artery, Three Arteries from Thoracic Artery, Open Approach
Ø212ØZF Bypass Coronary Artery, Three Arteries from Abdominal Artery, Open Approach
Ø212483 Bypass Coronary Artery, Three Arteries from Coronary Artery with Zooplastic Tissue, Percutaneous Endoscopic Approach
Ø212488 Bypass Coronary Artery, Three Arteries from Right Internal Mammary with Zooplastic Tissue, Percutaneous Endoscopic Approach
Ø212489 Bypass Coronary Artery, Three Arteries from Left Internal Mammary with Zooplastic Tissue, Percutaneous Endoscopic Approach
Ø21248C Bypass Coronary Artery, Three Arteries from Thoracic Artery with Zooplastic Tissue, Percutaneous Endoscopic Approach
Ø21248F Bypass Coronary Artery, Three Arteries from Abdominal Artery with Zooplastic Tissue, Percutaneous Endoscopic Approach
Ø21248W Bypass Coronary Artery, Three Arteries from Aorta with Zooplastic Tissue, Percutaneous Endoscopic Approach
Ø212493 Bypass Coronary Artery, Three Arteries from Coronary Artery with Autologous Venous Tissue, Percutaneous Endoscopic Approach
Ø212498 Bypass Coronary Artery, Three Arteries from Right Internal Mammary with Autologous Venous Tissue, Percutaneous Endoscopic Approach
Ø212499 Bypass Coronary Artery, Three Arteries from Left Internal Mammary with Autologous Venous Tissue, Percutaneous Endoscopic Approach
Ø21249C Bypass Coronary Artery, Three Arteries from Thoracic Artery with Autologous Venous Tissue, Percutaneous Endoscopic Approach
Ø21249F Bypass Coronary Artery, Three Arteries from Abdominal Artery with Autologous Venous Tissue, Percutaneous Endoscopic Approach
Ø21249W Bypass Coronary Artery, Three Arteries from Aorta with Autologous Venous Tissue, Percutaneous Endoscopic Approach
Ø2124A3 Bypass Coronary Artery, Three Arteries from Coronary Artery with Autologous Arterial Tissue, Percutaneous Endoscopic Approach
Ø2124A8 Bypass Coronary Artery, Three Arteries from Right Internal Mammary with Autologous Arterial Tissue, Percutaneous Endoscopic Approach
Ø2124A9 Bypass Coronary Artery, Three Arteries from Left Internal Mammary with Autologous Arterial Tissue, Percutaneous Endoscopic Approach

HAC 08: Surgical Site Infection of Mediastinitis After Coronary Bypass Graft (CABG) Procedures (continued)

Ø2124AC Bypass Coronary Artery, Three Arteries from Thoracic Artery with Autologous Arterial Tissue, Percutaneous Endoscopic Approach
Ø2124AF Bypass Coronary Artery, Three Arteries from Abdominal Artery with Autologous Arterial Tissue, Percutaneous Endoscopic Approach
Ø2124AW Bypass Coronary Artery, Three Arteries from Aorta with Autologous Arterial Tissue, Percutaneous Endoscopic Approach
Ø2124J3 Bypass Coronary Artery, Three Arteries from Coronary Artery with Synthetic Substitute, Percutaneous Endoscopic Approach
Ø2124J8 Bypass Coronary Artery, Three Arteries from Right Internal Mammary with Synthetic Substitute, Percutaneous Endoscopic Approach
Ø2124J9 Bypass Coronary Artery, Three Arteries from Left Internal Mammary with Synthetic Substitute, Percutaneous Endoscopic Approach
Ø2124JC Bypass Coronary Artery, Three Arteries from Thoracic Artery with Synthetic Substitute, Percutaneous Endoscopic Approach
Ø2124JF Bypass Coronary Artery, Three Arteries from Abdominal Artery with Synthetic Substitute, Percutaneous Endoscopic Approach
Ø2124JW Bypass Coronary Artery, Three Arteries from Aorta with Synthetic Substitute, Percutaneous Endoscopic Approach
Ø2124K3 Bypass Coronary Artery, Three Arteries from Coronary Artery with Nonautologous Tissue Substitute, Percutaneous Endoscopic Approach
Ø2124K8 Bypass Coronary Artery, Three Arteries from Right Internal Mammary with Nonautologous Tissue Substitute, Percutaneous Endoscopic Approach
Ø2124K9 Bypass Coronary Artery, Three Arteries from Left Internal Mammary with Nonautologous Tissue Substitute, Percutaneous Endoscopic Approach
Ø2124KC Bypass Coronary Artery, Three Arteries from Thoracic Artery with Nonautologous Tissue Substitute, Percutaneous Endoscopic Approach
Ø2124KF Bypass Coronary Artery, Three Arteries from Abdominal Artery with Nonautologous Tissue Substitute, Percutaneous Endoscopic Approach
Ø2124KW Bypass Coronary Artery, Three Arteries from Aorta with Nonautologous Tissue Substitute, Percutaneous Endoscopic Approach
Ø2124Z3 Bypass Coronary Artery, Three Arteries from Coronary Artery, Percutaneous Endoscopic Approach
Ø2124Z8 Bypass Coronary Artery, Three Arteries from Right Internal Mammary, Percutaneous Endoscopic Approach
Ø2124Z9 Bypass Coronary Artery, Three Arteries from Left Internal Mammary, Percutaneous Endoscopic Approach
Ø2124ZC Bypass Coronary Artery, Three Arteries from Thoracic Artery, Percutaneous Endoscopic Approach
Ø2124ZF Bypass Coronary Artery, Three Arteries from Abdominal Artery, Percutaneous Endoscopic Approach
Ø213Ø83 Bypass Coronary Artery, Four or More Arteries from Coronary Artery with Zooplastic Tissue, Open Approach
Ø213Ø88 Bypass Coronary Artery, Four or More Arteries from Right Internal Mammary with Zooplastic Tissue, Open Approach
Ø213Ø89 Bypass Coronary Artery, Four or More Arteries from Left Internal Mammary with Zooplastic Tissue, Open Approach
Ø213Ø8C Bypass Coronary Artery, Four or More Arteries from Thoracic Artery with Zooplastic Tissue, Open Approach
Ø213Ø8F Bypass Coronary Artery, Four or More Arteries from Abdominal Artery with Zooplastic Tissue, Open Approach
Ø213Ø8W Bypass Coronary Artery, Four or More Arteries from Aorta with Zooplastic Tissue, Open Approach
Ø213Ø93 Bypass Coronary Artery, Four or More Arteries from Coronary Artery with Autologous Venous Tissue, Open Approach
Ø213Ø98 Bypass Coronary Artery, Four or More Arteries from Right Internal Mammary with Autologous Venous Tissue, Open Approach
Ø213Ø99 Bypass Coronary Artery, Four or More Arteries from Left Internal Mammary with Autologous Venous Tissue, Open Approach
Ø213Ø9C Bypass Coronary Artery, Four or More Arteries from Thoracic Artery with Autologous Venous Tissue, Open Approach
Ø213Ø9F Bypass Coronary Artery, Four or More Arteries from Abdominal Artery with Autologous Venous Tissue, Open Approach
Ø213Ø9W Bypass Coronary Artery, Four or More Arteries from Aorta with Autologous Venous Tissue, Open Approach
Ø213ØA3 Bypass Coronary Artery, Four or More Arteries from Coronary Artery with Autologous Arterial Tissue, Open Approach
Ø213ØA8 Bypass Coronary Artery, Four or More Arteries from Right Internal Mammary with Autologous Arterial Tissue, Open Approach
Ø213ØA9 Bypass Coronary Artery, Four or More Arteries from Left Internal Mammary with Autologous Arterial Tissue, Open Approach
Ø213ØAC Bypass Coronary Artery, Four or More Arteries from Thoracic Artery with Autologous Arterial Tissue, Open Approach
Ø213ØAF Bypass Coronary Artery, Four or More Arteries from Abdominal Artery with Autologous Arterial Tissue, Open Approach
Ø213ØAW Bypass Coronary Artery, Four or More Arteries from Aorta with Autologous Arterial Tissue, Open Approach
Ø213ØJ3 Bypass Coronary Artery, Four or More Arteries from Coronary Artery with Synthetic Substitute, Open Approach
Ø213ØJ8 Bypass Coronary Artery, Four or More Arteries from Right Internal Mammary with Synthetic Substitute, Open Approach
Ø213ØJ9 Bypass Coronary Artery, Four or More Arteries from Left Internal Mammary with Synthetic Substitute, Open Approach
Ø213ØJC Bypass Coronary Artery, Four or More Arteries from Thoracic Artery with Synthetic Substitute, Open Approach
Ø213ØJF Bypass Coronary Artery, Four or More Arteries from Abdominal Artery with Synthetic Substitute, Open Approach
Ø213ØJW Bypass Coronary Artery, Four or More Arteries from Aorta with Synthetic Substitute, Open Approach
Ø213ØK3 Bypass Coronary Artery, Four or More Arteries from Coronary Artery with Nonautologous Tissue Substitute, Open Approach
Ø213ØK8 Bypass Coronary Artery, Four or More Arteries from Right Internal Mammary with Nonautologous Tissue Substitute, Open Approach
Ø213ØK9 Bypass Coronary Artery, Four or More Arteries from Left Internal Mammary with Nonautologous Tissue Substitute, Open Approach
Ø213ØKC Bypass Coronary Artery, Four or More Arteries from Thoracic Artery with Nonautologous Tissue Substitute, Open Approach
Ø213ØKF Bypass Coronary Artery, Four or More Arteries from Abdominal Artery with Nonautologous Tissue Substitute, Open Approach
Ø213ØKW Bypass Coronary Artery, Four or More Arteries from Aorta with Nonautologous Tissue Substitute, Open Approach
Ø213ØZ3 Bypass Coronary Artery, Four or More Arteries from Coronary Artery, Open Approach
Ø213ØZ8 Bypass Coronary Artery, Four or More Arteries from Right Internal Mammary, Open Approach
Ø213ØZ9 Bypass Coronary Artery, Four or More Arteries from Left Internal Mammary, Open Approach
Ø213ØZC Bypass Coronary Artery, Four or More Arteries from Thoracic Artery, Open Approach
Ø213ØZF Bypass Coronary Artery, Four or More Arteries from Abdominal Artery, Open Approach
Ø213483 Bypass Coronary Artery, Four or More Arteries from Coronary Artery with Zooplastic Tissue, Percutaneous Endoscopic Approach
Ø213488 Bypass Coronary Artery, Four or More Arteries from Right Internal Mammary with Zooplastic Tissue, Percutaneous Endoscopic Approach
Ø213489 Bypass Coronary Artery, Four or More Arteries from Left Internal Mammary with Zooplastic Tissue, Percutaneous Endoscopic Approach
Ø21348C Bypass Coronary Artery, Four or More Arteries from Thoracic Artery with Zooplastic Tissue, Percutaneous Endoscopic Approach
Ø21348F Bypass Coronary Artery, Four or More Arteries from Abdominal Artery with Zooplastic Tissue, Percutaneous Endoscopic Approach
Ø21348W Bypass Coronary Artery, Four or More Arteries from Aorta with Zooplastic Tissue, Percutaneous Endoscopic Approach
Ø213493 Bypass Coronary Artery, Four or More Arteries from Coronary Artery with Autologous Venous Tissue, Percutaneous Endoscopic Approach

HAC 08: Surgical Site Infection of Mediastinitis After Coronary Bypass Graft (CABG) Procedures (continued)

Ø213498 Bypass Coronary Artery, Four or More Arteries from Right Internal Mammary with Autologous Venous Tissue, Percutaneous Endoscopic Approach
Ø213499 Bypass Coronary Artery, Four or More Arteries from Left Internal Mammary with Autologous Venous Tissue, Percutaneous Endoscopic Approach
Ø21349C Bypass Coronary Artery, Four or More Arteries from Thoracic Artery with Autologous Venous Tissue, Percutaneous Endoscopic Approach
Ø21349F Bypass Coronary Artery, Four or More Arteries from Abdominal Artery with Autologous Venous Tissue, Percutaneous Endoscopic Approach
Ø21349W Bypass Coronary Artery, Four or More Arteries from Aorta with Autologous Venous Tissue, Percutaneous Endoscopic Approach
Ø2134A3 Bypass Coronary Artery, Four or More Arteries from Coronary Artery with Autologous Arterial Tissue, Percutaneous Endoscopic Approach
Ø2134A8 Bypass Coronary Artery, Four or More Arteries from Right Internal Mammary with Autologous Arterial Tissue, Percutaneous Endoscopic Approach
Ø2134A9 Bypass Coronary Artery, Four or More Arteries from Left Internal Mammary with Autologous Arterial Tissue, Percutaneous Endoscopic Approach
Ø2134AC Bypass Coronary Artery, Four or More Arteries from Thoracic Artery with Autologous Arterial Tissue, Percutaneous Endoscopic Approach
Ø2134AF Bypass Coronary Artery, Four or More Arteries from Abdominal Artery with Autologous Arterial Tissue, Percutaneous Endoscopic Approach
Ø2134AW Bypass Coronary Artery, Four or More Arteries from Aorta with Autologous Arterial Tissue, Percutaneous Endoscopic Approach
Ø2134J3 Bypass Coronary Artery, Four or More Arteries from Coronary Artery with Synthetic Substitute, Percutaneous Endoscopic Approach
Ø2134J8 Bypass Coronary Artery, Four or More Arteries from Right Internal Mammary with Synthetic Substitute, Percutaneous Endoscopic Approach
Ø2134J9 Bypass Coronary Artery, Four or More Arteries from Left Internal Mammary with Synthetic Substitute, Percutaneous Endoscopic Approach
Ø2134JC Bypass Coronary Artery, Four or More Arteries from Thoracic Artery with Synthetic Substitute, Percutaneous Endoscopic Approach
Ø2134JF Bypass Coronary Artery, Four or More Arteries from Abdominal Artery with Synthetic Substitute, Percutaneous Endoscopic Approach
Ø2134JW Bypass Coronary Artery, Four or More Arteries from Aorta with Synthetic Substitute, Percutaneous Endoscopic Approach
Ø2134K3 Bypass Coronary Artery, Four or More Arteries from Coronary Artery with Nonautologous Tissue Substitute, Percutaneous Endoscopic Approach
Ø2134K8 Bypass Coronary Artery, Four or More Arteries from Right Internal Mammary with Nonautologous Tissue Substitute, Percutaneous Endoscopic Approach
Ø2134K9 Bypass Coronary Artery, Four or More Arteries from Left Internal Mammary with Nonautologous Tissue Substitute, Percutaneous Endoscopic Approach
Ø2134KC Bypass Coronary Artery, Four or More Arteries from Thoracic Artery with Nonautologous Tissue Substitute, Percutaneous Endoscopic Approach
Ø2134KF Bypass Coronary Artery, Four or More Arteries from Abdominal Artery with Nonautologous Tissue Substitute, Percutaneous Endoscopic Approach
Ø2134KW Bypass Coronary Artery, Four or More Arteries from Aorta with Nonautologous Tissue Substitute, Percutaneous Endoscopic Approach
Ø2134Z3 Bypass Coronary Artery, Four or More Arteries from Coronary Artery, Percutaneous Endoscopic Approach
Ø2134Z8 Bypass Coronary Artery, Four or More Arteries from Right Internal Mammary, Percutaneous Endoscopic Approach
Ø2134Z9 Bypass Coronary Artery, Four or More Arteries from Left Internal Mammary, Percutaneous Endoscopic Approach
Ø2134ZC Bypass Coronary Artery, Four or More Arteries from Thoracic Artery, Percutaneous Endoscopic Approach
Ø2134ZF Bypass Coronary Artery, Four or More Arteries from Abdominal Artery, Percutaneous Endoscopic Approach

HAC 10: Deep Vein Thrombosis (DVT) or Pulmonary Embolism (PE) with Total Knee or Hip Replacement

Secondary diagnosis not POA:

I26.Ø2 Saddle embolus of pulmonary artery with acute cor pulmonale
I26.Ø9 Other pulmonary embolism with acute cor pulmonale
I26.92 Saddle embolus of pulmonary artery without acute cor pulmonale
I26.93 Single subsegmental pulmonary embolism without acute cor pulmonale
I26.94 Multiple subsegmental pulmonary emboli without acute cor pulmonale
I26.99 Other pulmonary embolism without acute cor pulmonale
I82.4Ø1 Acute embolism and thrombosis of unspecified deep veins of right lower extremity
I82.4Ø2 Acute embolism and thrombosis of unspecified deep veins of left lower extremity
I82.4Ø3 Acute embolism and thrombosis of unspecified deep veins of lower extremity, bilateral
I82.4Ø9 Acute embolism and thrombosis of unspecified deep veins of unspecified lower extremity
I82.411 Acute embolism and thrombosis of right femoral vein
I82.412 Acute embolism and thrombosis of left femoral vein
I82.413 Acute embolism and thrombosis of femoral vein, bilateral
I82.419 Acute embolism and thrombosis of unspecified femoral vein
I82.421 Acute embolism and thrombosis of right iliac vein
I82.422 Acute embolism and thrombosis of left iliac vein
I82.423 Acute embolism and thrombosis of iliac vein, bilateral
I82.429 Acute embolism and thrombosis of unspecified iliac vein
I82.431 Acute embolism and thrombosis of right popliteal vein
I82.432 Acute embolism and thrombosis of left popliteal vein
I82.433 Acute embolism and thrombosis of popliteal vein, bilateral
I82.439 Acute embolism and thrombosis of unspecified popliteal vein
I82.441 Acute embolism and thrombosis of right tibial vein
I82.442 Acute embolism and thrombosis of left tibial vein
I82.443 Acute embolism and thrombosis of tibial vein, bilateral
I82.449 Acute embolism and thrombosis of unspecified tibial vein
I82.451 Acute embolism and thrombosis of right peroneal vein
I82.452 Acute embolism and thrombosis of left peroneal vein
I82.453 Acute embolism and thrombosis of peroneal vein, bilateral
I82.459 Acute embolism and thrombosis of unspecified peroneal vein
I82.491 Acute embolism and thrombosis of other specified deep vein of right lower extremity
I82.492 Acute embolism and thrombosis of other specified deep vein of left lower extremity
I82.493 Acute embolism and thrombosis of other specified deep vein of lower extremity, bilateral
I82.499 Acute embolism and thrombosis of other specified deep vein of unspecified lower extremity
I82.4Y1 Acute embolism and thrombosis of unspecified deep veins of right proximal lower extremity
I82.4Y2 Acute embolism and thrombosis of unspecified deep veins of left proximal lower extremity
I82.4Y3 Acute embolism and thrombosis of unspecified deep veins of proximal lower extremity, bilateral
I82.4Y9 Acute embolism and thrombosis of unspecified deep veins of unspecified proximal lower extremity
I82.4Z1 Acute embolism and thrombosis of unspecified deep veins of right distal lower extremity
I82.4Z2 Acute embolism and thrombosis of unspecified deep veins of left distal lower extremity
I82.4Z3 Acute embolism and thrombosis of unspecified deep veins of distal lower extremity, bilateral
I82.4Z9 Acute embolism and thrombosis of unspecified deep veins of unspecified distal lower extremity

AND

Any of the following procedures:

ØSR9Ø19 Replacement of Right Hip Joint with Metal Synthetic Substitute, Cemented, Open Approach
ØSR9Ø1A Replacement of Right Hip Joint with Metal Synthetic Substitute, Uncemented, Open Approach
ØSR9Ø1Z Replacement of Right Hip Joint with Metal Synthetic Substitute, Open Approach
ØSR9Ø29 Replacement of Right Hip Joint with Metal on Polyethylene Synthetic Substitute, Cemented, Open Approach

HAC 10: Deep Vein Thrombosis (DVT) or Pulmonary Embolism (PE) with Total Knee or Hip Replacement (continued)

ØSR902A Replacement of Right Hip Joint with Metal on Polyethylene Synthetic Substitute, Uncemented, Open Approach
ØSR902Z Replacement of Right Hip Joint with Metal on Polyethylene Synthetic Substitute, Open Approach
ØSR9039 Replacement of Right Hip Joint with Ceramic Synthetic Substitute, Cemented, Open Approach
ØSR903A Replacement of Right Hip Joint with Ceramic Synthetic Substitute, Uncemented, Open Approach
ØSR903Z Replacement of Right Hip Joint with Ceramic Synthetic Substitute, Open Approach
ØSR9049 Replacement of Right Hip Joint with Ceramic on Polyethylene Synthetic Substitute, Cemented, Open Approach
ØSR904A Replacement of Right Hip Joint with Ceramic on Polyethylene Synthetic Substitute, Uncemented, Open Approach
ØSR904Z Replacement of Right Hip Joint with Ceramic on Polyethylene Synthetic Substitute, Open Approach
ØSR9069 Replacement of Right Hip Joint with Oxidized Zirconium on Polyethylene Synthetic Substitute, Cemented, Open Approach
ØSR906A Replacement of Right Hip Joint with Oxidized Zirconium on Polyethylene Synthetic Substitute, Uncemented, Open Approach
ØSR906Z Replacement of Right Hip Joint with Oxidized Zirconium on Polyethylene Synthetic Substitute, Open Approach
ØSR907Z Replacement of Right Hip Joint with Autologous Tissue Substitute, Open Approach
ØSR90EZ Replacement of Right Hip Joint with Articulating Spacer, Open Approach
ØSR90J9 Replacement of Right Hip Joint with Synthetic Substitute, Cemented, Open Approach
ØSR90JA Replacement of Right Hip Joint with Synthetic Substitute, Uncemented, Open Approach
ØSR90JZ Replacement of Right Hip Joint with Synthetic Substitute, Open Approach
ØSR90KZ Replacement of Right Hip Joint with Nonautologous Tissue Substitute, Open Approach
ØSRA009 Replacement of Right Hip Joint, Acetabular Surface with Polyethylene Synthetic Substitute, Cemented, Open Approach
ØSRA00A Replacement of Right Hip Joint, Acetabular Surface with Polyethylene Synthetic Substitute, Uncemented, Open Approach
ØSRA00Z Replacement of Right Hip Joint, Acetabular Surface with Polyethylene Synthetic Substitute, Open Approach
ØSRA019 Replacement of Right Hip Joint, Acetabular Surface with Metal Synthetic Substitute, Cemented, Open Approach
ØSRA01A Replacement of Right Hip Joint, Acetabular Surface with Metal Synthetic Substitute, Uncemented, Open Approach
ØSRA01Z Replacement of Right Hip Joint, Acetabular Surface with Metal Synthetic Substitute, Open Approach
ØSRA039 Replacement of Right Hip Joint, Acetabular Surface with Ceramic Synthetic Substitute, Cemented, Open Approach
ØSRA03A Replacement of Right Hip Joint, Acetabular Surface with Ceramic Synthetic Substitute, Uncemented, Open Approach
ØSRA03Z Replacement of Right Hip Joint, Acetabular Surface with Ceramic Synthetic Substitute, Open Approach
ØSRA07Z Replacement of Right Hip Joint, Acetabular Surface with Autologous Tissue Substitute, Open Approach
ØSRA0J9 Replacement of Right Hip Joint, Acetabular Surface with Synthetic Substitute, Cemented, Open Approach
ØSRA0JA Replacement of Right Hip Joint, Acetabular Surface with Synthetic Substitute, Uncemented, Open Approach
ØSRA0JZ Replacement of Right Hip Joint, Acetabular Surface with Synthetic Substitute, Open Approach
ØSRA0KZ Replacement of Right Hip Joint, Acetabular Surface with Nonautologous Tissue Substitute, Open Approach
ØSRB019 Replacement of Left Hip Joint with Metal Synthetic Substitute, Cemented, Open Approach
ØSRB01A Replacement of Left Hip Joint with Metal Synthetic Substitute, Uncemented, Open Approach
ØSRB01Z Replacement of Left Hip Joint with Metal Synthetic Substitute, Open Approach
ØSRB029 Replacement of Left Hip Joint with Metal on Polyethylene Synthetic Substitute, Cemented, Open Approach
ØSRB02A Replacement of Left Hip Joint with Metal on Polyethylene Synthetic Substitute, Uncemented, Open Approach
ØSRB02Z Replacement of Left Hip Joint with Metal on Polyethylene Synthetic Substitute, Open Approach
ØSRB039 Replacement of Left Hip Joint with Ceramic Synthetic Substitute, Cemented, Open Approach
ØSRB03A Replacement of Left Hip Joint with Ceramic Synthetic Substitute, Uncemented, Open Approach
ØSRB03Z Replacement of Left Hip Joint with Ceramic Synthetic Substitute, Open Approach
ØSRB049 Replacement of Left Hip Joint with Ceramic on Polyethylene Synthetic Substitute, Cemented, Open Approach
ØSRB04A Replacement of Left Hip Joint with Ceramic on Polyethylene Synthetic Substitute, Uncemented, Open Approach
ØSRB04Z Replacement of Left Hip Joint with Ceramic on Polyethylene Synthetic Substitute, Open Approach
ØSRB069 Replacement of Left Hip Joint with Oxidized Zirconium on Polyethylene Synthetic Substitute, Cemented, Open Approach
ØSRB06A Replacement of Left Hip Joint with Oxidized Zirconium on Polyethylene Synthetic Substitute, Uncemented, Open Approach
ØSRB06Z Replacement of Left Hip Joint with Oxidized Zirconium on Polyethylene Synthetic Substitute, Open Approach
ØSRB07Z Replacement of Left Hip Joint with Autologous Tissue Substitute, Open Approach
ØSRB0EZ Replacement of Left Hip Joint with Articulating Spacer, Open Approach
ØSRB0J9 Replacement of Left Hip Joint with Synthetic Substitute, Cemented, Open Approach
ØSRB0JA Replacement of Left Hip Joint with Synthetic Substitute, Uncemented, Open Approach
ØSRB0JZ Replacement of Left Hip Joint with Synthetic Substitute, Open Approach
ØSRB0KZ Replacement of Left Hip Joint with Nonautologous Tissue Substitute, Open Approach
ØSRC069 Replacement of Right Knee Joint with Oxidized Zirconium on Polyethylene Synthetic Substitute, Cemented, Open Approach
ØSRC06A Replacement of Right Knee Joint with Oxidized Zirconium on Polyethylene Synthetic Substitute, Uncemented, Open Approach
ØSRC06Z Replacement of Right Knee Joint with Oxidized Zirconium on Polyethylene Synthetic Substitute, Open Approach
ØSRC07Z Replacement of Right Knee Joint with Autologous Tissue Substitute, Open Approach
ØSRC0EZ Replacement of Right Knee Joint with Articulating Spacer, Open Approach
ØSRC0J9 Replacement of Right Knee Joint with Synthetic Substitute, Cemented, Open Approach
ØSRC0JA Replacement of Right Knee Joint with Synthetic Substitute, Uncemented, Open Approach
ØSRC0JZ Replacement of Right Knee Joint with Synthetic Substitute, Open Approach
ØSRC0KZ Replacement of Right Knee Joint with Nonautologous Tissue Substitute, Open Approach
ØSRC0L9 Replacement of Right Knee Joint with Medial Unicondylar Synthetic Substitute, Cemented, Open Approach
ØSRC0LA Replacement of Right Knee Joint with Medial Unicondylar Synthetic Substitute, Uncemented, Open Approach
ØSRC0LZ Replacement of Right Knee Joint with Medial Unicondylar Synthetic Substitute, Open Approach
ØSRC0M9 Replacement of Right Knee Joint with Lateral Unicondylar Synthetic Substitute, Cemented, Open Approach
ØSRC0MA Replacement of Right Knee Joint with Lateral Unicondylar Synthetic Substitute, Uncemented, Open Approach
ØSRC0MZ Replacement of Right Knee Joint with Lateral Unicondylar Synthetic Substitute, Open Approach
ØSRC0N9 Replacement of Right Knee Joint with Patellofemoral Synthetic Substitute, Cemented, Open Approach
ØSRC0NA Replacement of Right Knee Joint with Patellofemoral Synthetic Substitute, Uncemented, Open Approach
ØSRC0NZ Replacement of Right Knee Joint with Patellofemoral Synthetic Substitute, Open Approach
ØSRD069 Replacement of Left Knee Joint with Oxidized Zirconium on Polyethylene Synthetic Substitute, Cemented, Open Approach
ØSRD06A Replacement of Left Knee Joint with Oxidized Zirconium on Polyethylene Synthetic Substitute, Uncemented, Open Approach
ØSRD06Z Replacement of Left Knee Joint with Oxidized Zirconium on Polyethylene Synthetic Substitute, Open Approach
ØSRD07Z Replacement of Left Knee Joint with Autologous Tissue Substitute, Open Approach

HAC 10: Deep Vein Thrombosis (DVT) or Pulmonary Embolism (PE) with Total Knee or Hip Replacement (continued)

ØSRDØEZ Replacement of Left Knee Joint with Articulating Spacer, Open Approach
ØSRDØJ9 Replacement of Left Knee Joint with Synthetic Substitute, Cemented, Open Approach
ØSRDØJA Replacement of Left Knee Joint with Synthetic Substitute, Uncemented, Open Approach
ØSRDØJZ Replacement of Left Knee Joint with Synthetic Substitute, Open Approach
ØSRDØKZ Replacement of Left Knee Joint with Nonautologous Tissue Substitute, Open Approach
ØSRDØL9 Replacement of Left Knee Joint with Medial Unicondylar Synthetic Substitute, Cemented, Open Approach
ØSRDØLA Replacement of Left Knee Joint with Medial Unicondylar Synthetic Substitute, Uncemented, Open Approach
ØSRDØLZ Replacement of Left Knee Joint with Medial Unicondylar Synthetic Substitute, Open Approach
ØSRDØM9 Replacement of Left Knee Joint with Lateral Unicondylar Synthetic Substitute, Cemented, Open Approach
ØSRDØMA Replacement of Left Knee Joint with Lateral Unicondylar Synthetic Substitute, Uncemented, Open Approach
ØSRDØMZ Replacement of Left Knee Joint with Lateral Unicondylar Synthetic Substitute, Open Approach
ØSRDØN9 Replacement of Left Knee Joint with Patellofemoral Synthetic Substitute, Cemented, Open Approach
ØSRDØNA Replacement of Left Knee Joint with Patellofemoral Synthetic Substitute, Uncemented, Open Approach
ØSRDØNZ Replacement of Left Knee Joint with Patellofemoral Synthetic Substitute, Open Approach
ØSREØØ9 Replacement of Left Hip Joint, Acetabular Surface with Polyethylene Synthetic Substitute, Cemented, Open Approach
ØSREØØA Replacement of Left Hip Joint, Acetabular Surface with Polyethylene Synthetic Substitute, Uncemented, Open Approach
ØSREØØZ Replacement of Left Hip Joint, Acetabular Surface with Polyethylene Synthetic Substitute, Open Approach
ØSREØ19 Replacement of Left Hip Joint, Acetabular Surface with Metal Synthetic Substitute, Cemented, Open Approach
ØSREØ1A Replacement of Left Hip Joint, Acetabular Surface with Metal Synthetic Substitute, Uncemented, Open Approach
ØSREØ1Z Replacement of Left Hip Joint, Acetabular Surface with Metal Synthetic Substitute, Open Approach
ØSREØ39 Replacement of Left Hip Joint, Acetabular Surface with Ceramic Synthetic Substitute, Cemented, Open Approach
ØSREØ3A Replacement of Left Hip Joint, Acetabular Surface with Ceramic Synthetic Substitute, Uncemented, Open Approach
ØSREØ3Z Replacement of Left Hip Joint, Acetabular Surface with Ceramic Synthetic Substitute, Open Approach
ØSREØ7Z Replacement of Left Hip Joint, Acetabular Surface with Autologous Tissue Substitute, Open Approach
ØSREØJ9 Replacement of Left Hip Joint, Acetabular Surface with Synthetic Substitute, Cemented, Open Approach
ØSREØJA Replacement of Left Hip Joint, Acetabular Surface with Synthetic Substitute, Uncemented, Open Approach
ØSREØJZ Replacement of Left Hip Joint, Acetabular Surface with Synthetic Substitute, Open Approach
ØSREØKZ Replacement of Left Hip Joint, Acetabular Surface with Nonautologous Tissue Substitute, Open Approach
ØSRRØ19 Replacement of Right Hip Joint, Femoral Surface with Metal Synthetic Substitute, Cemented, Open Approach
ØSRRØ1A Replacement of Right Hip Joint, Femoral Surface with Metal Synthetic Substitute, Uncemented, Open Approach
ØSRRØ1Z Replacement of Right Hip Joint, Femoral Surface with Metal Synthetic Substitute, Open Approach
ØSRRØ39 Replacement of Right Hip Joint, Femoral Surface with Ceramic Synthetic Substitute, Cemented, Open Approach
ØSRRØ3A Replacement of Right Hip Joint, Femoral Surface with Ceramic Synthetic Substitute, Uncemented, Open Approach
ØSRRØ3Z Replacement of Right Hip Joint, Femoral Surface with Ceramic Synthetic Substitute, Open Approach
ØSRRØ7Z Replacement of Right Hip Joint, Femoral Surface with Autologous Tissue Substitute, Open Approach
ØSRRØJ9 Replacement of Right Hip Joint, Femoral Surface with Synthetic Substitute, Cemented, Open Approach
ØSRRØJA Replacement of Right Hip Joint, Femoral Surface with Synthetic Substitute, Uncemented, Open Approach
ØSRRØJZ Replacement of Right Hip Joint, Femoral Surface with Synthetic Substitute, Open Approach
ØSRRØKZ Replacement of Right Hip Joint, Femoral Surface with Nonautologous Tissue Substitute, Open Approach
ØSRSØ19 Replacement of Left Hip Joint, Femoral Surface with Metal Synthetic Substitute, Cemented, Open Approach
ØSRSØ1A Replacement of Left Hip Joint, Femoral Surface with Metal Synthetic Substitute, Uncemented, Open Approach
ØSRSØ1Z Replacement of Left Hip Joint, Femoral Surface with Metal Synthetic Substitute, Open Approach
ØSRSØ39 Replacement of Left Hip Joint, Femoral Surface with Ceramic Synthetic Substitute, Cemented, Open Approach
ØSRSØ3A Replacement of Left Hip Joint, Femoral Surface with Ceramic Synthetic Substitute, Uncemented, Open Approach
ØSRSØ3Z Replacement of Left Hip Joint, Femoral Surface with Ceramic Synthetic Substitute, Open Approach
ØSRSØ7Z Replacement of Left Hip Joint, Femoral Surface with Autologous Tissue Substitute, Open Approach
ØSRSØJ9 Replacement of Left Hip Joint, Femoral Surface with Synthetic Substitute, Cemented, Open Approach
ØSRSØJA Replacement of Left Hip Joint, Femoral Surface with Synthetic Substitute, Uncemented, Open Approach
ØSRSØJZ Replacement of Left Hip Joint, Femoral Surface with Synthetic Substitute, Open Approach
ØSRSØKZ Replacement of Left Hip Joint, Femoral Surface with Nonautologous Tissue Substitute, Open Approach
ØSRTØ7Z Replacement of Right Knee Joint, Femoral Surface with Autologous Tissue Substitute, Open Approach
ØSRTØJ9 Replacement of Right Knee Joint, Femoral Surface with Synthetic Substitute, Cemented, Open Approach
ØSRTØJA Replacement of Right Knee Joint, Femoral Surface with Synthetic Substitute, Uncemented, Open Approach
ØSRTØJZ Replacement of Right Knee Joint, Femoral Surface with Synthetic Substitute, Open Approach
ØSRTØKZ Replacement of Right Knee Joint, Femoral Surface with Nonautologous Tissue Substitute, Open Approach
ØSRUØ7Z Replacement of Left Knee Joint, Femoral Surface with Autologous Tissue Substitute, Open Approach
ØSRUØJ9 Replacement of Left Knee Joint, Femoral Surface with Synthetic Substitute, Cemented, Open Approach
ØSRUØJA Replacement of Left Knee Joint, Femoral Surface with Synthetic Substitute, Uncemented, Open Approach
ØSRUØJZ Replacement of Left Knee Joint, Femoral Surface with Synthetic Substitute, Open Approach
ØSRUØKZ Replacement of Left Knee Joint, Femoral Surface with Nonautologous Tissue Substitute, Open Approach
ØSRVØ7Z Replacement of Right Knee Joint, Tibial Surface with Autologous Tissue Substitute, Open Approach
ØSRVØJ9 Replacement of Right Knee Joint, Tibial Surface with Synthetic Substitute, Cemented, Open Approach
ØSRVØJA Replacement of Right Knee Joint, Tibial Surface with Synthetic Substitute, Uncemented, Open Approach
ØSRVØJZ Replacement of Right Knee Joint, Tibial Surface with Synthetic Substitute, Open Approach
ØSRVØKZ Replacement of Right Knee Joint, Tibial Surface with Nonautologous Tissue Substitute, Open Approach
ØSRWØ7Z Replacement of Left Knee Joint, Tibial Surface with Autologous Tissue Substitute, Open Approach
ØSRWØJ9 Replacement of Left Knee Joint, Tibial Surface with Synthetic Substitute, Cemented, Open Approach
ØSRWØJA Replacement of Left Knee Joint, Tibial Surface with Synthetic Substitute, Uncemented, Open Approach
ØSRWØJZ Replacement of Left Knee Joint, Tibial Surface with Synthetic Substitute, Open Approach
ØSRWØKZ Replacement of Left Knee Joint, Tibial Surface with Nonautologous Tissue Substitute, Open Approach
ØSU9ØBZ Supplement Right Hip Joint with Resurfacing Device, Open Approach
ØSUAØBZ Supplement Right Hip Joint, Acetabular Surface with Resurfacing Device, Open Approach
ØSUBØBZ Supplement Left Hip Joint with Resurfacing Device, Open Approach
ØSUEØBZ Supplement Left Hip Joint, Acetabular Surface with Resurfacing Device, Open Approach
ØSURØBZ Supplement Right Hip Joint, Femoral Surface with Resurfacing Device, Open Approach
ØSUSØBZ Supplement Left Hip Joint, Femoral Surface with Resurfacing Device, Open Approach

HAC 10: Deep Vein Thrombosis (DVT) or Pulmonary Embolism (PE) with Total Knee or Hip Replacement (continued)

XRRGØL8 Replacement of Right Knee Joint with Synthetic Substitute, Lateral Meniscus, Open Approach, New Technology Group 8
XRRGØM8 Replacement of Right Knee Joint with Synthetic Substitute, Medial Meniscus, Open Approach, New Technology Group 8
XRRHØL8 Replacement of Left Knee Joint with Synthetic Substitute, Lateral Meniscus, Open Approach, New Technology Group 8
XRRHØM8 Replacement of Left Knee Joint with Synthetic Substitute, Medial Meniscus, Open Approach, New Technology Group 8

HAC 11: Surgical Site Infection-Bariatric Surgery

Principal diagnosis of:
E66.Ø1 Morbid (severe) obesity due to excess calories

AND

Secondary diagnosis not POA:
K68.11 Postprocedural retroperitoneal abscess
K95.Ø1 Infection due to gastric band procedure
K95.81 Infection due to other bariatric procedure
T81.4ØXA Infection following a procedure, unspecified, initial encounter
T81.41XA Infection following a procedure, superficial incisional surgical site, initial encounter
T81.42XA Infection following a procedure, deep incisional surgical site, initial encounter
T81.43XA Infection following a procedure, organ and space surgical site, initial encounter
T81.44XA Sepsis following a procedure, initial encounter
T81.49XA Infection following a procedure, other surgical site, initial encounter

AND

Any of the following procedures:
ØD16Ø79 Bypass Stomach to Duodenum with Autologous Tissue Substitute, Open Approach
ØD16Ø7A Bypass Stomach to Jejunum with Autologous Tissue Substitute, Open Approach
ØD16Ø7B Bypass Stomach to Ileum with Autologous Tissue Substitute, Open Approach
ØD16Ø7L Bypass Stomach to Transverse Colon with Autologous Tissue Substitute, Open Approach
ØD16ØJ9 Bypass Stomach to Duodenum with Synthetic Substitute, Open Approach
ØD16ØJA Bypass Stomach to Jejunum with Synthetic Substitute, Open Approach
ØD16ØJB Bypass Stomach to Ileum with Synthetic Substitute, Open Approach
ØD16ØJL Bypass Stomach to Transverse Colon with Synthetic Substitute, Open Approach
ØD16ØK9 Bypass Stomach to Duodenum with Nonautologous Tissue Substitute, Open Approach
ØD16ØKA Bypass Stomach to Jejunum with Nonautologous Tissue Substitute, Open Approach
ØD16ØKB Bypass Stomach to Ileum with Nonautologous Tissue Substitute, Open Approach
ØD16ØKL Bypass Stomach to Transverse Colon with Nonautologous Tissue Substitute, Open Approach
ØD16ØZ9 Bypass Stomach to Duodenum, Open Approach
ØD16ØZA Bypass Stomach to Jejunum, Open Approach
ØD16ØZB Bypass Stomach to Ileum, Open Approach
ØD16ØZL Bypass Stomach to Transverse Colon, Open Approach
ØD16479 Bypass Stomach to Duodenum with Autologous Tissue Substitute, Percutaneous Endoscopic Approach
ØD1647A Bypass Stomach to Jejunum with Autologous Tissue Substitute, Percutaneous Endoscopic Approach
ØD1647B Bypass Stomach to Ileum with Autologous Tissue Substitute, Percutaneous Endoscopic Approach
ØD1647L Bypass Stomach to Transverse Colon with Autologous Tissue Substitute, Percutaneous Endoscopic Approach
ØD164J9 Bypass Stomach to Duodenum with Synthetic Substitute, Percutaneous Endoscopic Approach
ØD164JA Bypass Stomach to Jejunum with Synthetic Substitute, Percutaneous Endoscopic Approach
ØD164JB Bypass Stomach to Ileum with Synthetic Substitute, Percutaneous Endoscopic Approach
ØD164JL Bypass Stomach to Transverse Colon with Synthetic Substitute, Percutaneous Endoscopic Approach
ØD164K9 Bypass Stomach to Duodenum with Nonautologous Tissue Substitute, Percutaneous Endoscopic Approach
ØD164KA Bypass Stomach to Jejunum with Nonautologous Tissue Substitute, Percutaneous Endoscopic Approach
ØD164KB Bypass Stomach to Ileum with Nonautologous Tissue Substitute, Percutaneous Endoscopic Approach
ØD164KL Bypass Stomach to Transverse Colon with Nonautologous Tissue Substitute, Percutaneous Endoscopic Approach
ØD164Z9 Bypass Stomach to Duodenum, Percutaneous Endoscopic Approach
ØD164ZA Bypass Stomach to Jejunum, Percutaneous Endoscopic Approach
ØD164ZB Bypass Stomach to Ileum, Percutaneous Endoscopic Approach
ØD164ZL Bypass Stomach to Transverse Colon, Percutaneous Endoscopic Approach
ØD16879 Bypass Stomach to Duodenum with Autologous Tissue Substitute, Via Natural or Artificial Opening Endoscopic
ØD1687A Bypass Stomach to Jejunum with Autologous Tissue Substitute, Via Natural or Artificial Opening Endoscopic
ØD1687B Bypass Stomach to Ileum with Autologous Tissue Substitute, Via Natural or Artificial Opening Endoscopic
ØD1687L Bypass Stomach to Transverse Colon with Autologous Tissue Substitute, Via Natural or Artificial Opening Endoscopic
ØD168J9 Bypass Stomach to Duodenum with Synthetic Substitute, Via Natural or Artificial Opening Endoscopic
ØD168JA Bypass Stomach to Jejunum with Synthetic Substitute, Via Natural or Artificial Opening Endoscopic
ØD168JB Bypass Stomach to Ileum with Synthetic Substitute, Via Natural or Artificial Opening Endoscopic
ØD168JL Bypass Stomach to Transverse Colon with Synthetic Substitute, Via Natural or Artificial Opening Endoscopic
ØD168K9 Bypass Stomach to Duodenum with Nonautologous Tissue Substitute, Via Natural or Artificial Opening Endoscopic
ØD168KA Bypass Stomach to Jejunum with Nonautologous Tissue Substitute, Via Natural or Artificial Opening Endoscopic
ØD168KB Bypass Stomach to Ileum with Nonautologous Tissue Substitute, Via Natural or Artificial Opening Endoscopic
ØD168KL Bypass Stomach to Transverse Colon with Nonautologous Tissue Substitute, Via Natural or Artificial Opening Endoscopic
ØD168Z9 Bypass Stomach to Duodenum, Via Natural or Artificial Opening Endoscopic
ØD168ZA Bypass Stomach to Jejunum, Via Natural or Artificial Opening Endoscopic
ØD168ZB Bypass Stomach to Ileum, Via Natural or Artificial Opening Endoscopic
ØD168ZL Bypass Stomach to Transverse Colon, Via Natural or Artificial Opening Endoscopic
ØDV64CZ Restriction of Stomach with Extraluminal Device, Percutaneous Endoscopic Approach

HAC 12: Surgical Site Infection-Certain Orthopedic Procedures of the Spine, Shoulder, and Elbow

Secondary diagnosis not POA:
K68.11 Postprocedural retroperitoneal abscess
T81.4ØXA Infection following a procedure, unspecified, initial encounter
T81.41XA Infection following a procedure, superficial incisional surgical site, initial encounter
T81.42XA Infection following a procedure, deep incisional surgical site, initial encounter
T81.43XA Infection following a procedure, organ and space surgical site, initial encounter
T81.44XA Sepsis following a procedure, initial encounter
T81.49XA Infection following a procedure, other surgical site, initial encounter
T84.6ØXA Infection and inflammatory reaction due to internal fixation device of unspecified site, initial encounter
T84.61ØA Infection and inflammatory reaction due to internal fixation device of right humerus, initial encounter
T84.611A Infection and inflammatory reaction due to internal fixation device of left humerus, initial encounter
T84.612A Infection and inflammatory reaction due to internal fixation device of right radius, initial encounter
T84.613A Infection and inflammatory reaction due to internal fixation device of left radius, initial encounter
T84.614A Infection and inflammatory reaction due to internal fixation device of right ulna, initial encounter
T84.615A Infection and inflammatory reaction due to internal fixation device of left ulna, initial encounter
T84.619A Infection and inflammatory reaction due to internal fixation device of unspecified bone of arm, initial encounter
T84.63XA Infection and inflammatory reaction due to internal fixation device of spine, initial encounter
T84.69XA Infection and inflammatory reaction due to internal fixation device of other site, initial encounter
T84.7XXA Infection and inflammatory reaction due to other internal orthopedic prosthetic devices, implants and grafts, initial encounter

AND

Any of the following procedures:
ØRGØØ7Ø Fusion of Occipital-cervical Joint with Autologous Tissue Substitute, Anterior Approach, Anterior Column, Open Approach

HAC 12: Surgical Site Infection-Certain Orthopedic Procedures of the Spine, Shoulder, and Elbow (continued)

ØRGØØ71 Fusion of Occipital-cervical Joint with Autologous Tissue Substitute, Posterior Approach, Posterior Column, Open Approach
ØRGØØ7J Fusion of Occipital-cervical Joint with Autologous Tissue Substitute, Posterior Approach, Anterior Column, Open Approach
ØRGØØAØ Fusion of Occipital-cervical Joint with Interbody Fusion Device, Anterior Approach, Anterior Column, Open Approach
ØRGØØAJ Fusion of Occipital-cervical Joint with Interbody Fusion Device, Posterior Approach, Anterior Column, Open Approach
ØRGØØJØ Fusion of Occipital-cervical Joint with Synthetic Substitute, Anterior Approach, Anterior Column, Open Approach
ØRGØØJ1 Fusion of Occipital-cervical Joint with Synthetic Substitute, Posterior Approach, Posterior Column, Open Approach
ØRGØØJJ Fusion of Occipital-cervical Joint with Synthetic Substitute, Posterior Approach, Anterior Column, Open Approach
ØRGØØKØ Fusion of Occipital-cervical Joint with Nonautologous Tissue Substitute, Anterior Approach, Anterior Column, Open Approach
ØRGØØK1 Fusion of Occipital-cervical Joint with Nonautologous Tissue Substitute, Posterior Approach, Posterior Column, Open Approach
ØRGØØKJ Fusion of Occipital-cervical Joint with Nonautologous Tissue Substitute, Posterior Approach, Anterior Column, Open Approach
ØRGØ37Ø Fusion of Occipital-cervical Joint with Autologous Tissue Substitute, Anterior Approach, Anterior Column, Percutaneous Approach
ØRGØ371 Fusion of Occipital-cervical Joint with Autologous Tissue Substitute, Posterior Approach, Posterior Column, Percutaneous Approach
ØRGØ37J Fusion of Occipital-cervical Joint with Autologous Tissue Substitute, Posterior Approach, Anterior Column, Percutaneous Approach
ØRGØ3AØ Fusion of Occipital-cervical Joint with Interbody Fusion Device, Anterior Approach, Anterior Column, Percutaneous Approach
ØRGØ3AJ Fusion of Occipital-cervical Joint with Interbody Fusion Device, Posterior Approach, Anterior Column, Percutaneous Approach
ØRGØ3JØ Fusion of Occipital-cervical Joint with Synthetic Substitute, Anterior Approach, Anterior Column, Percutaneous Approach
ØRGØ3J1 Fusion of Occipital-cervical Joint with Synthetic Substitute, Posterior Approach, Posterior Column, Percutaneous Approach
ØRGØ3JJ Fusion of Occipital-cervical Joint with Synthetic Substitute, Posterior Approach, Anterior Column, Percutaneous Approach
ØRGØ3KØ Fusion of Occipital-cervical Joint with Nonautologous Tissue Substitute, Anterior Approach, Anterior Column, Percutaneous Approach
ØRGØ3K1 Fusion of Occipital-cervical Joint with Nonautologous Tissue Substitute, Posterior Approach, Posterior Column, Percutaneous Approach
ØRGØ3KJ Fusion of Occipital-cervical Joint with Nonautologous Tissue Substitute, Posterior Approach, Anterior Column, Percutaneous Approach
ØRGØ47Ø Fusion of Occipital-cervical Joint with Autologous Tissue Substitute, Anterior Approach, Anterior Column, Percutaneous Endoscopic Approach
ØRGØ471 Fusion of Occipital-cervical Joint with Autologous Tissue Substitute, Posterior Approach, Posterior Column, Percutaneous Endoscopic Approach
ØRGØ47J Fusion of Occipital-cervical Joint with Autologous Tissue Substitute, Posterior Approach, Anterior Column, Percutaneous Endoscopic Approach
ØRGØ4AØ Fusion of Occipital-cervical Joint with Interbody Fusion Device, Anterior Approach, Anterior Column, Percutaneous Endoscopic Approach
ØRGØ4AJ Fusion of Occipital-cervical Joint with Interbody Fusion Device, Posterior Approach, Anterior Column, Percutaneous Endoscopic Approach
ØRGØ4JØ Fusion of Occipital-cervical Joint with Synthetic Substitute, Anterior Approach, Anterior Column, Percutaneous Endoscopic Approach
ØRGØ4J1 Fusion of Occipital-cervical Joint with Synthetic Substitute, Posterior Approach, Posterior Column, Percutaneous Endoscopic Approach
ØRGØ4JJ Fusion of Occipital-cervical Joint with Synthetic Substitute, Posterior Approach, Anterior Column, Percutaneous Endoscopic Approach
ØRGØ4KØ Fusion of Occipital-cervical Joint with Nonautologous Tissue Substitute, Anterior Approach, Anterior Column, Percutaneous Endoscopic Approach
ØRGØ4K1 Fusion of Occipital-cervical Joint with Nonautologous Tissue Substitute, Posterior Approach, Posterior Column, Percutaneous Endoscopic Approach
ØRGØ4KJ Fusion of Occipital-cervical Joint with Nonautologous Tissue Substitute, Posterior Approach, Anterior Column, Percutaneous Endoscopic Approach
ØRG1Ø7Ø Fusion of Cervical Vertebral Joint with Autologous Tissue Substitute, Anterior Approach, Anterior Column, Open Approach
ØRG1Ø71 Fusion of Cervical Vertebral Joint with Autologous Tissue Substitute, Posterior Approach, Posterior Column, Open Approach
ØRG1Ø7J Fusion of Cervical Vertebral Joint with Autologous Tissue Substitute, Posterior Approach, Anterior Column, Open Approach
ØRG1ØAØ Fusion of Cervical Vertebral Joint with Interbody Fusion Device, Anterior Approach, Anterior Column, Open Approach
ØRG1ØAJ Fusion of Cervical Vertebral Joint with Interbody Fusion Device, Posterior Approach, Anterior Column, Open Approach
ØRG1ØJØ Fusion of Cervical Vertebral Joint with Synthetic Substitute, Anterior Approach, Anterior Column, Open Approach
ØRG1ØJ1 Fusion of Cervical Vertebral Joint with Synthetic Substitute, Posterior Approach, Posterior Column, Open Approach
ØRG1ØJJ Fusion of Cervical Vertebral Joint with Synthetic Substitute, Posterior Approach, Anterior Column, Open Approach
ØRG1ØKØ Fusion of Cervical Vertebral Joint with Nonautologous Tissue Substitute, Anterior Approach, Anterior Column, Open Approach
ØRG1ØK1 Fusion of Cervical Vertebral Joint with Nonautologous Tissue Substitute, Posterior Approach, Posterior Column, Open Approach
ØRG1ØKJ Fusion of Cervical Vertebral Joint with Nonautologous Tissue Substitute, Posterior Approach, Anterior Column, Open Approach
ØRG137Ø Fusion of Cervical Vertebral Joint with Autologous Tissue Substitute, Anterior Approach, Anterior Column, Percutaneous Approach
ØRG1371 Fusion of Cervical Vertebral Joint with Autologous Tissue Substitute, Posterior Approach, Posterior Column, Percutaneous Approach
ØRG137J Fusion of Cervical Vertebral Joint with Autologous Tissue Substitute, Posterior Approach, Anterior Column, Percutaneous Approach
ØRG13AØ Fusion of Cervical Vertebral Joint with Interbody Fusion Device, Anterior Approach, Anterior Column, Percutaneous Approach
ØRG13AJ Fusion of Cervical Vertebral Joint with Interbody Fusion Device, Posterior Approach, Anterior Column, Percutaneous Approach
ØRG13JØ Fusion of Cervical Vertebral Joint with Synthetic Substitute, Anterior Approach, Anterior Column, Percutaneous Approach
ØRG13J1 Fusion of Cervical Vertebral Joint with Synthetic Substitute, Posterior Approach, Posterior Column, Percutaneous Approach
ØRG13JJ Fusion of Cervical Vertebral Joint with Synthetic Substitute, Posterior Approach, Anterior Column, Percutaneous Approach
ØRG13KØ Fusion of Cervical Vertebral Joint with Nonautologous Tissue Substitute, Anterior Approach, Anterior Column, Percutaneous Approach
ØRG13K1 Fusion of Cervical Vertebral Joint with Nonautologous Tissue Substitute, Posterior Approach, Posterior Column, Percutaneous Approach
ØRG13KJ Fusion of Cervical Vertebral Joint with Nonautologous Tissue Substitute, Posterior Approach, Anterior Column, Percutaneous Approach
ØRG147Ø Fusion of Cervical Vertebral Joint with Autologous Tissue Substitute, Anterior Approach, Anterior Column, Percutaneous Endoscopic Approach
ØRG1471 Fusion of Cervical Vertebral Joint with Autologous Tissue Substitute, Posterior Approach, Posterior Column, Percutaneous Endoscopic Approach
ØRG147J Fusion of Cervical Vertebral Joint with Autologous Tissue Substitute, Posterior Approach, Anterior Column, Percutaneous Endoscopic Approach
ØRG14AØ Fusion of Cervical Vertebral Joint with Interbody Fusion Device, Anterior Approach, Anterior Column, Percutaneous Endoscopic Approach

HAC 12: Surgical Site Infection-Certain Orthopedic Procedures of the Spine, Shoulder, and Elbow (continued)

ØRG14AJ Fusion of Cervical Vertebral Joint with Interbody Fusion Device, Posterior Approach, Anterior Column, Percutaneous Endoscopic Approach
ØRG14JØ Fusion of Cervical Vertebral Joint with Synthetic Substitute, Anterior Approach, Anterior Column, Percutaneous Endoscopic Approach
ØRG14J1 Fusion of Cervical Vertebral Joint with Synthetic Substitute, Posterior Approach, Posterior Column, Percutaneous Endoscopic Approach
ØRG14JJ Fusion of Cervical Vertebral Joint with Synthetic Substitute, Posterior Approach, Anterior Column, Percutaneous Endoscopic Approach
ØRG14KØ Fusion of Cervical Vertebral Joint with Nonautologous Tissue Substitute, Anterior Approach, Anterior Column, Percutaneous Endoscopic Approach
ØRG14K1 Fusion of Cervical Vertebral Joint with Nonautologous Tissue Substitute, Posterior Approach, Posterior Column, Percutaneous Endoscopic Approach
ØRG14KJ Fusion of Cervical Vertebral Joint with Nonautologous Tissue Substitute, Posterior Approach, Anterior Column, Percutaneous Endoscopic Approach
ØRG2Ø7Ø Fusion of 2 or more Cervical Vertebral Joints with Autologous Tissue Substitute, Anterior Approach, Anterior Column, Open Approach
ØRG2Ø71 Fusion of 2 or more Cervical Vertebral Joints with Autologous Tissue Substitute, Posterior Approach, Posterior Column, Open Approach
ØRG2Ø7J Fusion of 2 or more Cervical Vertebral Joints with Autologous Tissue Substitute, Posterior Approach, Anterior Column, Open Approach
ØRG2ØAØ Fusion of 2 or more Cervical Vertebral Joints with Interbody Fusion Device, Anterior Approach, Anterior Column, Open Approach
ØRG2ØAJ Fusion of 2 or more Cervical Vertebral Joints with Interbody Fusion Device, Posterior Approach, Anterior Column, Open Approach
ØRG2ØJØ Fusion of 2 or more Cervical Vertebral Joints with Synthetic Substitute, Anterior Approach, Anterior Column, Open Approach
ØRG2ØJ1 Fusion of 2 or more Cervical Vertebral Joints with Synthetic Substitute, Posterior Approach, Posterior Column, Open Approach
ØRG2ØJJ Fusion of 2 or more Cervical Vertebral Joints with Synthetic Substitute, Posterior Approach, Anterior Column, Open Approach
ØRG2ØKØ Fusion of 2 or more Cervical Vertebral Joints with Nonautologous Tissue Substitute, Anterior Approach, Anterior Column, Open Approach
ØRG2ØK1 Fusion of 2 or more Cervical Vertebral Joints with Nonautologous Tissue Substitute, Posterior Approach, Posterior Column, Open Approach
ØRG2ØKJ Fusion of 2 or more Cervical Vertebral Joints with Nonautologous Tissue Substitute, Posterior Approach, Anterior Column, Open Approach
ØRG237Ø Fusion of 2 or more Cervical Vertebral Joints with Autologous Tissue Substitute, Anterior Approach, Anterior Column, Percutaneous Approach
ØRG2371 Fusion of 2 or more Cervical Vertebral Joints with Autologous Tissue Substitute, Posterior Approach, Posterior Column, Percutaneous Approach
ØRG237J Fusion of 2 or more Cervical Vertebral Joints with Autologous Tissue Substitute, Posterior Approach, Anterior Column, Percutaneous Approach
ØRG23AØ Fusion of 2 or more Cervical Vertebral Joints with Interbody Fusion Device, Anterior Approach, Anterior Column, Percutaneous Approach
ØRG23AJ Fusion of 2 or more Cervical Vertebral Joints with Interbody Fusion Device, Posterior Approach, Anterior Column, Percutaneous Approach
ØRG23JØ Fusion of 2 or more Cervical Vertebral Joints with Synthetic Substitute, Anterior Approach, Anterior Column, Percutaneous Approach
ØRG23J1 Fusion of 2 or more Cervical Vertebral Joints with Synthetic Substitute, Posterior Approach, Posterior Column, Percutaneous Approach
ØRG23JJ Fusion of 2 or more Cervical Vertebral Joints with Synthetic Substitute, Posterior Approach, Anterior Column, Percutaneous Approach
ØRG23KØ Fusion of 2 or more Cervical Vertebral Joints with Nonautologous Tissue Substitute, Anterior Approach, Anterior Column, Percutaneous Approach
ØRG23K1 Fusion of 2 or more Cervical Vertebral Joints with Nonautologous Tissue Substitute, Posterior Approach, Posterior Column, Percutaneous Approach
ØRG23KJ Fusion of 2 or more Cervical Vertebral Joints with Nonautologous Tissue Substitute, Posterior Approach, Anterior Column, Percutaneous Approach
ØRG247Ø Fusion of 2 or more Cervical Vertebral Joints with Autologous Tissue Substitute, Anterior Approach, Anterior Column, Percutaneous Endoscopic Approach
ØRG2471 Fusion of 2 or more Cervical Vertebral Joints with Autologous Tissue Substitute, Posterior Approach, Posterior Column, Percutaneous Endoscopic Approach
ØRG247J Fusion of 2 or more Cervical Vertebral Joints with Autologous Tissue Substitute, Posterior Approach, Anterior Column, Percutaneous Endoscopic Approach
ØRG24AØ Fusion of 2 or more Cervical Vertebral Joints with Interbody Fusion Device, Anterior Approach, Anterior Column, Percutaneous Endoscopic Approach
ØRG24AJ Fusion of 2 or more Cervical Vertebral Joints with Interbody Fusion Device, Posterior Approach, Anterior Column, Percutaneous Endoscopic Approach
ØRG24JØ Fusion of 2 or more Cervical Vertebral Joints with Synthetic Substitute, Anterior Approach, Anterior Column, Percutaneous Endoscopic Approach
ØRG24J1 Fusion of 2 or more Cervical Vertebral Joints with Synthetic Substitute, Posterior Approach, Posterior Column, Percutaneous Endoscopic Approach
ØRG24JJ Fusion of 2 or more Cervical Vertebral Joints with Synthetic Substitute, Posterior Approach, Anterior Column, Percutaneous Endoscopic Approach
ØRG24KØ Fusion of 2 or more Cervical Vertebral Joints with Nonautologous Tissue Substitute, Anterior Approach, Anterior Column, Percutaneous Endoscopic Approach
ØRG24K1 Fusion of 2 or more Cervical Vertebral Joints with Nonautologous Tissue Substitute, Posterior Approach, Posterior Column, Percutaneous Endoscopic Approach
ØRG24KJ Fusion of 2 or more Cervical Vertebral Joints with Nonautologous Tissue Substitute, Posterior Approach, Anterior Column, Percutaneous Endoscopic Approach
ØRG4Ø7Ø Fusion of Cervicothoracic Vertebral Joint with Autologous Tissue Substitute, Anterior Approach, Anterior Column, Open Approach
ØRG4Ø71 Fusion of Cervicothoracic Vertebral Joint with Autologous Tissue Substitute, Posterior Approach, Posterior Column, Open Approach
ØRG4Ø7J Fusion of Cervicothoracic Vertebral Joint with Autologous Tissue Substitute, Posterior Approach, Anterior Column, Open Approach
ØRG4ØAØ Fusion of Cervicothoracic Vertebral Joint with Interbody Fusion Device, Anterior Approach, Anterior Column, Open Approach
ØRG4ØAJ Fusion of Cervicothoracic Vertebral Joint with Interbody Fusion Device, Posterior Approach, Anterior Column, Open Approach
ØRG4ØJØ Fusion of Cervicothoracic Vertebral Joint with Synthetic Substitute, Anterior Approach, Anterior Column, Open Approach
ØRG4ØJ1 Fusion of Cervicothoracic Vertebral Joint with Synthetic Substitute, Posterior Approach, Posterior Column, Open Approach
ØRG4ØJJ Fusion of Cervicothoracic Vertebral Joint with Synthetic Substitute, Posterior Approach, Anterior Column, Open Approach
ØRG4ØKØ Fusion of Cervicothoracic Vertebral Joint with Nonautologous Tissue Substitute, Anterior Approach, Anterior Column, Open Approach
ØRG4ØK1 Fusion of Cervicothoracic Vertebral Joint with Nonautologous Tissue Substitute, Posterior Approach, Posterior Column, Open Approach
ØRG4ØKJ Fusion of Cervicothoracic Vertebral Joint with Nonautologous Tissue Substitute, Posterior Approach, Anterior Column, Open Approach
ØRG437Ø Fusion of Cervicothoracic Vertebral Joint with Autologous Tissue Substitute, Anterior Approach, Anterior Column, Percutaneous Approach
ØRG4371 Fusion of Cervicothoracic Vertebral Joint with Autologous Tissue Substitute, Posterior Approach, Posterior Column, Percutaneous Approach
ØRG437J Fusion of Cervicothoracic Vertebral Joint with Autologous Tissue Substitute, Posterior Approach, Anterior Column, Percutaneous Approach
ØRG43AØ Fusion of Cervicothoracic Vertebral Joint with Interbody Fusion Device, Anterior Approach, Anterior Column, Percutaneous Approach

HAC 12: Surgical Site Infection-Certain Orthopedic Procedures of the Spine, Shoulder, and Elbow (continued)

ØRG43AJ Fusion of Cervicothoracic Vertebral Joint with Interbody Fusion Device, Posterior Approach, Anterior Column, Percutaneous Approach
ØRG43JØ Fusion of Cervicothoracic Vertebral Joint with Synthetic Substitute, Anterior Approach, Anterior Column, Percutaneous Approach
ØRG43J1 Fusion of Cervicothoracic Vertebral Joint with Synthetic Substitute, Posterior Approach, Posterior Column, Percutaneous Approach
ØRG43JJ Fusion of Cervicothoracic Vertebral Joint with Synthetic Substitute, Posterior Approach, Anterior Column, Percutaneous Approach
ØRG43KØ Fusion of Cervicothoracic Vertebral Joint with Nonautologous Tissue Substitute, Anterior Approach, Anterior Column, Percutaneous Approach
ØRG43K1 Fusion of Cervicothoracic Vertebral Joint with Nonautologous Tissue Substitute, Posterior Approach, Posterior Column, Percutaneous Approach
ØRG43KJ Fusion of Cervicothoracic Vertebral Joint with Nonautologous Tissue Substitute, Posterior Approach, Anterior Column, Percutaneous Approach
ØRG447Ø Fusion of Cervicothoracic Vertebral Joint with Autologous Tissue Substitute, Anterior Approach, Anterior Column, Percutaneous Endoscopic Approach
ØRG4471 Fusion of Cervicothoracic Vertebral Joint with Autologous Tissue Substitute, Posterior Approach, Posterior Column, Percutaneous Endoscopic Approach
ØRG447J Fusion of Cervicothoracic Vertebral Joint with Autologous Tissue Substitute, Posterior Approach, Anterior Column, Percutaneous Endoscopic Approach
ØRG44AØ Fusion of Cervicothoracic Vertebral Joint with Interbody Fusion Device, Anterior Approach, Anterior Column, Percutaneous Endoscopic Approach
ØRG44AJ Fusion of Cervicothoracic Vertebral Joint with Interbody Fusion Device, Posterior Approach, Anterior Column, Percutaneous Endoscopic Approach
ØRG44JØ Fusion of Cervicothoracic Vertebral Joint with Synthetic Substitute, Anterior Approach, Anterior Column, Percutaneous Endoscopic Approach
ØRG44J1 Fusion of Cervicothoracic Vertebral Joint with Synthetic Substitute, Posterior Approach, Posterior Column, Percutaneous Endoscopic Approach
ØRG44JJ Fusion of Cervicothoracic Vertebral Joint with Synthetic Substitute, Posterior Approach, Anterior Column, Percutaneous Endoscopic Approach
ØRG44KØ Fusion of Cervicothoracic Vertebral Joint with Nonautologous Tissue Substitute, Anterior Approach, Anterior Column, Percutaneous Endoscopic Approach
ØRG44K1 Fusion of Cervicothoracic Vertebral Joint with Nonautologous Tissue Substitute, Posterior Approach, Posterior Column, Percutaneous Endoscopic Approach
ØRG44KJ Fusion of Cervicothoracic Vertebral Joint with Nonautologous Tissue Substitute, Posterior Approach, Anterior Column, Percutaneous Endoscopic Approach
ØRG607Ø Fusion of Thoracic Vertebral Joint with Autologous Tissue Substitute, Anterior Approach, Anterior Column, Open Approach
ØRG6071 Fusion of Thoracic Vertebral Joint with Autologous Tissue Substitute, Posterior Approach, Posterior Column, Open Approach
ØRG607J Fusion of Thoracic Vertebral Joint with Autologous Tissue Substitute, Posterior Approach, Anterior Column, Open Approach
ØRG6ØAØ Fusion of Thoracic Vertebral Joint with Interbody Fusion Device, Anterior Approach, Anterior Column, Open Approach
ØRG6ØAJ Fusion of Thoracic Vertebral Joint with Interbody Fusion Device, Posterior Approach, Anterior Column, Open Approach
ØRG6ØJØ Fusion of Thoracic Vertebral Joint with Synthetic Substitute, Anterior Approach, Anterior Column, Open Approach
ØRG6ØJ1 Fusion of Thoracic Vertebral Joint with Synthetic Substitute, Posterior Approach, Posterior Column, Open Approach
ØRG6ØJJ Fusion of Thoracic Vertebral Joint with Synthetic Substitute, Posterior Approach, Anterior Column, Open Approach
ØRG6ØKØ Fusion of Thoracic Vertebral Joint with Nonautologous Tissue Substitute, Anterior Approach, Anterior Column, Open Approach
ØRG6ØK1 Fusion of Thoracic Vertebral Joint with Nonautologous Tissue Substitute, Posterior Approach, Posterior Column, Open Approach
ØRG6ØKJ Fusion of Thoracic Vertebral Joint with Nonautologous Tissue Substitute, Posterior Approach, Anterior Column, Open Approach
ØRG637Ø Fusion of Thoracic Vertebral Joint with Autologous Tissue Substitute, Anterior Approach, Anterior Column, Percutaneous Approach
ØRG6371 Fusion of Thoracic Vertebral Joint with Autologous Tissue Substitute, Posterior Approach, Posterior Column, Percutaneous Approach
ØRG637J Fusion of Thoracic Vertebral Joint with Autologous Tissue Substitute, Posterior Approach, Anterior Column, Percutaneous Approach
ØRG63AØ Fusion of Thoracic Vertebral Joint with Interbody Fusion Device, Anterior Approach, Anterior Column, Percutaneous Approach
ØRG63AJ Fusion of Thoracic Vertebral Joint with Interbody Fusion Device, Posterior Approach, Anterior Column, Percutaneous Approach
ØRG63JØ Fusion of Thoracic Vertebral Joint with Synthetic Substitute, Anterior Approach, Anterior Column, Percutaneous Approach
ØRG63J1 Fusion of Thoracic Vertebral Joint with Synthetic Substitute, Posterior Approach, Posterior Column, Percutaneous Approach
ØRG63JJ Fusion of Thoracic Vertebral Joint with Synthetic Substitute, Posterior Approach, Anterior Column, Percutaneous Approach
ØRG63KØ Fusion of Thoracic Vertebral Joint with Nonautologous Tissue Substitute, Anterior Approach, Anterior Column, Percutaneous Approach
ØRG63K1 Fusion of Thoracic Vertebral Joint with Nonautologous Tissue Substitute, Posterior Approach, Posterior Column, Percutaneous Approach
ØRG63KJ Fusion of Thoracic Vertebral Joint with Nonautologous Tissue Substitute, Posterior Approach, Anterior Column, Percutaneous Approach
ØRG647Ø Fusion of Thoracic Vertebral Joint with Autologous Tissue Substitute, Anterior Approach, Anterior Column, Percutaneous Endoscopic Approach
ØRG6471 Fusion of Thoracic Vertebral Joint with Autologous Tissue Substitute, Posterior Approach, Posterior Column, Percutaneous Endoscopic Approach
ØRG647J Fusion of Thoracic Vertebral Joint with Autologous Tissue Substitute, Posterior Approach, Anterior Column, Percutaneous Endoscopic Approach
ØRG64AØ Fusion of Thoracic Vertebral Joint with Interbody Fusion Device, Anterior Approach, Anterior Column, Percutaneous Endoscopic Approach
ØRG64AJ Fusion of Thoracic Vertebral Joint with Interbody Fusion Device, Posterior Approach, Anterior Column, Percutaneous Endoscopic Approach
ØRG64JØ Fusion of Thoracic Vertebral Joint with Synthetic Substitute, Anterior Approach, Anterior Column, Percutaneous Endoscopic Approach
ØRG64J1 Fusion of Thoracic Vertebral Joint with Synthetic Substitute, Posterior Approach, Posterior Column, Percutaneous Endoscopic Approach
ØRG64JJ Fusion of Thoracic Vertebral Joint with Synthetic Substitute, Posterior Approach, Anterior Column, Percutaneous Endoscopic Approach
ØRG64KØ Fusion of Thoracic Vertebral Joint with Nonautologous Tissue Substitute, Anterior Approach, Anterior Column, Percutaneous Endoscopic Approach
ØRG64K1 Fusion of Thoracic Vertebral Joint with Nonautologous Tissue Substitute, Posterior Approach, Posterior Column, Percutaneous Endoscopic Approach
ØRG64KJ Fusion of Thoracic Vertebral Joint with Nonautologous Tissue Substitute, Posterior Approach, Anterior Column, Percutaneous Endoscopic Approach
ØRG707Ø Fusion of 2 to 7 Thoracic Vertebral Joints with Autologous Tissue Substitute, Anterior Approach, Anterior Column, Open Approach
ØRG7Ø71 Fusion of 2 to 7 Thoracic Vertebral Joints with Autologous Tissue Substitute, Posterior Approach, Posterior Column, Open Approach
ØRG707J Fusion of 2 to 7 Thoracic Vertebral Joints with Autologous Tissue Substitute, Posterior Approach, Anterior Column, Open Approach
ØRG7ØAØ Fusion of 2 to 7 Thoracic Vertebral Joints with Interbody Fusion Device, Anterior Approach, Anterior Column, Open Approach
ØRG7ØAJ Fusion of 2 to 7 Thoracic Vertebral Joints with Interbody Fusion Device, Posterior Approach, Anterior Column, Open Approach
ØRG7ØJØ Fusion of 2 to 7 Thoracic Vertebral Joints with Synthetic Substitute, Anterior Approach, Anterior Column, Open Approach

HAC 12: Surgical Site Infection-Certain Orthopedic Procedures of the Spine, Shoulder, and Elbow (continued)

ØRG70J1 Fusion of 2 to 7 Thoracic Vertebral Joints with Synthetic Substitute, Posterior Approach, Posterior Column, Open Approach
ØRG70JJ Fusion of 2 to 7 Thoracic Vertebral Joints with Synthetic Substitute, Posterior Approach, Anterior Column, Open Approach
ØRG70KØ Fusion of 2 to 7 Thoracic Vertebral Joints with Nonautologous Tissue Substitute, Anterior Approach, Anterior Column, Open Approach
ØRG70K1 Fusion of 2 to 7 Thoracic Vertebral Joints with Nonautologous Tissue Substitute, Posterior Approach, Posterior Column, Open Approach
ØRG70KJ Fusion of 2 to 7 Thoracic Vertebral Joints with Nonautologous Tissue Substitute, Posterior Approach, Anterior Column, Open Approach
ØRG737Ø Fusion of 2 to 7 Thoracic Vertebral Joints with Autologous Tissue Substitute, Anterior Approach, Anterior Column, Percutaneous Approach
ØRG7371 Fusion of 2 to 7 Thoracic Vertebral Joints with Autologous Tissue Substitute, Posterior Approach, Posterior Column, Percutaneous Approach
ØRG737J Fusion of 2 to 7 Thoracic Vertebral Joints with Autologous Tissue Substitute, Posterior Approach, Anterior Column, Percutaneous Approach
ØRG73AØ Fusion of 2 to 7 Thoracic Vertebral Joints with Interbody Fusion Device, Anterior Approach, Anterior Column, Percutaneous Approach
ØRG73AJ Fusion of 2 to 7 Thoracic Vertebral Joints with Interbody Fusion Device, Posterior Approach, Anterior Column, Percutaneous Approach
ØRG73JØ Fusion of 2 to 7 Thoracic Vertebral Joints with Synthetic Substitute, Anterior Approach, Anterior Column, Percutaneous Approach
ØRG73J1 Fusion of 2 to 7 Thoracic Vertebral Joints with Synthetic Substitute, Posterior Approach, Posterior Column, Percutaneous Approach
ØRG73JJ Fusion of 2 to 7 Thoracic Vertebral Joints with Synthetic Substitute, Posterior Approach, Anterior Column, Percutaneous Approach
ØRG73KØ Fusion of 2 to 7 Thoracic Vertebral Joints with Nonautologous Tissue Substitute, Anterior Approach, Anterior Column, Percutaneous Approach
ØRG73K1 Fusion of 2 to 7 Thoracic Vertebral Joints with Nonautologous Tissue Substitute, Posterior Approach, Posterior Column, Percutaneous Approach
ØRG73KJ Fusion of 2 to 7 Thoracic Vertebral Joints with Nonautologous Tissue Substitute, Posterior Approach, Anterior Column, Percutaneous Approach
ØRG747Ø Fusion of 2 to 7 Thoracic Vertebral Joints with Autologous Tissue Substitute, Anterior Approach, Anterior Column, Percutaneous Endoscopic Approach
ØRG7471 Fusion of 2 to 7 Thoracic Vertebral Joints with Autologous Tissue Substitute, Posterior Approach, Posterior Column, Percutaneous Endoscopic Approach
ØRG747J Fusion of 2 to 7 Thoracic Vertebral Joints with Autologous Tissue Substitute, Posterior Approach, Anterior Column, Percutaneous Endoscopic Approach
ØRG74AØ Fusion of 2 to 7 Thoracic Vertebral Joints with Interbody Fusion Device, Anterior Approach, Anterior Column, Percutaneous Endoscopic Approach
ØRG74AJ Fusion of 2 to 7 Thoracic Vertebral Joints with Interbody Fusion Device, Posterior Approach, Anterior Column, Percutaneous Endoscopic Approach
ØRG74JØ Fusion of 2 to 7 Thoracic Vertebral Joints with Synthetic Substitute, Anterior Approach, Anterior Column, Percutaneous Endoscopic Approach
ØRG74J1 Fusion of 2 to 7 Thoracic Vertebral Joints with Synthetic Substitute, Posterior Approach, Posterior Column, Percutaneous Endoscopic Approach
ØRG74JJ Fusion of 2 to 7 Thoracic Vertebral Joints with Synthetic Substitute, Posterior Approach, Anterior Column, Percutaneous Endoscopic Approach
ØRG74KØ Fusion of 2 to 7 Thoracic Vertebral Joints with Nonautologous Tissue Substitute, Anterior Approach, Anterior Column, Percutaneous Endoscopic Approach
ØRG74K1 Fusion of 2 to 7 Thoracic Vertebral Joints with Nonautologous Tissue Substitute, Posterior Approach, Posterior Column, Percutaneous Endoscopic Approach
ØRG74KJ Fusion of 2 to 7 Thoracic Vertebral Joints with Nonautologous Tissue Substitute, Posterior Approach, Anterior Column, Percutaneous Endoscopic Approach
ØRG8Ø7Ø Fusion of 8 or More Thoracic Vertebral Joints with Autologous Tissue Substitute, Anterior Approach, Anterior Column, Open Approach
ØRG8Ø71 Fusion of 8 or More Thoracic Vertebral Joints with Autologous Tissue Substitute, Posterior Approach, Posterior Column, Open Approach
ØRG8Ø7J Fusion of 8 or More Thoracic Vertebral Joints with Autologous Tissue Substitute, Posterior Approach, Anterior Column, Open Approach
ØRG8ØAØ Fusion of 8 or More Thoracic Vertebral Joints with Interbody Fusion Device, Anterior Approach, Anterior Column, Open Approach
ØRG8ØAJ Fusion of 8 or More Thoracic Vertebral Joints with Interbody Fusion Device, Posterior Approach, Anterior Column, Open Approach
ØRG8ØJØ Fusion of 8 or More Thoracic Vertebral Joints with Synthetic Substitute, Anterior Approach, Anterior Column, Open Approach
ØRG8ØJ1 Fusion of 8 or More Thoracic Vertebral Joints with Synthetic Substitute, Posterior Approach, Posterior Column, Open Approach
ØRG8ØJJ Fusion of 8 or More Thoracic Vertebral Joints with Synthetic Substitute, Posterior Approach, Anterior Column, Open Approach
ØRG8ØKØ Fusion of 8 or More Thoracic Vertebral Joints with Nonautologous Tissue Substitute, Anterior Approach, Anterior Column, Open Approach
ØRG8ØK1 Fusion of 8 or More Thoracic Vertebral Joints with Nonautologous Tissue Substitute, Posterior Approach, Posterior Column, Open Approach
ØRG8ØKJ Fusion of 8 or More Thoracic Vertebral Joints with Nonautologous Tissue Substitute, Posterior Approach, Anterior Column, Open Approach
ØRG837Ø Fusion of 8 or More Thoracic Vertebral Joints with Autologous Tissue Substitute, Anterior Approach, Anterior Column, Percutaneous Approach
ØRG8371 Fusion of 8 or More Thoracic Vertebral Joints with Autologous Tissue Substitute, Posterior Approach, Posterior Column, Percutaneous Approach
ØRG837J Fusion of 8 or More Thoracic Vertebral Joints with Autologous Tissue Substitute, Posterior Approach, Anterior Column, Percutaneous Approach
ØRG83AØ Fusion of 8 or More Thoracic Vertebral Joints with Interbody Fusion Device, Anterior Approach, Anterior Column, Percutaneous Approach
ØRG83AJ Fusion of 8 or More Thoracic Vertebral Joints with Interbody Fusion Device, Posterior Approach, Anterior Column, Percutaneous Approach
ØRG83JØ Fusion of 8 or More Thoracic Vertebral Joints with Synthetic Substitute, Anterior Approach, Anterior Column, Percutaneous Approach
ØRG83J1 Fusion of 8 or More Thoracic Vertebral Joints with Synthetic Substitute, Posterior Approach, Posterior Column, Percutaneous Approach
ØRG83JJ Fusion of 8 or More Thoracic Vertebral Joints with Synthetic Substitute, Posterior Approach, Anterior Column, Percutaneous Approach
ØRG83KØ Fusion of 8 or More Thoracic Vertebral Joints with Nonautologous Tissue Substitute, Anterior Approach, Anterior Column, Percutaneous Approach
ØRG83K1 Fusion of 8 or More Thoracic Vertebral Joints with Nonautologous Tissue Substitute, Posterior Approach, Posterior Column, Percutaneous Approach
ØRG83KJ Fusion of 8 or More Thoracic Vertebral Joints with Nonautologous Tissue Substitute, Posterior Approach, Anterior Column, Percutaneous Approach
ØRG847Ø Fusion of 8 or More Thoracic Vertebral Joints with Autologous Tissue Substitute, Anterior Approach, Anterior Column, Percutaneous Endoscopic Approach
ØRG8471 Fusion of 8 or More Thoracic Vertebral Joints with Autologous Tissue Substitute, Posterior Approach, Posterior Column, Percutaneous Endoscopic Approach
ØRG847J Fusion of 8 or More Thoracic Vertebral Joints with Autologous Tissue Substitute, Posterior Approach, Anterior Column, Percutaneous Endoscopic Approach
ØRG84AØ Fusion of 8 or More Thoracic Vertebral Joints with Interbody Fusion Device, Anterior Approach, Anterior Column, Percutaneous Endoscopic Approach
ØRG84AJ Fusion of 8 or More Thoracic Vertebral Joints with Interbody Fusion Device, Posterior Approach, Anterior Column, Percutaneous Endoscopic Approach
ØRG84JØ Fusion of 8 or More Thoracic Vertebral Joints with Synthetic Substitute, Anterior Approach, Anterior Column, Percutaneous Endoscopic Approach
ØRG84J1 Fusion of 8 or More Thoracic Vertebral Joints with Synthetic Substitute, Posterior Approach, Posterior Column, Percutaneous Endoscopic Approach

HAC 12: Surgical Site Infection-Certain Orthopedic Procedures of the Spine, Shoulder, and Elbow (continued)

ØRG84JJ Fusion of 8 or More Thoracic Vertebral Joints with Synthetic Substitute, Posterior Approach, Anterior Column, Percutaneous Endoscopic Approach
ØRG84KØ Fusion of 8 or More Thoracic Vertebral Joints with Nonautologous Tissue Substitute, Anterior Approach, Anterior Column, Percutaneous Endoscopic Approach
ØRG84K1 Fusion of 8 or More Thoracic Vertebral Joints with Nonautologous Tissue Substitute, Posterior Approach, Posterior Column, Percutaneous Endoscopic Approach
ØRG84KJ Fusion of 8 or More Thoracic Vertebral Joints with Nonautologous Tissue Substitute, Posterior Approach, Anterior Column, Percutaneous Endoscopic Approach
ØRGAØ7Ø Fusion of Thoracolumbar Vertebral Joint with Autologous Tissue Substitute, Anterior Approach, Anterior Column, Open Approach
ØRGAØ71 Fusion of Thoracolumbar Vertebral Joint with Autologous Tissue Substitute, Posterior Approach, Posterior Column, Open Approach
ØRGAØ7J Fusion of Thoracolumbar Vertebral Joint with Autologous Tissue Substitute, Posterior Approach, Anterior Column, Open Approach
ØRGAØAØ Fusion of Thoracolumbar Vertebral Joint with Interbody Fusion Device, Anterior Approach, Anterior Column, Open Approach
ØRGAØAJ Fusion of Thoracolumbar Vertebral Joint with Interbody Fusion Device, Posterior Approach, Anterior Column, Open Approach
ØRGAØJØ Fusion of Thoracolumbar Vertebral Joint with Synthetic Substitute, Anterior Approach, Anterior Column, Open Approach
ØRGAØJ1 Fusion of Thoracolumbar Vertebral Joint with Synthetic Substitute, Posterior Approach, Posterior Column, Open Approach
ØRGAØJJ Fusion of Thoracolumbar Vertebral Joint with Synthetic Substitute, Posterior Approach, Anterior Column, Open Approach
ØRGAØKØ Fusion of Thoracolumbar Vertebral Joint with Nonautologous Tissue Substitute, Anterior Approach, Anterior Column, Open Approach
ØRGAØK1 Fusion of Thoracolumbar Vertebral Joint with Nonautologous Tissue Substitute, Posterior Approach, Posterior Column, Open Approach
ØRGAØKJ Fusion of Thoracolumbar Vertebral Joint with Nonautologous Tissue Substitute, Posterior Approach, Anterior Column, Open Approach
ØRGA37Ø Fusion of Thoracolumbar Vertebral Joint with Autologous Tissue Substitute, Anterior Approach, Anterior Column, Percutaneous Approach
ØRGA371 Fusion of Thoracolumbar Vertebral Joint with Autologous Tissue Substitute, Posterior Approach, Posterior Column, Percutaneous Approach
ØRGA37J Fusion of Thoracolumbar Vertebral Joint with Autologous Tissue Substitute, Posterior Approach, Anterior Column, Percutaneous Approach
ØRGA3AØ Fusion of Thoracolumbar Vertebral Joint with Interbody Fusion Device, Anterior Approach, Anterior Column, Percutaneous Approach
ØRGA3AJ Fusion of Thoracolumbar Vertebral Joint with Interbody Fusion Device, Posterior Approach, Anterior Column, Percutaneous Approach
ØRGA3JØ Fusion of Thoracolumbar Vertebral Joint with Synthetic Substitute, Anterior Approach, Anterior Column, Percutaneous Approach
ØRGA3J1 Fusion of Thoracolumbar Vertebral Joint with Synthetic Substitute, Posterior Approach, Posterior Column, Percutaneous Approach
ØRGA3JJ Fusion of Thoracolumbar Vertebral Joint with Synthetic Substitute, Posterior Approach, Anterior Column, Percutaneous Approach
ØRGA3KØ Fusion of Thoracolumbar Vertebral Joint with Nonautologous Tissue Substitute, Anterior Approach, Anterior Column, Percutaneous Approach
ØRGA3K1 Fusion of Thoracolumbar Vertebral Joint with Nonautologous Tissue Substitute, Posterior Approach, Posterior Column, Percutaneous Approach
ØRGA3KJ Fusion of Thoracolumbar Vertebral Joint with Nonautologous Tissue Substitute, Posterior Approach, Anterior Column, Percutaneous Approach
ØRGA47Ø Fusion of Thoracolumbar Vertebral Joint with Autologous Tissue Substitute, Anterior Approach, Anterior Column, Percutaneous Endoscopic Approach
ØRGA471 Fusion of Thoracolumbar Vertebral Joint with Autologous Tissue Substitute, Posterior Approach, Posterior Column, Percutaneous Endoscopic Approach
ØRGA47J Fusion of Thoracolumbar Vertebral Joint with Autologous Tissue Substitute, Posterior Approach, Anterior Column, Percutaneous Endoscopic Approach
ØRGA4AØ Fusion of Thoracolumbar Vertebral Joint with Interbody Fusion Device, Anterior Approach, Anterior Column, Percutaneous Endoscopic Approach
ØRGA4AJ Fusion of Thoracolumbar Vertebral Joint with Interbody Fusion Device, Posterior Approach, Anterior Column, Percutaneous Endoscopic Approach
ØRGA4JØ Fusion of Thoracolumbar Vertebral Joint with Synthetic Substitute, Anterior Approach, Anterior Column, Percutaneous Endoscopic Approach
ØRGA4J1 Fusion of Thoracolumbar Vertebral Joint with Synthetic Substitute, Posterior Approach, Posterior Column, Percutaneous Endoscopic Approach
ØRGA4JJ Fusion of Thoracolumbar Vertebral Joint with Synthetic Substitute, Posterior Approach, Anterior Column, Percutaneous Endoscopic Approach
ØRGA4KØ Fusion of Thoracolumbar Vertebral Joint with Nonautologous Tissue Substitute, Anterior Approach, Anterior Column, Percutaneous Endoscopic Approach
ØRGA4K1 Fusion of Thoracolumbar Vertebral Joint with Nonautologous Tissue Substitute, Posterior Approach, Posterior Column, Percutaneous Endoscopic Approach
ØRGA4KJ Fusion of Thoracolumbar Vertebral Joint with Nonautologous Tissue Substitute, Posterior Approach, Anterior Column, Percutaneous Endoscopic Approach
ØRGEØ4Z Fusion of Right Sternoclavicular Joint with Internal Fixation Device, Open Approach
ØRGEØ7Z Fusion of Right Sternoclavicular Joint with Autologous Tissue Substitute, Open Approach
ØRGEØJZ Fusion of Right Sternoclavicular Joint with Synthetic Substitute, Open Approach
ØRGEØKZ Fusion of Right Sternoclavicular Joint with Nonautologous Tissue Substitute, Open Approach
ØRGE34Z Fusion of Right Sternoclavicular Joint with Internal Fixation Device, Percutaneous Approach
ØRGE37Z Fusion of Right Sternoclavicular Joint with Autologous Tissue Substitute, Percutaneous Approach
ØRGE3JZ Fusion of Right Sternoclavicular Joint with Synthetic Substitute, Percutaneous Approach
ØRGE3KZ Fusion of Right Sternoclavicular Joint with Nonautologous Tissue Substitute, Percutaneous Approach
ØRGE44Z Fusion of Right Sternoclavicular Joint with Internal Fixation Device, Percutaneous Endoscopic Approach
ØRGE47Z Fusion of Right Sternoclavicular Joint with Autologous Tissue Substitute, Percutaneous Endoscopic Approach
ØRGE4JZ Fusion of Right Sternoclavicular Joint with Synthetic Substitute, Percutaneous Endoscopic Approach
ØRGE4KZ Fusion of Right Sternoclavicular Joint with Nonautologous Tissue Substitute, Percutaneous Endoscopic Approach
ØRGFØ4Z Fusion of Left Sternoclavicular Joint with Internal Fixation Device, Open Approach
ØRGFØ7Z Fusion of Left Sternoclavicular Joint with Autologous Tissue Substitute, Open Approach
ØRGFØJZ Fusion of Left Sternoclavicular Joint with Synthetic Substitute, Open Approach
ØRGFØKZ Fusion of Left Sternoclavicular Joint with Nonautologous Tissue Substitute, Open Approach
ØRGF34Z Fusion of Left Sternoclavicular Joint with Internal Fixation Device, Percutaneous Approach
ØRGF37Z Fusion of Left Sternoclavicular Joint with Autologous Tissue Substitute, Percutaneous Approach
ØRGF3JZ Fusion of Left Sternoclavicular Joint with Synthetic Substitute, Percutaneous Approach
ØRGF3KZ Fusion of Left Sternoclavicular Joint with Nonautologous Tissue Substitute, Percutaneous Approach
ØRGF44Z Fusion of Left Sternoclavicular Joint with Internal Fixation Device, Percutaneous Endoscopic Approach
ØRGF47Z Fusion of Left Sternoclavicular Joint with Autologous Tissue Substitute, Percutaneous Endoscopic Approach
ØRGF4JZ Fusion of Left Sternoclavicular Joint with Synthetic Substitute, Percutaneous Endoscopic Approach
ØRGF4KZ Fusion of Left Sternoclavicular Joint with Nonautologous Tissue Substitute, Percutaneous Endoscopic Approach
ØRGGØ4Z Fusion of Right Acromioclavicular Joint with Internal Fixation Device, Open Approach

HAC 12: Surgical Site Infection-Certain Orthopedic Procedures of the Spine, Shoulder, and Elbow (continued)

ØRGGØ7Z Fusion of Right Acromioclavicular Joint with Autologous Tissue Substitute, Open Approach
ØRGGØJZ Fusion of Right Acromioclavicular Joint with Synthetic Substitute, Open Approach
ØRGGØKZ Fusion of Right Acromioclavicular Joint with Nonautologous Tissue Substitute, Open Approach
ØRGG34Z Fusion of Right Acromioclavicular Joint with Internal Fixation Device, Percutaneous Approach
ØRGG37Z Fusion of Right Acromioclavicular Joint with Autologous Tissue Substitute, Percutaneous Approach
ØRGG3JZ Fusion of Right Acromioclavicular Joint with Synthetic Substitute, Percutaneous Approach
ØRGG3KZ Fusion of Right Acromioclavicular Joint with Nonautologous Tissue Substitute, Percutaneous Approach
ØRGG44Z Fusion of Right Acromioclavicular Joint with Internal Fixation Device, Percutaneous Endoscopic Approach
ØRGG47Z Fusion of Right Acromioclavicular Joint with Autologous Tissue Substitute, Percutaneous Endoscopic Approach
ØRGG4JZ Fusion of Right Acromioclavicular Joint with Synthetic Substitute, Percutaneous Endoscopic Approach
ØRGG4KZ Fusion of Right Acromioclavicular Joint with Nonautologous Tissue Substitute, Percutaneous Endoscopic Approach
ØRGHØ4Z Fusion of Left Acromioclavicular Joint with Internal Fixation Device, Open Approach
ØRGHØ7Z Fusion of Left Acromioclavicular Joint with Autologous Tissue Substitute, Open Approach
ØRGHØJZ Fusion of Left Acromioclavicular Joint with Synthetic Substitute, Open Approach
ØRGHØKZ Fusion of Left Acromioclavicular Joint with Nonautologous Tissue Substitute, Open Approach
ØRGH34Z Fusion of Left Acromioclavicular Joint with Internal Fixation Device, Percutaneous Approach
ØRGH37Z Fusion of Left Acromioclavicular Joint with Autologous Tissue Substitute, Percutaneous Approach
ØRGH3JZ Fusion of Left Acromioclavicular Joint with Synthetic Substitute, Percutaneous Approach
ØRGH3KZ Fusion of Left Acromioclavicular Joint with Nonautologous Tissue Substitute, Percutaneous Approach
ØRGH44Z Fusion of Left Acromioclavicular Joint with Internal Fixation Device, Percutaneous Endoscopic Approach
ØRGH47Z Fusion of Left Acromioclavicular Joint with Autologous Tissue Substitute, Percutaneous Endoscopic Approach
ØRGH4JZ Fusion of Left Acromioclavicular Joint with Synthetic Substitute, Percutaneous Endoscopic Approach
ØRGH4KZ Fusion of Left Acromioclavicular Joint with Nonautologous Tissue Substitute, Percutaneous Endoscopic Approach
ØRGJØ4Z Fusion of Right Shoulder Joint with Internal Fixation Device, Open Approach
ØRGJØ7Z Fusion of Right Shoulder Joint with Autologous Tissue Substitute, Open Approach
ØRGJØJZ Fusion of Right Shoulder Joint with Synthetic Substitute, Open Approach
ØRGJØKZ Fusion of Right Shoulder Joint with Nonautologous Tissue Substitute, Open Approach
ØRGJ34Z Fusion of Right Shoulder Joint with Internal Fixation Device, Percutaneous Approach
ØRGJ37Z Fusion of Right Shoulder Joint with Autologous Tissue Substitute, Percutaneous Approach
ØRGJ3JZ Fusion of Right Shoulder Joint with Synthetic Substitute, Percutaneous Approach
ØRGJ3KZ Fusion of Right Shoulder Joint with Nonautologous Tissue Substitute, Percutaneous Approach
ØRGJ44Z Fusion of Right Shoulder Joint with Internal Fixation Device, Percutaneous Endoscopic Approach
ØRGJ47Z Fusion of Right Shoulder Joint with Autologous Tissue Substitute, Percutaneous Endoscopic Approach
ØRGJ4JZ Fusion of Right Shoulder Joint with Synthetic Substitute, Percutaneous Endoscopic Approach
ØRGJ4KZ Fusion of Right Shoulder Joint with Nonautologous Tissue Substitute, Percutaneous Endoscopic Approach
ØRGKØ4Z Fusion of Left Shoulder Joint with Internal Fixation Device, Open Approach
ØRGKØ7Z Fusion of Left Shoulder Joint with Autologous Tissue Substitute, Open Approach
ØRGKØJZ Fusion of Left Shoulder Joint with Synthetic Substitute, Open Approach
ØRGKØKZ Fusion of Left Shoulder Joint with Nonautologous Tissue Substitute, Open Approach
ØRGK34Z Fusion of Left Shoulder Joint with Internal Fixation Device, Percutaneous Approach
ØRGK37Z Fusion of Left Shoulder Joint with Autologous Tissue Substitute, Percutaneous Approach
ØRGK3JZ Fusion of Left Shoulder Joint with Synthetic Substitute, Percutaneous Approach
ØRGK3KZ Fusion of Left Shoulder Joint with Nonautologous Tissue Substitute, Percutaneous Approach
ØRGK44Z Fusion of Left Shoulder Joint with Internal Fixation Device, Percutaneous Endoscopic Approach
ØRGK47Z Fusion of Left Shoulder Joint with Autologous Tissue Substitute, Percutaneous Endoscopic Approach
ØRGK4JZ Fusion of Left Shoulder Joint with Synthetic Substitute, Percutaneous Endoscopic Approach
ØRGK4KZ Fusion of Left Shoulder Joint with Nonautologous Tissue Substitute, Percutaneous Endoscopic Approach
ØRGLØ3Z Fusion of Right Elbow Joint with Sustained Compression Internal Fixation Device, Open Approach
ØRGLØ4Z Fusion of Right Elbow Joint with Internal Fixation Device, Open Approach
ØRGLØ5Z Fusion of Right Elbow Joint with External Fixation Device, Open Approach
ØRGLØ7Z Fusion of Right Elbow Joint with Autologous Tissue Substitute, Open Approach
ØRGLØJZ Fusion of Right Elbow Joint with Synthetic Substitute, Open Approach
ØRGLØKZ Fusion of Right Elbow Joint with Nonautologous Tissue Substitute, Open Approach
ØRGL33Z Fusion of Right Elbow Joint with Sustained Compression Internal Fixation Device, Percutaneous Approach
ØRGL34Z Fusion of Right Elbow Joint with Internal Fixation Device, Percutaneous Approach
ØRGL35Z Fusion of Right Elbow Joint with External Fixation Device, Percutaneous Approach
ØRGL37Z Fusion of Right Elbow Joint with Autologous Tissue Substitute, Percutaneous Approach
ØRGL3JZ Fusion of Right Elbow Joint with Synthetic Substitute, Percutaneous Approach
ØRGL3KZ Fusion of Right Elbow Joint with Nonautologous Tissue Substitute, Percutaneous Approach
ØRGL43Z Fusion of Right Elbow Joint with Sustained Compression Internal Fixation Device, Percutaneous Endoscopic Approach
ØRGL44Z Fusion of Right Elbow Joint with Internal Fixation Device, Percutaneous Endoscopic Approach
ØRGL45Z Fusion of Right Elbow Joint with External Fixation Device, Percutaneous Endoscopic Approach
ØRGL47Z Fusion of Right Elbow Joint with Autologous Tissue Substitute, Percutaneous Endoscopic Approach
ØRGL4JZ Fusion of Right Elbow Joint with Synthetic Substitute, Percutaneous Endoscopic Approach
ØRGL4KZ Fusion of Right Elbow Joint with Nonautologous Tissue Substitute, Percutaneous Endoscopic Approach
ØRGMØ3Z Fusion of Left Elbow Joint with Sustained Compression Internal Fixation Device, Open Approach
ØRGMØ4Z Fusion of Left Elbow Joint with Internal Fixation Device, Open Approach
ØRGMØ5Z Fusion of Left Elbow Joint with External Fixation Device, Open Approach
ØRGMØ7Z Fusion of Left Elbow Joint with Autologous Tissue Substitute, Open Approach
ØRGMØJZ Fusion of Left Elbow Joint with Synthetic Substitute, Open Approach
ØRGMØKZ Fusion of Left Elbow Joint with Nonautologous Tissue Substitute, Open Approach
ØRGM33Z Fusion of Left Elbow Joint with Sustained Compression Internal Fixation Device, Percutaneous Approach
ØRGM34Z Fusion of Left Elbow Joint with Internal Fixation Device, Percutaneous Approach
ØRGM35Z Fusion of Left Elbow Joint with External Fixation Device, Percutaneous Approach
ØRGM37Z Fusion of Left Elbow Joint with Autologous Tissue Substitute, Percutaneous Approach
ØRGM3JZ Fusion of Left Elbow Joint with Synthetic Substitute, Percutaneous Approach
ØRGM3KZ Fusion of Left Elbow Joint with Nonautologous Tissue Substitute, Percutaneous Approach
ØRGM43Z Fusion of Left Elbow Joint with Sustained Compression Internal Fixation Device, Percutaneous Endoscopic Approach
ØRGM44Z Fusion of Left Elbow Joint with Internal Fixation Device, Percutaneous Endoscopic Approach
ØRGM45Z Fusion of Left Elbow Joint with External Fixation Device, Percutaneous Endoscopic Approach
ØRGM47Z Fusion of Left Elbow Joint with Autologous Tissue Substitute, Percutaneous Endoscopic Approach
ØRGM4JZ Fusion of Left Elbow Joint with Synthetic Substitute, Percutaneous Endoscopic Approach

HAC 12: Surgical Site Infection-Certain Orthopedic Procedures of the Spine, Shoulder, and Elbow (continued)

ØRGM4KZ Fusion of Left Elbow Joint with Nonautologous Tissue Substitute, Percutaneous Endoscopic Approach
ØRQEØZZ Repair Right Sternoclavicular Joint, Open Approach
ØRQE3ZZ Repair Right Sternoclavicular Joint, Percutaneous Approach
ØRQE4ZZ Repair Right Sternoclavicular Joint, Percutaneous Endoscopic Approach
ØRQEXZZ Repair Right Sternoclavicular Joint, External Approach
ØRQFØZZ Repair Left Sternoclavicular Joint, Open Approach
ØRQF3ZZ Repair Left Sternoclavicular Joint, Percutaneous Approach
ØRQF4ZZ Repair Left Sternoclavicular Joint, Percutaneous Endoscopic Approach
ØRQFXZZ Repair Left Sternoclavicular Joint, External Approach
ØRQGØZZ Repair Right Acromioclavicular Joint, Open Approach
ØRQG3ZZ Repair Right Acromioclavicular Joint, Percutaneous Approach
ØRQG4ZZ Repair Right Acromioclavicular Joint, Percutaneous Endoscopic Approach
ØRQGXZZ Repair Right Acromioclavicular Joint, External Approach
ØRQHØZZ Repair Left Acromioclavicular Joint, Open Approach
ØRQH3ZZ Repair Left Acromioclavicular Joint, Percutaneous Approach
ØRQH4ZZ Repair Left Acromioclavicular Joint, Percutaneous Endoscopic Approach
ØRQHXZZ Repair Left Acromioclavicular Joint, External Approach
ØRQJØZZ Repair Right Shoulder Joint, Open Approach
ØRQJ3ZZ Repair Right Shoulder Joint, Percutaneous Approach
ØRQJ4ZZ Repair Right Shoulder Joint, Percutaneous Endoscopic Approach
ØRQJXZZ Repair Right Shoulder Joint, External Approach
ØRQKØZZ Repair Left Shoulder Joint, Open Approach
ØRQK3ZZ Repair Left Shoulder Joint, Percutaneous Approach
ØRQK4ZZ Repair Left Shoulder Joint, Percutaneous Endoscopic Approach
ØRQKXZZ Repair Left Shoulder Joint, External Approach
ØRQLØZZ Repair Right Elbow Joint, Open Approach
ØRQL3ZZ Repair Right Elbow Joint, Percutaneous Approach
ØRQL4ZZ Repair Right Elbow Joint, Percutaneous Endoscopic Approach
ØRQLXZZ Repair Right Elbow Joint, External Approach
ØRQMØZZ Repair Left Elbow Joint, Open Approach
ØRQM3ZZ Repair Left Elbow Joint, Percutaneous Approach
ØRQM4ZZ Repair Left Elbow Joint, Percutaneous Endoscopic Approach
ØRQMXZZ Repair Left Elbow Joint, External Approach
ØRUEØ7Z Supplement Right Sternoclavicular Joint with Autologous Tissue Substitute, Open Approach
ØRUEØJZ Supplement Right Sternoclavicular Joint with Synthetic Substitute, Open Approach
ØRUEØKZ Supplement Right Sternoclavicular Joint with Nonautologous Tissue Substitute, Open Approach
ØRUE37Z Supplement Right Sternoclavicular Joint with Autologous Tissue Substitute, Percutaneous Approach
ØRUE3JZ Supplement Right Sternoclavicular Joint with Synthetic Substitute, Percutaneous Approach
ØRUE3KZ Supplement Right Sternoclavicular Joint with Nonautologous Tissue Substitute, Percutaneous Approach
ØRUE47Z Supplement Right Sternoclavicular Joint with Autologous Tissue Substitute, Percutaneous Endoscopic Approach
ØRUE4JZ Supplement Right Sternoclavicular Joint with Synthetic Substitute, Percutaneous Endoscopic Approach
ØRUE4KZ Supplement Right Sternoclavicular Joint with Nonautologous Tissue Substitute, Percutaneous Endoscopic Approach
ØRUFØ7Z Supplement Left Sternoclavicular Joint with Autologous Tissue Substitute, Open Approach
ØRUFØJZ Supplement Left Sternoclavicular Joint with Synthetic Substitute, Open Approach
ØRUFØKZ Supplement Left Sternoclavicular Joint with Nonautologous Tissue Substitute, Open Approach
ØRUF37Z Supplement Left Sternoclavicular Joint with Autologous Tissue Substitute, Percutaneous Approach
ØRUF3JZ Supplement Left Sternoclavicular Joint with Synthetic Substitute, Percutaneous Approach
ØRUF3KZ Supplement Left Sternoclavicular Joint with Nonautologous Tissue Substitute, Percutaneous Approach
ØRUF47Z Supplement Left Sternoclavicular Joint with Autologous Tissue Substitute, Percutaneous Endoscopic Approach
ØRUF4JZ Supplement Left Sternoclavicular Joint with Synthetic Substitute, Percutaneous Endoscopic Approach
ØRUF4KZ Supplement Left Sternoclavicular Joint with Nonautologous Tissue Substitute, Percutaneous Endoscopic Approach
ØRUGØ7Z Supplement Right Acromioclavicular Joint with Autologous Tissue Substitute, Open Approach
ØRUGØJZ Supplement Right Acromioclavicular Joint with Synthetic Substitute, Open Approach
ØRUGØKZ Supplement Right Acromioclavicular Joint with Nonautologous Tissue Substitute, Open Approach
ØRUG37Z Supplement Right Acromioclavicular Joint with Autologous Tissue Substitute, Percutaneous Approach
ØRUG3JZ Supplement Right Acromioclavicular Joint with Synthetic Substitute, Percutaneous Approach
ØRUG3KZ Supplement Right Acromioclavicular Joint with Nonautologous Tissue Substitute, Percutaneous Approach
ØRUG47Z Supplement Right Acromioclavicular Joint with Autologous Tissue Substitute, Percutaneous Endoscopic Approach
ØRUG4JZ Supplement Right Acromioclavicular Joint with Synthetic Substitute, Percutaneous Endoscopic Approach
ØRUG4KZ Supplement Right Acromioclavicular Joint with Nonautologous Tissue Substitute, Percutaneous Endoscopic Approach
ØRUHØ7Z Supplement Left Acromioclavicular Joint with Autologous Tissue Substitute, Open Approach
ØRUHØJZ Supplement Left Acromioclavicular Joint with Synthetic Substitute, Open Approach
ØRUHØKZ Supplement Left Acromioclavicular Joint with Nonautologous Tissue Substitute, Open Approach
ØRUH37Z Supplement Left Acromioclavicular Joint with Autologous Tissue Substitute, Percutaneous Approach
ØRUH3JZ Supplement Left Acromioclavicular Joint with Synthetic Substitute, Percutaneous Approach
ØRUH3KZ Supplement Left Acromioclavicular Joint with Nonautologous Tissue Substitute, Percutaneous Approach
ØRUH47Z Supplement Left Acromioclavicular Joint with Autologous Tissue Substitute, Percutaneous Endoscopic Approach
ØRUH4JZ Supplement Left Acromioclavicular Joint with Synthetic Substitute, Percutaneous Endoscopic Approach
ØRUH4KZ Supplement Left Acromioclavicular Joint with Nonautologous Tissue Substitute, Percutaneous Endoscopic Approach
ØRUJØ7Z Supplement Right Shoulder Joint with Autologous Tissue Substitute, Open Approach
ØRUJØJZ Supplement Right Shoulder Joint with Synthetic Substitute, Open Approach
ØRUJØKZ Supplement Right Shoulder Joint with Nonautologous Tissue Substitute, Open Approach
ØRUJ37Z Supplement Right Shoulder Joint with Autologous Tissue Substitute, Percutaneous Approach
ØRUJ3JZ Supplement Right Shoulder Joint with Synthetic Substitute, Percutaneous Approach
ØRUJ3KZ Supplement Right Shoulder Joint with Nonautologous Tissue Substitute, Percutaneous Approach
ØRUJ47Z Supplement Right Shoulder Joint with Autologous Tissue Substitute, Percutaneous Endoscopic Approach
ØRUJ4JZ Supplement Right Shoulder Joint with Synthetic Substitute, Percutaneous Endoscopic Approach
ØRUJ4KZ Supplement Right Shoulder Joint with Nonautologous Tissue Substitute, Percutaneous Endoscopic Approach
ØRUKØ7Z Supplement Left Shoulder Joint with Autologous Tissue Substitute, Open Approach
ØRUKØJZ Supplement Left Shoulder Joint with Synthetic Substitute, Open Approach
ØRUKØKZ Supplement Left Shoulder Joint with Nonautologous Tissue Substitute, Open Approach
ØRUK37Z Supplement Left Shoulder Joint with Autologous Tissue Substitute, Percutaneous Approach
ØRUK3JZ Supplement Left Shoulder Joint with Synthetic Substitute, Percutaneous Approach
ØRUK3KZ Supplement Left Shoulder Joint with Nonautologous Tissue Substitute, Percutaneous Approach
ØRUK47Z Supplement Left Shoulder Joint with Autologous Tissue Substitute, Percutaneous Endoscopic Approach
ØRUK4JZ Supplement Left Shoulder Joint with Synthetic Substitute, Percutaneous Endoscopic Approach
ØRUK4KZ Supplement Left Shoulder Joint with Nonautologous Tissue Substitute, Percutaneous Endoscopic Approach
ØRULØ7Z Supplement Right Elbow Joint with Autologous Tissue Substitute, Open Approach

HAC 12: Surgical Site Infection-Certain Orthopedic Procedures of the Spine, Shoulder, and Elbow (continued)

ØRULØJZ Supplement Right Elbow Joint with Synthetic Substitute, Open Approach
ØRULØKZ Supplement Right Elbow Joint with Nonautologous Tissue Substitute, Open Approach
ØRUL37Z Supplement Right Elbow Joint with Autologous Tissue Substitute, Percutaneous Approach
ØRUL3JZ Supplement Right Elbow Joint with Synthetic Substitute, Percutaneous Approach
ØRUL3KZ Supplement Right Elbow Joint with Nonautologous Tissue Substitute, Percutaneous Approach
ØRUL47Z Supplement Right Elbow Joint with Autologous Tissue Substitute, Percutaneous Endoscopic Approach
ØRUL4JZ Supplement Right Elbow Joint with Synthetic Substitute, Percutaneous Endoscopic Approach
ØRUL4KZ Supplement Right Elbow Joint with Nonautologous Tissue Substitute, Percutaneous Endoscopic Approach
ØRUMØ7Z Supplement Left Elbow Joint with Autologous Tissue Substitute, Open Approach
ØRUMØJZ Supplement Left Elbow Joint with Synthetic Substitute, Open Approach
ØRUMØKZ Supplement Left Elbow Joint with Nonautologous Tissue Substitute, Open Approach
ØRUM37Z Supplement Left Elbow Joint with Autologous Tissue Substitute, Percutaneous Approach
ØRUM3JZ Supplement Left Elbow Joint with Synthetic Substitute, Percutaneous Approach
ØRUM3KZ Supplement Left Elbow Joint with Nonautologous Tissue Substitute, Percutaneous Approach
ØRUM47Z Supplement Left Elbow Joint with Autologous Tissue Substitute, Percutaneous Endoscopic Approach
ØRUM4JZ Supplement Left Elbow Joint with Synthetic Substitute, Percutaneous Endoscopic Approach
ØRUM4KZ Supplement Left Elbow Joint with Nonautologous Tissue Substitute, Percutaneous Endoscopic Approach
ØSGØØ7Ø Fusion of Lumbar Vertebral Joint with Autologous Tissue Substitute, Anterior Approach, Anterior Column, Open Approach
ØSGØØ71 Fusion of Lumbar Vertebral Joint with Autologous Tissue Substitute, Posterior Approach, Posterior Column, Open Approach
ØSGØØ7J Fusion of Lumbar Vertebral Joint with Autologous Tissue Substitute, Posterior Approach, Anterior Column, Open Approach
ØSGØØAØ Fusion of Lumbar Vertebral Joint with Interbody Fusion Device, Anterior Approach, Anterior Column, Open Approach
ØSGØØAJ Fusion of Lumbar Vertebral Joint with Interbody Fusion Device, Posterior Approach, Anterior Column, Open Approach
ØSGØØJØ Fusion of Lumbar Vertebral Joint with Synthetic Substitute, Anterior Approach, Anterior Column, Open Approach
ØSGØØJ1 Fusion of Lumbar Vertebral Joint with Synthetic Substitute, Posterior Approach, Posterior Column, Open Approach
ØSGØØJJ Fusion of Lumbar Vertebral Joint with Synthetic Substitute, Posterior Approach, Anterior Column, Open Approach
ØSGØØKØ Fusion of Lumbar Vertebral Joint with Nonautologous Tissue Substitute, Anterior Approach, Anterior Column, Open Approach
ØSGØØK1 Fusion of Lumbar Vertebral Joint with Nonautologous Tissue Substitute, Posterior Approach, Posterior Column, Open Approach
ØSGØØKJ Fusion of Lumbar Vertebral Joint with Nonautologous Tissue Substitute, Posterior Approach, Anterior Column, Open Approach
ØSGØ37Ø Fusion of Lumbar Vertebral Joint with Autologous Tissue Substitute, Anterior Approach, Anterior Column, Percutaneous Approach
ØSGØ371 Fusion of Lumbar Vertebral Joint with Autologous Tissue Substitute, Posterior Approach, Posterior Column, Percutaneous Approach
ØSGØ37J Fusion of Lumbar Vertebral Joint with Autologous Tissue Substitute, Posterior Approach, Anterior Column, Percutaneous Approach
ØSGØ3AØ Fusion of Lumbar Vertebral Joint with Interbody Fusion Device, Anterior Approach, Anterior Column, Percutaneous Approach
ØSGØ3AJ Fusion of Lumbar Vertebral Joint with Interbody Fusion Device, Posterior Approach, Anterior Column, Percutaneous Approach
ØSGØ3JØ Fusion of Lumbar Vertebral Joint with Synthetic Substitute, Anterior Approach, Anterior Column, Percutaneous Approach
ØSGØ3J1 Fusion of Lumbar Vertebral Joint with Synthetic Substitute, Posterior Approach, Posterior Column, Percutaneous Approach
ØSGØ3JJ Fusion of Lumbar Vertebral Joint with Synthetic Substitute, Posterior Approach, Anterior Column, Percutaneous Approach
ØSGØ3KØ Fusion of Lumbar Vertebral Joint with Nonautologous Tissue Substitute, Anterior Approach, Anterior Column, Percutaneous Approach
ØSGØ3K1 Fusion of Lumbar Vertebral Joint with Nonautologous Tissue Substitute, Posterior Approach, Posterior Column, Percutaneous Approach
ØSGØ3KJ Fusion of Lumbar Vertebral Joint with Nonautologous Tissue Substitute, Posterior Approach, Anterior Column, Percutaneous Approach
ØSGØ47Ø Fusion of Lumbar Vertebral Joint with Autologous Tissue Substitute, Anterior Approach, Anterior Column, Percutaneous Endoscopic Approach
ØSGØ471 Fusion of Lumbar Vertebral Joint with Autologous Tissue Substitute, Posterior Approach, Posterior Column, Percutaneous Endoscopic Approach
ØSGØ47J Fusion of Lumbar Vertebral Joint with Autologous Tissue Substitute, Posterior Approach, Anterior Column, Percutaneous Endoscopic Approach
ØSGØ4AØ Fusion of Lumbar Vertebral Joint with Interbody Fusion Device, Anterior Approach, Anterior Column, Percutaneous Endoscopic Approach
ØSGØ4AJ Fusion of Lumbar Vertebral Joint with Interbody Fusion Device, Posterior Approach, Anterior Column, Percutaneous Endoscopic Approach
ØSGØ4JØ Fusion of Lumbar Vertebral Joint with Synthetic Substitute, Anterior Approach, Anterior Column, Percutaneous Endoscopic Approach
ØSGØ4J1 Fusion of Lumbar Vertebral Joint with Synthetic Substitute, Posterior Approach, Posterior Column, Percutaneous Endoscopic Approach
ØSGØ4JJ Fusion of Lumbar Vertebral Joint with Synthetic Substitute, Posterior Approach, Anterior Column, Percutaneous Endoscopic Approach
ØSGØ4KØ Fusion of Lumbar Vertebral Joint with Nonautologous Tissue Substitute, Anterior Approach, Anterior Column, Percutaneous Endoscopic Approach
ØSGØ4K1 Fusion of Lumbar Vertebral Joint with Nonautologous Tissue Substitute, Posterior Approach, Posterior Column, Percutaneous Endoscopic Approach
ØSGØ4KJ Fusion of Lumbar Vertebral Joint with Nonautologous Tissue Substitute, Posterior Approach, Anterior Column, Percutaneous Endoscopic Approach
ØSG1Ø7Ø Fusion of 2 or More Lumbar Vertebral Joints with Autologous Tissue Substitute, Anterior Approach, Anterior Column, Open Approach
ØSG1Ø71 Fusion of 2 or More Lumbar Vertebral Joints with Autologous Tissue Substitute, Posterior Approach, Posterior Column, Open Approach
ØSG1Ø7J Fusion of 2 or More Lumbar Vertebral Joints with Autologous Tissue Substitute, Posterior Approach, Anterior Column, Open Approach
ØSG1ØAØ Fusion of 2 or More Lumbar Vertebral Joints with Interbody Fusion Device, Anterior Approach, Anterior Column, Open Approach
ØSG1ØAJ Fusion of 2 or More Lumbar Vertebral Joints with Interbody Fusion Device, Posterior Approach, Anterior Column, Open Approach
ØSG1ØJØ Fusion of 2 or More Lumbar Vertebral Joints with Synthetic Substitute, Anterior Approach, Anterior Column, Open Approach
ØSG1ØJ1 Fusion of 2 or More Lumbar Vertebral Joints with Synthetic Substitute, Posterior Approach, Posterior Column, Open Approach
ØSG1ØJJ Fusion of 2 or More Lumbar Vertebral Joints with Synthetic Substitute, Posterior Approach, Anterior Column, Open Approach
ØSG1ØKØ Fusion of 2 or More Lumbar Vertebral Joints with Nonautologous Tissue Substitute, Anterior Approach, Anterior Column, Open Approach
ØSG1ØK1 Fusion of 2 or More Lumbar Vertebral Joints with Nonautologous Tissue Substitute, Posterior Approach, Posterior Column, Open Approach
ØSG1ØKJ Fusion of 2 or More Lumbar Vertebral Joints with Nonautologous Tissue Substitute, Posterior Approach, Anterior Column, Open Approach
ØSG137Ø Fusion of 2 or More Lumbar Vertebral Joints with Autologous Tissue Substitute, Anterior Approach, Anterior Column, Percutaneous Approach

HAC 12: Surgical Site Infection-Certain Orthopedic Procedures of the Spine, Shoulder, and Elbow (continued)

ØSG1371 Fusion of 2 or More Lumbar Vertebral Joints with Autologous Tissue Substitute, Posterior Approach, Posterior Column, Percutaneous Approach
ØSG137J Fusion of 2 or More Lumbar Vertebral Joints with Autologous Tissue Substitute, Posterior Approach, Anterior Column, Percutaneous Approach
ØSG13AØ Fusion of 2 or More Lumbar Vertebral Joints with Interbody Fusion Device, Anterior Approach, Anterior Column, Percutaneous Approach
ØSG13AJ Fusion of 2 or More Lumbar Vertebral Joints with Interbody Fusion Device, Posterior Approach, Anterior Column, Percutaneous Approach
ØSG13JØ Fusion of 2 or More Lumbar Vertebral Joints with Synthetic Substitute, Anterior Approach, Anterior Column, Percutaneous Approach
ØSG13J1 Fusion of 2 or More Lumbar Vertebral Joints with Synthetic Substitute, Posterior Approach, Posterior Column, Percutaneous Approach
ØSG13JJ Fusion of 2 or More Lumbar Vertebral Joints with Synthetic Substitute, Posterior Approach, Anterior Column, Percutaneous Approach
ØSG13KØ Fusion of 2 or More Lumbar Vertebral Joints with Nonautologous Tissue Substitute, Anterior Approach, Anterior Column, Percutaneous Approach
ØSG13K1 Fusion of 2 or More Lumbar Vertebral Joints with Nonautologous Tissue Substitute, Posterior Approach, Posterior Column, Percutaneous Approach
ØSG13KJ Fusion of 2 or More Lumbar Vertebral Joints with Nonautologous Tissue Substitute, Posterior Approach, Anterior Column, Percutaneous Approach
ØSG147Ø Fusion of 2 or More Lumbar Vertebral Joints with Autologous Tissue Substitute, Anterior Approach, Anterior Column, Percutaneous Endoscopic Approach
ØSG1471 Fusion of 2 or More Lumbar Vertebral Joints with Autologous Tissue Substitute, Posterior Approach, Posterior Column, Percutaneous Endoscopic Approach
ØSG147J Fusion of 2 or More Lumbar Vertebral Joints with Autologous Tissue Substitute, Posterior Approach, Anterior Column, Percutaneous Endoscopic Approach
ØSG14AØ Fusion of 2 or More Lumbar Vertebral Joints with Interbody Fusion Device, Anterior Approach, Anterior Column, Percutaneous Endoscopic Approach
ØSG14AJ Fusion of 2 or More Lumbar Vertebral Joints with Interbody Fusion Device, Posterior Approach, Anterior Column, Percutaneous Endoscopic Approach
ØSG14JØ Fusion of 2 or More Lumbar Vertebral Joints with Synthetic Substitute, Anterior Approach, Anterior Column, Percutaneous Endoscopic Approach
ØSG14J1 Fusion of 2 or More Lumbar Vertebral Joints with Synthetic Substitute, Posterior Approach, Posterior Column, Percutaneous Endoscopic Approach
ØSG14JJ Fusion of 2 or More Lumbar Vertebral Joints with Synthetic Substitute, Posterior Approach, Anterior Column, Percutaneous Endoscopic Approach
ØSG14KØ Fusion of 2 or More Lumbar Vertebral Joints with Nonautologous Tissue Substitute, Anterior Approach, Anterior Column, Percutaneous Endoscopic Approach
ØSG14K1 Fusion of 2 or More Lumbar Vertebral Joints with Nonautologous Tissue Substitute, Posterior Approach, Posterior Column, Percutaneous Endoscopic Approach
ØSG14KJ Fusion of 2 or More Lumbar Vertebral Joints with Nonautologous Tissue Substitute, Posterior Approach, Anterior Column, Percutaneous Endoscopic Approach
ØSG307Ø Fusion of Lumbosacral Joint with Autologous Tissue Substitute, Anterior Approach, Anterior Column, Open Approach
ØSG3Ø71 Fusion of Lumbosacral Joint with Autologous Tissue Substitute, Posterior Approach, Posterior Column, Open Approach
ØSG3Ø7J Fusion of Lumbosacral Joint with Autologous Tissue Substitute, Posterior Approach, Anterior Column, Open Approach
ØSG3ØAØ Fusion of Lumbosacral Joint with Interbody Fusion Device, Anterior Approach, Anterior Column, Open Approach
ØSG3ØAJ Fusion of Lumbosacral Joint with Interbody Fusion Device, Posterior Approach, Anterior Column, Open Approach
ØSG3ØJØ Fusion of Lumbosacral Joint with Synthetic Substitute, Anterior Approach, Anterior Column, Open Approach
ØSG3ØJ1 Fusion of Lumbosacral Joint with Synthetic Substitute, Posterior Approach, Posterior Column, Open Approach
ØSG3ØJJ Fusion of Lumbosacral Joint with Synthetic Substitute, Posterior Approach, Anterior Column, Open Approach
ØSG3ØKØ Fusion of Lumbosacral Joint with Nonautologous Tissue Substitute, Anterior Approach, Anterior Column, Open Approach
ØSG3ØK1 Fusion of Lumbosacral Joint with Nonautologous Tissue Substitute, Posterior Approach, Posterior Column, Open Approach
ØSG3ØKJ Fusion of Lumbosacral Joint with Nonautologous Tissue Substitute, Posterior Approach, Anterior Column, Open Approach
ØSG337Ø Fusion of Lumbosacral Joint with Autologous Tissue Substitute, Anterior Approach, Anterior Column, Percutaneous Approach
ØSG3371 Fusion of Lumbosacral Joint with Autologous Tissue Substitute, Posterior Approach, Posterior Column, Percutaneous Approach
ØSG337J Fusion of Lumbosacral Joint with Autologous Tissue Substitute, Posterior Approach, Anterior Column, Percutaneous Approach
ØSG33AØ Fusion of Lumbosacral Joint with Interbody Fusion Device, Anterior Approach, Anterior Column, Percutaneous Approach
ØSG33AJ Fusion of Lumbosacral Joint with Interbody Fusion Device, Posterior Approach, Anterior Column, Percutaneous Approach
ØSG33JØ Fusion of Lumbosacral Joint with Synthetic Substitute, Anterior Approach, Anterior Column, Percutaneous Approach
ØSG33J1 Fusion of Lumbosacral Joint with Synthetic Substitute, Posterior Approach, Posterior Column, Percutaneous Approach
ØSG33JJ Fusion of Lumbosacral Joint with Synthetic Substitute, Posterior Approach, Anterior Column, Percutaneous Approach
ØSG33KØ Fusion of Lumbosacral Joint with Nonautologous Tissue Substitute, Anterior Approach, Anterior Column, Percutaneous Approach
ØSG33K1 Fusion of Lumbosacral Joint with Nonautologous Tissue Substitute, Posterior Approach, Posterior Column, Percutaneous Approach
ØSG33KJ Fusion of Lumbosacral Joint with Nonautologous Tissue Substitute, Posterior Approach, Anterior Column, Percutaneous Approach
ØSG347Ø Fusion of Lumbosacral Joint with Autologous Tissue Substitute, Anterior Approach, Anterior Column, Percutaneous Endoscopic Approach
ØSG3471 Fusion of Lumbosacral Joint with Autologous Tissue Substitute, Posterior Approach, Posterior Column, Percutaneous Endoscopic Approach
ØSG347J Fusion of Lumbosacral Joint with Autologous Tissue Substitute, Posterior Approach, Anterior Column, Percutaneous Endoscopic Approach
ØSG34AØ Fusion of Lumbosacral Joint with Interbody Fusion Device, Anterior Approach, Anterior Column, Percutaneous Endoscopic Approach
ØSG34AJ Fusion of Lumbosacral Joint with Interbody Fusion Device, Posterior Approach, Anterior Column, Percutaneous Endoscopic Approach
ØSG34JØ Fusion of Lumbosacral Joint with Synthetic Substitute, Anterior Approach, Anterior Column, Percutaneous Endoscopic Approach
ØSG34J1 Fusion of Lumbosacral Joint with Synthetic Substitute, Posterior Approach, Posterior Column, Percutaneous Endoscopic Approach
ØSG34JJ Fusion of Lumbosacral Joint with Synthetic Substitute, Posterior Approach, Anterior Column, Percutaneous Endoscopic Approach
ØSG34KØ Fusion of Lumbosacral Joint with Nonautologous Tissue Substitute, Anterior Approach, Anterior Column, Percutaneous Endoscopic Approach
ØSG34K1 Fusion of Lumbosacral Joint with Nonautologous Tissue Substitute, Posterior Approach, Posterior Column, Percutaneous Endoscopic Approach
ØSG34KJ Fusion of Lumbosacral Joint with Nonautologous Tissue Substitute, Posterior Approach, Anterior Column, Percutaneous Endoscopic Approach
ØSG7Ø4Z Fusion of Right Sacroiliac Joint with Internal Fixation Device, Open Approach
ØSG7Ø7Z Fusion of Right Sacroiliac Joint with Autologous Tissue Substitute, Open Approach
ØSG7ØJZ Fusion of Right Sacroiliac Joint with Synthetic Substitute, Open Approach
ØSG7ØKZ Fusion of Right Sacroiliac Joint with Nonautologous Tissue Substitute, Open Approach

HAC 12: Surgical Site Infection-Certain Orthopedic Procedures of the Spine, Shoulder, and Elbow (continued)

ØSG734Z Fusion of Right Sacroiliac Joint with Internal Fixation Device, Percutaneous Approach
ØSG737Z Fusion of Right Sacroiliac Joint with Autologous Tissue Substitute, Percutaneous Approach
ØSG73JZ Fusion of Right Sacroiliac Joint with Synthetic Substitute, Percutaneous Approach
ØSG73KZ Fusion of Right Sacroiliac Joint with Nonautologous Tissue Substitute, Percutaneous Approach
ØSG744Z Fusion of Right Sacroiliac Joint with Internal Fixation Device, Percutaneous Endoscopic Approach
ØSG747Z Fusion of Right Sacroiliac Joint with Autologous Tissue Substitute, Percutaneous Endoscopic Approach
ØSG74JZ Fusion of Right Sacroiliac Joint with Synthetic Substitute, Percutaneous Endoscopic Approach
ØSG74KZ Fusion of Right Sacroiliac Joint with Nonautologous Tissue Substitute, Percutaneous Endoscopic Approach
ØSG8Ø4Z Fusion of Left Sacroiliac Joint with Internal Fixation Device, Open Approach
ØSG8Ø7Z Fusion of Left Sacroiliac Joint with Autologous Tissue Substitute, Open Approach
ØSG8ØJZ Fusion of Left Sacroiliac Joint with Synthetic Substitute, Open Approach
ØSG8ØKZ Fusion of Left Sacroiliac Joint with Nonautologous Tissue Substitute, Open Approach
ØSG834Z Fusion of Left Sacroiliac Joint with Internal Fixation Device, Percutaneous Approach
ØSG837Z Fusion of Left Sacroiliac Joint with Autologous Tissue Substitute, Percutaneous Approach
ØSG83JZ Fusion of Left Sacroiliac Joint with Synthetic Substitute, Percutaneous Approach
ØSG83KZ Fusion of Left Sacroiliac Joint with Nonautologous Tissue Substitute, Percutaneous Approach
ØSG844Z Fusion of Left Sacroiliac Joint with Internal Fixation Device, Percutaneous Endoscopic Approach
ØSG847Z Fusion of Left Sacroiliac Joint with Autologous Tissue Substitute, Percutaneous Endoscopic Approach
ØSG84JZ Fusion of Left Sacroiliac Joint with Synthetic Substitute, Percutaneous Endoscopic Approach
ØSG84KZ Fusion of Left Sacroiliac Joint with Nonautologous Tissue Substitute, Percutaneous Endoscopic Approach
XRGAØR7 Fusion of Thoracolumbar Vertebral Joint using Customizable Interbody Fusion Device, Open Approach, New Technology Group 7
XRGA3R7 Fusion of Thoracolumbar Vertebral Joint using Customizable Interbody Fusion Device, Percutaneous Approach, New Technology Group 7
XRGA4R7 Fusion of Thoracolumbar Vertebral Joint using Customizable Interbody Fusion Device, Percutaneous Endoscopic Approach, New Technology Group 7
XRGBØR7 Fusion of Lumbar Vertebral Joint using Customizable Interbody Fusion Device, Open Approach, New Technology Group 7
XRGB3R7 Fusion of Lumbar Vertebral Joint using Customizable Interbody Fusion Device, Percutaneous Approach, New Technology Group 7
XRGB4R7 Fusion of Lumbar Vertebral Joint using Customizable Interbody Fusion Device, Percutaneous Endoscopic Approach, New Technology Group 7
XRGCØR7 Fusion of 2 or more Lumbar Vertebral Joints using Customizable Interbody Fusion Device, Open Approach, New Technology Group 7
XRGC3R7 Fusion of 2 or more Lumbar Vertebral Joints using Customizable Interbody Fusion Device, Percutaneous Approach, New Technology Group 7
XRGC4R7 Fusion of 2 or more Lumbar Vertebral Joints using Customizable Interbody Fusion Device, Percutaneous Endoscopic Approach, New Technology Group 7
XRGDØR7 Fusion of Lumbosacral Joint using Customizable Interbody Fusion Device, Open Approach, New Technology Group 7
XRGD3R7 Fusion of Lumbosacral Joint using Customizable Interbody Fusion Device, Percutaneous Approach, New Technology Group 7
XRGD4R7 Fusion of Lumbosacral Joint using Customizable Interbody Fusion Device, Percutaneous Endoscopic Approach, New Technology Group 7
XRGEØ58 Fusion of Right Sacroiliac Joint using Internal Fixation Device with Tulip Connector, Open Approach, New Technology Group 8
XRGE358 Fusion of Right Sacroiliac Joint using Internal Fixation Device with Tulip Connector, Percutaneous Approach, New Technology Group 8
XRGFØ58 Fusion of Left Sacroiliac Joint using Internal Fixation Device with Tulip Connector, Open Approach, New Technology Group 8
XRGF358 Fusion of Left Sacroiliac Joint using Internal Fixation Device with Tulip Connector, Percutaneous Approach, New Technology Group 8

HAC 13: Surgical Site Infection (SSI) Following Cardiac Implantable Electronic Device (CIED) Procedures

Secondary diagnosis not POA:
K68.11 Postprocedural retroperitoneal abscess
T81.40XA Infection following a procedure, unspecified, initial encounter
T81.41XA Infection following a procedure, superficial incisional surgical site, initial encounter
T81.42XA Infection following a procedure, deep incisional surgical site, initial encounter
T81.43XA Infection following a procedure, organ and space surgical site, initial encounter
T81.44XA Sepsis following a procedure, initial encounter
T81.49XA Infection following a procedure, other surgical site, initial encounter
T82.7XXA Infection and inflammatory reaction due to other internal orthopedic prosthetic devices, implants and grafts, initial encounter

AND

Any of the following procedures:
Ø2H43JZ Insertion of Pacemaker Lead into Coronary Vein, Percutaneous Approach
Ø2H43KZ Insertion of Defibrillator Lead into Coronary Vein, Percutaneous Approach
Ø2H43MZ Insertion of Cardiac Lead into Coronary Vein, Percutaneous Approach
Ø2H63JZ Insertion of Pacemaker Lead into Right Atrium, Percutaneous Approach
Ø2H63MZ Insertion of Cardiac Lead into Right Atrium, Percutaneous Approach
Ø2H73JZ Insertion of Pacemaker Lead into Left Atrium, Percutaneous Approach
Ø2H73MZ Insertion of Cardiac Lead into Left Atrium, Percutaneous Approach
Ø2HK3JZ Insertion of Pacemaker Lead into Right Ventricle, Percutaneous Approach
Ø2HL3JZ Insertion of Pacemaker Lead into Left Ventricle, Percutaneous Approach
Ø2HNØJZ Insertion of Pacemaker Lead into Pericardium, Open Approach
Ø2HNØMZ Insertion of Cardiac Lead into Pericardium, Open Approach
Ø2HN3JZ Insertion of Pacemaker Lead into Pericardium, Percutaneous Approach
Ø2HN3MZ Insertion of Cardiac Lead into Pericardium, Percutaneous Approach
Ø2HN4JZ Insertion of Pacemaker Lead into Pericardium, Percutaneous Endoscopic Approach
Ø2HN4MZ Insertion of Cardiac Lead into Pericardium, Percutaneous Endoscopic Approach
Ø2PAØMZ Removal of Cardiac Lead from Heart, Open Approach
Ø2PA3MZ Removal of Cardiac Lead from Heart, Percutaneous Approach
Ø2PA4MZ Removal of Cardiac Lead from Heart, Percutaneous Endoscopic Approach
Ø2PAXMZ Removal of Cardiac Lead from Heart, External Approach
Ø2WAØMZ Revision of Cardiac Lead in Heart, Open Approach
Ø2WA3MZ Revision of Cardiac Lead in Heart, Percutaneous Approach
Ø2WA4MZ Revision of Cardiac Lead in Heart, Percutaneous Endoscopic Approach
ØJH6Ø4Z Insertion of Pacemaker, Single Chamber into Chest Subcutaneous Tissue and Fascia, Open Approach
ØJH6Ø5Z Insertion of Pacemaker, Single Chamber Rate Responsive into Chest Subcutaneous Tissue and Fascia, Open Approach
ØJH6Ø6Z Insertion of Pacemaker, Dual Chamber into Chest Subcutaneous Tissue and Fascia, Open Approach
ØJH6Ø7Z Insertion of Cardiac Resynchronization Pacemaker Pulse Generator into Chest Subcutaneous Tissue and Fascia, Open Approach
ØJH6Ø8Z Insertion of Defibrillator Generator into Chest Subcutaneous Tissue and Fascia, Open Approach
ØJH6Ø9Z Insertion of Cardiac Resynchronization Defibrillator Pulse Generator into Chest Subcutaneous Tissue and Fascia, Open Approach
ØJH6ØPZ Insertion of Cardiac Rhythm Related Device into Chest Subcutaneous Tissue and Fascia, Open Approach
ØJH634Z Insertion of Pacemaker, Single Chamber into Chest Subcutaneous Tissue and Fascia, Percutaneous Approach
ØJH635Z Insertion of Pacemaker, Single Chamber Rate Responsive into Chest Subcutaneous Tissue and Fascia, Percutaneous Approach
ØJH636Z Insertion of Pacemaker, Dual Chamber into Chest Subcutaneous Tissue and Fascia, Percutaneous Approach

HAC 13: Surgical Site Infection (SSI) Following Cardiac Implantable Electronic Device (CIED) Procedures (continued)

ØJH637Z Insertion of Cardiac Resynchronization Pacemaker Pulse Generator into Chest Subcutaneous Tissue and Fascia, Percutaneous Approach
ØJH638Z Insertion of Defibrillator Generator into Chest Subcutaneous Tissue and Fascia, Percutaneous Approach
ØJH639Z Insertion of Cardiac Resynchronization Defibrillator Pulse Generator into Chest Subcutaneous Tissue and Fascia, Percutaneous Approach
ØJH63PZ Insertion of Cardiac Rhythm Related Device into Chest Subcutaneous Tissue and Fascia, Percutaneous Approach
ØJH8Ø4Z Insertion of Pacemaker, Single Chamber into Abdomen Subcutaneous Tissue and Fascia, Open Approach
ØJH8Ø5Z Insertion of Pacemaker, Single Chamber Rate Responsive into Abdomen Subcutaneous Tissue and Fascia, Open Approach
ØJH8Ø6Z Insertion of Pacemaker, Dual Chamber into Abdomen Subcutaneous Tissue and Fascia, Open Approach
ØJH8Ø7Z Insertion of Cardiac Resynchronization Pacemaker Pulse Generator into Abdomen Subcutaneous Tissue and Fascia, Open Approach
ØJH8Ø8Z Insertion of Defibrillator Generator into Abdomen Subcutaneous Tissue and Fascia, Open Approach
ØJH8Ø9Z Insertion of Cardiac Resynchronization Defibrillator Pulse Generator into Abdomen Subcutaneous Tissue and Fascia, Open Approach
ØJH8ØPZ Insertion of Cardiac Rhythm Related Device into Abdomen Subcutaneous Tissue and Fascia, Open Approach
ØJH834Z Insertion of Pacemaker, Single Chamber into Abdomen Subcutaneous Tissue and Fascia, Percutaneous Approach
ØJH835Z Insertion of Pacemaker, Single Chamber Rate Responsive into Abdomen Subcutaneous Tissue and Fascia, Percutaneous Approach
ØJH836Z Insertion of Pacemaker, Dual Chamber into Abdomen Subcutaneous Tissue and Fascia, Percutaneous Approach
ØJH837Z Insertion of Cardiac Resynchronization Pacemaker Pulse Generator into Abdomen Subcutaneous Tissue and Fascia, Percutaneous Approach
ØJH838Z Insertion of Defibrillator Generator into Abdomen Subcutaneous Tissue and Fascia, Percutaneous Approach
ØJH839Z Insertion of Cardiac Resynchronization Defibrillator Pulse Generator into Abdomen Subcutaneous Tissue and Fascia, Percutaneous Approach
ØJH83PZ Insertion of Cardiac Rhythm Related Device into Abdomen Subcutaneous Tissue and Fascia, Percutaneous Approach
ØJPTØFZ Removal of Subcutaneous Defibrillator Lead from Trunk Subcutaneous Tissue and Fascia, Open Approach
ØJPTØPZ Removal of Cardiac Rhythm Related Device from Trunk Subcutaneous Tissue and Fascia, Open Approach
ØJPT3FZ Removal of Subcutaneous Defibrillator Lead from Trunk Subcutaneous Tissue and Fascia, Percutaneous Approach
ØJPT3PZ Removal of Cardiac Rhythm Related Device from Trunk Subcutaneous Tissue and Fascia, Percutaneous Approach
ØJWTØFZ Revision of Subcutaneous Defibrillator Lead in Trunk Subcutaneous Tissue and Fascia, Open Approach
ØJWTØPZ Revision of Cardiac Rhythm Related Device in Trunk Subcutaneous Tissue and Fascia, Open Approach
ØJWT3FZ Revision of Subcutaneous Defibrillator Lead in Trunk Subcutaneous Tissue and Fascia, Percutaneous Approach
ØJWT3PZ Revision of Cardiac Rhythm Related Device in Trunk Subcutaneous Tissue and Fascia, Percutaneous Approach

HAC 14: Iatrogenic Pneumothorax with Venous Catheterization

Secondary diagnosis not POA:
J95.811 Postprocedural pneumothorax
AND
Any of the following procedures:
Ø2H633Z Insertion of Infusion Device into Right Atrium, Percutaneous Approach
Ø2HK33Z Insertion of Infusion Device into Right Ventricle, Percutaneous Approach
Ø2HS33Z Insertion of Infusion Device into Right Pulmonary Vein, Percutaneous Approach
Ø2HS43Z Insertion of Infusion Device into Right Pulmonary Vein, Percutaneous Endoscopic Approach
Ø2HT33Z Insertion of Infusion Device into Left Pulmonary Vein, Percutaneous Approach
Ø2HT43Z Insertion of Infusion Device into Left Pulmonary Vein, Percutaneous Endoscopic Approach
Ø2HV33Z Insertion of Infusion Device into Superior Vena Cava, Percutaneous Approach
Ø2HV43Z Insertion of Infusion Device into Superior Vena Cava, Percutaneous Endoscopic Approach
Ø5HØ33Z Insertion of Infusion Device into Azygos Vein, Percutaneous Approach
Ø5HØ43Z Insertion of Infusion Device into Azygos Vein, Percutaneous Endoscopic Approach
Ø5H133Z Insertion of Infusion Device into Hemiazygos Vein, Percutaneous Approach
Ø5H143Z Insertion of Infusion Device into Hemiazygos Vein, Percutaneous Endoscopic Approach
Ø5H333Z Insertion of Infusion Device into Right Innominate Vein, Percutaneous Approach
Ø5H343Z Insertion of Infusion Device into Right Innominate Vein, Percutaneous Endoscopic Approach
Ø5H433Z Insertion of Infusion Device into Left Innominate Vein, Percutaneous Approach
Ø5H443Z Insertion of Infusion Device into Left Innominate Vein, Percutaneous Endoscopic Approach
Ø5H533Z Insertion of Infusion Device into Right Subclavian Vein, Percutaneous Approach
Ø5H543Z Insertion of Infusion Device into Right Subclavian Vein, Percutaneous Endoscopic Approach
Ø5H633Z Insertion of Infusion Device into Left Subclavian Vein, Percutaneous Approach
Ø5H643Z Insertion of Infusion Device into Left Subclavian Vein, Percutaneous Endoscopic Approach
Ø5HM33Z Insertion of Infusion Device into Right Internal Jugular Vein, Percutaneous Approach
Ø5HN33Z Insertion of Infusion Device into Left Internal Jugular Vein, Percutaneous Approach
Ø5HP33Z Insertion of Infusion Device into Right External Jugular Vein, Percutaneous Approach
Ø5HQ33Z Insertion of Infusion Device into Left External Jugular Vein, Percutaneous Approach
ØJH63XZ Insertion of Vascular Access Device into Chest Subcutaneous Tissue and Fascia, Percutaneous Approach

Appendix L: Procedure Combination Tables

The tables below were developed to help simplify the relationship between ICD-10-PCS coding and MS-DRG assignment. The Centers for Medicare & Medicaid Services (CMS) has identified in the MS-DRG Definitions Manual certain procedure combinations that must occur in order to assign a specific MS-DRG. There are many factors influencing MS-DRG assignment, including principal and secondary diagnoses, MCC or CC use, sex of the patient, and discharge status. These tables should be used only as a guide. These tables were created based on the proposed, version 40, MS-DRG Grouper software and Definitions Manual files published with the fiscal 2023 IPPS proposed rule. To view the most current files, refer to the following:
https://www.cms.gov/Medicare/Medicare-Fee-for-Service-Payment/AcuteInpatientPPS/MS-DRG-Classifications-and-Software.

DRG ØØ1-ØØ2 Heart Transplant or Implant of Heart Assist System

Heart Transplant

Replacement of Right and Left Ventricle Ø2RKØJZ and Ø2RLØJZ

Insertion With Removal of Heart Assist System

Type of Heart Assist System	Code as appropriate Insertion by approach	Code also as appropriate Removal of Heart Assist System by approach
Biventricular External	Ø2HA[Ø,3,4]RS	Ø2PA[Ø,3,4]RZ
External	Ø2HA[Ø,4]RZ	Ø2PA[Ø,3,4]RZ

Revision With Removal of Heart Assist System

Type of Heart Assist System	Code as appropriate Revision by approach	Code also as appropriate Removal of Heart Assist System by approach
Implantable	Ø2WA[Ø,3,4]QZ	Ø2PA[Ø,3,4]RZ
External	Ø2WA[Ø,3,4]RZ	Ø2PA[Ø,3,4]RZ

DRG ØØ8 Simultaneous Pancreas/Kidney Transplant

Transplanted Body Part	Code Transplant as appropriate by tissue type			Code also Pancreas Transplant as appropriate by tissue type		
	Allogeneic	Syngeneic	Zooplastic	Allogeneic	Syngeneic	Zooplastic
Kidney, Right	ØTYØØZØ	ØTYØØZ1	ØTYØØZ2	ØFYGØZØ	ØFYGØZ1	ØFYGØZ2
Kidney, Left	ØTY1ØZØ	ØTY1ØZ1	ØTY1ØZ2			

DRG Ø19 Simultaneous Pancreas/Kidney Transplant with Hemodialysis

Transplanted Body Part	Code Transplant as appropriate by tissue type			Code also Pancreas Transplant as appropriate by tissue type			Code also Hemodialysis		
	Allogeneic	Syngeneic	Zooplastic	Allogeneic	Syngeneic	Zooplastic	< 6 Hours	6-18 Hours	> 18 Hours
Kidney, Right	ØTYØØZØ	ØTYØØZ1	ØTYØØZ2	ØFYGØZØ	ØFYGØZ1	ØFYGØZ2	5A1D07Z	5A1D8ØZ	5A1D9ØZ
Kidney, Left	ØTY1ØZØ	ØTY1ØZ1	ØTY1ØZ2						

DRG Ø23-Ø27 Craniotomy

Site of Neurostimulator Lead	Code as appropriate Insertion of Lead by approach	Code also as appropriate Insertion of Device by type and subcutaneous site						
		Neuro-stimulator Generator	Stimulator Multiple Array Code as appropriate by approach			Stimulator Multiple Array, Rechargeable Code as appropriate by approach		
		Skull	Chest	Back	Abdomen	Chest	Back	Abdomen
Brain	ØØHØ[Ø,3,4]MZ	ØNHØØNZ	ØJH6[Ø,3]DZ	ØJH7[Ø,3]DZ	ØJH8[Ø,3]DZ	ØJH6[Ø,3]EZ	ØJH7[Ø,3]EZ	ØJH8[Ø,3]EZ
Cerebral Ventricle	ØØH6[Ø,3,4]MZ	ØNHØØNZ	ØJH6[Ø,3]DZ	ØJH7[Ø,3]DZ	ØJH8[Ø,3]DZ	ØJH6[Ø,3]EZ	ØJH7[Ø,3]EZ	ØJH8[Ø,3]EZ

DRG Ø28-Ø3Ø Spinal Procedures

Generator Type	Insertion of Generator by Site			Code also as appropriate Insertion of Neurostimulator Lead by approach	
	Chest	Abdomen	Back	Spinal Canal	Spinal Cord
Single Array	ØJH6[Ø,3]BZ	ØJH8[Ø,3]BZ	ØJH7[Ø,3]BZ	ØØHU[Ø,3,4]MZ	ØØHV[Ø,3,4]MZ
Single Array, Rechargeable	ØJH6[Ø,3]CZ	ØJH8[Ø,3]CZ	ØJH7[Ø,3]CZ	ØØHU[Ø,3,4]MZ	ØØHV[Ø,3,4]MZ
Multiple Array	ØJH6[Ø,3]DZ	ØJH8[Ø,3]DZ	ØJH7[Ø,3]DZ	ØØHU[Ø,3,4]MZ	ØØHV[Ø,3,4]MZ
Multiple Array, Rechargeable	ØJH6[Ø,3]EZ	—	ØJH7[Ø,3]EZ	ØØHU[Ø,3,4]MZ	ØØHV[Ø,3,4]MZ
Multiple Array, Rechargeable	—	ØJH8[Ø,3]EZ	—	ØØHU[Ø,3,4]MZ	ØØHV[Ø,3,4]MZ

DRG Ø4Ø-Ø42 Peripheral and Cranial Nerve and Other Nervous System Procedures

Insertion of Neurostimulator Generator and Lead

Insertion Single Array Generator, by Site		Code also Lead Insertion, by Site						
		Cranial Nerve	Peripheral Nerve	Azygos Vein	Innominate Vein, RT	Innominate Vein, LT	Stomach	Vagus Nerve
Chest	ØJH6[Ø,3]BZ	ØØHE[Ø,3,4]MZ	Ø1HY[Ø,3,4]MZ	Ø5HØ[Ø,3,4]MZ	Ø5H3[Ø,3,4]MZ	Ø5H4[Ø,3,4]MZ	ØDH6[Ø,3,4]MZ	XØHQ3R8
Back	ØJH7[Ø,3]BZ							
Abdomen	ØJH8[Ø,3]BZ							

Insertion Single Array, Rechargeable Generator, by Site		Code also Lead Insertion, by Site						
		Cranial Nerve	Peripheral Nerve	Azygos Vein	Innominate Vein, RT	Innominate Vein, LT	Stomach	Vagus Nerve
Chest	ØJH6[Ø,3]CZ	ØØHE[Ø,3,4]MZ	Ø1HY[Ø,3,4]MZ	Ø5HØ[Ø,3,4]MZ	Ø5H3[Ø,3,4]MZ	Ø5H4[Ø,3,4]MZ	ØDH6[Ø,3,4]MZ	XØHQ3R8
Back	ØJH7[Ø,3]CZ							
Abdomen	ØJH8[Ø,3]CZ							

Insertion Multiple Array Generator, by Site		Code also Lead Insertion, by Site						
		Cranial Nerve	Peripheral Nerve	Azygos Vein	Innominate Vein, RT	Innominate Vein, LT	Stomach	Vagus Nerve
Chest	ØJH6[Ø,3]DZ	ØØHE[Ø,3,4]MZ	Ø1HY[Ø,3,4]MZ	Ø5HØ[Ø,3,4]MZ	Ø5H3[Ø,3,4]MZ	Ø5H4[Ø,3,4]MZ	ØDH6[Ø,3,4]MZ	XØHQ3R8
Back	ØJH7[Ø,3]DZ							
Abdomen	ØJH8[Ø,3]DZ							

Insertion Multiple Array, Rechargeable Generator, by Site		Code also Lead Insertion, by Site						
		Cranial Nerve	Peripheral Nerve	Azygos Vein	Innominate Vein, RT	Innominate Vein, LT	Stomach	Vagus Nerve
Chest	ØJH6[Ø,3]EZ	ØØHE[Ø,3,4]MZ	Ø1HY[Ø,3,4]MZ	Ø5HØ[Ø,3,4]MZ	Ø5H3[Ø,3,4]MZ	Ø5H4[Ø,3,4]MZ	ØDH6[Ø,3,4]MZ	XØHQ3R8
Back	ØJH7[Ø,3]EZ							
Abdomen	ØJH8[Ø,3]EZ							

Insertion Stimulator Generator, by Site		Code also Lead Insertion, by Site						
		Cranial Nerve	Peripheral Nerve	Azygos Vein	Innominate Vein, RT	Innominate Vein, LT	Stomach	Vagus Nerve
Chest	ØJH6[Ø,3]MZ	ØØHE[Ø,3,4]MZ	Ø1HY[Ø,3,4]MZ	Ø5HØ[Ø,3,4]MZ	Ø5H3[Ø,3,4]MZ	Ø5H4[Ø,3,4]MZ	ØDH6[Ø,3,4]MZ	XØHQ3R8
Back	ØJH7[Ø,3]MZ							
Abdomen	ØJH8[Ø,3]MZ							

DRG 242-244 Permanent Cardiac Pacemaker Implant

Insertion of Generator and Lead(s) Only

Generator Type	Insertion of Generator by Site		Code also Insertion of Lead, by Site			
	Chest	Abdomen	Coronary Vein	Right Atrium (6)/Left Atrium (7)	Right Ventricle (K)/ Left Ventricle (L)	Pericardium
Single Chamber	ØJH6[Ø,3]4Z	ØJH8[Ø,3]4Z	Ø2H4[Ø,3,4][J,M]Z	Ø2H[6,7][Ø,3,4][J,M]Z	Ø2H[K,L][Ø,3,4][J,M]Z	Ø2HN[Ø,3,4][J,M]Z
Single Chamber RR	ØJH6[Ø,3]5Z	ØJH8[Ø,3]5Z	Ø2H4[Ø,3,4][J,M]Z	Ø2H[6,7][Ø,3,4][J,M]Z	Ø2H[K,L][Ø,3,4][J,M]Z	Ø2HN[Ø,3,4][J,M]Z
Dual Chamber	ØJH6[Ø,3]6Z	ØJH8[Ø,3]6Z	Ø2H4[Ø,3,4][J,M]Z	Ø2H[6,7][Ø,3,4][J,M]Z	Ø2H[K,L][Ø,3,4][J,M]Z	Ø2HN[Ø,3,4][J,M]Z
Cardiac Resynch	ØJH6[Ø,3]7Z	ØJH8[Ø,3]7Z	Ø2H4[Ø,3,4][J,M]Z	Ø2H[6,7][Ø,3,4][J,M]Z	Ø2H[K,L][Ø,3,4][J,M]Z	Ø2HN[Ø,3,4][J,M]Z
Cardiac Rhythm Related	ØJH6[Ø,3]PZ	ØJH8[Ø,3]PZ	Ø2H4[Ø,3,4][J,M]Z	Ø2H[6,7][Ø,3,4][J,M]Z	Ø2H[K,L][Ø,3,4][J,M]Z	Ø2HN[Ø,3,4][J,M]Z

DRG 275-277 Cardiac Defibrillator Implant

Insertion of Generator With Insertion of Lead(s) into Coronary Vein, Atrium or Ventricle

Generator Type	Insertion of Generator by Site		Code also as appropriate Insertion of Leads by site				
	Chest	Abdomen	Coronary Vein	Atrium		Ventricle	
				Right	Left	Right	Left
Defibrillator	ØJH6[Ø,3]8Z	ØJH8[Ø,3]8Z	Ø2H4[Ø,4]KZ	Ø2H6[Ø,3,4]KZ	Ø2H7[Ø,3,4]KZ	Ø2HK[Ø,3,4]KZ	Ø2HL[Ø,3,4]KZ
Cardiac Resynch Defibrillator Pulse Generator	ØJH6[Ø,3]9Z	ØJH8[Ø,3]9Z	Ø2H4[Ø,3,4]KZ or Ø2H43[J,M]Z	Ø2H6[Ø,3,4]KZ	Ø2H7[Ø,3,4]KZ	Ø2HK[Ø,3,4]KZ	Ø2HL[Ø,3,4]KZ
Contractility Modulation Device	ØJH6[Ø,3]AZ	ØJH8[Ø,3]AZ	—	Ø2H6[Ø,3,4]MZ	—	Ø2HK[Ø,3,4]MZ	—

Insertion of Generator with Insertion of Lead(s) into Pericardium or Chest

Generator Type	Insertion of Generator by Site		Code also as appropriate Insertion of Leads by Site and Type			
	Chest	Abdomen	Pericardium			Chest
			Pacemaker	Defibrillator	Cardiac	Subcutaneous
Defibrillator	ØJH6[Ø,3]8Z	ØJH8[Ø,3]8Z	Ø2HN[Ø,3,4]JZ	Ø2HN[Ø,3,4]KZ	Ø2HN[Ø,3,4]MZ	ØJH6[Ø,3]FZ
Cardiac Resynch Defibrillator Pulse Generator	ØJH6[Ø,3]9Z	ØJH8[Ø,3]9Z	Ø2HN[Ø,3,4]JZ	Ø2HN[Ø,3,4]KZ	Ø2HN[Ø,3,4]MZ	ØJH6[Ø,3]FZ

DRG 326-328 Stomach, Esophageal and Duodenal Procedures

Site	Resection by Open Approach	Code also as appropriate Resection of Pancreas by Open Approach
Duodenum	ØDT9ØZZ	ØFTGØZZ

DRG 344-346 Minor Small and Large Bowel Procedures

Site	Repair by Open Approach	Code also as appropriate Repair by external approach of Abdominal Wall Stoma
Small Intestine	ØDQ8ØZZ	ØWQFXZ2
Duodenum	ØDQ9ØZZ	ØWQFXZ2
Jejunum	ØDQAØZZ	ØWQFXZ2
Ileum	ØDQBØZZ	ØWQFXZ2
Large Intestine	ØDQEØZZ	ØWQFXZ2
Large Intestine, Right	ØDQFØZZ	ØWQFXZ2
Large Intestine, Left	ØDQGØZZ	ØWQFXZ2
Cecum	ØDQHØZZ	ØWQFXZ2
Ascending Colon	ØDQKØZZ	ØWQFXZ2
Transverse Colon	ØDQLØZZ	ØWQFXZ2
Descending Colon	ØDQMØZZ	ØWQFXZ2
Sigmoid Colon	ØDQNØZZ	ØWQFXZ2

DRG 456-458 Spinal Fusion Except Cervical with Spinal Curvature/Malignancy/ Infection or Extensive Fusions

Fusion of Thoracic and Lumbar Vertebra, Anterior Column

2 to 7 Thoracic Vertebra		Code also 2 or more Lumbar Vertebra	
ØRG[Ø,3,4][7,A,J,K]Ø	XRG7ØF3	ØSG1[Ø,3,4][7,A,J,K]Ø	XRGCØF3

Fusion of Thoracic and Lumbar Vertebra, Posterior Column

2 to 7 Thoracic Vertebra			Code also 2 or more Lumbar Vertebra		
Posterior Approach	Anterior Approach	New Technology	Posterior Approach	Anterior Approach	New Technology
ØRG7[Ø,3,4][7,J,K]1	ØRG7[Ø,3,4][7,A,J,K]J	XRG7Ø92 XRG7ØF3	ØSG1[Ø,3,4][7,J,K]1	ØSG1[Ø,3,4][7,A,J,K]J	XRGCØ92 XRGCØF3

DRG 461-462 Bilateral or Multiple Major Joint Procedures of Lower Extremity

For procedures to qualify as bilateral or multiple joint procedures, at least one replacement code or combination removal and replacement code from two different lower extremity sites from the following table(s) must be reported.

Examples: Left hip and right hip codes (bilateral); left hip and left knee codes (multiple); left hip and right ankle codes (multiple); left knee and right knee codes (bilateral); right hip removal and replacement, with right knee replacement

Hip, RT	Hip, LT	Knee, RT	Knee, LT	Ankle, RT	Ankle, LT
ØSR9Ø19	ØSRBØ19	ØSRCØ69	ØSRDØ69	ØSRFØ7Z	ØSRGØ7Z
ØSR9Ø1A	ØSRBØ1A	ØSRCØ6A	ØSRDØ6A	ØSRFØJ9	ØSRGØJ9
ØSR9Ø1Z	ØSRBØ1Z	ØSRCØ6Z	ØSRDØ6Z	ØSRFØJA	ØSRGØJA
ØSR9Ø29	ØSRBØ29	ØSRCØ7Z	ØSRDØ7Z	ØSRFØJZ	ØSRGØJZ
ØSR9Ø2A	ØSRBØ2A	ØSRCØJ9	ØSRDØJ9	ØSRFØKZ	ØSRGØKZ
ØSR9Ø2Z	ØSRBØ2Z	ØSRCØJA	ØSRDØJA		
ØSR9Ø39	ØSRBØ39	ØSRCØJZ	ØSRDØJZ		
ØSR9Ø3A	ØSRBØ3A	ØSRCØKZ	ØSRDØKZ		
ØSR9Ø3Z	ØSRBØ3Z	ØSRCØL9	ØSRDØL9		
ØSR9Ø49	ØSRBØ49	ØSRCØLA	ØSRDØLA		
ØSR9Ø4A	ØSRBØ4A	ØSRCØLZ	ØSRDØLZ		
ØSR9Ø4Z	ØSRBØ4Z	ØSRCØM9	ØSRDØM9		
ØSR9Ø69	ØSRBØ69	ØSRCØMA	ØSRDØMA		
ØSR9Ø6A	ØSRBØ6A	ØSRCØMZ	ØSRDØMZ		
ØSR9Ø6Z	ØSRBØ6Z	ØSRCØN9	ØSRDØN9		
ØSR9Ø7Z	ØSRBØ7Z	ØSRCØNA	ØSRDØNA		
ØSR9ØJ9	ØSRBØJ9	ØSRCØNZ	ØSRDØNZ		
ØSR9ØJA	ØSRBØJA	ØSRTØ7Z	ØSRUØ7Z		
ØSR9ØJZ	ØSRBØJZ	ØSRTØJ9	ØSRUØJ9		
ØSR9ØKZ	ØSRBØKZ	ØSRTØJA	ØSRUØJA		
ØSRAØØ9	ØSREØØ9	ØSRTØJZ	ØSRUØJZ		
ØSRAØØA	ØSREØØA	ØSRTØKZ	ØSRUØKZ		
ØSRAØØZ	ØSREØØZ	ØSRVØ7Z	ØSRWØ7Z		
ØSRAØ19	ØSREØ19	ØSRVØJ9	ØSRWØJ9		
ØSRAØ1A	ØSREØ1A	ØSRVØJA	ØSRWØJA		

Hip, RT	Hip, LT	Knee, RT	Knee, LT	Ankle, RT	Ankle, LT
ØSRAØ1Z	ØSREØ1Z	ØSRVØJZ	ØSRWØJZ		
ØSRAØ39	ØSREØ39	ØSRVØKZ	ØSRWØKZ		
ØSRAØ3A	ØSREØ3A	ØSPCØJZ	ØSPDØJZ		
ØSRAØ3Z	ØSREØ3Z				
ØSRAØ7Z	ØSREØ7Z				
ØSRAØJ9	ØSREØJ9				
ØSRAØJA	ØSREØJA				
ØSRAØJZ	ØSREØJZ				
ØSRAØKZ	ØSREØKZ				
ØSRRØ19	ØSRSØ19				
ØSRRØ1A	ØSRSØ1A				
ØSRRØ1Z	ØSRSØ1Z				
ØSRRØ39	ØSRSØ39				
ØSRRØ3A	ØSRSØ3A				
ØSRRØ3Z	ØSRSØ3Z				
ØSRRØ7Z	ØSRSØ7Z				
ØSRRØJ9	ØSRSØJ9				
ØSRRØJA	ØSRSØJA				
ØSRRØJZ	ØSRSØJZ				
ØSRRØKZ	ØSRSØKZ				
ØSU9ØBZ	ØSUBØBZ				
ØSUAØBZ	ØSUEØBZ				
ØSURØBZ	ØSUSØBZ				
ØSP9ØJZ	ØSPBØJZ				

Hip Procedure Combinations

Open Removal of Hip Spacer with Replacement

Removal of Spacer		Code also as appropriate Replacement by Device Type					
		Metal	Metal on Poly	Ceramic	Ceramic on Poly	Oxidized Zirc on Poly	Synth Subst
Hip, RT	ØSP9Ø8Z	ØSR9Ø1[9,A,Z]	ØSR9Ø2[9,A,Z]	ØSR9Ø3[9,A,Z]	ØSR9Ø4[9,A,Z]	ØSR9Ø6[9,A,Z]	ØSR9ØJ[9,A,Z]
Hip, LT	ØSPBØ8Z	ØSRBØ1[9,A,Z]	ØSRBØ2[9,A,Z]	ØSRBØ3[9,A,Z]	ØSRBØ4[9,A,Z]	ØSRBØ6[9,A,Z]	ØSRBØJ[9,A,Z]

Open Removal of Hip Spacer with Replacement

Removal of Spacer		Code also as appropriate Replacement by Device Type						
		Acetabular Surface				Femoral Surface		
		Poly	Metal	Ceramic	Synthetic	Metal	Ceramic	Synth
Hip, RT	ØSP9Ø8Z	ØSRAØØ[9,A,Z]	ØSRAØ1[9,A,Z]	ØSRAØ3[9,A,Z]	ØSRAØJ[9,A,Z]	ØSRRØ1[9,A,Z]	ØSRRØ3[9,A,Z]	ØSRRØJ[9,A,Z]
Hip, LT	ØSPBØ8Z	ØSREØØ[9,A,Z]	ØSREØ1[9,A,Z]	ØSREØ3[9,A,Z]	ØSREØJ[9,A,Z]	ØSRSØ1[9,A,Z]	ØSRSØ3[9,A,Z]	ØSRSØJ[9,A,Z]

Open Removal of Hip Liner with Replacement

Removal of Liner		Code also as appropriate Replacement by Device Type					
		Metal	Metal on Poly	Ceramic	Ceramic on Poly	Oxidized Zirc on Poly	Synth Subst
Hip, RT	ØSP9Ø9Z	ØSR9Ø1[9,A,Z]	ØSR9Ø2[9,A,Z]	ØSR9Ø3[9,A,Z]	ØSR9Ø4[9,A,Z]	ØSR9Ø6[9,A,Z]	ØSR9ØJ[9,A,Z]
Hip, LT	ØSPBØ9Z	ØSRBØ1[9,A,Z]	ØSRBØ2[9,A,Z]	ØSRBØ3[9,A,Z]	ØSRBØ4[9,A,Z]	ØSRBØ6[9,A,Z]	ØSRBØJ[9,A,Z]

Open Removal of Hip Liner with Replacement

Removal of Liner		Code also as appropriate Replacement by Device Type						
		Acetabular Surface				Femoral Surface		
		Poly	Metal	Ceramic	Synthetic	Metal	Ceramic	Synth
Hip, RT	ØSP9Ø9Z	ØSRAØØ[9,A,Z]	ØSRAØ1[9,A,Z]	ØSRAØ3[9,A,Z]	ØSRAØJ[9,A,Z]	ØSRRØ1[9,A,Z]	ØSRRØ3[9,A,Z]	ØSRRØJ[9,A,Z]
Hip, LT	ØSPBØ9Z	ØSREØØ[9,A,Z]	ØSREØ1[9,A,Z]	ØSREØ3[9,A,Z]	ØSREØJ[9,A,Z]	ØSRSØ1[9,A,Z]	ØSRSØ3[9,A,Z]	ØSRSØJ[9,A,Z]

Open Removal of Hip Resurfacing Device with Replacement

Removal of Resurfacing Device		Code also as appropriate Replacement by Device Type					
		Metal	Metal on Poly	Ceramic	Ceramic on Poly	Oxidized Zirc on Poly	Synth Subst
Hip, RT	ØSP9ØBZ	ØSR9Ø1[9,A,Z]	ØSR9Ø2[9,A,Z]	ØSR9Ø3[9,A,Z]	ØSR9Ø4[9,A,Z]	ØSR9Ø6[9,A,Z]	ØSR9ØJ[9,A,Z]
Hip, LT	ØSPBØBZ	ØSRBØ1[9,A,Z]	ØSRBØ2[9,A,Z]	ØSRBØ3[9,A,Z]	ØSRBØ4[9,A,Z]	ØSRBØ6[9,A,Z]	ØSRBØJ[9,A,Z]

Open Removal of Hip Resurfacing Device with Replacement

Removal of Resurfacing Device		Code also as appropriate Replacement by Device Type						
		Acetabular Surface				Femoral Surface		
		Poly	Metal	Ceramic	Synthetic	Metal	Ceramic	Synth
Hip, RT	ØSP9ØBZ	ØSRAØØ[9,A,Z]	ØSRAØ1[9,A,Z]	ØSRAØ3[9,A,Z]	ØSRAØJ[9,A,Z]	ØSRRØ1[9,A,Z]	ØSRRØ3[9,A,Z]	ØSRRØJ[9,A,Z]
Hip, LT	ØSPBØBZ	ØSREØØ[9,A,Z]	ØSREØ1[9,A,Z]	ØSREØ3[9,A,Z]	ØSREØJ[9,A,Z]	ØSRSØ1[9,A,Z]	ØSRSØ3[9,A,Z]	ØSRSØJ[9,A,Z]

Open Removal of Hip Articulating Spacer with Replacement

Removal of Articulating Spacer		Code also as appropriate Replacement by Device Type					
		Metal	Metal on Poly	Ceramic	Ceramic on Poly	Oxidized Zirc on Poly	Synth Subst
Hip, RT	ØSP9ØEZ	ØSR9Ø1[9,A,Z]	ØSR9Ø2[9,A,Z]	ØSR9Ø3[9,A,Z]	ØSR9Ø4[9,A,Z]	ØSR9Ø6[9,A,Z]	ØSR9ØJ[9,A,Z]
Hip, LT	ØSPBØEZ	ØSRBØ1[9,A,Z]	ØSRBØ2[9,A,Z]	ØSRBØ3[9,A,Z]	ØSRBØ4[9,A,Z]	ØSRBØ6[9,A,Z]	ØSRBØJ[9,A,Z]

Open Removal of Hip Articulating Spacer with Replacement

Removal of Articulating Spacer		Code also as appropriate Replacement by Device Type						
		Acetabular Surface				Femoral Surface		
		Poly	Metal	Ceramic	Synthetic	Metal	Ceramic	Synth
Hip, RT	ØSP9ØEZ	ØSRAØØ[9,A,Z]	ØSRAØ1[9,A,Z]	ØSRAØ3[9,A,Z]	ØSRAØJ[9,A,Z]	ØSRRØ1[9,A,Z]	ØSRRØ3[9,A,Z]	ØSRRØJ[9,A,Z]
Hip, LT	ØSPBØEZ	ØSREØØ[9,A,Z]	ØSREØ1[9,A,Z]	ØSREØ3[9,A,Z]	ØSREØJ[9,A,Z]	ØSRSØ1[9,A,Z]	ØSRSØ3[9,A,Z]	ØSRSØJ[9,A,Z]

Open Removal of Hip Synthetic Substitute with Replacement

Removal of Synthetic Substitute		Code also as appropriate Replacement by Device Type					
		Metal	Metal on Poly	Ceramic	Ceramic on Poly	Oxidized Zirc on Poly	Synth Subst
Hip, RT	ØSP[9,A,R]ØJZ	ØSR9Ø1[9,A,Z]	ØSR9Ø2[9,A,Z]	ØSR9Ø3[9,A,Z]	ØSR9Ø4[9,A,Z]	ØSR9Ø6[9,A,Z]	ØSR9ØJ[9,A,Z]
Hip, LT	ØSP[B,E,S]ØJZ	ØSRBØ1[9,A,Z]	ØSRBØ2[9,A,Z]	ØSRBØ3[9,A,Z]	ØSRBØ4[9,A,Z]	ØSRBØ6[9,A,Z]	ØSRBØJ[9,A,Z]

Open Removal of Hip Synthetic Substitute with Replacement

Removal of Synthetic Substitute		Code also as appropriate Replacement by Device Type						
		Acetabular Surface				Femoral Surface		
		Poly	Metal	Ceramic	Synthetic	Metal	Ceramic	Synth
Hip, RT	ØSP[9,A,R]ØJZ	ØSRAØØ[9,A,Z]	ØSRAØ1[9,A,Z]	ØSRAØ3[9,A,Z]	ØSRAØJ[9,A,Z]	ØSRRØ1[9,A,Z]	ØSRRØ3[9,A,Z]	ØSRRØJ[9,A,Z]
Hip, LT	ØSP[B,E,S]ØJZ	ØSREØØ[9,A,Z]	ØSREØ1[9,A,Z]	ØSREØ3[9,A,Z]	ØSREØJ[9,A,Z]	ØSRSØ1[9,A,Z]	ØSRSØ3[9,A,Z]	ØSRSØJ[9,A,Z]

Percutaneous Endoscopic Removal of Hip Spacer with Open Replacement

Removal of Spacer		Code also as appropriate Replacement by Device Type					
		Metal	Metal on Poly	Ceramic	Ceramic on Poly	Oxidized Zirc on Poly	Synth Subst
Hip, RT	ØSP948Z	ØSR9Ø1[9,A,Z]	ØSR9Ø2[9,A,Z]	ØSR9Ø3[9,A,Z]	ØSR9Ø4[9,A,Z]	ØSR9Ø6[9,A,Z]	ØSR9ØJ[9,A,Z]
Hip, LT	ØSPB48Z	ØSRBØ1[9,A,Z]	ØSRBØ2[9,A,Z]	ØSRBØ3[9,A,Z]	ØSRBØ4[9,A,Z]	ØSRBØ6[9,A,Z]	ØSRBØJ[9,A,Z]

Percutaneous Endoscopic Removal of Hip Spacer with Open Replacement

Removal of Spacer		Code also as appropriate Replacement by Device Type						
		Acetabular Surface				Femoral Surface		
		Poly	Metal	Ceramic	Synthetic	Metal	Ceramic	Synth
Hip, RT	ØSP948Z	ØSRAØØ[9,A,Z]	ØSRAØ1[9,A,Z]	ØSRAØ3[9,A,Z]	ØSRAØJ[9,A,Z]	ØSRRØ1[9,A,Z]	ØSRRØ3[9,A,Z]	ØSRRØJ[9,A,Z]
Hip, LT	ØSPB48Z	ØSREØØ[9,A,Z]	ØSREØ1[9,A,Z]	ØSREØ3[9,A,Z]	ØSREØJ[9,A,Z]	ØSRSØ1[9,A,Z]	ØSRSØ3[9,A,Z]	ØSRSØJ[9,A,Z]

Percutaneous Endoscopic Removal of Hip Synthetic Substitute with Open Replacement

Removal of Synthetic Substitute		Code also as appropriate Replacement by Device Type					
		Metal	Metal on Poly	Ceramic	Ceramic on Poly	Oxidized Zirc on Poly	Synth Subst
Hip, RT	ØSP[9,A,R]4JZ	ØSR9Ø1[9,A,Z]	ØSR9Ø2[9,A,Z]	ØSR9Ø3[9,A,Z]	ØSR9Ø4[9,A,Z]	ØSR9Ø6[9,A,Z]	ØSR9ØJ[9,A,Z]
Hip, LT	ØSP[B,E,S]4JZ	ØSRBØ1[9,A,Z]	ØSRBØ2[9,A,Z]	ØSRBØ3[9,A,Z]	ØSRBØ4[9,A,Z]	ØSRBØ6[9,A,Z]	ØSRBØJ[9,A,Z]

Percutaneous Endoscopic Removal of Hip Synthetic Substitute with Open Replacement

Removal of Synthetic Substitute		Code also as appropriate Replacement by Device Type						
		Acetabular Surface				Femoral Surface		
		Poly	Metal	Ceramic	Synthetic	Metal	Ceramic	Synth
Hip, RT	ØSP[9,A,R]4JZ	ØSRAØØ[9,A,Z]	ØSRAØ1[9,A,Z]	ØSRAØ3[9,A,Z]	ØSRAØJ[9,A,Z]	ØSRRØ1[9,A,Z]	ØSRRØ3[9,A,Z]	ØSRRØJ[9,A,Z]
Hip, LT	ØSP[B,E,S]4JZ	ØSREØØ[9,A,Z]	ØSREØ1[9,A,Z]	ØSREØ3[9,A,Z]	ØSREØJ[9,A,Z]	ØSRSØ1[9,A,Z]	ØSRSØ3[9,A,Z]	ØSRSØJ[9,A,Z]

Knee Procedure Combinations

Removal of Knee Spacer with Replacement

Removal of Spacer		Code also Replacement by Type of Synthetic Substitute					
		Oxidized Zirc on Poly	Synthetic Substitute	Patello-femoral	Femoral Surface	Tibial Surface	Medial (L)/Lateral (M) Meniscus
Knee, RT	ØSPC[Ø,3,4]8Z	ØSRCØ6[9,A,Z]	ØSRCØJ[9,A,Z]	ØSRCØN[9,A,Z]	ØSRTØJ[9,A,Z]	ØSRVØJ[9,A,Z]	XRRGØ[L,M]8
Knee, LT	ØSPD[Ø,3,4]8Z	ØSRDØ6[9,A,Z]	ØSRDØJ[9,A,Z]	ØSRDØN[9,A,Z]	ØSRUØJ[9,A,Z]	ØSRWØJ[9,A,Z]	XRRHØ[L,M]8

Removal of Knee Liner with Replacement

Removal of Liner		Code also Replacement by Type of Synthetic Substitute						
		Oxidized Zirc on Poly	Synthetic Substitute	Medial (L)/ Lateral (M) Unicondylar	Patello-femoral	Femoral Surface	Tibial Surface	Medial (L)/ Lateral (M) Meniscus
Knee, RT	ØSPCØ9Z	ØSRCØ6[9,A,Z]	ØSRCØJ[9,A,Z]	ØSRCØ[L,M][9,A,Z]	ØSRCØN[9,A,Z]	ØSRTØJ[9,A,Z]	ØSRVØJ[9,A,Z]	XRRGØ[L,M]8
Knee, LT	ØSPDØ9Z	ØSRDØ6[9,A,Z]	ØSRDØJ[9,A,Z]	ØSRDØ[L,M][9,A,Z]	ØSRDØN[9,A,Z]	ØSRUØJ[9,A,Z]	ØSRWØJ[9,A,Z]	XRRHØ[L,M]8

Removal of Knee Articulating Spacer with Replacement

Removal of Articulating Spacer		Code also Replacement by Type of Synthetic Substitute				
		Oxidized Zirc on Poly	Synthetic Substitute	Femoral Surface	Tibial Surface	Medial (L)/ Lateral (M) Meniscus
Knee, RT	ØSPCØEZ	ØSRCØ6[9,A,Z]	ØSRCØJ[9,A,Z]	ØSRTØJ[9,A,Z]	ØSRVØJ[9,A,Z]	XRRGØ[L,M]8
Knee, LT	ØSPDØEZ	ØSRDØ6[9,A,Z]	ØSRDØJ[9,A,Z]	ØSRUØJ[9,A,Z]	ØSRWØJ[9,A,Z]	XRRHØ[L,M]8

Removal of Knee Patellar Surface with Replacement

Removal of Patellar Surface		Code also Replacement by Type of Synthetic Substitute					
		Oxidized Zirc on Poly	Synthetic Substitute	Patello-femoral	Femoral Surface	Tibial Surface	Medial (L)/Lateral (M) Meniscus
Knee, RT	ØSPC[Ø,4]JC	ØSRCØ6[9,A,Z]	ØSRCØJ[9,A,Z]	ØSRCØN[9,A,Z]	ØSRTØJ[9,A,Z]	ØSRVØJ[9,A,Z]	XRRGØ[L,M]8
Knee, LT	ØSPD[Ø,4]JC	ØSRDØ6[9,A,Z]	ØSRDØJ[9,A,Z]	ØSRDØN[9,A,Z]	ØSRUØJ[9,A,Z]	ØSRWØJ[9,A,Z]	XRRHØ[L,M]8

Removal of Knee Synthetic Substitute with Replacement

Removal of Synthetic Substitute		Code also Replacement by Type of Synthetic Substitute						
		Oxidized Zirc on Poly	Synthetic Substitute	Medial (L)/ Lateral (M) Unicondylar	Patello-femoral	Femoral Surface	Tibial Surface	Medial (L)/ Lateral (M) Meniscus
Knee, RT	ØSPC[Ø,4]JZ	ØSRCØ6[9,A,Z]	ØSRCØJ[9,A,Z]	ØSRCØ[L,M][9,A,Z]	ØSRCØN[9,A,Z]	ØSRTØJ[9,A,Z]	ØSRVØJ[9,A,Z]	XRRGØ[L,M]8
Knee, LT	ØSPD[Ø,4]JZ	ØSRDØ6[9,A,Z]	ØSRDØJ[9,A,Z]	ØSRDØ[L,M][9,A,Z]	ØSRDØN[9,A,Z]	ØSRUØJ[9,A,Z]	ØSRWØJ[9,A,Z]	XRRHØ[L,M]8

Removal of Knee Unicondylar Device with Replacement

Removal of Medial (L)/ Lateral (M) Unicondylar Device		Code also Replacement by Type of Synthetic Substitute					
		Oxidized Zirc on Poly	Synthetic Substitute	Medial Unicondylar	Femoral Surface	Tibial Surface	Medial (L)/Lateral (M) Meniscus
Knee, RT	ØSPC[Ø,4][L,M]Z	ØSRCØ6[9,A,Z]	ØSRCØJ[9,A,Z]	ØSRCØL[9,A,Z]	ØSRTØJ[9,A,Z]	ØSRVØJ[9,A,Z]	XRRGØ[L,M]8
Knee, LT	ØSPD[Ø,4][L,M]Z	ØSRDØ6[9,A,Z]	ØSRDØJ[9,A,Z]	ØSRDØL[9,A,Z]	ØSRUØJ[9,A,Z]	ØSRWØJ[9,A,Z]	XRRHØ[L,M]8

Removal of Knee Patellofemoral Device with Replacement

Removal of Patellofemoral Device		Code also Replacement by Type of Synthetic Substitute					
		Oxidized Zirc on Poly	Synthetic Substitute	Medial Unicondylar	Femoral Surface	Tibial Surface	Medial (L)/Lateral (M) Meniscus
Knee, RT	ØSPC[Ø,4]NZ	ØSRCØ6[9,A,Z]	ØSRCØJ[9,A,Z]	ØSRCØL[9,A,Z]	ØSRTØJ[9,A,Z]	ØSRVØJ[9,A,Z]	XRRGØ[L,M]8
Knee, LT	ØSPD[Ø,4]NZ	ØSRDØ6[9,A,Z]	ØSRDØJ[9,A,Z]	ØSRDØL[9,A,Z]	ØSRUØJ[9,A,Z]	ØSRWØJ[9,A,Z]	XRRHØ[L,M]8

Removal of Knee Femoral/Tibial Surface Device with Replacement

Removal of Femoral (T,U)/ Tibial (V,W) Surface		Code also Replacement by Type of Synthetic Substitute						
		Oxidized Zirc on Poly	Synthetic Substitute	Articulating Spacer	Patello-femoral	Femoral Surface	Tibial Surface	Medial (L)/Lateral (M) Meniscus
Knee, RT	ØSP[T,V][Ø,4]JZ	ØSRCØ6[9,A,Z]	ØSRCØJ[9,A,Z]	ØSRCØEZ	ØSRCØN[9,A,Z]	ØSRTØJ[9,A,Z]	ØSRVØJ[9,A,Z]	XRRGØ[L,M]8
Knee, LT	ØSP[U,W][Ø,4]JZ	ØSRDØ6[9,A,Z]	ØSRDØJ[9,A,Z]	ØSRDØEZ	ØSRDØN[9,A,Z]	ØSRUØJ[9,A,Z]	ØSRWØJ[9,A,Z]	XRRHØ[L,M]8

466-468 Revision of Hip or Knee Replacement

Hip Procedure Combinations

Open Removal of Hip Spacer with Replacement

Removal of Spacer		Code also as appropriate Replacement by Device Type						
		Metal	Metal on Poly	Ceramic	Ceramic on Poly	Oxidized Zirc on Poly	Articulating Spacer	Synth Subst
Hip, RT	ØSP9Ø8Z	ØSR9Ø1[9,A,Z]	ØSR9Ø2[9,A,Z]	ØSR9Ø3[9,A,Z]	ØSR9Ø4[9,A,Z]	ØSR9Ø6[9,A,Z]	ØSR9ØEZ	ØSR9ØJ[9,A,Z]
Hip, LT	ØSPBØ8Z	ØSRBØ1[9,A,Z]	ØSRBØ2[9,A,Z]	ØSRBØ3[9,A,Z]	ØSRBØ4[9,A,Z]	ØSRBØ6[9,A,Z]	ØSRBØEZ	ØSRBØJ[9,A,Z]

Open Removal of Hip Spacer with Replacement

Removal of Spacer		Code also as appropriate Replacement by Device Type						
		Acetabular Surface				Femoral Surface		
		Poly	Metal	Ceramic	Synthetic	Metal	Ceramic	Synth
Hip, RT	ØSP9Ø8Z	ØSRAØØ[9,A,Z]	ØSRAØ1[9,A,Z]	ØSRAØ3[9,A,Z]	ØSRAØJ[9,A,Z]	ØSRRØ1[9,A,Z]	ØSRRØ3[9,A,Z]	ØSRRØJ[9,A,Z]
Hip, LT	ØSPBØ8Z	ØSREØØ[9,A,Z]	ØSREØ1[9,A,Z]	ØSREØ3[9,A,Z]	ØSREØJ[9,A,Z]	ØSRSØ1[9,A,Z]	ØSRSØ3[9,A,Z]	ØSRSØJ[9,A,Z]

Open Removal of Hip Spacer with Liner Insertion (supplement)

Removal of Spacer		Code also as appropriate Supplement of Body Part by Site		
		Joint	Acetabular Surface	Femoral Surface
Hip, RT	ØSP9Ø8Z	ØSU9Ø9Z	ØSUAØ9Z	ØSURØ9Z
Hip, LT	ØSPBØ8Z	ØSUBØ9Z	ØSUEØ9Z	ØSUSØ9Z

Open Removal of Hip Liner with Replacement

Removal of Liner		Code also as appropriate Replacement by Device Type						
		Metal	Metal on Poly	Ceramic	Ceramic on Poly	Oxidized Zirc on Poly	Articulating Spacer	Synth Subst
Hip, RT	ØSP9Ø9Z	ØSR9Ø1[9,A,Z]	ØSR9Ø2[9,A,Z]	ØSR9Ø3[9,A,Z]	ØSR9Ø4[9,A,Z]	ØSR9Ø6[9,A,Z]	ØSR9ØEZ	ØSR9ØJ[9,A,Z]
Hip, LT	ØSPBØ9Z	ØSRBØ1[9,A,Z]	ØSRBØ2[9,A,Z]	ØSRBØ3[9,A,Z]	ØSRBØ4[9,A,Z]	ØSRBØ6[9,A,Z]	ØSRBØEZ	ØSRBØJ[9,A,Z]

Open Removal of Hip Liner with Replacement

Removal of Liner		Code also as appropriate Replacement by Device Type						
		Acetabular Surface				Femoral Surface		
		Poly	Metal	Ceramic	Synthetic	Metal	Ceramic	Synth
Hip, RT	ØSP9Ø9Z	ØSRAØØ[9,A,Z]	ØSRAØ1[9,A,Z]	ØSRAØ3[9,A,Z]	ØSRAØJ[9,A,Z]	ØSRRØ1[9,A,Z]	ØSRRØ3[9,A,Z]	ØSRRØJ[9,A,Z]
Hip, LT	ØSPBØ9Z	ØSREØØ[9,A,Z]	ØSREØ1[9,A,Z]	ØSREØ3[9,A,Z]	ØSREØJ[9,A,Z]	ØSRSØ1[9,A,Z]	ØSRSØ3[9,A,Z]	ØSRSØJ[9,A,Z]

Open Removal of Hip Liner with Liner Insertion (supplement)

Removal of Liner		Code also as appropriate Supplement of Body Part by Site		
		Joint	Acetabular Surface	Femoral Surface
Hip, RT	ØSP9Ø9Z	ØSU9Ø9Z	ØSUAØ9Z	ØSURØ9Z
Hip, LT	ØSPBØ9Z	ØSUBØ9Z	ØSUEØ9Z	ØSUSØ9Z

Open Removal of Hip Resurfacing Device with Replacement

Removal of Resurfacing Device		Code also as appropriate Replacement by Device Type						
		Metal	Metal on Poly	Ceramic	Ceramic on Poly	Oxidized Zirc on Poly	Articulating Spacer	Synth Subst
Hip, RT	ØSP9ØBZ	ØSR9Ø1[9,A,Z]	ØSR9Ø2[9,A,Z]	ØSR9Ø3[9,A,Z]	ØSR9Ø4[9,A,Z]	ØSR9Ø6[9,A,Z]	ØSR9ØEZ	ØSR9ØJ[9,A,Z]
Hip, LT	ØSPBØBZ	ØSRBØ1[9,A,Z]	ØSRBØ2[9,A,Z]	ØSRBØ3[9,A,Z]	ØSRBØ4[9,A,Z]	ØSRBØ6[9,A,Z]	ØSRBØEZ	ØSRBØJ[9,A,Z]

Open Removal of Hip Resurfacing Device with Replacement

Removal of Resurfacing Device		Code also as appropriate Replacement by Device Type						
		Acetabular Surface				Femoral Surface		
		Poly	Metal	Ceramic	Synthetic	Metal	Ceramic	Synth
Hip, RT	ØSP9ØBZ	ØSRAØØ[9,A,Z]	ØSRAØ1[9,A,Z]	ØSRAØ3[9,A,Z]	ØSRAØJ[9,A,Z]	ØSRRØ1[9,A,Z]	ØSRRØ3[9,A,Z]	ØSRRØJ[9,A,Z]
Hip, LT	ØSPBØBZ	ØSREØØ[9,A,Z]	ØSREØ1[9,A,Z]	ØSREØ3[9,A,Z]	ØSREØJ[9,A,Z]	ØSRSØ1[9,A,Z]	ØSRSØ3[9,A,Z]	ØSRSØJ[9,A,Z]

Open Removal of Hip Resurfacing Device with Liner Insertion (supplement)

Removal of Resurfacing Device		Code also as appropriate Supplement of Body Part by Site		
		Joint	Acetabular Surface	Femoral Surface
Hip, RT	ØSP9ØBZ	ØSU9Ø9Z	ØSUAØ9Z	ØSURØ9Z
Hip, LT	ØSPBØBZ	ØSUBØ9Z	ØSUEØ9Z	ØSUSØ9Z

Open Removal of Hip Articulating Spacer with Replacement

Removal of Articulating Spacer		Code also as appropriate Replacement by Device Type					
		Metal	Metal on Poly	Ceramic	Ceramic on Poly	Oxidized Zirc on Poly	Synth Subst
Hip, RT	ØSP9ØEZ	ØSR9Ø1[9,A,Z]	ØSR9Ø2[9,A,Z]	ØSR9Ø3[9,A,Z]	ØSR9Ø4[9,A,Z]	ØSR9Ø6[9,A,Z]	ØSR9ØJ[9,A,Z]
Hip, LT	ØSPBØEZ	ØSRBØ1[9,A,Z]	ØSRBØ2[9,A,Z]	ØSRBØ3[9,A,Z]	ØSRBØ4[9,A,Z]	ØSRBØ6[9,A,Z]	ØSRBØJ[9,A,Z]

Open Removal of Hip Articulating Spacer with Replacement

Removal of Articulating Spacer		Code also as appropriate Replacement by Device Type						
		Acetabular Surface				Femoral Surface		
		Poly	Metal	Ceramic	Synthetic	Metal	Ceramic	Synth
Hip, RT	ØSP9ØEZ	ØSRAØØ[9,A,Z]	ØSRAØ1[9,A,Z]	ØSRAØ3[9,A,Z]	ØSRAØJ[9,A,Z]	ØSRRØ1[9,A,Z]	ØSRRØ3[9,A,Z]	ØSRRØJ[9,A,Z]
Hip, LT	ØSPBØEZ	ØSREØØ[9,A,Z]	ØSREØ1[9,A,Z]	ØSREØ3[9,A,Z]	ØSREØJ[9,A,Z]	ØSRSØ1[9,A,Z]	ØSRSØ3[9,A,Z]	ØSRSØJ[9,A,Z]

Open Removal of Hip Articulating Spacer with Liner Insertion (supplement)

Removal of Articulating Spacer		Code also as appropriate Supplement of Body Part by Site		
		Joint	Acetabular Surface	Femoral Surface
Hip, RT	ØSP9ØEZ	ØSU9Ø9Z	ØSUAØ9Z	ØSURØ9Z
Hip, LT	ØSPBØEZ	ØSUBØ9Z	ØSUEØ9Z	ØSUSØ9Z

Open Removal of Hip Synthetic Substitute with Replacement

Removal of Synthetic Substitute		Code also as appropriate Replacement by Device Type						
		Metal	Metal on Poly	Ceramic	Ceramic on Poly	Oxidized Zirc on Poly	Articulating Spacer	Synth Subst
Hip, RT	ØSP[9,A,R]ØJZ	ØSR9Ø1[9,A,Z]	ØSR9Ø2[9,A,Z]	ØSR9Ø3[9,A,Z]	ØSR9Ø4[9,A,Z]	ØSR9Ø6[9,A,Z]	ØSR9ØEZ	ØSR9ØJ[9,A,Z]
Hip, LT	ØSP[B,E,S]ØJZ	ØSRBØ1[9,A,Z]	ØSRBØ2[9,A,Z]	ØSRBØ3[9,A,Z]	ØSRBØ4[9,A,Z]	ØSRBØ6[9,A,Z]	ØSRBØEZ	ØSRBØJ[9,A,Z]

Open Removal of Hip Synthetic Substitute with Replacement

Removal of Synthetic Substitute		Code also as appropriate Replacement by Device Type						
		Acetabular Surface				Femoral Surface		
		Poly	Metal	Ceramic	Synthetic	Metal	Ceramic	Synth
Hip, RT	ØSP[9,A,R]ØJZ	ØSRAØØ[9,A,Z]	ØSRAØ1[9,A,Z]	ØSRAØ3[9,A,Z]	ØSRAØJ[9,A,Z]	ØSRRØ1[9,A,Z]	ØSRRØ3[9,A,Z]	ØSRRØJ[9,A,Z]
Hip, LT	ØSP[B,E,S]ØJZ	ØSREØØ[9,A,Z]	ØSREØ1[9,A,Z]	ØSREØ3[9,A,Z]	ØSREØJ[9,A,Z]	ØSRSØ1[9,A,Z]	ØSRSØ3[9,A,Z]	ØSRSØJ[9,A,Z]

Percutaneous Endoscopic Removal of Hip Spacer with Open Replacement

Removal of Spacer		Code also as appropriate Replacement by Device Type						
		Metal	Metal on Poly	Ceramic	Ceramic on Poly	Oxidized Zirc on Poly	Articulating Spacer	Synth Subst
Hip, RT	ØSP948Z	ØSR9Ø1[9,A,Z]	ØSR9Ø2[9,A,Z]	ØSR9Ø3[9,A,Z]	ØSR9Ø4[9,A,Z]	ØSR9Ø6[9,A,Z]	ØSR9ØEZ	ØSR9ØJ[9,A,Z]
Hip, LT	ØSPB48Z	ØSRBØ1[9,A,Z]	ØSRBØ2[9,A,Z]	ØSRBØ3[9,A,Z]	ØSRBØ4[9,A,Z]	ØSRBØ6[9,A,Z]	ØSRBØEZ	ØSRBØJ[9,A,Z]

Percutaneous Endoscopic Removal of Hip Spacer with Open Replacement

Removal of Spacer		Code also as appropriate Replacement by Device Type						
		Acetabular Surface				Femoral Surface		
		Poly	Metal	Ceramic	Synthetic	Metal	Ceramic	Synth
Hip, RT	ØSP948Z	ØSRAØØ[9,A,Z]	ØSRAØ1[9,A,Z]	ØSRAØ3[9,A,Z]	ØSRAØJ[9,A,Z]	ØSRRØ1[9,A,Z]	ØSRRØ3[9,A,Z]	ØSRRØJ[9,A,Z]
Hip, LT	ØSPB48Z	ØSREØØ[9,A,Z]	ØSREØ1[9,A,Z]	ØSREØ3[9,A,Z]	ØSREØJ[9,A,Z]	ØSRSØ1[9,A,Z]	ØSRSØ3[9,A,Z]	ØSRSØJ[9,A,Z]

Percutaneous Endoscopic Removal of Hip Spacer with Open Liner Insertion (supplement)

Removal of Spacer		Code also as appropriate Supplement of Body Part by Site		
		Joint	Acetabular Surface	Femoral Surface
Hip, RT	ØSP948Z	ØSU9Ø9Z	ØSUAØ9Z	ØSURØ9Z
Hip, LT	ØSPB48Z	ØSUBØ9Z	ØSUEØ9Z	ØSUSØ9Z

Percutaneous Endoscopic Removal of Hip Synthetic Substitute with Open Replacement

Removal of Synthetic Substitute		Code also as appropriate Replacement by Device Type						
		Metal	Metal on Poly	Ceramic	Ceramic on Poly	Oxidized Zirc on Poly	Articulating Spacer	Synth Subst
Hip, RT	ØSP[9,A,R]4JZ	ØSR9Ø1[9,A,Z]	ØSR9Ø2[9,A,Z]	ØSR9Ø3[9,A,Z]	ØSR9Ø4[9,A,Z]	ØSR9Ø6[9,A,Z]	ØSR9ØEZ	ØSR9ØJ[9,A,Z]
Hip, LT	ØSP[B,E,S]4JZ	ØSRBØ1[9,A,Z]	ØSRBØ2[9,A,Z]	ØSRBØ3[9,A,Z]	ØSRBØ4[9,A,Z]	ØSRBØ6[9,A,Z]	ØSRBØEZ	ØSRBØJ[9,A,Z]

Percutaneous Endoscopic Removal of Hip Synthetic Substitute with Open Replacement

Removal of Synthetic Substitute		Code also as appropriate Replacement by Device Type						
		Acetabular Surface				Femoral Surface		
		Poly	Metal	Ceramic	Synthetic	Metal	Ceramic	Synth
Hip, RT	ØSP[9,A,R]4JZ	ØSRAØØ[9,A,Z]	ØSRAØ1[9,A,Z]	ØSRAØ3[9,A,Z]	ØSRAØJ[9,A,Z]	ØSRRØ1[9,A,Z]	ØSRRØ3[9,A,Z]	ØSRRØJ[9,A,Z]
Hip, LT	ØSP[B,E,S]4JZ	ØSREØØ[9,A,Z]	ØSREØ1[9,A,Z]	ØSREØ3[9,A,Z]	ØSREØJ[9,A,Z]	ØSRSØ1[9,A,Z]	ØSRSØ3[9,A,Z]	ØSRSØJ[9,A,Z]

Percutaneous Endoscopic Removal of Hip Synthetic Substitute with Open Liner Insertion (supplement)

Removal of Synthetic Substitute		Code also as appropriate Supplement of Body Part by Site		
		Joint	Acetabular Surface	Femoral Surface
Hip, RT	ØSP[9,A,R]4JZ	ØSU9Ø9Z	ØSUAØ9Z	ØSURØ9Z
Hip, LT	ØSP[B,E,S]4JZ	ØSUBØ9Z	ØSUEØ9Z	ØSUSØ9Z

Knee Procedure Combinations

Removal of Knee Spacer with Replacement

Removal of Spacer		Code also Replacement by Type of Synthetic Substitute						
		Oxidized Zirc on Poly	Synthetic Substitute	Articulating Spacer	Patello-femoral	Femoral Surface	Tibial Surface	Medial (L)/ Lateral (M) Meniscus
Knee, RT	ØSPC[Ø,3,4]8Z	ØSRCØ6[9,A,Z]	ØSRCØJ[9,A,Z]	ØSRCØEZ	ØSRCØN[9,A,Z]	ØSRTØJ[9,A,Z]	ØSRVØJ[9,A,Z]	XRRGØ[L,M]8
Knee, LT	ØSPD[Ø,3,4]8Z	ØSRDØ6[9,A,Z]	ØSRDØJ[9,A,Z]	ØSRDØEZ	ØSRDØN[9,A,Z]	ØSRUØJ[9,A,Z]	ØSRWØJ[9,A,Z]	XRRHØ[L,M]8

Removal of Knee Liner with Replacement

Removal of Liner		Code also Replacement by Type of Synthetic Substitute							
		Oxidized Zirc on Poly	Synthetic Substitute	Articulating Spacer	Medial (L)/ Lateral (M) Unicondylar	Patello-femoral	Femoral Surface	Tibial Surface	Medial (L)/Lateral (M) Meniscus
Knee, RT	ØSPCØ9Z	ØSRCØ6[9,A,Z]	ØSRCØJ[9,A,Z]	ØSRCØEZ	ØSRCØ[L,M][9,A,Z]	ØSRCØN[9,A,Z]	ØSRTØJ[9,A,Z]	ØSRVØJ[9,A,Z]	XRRGØ[L,M]8
Knee, LT	ØSPDØ9Z	ØSRDØ6[9,A,Z]	ØSRDØJ[9,A,Z]	ØSRDØEZ	ØSRDØ[L,M][9,A,Z]	ØSRDØN[9,A,Z]	ØSRUØJ[9,A,Z]	ØSRWØJ[9,A,Z]	XRRHØ[L,M]8

Removal of Knee Articulating Spacer with Replacement

Removal of Articulating Spacer		Code also Replacement by Type of Synthetic Substitute				
		Oxidized Zirc on Poly	Synthetic Substitute	Femoral Surface	Tibial Surface	Medial (L)/Lateral (M) Meniscus
Knee, RT	ØSPCØEZ	ØSRCØ6[9,A,Z]	ØSRCØJ[9,A,Z]	ØSRTØJ[9,A,Z]	ØSRVØJ[9,A,Z]	XRRGØ[L,M]8
Knee, LT	ØSPDØEZ	ØSRDØ6[9,A,Z]	ØSRDØJ[9,A,Z]	ØSRUØJ[9,A,Z]	ØSRWØJ[9,A,Z]	XRRHØ[L,M]8

Removal of Knee Patellar Surface with Replacement

Removal of Patellar Surface		Code also Replacement by Type of Synthetic Substitute						
		Oxidized Zirc on Poly	Synthetic Substitute	Articulating Spacer	Patello-femoral	Femoral Surface	Tibial Surface	Medial (L)/Lateral (M) Meniscus
Knee, RT	ØSPC[Ø,4]JC	ØSRCØ6[9,A,Z]	ØSRCØJ[9,A,Z]	ØSRCØEZ	ØSRCØN[9,A,Z]	ØSRTØJ[9,A,Z]	ØSRVØJ[9,A,Z]	XRRGØ[L,M]8
Knee, LT	ØSPD[Ø,4]JC	ØSRDØ6[9,A,Z]	ØSRDØJ[9,A,Z]	ØSRDØEZ	ØSRDØN[9,A,Z]	ØSRUØJ[9,A,Z]	ØSRWØJ[9,A,Z]	XRRHØ[L,M]8

Removal of Knee Synthetic Substitute with Replacement

Removal of Synthetic Substitute		Code also Replacement by Type of Synthetic Substitute							
		Oxidized Zirc on Poly	Synthetic Substitute	Articulatin g Spacer	Medial (L)/ Lateral (M) Unicondylar	Patello-femoral	Femoral Surface	Tibial Surface	Medial (L)/ Lateral (M) Meniscus
Knee, RT	ØSPC[Ø,4]JZ	ØSRCØ6[9,A,Z]	ØSRCØJ[9,A,Z]	ØSRCØEZ	ØSRCØ[L,M][9,A,Z]	ØSRCØN[9,A,Z]	ØSRTØJ[9,A,Z]	ØSRVØJ[9,A,Z]	XRRGØ[L,M]8
Knee, LT	ØSPD[Ø,4]JZ	ØSRDØ6[9,A,Z]	ØSRDØJ[9,A,Z]	ØSRDØEZ	ØSRDØ[L,M][9,A,Z]	ØSRDØN[9,A,Z]	ØSRUØJ[9,A,Z]	ØSRWØJ[9,A,Z]	XRRHØ[L,M]8

Removal of Knee Unicondylar Device with Replacement

Removal of Medial (L)/ Lateral (M) Unicondylar Device		Code also Replacement by Type of Synthetic Substitute					
		Oxidized Zirc on Poly	Synthetic Substitute	Medial Unicondylar	Femoral Surface	Tibial Surface	Medial (L)/Lateral (M) Meniscus
Knee, RT	ØSPC[Ø,4][L,M]Z	ØSRCØ6[9,A,Z]	ØSRCØJ[9,A,Z]	ØSRCØL[9,A,Z]	ØSRTØJ[9,A,Z]	ØSRVØJ[9,A,Z]	XRRGØ[L,M]8
Knee, LT	ØSPD[Ø,4][L,M]Z	ØSRDØ6[9,A,Z]	ØSRDØJ[9,A,Z]	ØSRDØL[9,A,Z]	ØSRUØJ[9,A,Z]	ØSRWØJ[9,A,Z]	XRRHØ[L,M]8

Removal of Knee Patellofemoral Device with Replacement

Removal of Patellofemoral Device		Code also Replacement by Type of Synthetic Substitute					
		Oxidized Zirc on Poly	Synthetic Substitute	Medial Unicondylar	Femoral Surface	Tibial Surface	Medial (L)/Lateral (M) Meniscus
Knee, RT	ØSPC[Ø,4]NZ	ØSRCØ6[9,A,Z]	ØSRCØJ[9,A,Z]	ØSRCØL[9,A,Z]	ØSRTØJ[9,A,Z]	ØSRVØJ[9,A,Z]	XRRGØ[L,M]8
Knee, LT	ØSPD[Ø,4]NZ	ØSRDØ6[9,A,Z]	ØSRDØJ[9,A,Z]	ØSRDØL[9,A,Z]	ØSRUØJ[9,A,Z]	ØSRWØJ[9,A,Z]	XRRHØ[L,M]8

Removal of Knee Femoral/Tibial Surface Device with Replacement

Removal of Femoral (T,U)/ Tibial (V,W) Surface		Code also Replacement by Type of Synthetic Substitute						
		Oxidized Zirc on Poly	Synthetic Substitute	Articulating Spacer	Patello-femoral	Femoral Surface	Tibial Surface	Medial (L)/Lateral (M) Meniscus
Knee, RT	ØSP[T,V][Ø,4]JZ	ØSRCØ6[9,A,Z]	ØSRCØJ[9,A,Z]	ØSRCØEZ	ØSRCØN[9,A,Z]	ØSRTØJ[9,A,Z]	ØSRVØJ[9,A,Z]	XRRGØ[L,M]8
Knee, LT	ØSP[U,W][Ø,4]JZ	ØSRDØ6[9,A,Z]	ØSRDØJ[9,A,Z]	ØSRDØEZ	ØSRDØN[9,A,Z]	ØSRUØJ[9,A,Z]	ØSRWØJ[9,A,Z]	XRRHØ[L,M]8

DRG 485-489 Knee Procedures

Joint	Removal of Liner by open approach	Code also as appropriate Supplement of Tibial Surface by Site
Knee, RT	ØSPCØ9Z	ØSUVØ9Z
Knee, LT	ØSPDØ9Z	ØSUWØ9Z

DRG 515-517 Other Musculoskeletal System and Connective Tissue Procedures

Site	Reposition of Vertebra by percutaneous approach	Code also as appropriate Supplement With Synthetic Substitute by Percutaneous Approach at site of Repositioned Vertebra
Cervical	ØPS33ZZ	ØPU33JZ
Coccyx	ØQSS3ZZ	ØQUS3JZ
Lumbar	ØQSØ3ZZ	ØQUØ3JZ
Sacrum	ØQS13ZZ	ØQU13JZ
Thoracic	ØPS43ZZ	ØPU43JZ

DRG 518-52Ø Back and Neck Procedures, Except Spinal Fusion, or Disc Devices/Neurostimulators

Generator Type	Insertion of Generator by Site			Code also as appropriate Insertion Neurostimulator Lead by approach and Site	
	Chest	Abdomen	Back	Spinal Canal	Spinal Cord
Single Array	ØJH6[Ø,3]BZ	ØJH8[Ø,3]BZ	ØJH7[Ø,3]BZ	ØØHU[Ø,3,4]MZ	ØØHV[Ø,3,4]MZ
Single Array, Rechargeable	ØJH6[Ø,3]CZ	ØJH8[Ø,3]CZ	ØJH7[Ø,3]CZ	ØØHU[Ø,3,4]MZ	ØØHV[Ø,3,4]MZ
Multiple Array	ØJH6[Ø,3]DZ	ØJH8[Ø,3]DZ	ØJH7[Ø,3]DZ	ØØHU[Ø,3,4]MZ	ØØHV[Ø,3,4]MZ
Multiple Array, Rechargeable	ØJH6[Ø,3]EZ	—	ØJH7[Ø,3]EZ	ØØHU[Ø,3,4]MZ	ØØHV[Ø,3,4]MZ
Multiple Array, Rechargeable	—	ØJH8[Ø,3]EZ	—	ØØHU[Ø,3,4]MZ	ØØHV[Ø,3,4]MZ

DRG 582-583 Mastectomy for Malignancy

Site	Resection by Open approach	Code also as appropriate Resection of Lymph Nodes by Open approach by site			Code also as appropriate Resection of Thorax Muscle by Open approach	
		Axillary	Internal Mammary	Thorax	Right	Left
Breast, Right	ØHTTØZZ	Ø7T5ØZZ	Ø7T8ØZZ	Ø7T7ØZZ	ØKTHØZZ	—
Breast, Left	ØHTUØZZ	Ø7T6ØZZ	Ø7T9ØZZ	Ø7T7ØZZ	—	ØKTJØZZ
Breast, Bilateral	ØHTVØZZ	Ø7T5ØZZ and Ø7T6ØZZ	Ø7T8ØZZ and Ø7T9ØZZ	Ø7T7ØZZ	ØKTHØZZ	ØKTJØZZ

DRG 584-585 Breast Biopsy, Local Excision and Other Breast Procedures

Resection of Breast With Resection of Lymph Nodes and Thorax Muscle

Site	Resection by Open approach	Code also as appropriate Resection of Lymph Nodes by Open approach by site			Code also as appropriate Resection of Thorax Muscle by Open approach	
		Axillary	Internal Mammary	Thorax	Right	Left
Breast, Right	ØHTTØZZ	Ø7T5ØZZ	Ø7T8ØZZ	Ø7T7ØZZ	ØKTHØZZ	—
Breast, Left	ØHTUØZZ	Ø7T6ØZZ	Ø7T9ØZZ	Ø7T7ØZZ	—	ØKTJØZZ
Breast, Bilateral	ØHTVØZZ	Ø7T5ØZZ and Ø7T6ØZZ	Ø7T8ØZZ and Ø7T9ØZZ	Ø7T7ØZZ	ØKTHØZZ	ØKTJØZZ

Replacement of Breast Tissue

Site	Replacement by Percutaneous approach with Autologous Tissue	Code also as appropriate Extraction of Subcutaneous Tissue by Percutaneous approach					
		Abdomen	Back	Buttock	Chest	Leg, Upper, Right	Leg, Upper, Left
Breast, Right	ØHRT37Z	ØJD83ZZ	ØJD73ZZ	ØJD93ZZ	ØJD63ZZ	ØJDL3ZZ	ØJDM3ZZ
Breast, Left	ØHRU37Z	ØJD83ZZ	ØJD73ZZ	ØJD93ZZ	ØJD63ZZ	ØJDL3ZZ	ØJDM3ZZ
Breast, Bilateral	ØHRV37Z	ØJD83ZZ	ØJD73ZZ	ØJD93ZZ	ØJD63ZZ	ØJDL3ZZ	ØJDM3ZZ

DRG 628-63Ø Other Endocrine, Nutritional and Metabolic Procedures

Hip Procedure Combinations

Open Removal of Hip Spacer with Replacement

Removal of Spacer		Code also as appropriate Replacement by Device Type					
		Metal	Metal on Poly	Ceramic	Ceramic on Poly	Oxidized Zirc on Poly	Synthetic Substitute
Hip, RT	ØSP9Ø8Z	ØSR9Ø1[9,A,Z]	ØSR9Ø2[9,A,Z]	ØSR9Ø3[9,A,Z]	ØSR9Ø4[9,A,Z]	ØSR9Ø6[9,A,Z]	ØSR9ØJ[9,A,Z]
Hip, LT	ØSPBØ8Z	ØSRBØ1[9,A,Z]	ØSRBØ2[9,A,Z]	ØSRBØ3[9,A,Z]	ØSRBØ4[9,A,Z]	ØSRBØ6[9,A,Z]	ØSRBØJ[9,A,Z]

Open Removal of Hip Spacer with Replacement

Removal of Spacer		Code also as appropriate Replacement by Device Type						
		Acetabular Surface				Femoral Surface		
		Poly	Metal	Ceramic	Synthetic	Metal	Ceramic	Synthetic
Hip, RT	ØSP9Ø8Z	ØSRAØØ[9,A,Z]	ØSRAØ1[9,A,Z]	ØSRAØ3[9,A,Z]	ØSRAØJ[9,A,Z]	ØSRRØ1[9,A,Z]	ØSRRØ3[9,A,Z]	ØSRRØJ[9,A,Z]
Hip, LT	ØSPBØ8Z	ØSREØØ[9,A,Z]	ØSREØ1[9,A,Z]	ØSREØ3[9,A,Z]	ØSREØJ[9,A,Z]	ØSRSØ1[9,A,Z]	ØSRSØ3[9,A,Z]	ØSRSØJ[9,A,Z]

Open Removal of Hip Spacer with Liner Insertion (supplement)

Removal of Spacer		Code also as appropriate Supplement of Body Part by Site		
		Joint	Acetabular Surface	Femoral Surface
Hip, RT	ØSP9Ø8Z	ØSU9Ø9Z	ØSUAØ9Z	ØSURØ9Z
Hip, LT	ØSPBØ8Z	ØSUBØ9Z	ØSUEØ9Z	ØSUSØ9Z

Open Removal of Hip Liner with Replacement

Removal of Liner		Code also as appropriate Replacement by Device Type					
		Metal	Metal on Poly	Ceramic	Ceramic on Poly	Oxidized Zirc on Poly	Synthetic Substitute
Hip, RT	ØSP9Ø9Z	ØSR9Ø1[9,A,Z]	ØSR9Ø2[9,A,Z]	ØSR9Ø3[9,A,Z]	ØSR9Ø4[9,A,Z]	ØSR9Ø6[9,A,Z]	ØSR9ØJ[9,A,Z]
Hip, LT	ØSPBØ9Z	ØSRBØ1[9,A,Z]	ØSRBØ2[9,A,Z]	ØSRBØ3[9,A,Z]	ØSRBØ4[9,A,Z]	ØSRBØ6[9,A,Z]	ØSRBØJ[9,A,Z]

Open Removal of Hip Liner with Replacement

Removal of Liner		Code also as appropriate Replacement by Device Type						
		Acetabular Surface				Femoral Surface		
		Poly	Metal	Ceramic	Synthetic	Metal	Ceramic	Synthetic
Hip, RT	ØSP9Ø9Z	ØSRAØØ[9,A,Z]	ØSRAØ1[9,A,Z]	ØSRAØ3[9,A,Z]	ØSRAØJ[9,A,Z]	ØSRRØ1[9,A,Z]	ØSRRØ3[9,A,Z]	ØSRRØJ[9,A,Z]
Hip, LT	ØSPBØ9Z	ØSREØØ[9,A,Z]	ØSREØ1[9,A,Z]	ØSREØ3[9,A,Z]	ØSREØJ[9,A,Z]	ØSRSØ1[9,A,Z]	ØSRSØ3[9,A,Z]	ØSRSØJ[9,A,Z]

Open Removal of Hip Liner with Liner Insertion (supplement)

Removal of Liner		Code also as appropriate Supplement of Body Part by Site		
		Joint	Acetabular Surface	Femoral Surface
Hip, RT	ØSP9Ø9Z	ØSU9Ø9Z	ØSUAØ9Z	ØSURØ9Z
Hip, LT	ØSPBØ9Z	ØSUBØ9Z	ØSUEØ9Z	ØSUSØ9Z

Open Removal of Hip Resurfacing Device with Replacement

Removal of Resurfacing Device		Code also as appropriate Replacement by Device Type					
		Metal	Metal on Poly	Ceramic	Ceramic on Poly	Oxidized Zirc on Poly	Synthetic Substitute
Hip, RT	ØSP9ØBZ	ØSR9Ø1[9,A,Z]	ØSR9Ø2[9,A,Z]	ØSR9Ø3[9,A,Z]	ØSR9Ø4[9,A,Z]	ØSR9Ø6[9,A,Z]	ØSR9ØJ[9,A,Z]
Hip, LT	ØSPBØBZ	ØSRBØ1[9,A,Z]	ØSRBØ2[9,A,Z]	ØSRBØ3[9,A,Z]	ØSRBØ4[9,A,Z]	ØSRBØ6[9,A,Z]	ØSRBØJ[9,A,Z]

Open Removal of Hip Resurfacing Device with Replacement

Removal of Resurfacing Device		Code also as appropriate Replacement by Device Type						
		Acetabular Surface				Femoral Surface		
		Poly	Metal	Ceramic	Synthetic	Metal	Ceramic	Synthetic
Hip, RT	ØSP9ØBZ	ØSRAØØ[9,A,Z]	ØSRAØ1[9,A,Z]	ØSRAØ3[9,A,Z]	ØSRAØJ[9,A,Z]	ØSRRØ1[9,A,Z]	ØSRRØ3[9,A,Z]	ØSRRØJ[9,A,Z]
Hip, LT	ØSPBØBZ	ØSREØØ[9,A,Z]	ØSREØ1[9,A,Z]	ØSREØ3[9,A,Z]	ØSREØJ[9,A,Z]	ØSRSØ1[9,A,Z]	ØSRSØ3[9,A,Z]	ØSRSØJ[9,A,Z]

Open Removal of Hip Resurfacing Device with Liner Insertion (supplement)

Removal of Resurfacing Device		Code also as appropriate Supplement of Body Part by Site		
		Joint	Acetabular Surface	Femoral Surface
Hip, RT	ØSP9ØBZ	ØSU9Ø9Z	ØSUAØ9Z	ØSURØ9Z
Hip, LT	ØSPBØBZ	ØSUBØ9Z	ØSUEØ9Z	ØSUSØ9Z

Open Removal of Hip Synthetic Substitute with Replacement

Removal of Synthetic Substitute		Code also as appropriate Replacement by Device Type					
		Metal	Metal on Poly	Ceramic	Ceramic on Poly	Oxidized Zirc on Poly	Synthetic Substitute
Hip, RT	ØSP9ØJZ	ØSR9Ø1[9,A,Z]	ØSR9Ø2[9,A,Z]	ØSR9Ø3[9,A,Z]	ØSR9Ø4[9,A,Z]	ØSR9Ø6[9,A,Z]	ØSR9ØJ[9,A,Z]
Hip, LT	ØSPBØJZ	ØSRBØ1[9,A,Z]	ØSRBØ2[9,A,Z]	ØSRBØ3[9,A,Z]	ØSRBØ4[9,A,Z]	ØSRBØ6[9,A,Z]	ØSRBØJ[9,A,Z]

Open Removal of Hip Synthetic Substitute with Replacement

Removal of Synthetic Substitute		Code also as appropriate Replacement by Device Type						
		Acetabular Surface				Femoral Surface		
		Poly	Metal	Ceramic	Synthetic	Metal	Ceramic	Synthetic
Hip, RT	ØSP9ØJZ	ØSRAØØ[9,A,Z]	ØSRAØ1[9,A,Z]	ØSRAØ3[9,A,Z]	ØSRAØJ[9,A,Z]	ØSRRØ1[9,A,Z]	ØSRRØ3[9,A,Z]	ØSRRØJ[9,A,Z]
Hip, LT	ØSPBØJZ	ØSREØØ[9,A,Z]	ØSREØ1[9,A,Z]	ØSREØ3[9,A,Z]	ØSREØJ[9,A,Z]	ØSRSØ1[9,A,Z]	ØSRSØ3[9,A,Z]	ØSRSØJ[9,A,Z]

Open Removal of Hip Acetabular/Femoral Surface with Replacement

Removal of Acetabular/Femoral Surface		Code also as appropriate Replacement by Device Type					
		Metal	Metal on Poly	Ceramic	Ceramic on Poly	Oxidized Zirc on Poly	Synthetic Substitute
Hip, RT	ØSP[A,R]ØJZ	ØSR9Ø1[9,A,Z]	ØSR9Ø2[9,A,Z]	ØSR9Ø3[9,A,Z]	ØSR9Ø4[9,A,Z]	ØSR9Ø6[9,A,Z]	ØSR9ØJ[9,A,Z]
Hip, LT	ØSP[E,S]ØJZ	ØSRBØ1[9,A,Z]	ØSRBØ2[9,A,Z]	ØSRBØ3[9,A,Z]	ØSRBØ4[9,A,Z]	ØSRBØ6[9,A,Z]	ØSRBØJ[9,A,Z]

Open Removal of Hip Acetabular/Femoral Surface with Replacement

Removal of Acetabular/Femoral Surface		Code also as appropriate Replacement by Device Type						
		Acetabular Surface				Femoral Surface		
		Poly	Metal	Ceramic	Synthetic	Metal	Ceramic	Synthetic
Hip, RT	ØSP[A,R]ØJZ	ØSRAØØ[9,A,Z]	ØSRAØ1[9,A,Z]	ØSRAØ3[9,A,Z]	ØSRAØJ[9,A,Z]	ØSRRØ1[9,A,Z]	ØSRRØ3[9,A,Z]	ØSRRØJ[9,A,Z]
Hip, LT	ØSP[E,S]ØJZ	ØSREØØ[9,A,Z]	ØSREØ1[9,A,Z]	ØSREØ3[9,A,Z]	ØSREØJ[9,A,Z]	ØSRSØ1[9,A,Z]	ØSRSØ3[9,A,Z]	ØSRSØJ[9,A,Z]

Percutaneous Endoscopic Removal of Hip Spacer with Replacement

Removal of Spacer		Code also as appropriate Replacement by Device Type					
		Metal	Metal on Poly	Ceramic	Ceramic on Poly	Oxidized Zirc on Poly	Synthetic Substitute
Hip, RT	ØSP948Z	ØSR9Ø1[9,A,Z]	ØSR9Ø2[9,A,Z]	ØSR9Ø3[9,A,Z]	ØSR9Ø4[9,A,Z]	ØSR9Ø6[9,A,Z]	ØSR9ØJ[9,A,Z]
Hip, LT	ØSPB48Z	ØSRBØ1[9,A,Z]	ØSRBØ2[9,A,Z]	ØSRBØ3[9,A,Z]	ØSRBØ4[9,A,Z]	ØSRBØ6[9,A,Z]	ØSRBØJ[9,A,Z]

Percutaneous Endoscopic Removal of Hip Spacer with Replacement

Removal of Spacer		Code also as appropriate Replacement by Device Type						
		Acetabular Surface				Femoral Surface		
		Poly	Metal	Ceramic	Synthetic	Metal	Ceramic	Synthetic
Hip, RT	ØSP948Z	ØSRAØØ[9,A,Z]	ØSRAØ1[9,A,Z]	ØSRAØ3[9,A,Z]	ØSRAØJ[9,A,Z]	ØSRRØ1[9,A,Z]	ØSRRØ3[9,A,Z]	ØSRRØJ[9,A,Z]
Hip, LT	ØSPB48Z	ØSREØØ[9,A,Z]	ØSREØ1[9,A,Z]	ØSREØ3[9,A,Z]	ØSREØJ[9,A,Z]	ØSRSØ1[9,A,Z]	ØSRSØ3[9,A,Z]	ØSRSØJ[9,A,Z]

Percutaneous Endoscopic Removal of Hip Spacer with Liner Insertion (supplement)

Removal of Spacer		Code also as appropriate Supplement of Body Part by Site		
		Joint	Acetabular Surface	Femoral Surface
Hip, RT	ØSP948Z	ØSU9Ø9Z	ØSUAØ9Z	ØSURØ9Z
Hip, LT	ØSPB48Z	ØSUBØ9Z	ØSUEØ9Z	ØSUSØ9Z

Percutaneous Endoscopic Removal of Hip Synthetic Substitute with Replacement

Removal of Synthetic Substitute		Code also as appropriate Replacement by Device Type					
		Metal	Metal on Poly	Ceramic	Ceramic on Poly	Oxidized Zirc on Poly	Synthetic Substitute
Hip, RT	ØSP94JZ	ØSR9Ø1[9,A,Z]	ØSR9Ø2[9,A,Z]	ØSR9Ø3[9,A,Z]	ØSR9Ø4[9,A,Z]	ØSR9Ø6[9,A,Z]	ØSR9ØJ[9,A,Z]
Hip, LT	ØSPB4JZ	ØSRBØ1[9,A,Z]	ØSRBØ2[9,A,Z]	ØSRBØ3[9,A,Z]	ØSRBØ4[9,A,Z]	ØSRBØ6[9,A,Z]	ØSRBØJ[9,A,Z]

Percutaneous Endoscopic of Hip Synthetic Substitute with Replacement

Removal of Synthetic Substitute		Code also as appropriate Replacement by Device Type						
		Acetabular Surface				Femoral Surface		
		Poly	Metal	Ceramic	Synthetic	Metal	Ceramic	Synthetic
Hip, RT	ØSP94JZ	ØSRAØØ[9,A,Z]	ØSRAØ1[9,A,Z]	ØSRAØ3[9,A,Z]	ØSRAØJ[9,A,Z]	ØSRRØ1[9,A,Z]	ØSRRØ3[9,A,Z]	ØSRRØJ[9,A,Z]
Hip, LT	ØSPB4JZ	ØSREØØ[9,A,Z]	ØSREØ1[9,A,Z]	ØSREØ3[9,A,Z]	ØSREØJ[9,A,Z]	ØSRSØ1[9,A,Z]	ØSRSØ3[9,A,Z]	ØSRSØJ[9,A,Z]

Percutaneous Endoscopic Removal of Hip Synthetic Substitute with Liner Insertion (supplement)

Removal of Synthetic Substitute		Code also as appropriate Supplement of Body Part by Site		
		Joint	Acetabular Surface	Femoral Surface
Hip, RT	ØSP94JZ	ØSU9Ø9Z	ØSUAØ9Z	ØSURØ9Z
Hip, LT	ØSPB4JZ	ØSUBØ9Z	ØSUEØ9Z	ØSUSØ9Z

Percutaneous Endoscopic Removal of Hip Acetabular/Femoral Surface with Replacement

Removal of Acetabular/Femoral Surface		Code also as appropriate Replacement by Device Type					
		Metal	Metal on Poly	Ceramic	Ceramic on Poly	Oxidized Zirc on Poly	Synthetic Substitute
Hip, RT	ØSP[A,R]4JZ	ØSR9Ø1[9,A,Z]	ØSR9Ø2[9,A,Z]	ØSR9Ø3[9,A,Z]	ØSR9Ø4[9,A,Z]	ØSR9Ø6[9,A,Z]	ØSR9ØJ[9,A,Z]
Hip, LT	ØSP[E,S]4JZ	ØSRBØ1[9,A,Z]	ØSRBØ2[9,A,Z]	ØSRBØ3[9,A,Z]	ØSRBØ4[9,A,Z]	ØSRBØ6[9,A,Z]	ØSRBØJ[9,A,Z]

Percutaneous Endoscopic of Hip Acetabular/Femoral Surface with Replacement

Removal of Acetabular/Femoral Surface		Code also as appropriate Replacement by Device Type						
		Acetabular Surface				Femoral Surface		
		Poly	Metal	Ceramic	Synthetic	Metal	Ceramic	Synthetic
Hip, RT	ØSP[A,R]4JZ	ØSRAØØ[9,A,Z]	ØSRAØ1[9,A,Z]	ØSRAØ3[9,A,Z]	ØSRAØJ[9,A,Z]	ØSRRØ1[9,A,Z]	ØSRRØ3[9,A,Z]	ØSRRØJ[9,A,Z]
Hip, LT	ØSP[E,S]4JZ	ØSREØØ[9,A,Z]	ØSREØ1[9,A,Z]	ØSREØ3[9,A,Z]	ØSREØJ[9,A,Z]	ØSRSØ1[9,A,Z]	ØSRSØ3[9,A,Z]	ØSRSØJ[9,A,Z]

Percutaneous Endoscopic Removal of Hip Acetabular/Femoral Surface with Liner Insertion (supplement)

Removal of Acetabular/Femoral Surface		Code also as appropriate Supplement of Body Part by Site		
		Joint	Acetabular Surface	Femoral Surface
Hip, RT	ØSP[A,R]4JZ	ØSU9Ø9Z	ØSUAØ9Z	ØSURØ9Z
Hip, LT	ØSP[E,S]4JZ	ØSUBØ9Z	ØSUEØ9Z	ØSUSØ9Z

Knee Procedure Combinations

Removal of Knee Liner with Replacement

Removal of Liner		Code also Replacement by Device Type						
		Oxidized Zirc on Poly	Synthetic Substitute	Medial (L)/ Lateral (M) Unicondylar	Patello-femoral	Femoral Surface	Tibial Surface	Medial (L)/ Lateral (M) Meniscus
Knee, RT	ØSPCØ9Z	ØSRCØ6[9,A,Z]	ØSRCØJ[9,A,Z]	ØSRCØ[L,M][9,A,Z]	ØSRCØN[9,A,Z]	ØSRTØJ[9,A,Z]	ØSRVØJ[9,A,Z]	XRRGØ[L,M]8
Knee, LT	ØSPDØ9Z	ØSRDØ6[9,A,Z]	ØSRDØJ[9,A,Z]	ØSRDØ[L,M][9,A,Z]	ØSRDØN[9,A,Z]	ØSRUØJ[9,A,Z]	ØSRWØJ[9,A,Z]	XRRHØ[L,M]8

Removal of Knee Patellar Surface with Replacement

Removal of Patellar Surface		Code also Replacement by Device Type	
		Femoral Surface	Tibial Surface
Knee, RT	ØSPC[Ø,4]JC	ØSRTØJ[9,A,Z]	ØSRVØJ[9,A,Z]
Knee, LT	ØSPD[Ø,4]JC	ØSRUØJ[9,A,Z]	ØSRWØJ[9,A,Z]

Removal of Knee Synthetic Substitute with Replacement

Removal of Synthetic Substitute		Code also Replacement by Device Type	
		Femoral Surface	Tibial Surface
Knee, RT	ØSPC[Ø,4]JZ	ØSRTØJ[9,A,Z]	ØSRVØJ[9,A,Z]
Knee, LT	ØSPD[Ø,4]JZ	ØSRUØJ[9,A,Z]	ØSRWØJ[9,A,Z]

Removal of Knee Unicondylar Device with Replacement

Removal of Medial (L)/ Lateral (M) Unicondylar Device		Code also Replacement by Device Type	
		Femoral Surface	Tibial Surface
Knee, RT	ØSPC[Ø,4][L,M]Z	ØSRTØJ[9,A,Z]	ØSRVØJ[9,A,Z]
Knee, LT	ØSPD[Ø,4][L,M]Z	ØSRUØJ[9,A,Z]	ØSRWØJ[9,A,Z]

Removal of Knee Patellofemoral Device with Replacement

Removal of Patellofemoral Device		Code also Replacement by Device Type	
		Femoral Surface	Tibial Surface
Knee, RT	ØSPC[Ø,4]NZ	ØSRTØJ[9,A,Z]	ØSRVØJ[9,A,Z]
Knee, LT	ØSPD[Ø,4]NZ	ØSRUØJ[9,A,Z]	ØSRWØJ[9,A,Z]

Removal of Knee Femoral/Tibial Surface Device with Replacement

Removal of Femoral (T,U)/Tibial (V,W) Surface		Code also Replacement by Device Type	
		Femoral Surface	Tibial Surface
Knee, RT	ØSP[T,V][Ø,4]JZ	ØSRTØJ[9,A,Z]	ØSRVØJ[9,A,Z]
Knee, LT	ØSP[U,W][Ø,4]JZ	ØSRUØJ[9,A,Z]	ØSRWØJ[9,A,Z]

DRG 662-664 Minor Bladder Procedure

Repair of Bladder	Code also as appropriate Repair of Abdominal Wall	
	with Stoma	without Stoma
ØTQB[Ø,3,4]ZZ	ØWQFXZ2	ØWQFXZZ

DRG 665-667 Prostatectomy

Site	Resection by approach				Code also as appropriate Resection of Seminal Vesicles, Bilateral by approach	
	Open	Percutaneous Endoscopic	Via Natural or Artificial Opening	Via Natural or Artificial Opening Endoscopic	Open	Percutaneous Endoscopic
Prostate	ØVTØØZZ	ØVTØ4ZZ	ØVTØ7ZZ	ØVTØ8ZZ	ØVT3ØZZ	ØVT34ZZ

DRG 7Ø7-7Ø8 Major Male Pelvic Procedures

Site	Resection by approach				Code also as appropriate Resection of Seminal Vesicles, Bilateral by approach	
	Open	Percutaneous Endoscopic	Via Natural or Artificial Opening	Via Natural or Artificial Opening Endoscopic	Open	Percutaneous Endoscopic
Prostate	ØVTØØZZ	ØVTØ4ZZ	ØVTØ7ZZ	ØVTØ8ZZ	ØVT3ØZZ	ØVT34ZZ

DRG 734-735 Pelvic Evisceration, Radical Hysterectomy and Radical Vulvectomy

Pelvic Evisceration

Resection by Site						
Bladder	Cervix	Fallopian Tubes, Bilateral	Ovaries, Bilateral	Urethra	Uterus	Vagina
ØTTBØZZ	ØUTCØZZ	ØUT7ØZZ	ØUT2ØZZ	ØTTDØZZ	ØUT9ØZZ	ØUTGØZZ

Radical Hysterectomy

Approach	Resection by Site		
	Cervix	Uterus	Uterine Support Structure
Vaginal	ØUTC[7,8]ZZ	ØUT9[7,8]ZZ	ØUT4[7,8]ZZ
Abdominal, Endoscopic	ØUTC4ZZ	ØUT9[4,F]ZZ	ØUT44ZZ
Abdominal, Open	ØUTCØZZ	ØUT9ØZZ	ØUT4ØZZ

Radical Vulvectomy

Resection by Site	Code also as appropriate Excision of Inguinal Lymph Nodes by Approach	
Vulva	Right	Left
ØUTM[Ø,X]ZZ	Ø7BH[Ø,4]ZZ	Ø7BJ[Ø,4]ZZ

Non-OR procedure combinations

Note: The following table identifies procedure combinations that are considered Non-OR even though one or more procedures of the combination are considered valid DRG OR procedures

Insertion With Removal of Intraluminal Device

Code as appropriate Insertion of Intraluminal Device into Hepatobiliary Duct	Code also as appropriate Removal of Intraluminal Device by Approach and Site			
	Via Natural or Artificial Opening		External	
	Hepatobiliary Duct	Pancreatic Duct	Hepatobiliary Duct	Pancreatic Duct
ØFHB7DZ	ØFPB[7,8]DZ	ØFPD[7,8]DZ	ØFPBXDZ	ØFPDXDZ

Appendix M: Coding Exercises and Answers

Using the ICD-10-PCS tables construct the code that accurately represents the procedure performed.

Medical Surgical Section

Procedure	Code
1. Excision of malignant melanoma from skin of right ear	
2. Laparoscopy with excision of endometrial implant from left ovary	
3. Percutaneous needle core biopsy of right kidney	
4. EGD with excisional gastric biopsy	
5. Open endarterectomy of left common carotid artery	
6. Excision of basal cell carcinoma of lower lip	
7. Open excision of tail of pancreas	
8. Percutaneous biopsy of right gastrocnemius muscle	
9. Sigmoidoscopy with sigmoid polypectomy	
10. Open excision of lesion from right Achilles tendon	
11. Open resection of cecum	
12. Total excision of pituitary gland, open	
13. Explantation of left failed kidney, open	
14. Open left axillary total lymphadenectomy	
15. Laparoscopic-assisted vaginal hysterectomy	
16. Right total mastectomy, open	
17. Open resection of papillary muscle	
18. Total retropubic prostatectomy, open	
19. Laparoscopic cholecystectomy	
20. Endoscopic bilateral total maxillary sinusectomy	
21. Amputation at right elbow level	
22. Right below-knee amputation, proximal tibia/fibula	
23. Fifth ray carpometacarpal joint amputation, left hand	
24. Right leg and hip amputation through ischium	
25. DIP joint amputation of right thumb	
26. Right wrist joint amputation	
27. Trans-metatarsal amputation of foot at left big toe	
28. Mid-shaft amputation, right humerus	
29. Left fourth toe amputation, mid-proximal phalanx	
30. Right above-knee amputation, distal femur	
31. Cryotherapy of wart on left hand	
32. Percutaneous radiofrequency ablation of right vocal cord lesion	
33. Left heart catheterization with laser destruction of arrhythmogenic focus, A-V node	
34. Cautery of nosebleed	
35. Transurethral endoscopic laser ablation of prostate	
36. Percutaneous cautery of oozing varicose vein, left calf	
37. Laparoscopy with destruction of endometriosis, bilateral ovaries	
38. Laser coagulation of right retinal vessel, percutaneous	
39. Thoracoscopic pleurodesis, left side	
40. Percutaneous insertion of Greenfield IVC filter	
41. Forceps total mouth extraction, upper and lower teeth	
42. Removal of left thumbnail	
43. Extraction of right intraocular lens without replacement, percutaneous	
44. Laparoscopy with needle aspiration of ova for in vitro fertilization	
45. Nonexcisional debridement of skin ulcer, right foot	
46. Open stripping of abdominal fascia, right side	
47. Hysteroscopy with D&C, diagnostic	
48. Liposuction for medical purposes, left upper arm	
49. Removal of tattered right ear drum fragments with tweezers	
50. Microincisional phlebectomy of spider veins, right lower leg	
51. Routine Foley catheter placement	
52. Incision and drainage of external anal abscess	
53. Percutaneous drainage of ascites	
54. Laparoscopy with left ovarian cystotomy and drainage	
55. Laparotomy and drain placement for liver abscess, right lobe	
56. Right knee arthrotomy with drain placement	
57. Thoracentesis of left pleural effusion	
58. Phlebotomy of left median cubital vein for polycythemia vera	
59. Percutaneous chest tube placement for right pneumothorax	
60. Endoscopic drainage of left ethmoid sinus	
61. External ventricular CSF drainage catheter placement via burr hole	
62. Removal of foreign body, right cornea	
63. Percutaneous mechanical thrombectomy, left brachial artery	
64. Esophagogastroscopy with removal of bezoar from stomach	
65. Foreign body removal, skin of left thumb	
66. Transurethral cystoscopy with removal of bladder stone	
67. Forceps removal of foreign body in right nostril	
68. Laparoscopy with excision of old suture from mesentery	
69. Incision and removal of right lacrimal duct stone	
70. Nonincisional removal of intraluminal foreign body from vagina	
71. Right common carotid endarterectomy, open	
72. Open excision of retained sliver, subcutaneous tissue of left foot	
73. Extracorporeal shockwave lithotripsy (ESWL), bilateral ureters	
74. Endoscopic retrograde cholangiopancreatography (ERCP) with lithotripsy of common bile duct stone	
75. Thoracotomy with crushing of pericardial calcifications	
76. Transurethral cystoscopy with fragmentation of bladder calculus	
77. Hysteroscopy with intraluminal lithotripsy of left fallopian tube calcification	
78. Division of right foot tendon, percutaneous	

Procedure	Code
79. Left heart catheterization with division of bundle of HIS	
80. Open osteotomy of capitate, left hand	
81. EGD with esophagotomy of esophagogastric junction	
82. Sacral rhizotomy for pain control, percutaneous	
83. Laparotomy with exploration and adhesiolysis of right ureter	
84. Incision of scar contracture, right elbow	
85. Frenulotomy for treatment of tongue-tie syndrome	
86. Right shoulder arthroscopy with coracoacromial ligament release	
87. Mitral valvulotomy for release of fused leaflets, open approach	
88. Percutaneous left Achilles tendon release	
89. Laparoscopy with lysis of peritoneal adhesions	
90. Manual rupture of right shoulder joint adhesions under general anesthesia	
91. Open posterior tarsal tunnel release	
92. Laparoscopy with freeing of left ovary and fallopian tube	
93. Liver transplant with donor matched liver	
94. Orthotopic heart transplant using porcine heart	
95. Right lung transplant, open, using organ donor match	
96. Transplant of large intestine, organ donor match	
97. Left kidney/pancreas organ bank transplant	
98. Replantation of avulsed scalp	
99. Reattachment of severed right ear	
100. Reattachment of traumatic left gastrocnemius avulsion, open	
101. Closed replantation of three avulsed teeth, lower jaw	
102. Reattachment of severed left hand	
103. Right open palmaris longus tendon transfer	
104. Endoscopic radial to median nerve transfer	
105. Fasciocutaneous flap closure of left thigh, open	
106. Transfer left index finger to left thumb position, open	
107. Percutaneous fascia transfer to fill defect, right neck	
108. Trigeminal to facial nerve transfer, percutaneous endoscopic	
109. Endoscopic left leg flexor hallucis longus tendon transfer	
110. Right scalp advancement flap to right temple	
111. Resection right breast with TRAM flap reconstruction, open	
112. Skin transfer flap closure of complex open wound, left lower back	
113. Open fracture reduction, right tibia	
114. Laparoscopy with gastropexy for malrotation	
115. Left knee arthroscopy with reposition of anterior cruciate ligament	
116. Open transposition of ulnar nerve	
117. Closed reduction with percutaneous internal fixation of right femoral neck fracture	
118. Trans-vaginal intraluminal cervical cerclage	
119. Cervical cerclage using Shirodkar technique	
120. Thoracotomy with banding of left pulmonary artery using extraluminal device	
121. Restriction of thoracic duct with intraluminal stent, percutaneous	

Procedure	Code
122. Craniotomy with clipping of cerebral aneurysm	
123. Nonincisional, transnasal placement of restrictive stent in right lacrimal duct	
124. Catheter-based temporary restriction of blood flow in abdominal aorta for treatment of cerebral ischemia	
125. Percutaneous ligation of esophageal vein	
126. Percutaneous embolization of left internal carotid-cavernous fistula	
127. Laparoscopy with bilateral occlusion of fallopian tubes using Hulka extraluminal clips	
128. Open suture ligation of failed AV graft, left brachial artery	
129. Percutaneous embolization of vascular supply, intracranial meningioma	
130. Percutaneous embolization of right uterine artery, using coils	
131. Open occlusion of left atrial appendage, using extraluminal pressure clips	
132. Percutaneous suture exclusion of left atrial appendage, via femoral artery access	
133. ERCP with balloon dilation of common bile duct	
134. PTCA of two coronary arteries, LAD with stent placement, RCA with no stent	
135. Cystoscopy with intraluminal dilation of bladder neck stricture	
136. Open dilation of old anastomosis, left femoral artery	
137. Dilation of upper esophageal stricture, direct visualization, with Bougie sound	
138. PTA of right brachial artery stenosis	
139. Transnasal dilation and stent placement in right lacrimal duct	
140. Hysteroscopy with balloon dilation of bilateral fallopian tubes	
141. Tracheoscopy with intraluminal dilation of tracheal stenosis	
142. Cystoscopy with dilation of left ureteral stricture, with stent placement	
143. Open gastric bypass with Roux-en-Y limb to jejunum	
144. Right temporal artery to intracranial artery bypass using Gore-Tex graft, open	
145. Tracheostomy formation with tracheostomy tube placement, percutaneous	
146. PICVA (percutaneous in situ coronary venous arterialization) of single coronary artery	
147. Open left femoral-popliteal artery bypass using cadaver vein graft	
148. Shunting of intrathecal cerebrospinal fluid to peritoneal cavity using synthetic shunt	
149. Colostomy formation, open, transverse colon to abdominal wall	
150. Open urinary diversion, left ureter, using ileal conduit to skin	
151. CABG of LAD using pedicled left internal mammary artery, open off-bypass	
152. Open pleuroperitoneal shunt, right pleural cavity, using synthetic device	
153. Percutaneous placement of ventriculoperitoneal shunt for treatment of hydrocephalus	
154. End-of-life replacement of spinal neurostimulator generator, multiple array, in lower abdomen	
155. Percutaneous insertion of spinal neurostimulator lead, lumbar spinal cord	

Procedure	Code
156. Percutaneous replacement of broken pacemaker lead in left atrium	
157. Open placement of dual chamber pacemaker generator in chest wall	
158. Percutaneous placement of venous central line in right internal jugular, with tip in superior vena cava	
159. Open insertion of multiple channel cochlear implant, left ear	
160. Percutaneous placement of Swan-Ganz catheter in pulmonary trunk	
161. Bronchoscopy with insertion of Low Dose, Pd-103 brachytherapy seeds, right lung	
162. Open insertion of interspinous process device into lumbar vertebral joint	
163. Open placement of bone growth stimulator, left femoral shaft	
164. Cystoscopy with placement of brachytherapy seeds in prostate gland	
165. Percutaneous insertion of Greenfield IVC filter	
166. Full-thickness skin graft to right lower arm, autograft (do not code graft harvest for this exercise)	
167. Excision of necrosed left femoral head with bone bank bone graft to fill the defect, open	
168. Penetrating keratoplasty of right cornea with donor matched cornea, percutaneous approach	
169. Excision of abdominal aorta with Gore-Tex graft replacement, open	
170. Total right knee arthroplasty with insertion of total knee prosthesis	
171. Tenonectomy with graft to right ankle using cadaver graft, open	
172. Mitral valve replacement using porcine valve, open	
173. Percutaneous phacoemulsification of right eye cataract with prosthetic lens insertion	
174. Transcatheter replacement of pulmonary valve using of bovine jugular vein valve	
175. Total left hip replacement using ceramic on ceramic prosthesis, without bone cement	
176. Aortic valve annuloplasty using ring, open	
177. Laparoscopic repair of left inguinal hernia with marlex plug	
178. Autograft nerve graft to right median nerve, percutaneous endoscopic (do not code graft harvest for this exercise)	
179. Exchange of liner in femoral component of previous left hip replacement, open approach	
180. Anterior colporrhaphy with polypropylene mesh reinforcement, open approach	
181. Implantation of CorCap cardiac support device, open approach	
182. Abdominal wall herniorrhaphy, open, using synthetic mesh	
183. Tendon graft to strengthen injured left shoulder using autograft, open (do not code graft harvest for this exercise)	
184. Onlay lamellar keratoplasty of left cornea using autograft, external approach	
185. Resurfacing procedure on right femoral head, open approach	
186. Exchange of drainage tube from right hip joint	
187. Tracheostomy tube exchange	
188. Change chest tube for left pneumothorax	

Procedure	Code
189. Exchange of cerebral ventriculostomy drainage tube	
190. Foley urinary catheter exchange	
191. Open removal of lumbar sympathetic neurostimulator lead	
192. Nonincisional removal of Swan-Ganz catheter from right pulmonary artery	
193. Laparotomy with removal of pancreatic drain	
194. Extubation, endotracheal tube	
195. Nonincisional PEG tube removal	
196. Transvaginal removal of brachytherapy seeds	
197. Transvaginal removal of extraluminal cervical cerclage	
198. Incision with removal of K-wire fixation, right first metatarsal	
199. Cystoscopy with retrieval of left ureteral stent	
200. Removal of nasogastric drainage tube for decompression	
201. Removal of external fixator, left radial fracture	
202. Trimming and reanastomosis of stenosed femorofemoral synthetic bypass graft, open	
203. Open revision of right hip replacement, with readjustment of prosthesis	
204. Adjustment of position, pacemaker lead in left ventricle, percutaneous	
205. External repositioning of Foley catheter to bladder	
206. Taking out loose screw and putting larger screw in fracture repair plate, left tibia	
207. Revision of totally implantable VAD port placement in chest wall, causing patient discomfort, open	
208. Thoracotomy with exploration of right pleural cavity	
209. Diagnostic laryngoscopy	
210. Exploratory arthrotomy of left knee	
211. Colposcopy with diagnostic hysteroscopy	
212. Digital rectal exam	
213. Diagnostic arthroscopy of right shoulder	
214. Endoscopy of maxillary sinus	
215. Laparotomy with palpation of liver	
216. Transurethral diagnostic cystoscopy	
217. Colonoscopy, discontinued at sigmoid colon	
218. Percutaneous mapping of basal ganglia	
219. Heart catheterization with cardiac mapping	
220. Intraoperative whole brain mapping via craniotomy	
221. Mapping of left cerebral hemisphere, percutaneous endoscopic	
222. Intraoperative cardiac mapping during open heart surgery	
223. Hysteroscopy with cautery of post-hysterectomy oozing and evacuation of clot	
224. Open exploration and ligation of post-op arterial bleeder, left forearm	
225. Control of post-operative retroperitoneal bleeding via laparotomy	
226. Reopening of thoracotomy site with drainage and control of post-op hemopericardium	
227. Arthroscopy with drainage of hemarthrosis at previous operative site, right knee	
228. Radiocarpal fusion of left hand with internal fixation, open	
229. Posterior approach spinal fusion at L1-L3 level with BAK cage interbody fusion device, open	

Appendix M: Coding Exercises and Answers

Procedure	Code
230. Intercarpal fusion of right hand with bone bank bone graft, open	
231. Sacrococcygeal fusion with bone graft from same operative site, open	
232. Interphalangeal fusion of left great toe, percutaneous pin fixation	
233. Suture repair of left radial nerve laceration	
234. Laparotomy with suture repair of blunt force duodenal laceration	
235. Perineoplasty with repair of old obstetric laceration, open	
236. Suture repair of right biceps tendon (upper arm) laceration, open	
237. Closure of abdominal wall stab wound	
238. Cosmetic face lift, open, no other information available	
239. Bilateral breast augmentation with silicone implants, open	
240. Cosmetic rhinoplasty with septal reduction and tip elevation using local tissue graft, open	
241. Abdominoplasty (tummy tuck), open	
242. Liposuction of bilateral thighs	
243. Creation of penis in female patient using tissue bank donor graft	
244. Creation of vagina in male patient using synthetic material	
245. Laparoscopic vertical (sleeve) gastrectomy	
246. Left uterine artery embolization with intraluminal biosphere injection	

Obstetrics

Procedure	Code
1. Abortion by dilation and evacuation following laminaria insertion	
2. Manually assisted spontaneous abortion	
3. Abortion by abortifacient insertion	
4. Bimanual pregnancy examination	
5. Extraperitoneal C-section, low transverse incision	
6. Fetal spinal tap, percutaneous	
7. Fetal kidney transplant, laparoscopic	
8. Open in utero repair of congenital diaphragmatic hernia	
9. Laparoscopy with total excision of tubal pregnancy	
10. Transvaginal removal of fetal monitoring electrode	

Placement

Procedure	Code
1. Placement of packing material, right ear	
2. Mechanical traction of entire left leg	
3. Removal of splint, right shoulder	
4. Placement of neck brace	
5. Change of vaginal packing	
6. Packing of wound, chest wall	
7. Sterile dressing placement to left groin region	
8. Removal of packing material from pharynx	
9. Placement of intermittent pneumatic compression device, covering entire right arm	
10. Exchange of pressure dressing to left thigh	

Administration

Procedure	Code
1. Peritoneal dialysis via indwelling catheter	
2. Transvaginal artificial insemination	
3. Infusion of total parenteral nutrition via central venous catheter	
4. Esophagogastroscopy with Botox injection into esophageal sphincter	
5. Percutaneous irrigation of knee joint	
6. Systemic infusion of recombinant tissue plasminogen activator (r-tPA) via peripheral venous catheter	
7. Transabdominal in vitro fertilization, implantation of donor ovum	
8. Autologous bone marrow transplant via central venous line	
9. Implantation of anti-microbial envelope with cardiac defibrillator placement, open	
10. Sclerotherapy of brachial plexus lesion, alcohol injection	
11. Percutaneous peripheral vein injection, glucarpidase	
12. Introduction of anti-infective envelope into subcutaneous tissue, open	

Measurement and Monitoring

Procedure	Code
1. Cardiac stress test, single measurement	
2. EGD with biliary flow measurement	
3. Right and left heart cardiac catheterization with bilateral sampling and pressure measurements	
4. Temperature monitoring, rectal	
5. Peripheral venous pulse, external, single measurement	
6. Holter monitoring	
7. Respiratory rate, external, single measurement	
8. Fetal heart rate monitoring, transvaginal	
9. Visual mobility test, single measurement	
10. Left ventricular cardiac output monitoring from pulmonary artery wedge (Swan-Ganz) catheter	
11. Olfactory acuity test, single measurement	

Extracorporeal or Systemic Assistance and Performance

Procedure	Code
1. Intermittent mechanical ventilation, 16 hours	
2. Intubated patient on mechanical ventilation, positioned prone for 14 hrs	
3. Cardiac countershock with successful conversion to sinus rhythm	
4. IPPB (intermittent positive pressure breathing) for mobilization of secretions, 22 hours	
5. Renal dialysis, 12 hours	
6. IABP (intra-aortic balloon pump) continuous	
7. Intraoperative cardiac pacing, continuous	
8. Intraoperative ECMO (extracorporeal membrane oxygenation), central	
9. Controlled mechanical ventilation (CMV), 45 hours	
10. Pulsatile compression boot with intermittent inflation	

Extracorporeal or Systemic Therapies

Procedure	Code
1. Donor thrombocytapheresis, single encounter	
2. Bili-lite phototherapy, series treatment	
3. Whole body hypothermia, single treatment	
4. Circulatory phototherapy, single encounter	
5. Shock wave therapy of plantar fascia, single treatment	
6. Antigen-free air conditioning, series treatment	
7. TMS (transcranial magnetic stimulation), series treatment	
8. Therapeutic ultrasound of peripheral vessels, single treatment	
9. Plasmapheresis, series treatment	
10. Extracorporeal electromagnetic stimulation (EMS) for urinary incontinence, single treatment	

Osteopathic

Procedure	Code
1. Isotonic muscle energy treatment of right leg	
2. Low velocity-high amplitude osteopathic treatment of head	
3. Lymphatic pump osteopathic treatment of left axilla	
4. Indirect osteopathic treatment of sacrum	
5. Articulatory osteopathic treatment of cervical region	

Other Procedures

Procedure	Code
1. Near infrared spectroscopy of leg vessels	
2. CT computer assisted sinus surgery	
3. Suture removal, abdominal wall	
4. Isolation after infectious disease exposure	
5. Robotic assisted open prostatectomy	
6. CSF extracted from LP shunt	

Chiropractic

Procedure	Code
1. Chiropractic treatment of lumbar region using long lever specific contact	
2. Chiropractic manipulation of abdominal region, indirect visceral	
3. Chiropractic extra-articular treatment of hip region	
4. Chiropractic treatment of sacrum using long and short lever specific contact	
5. Mechanically-assisted chiropractic manipulation of head	

Imaging

Procedure	Code
1. Noncontrast CT of abdomen and pelvis	
2. Intravascular ultrasound, left subclavian artery	
3. Fluoroscopic guidance for insertion of central venous catheter in SVC, low osmolar contrast	
4. Chest x-ray, AP/PA and lateral views	
5. Endoluminal ultrasound of gallbladder and bile ducts	
6. MRI of thyroid gland, contrast unspecified	
7. Esophageal videofluoroscopy study with oral barium contrast	
8. Portable x-ray study of right radius/ulna shaft, standard series	
9. Routine fetal ultrasound, second trimester twin gestation	
10. CT scan of bilateral lungs, high osmolar contrast with densitometry	
11. Fluoroscopic guidance for percutaneous transluminal angioplasty (PTA) of left common femoral artery, low osmolar contrast	

Nuclear Medicine

Procedure	Code
1. Tomo scan of right and left heart, unspecified radiopharmaceutical, qualitative gated rest	
2. Technetium pentetate assay of kidneys, ureters, and bladder	
3. Uniplanar scan of spine using technetium oxidronate, with first-pass study	
4. Thallous chloride tomographic scan of bilateral breasts	
5. PET scan of myocardium using rubidium	
6. Gallium citrate scan of head and neck, single plane imaging	
7. Xenon gas nonimaging probe of brain	
8. Upper GI scan, radiopharmaceutical unspecified, for gastric emptying	
9. Carbon 11 PET scan of brain with quantification	
10. Iodinated albumin nuclear medicine assay, blood plasma volume study	

Radiation Therapy

Procedure	Code
1. Plaque radiation of left eye, single port	
2. 8 MeV photon beam radiation to brain	
3. IORT of colon, 3 ports	
4. HDR brachytherapy of prostate using low dose palladium-103, unidirectional source	
5. Electron radiation treatment of right breast, with custom device	
6. Hyperthermia oncology treatment of pelvic region	
7. Contact radiation of tongue	
8. Heavy particle radiation treatment of pancreas, four risk sites	
9. LDR brachytherapy to spinal cord using iodine	
10. Whole body Phosphorus 32 administration with risk to hematopoietic system	

Physical Rehabilitation and Diagnostic Audiology

Procedure	Code
1. Bekesy assessment using audiometer	
2. Individual fitting of left eye prosthesis	
3. Physical therapy for range of motion and mobility, patient right hip, no special equipment	
4. Bedside swallow assessment using assessment kit	
5. Caregiver training in airway clearance techniques	
6. Application of short arm cast in rehabilitation setting	
7. Verbal assessment of patient's pain level	
8. Caregiver training in communication skills using manual communication board	
9. Group musculoskeletal balance training exercises, whole body, no special equipment	
10. Individual therapy for auditory processing using tape recorder	

Mental Health

Procedure	Code
1. Cognitive-behavioral psychotherapy, individual	
2. Narcosynthesis	
3. Light therapy	
4. ECT (electroconvulsive therapy), unilateral, multiple seizure	
5. Crisis intervention	
6. Neuropsychological testing	
7. Hypnosis	
8. Developmental testing	
9. Vocational counseling	
10. Family psychotherapy	

Substance Abuse Treatment

Procedure	Code
1. Naltrexone treatment for drug dependency	
2. Substance abuse treatment family counseling	
3. Medication monitoring of patient on methadone maintenance	
4. Individual interpersonal psychotherapy for drug abuse	
5. Patient in for alcohol detoxification treatment	
6. Group motivational counseling	
7. Individual 12-step psychotherapy for substance abuse	
8. Post-test infectious disease counseling for IV drug abuser	
9. Psychodynamic psychotherapy for drug dependent patient	
10. Group cognitive-behavioral counseling for substance abuse	

New Technology

Procedure	Code
1. Infusion of terlipressin via peripheral venous catheter	
2. Transcatheter dilation of left peroneal artery with 2 SAVAL stents	
3. Cranial reconstruction using Longeviti ClearFit® cranial implant	

Answers to Coding Exercises

Medical Surgical Section

Procedure	Code
1. Excision of malignant melanoma from skin of right ear	ØHB2XZZ
2. Laparoscopy with excision of endometrial implant from left ovary	ØUB14ZZ
3. Percutaneous needle core biopsy of right kidney	ØTBØ3ZX
4. EGD with excisional gastric biopsy	ØDB68ZX
5. Open endarterectomy of left common carotid artery	Ø3CJØZZ
6. Excision of basal cell carcinoma of lower lip	ØCB1XZZ
7. Open excision of tail of pancreas	ØFBGØZZ
8. Percutaneous biopsy of right gastrocnemius muscle	ØKBS3ZX
9. Sigmoidoscopy with sigmoid polypectomy	ØDBN8ZZ
10. Open excision of lesion from right Achilles tendon	ØLBNØZZ
11. Open resection of cecum	ØDTHØZZ
12. Total excision of pituitary gland, open	ØGTØØZZ
13. Explantation of left failed kidney, open	ØTT1ØZZ
14. Open left axillary total lymphadenectomy	Ø7T6ØZZ (RESECTION is coded for cutting out a chain of lymph nodes.)
15. Laparoscopic-assisted vaginal hysterectomy	ØUT9FZZ
16. Right total mastectomy, open	ØHTTØZZ
17. Open resection of papillary muscle	Ø2TDØZZ (The papillary muscle refers to the heart and is found in the *Heart and Great Vessels* body system.)
18. Total retropubic prostatectomy, open	ØVTØØZZ
19. Laparoscopic cholecystectomy	ØFT44ZZ
20. Endoscopic bilateral total maxillary sinusectomy	Ø9TQ8ZZ, Ø9TR8ZZ
21. Amputation at right elbow level	ØX6BØZZ
22. Right below-knee amputation, proximal tibia/fibula	ØY6HØZ1 (The qualifier *High* here means the portion of the tib/fib closest to the knee.)
23. Fifth ray carpometacarpal joint amputation, left hand	ØX6KØZ8 (A *complete* ray amputation is through the carpometacarpal joint.)
24. Right leg and hip amputation through ischium	ØY62ØZZ (The *Hindquarter* body part includes amputation along any part of the hip bone.)
25. DIP joint amputation of right thumb	ØX6LØZ3 (The qualifier *Low* here means through the distal interphalangeal joint.)
26. Right wrist joint amputation	ØX6JØZØ (Amputation at the wrist joint is considered a complete amputation of the hand.)
27. Trans-metatarsal amputation of foot at left big toe	ØY6NØZ9 (A *partial* amputation is through the shaft of the metatarsal bone.)
28. Mid-shaft amputation, right humerus	ØX68ØZ2
29. Left fourth toe amputation, mid-proximal phalanx	ØY6WØZ1 (The qualifier *High* here means anywhere along the proximal phalanx.)
30. Right above-knee amputation, distal femur	ØY6CØZ3
31. Cryotherapy of wart on left hand	ØH5GXZZ
32. Percutaneous radiofrequency ablation of right vocal cord lesion	ØC5T3ZZ
33. Left heart catheterization with laser destruction of arrhythmogenic focus, A-V node	Ø2583ZZ
34. Cautery of nosebleed	Ø93K7ZZ
35. Transurethral endoscopic laser ablation of prostate	ØV5Ø8ZZ
36. Percutaneous cautery of oozing varicose vein, left calf	ØY3J3ZZ
37. Laparoscopy with destruction of endometriosis, bilateral ovaries	ØU524ZZ
38. Laser coagulation of right retinal vessel, percutaneous	Ø85G3ZZ (The *Retinal Vessel* body-part values are in the *Eye* body system.)
39. Thoracoscopic pleurodesis, left side	ØB5P4ZZ
40. Percutaneous insertion of Greenfield IVC filter	Ø6HØ3DZ
41. Forceps total mouth extraction, upper and lower teeth	ØCDWXZ2, ØCDXXZ2
42. Removal of left thumbnail	ØHDQXZZ (No separate body-part value is given for thumbnail, so this is coded to *Fingernail*.)
43. Extraction of right intraocular lens without replacement, percutaneous	Ø8DJ3ZZ
44. Laparoscopy with needle aspiration of ova for in vitro fertilization	ØUDN4ZZ
45. Nonexcisional debridement of skin ulcer, right foot	ØHDMXZZ
46. Open stripping of abdominal fascia, right side	ØJD8ØZZ
47. Hysteroscopy with D&C, diagnostic	ØUDB8ZX
48. Liposuction for medical purposes, left upper arm	ØJDF3ZZ (The *Percutaneous* approach is inherent in the liposuction technique.)
49. Removal of tattered right ear drum fragments with tweezers	Ø9D77ZZ
50. Microincisional phlebectomy of spider veins, right lower leg	Ø6DY3ZZ
51. Routine Foley catheter placement	ØT9B7ØZ
52. Incision and drainage of external anal abscess	ØD9QXZZ
53. Percutaneous drainage of ascites	ØW9G3ZZ (This is drainage of the cavity and not the peritoneal membrane itself.)
54. Laparoscopy with left ovarian cystotomy and drainage	ØU914ZZ
55. Laparotomy and drain placement for liver abscess, right lobe	ØF91ØØZ
56. Right knee arthrotomy with drain placement	ØS9CØØZ
57. Thoracentesis of left pleural effusion	ØW9B3ZZ (This is drainage of the pleural cavity)
58. Phlebotomy of left median cubital vein for polycythemia vera	Ø59C3ZZ (The median cubital vein is a branch of the basilic vein)
59. Percutaneous chest tube placement for right pneumothorax	ØW993ØZ
60. Endoscopic drainage of left ethmoid sinus	Ø99V4ZZ
61. External ventricular CSF drainage catheter placement via burr hole	ØØ963ØZ

Procedure	Code
62. Removal of foreign body, right cornea	Ø8C8XZZ
63. Percutaneous mechanical thrombectomy, left brachial artery	Ø3C83ZZ
64. Esophagogastroscopy with removal of bezoar from stomach	ØDC68ZZ
65. Foreign body removal, skin of left thumb	ØHCGXZZ (There is no specific value for thumb skin, so the procedure is coded to *Hand*.)
66. Transurethral cystoscopy with removal of bladder stone	ØTCB8ZZ
67. Forceps removal of foreign body in right nostril	Ø9CKXZZ (Nostril is coded to the *Nasal mucosa and soft tissue* body-part value.)
68. Laparoscopy with excision of old suture from mesentery	ØDCV4ZZ
69. Incision and removal of right lacrimal duct stone	Ø8CXØZZ
70. Nonincisional removal of intraluminal foreign body from vagina	ØUCG7ZZ (The approach *External* is also a possibility. It is assumed here that since the patient went to the doctor to have the object removed, that it was not in the vaginal orifice.)
71. Right common carotid endarterectomy, open	Ø3CHØZZ
72. Open excision of retained sliver, subcutaneous tissue of left foot	ØJCRØZZ
73. Extracorporeal shockwave lithotripsy (ESWL), bilateral ureters	ØTF6XZZ, ØTF7XZZ (The *Bilateral Ureter* body-part value is not available for the root operation FRAGMENTATION, so the procedures are coded separately.)
74. Endoscopic retrograde cholangiopancreatography (ERCP) with lithotripsy of common bile duct stone	ØFF98ZZ (ERCP is performed through the mouth to the biliary system via the duodenum, so the approach value is *Via Natural or Artificial Opening Endoscopic*.)
75. Thoracotomy with crushing of pericardial calcifications	Ø2FNØZZ
76. Transurethral cystoscopy with fragmentation of bladder calculus	ØTFB8ZZ
77. Hysteroscopy with intraluminal lithotripsy of left fallopian tube calcification	ØUF68ZZ
78. Division of right foot tendon, percutaneous	ØL8V3ZZ
79. Left heart catheterization with division of bundle of HIS	Ø2883ZZ
80. Open osteotomy of capitate, left hand	ØP8NØZZ (The capitate is one of the carpal bones of the hand.)
81. EGD with esophagotomy of esophagogastric junction	ØD948ZZ
82. Sacral rhizotomy for pain control, percutaneous	Ø18R3ZZ
83. Laparotomy with exploration and adhesiolysis of right ureter	ØTN6ØZZ
84. Incision of scar contracture, right elbow	ØHNDXZZ (The skin of the elbow region is coded to *Lower Arm*.)
85. Frenulotomy for treatment of tongue-tie syndrome	ØCN7XZZ (The frenulum is coded to the body-part value *Tongue*.)

Procedure	Code
86. Right shoulder arthroscopy with coracoacromial ligament release	ØMN14ZZ
87. Mitral valvulotomy for release of fused leaflets, open approach	Ø2NGØZZ
88. Percutaneous left Achilles tendon release	ØLNP3ZZ
89. Laparoscopy with lysis of peritoneal adhesions	ØDNW4ZZ
90. Manual rupture of right shoulder joint adhesions under general anesthesia	ØRNJXZZ
91. Open posterior tarsal tunnel release	Ø1NGØZZ (The nerve released in the posterior tarsal tunnel is the tibial nerve.)
92. Laparoscopy with freeing of left ovary and fallopian tube	ØUN14ZZ, ØUN64ZZ
93. Liver transplant with donor matched liver	ØFYØØZØ
94. Orthotopic heart transplant using porcine heart	Ø2YAØZ2 (The donor heart comes from an animal [pig], so the qualifier value is *Zooplastic*.)
95. Right lung transplant, open, using organ donor match	ØBYKØZØ
96. Transplant of large intestine, organ donor match	ØDYEØZØ
97. Left kidney/pancreas organ bank transplant	ØFYGØZØ, ØTY1ØZØ
98. Replantation of avulsed scalp	ØHMØXZZ
99. Reattachment of severed right ear	Ø9MØXZZ
100. Reattachment of traumatic left gastrocnemius avulsion, open	ØKMTØZZ
101. Closed replantation of three avulsed teeth, lower jaw	ØCMXXZ1
102. Reattachment of severed left hand	ØXMKØZZ
103. Right open palmaris longus tendon transfer	ØLX5ØZZ
104. Endoscopic radial to median nerve transfer	Ø1X64Z5
105. Fasciocutaneous flap closure of left thigh, open	ØJXMØZC (The qualifier identifies the body layers in addition to fascia included in the procedure.)
106. Transfer left index finger to left thumb position, open	ØXXPØZM
107. Percutaneous fascia transfer to fill defect, right neck	ØJX43ZZ
108. Trigeminal to facial nerve transfer, percutaneous endoscopic	ØØXK4ZM
109. Endoscopic left leg flexor hallucis longus tendon transfer	ØLXP4ZZ
110. Right scalp advancement flap to right temple	ØHXØXZZ
111. Resection right breast with TRAM flap reconstruction, open	ØHTTØZZ, ØHRTØ76 (Code both the resection and the replacement per guideline B3.18)
112. Skin transfer flap closure of complex open wound, left lower back	ØHX6XZZ
113. Open fracture reduction, right tibia	ØQSGØZZ
114. Laparoscopy with gastropexy for malrotation	ØDS64ZZ
115. Left knee arthroscopy with reposition of anterior cruciate ligament	ØMSP4ZZ
116. Open transposition of ulnar nerve	Ø1S4ØZZ
117. Closed reduction with percutaneous internal fixation of right femoral neck fracture	ØQS634Z
118. Trans-vaginal intraluminal cervical cerclage	ØUVC7DZ
119. Cervical cerclage using Shirodkar technique	ØUVC7ZZ
120. Thoracotomy with banding of left pulmonary artery using extraluminal device	Ø2VRØCZ

Procedure	Code
121. Restriction of thoracic duct with intraluminal stent, percutaneous	Ø7VK3DZ
122. Craniotomy with clipping of cerebral aneurysm	Ø3VGØCZ (The clip is placed lengthwise on the outside wall of the widened portion of the vessel.)
123. Nonincisional, transnasal placement of restrictive stent in right lacrimal duct	Ø8VX7DZ
124. Catheter-based temporary restriction of blood flow in abdominal aorta for treatment of cerebral ischemia	Ø4VØ3DJ
125. Percutaneous ligation of esophageal vein	Ø6L33ZZ
126. Percutaneous embolization of left internal carotid-cavernous fistula	Ø3LL3DZ
127. Laparoscopy with bilateral occlusion of fallopian tubes using Hulka extraluminal clips	ØUL74CZ
128. Open suture ligation of failed AV graft, left brachial artery	Ø3L8ØZZ
129. Percutaneous embolization of vascular supply, intracranial meningioma	Ø3LG3DZ
130. Percutaneous embolization of right uterine artery, using coils	Ø4LE3DT
131. Open occlusion of left atrial appendage, using extraluminal pressure clips	Ø2L7ØCK
132. Percutaneous suture exclusion of left atrial appendage, via femoral artery access	Ø2L73ZK
133. ERCP with balloon dilation of common bile duct	ØF798ZZ
134. PTCA of two coronary arteries, LAD with stent placement, RCA with no stent	Ø27Ø3DZ, Ø27Ø3ZZ (A separate procedure is coded for each artery dilated, since the device value differs for each artery.)
135. Cystoscopy with intraluminal dilation of bladder neck stricture	ØT7C8ZZ
136. Open dilation of old anastomosis, left femoral artery	Ø47LØZZ
137. Dilation of upper esophageal stricture, direct visualization, with Bougie sound	ØD717ZZ
138. PTA of right brachial artery stenosis	Ø3773ZZ
139. Transnasal dilation and stent placement in right lacrimal duct	Ø87X7DZ
140. Hysteroscopy with balloon dilation of bilateral fallopian tubes	ØU778ZZ
141. Tracheoscopy with intraluminal dilation of tracheal stenosis	ØB718ZZ
142. Cystoscopy with dilation of left ureteral stricture, with stent placement	ØT778DZ
143. Open gastric bypass with Roux-en-Y limb to jejunum	ØD16ØZA
144. Right temporal artery to intracranial artery bypass using Gore-Tex graft, open	Ø31SØJG
145. Tracheostomy formation with tracheostomy tube placement, percutaneous	ØB113F4
146. PICVA (percutaneous in situ coronary venous arterialization) of single coronary artery	Ø21Ø3D4
147. Open left femoral-popliteal artery bypass using cadaver vein graft	Ø41LØKL
148. Shunting of intrathecal cerebrospinal fluid to peritoneal cavity using synthetic shunt	ØØ16ØJ6
149. Colostomy formation, open, transverse colon to abdominal wall	ØD1LØZ4
150. Open urinary diversion, left ureter, using ileal conduit to skin	ØT17ØZC

Procedure	Code
151. CABG of LAD using pedicled left internal mammary artery, open off-bypass	Ø21ØØZ9
152. Open pleuroperitoneal shunt, right pleural cavity, using synthetic device	ØW19ØJG
153. Percutaneous placement of ventriculoperitoneal shunt for treatment of hydrocephalus	ØØ163J6
154. End-of-life replacement of spinal neurostimulator generator, multiple array, in lower abdomen	ØJH8ØDZ (Taking out of the old generator is coded separately to the root operation *Removal*)
155. Percutaneous insertion of spinal neurostimulator lead, lumbar spinal cord	ØØHV3MZ
156. Percutaneous replacement of broken pacemaker lead in left atrium	Ø2H73JZ (Taking out the broken pacemaker lead is coded separately to the root operation *Removal*.)
157. Open placement of dual chamber pacemaker generator in chest wall	ØJH6Ø6Z
158. Percutaneous placement of venous central line in right internal jugular, with tip in superior vena cava	Ø2HV33Z
159. Open insertion of multiple channel cochlear implant, left ear	Ø9HEØ6Z
160. Percutaneous placement of Swan-Ganz catheter in pulmonary trunk	Ø2HP32Z (The Swan-Ganz catheter is coded to the device value *Monitoring Device* because it monitors pulmonary artery output.)
161. Bronchoscopy with insertion of Low Dose Pd-103 brachytherapy seeds, right lung	ØBHK81Z, DB11BBZ
162. Open insertion of interspinous process device into lumbar vertebral joint	ØSHØØBZ
163. Open placement of bone growth stimulator, left femoral shaft	ØQHYØMZ
164. Cystoscopy with placement of brachytherapy seeds in prostate gland	ØVHØ81Z
165. Percutaneous insertion of Greenfield IVC filter	Ø6HØ3DZ
166. Full-thickness skin graft to right lower arm, autograft (do not code graft harvest for this exercise)	ØHRDX73
167. Excision of necrosed left femoral head with bone bank bone graft to fill the defect, open	ØQR7ØKZ
168. Penetrating keratoplasty of right cornea with donor matched cornea, percutaneous approach	Ø8R83KZ
169. Excision of abdominal aorta with Gore-Tex graft replacement, open	Ø4RØØJZ
170. Total right knee arthroplasty with insertion of total knee prosthesis	ØSRCØJZ
171. Tenonectomy with graft to right ankle using cadaver graft, open	ØLRSØKZ
172. Mitral valve replacement using porcine valve, open	Ø2RGØ8Z
173. Percutaneous phacoemulsification of right eye cataract with prosthetic lens insertion	Ø8RJ3JZ
174. Transcatheter replacement of pulmonary valve using of bovine jugular vein valve	Ø2RH38Z
175. Total left hip replacement using ceramic on ceramic prosthesis, without bone cement	ØSRBØ3A
176. Aortic valve annuloplasty using ring, open	Ø2UFØJZ
177. Laparoscopic repair of left inguinal hernia with marlex plug	ØYU64JZ
178. Autograft nerve graft to right median nerve, percutaneous endoscopic (do not code graft harvest for this exercise)	Ø1U547Z

Procedure	Code
179. Exchange of liner in femoral component of previous left hip replacement, open approach	ØSUSØ9Z (Taking out of the old liner is coded separately to the root operation *Removal*)
180. Anterior colporrhaphy with polypropylene mesh reinforcement, open approach	ØJUCØJZ
181. Implantation of CorCap cardiac support device, open approach	Ø2UAØJZ
182. Abdominal wall herniorrhaphy, open, using synthetic mesh	ØWUFØJZ
183. Tendon graft to strengthen injured left shoulder using autograft, open (do not code graft harvest for this exercise)	ØLU2Ø7Z
184. Onlay lamellar keratoplasty of left cornea using autograft, external approach	Ø8U9X7Z
185. Resurfacing procedure on right femoral head, open approach	ØSURØBZ
186. Exchange of drainage tube from right hip joint	ØS2YXØZ
187. Tracheostomy tube exchange	ØB21XFZ
188. Change chest tube for left pneumothorax	ØW2BXØZ
189. Exchange of cerebral ventriculostomy drainage tube	ØØ2ØXØZ
190. Foley urinary catheter exchange	ØT2BXØZ (This is coded to *Drainage Device* because urine is being drained.)
191. Open removal of lumbar sympathetic neurostimulator lead	Ø1PYØMZ
192. Nonincisional removal of Swan-Ganz catheter from right pulmonary artery	Ø2PYX2Z
193. Laparotomy with removal of pancreatic drain	ØFPGØØZ
194. Extubation, endotracheal tube	ØBP1XDZ
195. Nonincisional PEG tube removal	ØDP6XUZ
196. Transvaginal removal of brachytherapy seeds	ØUPH71Z
197. Transvaginal removal of extraluminal cervical cerclage	ØUPD7CZ
198. Incision with removal of K-wire fixation, right first metatarsal	ØQPNØ4Z
199. Cystoscopy with retrieval of left ureteral stent	ØTP98DZ
200. Removal of nasogastric drainage tube for decompression	ØDP6XØZ
201. Removal of external fixator, left radial fracture	ØPPJX5Z
202. Trimming and reanastomosis of stenosed femorofemoral synthetic bypass graft, open	Ø4WYØJZ
203. Open revision of right hip replacement, with readjustment of prosthesis	ØSW9ØJZ
204. Adjustment of position, pacemaker lead in left ventricle, percutaneous	Ø2WA3MZ
205. External repositioning of Foley catheter to bladder	ØTWBXØZ
206. Taking out loose screw and putting larger screw in fracture repair plate, left tibia	ØQWHØ4Z
207. Revision of totally implantable VAD port placement in chest wall, causing patient discomfort, open	ØJWTØWZ
208. Thoracotomy with exploration of right pleural cavity	ØWJ9ØZZ
209. Diagnostic laryngoscopy	ØCJS8ZZ
210. Exploratory arthrotomy of left knee	ØSJDØZZ
211. Colposcopy with diagnostic hysteroscopy	ØUJD8ZZ
212. Digital rectal exam	ØDJD7ZZ
213. Diagnostic arthroscopy of right shoulder	ØRJJ4ZZ
214. Endoscopy of maxillary sinus	Ø9JY4ZZ
215. Laparotomy with palpation of liver	ØFJØØZZ
216. Transurethral diagnostic cystoscopy	ØTJB8ZZ
217. Colonoscopy, discontinued at sigmoid colon	ØDJD8ZZ

Procedure	Code
218. Percutaneous mapping of basal ganglia	ØØK83ZZ
219. Heart catheterization with cardiac mapping	Ø2K83ZZ
220. Intraoperative whole brain mapping via craniotomy	ØØKØØZZ
221. Mapping of left cerebral hemisphere, percutaneous endoscopic	ØØK74ZZ
222. Intraoperative cardiac mapping during open heart surgery	Ø2K8ØZZ
223. Hysteroscopy with cautery of post-hysterectomy oozing and evacuation of clot	ØW3R8ZZ
224. Open exploration and ligation of post-op arterial bleeder, left forearm	ØX3FØZZ
225. Control of post-operative retroperitoneal bleeding via laparotomy	ØW3HØZZ
226. Reopening of thoracotomy site with drainage and control of post-op hemopericardium	ØW3DØZZ
227. Arthroscopy with drainage of hemarthrosis at previous operative site, right knee	ØY3F4ZZ
228. Radiocarpal fusion of left hand with internal fixation, open	ØRGPØ4Z
229. Posterior approach spinal fusion at L1-L3 level with BAK cage interbody fusion device, open	ØSG1ØAJ
230. Intercarpal fusion of right hand with bone bank bone graft, open	ØRGQØKZ
231. Sacrococcygeal fusion with bone graft from same operative site, open	ØSG5Ø7Z
232. Interphalangeal fusion of left great toe, percutaneous pin fixation	ØSGQ34Z
233. Suture repair of left radial nerve laceration	Ø1Q6ØZZ (The approach value is *Open*, though the surgical exposure may have been created by the wound itself.)
234. Laparotomy with suture repair of blunt force duodenal laceration	ØDQ9ØZZ
235. Perineoplasty with repair of old obstetric laceration, open	ØWQNØZZ
236. Suture repair of right biceps tendon (upper arm) laceration, open	ØLQ3ØZZ
237. Closure of abdominal wall stab wound	ØWQFØZZ
238. Cosmetic face lift, open, no other information available	ØWØ2ØZZ
239. Bilateral breast augmentation with silicone implants, open	ØHØVØJZ
240. Cosmetic rhinoplasty with septal reduction and tip elevation using local tissue graft, open	Ø9ØKØ7Z
241. Abdominoplasty (tummy tuck), open	ØWØFØZZ
242. Liposuction of bilateral thighs	ØJØL3ZZ, ØJØM3ZZ
243. Creation of penis in female patient using tissue bank donor graft	ØW4NØK1
244. Creation of vagina in male patient using synthetic material	ØW4MØJØ
245. Laparoscopic vertical (sleeve) gastrectomy	ØDB64Z3
246. Left uterine artery embolization with intraluminal biosphere injection	Ø4LF3DU

Obstetrics

Procedure	Code
1. Abortion by dilation and evacuation following laminaria insertion	1ØAØ7ZW
2. Manually assisted spontaneous abortion	1ØEØXZZ (Since the pregnancy was not artificially terminated, this is coded to *Delivery* because it captures the procedure objective. The fact that it was an abortion will be identified in the diagnosis code.)
3. Abortion by abortifacient insertion	1ØAØ7ZX
4. Bimanual pregnancy examination	1ØJØ7ZZ
5. Extraperitoneal C-section, low transverse incision	1ØDØØZ1
6. Fetal spinal tap, percutaneous	1Ø9Ø3ZA
7. Fetal kidney transplant, laparoscopic	1ØYØ4ZS
8. Open in utero repair of congenital diaphragmatic hernia	1ØQØØZK (Diaphragm is classified to the *Respiratory* body system in the *Medical and Surgical* section.)
9. Laparoscopy with total excision of tubal pregnancy	1ØT24ZZ
10. Transvaginal removal of fetal monitoring electrode	1ØPØ73Z

Placement

Procedure	Code
1. Placement of packing material, right ear	2Y42X5Z
2. Mechanical traction of entire left leg	2W6MXØZ
3. Removal of splint, right shoulder	2W5AX1Z
4. Placement of neck brace	2W32X3Z
5. Change of vaginal packing	2YØ4X5Z
6. Packing of wound, chest wall	2W44X5Z
7. Sterile dressing placement to left groin region	2W27X4Z
8. Removal of packing material from pharynx	2Y5ØX5Z
9. Placement of intermittent pneumatic compression device, covering entire right arm	2W18X7Z
10. Exchange of pressure dressing to left thigh	2WØPX6Z

Administration

Procedure	Code
1. Peritoneal dialysis via indwelling catheter	3E1M39Z
2. Transvaginal artificial insemination	3EØP7LZ
3. Infusion of total parenteral nutrition via central venous catheter	3EØ436Z
4. Esophagogastroscopy with Botox injection into esophageal sphincter	3EØG8GC (Botulinum toxin is a paralyzing agent with temporary effects; it does not sclerose or destroy the nerve.)
5. Percutaneous irrigation of knee joint	3E1U38Z
6. Systemic infusion of recombinant tissue plasminogen activator (r-tPA) via peripheral venous catheter	3EØ3317
7. Transabdominal in vitro fertilization, implantation of donor ovum	3EØP3Q1
8. Autologous bone marrow transplant via central venous line	3Ø243GØ
9. Implantation of anti-microbial envelope with cardiac defibrillator placement, open	3EØ1Ø2A
10. Sclerotherapy of brachial plexus lesion, alcohol injection	3EØT3TZ
11. Percutaneous peripheral vein injection, glucarpidase	3EØ33GQ
12. Introduction of anti-infective envelope into subcutaneous tissue, open	3EØ1Ø2A

Measurement and Monitoring

Procedure	Code
1. Cardiac stress test, single measurement	4AØ2XM4
2. EGD with biliary flow measurement	4AØC85Z
3. Right and left heart cardiac catheterization with bilateral sampling and pressure measurements	4AØ23N8
4. Temperature monitoring, rectal	4A1Z7KZ
5. Peripheral venous pulse, external, single measurement	4AØ4XJ1
6. Holter monitoring	4A12X45
7. Respiratory rate, external, single measurement	4AØ9XCZ
8. Fetal heart rate monitoring, transvaginal	4A1H7CZ
9. Visual mobility test, single measurement	4AØ7X7Z
10. Left ventricular cardiac output monitoring from pulmonary artery wedge (Swan-Ganz) catheter	4A1239Z
11. Olfactory acuity test, single measurement	4AØ8XØZ

Extracorporeal or Systemic Assistance and Performance

Procedure	Code
1. Intermittent mechanical ventilation, 16 hours	5A1935Z
2. Intubated patient on mechanical ventilation, positioned prone for 14 hrs	5AØ9C5K
3. Cardiac countershock with successful conversion to sinus rhythm	5A22Ø4Z
4. IPPB (intermittent positive pressure breathing) for mobilization of secretions, 22 hours	5AØ9358
5. Renal dialysis, 12 hours	5A1D8ØZ
6. IABP (intra-aortic balloon pump) continuous	5AØ221Ø
7. Intra-operative cardiac pacing, continuous	5A1223Z
8. Intraoperative ECMO (extracorporeal membrane oxygenation), central	5A15A2F
9. Controlled mechanical ventilation (CMV), 45 hours	5A1945Z
10. Pulsatile compression boot with intermittent inflation	5AØ2115 (This is coded to the function value *Cardiac Output*, because the purpose of such compression devices is to return blood to the heart faster.)

Extracorporeal or Systemic Therapies

Procedure	Code
1. Donor thrombocytapheresis, single encounter	6A55ØZ2
2. Bili-lite phototherapy, series treatment	6A6Ø1ZZ
3. Whole body hypothermia, single treatment	6A4ZØZZ
4. Circulatory phototherapy, single encounter	6A65ØZZ
5. Shock wave therapy of plantar fascia, single treatment	6A93ØZZ
6. Antigen-free air conditioning, series treatment	6AØZ1ZZ
7. TMS (transcranial magnetic stimulation), series treatment	6A221ZZ

Procedure	Code
8. Therapeutic ultrasound of peripheral vessels, single treatment	6A75ØZ6
9. Plasmapheresis, series treatment	6A551Z3
10. Extracorporeal electromagnetic stimulation (EMS) for urinary incontinence, single treatment	6A21ØZZ

Osteopathic

Procedure	Code
1. Isotonic muscle energy treatment of right leg	7WØ6X8Z
2. Low velocity-high amplitude osteopathic treatment of head	7WØØX5Z
3. Lymphatic pump osteopathic treatment of left axilla	7WØ7X6Z
4. Indirect osteopathic treatment of sacrum	7WØ4X4Z
5. Articulatory osteopathic treatment of cervical region	7WØ1XØZ

Other Procedures

Procedure	Code
1. Near infrared spectroscopy of leg vessels	8EØ23DZ
2. CT computer assisted sinus surgery	8EØ9XBG (The primary procedure is coded separately.)
3. Suture removal, abdominal wall	8EØWXY8
4. Isolation after infectious disease exposure	8EØZXY6
5. Robotic assisted open prostatectomy	8EØWØCZ (The primary procedure is coded separately.)
6. CSF extracted from LP shunt	8CØ1X6J

Chiropractic

Procedure	Code
1. Chiropractic treatment of lumbar region using long lever specific contact	9WB3XGZ
2. Chiropractic manipulation of abdominal region, indirect visceral	9WB9XCZ
3. Chiropractic extra-articular treatment of hip region	9WB6XDZ
4. Chiropractic treatment of sacrum using long and short lever specific contact	9WB4XJZ
5. Mechanically-assisted chiropractic manipulation of head	9WBØXKZ

Imaging

Procedure	Code
1. Noncontrast CT of abdomen and pelvis	BW21ZZZ
2. Intravascular ultrasound, left subclavian artery	B342ZZ3
3. Fluoroscopic guidance for insertion of central venous catheter in SVC, low osmolar contrast	B5181ZA
4. Chest x-ray, AP/PA and lateral views	BWØ3ZZZ
5. Endoluminal ultrasound of gallbladder and bile ducts	BF43ZZZ
6. MRI of thyroid gland, contrast unspecified	BG34YZZ
7. Esophageal videofluoroscopy study with oral barium contrast	BD11YZZ
8. Portable x-ray study of right radius/ulna shaft, standard series	BPØJZZZ
9. Routine fetal ultrasound, second trimester twin gestation	BY4DZZZ

Procedure	Code
10. CT scan of bilateral lungs, high osmolar contrast with densitometry	BB24ØZZ
11. Fluoroscopic guidance for percutaneous transluminal angioplasty (PTA) of left common femoral artery, low osmolar contrast	B41G1ZZ

Nuclear Medicine

Procedure	Code
1. Tomo scan of right and left heart, unspecified radiopharmaceutical, qualitative gated rest	C226YZZ
2. Technetium pentetate assay of kidneys, ureters, and bladder	CT631ZZ
3. Uniplanar scan of spine using technetium oxidronate, with first-pass study	CP151ZZ
4. Thallous chloride tomographic scan of bilateral breasts	CH22SZZ
5. PET scan of myocardium using rubidium	C23GQZZ
6. Gallium citrate scan of head and neck, single plane imaging	CW1BLZZ
7. Xenon gas nonimaging probe of brain	CØ5ØVZZ
8. Upper GI scan, radiopharmaceutical unspecified, for gastric emptying	CD15YZZ
9. Carbon 11 PET scan of brain with quantification	CØ3ØBZZ
10. Iodinated albumin nuclear medicine assay, blood plasma volume study	C763HZZ

Radiation Therapy

Procedure	Code
1. Plaque radiation of left eye, single port	D8YØFZZ
2. 8 MeV photon beam radiation to brain	DØØ11ZZ
3. IORT of colon, 3 ports	DDY5CZZ
4. HDR brachytherapy of prostate using low dose palladium-103, unidirectional source	DV1ØBB1
5. Electron radiation treatment of right breast, with custom device	DMØ13ZZ
6. Hyperthermia oncology treatment of pelvic region	DWY68ZZ
7. Contact radiation of tongue	D9Y57ZZ
8. Heavy particle radiation treatment of pancreas, four risk sites	DFØ34ZZ
9. LDR brachytherapy to spinal cord using iodine	DØ16B9Z
10. Whole body Phosphorus 32 administration with risk to hematopoietic system	DWY5GFZ

Physical Rehabilitation and Diagnostic Audiology

Procedure	Code
1. Bekesy assessment using audiometer	F13Z31Z
2. Individual fitting of left eye prosthesis	FØDZ8UZ
3. Physical therapy for range of motion and mobility, patient right hip, no special equipment	FØ7LØZZ
4. Bedside swallow assessment using assessment kit	FØØZHYZ
5. Caregiver training in airway clearance techniques	FØFZ8ZZ
6. Application of short arm cast in rehabilitation setting	FØDZ7EZ (Inhibitory cast is listed in the equipment reference table under E, *Orthosis*.)
7. Verbal assessment of patient's pain level	FØ2ZFZZ

Procedure	Code
8. Caregiver training in communication skills using manual communication board	FØFZJMZ (Manual communication board is listed in the equipment reference table under M, *Augmentative/ Alternative Communication*.)
9. Group musculoskeletal balance training exercises, whole body, no special equipment	FØ7M6ZZ (Balance training is included in the motor treatment reference table under *Therapeutic Exercise*.)
10. Individual therapy for auditory processing using tape recorder	FØ9Z2KZ (Tape recorder is listed in the equipment reference table under *Audiovisual Equipment*.)

Mental Health

Procedure	Code
1. Cognitive-behavioral psychotherapy, individual	GZ58ZZZ
2. Narcosynthesis	GZGZZZZ
3. Light therapy	GZJZZZZ
4. ECT (electroconvulsive therapy), unilateral, multiple seizure	GZB1ZZZ
5. Crisis intervention	GZ2ZZZZ
6. Neuropsychological testing	GZ13ZZZ
7. Hypnosis	GZFZZZZ
8. Developmental testing	GZ1ØZZZ
9. Vocational counseling	GZ61ZZZ
10. Family psychotherapy	GZ72ZZZ

Substance Abuse Treatment

Procedure	Code
1. Naltrexone treatment for drug dependency	HZ94ZZZ
2. Substance abuse treatment family counseling	HZ63ZZZ
3. Medication monitoring of patient on methadone maintenance	HZ81ZZZ
4. Individual interpersonal psychotherapy for drug abuse	HZ54ZZZ
5. Patient in for alcohol detoxification treatment	HZ2ZZZZ
6. Group motivational counseling	HZ47ZZZ
7. Individual 12-step psychotherapy for substance abuse	HZ53ZZZ
8. Post-test infectious disease counseling for IV drug abuser	HZ3CZZZ
9. Psychodynamic psychotherapy for drug dependent patient	HZ5CZZZ
10. Group cognitive-behavioral counseling for substance abuse	HZ42ZZZ

New Technology

Procedure	Code
1. Infusion of terlipressin via peripheral venous catheter	XWØ3367
2. Transcatheter dilation of left peroneal artery with 2 SAVAL stents	X27U395
3. Cranial reconstruction using Longeviti ClearFit® cranial implant	XNR8ØD9

Notes

Notes

Notes

Notes